Oral and Maxillofacial
PATHOLOGY

evolve

To access your Student Resources, visit:

http://evolve.elsevier.com/Neville/OMP

Evolve® Student Learning Resources for **Neville/Damm/Allen/Bouquot:**
Oral and Maxillofacial Pathology, **third edition,** offers the following features:

- **Differential Diagnosis of Clinical Cases**
  These cases include an image or images of a specific disease or condition. Multiple choice questions test the student's identification skills and diagnostic competency pertaining to the disease or condition shown. The correct answer and a rationale are provided for each case.

- **Selected Questions from** *Mosby's Review for the NBDE, Part II*
  35 multiple choice questions taken from *Mosby's Review for the NBDE, Part II,* are designed to familiarize students with the format of the NBDE, Part II, examination as well as test their oral diagnosis knowledge. Rationales are provided for the correct answer.

- **Appendix: Differential Diagnosis of Oral and Maxillofacial Diseases**
  The entire appendix as it appears in the book is included in a printable format.

- **Weblinks**
  A variety of weblinks provides additional means of study and research.

Oral and Maxillofacial
PATHOLOGY

THIRD EDITION

BRAD W. NEVILLE, DDS

Distinguished University Professor
Director, Division of Oral and Maxillofacial Pathology
Department of Stomatology
College of Dental Medicine
Medical University of South Carolina
Charleston, South Carolina

DOUGLAS D. DAMM, DDS

Professor
Division of Oral and Maxillofacial Pathology
College of Dentistry
University of Kentucky
Lexington, Kentucky

CARL M. ALLEN, DDS, MSD

Professor and Director
Oral and Maxillofacial Pathology
College of Dentistry
The Ohio State University
Columbus, Ohio

Professor
Department of Pathology
College of Medicine and Public Health
The Ohio State University
Columbus, Ohio

JERRY E. BOUQUOT, DDS, MSD

Professor and Chair
Department of Diagnostic Sciences
University of Texas
Dental Branch at Houston
Houston, Texas

Consultant in Pediatric Oral Pathology
Division of Dentistry
Pittsburgh Children's Hospital
Pittsburgh, Pennsylvania

Consultant in Oral Pathology
Department of Pathology
New York Eye and Ear Infirmary
New York, New York

Adjunct Professor
Department of Rural Health and Community
  Dentistry
School of Dentistry
West Virginia University
Morgantown, West Virginia

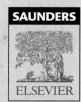

SAUNDERS

ELSEVIER

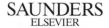

11830 Westline Industrial Drive
St. Louis, Missouri 63146

ORAL AND MAXILLOFACIAL PATHOLOGY   ISBN: 978-1-4160-3435-3
Third Edition
Copyright © 2009, 2002 by Saunders, an imprint of Elsevier Inc.

Notice

Knowledge and best practice in this field are constantly changing. As new research and experience broaden our knowledge, changes in practice, treatment and drug therapy may become necessary or appropriate. Readers are advised to check the most current information provided (i) on procedures featured or (ii) by the manufacturer of each product to be administered, to verify the recommended dose or formula, the method and duration of administration, and contraindications. It is the responsibility of the practitioner, relying on their own experience and knowledge of the patient, to make diagnoses, to determine dosages and the best treatment for each individual patient, and to take all appropriate safety precautions. To the fullest extent of the law, neither the Publisher nor the Authors assume any liability for any injury and/or damage to persons or property arising out of or related to any use of the material contained in this book.

The Publisher

Library of Congress Cataloging-in-Publication Data

Oral and maxillofacial pathology / Brad W. Neville . . . [et al.]. – 3rd ed.
    p. ; cm.
    Includes bibliographical references and index.
    ISBN 978-1-4160-3435-3 (hardcover : alk. paper)   1. Mouth–Diseases.   2. Teeth–Diseases.
3. Maxilla–Diseases.   I. Neville, Brad W.
    [DNLM: 1. Mouth Diseases–pathology.   2. Jaw Diseases–pathology.   3. Maxillofacial
Injuries–pathology.   4. Tooth Diseases–pathology.   WU 140 O6253 2009]
    RK307.O73 2009
    617.5′2207–dc22

                                                                    2008006904

Vice President and Publisher: Linda Duncan
Senior Editor: John Dolan
Developmental Editor: Courtney Sprehe
Publishing Services Manager: Patricia Tannian
Project Manager: Jonathan M. Taylor
Design Direction: Teresa McBryan

Printed in China

Last digit is the print number: 9   8   7   6   5   4   3   2   1

This book is dedicated to three of our mentors:

CHARLES A. WALDRON
WILLIAM G. SHAFER
ROBERT J. GORLIN

in appreciation for all that they taught us
and in recognition of their contributions to the field
of oral and maxillofacial pathology.

Contributors

ANGELA C. CHI, DMD

Assistant Professor
Division of Oral and Maxillofacial Pathology
Department of Stomatology
College of Dental Medicine
Medical University of South Carolina
Charleston, South Carolina

THERESA S. GONZALES, DMD, MS, MS

Consultant in Orofacial Pain

Consultant in Oral and Maxillofacial Pathology

Consultant in Forensic Odontology
Carl R. Darnall Army Medical Center
Fort Hood, Texas

Diplomate, American Board of Orofacial Pain

**Diplomate, American Board of Oral and Maxillofacial
    Pathology**

**EDWARD E. HERSCHAFT, DDS, MA,
FACD, FICD**

Professor
Department of Biomedical Sciences
University of Nevada-Las Vegas
School of Dental Medicine
Las Vegas, Nevada

Professor Emeritus
Department of Stomatology
College of Dental Medicine
Medical University of South Carolina
Charleston, South Carolina

**Diplomate, American Board of Forensic Odontology and
    Oral Medicine**

Fellow, American Academy of Forensic Sciences

Consulting Forensic Odontologist
Office of the Coroner/Medical Examiner, Clark County
Las Vegas, Nevada

Preface

Oral and maxillofacial pathology is the specialty of dentistry and the discipline of pathology that addresses the nature, identification, and management of diseases affecting the oral and maxillofacial regions. As such, it occupies a unique position in the health care community for both the dental and medical professions. Naturally, members of the dental profession (including general practitioners, specialists, and dental hygienists) must have a good knowledge of the pathogenesis, clinical features, treatment, and prognosis for oral and paraoral diseases. Likewise, such knowledge is important for those in the medical profession, especially for physicians who specialize in such areas as otolaryngology, dermatology, and pathology.

ORGANIZATION

The purpose of the third edition of this text remains the same: to provide the reader with a comprehensive discussion of the wide variety of diseases that may affect the oral and maxillofacial region. *Oral and Maxillofacial Pathology* has been organized to serve as a primary teaching text, although it should also be a valuable reference source for the practicing clinician. Chapters have been created that include disease processes of a similar source (e.g., "Bacterial Infections," "Salivary Gland Pathology," "Bone Pathology," "Dermatologic Diseases"), because the basic understanding of pathology is facilitated by discussing diseases of a similar nature at the same time. Only after attaining this basic understanding can the clinician tackle the difficult task of clinical diagnosis and treatment. With this in mind, a comprehensive appendix is included at the end of the book to help the clinician with the differential diagnosis of oral and maxillofacial disease processes.

It is impossible to write a book that perfectly matches the requirements of every reader. Because all the authors are involved in teaching, the subjects selected for inclusion in this text primarily reflect what is taught in courses on oral and maxillofacial pathology. Although dental caries is undeniably a common and important disease affecting the oral cavity, it is usually not taught in an oral and maxillofacial pathology course; rather, it is taught elsewhere in most dental schools' curricula. Therefore, we have not included a chapter on dental caries. Similarly, our discussion on common gingivitis and periodontitis is limited in scope, although a more in-depth discussion is provided for other conditions that affect the periodontium. In other areas, the text offers greater detail than necessary for some primary courses in oral and maxillofacial pathology. However, because this book is also intended as a reference source for the practicing clinician, this additional material has been included.

NEW TO THIS EDITION

It has been seven years since the publication of the second edition of this text. Although this is seemingly a short time, many significant advances have been made in our understanding of various oral diseases during this period. We have added a number of new topics, including:

- Bisphosphonate-associated osteonecrosis
- Hemangiopericytoma–solitary fibrous tumor
- Transient lingual papillitis
- Tongue splitting and charm needles
- Hereditary mucoepithelial dysplasia
- Chronic ulcerative stomatitis
- Plasminogen deficiency
- Oral manifestions of methamphetamine abuse

We also have included more than 200 new illustrations in this latest edition.

This new edition features an accompanying Evolve site. A specific listing of the Evolve assets for students can be found in the front of the book.

ACKNOWLEDGMENTS

Obviously, this book could not have been accomplished without the help of many individuals. We wish to thank Dr. Edward E. Herschaft, who thoroughly updated his excellent chapter on forensic dentistry. For this third edition, we are deeply indebted to Dr. Angela C. Chi, who revised the chapters on Epithelial Pathology and Bone Pathology. We are also grateful to Dr. Theresa S. Gonzales, who updated the chapter on Facial Pain and Neuromuscular Diseases. We must thank our many colleagues who shared cases with us, and they have been credited in the legends of the illustrations. Although these individuals are too numerous to cite here, one person in particular, Dr. George Blozis, deserves special recognition for his generosity in sharing his excellent teaching collection. We have attempted to be as thorough as possible in listing credit for all the cases shared with us. However, if someone's name has been inadvertently omitted, please accept our apologies.

Since its inception, this book has been dedicated to three of our mentors: Drs. Charles Waldron, William Shafer, and Robert Gorlin. For the first edition of this text, we were fortunate to have Dr. Waldron write two outstanding chapters on areas of his special interest and expertise, "Bone Pathology" and "Odontogenic Cysts and Tumors." We and those in the oral pathology community were tremendously saddened by his death in 1995. Chuck's unique expertise has been greatly missed during the revision of these chapters, but their content still reflects much of his basic philosophy. In 2000, we were sorry to learn of the death of Dr. Shafer, who was the principal author of the well-known and respected book, *A Textbook of Oral Pathology*. This valuable resource was the "bible" that we all used for many years to learn about and teach our specialty. We also mourn the death in 2006 of Dr. Robert Gorlin, one of the true geniuses in the fields of oral pathology and genetics. Dr. Gorlin, who was still active in patient care and research at the time of his death at the age of 83, offered numerous excellent suggestions for improvements in the second and third editions of our

book. We truly have stood on the shoulders of giants.

We would like to acknowledge the people at Elsevier Health Sciences for their hard work in making this book a success. We must praise Courtney Sprehe and John Dolan, who helped us at every step and did an excellent job coordinating the many aspects of the publishing process. Tripp Narup provided valuable guidance to help us with the digitization of the illustrations. Many thanks go to Jonathan Taylor, who was responsible for the primary editing of the manuscript and correcting our many mistakes. In addition, even though she has now moved on to more important responsibilities, we still must recognize Penny Rudolph, who handled us with aplomb through the first two editions of the book.

Finally, our deepest thanks must go to our families for their support during the writing of this book. They have had to endure our neglect during the long hours of work, and this project could never have been completed without their love and encouragement.

BRAD W. NEVILLE
DOUGLAS D. DAMM
CARL M. ALLEN
JERRY E. BOUQUOT

Contents

CHAPTER 5
Bacterial Infections, 181

CHAPTER 6
Fungal and Protozoal Diseases, 213

CHAPTER 7
Viral Infections, 240

CHAPTER 8
Physical and Chemical Injuries, 285

CHAPTER 9
Allergies and Immunologic Diseases, 330

CHAPTER 10
Epithelial Pathology, 362

Revised by ANGELA C. CHI

Contents

CHAPTER 11
Salivary Gland Pathology, 453

Salivary Gland Tumors, 473

CHAPTER 12
Soft Tissue Tumors, 507

Soft Tissue Sarcomas, 552

CHAPTER 13
Hematologic Disorders, 571

CHAPTER 14
Bone Pathology, 613

Revised By ANGELA C. CHI

Fibro-Osseous Lesions of the Jaws, 635

CHAPTER 15
Odontogenic Cysts and Tumors, 678

Odontogenic Cysts, 678

Odontogenic Tumors, 701
Tumors of Odontogenic Epithelium, 702

Mixed Odontogenic Tumors, 719

Tumors of Odontogenic Ectomesenchyme, 726

Developmental Defects of the Oral and Maxillofacial Region

CHAPTER OUTLINE

OROFACIAL CLEFTS

The formation of the face and oral cavity is complex in nature and involves the development of multiple tissue processes that must merge and fuse in a highly orchestrated fashion. Disturbances in the growth of these tissue processes or their fusion may result in the formation of **orofacial clefts.**

Development of the central face begins around the end of the fourth week of human development, with the appearance of the nasal (olfactory) placodes on either side of the inferior aspect of the frontonasal process. Proliferation of ectomesenchyme on both sides of each placode results in the formation of the medial and lateral nasal processes. Between each pair of processes is a depression, or nasal pit, that represents the primitive nostril.

During the sixth and seventh weeks of development, the upper lip forms when the medial nasal processes merge with each other and with the maxillary processes of the first branchial arches. Thus the midportion of the upper lip is derived from the medial nasal processes, and the lateral portions are derived from the maxillary processes. The lateral nasal processes are not involved in the formation of the upper lip, but they give rise to the alae of the nose.

The **primary palate** also is formed by the merger of the medial nasal processes to form the intermaxillary segment. This segment gives rise to the premaxilla, a triangular-shaped piece of bone that will include the four incisor teeth. The **secondary palate,** which makes up 90% of the hard and soft palates, is formed from the maxillary processes of the first branchial arches.

During the sixth week, bilateral projections emerge from the medial aspects of the maxillary processes to form the palatal shelves. Initially, these shelves are oriented in a vertical position on each side of the developing tongue. As the mandible grows, the tongue drops down, allowing the palatal shelves to rotate to a horizontal position and grow toward one another. By the eighth week, sufficient growth has occurred to allow the anterior aspects of these shelves to begin fusion with one another. The palatal shelves also fuse with the primary palate and the nasal septum. The fusion of the palatal shelves begins in the anterior palate and progresses posteriorly; it is completed by the twelfth week.

Defective fusion of the medial nasal process with the maxillary process leads to **cleft lip** (CL). Likewise, failure of the palatal shelves to fuse results in **cleft palate** (CP). Frequently, CL and CP occur together. Approximately 45% of cases are CL + CP, with 30% being CP only (CPO) and 25% being isolated CL. Both isolated CL and CL associated with CP are thought to be etiologically related conditions and can be considered as a group: CL, with or without CP (i.e., CL ± CP). Isolated CPO appears to represent a separate entity from CL ± CP.

The cause of CL ± CP and CPO is still being debated. First of all, distinguishing isolated clefts from cases associated with specific syndromes is important. Although many facial clefts are isolated anomalies, more than 350 developmental syndromes have been identified that may be associated with CL ± CP or CPO. Recent studies have suggested that up to 30% of patients with CL ± CP and 50% of those with CPO have associated anomalies. Some of these cases are single-gene syndromes that may follow autosomal dominant, autosomal recessive, or X-linked inheritance patterns. Other syndromes are the result of chromosome anomalies or are idiopathic.

Box 1-1

Genetic and Environmental Causes of Nonsyndromic Orofacial Clefts

GENETIC FACTORS

Gene	Locus
SKI/MTHFR	1p36
TGFB2	1q41
TGFA	2p13
MSX1	4p16, 4q31, 6p23
PVRL1	11q23
TGFB3	14q24
GABRB3	15q11
RARA	17q21
BCL3	19q13

ENVIRONMENTAL FACTORS

- Maternal alcohol consumption
- Maternal cigarette smoking
- Folic acid deficiency
- Corticosteroid use
- Anticonvulsant therapy

Adapted from Murray JC: Gene/environment causes of cleft lip and/or palate, *Clin Genet* 61:248-256, 2002; Eppley BL, van Aalst JA, Robey A et al: The spectrum of orofacial clefting, *Plast Reconstr Surg* 115:101e-114e, 2005.

The cause of nonsyndromic clefts does not follow any simple mendelian pattern of inheritance but appears to be heterogeneous (Box 1-1). Thus the propensity for cleft development may be related to a number of major genes, minor genes, and environmental factors that can combine to surpass a developmental threshold. A number of candidate clefting genes and loci have been identified on different chromosome regions, such as 1q, 2p, 4q, 6p, 14q, 17q, and 19q. Maternal alcohol consumption has been associated with an increased risk for both syndromic and nonsyndromic clefts. Maternal cigarette smoking at least doubles the frequency of cleft development compared with nonsmoking mothers. Multiple studies have demonstrated that a deficiency of folic acid increases the risk for CL and CP. Maternal corticosteroid use has been associated with a 3.4 times greater risk of orofacial clefting. An increased frequency also has been related to anticonvulsant therapy, especially phenytoin, which causes a nearly tenfold greater risk of cleft formation.

CL ± CP and CPO represent the vast majority of orofacial clefts. However, other rare clefts also may occur.

The **lateral facial cleft** is caused by lack of fusion of the maxillary and mandibular processes and represents 0.3% of all facial clefts. This cleft may be unilateral or bilateral, extending from the commissure toward the ear, resulting in macrostomia. The lateral facial cleft may occur as an isolated defect, but more often it is associated with other disorders, such as the following:

- Mandibulofacial dysostosis (see page 45)
- Oculo-auriculo-vertebral spectrum (hemifacial microsomia)
- Nager acrofacial dysostosis
- Amniotic rupture sequence

The **oblique facial cleft** extends from the upper lip to the eye. It is nearly always associated with CP, and severe forms often are incompatible with life. The oblique facial cleft may involve the nostril, as in CL, or it may bypass the nose laterally as it extends to the eye. This cleft is rare, representing only 1 in 1300 facial clefts. Some of these clefts may represent failure of fusion of the lateral nasal process with the maxillary process; amniotic bands may cause others.

Median cleft of the upper lip is an extremely rare anomaly that results from failure of fusion of the medial nasal processes. It may be associated with a number of syndromes, including the oral-facial-digital syndromes and Ellis-van Creveld syndrome. Most apparent median clefts of the upper lip actually represent agenesis of the primary palate associated with holoprosencephaly.

CLINICAL AND RADIOGRAPHIC FEATURES

Clefting is one of the most common major congenital defects in humans. Considerable racial variation in prevalence is seen. In whites, CL ± CP occurs in 1 of every 700 to 1000 births. The frequency of CL ± CP in Asian populations is about 1.5 times higher than in whites. In contrast, the prevalence of CL ± CP in blacks is much lower, occurring in 0.4 of 1000 births. Native Americans appear to have the highest frequency, around 3.6 of 1000 births. CPO is less common than CL ± CP, with a frequency of 0.4 of 1000 births in whites and blacks.

CL ± CP is more common in males than in females. The more severe the defect, the greater the male predilection; the male-to-female ratio for isolated CL is 1.5:1; the ratio for CL + CP is 2:1. In contrast, CPO is more common in females. Likewise, the more severe the cleft, the greater the female predilection. Clefts of both the hard and soft palates are twice as common in females, but the ratio is nearly equal for clefts of the soft palate only.

Approximately 80% of cases of CL will be unilateral, with 20% bilateral (Fig. 1-1). Approximately 70% of unilateral CLs occur on the left side. In addition, about 70% of unilateral CLs will be associated with CP, whereas the frequency of concomitant CP increases to 85% for patients with bilateral CL. A complete CL

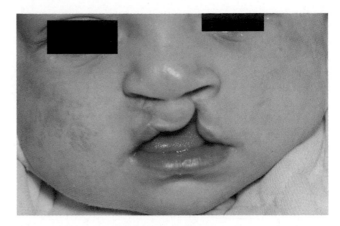

Fig. 1-1   Cleft lip (CL). Infant with bilateral cleft of the upper lip. *(Courtesy of Dr. William Bruce.)*

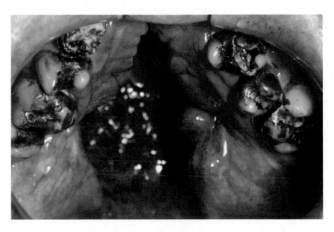

Fig. 1-2   Cleft palate (CP). Palatal defect resulting in communication with the nasal cavity.

extends upward into the nostril, but an incomplete CL does not involve the nose. Complete clefts involving the alveolus usually occur between the lateral incisor and cuspid. It is not unusual for teeth, especially the lateral incisor, to be missing in the cleft area. Conversely, supernumerary teeth may be discovered. The bony defect can be observed on radiographs.

A CP shows considerable range in severity (Fig. 1-2). The defect may involve the hard and soft palates or the soft palate alone. The minimal manifestation of CP is a **cleft** or **bifid uvula** (Fig. 1-3). The prevalence of cleft uvula is much higher than that of CP, with a frequency of 1 in every 80 white individuals. The frequency in Asian and Native American populations is as high as 1 in 10. Cleft uvula is less common in blacks, occurring in 1 out of every 250 persons.

In some instances a **submucous palatal cleft** develops. The surface mucosa is intact, but a defect exists in the underlying musculature of the soft palate (Fig. 1-4). Frequently a notch in the bone is present along the

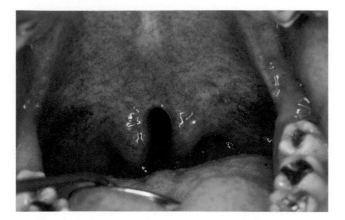

Fig. 1-3   Bifid uvula.

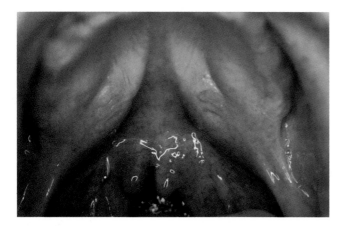

Fig. 1-4   Submucous palatal cleft. A cleft of the midline palatal bone exists, but the overlying mucosa is intact. A bifid uvula also is present.

posterior margin of the hard palate. This incomplete cleft occasionally appears as a bluish midline discoloration but is best identified by palpation with a blunt instrument. An associated cleft uvula is also usually seen.

The **Pierre Robin sequence** (Pierre Robin anomalad) (Fig. 1-5) is a well-recognized presentation characterized by CP, mandibular micrognathia, and glossoptosis (airway obstruction caused by lower, posterior displacement of the tongue). The Pierre Robin sequence may occur as an isolated phenomenon, or it may be associated with a wide variety of syndromes or other anomalies. Stickler syndrome and velocardiofacial syndrome are the two most frequently associated genetic disorders. Researchers have theorized that constraint of mandibular growth *in utero* results in failure of the tongue to descend, thus preventing fusion of the palatal shelves. The retruded mandible results in the following:

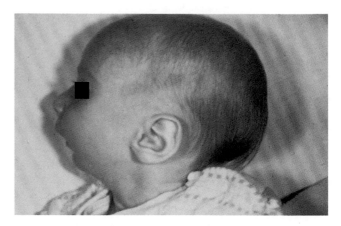

Fig. 1-5   Pierre Robin sequence. Micrognathic mandible in an infant with cleft palate (CP). *(Courtesy of Dr. Robert Gorlin.)*

- Posterior displacement of the tongue
- Lack of support of the tongue musculature
- Airway obstruction

Respiratory difficulty, especially when the child is in a supine position, is usually noted from birth and can cause asphyxiation. The palatal cleft is often U-shaped and wider than isolated CP.

The patient with a cleft is burdened with a variety of problems, some obvious and some less so. The most obvious problem is the clinical appearance, which may lead to psychosocial difficulties. Feeding and speech difficulties are inherent, especially with CP. Malocclusion is caused by collapse of the maxillary arch, possibly along with missing teeth, supernumerary teeth, or both.

TREATMENT AND PROGNOSIS

The management of the patient with an orofacial cleft is challenging. Ideally, treatment should involve a multidisciplinary approach, including (but not limited to) a pediatrician, oral and maxillofacial surgeon, otolaryngologist, plastic surgeon, pediatric dentist, orthodontist, prosthodontist, speech pathologist, and geneticist.

Surgical repair often involves multiple primary and secondary procedures throughout childhood. The specific types of surgical procedures and their timing will vary, depending on the severity of the defect and the philosophy of the treatment team. A detailed discussion of these procedures is beyond the scope of this text. However, primary lip closure is usually accomplished during the first few months of life, followed later by repair of the palate. Prosthetic and orthopedic appliances often are used to mold or expand the maxillary segments before closure of the palatal defect. Later in childhood, autogenous bone grafts can be placed in the area of the alveolar bone defect. Secondary soft tissue and orthognathic procedures may be used to improve function and cosmetic appearance. Distraction osteogenesis of the maxilla can prove useful in patients in whom palatal scarring limits the amount of advancement possible at the time of osteotomy.

Genetic counseling is important for the patient and family. In nonsyndromic cases, the risk for cleft development in a sibling or offspring of an affected person is 3% to 5% if no other first-degree relatives also are affected. The risk increases to 10% to 20% if other first-degree relatives are affected. The risk may be even higher for those with clefts that are associated with syndromes, depending on the possible inheritance pattern.

COMMISSURAL LIP PITS

Commissural lip pits are small mucosal invaginations that occur at the corners of the mouth on the vermilion border. Their location suggests that they may represent a failure of normal fusion of the embryonal maxillary and mandibular processes.

Commissural lip pits appear to be common in adults, where they have been reported in 12% to 20% of the population. Their prevalence in children is considerably lower, ranging from 0.2% to 0.7% of those examined.

Although commissural lip pits are generally considered to be congenital lesions, these figures suggest that these invaginations often develop later in life. Commissural pits are seen more often in males than in females. A family history suggestive of autosomal dominant transmission has been noted in some cases.

CLINICAL FEATURES

Commissural lip pits are usually discovered on routine examination, and the patient often is unaware of their presence. These pits may be unilateral or bilateral. They manifest as blind fistulas that may extend to a depth of 1 to 4 mm (Fig. 1-6). In some cases a small amount of fluid may be expressed from the pit when the pit is squeezed, presumably representing saliva from minor salivary glands that drain into the depth of the invagination.

Unlike **paramedian lip pits** (described in the following section), commissural lip pits are not associated with facial or palatal clefts. However, there does appear to be a significantly higher prevalence of preauricular pits (aural sinuses) in these patients.

HISTOPATHOLOGIC FEATURES

Although biopsy rarely is performed for patients with commissural lip pits, microscopic examination reveals a narrow invagination lined by stratified squamous epi-

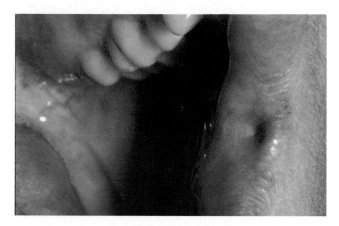

Fig. 1-6   Commissural lip pit. Depression at the labial commissure.

thelium. Ducts from minor salivary glands may drain into this invagination.

TREATMENT AND PROGNOSIS

Because commissural lip pits are virtually always asymptomatic and innocuous, no treatment is usually necessary. In extremely rare instances, salivary secretions may be excessive or secondary infection may occur, necessitating surgical excision of the pit.

PARAMEDIAN LIP PITS (CONGENITAL FISTULAS OF THE LOWER LIP; CONGENITAL LIP PITS)

Paramedian lip pits are rare congenital invaginations of the lower lip. They are believed to arise from persistent lateral sulci on the embryonic mandibular arch. These sulci normally disappear by 6 weeks of embryonic age.

CLINICAL FEATURES

Paramedian lip pits typically appear as bilateral and symmetric fistulas on either side of the midline of the vermilion of the lower lip (Fig. 1-7). Their appearance can range from subtle depressions to prominent humps. These blind sinuses can extend down to a depth of 1.5 cm and may express salivary secretions. Occasionally, only a single pit is present that may be centrally located or lateral to the midline.

The greatest significance of paramedian lip pits is that they are usually inherited as an autosomal dominant trait in combination with cleft lip (CL) and/or cleft palate (CP) **(van der Woude syndrome)**. Van der Woude syndrome is the most common form of syndromic clefting and accounts for 2% of all cases of CL

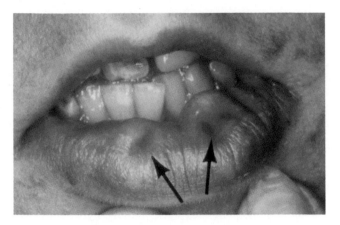

Fig. 1-7   Paramedian lip pits. Bilateral pits (*arrows*) on the lower lip in a patient with van der Woude syndrome.

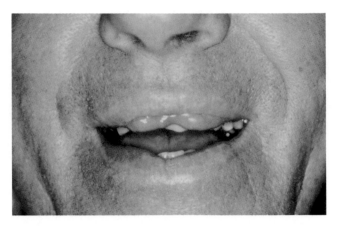

Fig. 1-8   Double lip. Redundant fold of tissue on the upper lip in a patient with Ascher syndrome. *(Courtesy of Dr. R.C. Zeigler.)*

and CP. Associated hypodontia also may be observed. Genetic studies have shown that this condition is caused by mutations in the gene that encodes interferon regulatory factor 6, which has been mapped to chromosome locus 1q32-q41. Some people who carry the trait may not demonstrate clefts or may have a submucous CP; however, they may pass the full syndrome to their offspring.

Paramedian lip pits also may be a feature of the **popliteal pterygium syndrome** and **Kabuki syndrome.** Popliteal webbing **(pterygia),** CL and/or CP, genital abnormalities, and congenital bands connecting the upper and lower jaws **(syngnathia)** characterize popliteal pterygium syndrome, which is closely related to van der Woude syndrome. Kabuki syndrome received its name because affected patients exhibit eversion of the lower lateral eyelids, which is reminiscent of the makeup used by actors in Kabuki, the traditional form of Japanese theater. Other common findings include mental retardation, large ears, CL and/or CP, hypodontia, joint laxity, and various skeletal abnormalities.

HISTOPATHOLOGIC FEATURES

Microscopic examination of a paramedian lip pit shows a tract that is lined by stratified squamous epithelium. Minor salivary glands may communicate with the sinus. A chronic inflammatory cell infiltrate often is noted in the surrounding connective tissue.

TREATMENT AND PROGNOSIS

If necessary, the labial pits may be excised for cosmetic reasons. The most significant problems are related to associated congenital anomalies, such as CL and/or

CP, and the potential for transmission of the trait to subsequent generations.

DOUBLE LIP

Double lip is a rare oral anomaly characterized by a redundant fold of tissue on the mucosal side of the lip. It is most often congenital in nature, but it may be acquired later in life. Congenital cases are believed to arise during the second to third month of gestation as a result of the persistence of the sulcus between the pars glabrosa and pars villosa of the lip. Acquired double lip may be a component of **Ascher syndrome,** or it may result from trauma or oral habits, such as sucking on the lip.

CLINICAL FEATURES

In a patient with double lip, the upper lip is affected much more often than the lower lip; occasionally, both lips are involved. With the lips at rest, the condition is usually unnoticeable, but when the patient smiles or when the lips are tensed, the excess fold of tissue is visible (Fig. 1-8).

Ascher syndrome is characterized by a triad of features:
- Double lip
- Blepharochalasis
- Nontoxic thyroid enlargement

In a person with blepharochalasis, recurring edema of the upper eyelid leads to sagging of the lid at the outer canthus of the eye (Fig. 1-9). This drooping may be severe enough to interfere with vision. Both the double lip and blepharochalasis usually occur abruptly and simultaneously, but in some cases they develop more gradually.

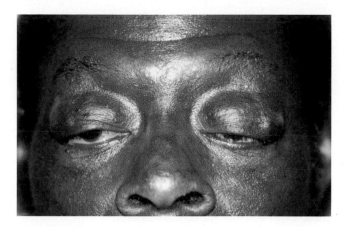

Fig. 1-9   Ascher syndrome. Edema of the upper eyelids (blepharochalasis).

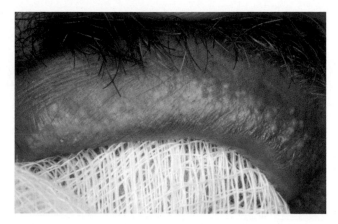

Fig. 1-10   Fordyce granules. Yellow papules on the vermilion of the upper lip.

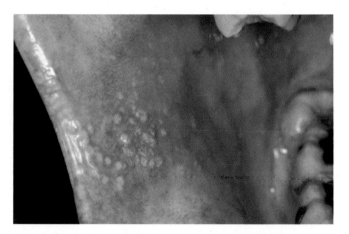

Fig. 1-11   Fordyce granules. Lesions at the commissure.

The nontoxic thyroid enlargement occurs in as many as 50% of patients with Ascher syndrome and may be mild in degree. The cause of Ascher syndrome is not certain; autosomal dominant inheritance has been suggested in some cases.

HISTOPATHOLOGIC FEATURES

On microscopic examination, double lip shows essentially normal structures. Often there is an abundance of minor salivary glands. The blepharochalasis of Ascher syndrome usually shows hyperplasia of the lacrimal glands or prolapse of orbital fat.

TREATMENT AND PROGNOSIS

In mild cases of double lip, no treatment may be required. In more severe cases, simple surgical excision of the excess tissue can be performed for aesthetic purposes.

FORDYCE GRANULES

Fordyce granules are sebaceous glands that occur on the oral mucosa. Similar lesions also have been reported on the genital mucosa. Because sebaceous glands are typically considered to be dermal adnexal structures, those found in the oral cavity often have been considered to be "ectopic." However, because Fordyce granules have been reported in more than 80% of the population, their presence must be considered a normal anatomic variation.

CLINICAL FEATURES

Fordyce granules appear as multiple yellow or yellow-white papular lesions that are most common on the buccal mucosa and the lateral portion of the vermilion of the upper lip (Figs. 1-10 and 1-11). Occasionally, these glands also may appear in the retromolar area and anterior tonsillar pillar. They are more common in adults than in children, probably as a result of hormonal factors; puberty appears to stimulate their development. The lesions are typically asymptomatic, although patients may be able to feel a slight roughness to the mucosa. Considerable clinical variation may exist; some patients may have only a few lesions, whereas others may have literally hundreds of these "granules."

HISTOPATHOLOGIC FEATURES

Except for the absence of associated hair follicles, Fordyce granules are closely similar to normal sebaceous glands found in the skin. Acinar lobules can be seen immediately beneath the epithelial surface, often communicating with the surface through a central duct (Fig. 1-12). The sebaceous cells in these lobules are

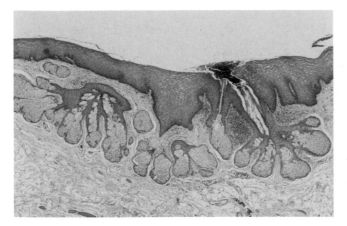

Fig. 1-12 **Fordyce granules.** Multiple sebaceous glands below the surface epithelium.

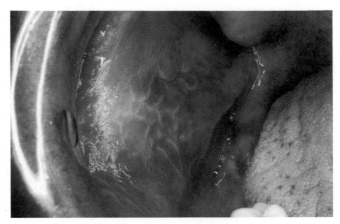

Fig. 1-13 **Leukoedema.** White, wrinkled appearance of the buccal mucosa.

polygonal in shape, containing centrally located nuclei and abundant foamy cytoplasm.

TREATMENT AND PROGNOSIS

Because Fordyce granules represent a normal anatomic variation and are asymptomatic, no treatment is indicated. Usually, the clinical appearance is characteristic and biopsy is not necessary for diagnosis.

On occasion, Fordyce granules may become hyperplastic or may form keratin-filled pseudocysts. Tumors arising from these glands are exceedingly rare.

LEUKOEDEMA

Leukoedema is a common oral mucosal condition of unknown cause. It occurs more commonly in blacks than in whites, supporting the likelihood of an ethnic predisposition to its development. Leukoedema has been reported in 70% to 90% of black adults and in 50% of black children. The prevalence in whites is considerably less, although published reports have ranged from less than 10% to more than 90%. This variation may reflect differing population groups, examination conditions, and stringency of criteria used to make the diagnosis. At any rate, leukoedema shows a much milder presentation in whites and often is hardly noticeable. The difference in racial predilection may be explained by the presence of background mucosal pigmentation in blacks that makes the edematous changes more noticeable.

Because leukoedema is so common, it can reasonably be argued that it represents a *variation of normal* rather than a disease. The finding of similar edematous mucosa in the vagina and larynx further supports this argument. Although leukoedema appears to be developmental in nature, some studies have indicated that it is more common and more severe in smokers and becomes less pronounced with cessation of smoking.

CLINICAL FEATURES

Leukoedema is characterized by a diffuse, gray-white, milky, opalescent appearance of the mucosa (Fig. 1-13). The surface frequently appears folded, resulting in wrinkles or whitish streaks. The lesions do not rub off. Leukoedema typically occurs bilaterally on the buccal mucosa and may extend forward onto the labial mucosa. On rare occasions, it can also involve the floor of the mouth and palatopharyngeal tissues. Leukoedema can be easily diagnosed clinically because the white appearance greatly diminishes or disappears when the cheek is everted and stretched (Fig. 1-14).

HISTOPATHOLOGIC FEATURES

Biopsy specimens of leukoedema demonstrate an increase in thickness of the epithelium, with striking intracellular edema of the spinous layer (Fig. 1-15). These vacuolated cells appear large and have pyknotic nuclei. The epithelial surface is frequently parakeratinized, and the rete ridges are broad and elongated.

TREATMENT AND PROGNOSIS

Leukoedema is a benign condition, and no treatment is required. The characteristic milky-white, opalescent lesions of the buccal mucosa that disappear when stretched help distinguish it from other common white lesions, such as leukoplakia, candidiasis, and lichen

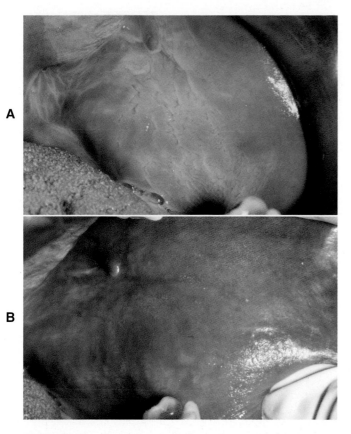

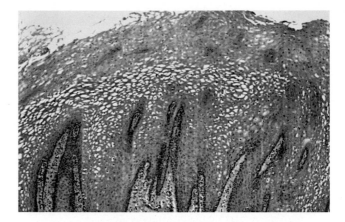

Fig. 1-15   Leukoedema. Parakeratosis and intracellular edema of the spinous layer.

Fig. 1-14   Leukoedema. A, Diffuse white appearance of the buccal mucosa. **B,** Whiteness disappears when the cheek is stretched.

planus. The affected mucosa always should be stretched during clinical examination to rule out any underlying lesions that may be hidden by the edematous change.

MICROGLOSSIA (HYPOGLOSSIA)

CLINICAL FEATURES

Microglossia is an uncommon developmental condition of unknown cause that is characterized by an abnormally small tongue. In rare instances, virtually the entire tongue may be missing **(aglossia).** Isolated microglossia is known to occur, and mild degrees of microglossia may be difficult to detect and may go unnoticed. However, most reported cases have been associated with one of a group of overlapping conditions known as **oromandibular-limb hypogenesis syndromes.** These syndromes feature associated limb anomalies, such as **hypodactylia** (i.e., absence of digits) and **hypomelia** (i.e., hypoplasia of part or all of a limb). Other patients have had coexisting anomalies, such as cleft palate, intraoral bands, and situs inversus. Microglossia frequently is associated with hypoplasia of the mandible, and the lower incisors may be missing (Fig. 1-16).

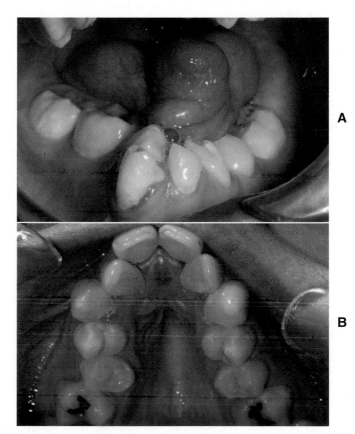

Fig. 1-16   Microglossia. A, Abnormally small tongue associated with constricted mandibular arch. **B,** Same patient with associated constriction of the maxillary arch.

TREATMENT AND PROGNOSIS

Treatment of the patient with microglossia depends on the nature and severity of the condition. Surgery and orthodontics may improve oral function. Surprisingly, speech development often is quite good but depends on tongue size.

Box 1-2

Causes of Macroglossia

CONGENITAL AND HEREDITARY
- Vascular malformations
- Lymphangioma
- Hemangioma
- Hemihyperplasia
- Cretinism
- Beckwith-Wiedemann syndrome
- Down syndrome
- Mucopolysaccharidoses
- Neurofibromatosis type I
- Multiple endocrine neoplasia, type 2B

ACQUIRED
- Edentulous patients
- Amyloidosis
- Myxedema
- Acromegaly
- Angioedema
- Carcinoma and other tumors

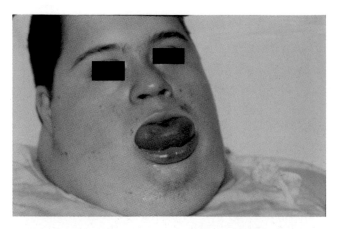

Fig. 1-17   Macroglossia. Large tongue in a patient with Down syndrome. *(Courtesy of Dr. Sanford Fenton.)*

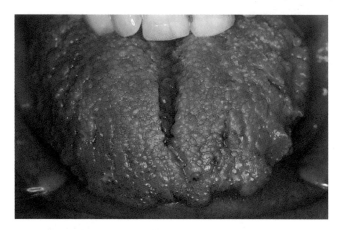

Fig. 1-18   Macroglossia. The tongue enlargement has resulted in a crenated border that corresponds to the embrasures between the teeth.

MACROGLOSSIA

Macroglossia is an uncommon condition characterized by enlargement of the tongue. The enlargement may be caused by a wide variety of conditions, including congenital malformations and acquired diseases. The most frequent causes are vascular malformations and muscular hypertrophy. Box 1-2 lists the most common and important causes of macroglossia. Many of these diseases are discussed in greater detail in subsequent chapters of this book.

CLINICAL FEATURES

Macroglossia most commonly occurs in children and can range from mild to severe (Fig. 1-17). In infants, macroglossia may be manifested first by noisy breathing, drooling, and difficulty in eating. The tongue enlargement may result in a lisping speech. The pressure of the tongue against the mandible and teeth can produce a crenated lateral border to the tongue (Fig. 1-18), open bite, and mandibular prognathism. If the tongue constantly protrudes from the mouth, it may ulcerate and become secondarily infected or may even undergo necrosis. Severe macroglossia can produce airway obstruction.

Macroglossia is a characteristic feature of **Beck-with-Wiedemann syndrome,** a rare hereditary condition that includes many other possible defects, such as the following:

- Omphalocele (i.e., protrusion of part of the intestine through a defect in the abdominal wall at the umbilicus)
- Visceromegaly
- Gigantism
- Neonatal hypoglycemia

Individuals with Beckwith-Wiedemann syndrome have an increased risk for several childhood visceral tumors, including Wilms' tumor, adrenal carcinoma, hepatoblastoma, rhabdomyosarcoma, and neuroblastoma. Facial features may include nevus flammeus of the forehead and eyelids, linear indentations of the earlobes, and maxillary hypoplasia (resulting in relative mandibular prognathism). Most examples of Beckwith-Wiedemann syndrome are sporadic, but 10% to 15% of cases show autosomal dominant inheritance with preferential maternal transmission. The genetic basis is complex, involving a variety of alterations within two domains of imprinted growth-regulatory genes on chromosome 11p15.

In patients with **hypothyroidism** (see page 843) or Beckwith-Wiedemann syndrome, the tongue usually shows a diffuse, smooth, generalized enlargement. In those with other forms of macroglossia, the tongue usually has a multinodular appearance. Examples of this nodular type include **amyloidosis** (see page 822) and neoplastic conditions, such as **neurofibromatosis** (see page 529) and **multiple endocrine neoplasia, type 2B** (see page 532).

In patients with **lymphangiomas** (see page 547), the tongue surface is characteristically pebbly and exhibits multiple vesicle-like blebs that represent superficial dilated lymphatic channels. The enlarged tongue in those with **Down syndrome** typically demonstrates a papillary, fissured surface.

In patients with **hemifacial hyperplasia** (see page 38), the enlargement will be unilateral. Some patients with neurofibromatosis also can have unilateral lingual enlargement.

In edentulous patients, the tongue often appears elevated and tends to spread out laterally because of loss of the surrounding teeth; as a result, wearing a denture may become difficult.

HISTOPATHOLOGIC FEATURES

The microscopic appearance of macroglossia depends on the specific cause. In some cases, such as the tongue enlargement seen with Down syndrome or in edentulous patients, no histologic abnormality can be detected. When macroglossia is due to tumor, a neoplastic proliferation of a particular tissue can be found (e.g., lymphatic vessels, blood vessels, neural tissue). Muscular enlargement occurs in those with hemihyperplasia and Beckwith-Wiedemann syndrome. In the patient with amyloidosis, an abnormal protein material is deposited in the tongue.

TREATMENT AND PROGNOSIS

The treatment and prognosis of macroglossia depend on the cause and severity of the condition. In mild cases, surgical treatment may not be necessary, although speech therapy may be helpful if speech is affected. In symptomatic patients, reduction glossectomy may be needed.

ANKYLOGLOSSIA (TONGUE-TIE)

Ankyloglossia is a developmental anomaly of the tongue characterized by a short, thick lingual frenum resulting in limitation of tongue movement. It has been reported to occur in 1.7% to 4.4% of neonates and is four times more common in boys than in girls. In adults, mild forms are not unusual, but severe ankyloglossia

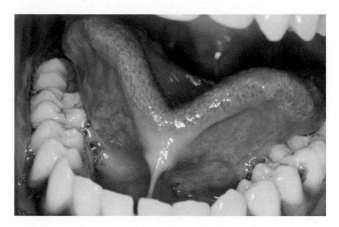

Fig. 1-19   Ankyloglossia. Abnormal attachment of the lingual frenum, limiting tongue mobility.

is a relatively uncommon condition that has been estimated to occur in about 2 to 3 of every 10,000 people.

CLINICAL FEATURES

Ankyloglossia can range in severity from mild cases with little clinical significance to rare examples of complete ankyloglossia in which the tongue is actually fused to the floor of the mouth (Fig. 1-19). Sometimes the frenum extends forward and attaches to the tip of the tongue, and slight clefting of the tip may be seen.

Some investigators have speculated that ankyloglossia may contribute to the development of an anterior open bite because the inability to raise the tongue to the roof of the mouth prevents development of the normal adult swallowing pattern. However, others have questioned this theory. It also is possible that a high mucogingival attachment of the lingual frenum may lead to periodontal problems.

It has been suggested that tongue-tie may result in speech defects. Usually, however, the shortened frenum results in only minor difficulties because most people can compensate for the limitation in tongue movement. Yet there are rare examples of patients who have experienced an immediate noticeable improvement in speech after surgical correction of ankyloglossia. With the increase in popularity of breast-feeding over the past several decades, some clinicians have related tongue-tie with feeding problems, such as nipple pain or difficulty in the baby attaching to the breast. Recent reports from Japan have theorized that some ankyloglossia cases can be associated with an upward and forward displacement of the epiglottis and larynx, resulting in various degrees of dyspnea.

TREATMENT AND PROGNOSIS

Because most cases of ankyloglossia result in few or no clinical problems, treatment is often unnecessary. For infants with specific breast-feeding problems, a frenotomy ("clipping" or simple release of the frenulum) can be performed. In children or adults with associated functional or periodontal difficulties, a frenuloplasty (release with plastic repair) may allow greater freedom of tongue movement. In young children it often is recommended that surgery be postponed until age 4 or 5. Because the tongue is always short at birth, assessing the degree of tongue limitation caused by ankyloglossia is difficult in the infant's early life. As the infant grows, the tongue becomes longer and thinner at the tip, often decreasing the severity of the tongue-tie. The condition probably is self-correcting in many cases because it is less common in adults.

LINGUAL THYROID

During the third to fourth week of fetal life, the thyroid gland begins as an epithelial proliferation in the floor of the pharyngeal gut. By the seventh embryonic week, this thyroid bud normally descends into the neck to its final resting position anterior to the trachea and larynx. The site where this descending bud invaginates later becomes the foramen cecum, located at the junction of the anterior two thirds and posterior third of the tongue in the midline. If the primitive gland does not descend normally, ectopic thyroid tissue may be found between the foramen cecum and the epiglottis. Of all ectopic thyroids, 90% are found in this region.

CLINICAL FEATURES

Based on autopsy studies, small asymptomatic remnants of thyroid tissue can be discovered on the posterior dorsal tongue in about 10% of both men and women. However, clinically evident or symptomatic **lingual thyroids** are much less common and are four to seven times more frequent in females, presumably because of hormonal influences. Symptoms most often develop during puberty, adolescence, pregnancy, or menopause. In 70% of cases, this ectopic gland is the patient's only thyroid tissue.

Lingual thyroids may range from small, asymptomatic, nodular lesions to large masses that can block the airway (Fig. 1-20). The most common clinical symptoms are dysphagia, dysphonia, and dyspnea. The mass often is vascular, but the physical appearance is variable and there are no reliable features to distinguish it from other masses that might develop in this area. Hypothyroidism has been reported in up to 33% of patients. Many authors say that lingual thyroid enlarge-

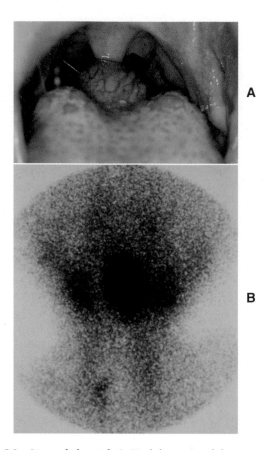

Fig. 1-20 Lingual thyroid. A, Nodular mass of the posterior dorsal midline of the tongue in a 4-year-old girl. **B,** Thyroid scan of the same patient. The scan shows localization (*central dark zone*) of iodine isotope in the tongue mass and minimal uptake in the neck.

ment is a secondary phenomenon, compensating for thyroid hypofunction. Interestingly, as many as 75% of patients with infantile hypothyroidism have some ectopic thyroid tissue.

Diagnosis is best established by thyroid scan using iodine isotopes or technetium-99m. Computed tomography (CT) and magnetic resonance imaging (MRI) can be helpful in delineating the size and extent of the lesion. Biopsy is often avoided because of the risk of hemorrhage and because the mass may represent the patient's only functioning thyroid tissue. In some cases, incisional biopsy may be needed to confirm the diagnosis or to rule out malignant changes.

TREATMENT AND PROGNOSIS

No treatment except periodic follow-up is required for patients with asymptomatic lingual thyroids. In symptomatic patients, suppressive therapy with supplemental thyroid hormone often can reduce the size of the lesion. Some authors advise that this treatment also should be tried in asymptomatic patients to prevent possible subsequent enlargement. If hormone therapy does not eliminate symptoms, surgical removal or ablation with radioactive iodine-131 can be performed. If the mass is surgically excised, autotransplantation to another body site can be attempted to maintain functional thyroid tissue and to prevent hypothyroidism.

Rare examples of carcinomas arising in lingual thyroids have been reported; malignancy develops in about 1% of identified cases. Although lingual thyroids are decidedly more common in females, this predilection for females is less pronounced for lingual thyroid carcinomas. Because a disproportionate number of these malignancies have been documented in males, some authors have advocated prophylactic excision of lingual thyroids in men older than 30 years of age.

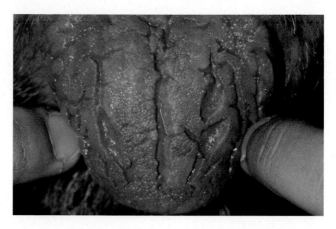

Fig. 1-21   Fissured tongue. Extensive fissuring involving the entire dorsal tongue surface. (*Courtesy of Chris Neville.*)

FISSURED TONGUE (SCROTAL TONGUE)

Fissured tongue is a relatively common condition that is characterized by the presence of numerous grooves, or fissures, on the dorsal tongue surface. The cause is uncertain, but heredity appears to play a significant role. Evidence indicates that the condition may be either a polygenic trait or an autosomal dominant trait with incomplete penetrance. Aging or local environmental factors also may contribute to its development.

CLINICAL FEATURES

Patients with fissured tongue exhibit multiple grooves, or furrows, on the surface of the tongue, ranging from 2 to 6 mm in depth (Fig. 1-21). Considerable variation can be seen. In the most severe cases, numerous fissures cover the entire dorsal surface and divide the tongue papillae into multiple separate "islands." Some patients have fissures that are located mostly on the dorsolateral areas of the tongue. Other patients exhibit a large central fissure, with smaller fissures branching outward at right angles. The condition is usually asymptomatic, although some patients may complain of mild burning or soreness.

Most studies have shown that the prevalence of fissured tongue ranges from 2% to 5% of the overall population. The condition may be seen in children or adults, but the prevalence and severity appear to increase with age, with some studies noting the presence of fissured tongue in as many as 30% of older adults. In some investigations, a male predilection has been noted.

A strong association has been found between fissured tongue and **geographic tongue** (see page 779), with many patients having both conditions. A hereditary basis also has been suggested for geographic

tongue, and the same gene or genes may possibly be linked to both conditions. In fact, it even has been suggested that geographic tongue may *cause* fissured tongue. Fissured tongue also may be a component of **Melkersson-Rosenthal syndrome** (see page 342).

HISTOPATHOLOGIC FEATURES

Microscopic examination of fissured tongue reveals hyperplasia of the rete ridges and loss of the keratin "hairs" on the surface of the filiform papillae. The papillae vary in size and often are separated by deep grooves. Polymorphonuclear leukocytes can be seen migrating into the epithelium, often forming microabscesses in the upper epithelial layers. A mixed inflammatory cell infiltrate is present in the lamina propria.

TREATMENT AND PROGNOSIS

Fissured tongue is a benign condition, and no specific treatment is indicated. The patient should be encouraged to brush the tongue, because food or debris entrapped in the grooves may act as a source of irritation.

HAIRY TONGUE (BLACK HAIRY TONGUE; COATED TONGUE)

Hairy tongue is characterized by marked accumulation of keratin on the filiform papillae of the dorsal tongue, resulting in a hairlike appearance. The condition apparently represents an increase in keratin production or a decrease in normal keratin desquamation. Hairy tongue is found in about 0.5% of adults. Although the cause is uncertain, many affected people are heavy smokers. Other possible associated factors include

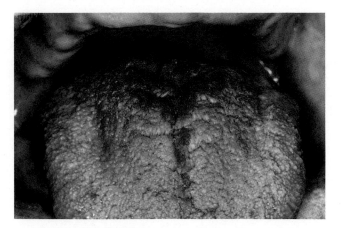

Fig. 1-22   Hairy tongue. Elongated, yellow-brown filiform papillae on the posterior dorsal surface of the tongue.

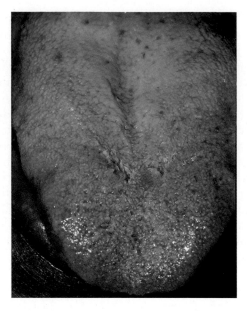

Fig. 1-24   Coated tongue. The dorsal tongue appears white and thickened from the accumulation of keratin and bacteria on the surface.

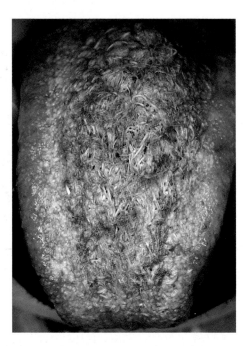

Fig. 1-23   Hairy tongue. Marked elongation and brown staining of the filiform papillae, resulting in a hairlike appearance.

general debilitation, poor oral hygiene, and a history of radiation therapy to the head and neck.

CLINICAL FEATURES

Hairy tongue most commonly affects the midline just anterior to the circumvallate papillae, sparing the lateral and anterior borders (Fig. 1-22). The elongated papillae are usually brown, yellow, or black as a result of growth of pigment-producing bacteria or staining from tobacco and food. Sometimes most of the dorsal tongue may be involved, resulting in a thick, matted appearance (Fig. 1-23). Multiple individual elongated

filiform papillae may be elevated by using gauze or a dental instrument. The condition is typically asymptomatic, although occasionally patients complain of a gagging sensation or a bad taste in the mouth. Because the diagnosis usually can be made from the clinical appearance, biopsy is unnecessary in most instances.

Because of the similarity in names, care should be taken to avoid confusing hairy tongue with **hairy leukoplakia** (see page 268), which typically occurs on the lateral border of the tongue. Hairy leukoplakia is caused by the Epstein-Barr virus and is usually associated with human immunodeficiency virus (HIV) infection or other immunosuppressive conditions.

In some individuals, numerous bacteria and desquamated epithelial cells accumulate on the dorsal tongue surface, but without the hairlike filiform projections (Fig. 1-24). Such cases, which are often designated as a **coated tongue,** also may be the source of oral malodor.

HISTOPATHOLOGIC FEATURES

On histopathologic examination, hairy tongue is characterized by marked elongation and hyperparakeratosis of the filiform papillae (Fig. 1-25). Usually, numerous bacteria can be seen growing on the epithelial surface.

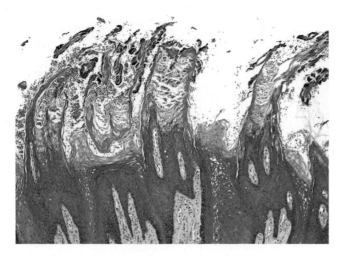

Fig. 1-25   Hairy tongue. Elongation and marked hyperkeratosis of the filiform papillae, with bacterial accumulation on the surface.

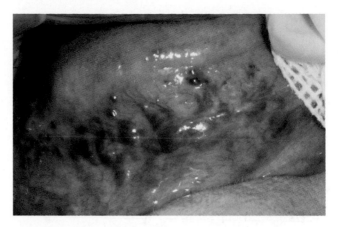

Fig. 1-26   Varicosities. Multiple purple dilated veins on the ventral and lateral surface of the tongue.

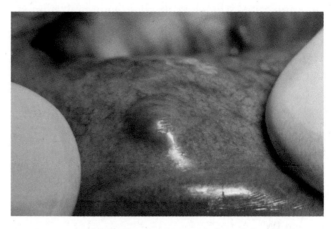

Fig. 1-27   Varicosity. Firm, thrombosed varix on the lower lip.

TREATMENT AND PROGNOSIS

Hairy or coated tongue is a benign condition with no serious sequelae. The major concern is often the aesthetic appearance of the tongue along with possible associated bad breath. Any predisposing factors, such as tobacco, antibiotics, or mouthwashes, should be eliminated, and excellent oral hygiene should be encouraged. Periodic scraping or brushing with a toothbrush or tongue scraper can promote desquamation of the hyperkeratotic papillae and surface debris. Keratolytic agents, such as podophyllin, also have been tried with success, but for safety reasons their use probably should not be encouraged.

VARICOSITIES (VARICES)

Varicosities, or **varices,** are abnormally dilated and tortuous veins. Age appears to be an important etiologic factor because varices are rare in children but common in older adults. This suggests that their development may be an age-related degeneration, in which a loss of connective tissue tone supporting the vessels occurs. Oral varices have not been associated with systemic hypertension or other cardiopulmonary diseases, although one study did find that people with varicose veins of the legs were more likely to have varicosities of the tongue.

CLINICAL FEATURES

The most common type of oral varicosity is the **sublingual varix,** which occurs in two thirds of people older than 60 years of age. Sublingual varicosities classically present as multiple blue-purple, elevated or papular blebs on the ventral and lateral border of the tongue (Fig. 1-26). The lesions are usually asymptomatic, except in rare instances when secondary thrombosis occurs.

Less frequently, solitary varices occur in other areas of the mouth, especially the lips and buccal mucosa. These isolated varicosities often are first noticed after they have become thrombosed (Fig. 1-27). Clinically, a thrombosed varix presents as a firm, nontender, blue-purple nodule that may feel like a piece of buckshot beneath the mucosal surface.

HISTOPATHOLOGIC FEATURES

Microscopic examination of a varix reveals a dilated vein, the wall of which shows little smooth muscle and poorly developed elastic tissue. If secondary thrombosis has occurred, then the lumen may contain concentrically layered zones of platelets and erythrocytes

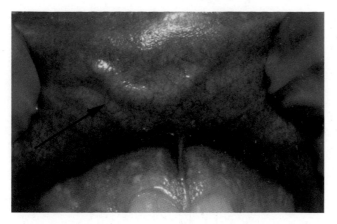

Fig. 1-28 Caliber-persistent artery. Linear, arcuate lesion on the upper labial mucosa (*arrow*). (*Courtesy of Dr. John Lovas.*)

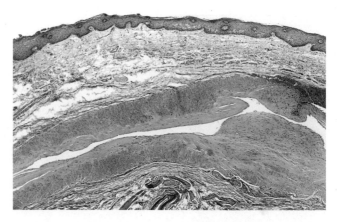

Fig. 1-29 Caliber-persistent artery. Thick-walled artery located just beneath the mucosal surface.

(lines of Zahn). The clot can undergo organization via granulation tissue, with subsequent recanalization. Older thrombi may exhibit dystrophic calcification, resulting in formation of a **phlebolith** (*phlebo* = vein; *lith* = stone).

TREATMENT AND PROGNOSIS

Sublingual varicosities are typically asymptomatic, and no treatment is indicated. Solitary varicosities of the lips and buccal mucosa may need to be surgically removed to confirm the diagnosis, because of secondary thrombus formation or for aesthetic purposes.

CALIBER-PERSISTENT ARTERY

A **caliber-persistent artery** is a common vascular anomaly in which a main arterial branch extends up into the superficial submucosal tissues without a reduction in its diameter. Similar to oral varices, caliber-persistent arteries are seen more frequently in older adults. This suggests that their development may be an age-related degenerative phenomenon in which there is a loss of tone in the surrounding supporting connective tissue.

CLINICAL FEATURES

The caliber-persistent artery occurs almost exclusively on the lip mucosa. Either lip may be affected, and some patients have bilateral lesions or lesions on both lips. The average patient age is 58 years, and the gender ratio is nearly equal. The lesion presents as a linear, arcuate, or papular elevation that ranges from pale to normal to bluish in color (Fig. 1-28). Stretching the lip usually causes the artery to become inconspicuous. The unique feature is pulsation—not only vertically but also in a lateral direction. However, usually it is not possible

to feel a pulse in a caliber-persistent artery with gloved fingers.

The lesion is usually asymptomatic, being discovered as an incidental finding during an oral examination; rarely a patient may notice a pulsatile lip nodule. A few cases have been associated with ulceration of the overlying mucosa. In addition, a couple of examples have been found adjacent to labial squamous cell carcinomas, although this is probably coincidental.

HISTOPATHOLOGIC FEATURES

Microscopic examination shows a thick-walled artery situated close to the mucosal surface (Fig. 1-29).

TREATMENT AND PROGNOSIS

If the true nature of the caliber-persistent artery can be recognized clinically, no treatment is necessary. Oftentimes a biopsy is performed when the lesion is mistaken for a mucocele or another vascular lesion, such as a varix or hemangioma. Brisk bleeding is typically encountered if the lesion is removed.

LATERAL SOFT PALATE FISTULAS

Lateral soft palate fistulas are rare anomalies of uncertain pathogenesis. Many cases appear to be congenital, possibly related to a defect in the development of the second pharyngeal pouch. Some fistulas may be the result of infection or surgery of the tonsillar region.

CLINICAL FEATURES

Lateral soft palate fistulas are usually bilateral, but they may occur only on one side. They are more common on the anterior tonsillar pillar (Fig. 1-30), but they also may

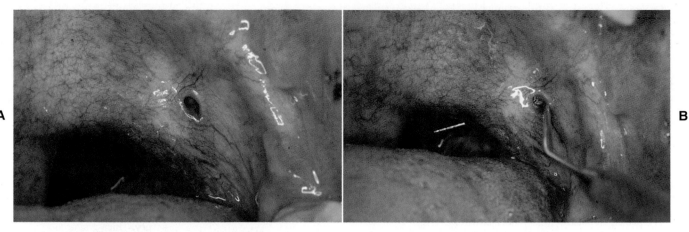

Fig. 1-30   Lateral palatal fistula. A, Asymptomatic "hole" in the anterior tonsillar pillar. **B,** Periodontal probe has been used to demonstrate the communication of the lesion with the tonsillar fossa.

involve the posterior pillar. The perforations are typically asymptomatic, ranging from a few millimeters to more than 1 cm. A few cases have been associated with other anomalies, such as absence or hypoplasia of the palatine tonsils, hearing loss, and preauricular fistulas.

TREATMENT AND PROGNOSIS

The lesions are innocuous, and no treatment is necessary.

CORONOID HYPERPLASIA

Hyperplasia of the coronoid process of the mandible is a rare developmental anomaly that may result in limitation of mandibular movement. The cause of **coronoid hyperplasia** is unknown, but the overall male-to-female ratio is 5:1. Because most cases have been seen in pubertal males, an endocrine influence has been suggested. Heredity also may play a role, because cases have been noted in siblings.

Coronoid hyperplasia may be unilateral or bilateral, although bilateral cases are nearly five times more common than unilateral examples. Unilateral enlargement of the coronoid process also can result from a true tumor, such as an osteoma or osteochondroma, and such cases should be distinguished from pure coronoid hyperplasia. However, some cases reported as tumors of the coronoid process actually may have been hyperplastic processes rather than true neoplasms.

CLINICAL AND RADIOGRAPHIC FEATURES

In a person with **unilateral coronoid hyperplasia,** the enlarged coronoid process impinges on the posterior surface of the zygoma, restricting mandibular opening. In addition, the mandible may deviate toward the affected side. Usually, there is no pain or associated abnormality in occlusion. Radiographs may reveal an irregular, nodular growth of the tip of the coronoid process.

In bilateral coronoid hyperplasia, the limitation of mandibular opening may progressively worsen over several years during childhood, reaching maximum severity during the late teens. The radiographic appearance is characterized by regular elongation of both processes. Because the coronoid process is often superimposed on the zygoma on conventional radiographs, tomograms or CT scans often demonstrate the hyperplasia more effectively.

TREATMENT AND PROGNOSIS

Treatment of coronoid hyperplasia consists of surgical removal of the elongated coronoid process or processes to allow freedom of mandibular motion. Coronoidectomy or coronoidotomy is usually accomplished via an intraoral approach. Although initial improvement in oral opening can be effected, the long-term results sometimes can be disappointing because of surgically induced fibrosis and the tendency for coronoid regrowth. Postoperative physiotherapy is important for reestablishing normal function.

CONDYLAR HYPERPLASIA

Condylar hyperplasia is an uncommon malformation of the mandible created by excessive growth of one of the condyles. The cause of this hyperplasia is unknown, but local circulatory problems, endocrine disturbances, and trauma have been suggested as possible etiologic factors.

Condylar hyperplasia can be difficult to distinguish from **hemifacial hyperplasia** (see page 38); however, in the latter condition the associated soft tissues and teeth also may be enlarged.

CLINICAL AND RADIOGRAPHIC FEATURES

Condylar hyperplasia may manifest itself in a variety of ways, including facial asymmetry, prognathism, crossbite, and open bite (Fig. 1-31). Sometimes compensatory maxillary growth and tilting of the occlusal plane occurs. The condition most commonly is discovered in adolescents and young adults.

The radiographic features are quite variable. Some patients have an enlargement of the condylar head, and others show elongation of the condylar neck (Fig. 1-32). Many cases also demonstrate hyperplasia of the entire ramus, suggesting that the condition sometimes affects more than just the condyle. Scintigraphy using ^{99m}Tc-MDP has been advocated as a useful method for assessing the degree of bone activity in condylar hyperplasia.

HISTOPATHOLOGIC FEATURES

During active growth, proliferation of the condylar cartilage is noted. Once condylar growth has ceased, the condyle has a normal histologic appearance.

TREATMENT AND PROGNOSIS

Condylar hyperplasia is a self-limiting condition, and treatment is determined by the degree of functional difficulty and aesthetic change. Some patients can be treated with unilateral condylectomy, whereas others require unilateral or bilateral mandibular osteotomies. In patients with compensatory maxillary growth, a maxillary osteotomy also may be needed. Concomitant orthodontic therapy frequently is necessary.

CONDYLAR HYPOPLASIA

Condylar hypoplasia, or underdevelopment of the mandibular condyle, can be either congenital or acquired. **Congenital condylar hypoplasia** often is

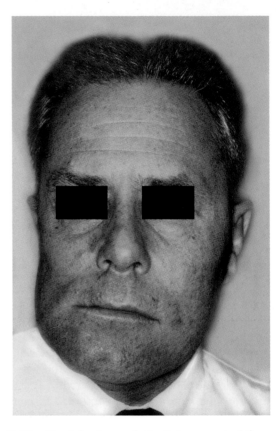

Fig. 1-31 Condylar hyperplasia. Enlargement of the patient's left condyle has displaced the mandible to the right and resulted in facial asymmetry.

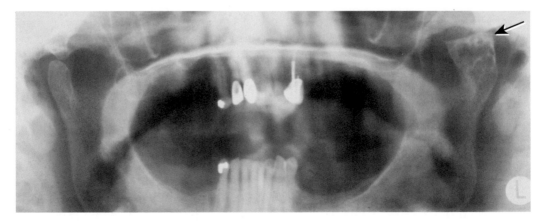

Fig. 1-32 Condylar hyperplasia. Enlargement of the left mandibular condyle (*arrow*).
(Courtesy of Dr. Gary Reinhart.)

associated with head and neck syndromes, including **mandibulofacial dysostosis** (see page 45), **oculoauriculovertebral syndrome (Goldenhar syndrome),** and **hemifacial microsomia.** In the most severe cases, complete agenesis of the condyle or ramus **(condylar aplasia)** is seen.

Acquired condylar hypoplasia results from disturbances of the growth center of the developing condyle. The most frequent cause is trauma to the condylar region during infancy or childhood. Other causes include infections, radiation therapy, and rheumatoid or degenerative arthritis.

CLINICAL AND RADIOGRAPHIC FEATURES

Condylar hypoplasia can be unilateral or bilateral, producing a small mandible with a Class II malocclusion. Unilateral hypoplasia results in distortion and depression of the face on the affected side. The mandibular midline shifts to the involved side when the mouth is opened, accentuating the deformity. Ankylosis of the temporomandibular joint (TMJ) can develop in cases caused by trauma.

The deformity is observed easily on panoramic films and can range in severity. In severe cases the condyle or ramus may be totally absent. Milder types demonstrate a short condylar process, shallow sigmoid notch, and poorly formed condylar head. A prominent antegonial notch may be present. CT scans may be helpful in evaluating the condyles.

TREATMENT AND PROGNOSIS

Treatment of the patient with condylar hypoplasia depends on the cause and severity of the defect, but surgery often is required. If the condyle is missing, then a costochondral rib graft can be placed to help establish an active growth center. In addition, osteotomies sometimes provide a cosmetically acceptable result. In certain instances, distraction osteogenesis can be used to stimulate new bone formation.

BIFID CONDYLE

A **bifid condyle** is a rare developmental anomaly characterized by a double-headed mandibular condyle. Most bifid condyles have a medial and lateral head divided by an anteroposterior groove. Some condyles may be divided into an anterior and posterior head.

The cause of bifid condyle is uncertain. Anteroposterior bifid condyles may be of traumatic origin, such as a childhood fracture. Mediolaterally divided condyles may result from trauma, abnormal muscle attach-

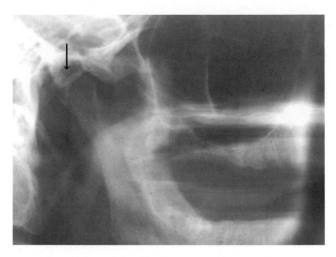

Fig. 1-33 Bifid condyle. Radiograph of the mandibular condyle showing a double head (*arrow*).

ment, teratogenic agents, or persistence of a fibrous septum within the condylar cartilage.

CLINICAL AND RADIOGRAPHIC FEATURES

A bifid condyle is usually unilateral, but occasionally both sides may be affected. The malformation is often asymptomatic and may be discovered on routine radiographs, although some patients may have a "pop" or "click" of the TMJ when opening their mouths. Panoramic radiographs and CT scans will demonstrate a bilobed appearance of the condylar head (Fig. 1-33).

TREATMENT AND PROGNOSIS

Because a bifid condyle is usually asymptomatic, most of the time no treatment is necessary. If the patient has joint complaints, the appropriate temporomandibular therapy may be required.

EXOSTOSES

Exostoses are localized bony protuberances that arise from the cortical plate. These benign growths frequently affect the jaws. The best-known oral exostoses, the **torus palatinus** and the **torus mandibularis,** are described later in the chapter. Other types of exostoses also may affect the jaws and are considered here.

CLINICAL AND RADIOGRAPHIC FEATURES

Exostoses are discovered most often in adults. **Buccal exostoses** occur as a bilateral row of bony hard nodules along the facial aspect of the maxillary and/or

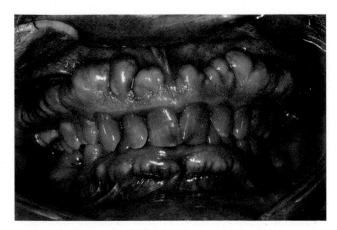

Fig. 1-34   Exostoses. Multiple buccal exostoses of the maxillary and mandibular alveolar ridges.

mandibular alveolar ridge (Fig. 1-34). They are usually asymptomatic, unless the thin overlying mucosa becomes ulcerated from trauma. One study reported that buccal exostoses were found in nearly 1 of every 1000 adults (0.09%); however, a more recent survey found a much higher prevalence of nearly 19%. This variation may be due to the different populations being studied or to the clinical criteria used to make the diagnosis.

Palatal exostoses (palatal tubercles) are similar bony protuberances that develop from the lingual aspect of the maxillary tuberosities. These lesions are usually bilateral but may affect only one side (Fig. 1-35). They are more common in males and have been reported in 8% to 69% of various populations. Many patients with buccal or palatal exostoses also will have palatal or mandibular tori.

Less commonly, **solitary exostoses** may occur, possibly in response to local irritation. Such lesions may develop from the alveolar bone beneath free gingival grafts and skin grafts. Presumably placement of the graft acts as a stimulant to the periosteum to form new bone.

Another uncommon, interesting variant is the **reactive subpontine exostosis (subpontic osseous proliferation, subpontic osseous hyperplasia)**, which may develop from the alveolar crestal bone beneath the pontic of a posterior bridge (Fig. 1-36).

If enough excess bone is present, exostoses may exhibit a relative radiopacity on dental radiographs (see Fig. 1-35, *B*). In rare instances an exostosis may become so large that distinguishing it from a tumor, such as an osteoma, is difficult (see page 650).

HISTOPATHOLOGIC FEATURES

Microscopic examination reveals a mass of dense, lamellar, cortical bone with a small amount of fibro-

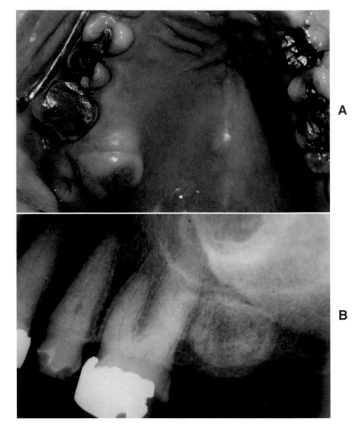

A

B

Fig. 1-35   Exostosis. A, Secondarily ulcerated palatal exostosis. **B,** Radiograph shows an ovoid radiopacity distal to the molar.

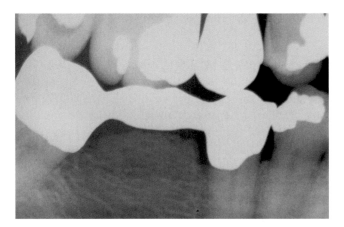

Fig. 1-36   Reactive subpontine exostosis. Nodular growth of bone beneath the pontic of a posterior mandibular bridge.

fatty marrow. In some cases an inner zone of trabecular bone also is present.

TREATMENT AND PROGNOSIS

Most exostoses are distinctive enough clinically to make biopsy unnecessary. If the diagnosis is uncertain, biopsy should be performed to rule out other bony pathosis. Sometimes the exostosis must be removed if it repeatedly has been exposed to trauma or has become ulcerated and painful. In addition, surgical removal may be required to accommodate a dental prosthesis or to allow for proper flap adaptation during periodontal surgery. Reactive subpontine exostoses may need to be removed if they interfere with oral hygiene or are associated with adjacent periodontal disease.

TORUS PALATINUS

The **torus palatinus** is a common exostosis that occurs in the midline of the vault of the hard palate. The pathogenesis of these tori has long been debated, with arguments centering on genetic versus environmental factors, such as masticatory stress. Some authorities have suggested that the torus palatinus is inherited as an autosomal dominant trait. However, others believe that the development of this lesion is multifactorial, including both genetic and environmental influences. In this model, patients are affected by a variety of hereditary and local environmental factors. If enough of these factors are present, then a "threshold" is surpassed and the trait (torus palatinus) will be expressed.

CLINICAL AND RADIOGRAPHIC FEATURES

The torus palatinus presents as a bony hard mass that arises along the midline suture of the hard palate (Figs. 1-37 to 1-39). Tori sometimes are classified according to their morphologic appearance:

- The **flat torus** has a broad base and a slightly convex, smooth surface. It extends symmetrically onto both sides of the midline raphe.

- The **spindle torus** has a midline ridge along the palatal raphe. A median groove is sometimes present.
- The **nodular torus** arises as multiple protuberances, each with an individual base. These protuberances may coalesce, forming grooves between them.
- The **lobular torus** is also a lobulated mass, but it rises from a single base. Lobular tori can be either sessile or pedunculated.

Most palatal tori are small, measuring less than 2 cm in diameter; however, they can slowly increase in size throughout life, sometimes to the extent that they fill the entire palatal vault. Most tori cause no symptoms, but in some cases the thin overlying mucosa may become ulcerated secondary to trauma.

The torus palatinus does not usually appear on routine dental radiographs. Rarely it may be seen as a radiopacity on periapical films if the film is placed behind the torus when the radiograph is taken.

The prevalence of palatal tori has varied widely in a number of population studies, ranging from 9% to 60%.

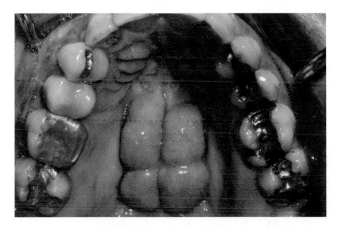

Fig. 1-38   Torus palatinus. Large, lobulated palatal mass.

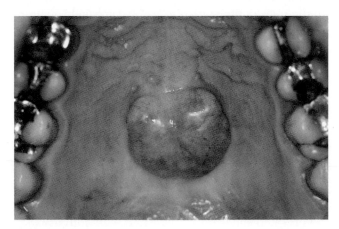

Fig. 1-37   Torus palatinus. Midline bony nodule of the palatal vault.

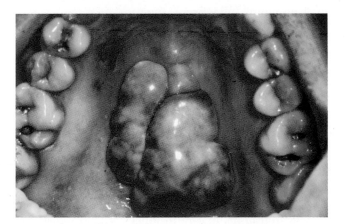

Fig. 1-39   Torus palatinus. Asymmetric, lobulated bony mass.

Some of this variation may be due to the criteria used to make the diagnosis and also may be based on whether the study was conducted on live patients or skulls. There appear to be significant racial differences, however, with a higher prevalence in Asian and Inuit (i.e., Eskimo) populations. In the United States, most studies have shown a prevalence of 20% to 35%, with little difference between whites and blacks. Almost all studies from around the world have shown a pronounced female-to-male ratio of 2:1. The prevalence peaks during early adult life, tapering off in later years. This finding supports the theory that tori are dynamic lesions that are related, in part, to environmental factors; in later life, some may undergo resorption remodeling in response to decreased functional stresses.

HISTOPATHOLOGIC FEATURES

Microscopic examination of the torus shows a mass of dense, lamellar, cortical bone. An inner zone of trabecular bone sometimes is seen.

TREATMENT AND PROGNOSIS

Most palatal tori can be diagnosed clinically based on their characteristic appearance; therefore biopsy rarely is necessary. In edentulous patients, the torus may need to be removed surgically to accommodate a denture base. Surgical removal may also be indicated for palatal tori that become repeatedly ulcerated or that interfere with oral function.

TORUS MANDIBULARIS

The **torus mandibularis** is a common exostosis that develops along the lingual aspect of the mandible. As with torus palatinus, the cause of mandibular tori is probably multifactorial, including both genetic and environmental influences.

CLINICAL AND RADIOGRAPHIC FEATURES

The mandibular torus presents as a bony protuberance along the lingual aspect of the mandible above the mylohyoid line in the region of the premolars (Fig. 1-40). Bilateral involvement occurs in more than 90% of cases. Most mandibular tori occur as single nodules, although multiple lobules paralleling the teeth are not unusual. Patients often are unaware of their presence unless the overlying mucosa becomes ulcerated secondary to trauma. In rare instances, bilateral tori may become so large that they almost meet in the midline (Fig. 1-41). A large mandibular torus may appear on

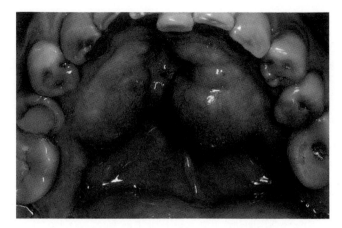

Fig. 1-40   Torus mandibularis. Bilateral lobulated bony protuberances of the mandibular lingual alveolar ridge.

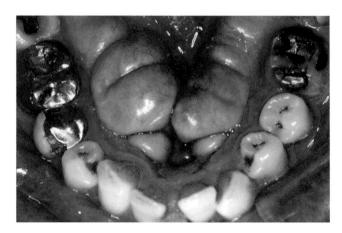

Fig. 1-41   Torus mandibularis. Massive "kissing" tori meet in the midline.

periapical radiographs as a radiopacity superimposed on the roots of the teeth (Fig. 1-42), especially on anterior films. Mandibular tori are easily visualized on occlusal radiographs (Fig. 1-43).

Most studies indicate that the torus mandibularis is not as common as the torus palatinus; the prevalence ranges from 5% to 40%. Like the torus palatinus, the mandibular torus appears to be more common in Asians and the Inuit. The prevalence in the United States ranges from 7% to 10%, with little difference between blacks and whites. A slight male predilection has been noted.

The prevalence of mandibular torus peaks in early adult life, tapering slightly in later years. In addition, the prevalence has been correlated with both bruxism and the number of teeth remaining present. These findings support the theory that the torus mandibularis

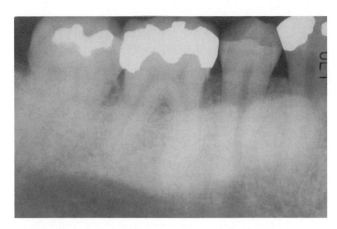

Fig. 1-42   Torus mandibularis. Torus is causing a radiopacity that is superimposed over the roots of the mandibular teeth.

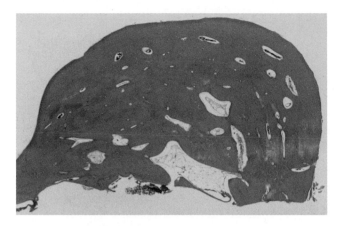

Fig. 1-44   Torus mandibularis. Nodular mass of dense, cortical bone. Some fatty marrow is visible at the base of the specimen.

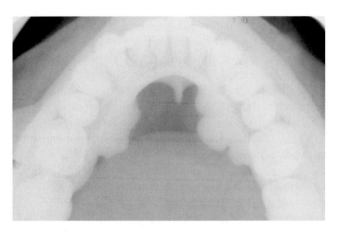

Fig. 1-43   Torus mandibularis. Occlusal radiograph showing bilateral mandibular tori.

is multifactorial in development and responds to functional stresses.

HISTOPATHOLOGIC FEATURES

The histopathologic appearance of the torus mandibularis is similar to that of other exostoses, consisting primarily of a nodular mass of dense, cortical lamellar bone (Fig. 1-44). An inner zone of trabecular bone with associated fatty marrow sometimes is visible.

TREATMENT AND PROGNOSIS

Most mandibular tori are easily diagnosed clinically, and no treatment is necessary. However, surgical removal may be required to accommodate a lower full or partial denture. Occasionally, tori may recur if teeth are still present in the area.

EAGLE SYNDROME (STYLOHYOID SYNDROME; CAROTID ARTERY SYNDROME; STYLALGIA)

The styloid process is a slender bony projection that originates from the inferior aspect of the temporal bone, anterior and medial to the stylomastoid foramen. It is connected to the lesser cornu of the hyoid bone by the stylohyoid ligament. The external and internal carotid arteries lie on either side. Elongation of the styloid process or mineralization of the stylohyoid ligament complex is not unusual, having been reported in 18% to 40% of the population in some radiographic reviews. Such mineralization is usually bilateral, but it may affect only one side. Most cases are asymptomatic; however, a small number of such patients experience symptoms of **Eagle syndrome,** caused by impingement or compression of adjacent nerves or blood vessels.

CLINICAL AND RADIOGRAPHIC FEATURES

Eagle syndrome most commonly affects adults. The patient experiences vague facial pain, especially while swallowing, turning the head, or opening the mouth. Other symptoms may include dysphagia, dysphonia, otalgia, headache, dizziness, and transient syncope.

Elongation of the styloid process or mineralization of the stylohyoid ligament complex can be seen on panoramic or lateral-jaw radiographs (Fig. 1-45). The mineralized stylohyoid complex may be palpated in the tonsillar fossa area, and pain often is elicited.

Classic Eagle syndrome occurs after a tonsillectomy. Development of scar tissue in the area of a mineralized stylohyoid complex then results in cervicopharyngeal

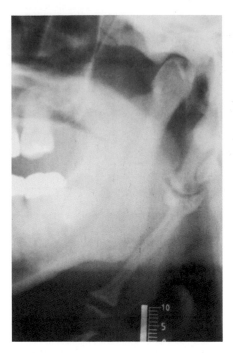

Fig. 1-45 Eagle syndrome. Mineralization of the stylohyoid ligament is visible posterior to the mandibular ramus.

pain in the region of cranial nerves V, VII, IX, and X, especially during swallowing. Some authors reserve the term *Eagle syndrome* only for those cases in which the ossification of the stylohyoid chain occurs as a result of the tonsillectomy or other neck trauma.

A second form of this condition unrelated to tonsillectomy is sometimes known as **carotid artery syndrome** or **stylohyoid syndrome.** The elongated, mineralized complex is thought to impinge on the internal or external carotid arteries and associated sympathetic nerve fibers. The patient may complain of pain in the neck when turning the head, and this pain may radiate to other sites in the head or neck.

Traumatic Eagle syndrome also has been reported, in which symptoms develop after fracture of a mineralized stylohyoid ligament.

TREATMENT AND PROGNOSIS

Treatment of Eagle syndrome depends on the severity of the symptoms. For mild cases, no treatment may be necessary (except reassurance of the patient). Local injection of corticosteroids sometimes provides relief. In more severe cases, partial surgical excision of the elongated styloid process or mineralized stylohyoid ligament is required. Usually, this is accomplished via an intraoral approach, although an extraoral approach also can be used. The prognosis is good.

STAFNE DEFECT (STAFNE BONE CYST; LINGUAL MANDIBULAR SALIVARY GLAND DEPRESSION; LATENT BONE CYST; STATIC BONE CYST; STATIC BONE DEFECT; LINGUAL CORTICAL MANDIBULAR DEFECT)

In 1942, Stafne described a series of asymptomatic radiolucent lesions located near the angle of the mandible. Subsequent reports of similar lesions have shown that this condition represents a focal concavity of the cortical bone on the lingual surface of the mandible. In most cases, biopsy has revealed histologically normal salivary gland tissue, suggesting that these lesions represent developmental defects containing a portion of the submandibular gland. However, a few of these defects have been reported to be devoid of contents or to contain muscle, fibrous connective tissue, blood vessels, fat, or lymphoid tissue.

Similar lingual cortical defects also have been noted more anteriorly in the mandible, in the area of the incisor, canine, or premolar teeth. These rare defects have been related to the sublingual gland or to aberrant salivary gland tissue. In addition, one report has implicated the parotid gland as the cause of an apparent cortical defect in the upper mandibular ramus. Therefore, all of the major salivary glands appear to be capable of causing such cortical concavities.

In rare examples, the radiolucent defect has been reported to be totally surrounded by intact bone. Such cases might be explained by entrapment of embryonic salivary gland tissue within the jawbone.

CLINICAL AND RADIOGRAPHIC FEATURES

The classic **Stafne defect** presents as an asymptomatic radiolucency below the mandibular canal in the posterior mandible, between the molar teeth and the angle of the mandible (Fig. 1-46). The lesion is typically well circumscribed and has a sclerotic border. Sometimes the defect may interrupt the continuity of the inferior border of the mandible, with a palpable notch observed clinically in this area. Most Stafne defects are unilateral, although bilateral cases may be seen. Anterior lingual salivary defects associated with the sublingual gland present as well-defined radiolucencies that may appear superimposed over the apices of the anterior teeth (Figs. 1-47 and 1-48).

Posterior Stafne defects are not rare, having been reported in 0.3% of panoramic radiographs. A striking male predilection is observed, with 80% to 90% of all cases seen in men.

Although the defect is believed to be developmental in nature, it does not appear to be present from birth.

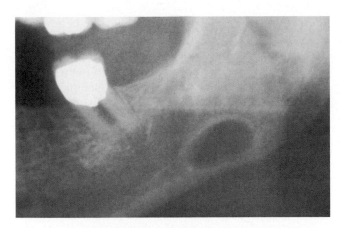

Fig. 1-46   **Stafne defect.** Radiolucency of the posterior mandible below the mandibular canal.

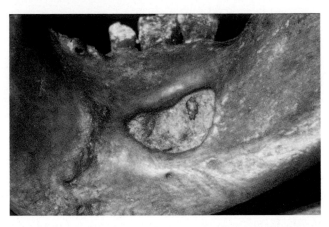

Fig. 1-48   **Stafne defect.** Lingual surface of the mandible showing an anterior cortical defect caused by the sublingual gland.

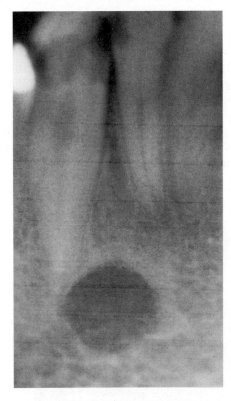

Fig. 1-47   **Stafne defect.** Anterior radiolucent lesion of the body of the mandible associated with the sublingual gland.

Most cases have been reported in middle-aged and older adults, with children rarely affected; this implies that the lesion usually "develops" at a later age. Stafne defects typically remain stable in size; hence the name **static bone cyst.** In a few cases, however, the lesion has increased in size over time (Fig. 1-49). This also indicates that these lesions are not congenital.

The diagnosis can usually be made on a clinical basis by the typical radiographic location and lack of symp-

toms. If the clinical diagnosis is in doubt, then it can be confirmed by CT scans, MRI, or sialography. CT scans and MRIs show a well-defined concavity on the lingual surface of the mandible. Sialograms may be able to demonstrate the presence of salivary gland tissue in the area of the defect.

HISTOPATHOLOGIC FEATURES

Because of the typical radiographic appearance, biopsy is usually not necessary to establish the diagnosis of Stafne defects of the posterior mandible. If biopsy is performed, normal submandibular gland tissue is usually seen. However, some defects are devoid of tissue or contain muscle, blood vessels, fat, connective tissue, or lymphoid tissue. In cases reported to be devoid of contents, it is possible that the gland was simply displaced at the time of biopsy.

TREATMENT AND PROGNOSIS

No treatment is necessary for patients with Stafne defects of the posterior mandible, and the prognosis is excellent. Because anterior lingual salivary defects may be difficult to recognize, biopsy may be necessary to rule out other pathologic lesions.

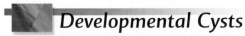

Developmental Cysts

By definition, a **cyst** is a pathologic cavity (often fluid-filled) that is lined by epithelium. A number of different developmental cysts of the head and neck have been described. Some of these have been considered historically as "fissural" cysts because they were thought to arise from epithelium entrapped along embryonal lines of fusion. However, the concept of a fissural origin for many of these cysts has been questioned in more recent years. In many instances the exact pathogenesis of these lesions is still uncertain. Regardless of their origin, once cysts develop in the oral and maxillofacial region, they tend to slowly increase in size, possibly in response to a slightly elevated hydrostatic luminal pressure.

PALATAL CYSTS OF THE NEWBORN (EPSTEIN'S PEARLS; BOHN'S NODULES)

Small developmental cysts are a common finding on the palate of newborn infants. Researchers have theorized that these "inclusion" cysts may arise in one of two ways. First, as the palatal shelves meet and fuse in the midline during embryonic life to form the secondary palate, small islands of epithelium may become entrapped below the surface along the median palatal raphe and form cysts. Second, these cysts may arise from epithelial remnants derived from the development of the minor salivary glands of the palate.

As originally described, **Epstein's pearls** occur along the median palatal raphe and presumably arise from epithelium entrapped along the line of fusion. **Bohn's nodules** are scattered over the hard palate,

often near the soft palate junction and are believed to be derived from the minor salivary glands. However, these two terms have been used almost interchangeably in the literature and also have often been used to describe gingival cysts of the newborn (see page 691), similar-appearing lesions of dental lamina origin. Therefore, the term **palatal cysts of the newborn** may be preferable to help distinguish them from gingival cysts of the newborn. In addition, because these cysts are most common near the midline at the junction of the hard and soft palates, it is usually difficult to ascertain clinically whether they are arising from epithelium entrapped by fusion of the palate or from the developing minor salivary glands.

CLINICAL FEATURES

Palatal cysts of the newborn are quite common and have been reported in as many as 65% to 85% of neonates. The cysts are small, 1- to 3-mm, white or yellow-white papules that appear most often along the midline near the junction of the hard and soft palates (Fig. 1-50). Occasionally, they may occur in a more anterior location along the raphe or on the posterior palate lateral to the midline. Frequently a cluster of two to six cysts is observed, although the lesions also can occur singly.

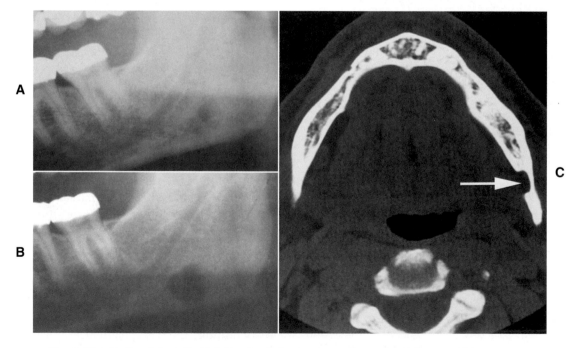

Fig. 1-49   Stafne defect. A, Ill-defined radiolucency near the angle of the mandible.
B, Appearance of the same defect several years later showing enlargement of the lesion.
C, Computed tomography (CT) image of the same lesion showing a left lingual cortical defect
(**arrow**). (*Courtesy of Dr. Carroll Gallagher.*)

HISTOPATHOLOGIC FEATURES

Microscopic examination reveals keratin-filled cysts that are lined by stratified squamous epithelium. Sometimes these cysts demonstrate a communication with the mucosal surface.

TREATMENT AND PROGNOSIS

Palatal cysts of the newborn are innocuous lesions, and no treatment is required. They are self-healing and rarely observable several weeks after birth. Presumably the epithelium degenerates, or the cysts rupture onto the mucosal surface and eliminate their keratin contents.

NASOLABIAL CYST (NASOALVEOLAR CYST; KLESTADT CYST)

The **nasolabial cyst** is a rare developmental cyst that occurs in the upper lip lateral to the midline. The

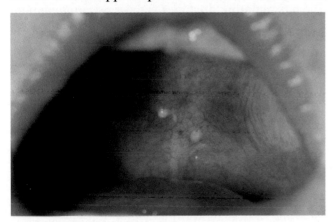

Fig. 1-50   Epstein's pearls. Small keratin-filled cysts at the junction of the hard and soft palates. *(Courtesy of Tristan Neville.)*

pathogenesis is uncertain, although there are two major theories. One theory considers the nasolabial cyst to be a "fissural" cyst arising from epithelial remnants entrapped along the line of fusion of the maxillary, medial nasal, and lateral nasal processes. A second theory suggests that these cysts develop from misplaced epithelium of the nasolacrimal duct because of their similar location and histologic appearance.

CLINICAL AND RADIOGRAPHIC FEATURES

The nasolabial cyst usually appears as a swelling of the upper lip lateral to the midline, resulting in elevation of the ala of the nose. The enlargement often elevates the mucosa of the nasal vestibule and obliterates the maxillary mucolabial fold (Fig. 1-51). On occasion, this expansion may result in nasal obstruction or may interfere with the wearing of a denture. Pain is uncommon unless the lesion is secondarily infected. The cyst may rupture spontaneously and may drain into the oral cavity or nose.

Nasolabial cysts are most commonly seen in adults, with a peak prevalence in the fourth and fifth decades of life. A significant predilection exists for women, with a female-to-male ratio of 3:1. Approximately 10% of the reported cases have been bilateral.

Because the nasolabial cyst arises in soft tissues, in most cases no radiographic changes are seen. Occasionally, pressure resorption of the underlying bone may occur.

HISTOPATHOLOGIC FEATURES

The nasolabial cyst is characteristically lined by pseudostratified columnar epithelium, often demonstrating goblet cells and cilia (Fig. 1-52). Areas of cuboidal

A   B

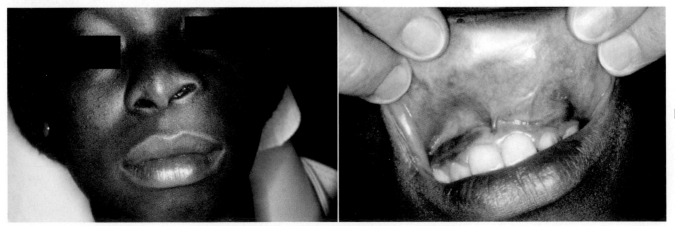

Fig. 1-51   Nasolabial cyst. A, Enlargement of the left upper lip with elevation of the ala of the nose. **B,** Intraoral swelling fills the maxillary labial fold. *(Courtesy of Dr. Jim Weir.)*

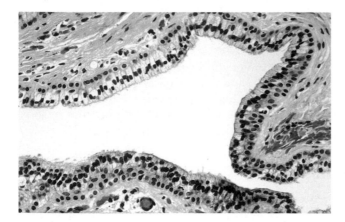

Fig. 1-52   Nasolabial cyst. Pseudostratified columnar epithelial lining.

epithelium and squamous metaplasia are not unusual. Apocrine changes also have been reported. The cyst wall is composed of fibrous connective tissue with adjacent skeletal muscle. Inflammation may be seen if the lesion is secondarily infected.

TREATMENT AND PROGNOSIS

Complete surgical excision of the cyst via an intraoral approach has been the treatment of choice. Because the lesion is often close to the floor of the nose, it is sometimes necessary to sacrifice a portion of the nasal mucosa to ensure total removal. Recurrence is rare. Recently an alternative transnasal approach has been suggested that allows endoscopic marsupialization of the cystic cavity.

"GLOBULOMAXILLARY CYST"

As originally described, the "**globulomaxillary cyst**" was purported to be a fissural cyst that arose from epithelium entrapped during fusion of the globular portion of the medial nasal process with the maxillary process. This concept has been questioned, however, because the globular portion of the medial nasal process is primarily united with the maxillary process and a fusion does not occur. Therefore, epithelial entrapment should not occur during embryologic development of this area.

Virtually all cysts in the globulomaxillary region (between the lateral incisor and canine teeth) can be explained on an odontogenic basis. Many are lined by inflamed stratified squamous epithelium and are consistent with **periapical cysts** (see page 130). Some exhibit specific histopathologic features of an **odontogenic keratocyst** (see page 683) or developmental **lateral periodontal cyst** (see page 692). Researchers

have also theorized that some of these lesions may arise from inflammation of the reduced enamel epithelium at the time of eruption of the teeth.

On rare occasions, cysts in the globulomaxillary area may be lined by pseudostratified, ciliated, columnar epithelium. Such cases may lend credence to the fissural theory of origin. However, this epithelium may be explained by the close proximity of the sinus lining. In addition, respiratory epithelium also has been reported in periapical cysts, dentigerous cysts, and glandular odontogenic cysts found in other locations.

Because a fissural cyst in this region probably does not exist, the term *globulomaxillary cyst* should no longer be used. When a radiolucency between the maxillary lateral incisor and canine is encountered, the clinician should first consider an odontogenic origin for the lesion.

NASOPALATINE DUCT CYST (INCISIVE CANAL CYST)

The **nasopalatine duct cyst** is the most common non-odontogenic cyst of the oral cavity, occurring in about 1% of the population. The cyst is believed to arise from remnants of the **nasopalatine duct,** an embryologic structure connecting the oral and nasal cavities in the area of the incisive canal.

In the 7-week-old fetus, the developing palate consists of the **primary palate,** which is formed by the fusion of the medial nasal processes. Behind the primary palate, downgrowth of the nasal septum produces two communications between the oral and nasal cavities, the primitive nasal choanae. Formation of the **secondary palate** begins around the eighth intrauterine week, with downward growth of the medial parts of the maxillary processes (palatine processes) to a location on either side of the tongue.

As the mandible develops and the tongue drops down, these palatine processes grow horizontally, fusing with the nasal septum in the midline and with the primary palate along their anterior aspect. Two passageways persist in the midline between the primary and secondary palates (the **incisive canals**). Also formed by this fusion and found within the incisive canals are epithelial structures–the **nasopalatine ducts.** These ducts normally degenerate in humans but may leave epithelial remnants behind in the incisive canals.

The incisive canals begin on the floor of the nasal cavity on either side of the nasal septum, coursing downward and forward to exit the palatal bone via a common foramen in the area of the incisive papilla. In addition to the nasopalatine ducts, these canals contain the nasopalatine nerve plus anastomosing branches of the descending palatine and sphenopalatine arteries.

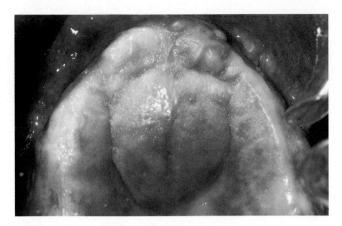

Fig. 1-53 Nasopalatine duct cyst. Fluctuant swelling of the anterior hard palate.

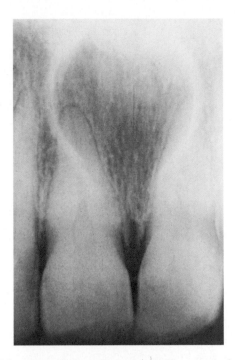

Fig. 1-54 Nasopalatine duct cyst. Well-circumscribed radiolucency between and apical to the roots of the maxillary central incisors.

Occasionally, two smaller foramina carrying the nasopalatine nerves—the **canals of Scarpa**—are found within the incisive foramen.

In some mammals the nasopalatine ducts remain patent and provide communication between the oral and nasal cavities. On rare occasions, patent or partially patent nasopalatine ducts may be encountered in humans. In mammals the nasopalatine ducts may communicate with the vomer-nasal **organ of Jacobson,** acting as an accessory olfactory organ. However, in humans, Jacobson's organ usually recedes in uterine life to become a vestigial structure.

Researchers have suggested that the nasopalatine duct cyst may arise from the epithelium of Jacobson's organ, but this appears highly unlikely. Trauma or infection of the duct and mucous retention of adjacent minor salivary glands also have been mentioned as possible etiologic factors, but the role of each has been questioned. Although the pathogenesis of this lesion is still uncertain, the lesion most likely represents a spontaneous cystic degeneration of remnants of the nasopalatine duct.

CLINICAL AND RADIOGRAPHIC FEATURES

The nasopalatine duct cyst may develop at almost any age but is most common in the fourth to sixth decades of life. In spite of its being a "developmental" cyst, the nasopalatine duct cyst is rarely seen during the first decade. Most studies have shown a male predilection.

The most common presenting symptoms include swelling of the anterior palate, drainage, and pain (Fig. 1-53). Patients sometimes relate a long history of these symptoms, probably because of their intermittent nature. However, many lesions are asymptomatic and are discovered on routine radiographs. Rarely a large

cyst may produce a "through-and-through" fluctuant expansion involving the anterior palate and labial alveolar mucosa.

Radiographs usually demonstrate a well-circumscribed radiolucency in or near the midline of the anterior maxilla, between and apical to the central incisor teeth (Figs. 1-54 and 1-55). Root resorption is rarely noted. The lesion most often is round or oval with a sclerotic border. Some cysts may have an inverted pear shape, presumably because of resistance of adjacent tooth roots. Other examples may show a classic heart shape as a result of superimposition of the nasal spine or because they are notched by the nasal septum.

The radiographic diameter of nasopalatine duct cysts can range from small lesions, less than 6 mm, to destructive lesions as large as 6 cm. However, most cysts are in the range of 1.0 to 2.5 cm, with an average diameter of 1.5 to 1.7 cm. It may be difficult to distinguish a small nasopalatine duct cyst from a large incisive foramen. It is generally accepted that a diameter of 6 mm is the upper limit of normal size for the incisive foramen. Therefore, a radiolucency that is 6 mm or smaller in this area is usually considered a normal foramen unless other clinical signs or symptoms are present.

In rare instances, a nasopalatine duct cyst may develop in the soft tissues of the incisive papilla area without any bony involvement. Such lesions often are

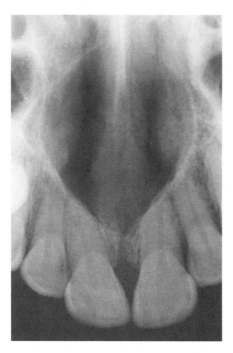

Fig. 1-55   Nasopalatine duct cyst. Large destructive cyst of the palate.

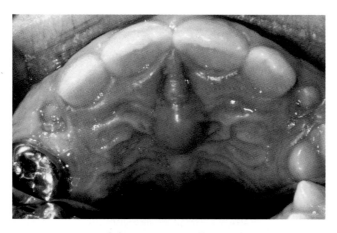

Fig. 1-56   Cyst of the incisive papilla. Swelling of the incisive papilla.

called **cysts of the incisive papilla.** These cysts frequently demonstrate bluish discoloration as a result of the fluid contents in the cyst lumen (Fig. 1-56).

HISTOPATHOLOGIC FEATURES

The epithelial lining of nasopalatine duct cysts is highly variable (Figs. 1-57 and 1-58). It may be composed of the following:

- Stratified squamous epithelium
- Pseudostratified columnar epithelium
- Simple columnar epithelium
- Simple cuboidal epithelium

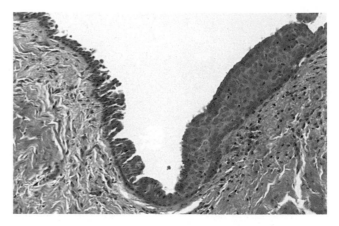

Fig. 1-57   Nasopalatine duct cyst. Cystic lining showing transition from pseudostratified columnar to stratified squamous epithelium.

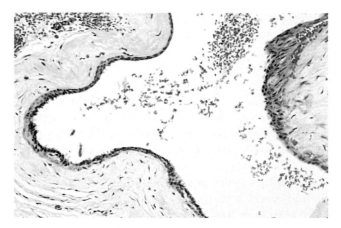

Fig. 1-58   Nasopalatine duct cyst. Flattened cuboidal epithelial lining.

Frequently, more than one epithelial type is found in the same cyst. Stratified squamous epithelium is most common, present in at least three fourths of all cysts. Pseudostratified columnar epithelium has been reported in from one third to three fourths of all cases. Simple cuboidal and columnar epithelium are discovered less frequently.

Cilia and goblet cells may be found in association with columnar linings. The type of epithelium may be related to the vertical position of the cyst within the incisive canal. Cysts developing within the superior aspect of the canal near the nasal cavity are more likely to demonstrate respiratory epithelium; those in an inferior position near the oral cavity are more likely to exhibit squamous epithelium.

The contents of the cyst wall can be a helpful diagnostic aid. Because the nasopalatine duct cyst arises within the incisive canal, moderate-sized nerves and small muscular arteries and veins are usually found in

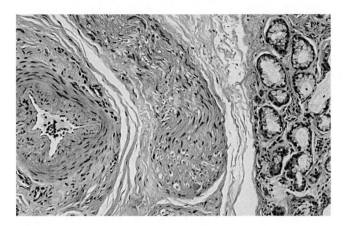

Fig. 1-59   Nasopalatine duct cyst. Cyst wall showing blood vessels, nerve bundles, and minor salivary glands.

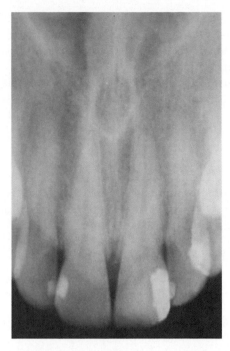

Fig. 1-60   Median palatal cyst. Well-circumscribed radiolucency apical to the maxillary incisors in the midline. At surgery the lesion was unrelated to the incisive canal. *(Courtesy of Dr. Timothy Armanini.)*

the wall of the cyst (Fig. 1-59). Small mucous glands have been reported in as many as one third of cases. Occasionally, the clinician may see small islands of hyaline cartilage. Frequently, an inflammatory response is noted in the cyst wall and may range from mild to heavy. This inflammation is usually chronic in nature and is composed of lymphocytes, plasma cells, and histiocytes. Associated acute inflammatory cells (neutrophils) sometimes may be seen.

TREATMENT AND PROGNOSIS

Nasopalatine duct cysts are treated by surgical enucleation. Biopsy is recommended because the lesion is not diagnostic radiographically; other benign and malignant lesions have been known to mimic the nasopalatine duct cyst. The lesion is best approached with a palatal flap that is reflected after an incision is made along the lingual gingival margin of the anterior maxillary teeth. Recurrence is rare. Malignant transformation has been reported in a couple of cases, but this is an extremely rare complication.

MEDIAN PALATAL (PALATINE) CYST

The median palatal cyst is a rare fissural cyst that theoretically develops from epithelium entrapped along the embryonic line of fusion of the lateral palatal shelves of the maxilla. This cyst may be difficult to distinguish from a nasopalatine duct cyst. In fact, most "median palatal cysts" may represent posteriorly positioned nasopalatine duct cysts. Because the nasopalatine ducts course posteriorly and superiorly as they extend from the incisive canal to the nasal cavity, a nasopalatine duct cyst that arises from posterior remnants of this duct near the nasal cavity might be mistaken for a median palatal cyst. On the other hand, if

a true median palatal cyst were to develop toward the anterior portion of the hard palate, then it could easily be mistaken for a nasopalatine duct cyst.

CLINICAL AND RADIOGRAPHIC FEATURES

The median palatal cyst presents as a firm or fluctuant swelling of the midline of the hard palate posterior to the palatine papilla. The lesion appears most frequently in young adults. Often it is asymptomatic, but some patients complain of pain or expansion. The average size of this cyst is 2 × 2 cm, but sometimes it can become quite large. Occlusal radiographs demonstrate a well-circumscribed radiolucency in the midline of the hard palate (Fig. 1-60). Occasional reported cases have been associated with divergence of the central incisors, although it may be difficult to rule out a nasopalatine duct cyst in these instances.

To differentiate the median palatal cyst from other cystic lesions of the maxilla, Gingell and associates suggested the following diagnostic criteria:
- Grossly appears symmetrical along the midline of the hard palate
- Located posterior to the palatine papilla
- Appears ovoid or circular radiographically
- Not intimately associated with a nonvital tooth

- Does not communicate with the incisive canal
- Shows no microscopic evidence of large neurovascular bundles, hyaline cartilage, or minor salivary glands in the cyst wall

It must be stressed that a true median palatal cyst should exhibit clinical enlargement of the palate. A midline radiolucency without clinical evidence of expansion is probably a nasopalatine duct cyst.

HISTOPATHOLOGIC FEATURES

Microscopic examination shows a cyst that is usually lined by stratified squamous epithelium. Areas of ciliated pseudostratified columnar epithelium have been reported in some cases. Chronic inflammation may be present in the cyst wall.

TREATMENT AND PROGNOSIS

The median palatal cyst is treated by surgical removal. Recurrence should not be expected.

"MEDIAN MANDIBULAR CYST"

The **"median mandibular cyst"** is a controversial lesion of questionable existence. Theoretically, it represents a fissural cyst in the anterior midline of the mandible that develops from epithelium entrapped during fusion of the halves of the mandible during embryonic life. However, the mandible actually develops as a single bilobed proliferation of mesenchyme with a central isthmus in the midline. As the mandible grows, this isthmus is eliminated. Therefore, because no fusion of epithelium-lined processes occurs, entrapment of epithelium should not be possible.

Because respiratory prosoplasia is not uncommon in odontogenic cysts, it appears likely that most (if not all) of these midline cysts are of odontogenic origin. Many purported cases would be classified today as examples of the *glandular odontogenic cyst* (see page 697), which has a propensity for occurrence in the midline mandibular region. Others could be classified as *periapical cysts, odontogenic keratocysts*, or *lateral periodontal cysts*. Because a fissural cyst in this region probably does not exist, the term *median mandibular cyst* should no longer be used.

FOLLICULAR CYSTS OF THE SKIN

Follicular cysts of the skin are common keratin-filled lesions that arise from one or more portions of the hair follicle. The most common type, which is derived from the follicular infundibulum, is known as an **epidermoid** or **infundibular cyst**. These cysts often arise after localized inflammation of the hair follicle and probably represent a nonneoplastic proliferation of the

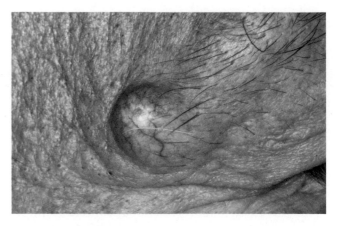

Fig. 1-61 Epidermoid cyst. Fluctuant nodule at the lateral edge of the eyebrow.

infundibular epithelium resulting from the healing process. The term **sebaceous cyst** sometimes is used mistakenly as a synonym for both the epidermoid cyst and another cyst of the scalp known as a **pilar, tricholemmal,** or **isthmus-catagen cyst.** However, because both the epidermoid cyst and pilar cyst are derived from the hair follicle rather than the sebaceous gland, the term *sebaceous cyst* should be avoided.

Keratin-filled cysts of the skin may occasionally arise after traumatic implantation of epithelium, although such lesions may be difficult to distinguish from an infundibular cyst. Rarely, such **epidermal inclusion (implantation) cysts** also can develop in the mouth. These small inclusion cysts should be distinguished from oral epidermoid cysts that occur in the midline floor of mouth region and represent the minimal manifestation of the teratoma-dermoid cyst-epidermoid cyst spectrum (see page 33).

CLINICAL FEATURES

Epidermoid (infundibular) cysts account for approximately 80% of follicular cysts of the skin and are most common in the acne-prone areas of the head, neck, and back. They are unusual before puberty unless they are associated with **Gardner syndrome** (see page 651). Young adults are more likely to have cysts on the face, whereas older adults are more likely to have cysts on the back. Males are affected more frequently than females.

Epidermoid cysts present as nodular, fluctuant subcutaneous lesions that may or may not be associated with inflammation (Figs. 1-61 and 1-62). If a noninflamed lesion presents in an area of thin skin, such as the earlobe, then it may be white or yellow.

Pilar (tricholemmal) cysts comprise approximately 10% to 15% of skin cysts, occurring most frequently on

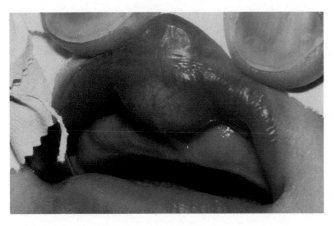

Fig. 1-62   Epidermoid cyst. Infant with a mass in the upper lip.

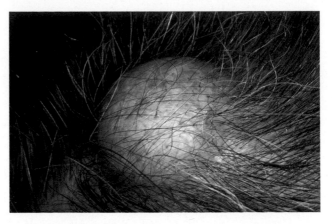

Fig. 1-63   Pilar cyst. Nodular mass on the scalp.

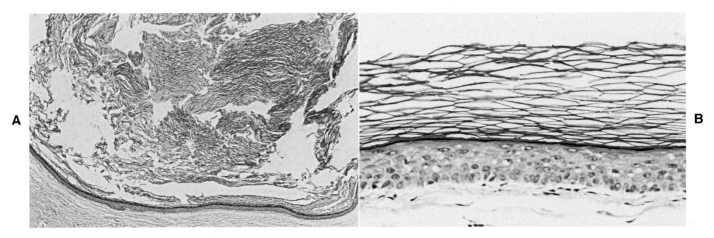

A   **B**

Fig. 1-64   Epidermoid cyst. A, Low-power view showing a keratin-filled cystic cavity.
B, High-power view showing stratified squamous epithelial lining with orthokeratin production.

the scalp (Fig. 1-63). They are twice as common in women as in men. The lesion is usually movable and shells out easily.

HISTOPATHOLOGIC FEATURES

Microscopic examination of an epidermoid cyst reveals a cavity that is lined by stratified squamous epithelium resembling epidermis (Fig. 1-64). A well-developed granular cell layer is seen, and the lumen is filled with degenerating orthokeratin. Not infrequently, the epithelial lining will be disrupted. When this occurs, a prominent granulomatous inflammatory reaction, including multinucleated giant cells, can be present in the cyst wall because the exposed keratin is recognized as a foreign material.

The pilar cyst is also lined by stratified squamous epithelium, although a granular cell layer is usually absent or greatly diminished (Fig. 1-65). The keratino-

cytes remain large in the upper epithelial layers with an abrupt transition to dense, compact keratin that fills the cyst lumen.

TREATMENT AND PROGNOSIS

Epidermoid and pilar cysts are usually treated by conservative surgical excision, and recurrence is uncommon. Malignant transformation has been reported but is exceedingly rare.

DERMOID CYST

The **dermoid cyst** is an uncommon developmental cystic malformation. The cyst is lined by epidermis-like epithelium and contains dermal adnexal structures in the cyst wall. It is generally classified as a benign cystic form of **teratoma.**

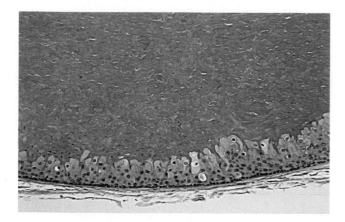

Fig. 1-65 **Pilar cyst.** Medium-power view showing an abrupt transition between the stratified squamous epithelial lining and compact keratin without the presence of a transitional granular cell layer.

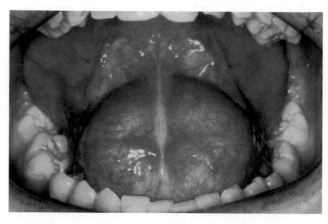

Fig. 1-66 **Dermoid cyst.** Fluctuant midline swelling in the floor of the mouth. *(From Budnick SD:* Handbook of pediatric oral pathology, *Chicago, 1981, Year Book Medical.)*

By definition, a true teratoma is a developmental tumor composed of tissue from all three germ layers: (1) ectoderm, (2) mesoderm, and (3) endoderm. Such tumors are believed to arise from germ cells or entrapped totipotent blastomeres, which can produce derivatives of all three germ layers.

Teratomatous malformations have a spectrum of complexity. In their most complex form, these lesions produce multiple types of tissue that are arranged in a disorganized fashion. These "complex" teratomas are most common in the ovaries or testes and can be benign or malignant. Occasionally, ovarian teratomas (or "dermoids") produce well-formed teeth, or even partially complete jaws. Complex teratomas of the oral cavity are rare and are usually congenital in nature. When they occur, they usually extend through a cleft palate from the pituitary area via Rathke's pouch. Cervical teratomas also have been reported.

The term **teratoid cyst** has been used to describe a cystic form of teratoma that contains a variety of germ layer derivatives:

1. Skin appendages, including hair follicles, sebaceous glands, and sweat glands
2. Connective tissue elements, such as muscle, blood vessels, and bone
3. Endodermal structures, such as gastrointestinal lining

Rarely, oral cysts may be lined entirely by gastrointestinal epithelium. These **heterotopic oral gastrointestinal cysts (enterocystomas, enteric duplication cysts)** are usually considered to be choristomas, or histologically normal tissue found in an abnormal location. However, these lesions probably can be included under the broad umbrella of teratomatous lesions,

especially because they are occasionally found in combination with dermoid cysts.

Dermoid cysts are simpler in structure than complex teratomas or teratoid cysts. Although they do not contain tissue from all three germ layers, they probably represent a *forme fruste* of a teratoma. Similar cysts of the oral cavity can be seen that are lined by epidermis-like epithelium, but they contain no dermal appendages in the cyst wall. These lesions have been called **epidermoid cysts** and represent the simplest expression of the teratoma spectrum. These intraoral epidermoid cysts should not be confused with the more common **epidermoid cyst of the skin** (see page 32), a nonteratomatous lesion that arises from the hair follicle.

CLINICAL AND RADIOGRAPHIC FEATURES

Dermoid cysts most commonly occur in the midline of the floor of the mouth (Fig. 1-66), although occasionally they are displaced laterally or develop in other locations. If the cyst develops above the geniohyoid muscle, then a sublingual swelling may displace the tongue toward the roof of the mouth and create difficulty in eating, speaking, or even breathing. Cysts that occur below the geniohyoid muscle often produce a submental swelling, with a "double-chin" appearance.

Oral dermoid cysts can vary in size from a few millimeters to 12 cm in diameter. They are most common in children and young adults; 15% of reported cases have been congenital. The lesion is usually slow growing and painless, presenting as a doughy or rubbery mass that frequently retains pitting after application of pres-

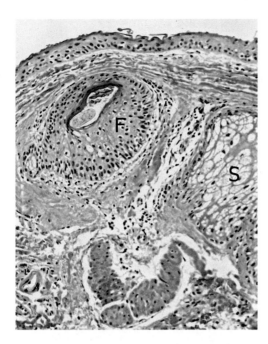

Fig. 1-67   Dermoid cyst. Squamous epithelial lining (*top*), with hair follicle (*F*), sebaceous glands (*S*) in the cyst wall.

sure. Secondary infection can occur, and the lesion may drain intraorally or onto the skin. MRIs, CT scans, or contrast medium radiographs may be helpful in delineating the extent of the lesion.

HISTOPATHOLOGIC FEATURES

Dermoid cysts are lined by orthokeratinized stratified squamous epithelium, with a prominent granular cell layer. Abundant keratin often is found within the cyst lumen. On rare occasions, areas of respiratory epithelium can be seen. The cyst wall is composed of fibrous connective tissue that contains one or more skin appendages, such as sebaceous glands, hair follicles, or sweat glands (Fig. 1-67).

TREATMENT AND PROGNOSIS

Dermoid cysts are treated by surgical removal. Those located above the geniohyoid muscle can be removed by an intraoral incision, and those below the geniohyoid muscle may require an extraoral approach. Recurrence is uncommon. Malignant transformation into squamous cell carcinoma has been reported only rarely.

THYROGLOSSAL DUCT CYST (THYROGLOSSAL TRACT CYST)

The thyroid gland begins its development at the end of the third week of embryonic life as a proliferation of endodermal cells from the ventral floor of the pharynx,

between the tuberculum impar and copula of the developing tongue—a point that later becomes the foramen cecum. This thyroid anlage descends into the neck as a bilobed diverticulum anterior to the developing hyoid bone and reaches its definitive level below the thyroid cartilage by the seventh embryonic week. Along this path of descent, an epithelial tract or duct is formed, maintaining an attachment to the base of the tongue. This thyroglossal duct becomes intimately associated with the developing hyoid bone. As the hyoid matures and rotates to its adult position, the thyroglossal duct passes in front and beneath the hyoid, looping upward and behind it before curving downward again into the lower neck. The caudal segment of this duct often persists, forming the pyramidal lobe of the thyroid gland.

The thyroglossal duct epithelium normally undergoes atrophy and is obliterated. However, remnants of this epithelium may persist and give rise to cysts along this tract known as **thyroglossal duct cysts.** The impetus for cystic degeneration is uncertain. Inflammation is the most frequently suggested stimulus, especially from adjacent lymphoid tissue that may react to draining infections of the head and neck. Retention of secretions within the duct is another possible factor. In addition, there are several reports of familial occurrence of such cysts.

CLINICAL FEATURES

Thyroglossal duct cysts classically develop in the midline and may occur anywhere from the foramen cecum area of the tongue to the suprasternal notch. Suprahyoid cysts may be submental in location. In 60% to 80% of cases, the cyst develops below the hyoid bone. Intralingual cysts are rare. Cysts that develop in the area of the thyroid cartilage often are deflected lateral to the midline because of the sharp anterior margin of the thyroid cartilage.

Thyroglossal duct cysts may develop at any age, but they are most commonly diagnosed in the first two decades of life; about 50% of cases occur before the age of 20. There is no sex predilection. The cyst usually presents as a painless, fluctuant, movable swelling unless it is complicated by secondary infection (Fig. 1-68). Lesions that develop at the base of the tongue may cause laryngeal obstruction. Most thyroglossal duct cysts are smaller than 3 cm in diameter, but occasional cysts may reach 10 cm in size. If the cyst maintains an attachment to the hyoid bone or tongue, it will move vertically during swallowing or protrusion of the tongue. Fistulous tracts to the skin or mucosa develop in as many as one third of cases, usually from rupture of an infected cyst or as a sequela of surgery.

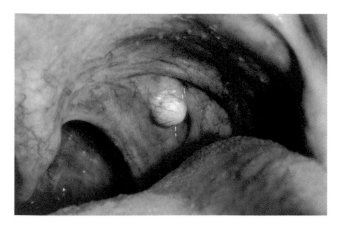

Fig. 1-73 Oral lymphoepithelial cyst. Small yellow-white nodule of the tonsillar fossa.

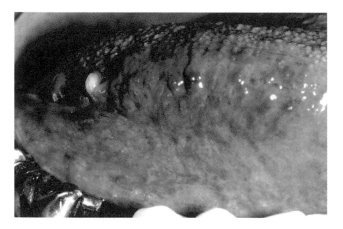

Fig. 1-74 Oral lymphoepithelial cyst. Small white nodule of the posterior lateral border of the tongue.

become obstructed or pinched off from the surface, producing a keratin-filled cyst within the lymphoid tissue just below the mucosal surface. It also is possible that oral lymphoepithelial cysts may develop from salivary or surface mucosal epithelium that becomes enclaved in lymphoid tissue during embryogenesis. It even has been suggested that these cysts may arise from the excretory ducts of the sublingual gland or minor salivary glands, and that the associated lymphoid tissue represents a secondary immune response.

CLINICAL FEATURES

The oral lymphoepithelial cyst presents as a small submucosal mass that is usually less than 1 cm in diameter; rarely will the lesion be greater than 1.5 cm (Figs. 1-73 and 1-74). The cyst may feel firm or soft to palpation, and the overlying mucosa is smooth and nonulcerated. The lesion is typically white or yellow and often con-

tains creamy or cheesy keratinous material in the lumen. The cyst is usually asymptomatic, although occasionally, patients may complain of swelling or drainage. Pain is rare but may occur secondary to trauma.

Oral lymphoepithelial cysts may develop in people of almost any age, but they are most common in young adults. The most frequent location is the floor of the mouth, with at least half of all cases found there. The ventral surface and posterior lateral border of the tongue are the next most common sites. These cysts also may develop in the area of the palatine tonsil or soft palate. All of these locations represent sites of normal or accessory oral lymphoid tissue.

HISTOPATHOLOGIC FEATURES

Microscopic examination of the oral lymphoepithelial cyst demonstrates a cystic cavity that is lined by stratified squamous epithelium without rete ridges (Fig. 1-75). This epithelium is typically parakeratinized, with desquamated epithelial cells seen filling the cyst lumen. In rare instances the epithelial lining also may contain mucous cells. Occasional cysts may communicate with the overlying mucosal surface.

The most striking feature is the presence of lymphoid tissue in the cyst wall. In most instances, this lymphoid tissue encircles the cyst, but sometimes it involves only a portion of the cyst wall. Germinal centers are usually, but not always, present.

TREATMENT AND PROGNOSIS

The oral lymphoepithelial cyst is usually treated with surgical excision and should not recur. Because the lesion is typically asymptomatic and innocuous, biopsy may not always be necessary if the lesion is distinctive enough to make the diagnosis on a clinical basis.

Other Rare Developmental Anomalies

HEMIHYPERPLASIA (HEMIHYPERTROPHY)

Hemihyperplasia is a rare developmental anomaly characterized by asymmetric overgrowth of one or more body parts. Although the condition is known more commonly as **hemihypertrophy,** it actually represents a hyperplasia of the tissues rather than a hypertrophy. Hemihyperplasia can be an isolated finding, but it also may be associated with a variety of malformation syndromes (Box 1-3).

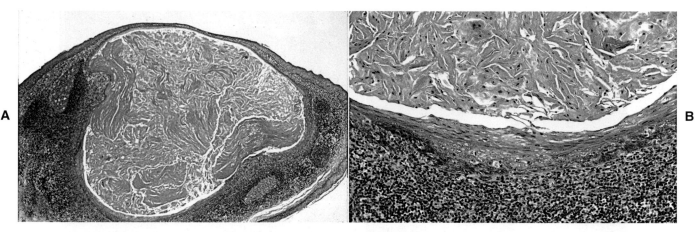

Fig. 1-75   Oral lymphoepithelial cyst. A, Low-power view showing a keratin-filled cyst below the mucosal surface. Lymphoid tissue is present in the cyst wall. **B,** High-power view showing lymphoid tissue adjacent to the cystic lining.

Box 1-3

Malformation Syndromes Associated with Hemihyperplasia

- Beckwith-Wiedemann syndrome
- Neurofibromatosis
- Klippel-Trénaunay-Weber syndrome
- Proteus syndrome
- McCune-Albright syndrome
- Epidermal nevus syndrome
- Triploid/diploid mixoploidy
- Langer-Giedion syndrome
- Multiple exostoses syndrome
- Maffucci syndrome
- Ollier syndrome
- Segmental odontomaxillary dysplasia

Almost all cases of isolated hemihyperplasia are sporadic. A number of possible etiologic factors have been suggested, but the cause remains obscure. Various theories include vascular or lymphatic abnormalities, central nervous system disturbances, endocrine dysfunctions, and aberrant twinning mechanisms. Occasionally, chromosomal anomalies have been documented.

CLINICAL AND RADIOGRAPHIC FEATURES

In a person with hemihyperplasia, one entire side of the body **(complex hemihyperplasia)** may be affected or the enlargement may be limited to a single limb **(simple hemihyperplasia).** If the enlargement is confined to one side of the face, the term **hemifacial hyperplasia** (or **hemifacial hypertrophy**) may apply. The condition can occasionally be crossed, involving different areas on both sides of the body. Hemihyperplasia shows a 2:1 female-to-male predilection, and it occurs more often on the right side of the body.

Asymmetry often is noted at birth, although in some cases the condition may not become evident until later in childhood (Fig. 1-76). The enlargement becomes more accentuated with age, especially at puberty. This disproportionate growth continues until the patient's overall growth ceases, resulting in permanent asymmetry.

The changes may involve all the tissues on the affected side, including the underlying bone. Often the skin is thickened and may demonstrate increased pigmentation, hypertrichosis, telangiectasias, or nevus flammeus. About 20% of those affected are mentally retarded. One of the most significant features is an increased prevalence of abdominal tumors, especially Wilms' tumor, adrenal cortical carcinoma, and hepatoblastoma. These tumors have been reported in 5.9% of patients with isolated hemihyperplasia, and they do not necessarily occur on the same side as the somatic enlargement.

Unilateral **macroglossia,** featuring prominent tongue papillae, is common. Enlargement of other oral soft tissues and bone can occur. The mandibular canal may be increased in size on radiographs. The crowns of the teeth on the affected side, especially the permanent cuspids, premolars, and first molars, can be larger. Premature development of these teeth, along with precocious eruption, may be obvious. The roots also may be larger, but some reports have described root resorption. Malocclusion with open bite is not unusual.

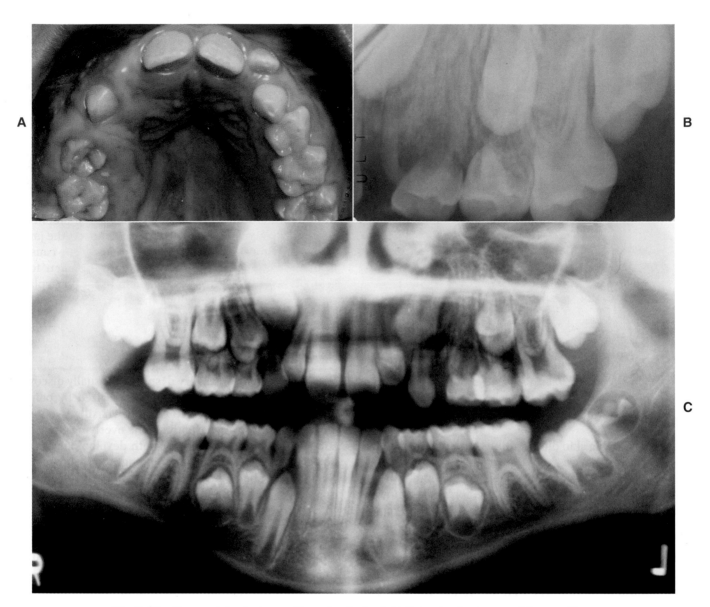

Fig. 1-78   Segmental odontomaxillary dysplasia. A, Unilateral enlargement of the maxilla and overlying gingival soft tissues. **B,** Periapical radiograph showing coarse trabecular pattern with absence of the first premolar. **C,** Panoramic radiograph showing irregular bone pattern of the left maxilla expanding into the maxillary sinus.

the condition seems to remain stable and may not require surgical intervention. However, orthodontic therapy and orthognathic surgery may be considered in some cases.

CROUZON SYNDROME (CRANIOFACIAL DYSOSTOSIS)

Crouzon syndrome is one of a rare group of syndromes characterized by craniosynostosis, or premature closing of the cranial sutures. It is believed to be caused by one of a variety of mutations of the fibroblast growth factor receptor 2 *(FGFR2)* gene on chromosome 10q26. The condition occurs in about 1 of every

65,000 births and is inherited as an autosomal dominant trait. A significant number of cases, however, represent new mutations, often apparently related to increased paternal age.

CLINICAL AND RADIOGRAPHIC FEATURES

Crouzon syndrome exhibits a wide variability in expression. The premature sutural closing leads to cranial malformations, such as **brachycephaly** (short head), **scaphocephaly** (boat-shaped head), or **trigonocephaly** (triangle-shaped head). The most severely affected patients can demonstrate a "cloverleaf" skull (*kleeblatt-*

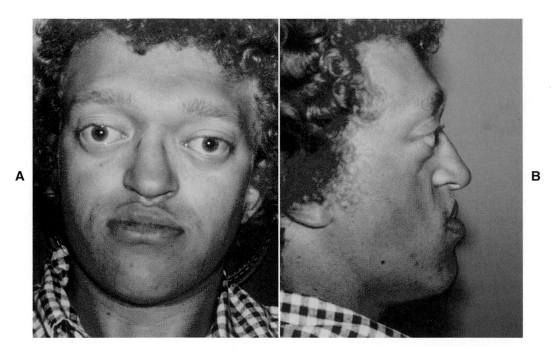

Fig. 1-79   **Crouzon syndrome.** Ocular proptosis and midface hypoplasia. *(Courtesy of Dr. Robert Gorlin.)*

schädel deformity). The orbits are shallow, resulting in characteristic ocular proptosis (Fig. 1-79). Visual impairment or total blindness and a hearing deficit may occur. Some patients report headaches, attributable to increased intracranial pressure. Marked mental deficiency is rarely seen. Skull radiographs typically show increased digital markings (i.e., "beaten-metal" pattern).

The maxilla is underdeveloped, resulting in midface hypoplasia. Often the maxillary teeth are crowded, and occlusal disharmony usually occurs. Cleft lip and cleft palate are rare, but lateral palatal swellings may produce a midline maxillary pseudocleft.

TREATMENT AND PROGNOSIS

The clinical defects of Crouzon syndrome can be treated surgically, but multiple procedures may be necessary. Early craniectomy often is needed to alleviate the raised intracranial pressure. Frontoorbital advancement can be performed to correct the ocular defects, with midfacial advancement used to correct the maxillary hypoplasia.

APERT SYNDROME (ACROCEPHALOSYNDACTYLY)

Like Crouzon syndrome, **Apert syndrome** is a rare condition that is characterized by craniosynostosis. It occurs in about 1 of every 65,000 births and is caused by one of two point mutations in the fibroblast growth factor receptor 2 (*FGFR2*) gene, which is located on chromosome 10q26. Although it is inherited as an autosomal dominant trait, most cases represent sporadic new mutations, which are thought to be exclusively of paternal origin and often associated with increased paternal age.

CLINICAL AND RADIOGRAPHIC FEATURES

Craniosynostosis typically produces **acrobrachycephaly** (tower skull); severe cases may demonstrate the *kleeblattschädel* deformity (cloverleaf skull). The occiput is flattened, and a tall appearance to the forehead is noted. Ocular proptosis is a characteristic finding, along with hypertelorism and downward-slanting lateral palpebral fissures (Fig. 1-80). Visual loss can result from the following:

- Chronic exposure of the unprotected eyes
- Increased intracranial pressure
- Compression of the optic nerves

Skull films may demonstrate digital impressions similar to those of Crouzon syndrome (Fig. 1-81).

The middle third of the face is significantly retruded and hypoplastic, resulting in a relative mandibular prognathism. The reduced size of the nasopharynx and narrowing of the posterior choanae can lead to respiratory distress in the young child. To compensate for this, most infants become mouth breathers, contributing to an "open-mouth" appearance. Sleep apnea may processes, with prominent antegonial notching. The mouth is downturned, and about 15% of patients have lateral facial clefting (see page 2) that produces macrostomia. Cleft palate is seen in about one third of cases. The parotid glands may be hypoplastic or may be totally absent (see page 453).

A number of infants may experience respiratory and feeding difficulties because of hypoplasia of the nasopharynx, oropharynx, and hypopharynx. Choanal atresia is a common finding, and the larynx and trachea are often narrow. Combined with the mandibular hypoplasia and resultant improper tongue position, these defects can lead to the infant's death from respiratory complications.

TREATMENT AND PROGNOSIS

Patients with mild forms of mandibulofacial dysostosis may not require treatment. In more severe cases the clinical appearance can be improved with cosmetic surgery. Because of the extent of facial reconstruction required, multiple surgical procedures are usually necessary. Individual operations may be needed for the eyes, zygomas, jaws, ears, and nose. Combined orthodontic therapy is needed along with the orthognathic surgery.

BIBLIOGRAPHY

Orofacial Clefts

Avery JK, Chiego DJ Jr: Development of the face and palate. In *Essentials of oral histology and embryology: a clinical approach*, ed 3, pp 51-61, St Louis, 2006, Mosby.

Berkovitz BK, Holland GR, Moxham BJ: Development of the face and development of the palate. In *Oral anatomy, histology and embryology*, ed 3, pp 269-283, St Louis, 2002, Mosby.

Carinci F, Pezzetti F, Scapoli L et al: Recent developments in orofacial cleft genetics, *J Craniofac Surg* 14:130-143, 2003.

Derijcke A, Eerens A, Carels C: The incidence of oral clefts: a review, *Br J Oral Maxillofac Surg* 34:488-494, 1996.

Eppley BL, van Aalst JA, Robey A et al: The spectrum of orofacial clefting, *Plast Reconstr Surg* 115:101e-114e, 2005.

Evans CA: Orthodontic treatment for patients with clefts, *Clin Plast Surg* 31:271-290, 2004.

Gorlin RJ, Cohen MM Jr, Hennekam RCM: Orofacial clefting syndromes: general aspects. In *Syndromes of the head and neck*, ed 4, pp 850-876, New York, 2001, Oxford University Press.

Gosain AK, Conley SF, Marks S et al: Submucous cleft palate: diagnostic methods and outcomes of surgical treatment, *Plast Reconstr Surg* 97:1497-1509, 1996.

Harada K, Sato M, Omura K: Long-term maxillomandibular skeletal and dental changes in children with cleft lip and palate after maxillary distraction, *Oral Surg Oral Med Oral Pathol Oral Radiol Endod* 102:292-299, 2006.

Krapels IP, Vermeij-Keers C, Müller M et al: Nutrition and genes in the development of orofacial clefting, *Nutr Rev* 64:280-288, 2006.

Marazita ML, Mooney MP: Current concepts in the embryology and genetics of cleft lip and cleft palate, *Clin Plast Surg* 31:125-140, 2004.

Millard DR Jr, Latham RA: Improved primary surgical and dental treatment of clefts, *Plast Reconstr Surg* 86:856-871, 1990.

Murray JC: Gene/environment causes of cleft lip and/or palate, *Clin Genet* 61:248-256, 2002.

Rintala A, Leisti J, Liesmaa M et al: Oblique facial clefts, *Scand J Plast Reconstr Surg* 14:291-297, 1980.

Shprintzen RJ: Pierre Robin, micrognathia, and airway obstruction: the dependency of treatment on accurate diagnosis, *Int Anesthesiol Clin* 26:64-71, 1988.

St-Hilaire H, Buchbinder D: Maxillofacial pathology and management of Pierre Robin sequence, *Otolaryngol Clin North Am* 33:1241-1256, 2000.

Stoll C, Alembik Y, Dott B et al: Associated malformations in cases with oral clefts, *Cleft Palate Craniofac J* 37:41-47, 2000.

Ten Cate AR, Nanci A: Embryology of the head, face, and oral cavity. In Nanci A: *Ten Cate's oral histology: development, structure, and function*, ed 6, pp 30-53, St Louis, 2003, Mosby.

Thornton JB, Nimer S, Howard PS: The incidence, classification, etiology, and embryology of oral clefts, *Semin Orthod* 2:162-168, 1996.

van den Elzen AP, Semmekrot BA, Bongers EM et al: Diagnosis and treatment of the Pierre Robin sequence: results of a retrospective clinical study and review of the literature, *Eur J Pediatr* 160:47-53, 2001.

Vanderas AP: Incidence of cleft lip, cleft palate, and cleft lip and palate among races: a review, *Cleft Palate J* 24:216-225, 1987.

Weinberg SM, Neiswanger K, Martin RA et al: The Pittsburgh oral-facial cleft study: expanding the cleft phenotype. Background and justification, *Cleft Palate Craniofac J* 43:7-20, 2006.

Commissural Lip Pits

Baker BR: Pits of the lip commissures in caucasoid males, *Oral Surg Oral Med Oral Pathol* 21:56-60, 1966.

Everett FG, Wescott WB: Commissural lip pits, *Oral Surg Oral Med Oral Pathol* 14:202-209, 1961.

Gorsky M, Buchner A, Cohen C: Commissural lip pits in Israeli Jews of different ethnic origin, *Community Dent Oral Epidemiol* 13:195-196, 1985.

Paramedian Lip Pits

Burdick AB, Bixler D, Puckett CL: Genetic analysis in families with van der Woude syndrome, *J Craniofac Genet Dev Biol* 5:181-208, 1985.

Cervenka J, Gorlin RJ, Anderson VE: The syndrome of pits of the lower lip and cleft lip and/or palate: genetic considerations, *Am J Hum Genet* 19:416-432, 1967.

Gorlin RJ, Cohen MM Jr, Hennekam RCM: Popliteal pterygium syndrome (facio-genito-popliteal syndrome). In *Syndromes of the head and neck*, ed 4, pp 775-778, New York, 2001, Oxford University Press.

Kondo S, Schutte BC, Richardson RJ et al: Mutations in IRF6 cause Van der Woude and popliteal pterygium syndromes, *Nat Genet* 32:285-289, 2002.

Matsumoto N, Niikawa N: Kabuki make-up syndrome: a review, *Am J Med Genet C Semin Med Genet* 117:57-65, 2003.

Onofre MA, Brosco HB, Brosco JU et al: Congenital fistulae of the lower lip in van der Woude syndrome: a histomorphological study, *Cleft Palate Craniofac J* 36:79-85, 1999.

Onofre MA, Brosco HB, Taga R: Relationship between lower-lip fistulae and cleft lip and/or palate in van der Woude syndrome, *Cleft Palate Craniofac J* 34:261-265, 1997.

Rizos M, Spyropoulos MN: Van der Woude syndrome: a review. Cardinal signs, epidemiology, associated features, differential diagnosis, expressivity, genetic counseling and treatment, *Eur J Orthod* 26:17-24, 2004.

Schutte BC, Basart AM, Watanabe Y et al: Microdeletions at chromosome bands 1q32-q41 as a cause of van der Woude syndrome, *Am J Med Genet* 84:145-150, 1999.

Shotelersuk V, Punyashthiti R, Srivuthana S et al: Kabuki syndrome: report of six Thai children and further phenotypic and genetic delineation, *Am J Med Genet* 110:384-390, 2002.

Double Lip

Barnett ML, Bosshardt LL, Morgan AF: Double lip and double lip with blepharochalasis (Ascher's syndrome), *Oral Surg Oral Med Oral Pathol* 34:727-733, 1972.

Eski M, Nisanci M, Atkas A et al: Congenital double lip: review of 5 cases, *Br J Oral Maxillofac Surg* 45:68-70, 2007.

Gomez-Duaso AJ, Seoane J, Vazquez-Garcia J et al: Ascher syndrome: report of two cases, *J Oral Maxillofac Surg* 55:88-90, 1997.

Kenny KF, Hreha JP, Dent CD: Bilateral redundant mucosal tissue of the upper lip, *J Am Dent Assoc* 120:193-194, 1990.

Fordyce Granules

Daley TD: Pathology of intraoral sebaceous glands, *J Oral Pathol Med* 22:241-245, 1993.

Fordyce JA: A peculiar affection of the mucous membrane of the lips and oral cavity, *J Cutan Genito-Urin Dis* 14:413-419, 1896.

Halperin V, Kolas S, Jefferis KR et al: The occurrence of Fordyce spots, benign migratory glossitis, median rhomboid glossitis, and fissured tongue in 2,478 dental patients, *Oral Surg Oral Med Oral Pathol* 6:1072-1077, 1953.

Miles AEW: Sebaceous glands in the lip and cheek mucosa of man, *Br Dent J* 105:235-248, 1958.

Sewerin I: The sebaceous glands in the vermilion border of the lips and in the oral mucosa of man, *Acta Odontol Scand* 33(suppl 68):13-226, 1975.

Sewerin I, Prætorius F: Keratin-filled pseudocysts of ducts of sebaceous glands in the vermilion border of the lip, *J Oral Pathol* 3:279-283, 1974.

Leukoedema

Archard HO, Carlson KP, Stanley HR: Leukoedema of the human oral mucosa, *Oral Surg Oral Med Oral Pathol* 25:717-728, 1968.

Axéll T, Henricsson V: Leukoedema—an epidemiologic study with special reference to the influence of tobacco habits, *Community Dent Oral Epidemiol* 9:142-146, 1981.

Durocher RT, Thalman R, Fiore-Donno G: Leukoedema of the oral mucosa, *J Am Dent Assoc* 85:1105-1109, 1972.

Martin JL: Leukoedema: an epidemiological study in white and African Americans, *J Tenn Dent Assoc* 77:18-21, 1997.

Martin JL, Crump EP: Leukoedema of the buccal mucosa in Negro children and youth, *Oral Surg Oral Med Oral Pathol* 34:49-58, 1972.

Sandstead HR, Lowe JW: Leukoedema and keratosis in relation to leukoplakia of the buccal mucosa in man, *J Natl Cancer Inst* 14:423-437, 1953.

van Wyk CW, Ambrosio SC: Leukoedema: ultrastructural and histochemical observations, *J Oral Pathol* 12:319-329, 1983.

Microglossia

Dunham ME, Austin TL: Congenital aglossia and situs inversus, *Int J Pediatr Otorhinolaryngol* 19:163-168, 1990.

Gorlin RJ, Cohen MM Jr, Hennekam RCM: Oromandibular-limb hypogenesis syndromes. In *Syndromes of the head and neck*, ed 4, pp 822-826, New York, 2001, Oxford University Press.

Hall BD: Aglossa-adactylia, *Birth Defects Orig Artic Ser* 7:233-236, 1971.

Shah RM: Palatomandibular and maxillo-mandibular fusion, partial aglossia and cleft palate in a human embryo: report of a case, *Teratology* 15:261-272, 1977.

Yasuda Y, Kitai N, Fujii Y et al: Report of a patient with hypoglossia-hypodactylia syndrome and a review of the literature, *Cleft Palate Craniofac J* 40:196-202, 2003.

Macroglossia

Cohen MM Jr: Beckwith-Wiedemann syndrome: historical, clinicopathological, and etiopathogenetic perspectives, *Pediatr Dev Pathol* 8:287-304, 2005.

Engström W, Lindham S, Schofield P: Wiedemann-Beckwith syndrome, *Eur J Pediatr* 147:450-457, 1988.

Maturo SC, Mair EA: Submucosal minimally invasive lingual excision: an effective, novel surgery for pediatric tongue base reduction, *Ann Otol Rhinol Laryngol* 115:624-630, 2006.

Morgan WE, Friedman EM, Duncan NO et al: Surgical management of macroglossia in children, *Arch Otolaryngol Head Neck Surg* 122:326-329, 1996.

Myer CM III, Hotaling AJ, Reilly JS: The diagnosis and treatment of macroglossia in children, *Ear Nose Throat J* 65:444-448, 1986.

Rimell FL, Shapiro AM, Shoemaker DL et al: Head and neck manifestations of Beckwith-Wiedemann syndrome, *Otolaryngol Head Neck Surg* 113:262-265, 1995.

Siddiqui A, Pensler JM: The efficacy of tongue resection in treatment of symptomatic macroglossia in the child, *Ann Plast Surg* 25:14-17, 1990.

Vogel JE, Mulliken JB, Kaban LB: Macroglossia: a review of the condition and a new classification, *Plast Reconstr Surg* 78:715-723, 1986.

Wang J, Goodger NM, Pogrel MA: The role of tongue reduction, *Oral Surg Oral Med Oral Pathol Oral Radiol Endod* 95:269-273, 2003.

Weksberg R, Shuman C, Smith AC: Beckwith-Wiedemann syndrome, *Am J Med Genet C Semin Med Genet* 137:12-23, 2005.

Wolford LM, Cottrell DA: Diagnosis of macroglossia and indications for reduction glossectomy, *Am J Orthod Dentofac Orthop* 110:170-177, 1996.

Ankyloglossia

Dollberg S, Botzer E, Grunis E et al: Immediate nipple pain relief after frenotomy in breast-fed infants with ankyloglossia: a randomized, prospective study, *J Pediatr Surg* 41:1598-1600, 2006.

Ewart NP: A lingual mucogingival problem associated with ankyloglossia: a case report, *N Z Dent J* 86:16-17, 1990.

Flinck A, Paludan A, Matsson L et al: Oral findings in a group of newborn Swedish children, *Int J Paediatr Dent* 4:67-73, 1994.

Hall DMB, Renfrew MJ: Tongue tie, *Arch Dis Child* 90:1211-1215, 2005.

Lalakea ML, Messner AH: Ankyloglossia: does it matter? *Pediatr Clin N Am* 50:381-397, 2003.

Lalakea ML, Messner AH: Ankyloglossia: the adolescent and adult perspective, *Otolaryngol Head Neck Surg* 128:746-752, 2003.

Mukai S, Mukai C, Asaoka K: Ankyloglossia with deviation of the epiglottis and larynx, *Ann Otol Rhinol Laryngol* 100:3-20, 1991.

Camarda AJ, Deschamps C, Forest D: II. Stylohyoid chain ossification: a discussion of etiology, *Oral Surg Oral Med Oral Pathol* 67:515-520, 1989.

Correll RW, Jensen JL, Taylor JB et al: Mineralization of the stylohyoid-stylomandibular ligament complex: a radiographic incidence study, *Oral Surg Oral Med Oral Pathol* 48:286-291, 1979.

Eagle WW: Elongated styloid processes: report of two cases, *Arch Otolaryngol* 25:584-587, 1937.

Montalbetti L, Ferrandi D, Pergami P et al: Elongated styloid process and Eagle's syndrome, *Cephalalgia* 15:80-93, 1995.

Rechtweg JS, Wax MK: Eagle's syndrome: a review, *Am J Otolaryngol* 19:316-321, 1998.

Smith RG, Cherry JE: Traumatic Eagle's syndrome: report of a case and review of the literature, *J Oral Maxillofac Surg* 46:606-609, 1988.

Stafne Defect

Apruzzese D, Longoni S: Stafne cyst in an anterior location, *J Oral Maxillofac Surg* 57:333-338, 1999.

Ariji E, Fujiwara N, Tabata O et al: Stafne's bone cavity: classification based on outline and content determined by computed tomography, *Oral Surg Oral Med Oral Pathol* 76:375-380, 1993.

Barker GR: A radiolucency of the ascending ramus of the mandible associated with invested parotid salivary gland material and analogous with a Stafne bone cavity, *Br J Oral Maxillofac Surg* 26:81-84, 1988.

Bouquot JE, Gnepp DR, Dardick I et al: Intraosseous salivary tissue: jawbone examples of choristomas, hamartomas, embryonic rests, and inflammatory entrapment: another histogenetic source for intraosseous adenocarcinoma, *Oral Surg Oral Med Oral Pathol Oral Radiol Endod* 90:205-217, 2000.

Branstetter BF, Weissman JL, Kaplan SB: Imaging of a Stafne bone cavity: what MR adds and why a new name is needed, *AJNR Am J Neuroradiol* 20:587, 1999.

Buchner A, Carpenter WM, Merrell PW et al: Anterior lingual mandibular salivary gland defect. Evaluation of twenty-four cases, *Oral Surg Oral Med Oral Pathol* 71:131-136, 1991.

Correll RW, Jensen JL, Rhyne RR: Lingual cortical mandibular defects: a radiographic incidence study, *Oral Surg Oral Med Oral Pathol* 50:287-291, 1980.

de Courten A, Küffer R, Samson J et al: Anterior lingual mandibular salivary gland defect (Stafne defect) presenting as a residual cyst, *Oral Surg Oral Med Oral Pathol Oral Radiol Endod* 94:460-464, 2002.

Miller AS, Winnick M: Salivary gland inclusion in the anterior mandible: report of a case with a review of the literature on aberrant salivary gland tissue and neoplasms, *Oral Surg Oral Med Oral Pathol* 31:790-797, 1971.

Oikarinen VJ, Wolf J, Julku M: A stereosialographic study of developmental mandibular bone defects (Stafne's idiopathic bone cavities), *Int J Oral Surg* 4:51-54, 1975.

Stafne EC: Bone cavities situated near the angle of the mandible, *J Am Dent Assoc* 29:1969-1972, 1942.

Palatal Cysts of the Newborn

Burke GW Jr, Feagans WM, Elzay RP et al: Some aspects of the origin and fate of midpalatal cysts in human fetuses, *J Dent Res* 45:159-164, 1966.

Cataldo E, Berkman MD: Cysts of the oral mucosa in newborns, *Am J Dis Child* 116:44-48, 1968.

Donley CL, Nelson, LP: Comparison of palatal and alveolar cysts of the newborn in premature and full term infants, *Pediatr Dent* 22:321-324, 2000.

Flinck A, Paludan A, Matsson L et al: Oral findings in a group of newborn Swedish children, *Int J Paediatr Dent* 4:67-73, 1994.

Fromm A: Epstein's pearls, Bohn's nodules and inclusion-cysts of the oral cavity, *J Dent Child* 34:275-287, 1967.

Jorgenson RJ, Shapiro SD, Salinas CF et al: Intraoral findings and anomalies in neonates, *Pediatrics* 69:577-582, 1982.

Liu MH, Huang WH: Oral abnormalities in Taiwanese newborns, *J Dent Child* 71:118-120, 2004.

Monteleone L, McLellan MS: Epstein's pearls (Bohn's nodules) of the palate, *J Oral Surg* 22:301-304, 1964.

Moreillon MC, Schroeder HE: Numerical frequency of epithelial abnormalities, particularly microkeratocysts, in the developing human oral mucosa, *Oral Surg Oral Med Oral Pathol* 53:44-55, 1982.

Nasolabial Cyst

Allard RHB: Nasolabial cyst: review of the literature and report of 7 cases, *Int J Oral Surg* 11:351-359, 1982.

Choi JH, Cho JH, Kang HJ et al: Nasolabial cyst: a retrospective analysis of 18 cases, *Ear Nose Throat J* 81:94-96, 2002.

Kuriloff DB: The nasolabial cyst—nasal hamartoma, *Otolaryngol Head Neck Surg* 96:268-272, 1987.

López-Ríos F, Lassaletta-Atienza L, Domingo-Carrasco C et al: Nasolabial cyst. Report of a case with extensive apocrine change, *Oral Surg Oral Med Oral Pathol Oral Radiol Endod* 84:404-406, 1997.

Roed-Petersen B: Nasolabial cysts: a presentation of five patients with a review of the literature, *Br J Oral Surg* 7:84-95, 1969.

Su C-Y, Chien C-Y, Hwang C-F: A new transnasal approach to endoscopic marsupialization of the nasolabial cyst, *Laryngoscope* 109:1116-1118, 1999.

Vasconcelos RF, Souza PE, Mesquita RA: Retrospective analysis of 15 cases of nasolabial cyst, *Quintessence Int* 30:629-632, 1999

"Globulomaxillary Cyst"

Christ TF: The globulomaxillary cyst: an embryologic misconception, *Oral Surg Oral Med Oral Pathol* 30:515-526, 1970.

D'Silva NJ, Anderson L: Globulomaxillary cyst revisited, *Oral Surg Oral Med Oral Pathol* 76:182-184, 1993.

Ferenczy K: The relationship of globulomaxillary cysts to the fusion of embryonal processes and to cleft palates, *Oral Surg Oral Med Oral Pathol* 11:1388-1393, 1958.

Little JW, Jakobsen J: Origin of the globulomaxillary cyst, *J Oral Surg* 31:188-195, 1973.

Steiner DR: A lesion of endodontic origin misdiagnosed as a globulomaxillary cyst, *J Endod* 25:277-281, 1999.

Vedtofte P, Holmstrup P: Inflammatory paradental cysts in the globulomaxillary region, *J Oral Pathol Med* 18:125-127, 1989.

Wysocki GP: The differential diagnosis of globulomaxillary radiolucencies, *Oral Surg Oral Med Oral Pathol* 51:281-286, 1981.

Wysocki GP, Goldblatt LI: The so-called "globulomaxillary cyst" is extinct, *Oral Surg Oral Med Oral Pathol* 76:185-186, 1993.

Nasopalatine Duct Cyst

Abrams AM, Howell FV, Bullock WK: Nasopalatine cysts, *Oral Surg Oral Med Oral Pathol* 16:306-332, 1963.

Allard RHB, van der Kwast WAM, van der Waal I: Nasopalatine duct cyst: review of the literature and report of 22 cases, *Int J Oral Surg* 10:447-461, 1981.

Anneroth G, Hall G, Stuge U: Nasopalatine duct cyst, *Int J Oral Maxillofac Surg* 15:572-580, 1986.

Brown FH, Houston GD, Lubow RM et al: Cyst of the incisive (palatine) papilla: report of a case, *J Periodontol* 58:274-275, 1987.

Chapple IL, Ord RA: Patent nasopalatine ducts: four case presentations and review of the literature, *Oral Surg Oral Med Oral Pathol* 69:554-558, 1990.

Hisatomi M, Asaumi J, Konouchi H et al: MR imaging of nasopalatine duct cysts, *Eur J Radiol* 39:73-76, 2001.

Swanson KS, Kaugars GE, Gunsolley JC: Nasopalatine duct cyst: an analysis of 334 cases, *J Oral Maxillofac Surg* 49:268-271, 1991.

Takagi R, Ohashi Y, Suzuki M: Squamous cell carcinoma in the maxilla probably originating from a nasopalatine duct cyst: report of case, *J Oral Maxillofac Surg* 54:112-115, 1996.

Vasconcelos RF, de Aguiar MF, Castro WH et al: Retrospective analysis of 31 cases of nasopalatine duct cyst, *Oral Dis* 5:325-328, 1999.

Median Palatal Cyst

Courage GR, North AF, Hansen LS: Median palatine cysts, *Oral Surg Oral Med Oral Pathol* 37:745-753, 1974.

Donnelly JC, Koudelka BM, Hartwell GR: Median palatal cyst, *J Endod* 12:546-549, 1986.

Gingell JC, Levy BA, DePaola LG: Median palatine cyst, *J Oral Maxillofac Surg* 43:47-51, 1985.

Gordon NC, Swann NP, Hansen LS: Median palatine cyst and maxillary antral osteoma: report of an unusual case, *J Oral Surg* 38:361-365, 1980.

"Median Mandibular Cyst"

Gardner DG: An evaluation of reported cases of median mandibular cysts, *Oral Surg Oral Med Oral Pathol* 65:208-213, 1988.

Soskolne WA, Shteyer A: Median mandibular cyst, *Oral Surg Oral Med Oral Pathol* 44:84-88, 1977.

White DK, Lucas RM, Miller AS: Median mandibular cyst: review of the literature and report of two cases, *J Oral Surg* 33:372-375, 1975.

Epidermoid Cyst

Boatman BW, Headington JT: Epidermoid and tricholemmal cysts. In Demis DJ: *Clinical dermatology*, chapter 4-57, Philadelphia, 1996, Lippincott-Raven.

Golden BA, Zide MF: Cutaneous cysts of the head and neck, *J Oral Maxillofac Surg* 63:1613-1619, 2005.

Kligman AM: The myth of the sebaceous cyst, *Arch Dermatol* 89:253-256, 1964.

López-Ríos F, Rodríguez-Peralto JL, Castaño E et al: Squamous cell carcinoma arising in a cutaneous epidermal cyst, *Am J Dermatopathol* 21:174-177, 1999.

Maize JC, Burgdorf WHC, Hurt MA et al: Follicular cysts. In *Cutaneous pathology*, pp 540-541, Philadelphia, 1998, Churchill Livingstone.

McGavran MH, Binnington B: Keratinous cysts of the skin, *Arch Dermatol* 94:499-508, 1966.

Rajayogeswaran V, Eveson JW: Epidermoid cyst of the buccal mucosa, *Oral Surg Oral Med Oral Pathol* 67:181-184, 1989.

Dermoid Cyst

Arcand P, Granger J, Brochu P: Congenital dermoid cyst of the oral cavity with gastric choristoma, *J Otolaryngol* 17:219-222, 1988.

Crivelini MM, Soubhia AM, Biazolla ÉR et al: Heterotopic gastrointestinal cyst partially lined with dermoid cyst epithelium, *Oral Surg Oral Med Oral Pathol Oral Radiol Endod* 91:686-688, 2001.

Edwards PC, Lustrin L, Valderrama E: Dermoid cysts of the tongue: report of five cases and review of the literature, *Pediatr Dev Pathol* 6:531-535, 2003.

King RC, Smith BR, Burk JL: Dermoid cyst in the floor of the mouth. Review of the literature and case reports, *Oral Surg Oral Med Oral Pathol* 78:567-576, 1994.

Lipsett J, Sparnon AL, Byard RW: Embryogenesis of enterocystomas-enteric duplication cysts of the tongue, *Oral Surg Oral Med Oral Pathol* 75:626-630, 1993.

Meyer I: Dermoid cysts (dermoids) of the floor of the mouth, *Oral Surg Oral Med Oral Pathol* 8:1149-1164, 1955.

Said-Al-Naief N, Fantasia JE, Sciubba JJ et al: Heterotopic oral gastrointestinal cyst. Report of 2 cases and review of the literature, *Oral Surg Oral Med Oral Pathol Oral Radiol Endod* 88:80-86, 1999.

Shigematsu H, Dobashi A, Suzuki S et al: Delayed recurrence of teratoid cyst 17 years after enucleation, *Oral Surg Oral Med Oral Pathol Oral Radiol Endod* 92:539-542, 2001.

Thyroglossal Duct Cyst

Allard RHB: The thyroglossal cyst, *Head Neck Surg* 5:134-146, 1982.

Brousseau VJ, Solares CA, Xu M et al: Thyroglossal duct cysts: presentation and management in children versus adults, *Int J Pediatr Otorhinolaryngol* 67:1285-1290, 2003.

Dedivitis RA, Camargo DL, Peixoto GL et al: Thyroglossal duct: a review of 55 cases, *J Am Coll Surg* 194:274-277, 2002.

Fernandez JF, Ordoñez NG, Schultz NA et al: Thyroglossal duct carcinoma, *Surgery* 110:928-935, 1991.

Katz AD, Hachigian M: Thyroglossal duct cysts: a thirty-year experience with emphasis on occurrence in older patients, *Am J Surg* 155:741-744, 1988.

Kuint J, Horowitz Z, Kugel C et al: Laryngeal obstruction caused by lingual thyroglossal duct cyst presenting at birth, *Am J Perinatol* 14:353-356, 1997.

Patel SG, Escrig M, Shaha AR et al: Management of well-differentiated thyroid carcinoma presenting within a thyroglossal duct cyst, *J Surg Oncol* 79:134-139, 2002.

Plaza CP, López ME, Carrasco CE et al: Management of well-differentiated thyroglossal remnant thyroid carcinoma: time to close the debate? Report of five new cases and proposal of a definitive algorithm for treatment, *Ann Surg Oncol* 13:745-752, 2006.

Schader I, Robertson S, Maoate K et al: Hereditary thyroglossal duct cysts, *Pediatr Surg Int* 21:593-594, 2005.

Branchial Cleft Cyst

Bhaskar SN, Bernier JL: Histogenesis of branchial cysts: a report of 468 cases, *Am J Pathol* 35:407-423, 1959.

Elliott JN, Oertel YC: Lymphoepithelial cysts of the salivary glands, *Am J Clin Pathol* 93:39-43, 1990.

Foss RD, Warnock GR, Clark WB et al: Malignant cyst of the lateral aspect of the neck: branchial cleft carcinoma or metastasis? *Oral Surg Oral Med Oral Pathol* 71:214-217, 1991.

Goldenberg D, Sciubba J, Koch WM: Cystic metastasis from head and neck squamous cell cancer: a distinct disease variant? *Head Neck* 28:633-638, 2006.

Kadhim AL, Sheahan P, Colreavy MP et al: Pearls and pitfalls in the management of branchial cyst, *J Laryngol Otol* 118:946-950, 2004.

Little JW, Rickles NH: The histogenesis of the branchial cyst, *Am J Pathol* 50:533-547, 1967.

Mandel L, Reich R: HIV parotid gland lymphoepithelial cysts: review and case reports, *Oral Surg Oral Med Oral Pathol* 74:273-278, 1992.

Regauer S, Gogg-Kamerer M, Braun H et al: Lateral neck cysts–the branchial theory revisited, *APMIS* 105:623-630, 1997.

Skouteris CA, Patterson GT, Sotereanos GC: Benign cervical lymphoepithelial cyst: report of cases, *J Oral Maxillofac Surg* 47:1106-1112, 1989.

Thompson LD, Heffner DK: The clinical importance of cystic squamous cell carcinomas in the neck: a study of 136 cases, *Cancer* 82:944-956, 1998.

Oral Lymphoepithelial Cyst

Bhaskar SN: Lymphoepithelial cysts of the oral cavity: report of twenty-four cases, *Oral Surg Oral Med Oral Pathol* 21:120-128, 1966.

Buchner A, Hansen LS: Lymphoepithelial cysts of the oral cavity, *Oral Surg Oral Med Oral Pathol* 50:441-449, 1980.

Chaudhry AP, Yamane GM, Scharlock SE et al: A clinico-pathological study of intraoral lymphoepithelial cysts, *J Oral Med* 39:79-84, 1984.

Giunta J, Cataldo E: Lymphoepithelial cysts of the oral mucosa, *Oral Surg Oral Med Oral Pathol* 35:77-84, 1973.

Hemihyperplasia

Ballock RT, Wiesner GL, Myers MT et al: Hemihypertrophy. Concepts and controversies, *J Bone Joint Surg* 79:1731-1738, 1997.

Bell RA, McTigue DJ: Complex congenital hemihypertrophy: a case report and literature review, *J Pedod* 8:300-313, 1984.

Dalal AB, Phadke SR, Pradhan M et al: Hemihyperplasia syndromes, *Indian J Pediatr* 73:609-615, 2006.

Elliott M, Bayly R, Cole T et al: Clinical features and natural history of Beckwith-Wiedemann syndrome: presentation of 74 new cases, *Clin Genet* 46:168-174, 1994.

Gorlin RJ, Cohen MM Jr, Hennekam RCM: Hemihyperplasia (hemihypertrophy). In *Syndromes of the head and neck*, ed 4, pp 405-408, New York, 2001, Oxford University Press.

Horswell BB, Holmes AD, Barnett JS et al: Primary hemihypertrophy of the face: review and report of two cases, *J Oral Maxillofac Surg* 45:217-222, 1987.

Hoyme HE, Seaver LH, Jones KL et al: Isolated hemihyperplasia (hemihypertrophy): report of a prospective multicenter study of the incidence of neoplasia and review, *Am J Med Genet* 79:274-278, 1998.

Progressive Hemifacial Atrophy

Abele DC, Bedingfield RB, Chandler FW et al: Progressive facial hemiatrophy (Parry-Romberg syndrome) and borreliosis, *J Am Acad Dermatol* 22:531-533, 1990.

Blaszczyk M, Królicki L, Krasu M et al: Progressive facial hemiatrophy: central nervous system involvement and relationship with scleroderma en coup de sabre, *J Rheumatol* 30:1997-2004, 2003.

Fayad S, Steffensen B: Root resorptions in a patient with hemifacial atrophy, *J Endod* 20:299-303, 1994.

Foster TD: The effects of hemifacial atrophy on dental growth, *Br Dent J* 146:148-150, 1979.

Iñigo F, Rojo P, Ysunza A: Aesthetic treatment of Romberg's disease: experience with 35 cases, *Br J Plast Surg* 46:194-200, 1993.

Orozco-Covarrubias L, Guzmán-Meza A, Ridaura-Sanz C et al: Scleroderma "en coup de sabre" and progressive facial hemiatrophy. Is it possible to differentiate them? *J Eur Acad Dermatol Venereol* 16:361-366, 2002.

Pensler JM, Murphy GF, Mulliken JB: Clinical and ultrastructural studies of Romberg's hemifacial atrophy, *Plast Reconstr Surg* 85:669-674, 1990.

Roddi R, Riggio E, Gilbert PM et al: Clinical evaluation of techniques used in the surgical treatment of progressive hemifacial atrophy, *J Craniomaxillofac Surg* 22:23-32, 1994.

Sommer A, Gambichler T, Bacharach-Buhles M et al: Clinical and serological characteristics of progressive facial hemiatrophy: a case series of 12 patients, *J Am Acad Dermatol* 54:227-223, 2006.

Segmental Odontomaxillary Dysplasia

Armstrong C, Napier SS, Boyd RC et al: Histopathology of the teeth in segmental odontomaxillary dysplasia: new findings, *J Oral Pathol Med* 33:246-248, 2004.

Becktor KB, Reibel J, Vedel B et al: Segmental odontomaxillary dysplasia: clinical, radiological and histological aspects of four cases, *Oral Dis* 8:106-110, 2002.

Danforth RA, Melrose RJ, Abrams AM, et al: Segmental odontomaxillary dysplasia. Report of eight cases and comparison with hemimaxillofacial dysplasia, *Oral Surg Oral Med Oral Pathol* 70:81-85, 1990.

Jones AC, Ford MJ: Simultaneous occurrence of segmental odontomaxillary dysplasia and Becker's nevus, *J Oral Maxillofac Surg* 57:1251-1254, 1999.

Miles DA, Lovas JL, Cohen MM Jr: Hemimaxillofacial dysplasia: a newly recognized disorder of facial asymmetry, hypertrichosis of the facial skin, unilateral enlargement of the maxilla, and hypoplastic teeth in two patients, *Oral Surg Oral Med Oral Pathol* 64:445-448, 1987.

Packota GV, Pharoah MJ, Petrikowski CG: Radiographic features of segmental odontomaxillary dysplasia. A study of 12 cases, *Oral Surg Oral Med Oral Pathol Oral Radiol Endod* 82:577-584, 1996.

Paticoff K, Marion RW, Shprintzen RJ et al: Hemimaxillofacial dysplasia. A report of two new cases and further delineation of the disorder, *Oral Surg Oral Med Oral Pathol Oral Radiol Endod* 83:484-488, 1997.

Crouzon Syndrome

David DJ, Sheen R: Surgical correction of Crouzon syndrome, *Plast Reconstr Surg* 85:344-354, 1990.

Gorlin RJ, Cohen MM Jr, Hennekam RCM: Crouzon syndrome (craniofacial dysostosis). In *Syndromes of the head and neck*, ed 4, pp 658-659, New York, 2001, Oxford University Press.

Katzen JT, McCarthy JG: Syndromes involving craniosynostosis and midface hypoplasia, *Otolaryngol Clin North Am* 33:1257-1284, 2000.

Kreiborg S: Crouzon syndrome, *Scand J Plast Reconstr Surg Suppl* 18:1-198, 1981.

Mulliken JB, Steinberger D, Kunze S et al: Molecular diagnosis of bilateral coronal synostosis, *Plast Reconstr Surg* 104:1603-1615, 1999.

Posnick JC: The craniofacial dysostosis syndromes. Staging of reconstruction and management of secondary deformities, *Clin Plast Surg* 24:429-446, 1997.

Singer SL, Walpole I, Brogan WF et al: Dentofacial features of a family with Crouzon syndrome. Case reports, *Aust Dent J* 42:11-17, 1997.

Apert Syndrome

Cohen MM Jr, Kreiborg S: A clinical study of the craniofacial features in Apert syndrome, *Int J Oral Maxillofac Surg* 25:45-53, 1996.

Ferraro NF: Dental, orthodontic, and oral/maxillofacial evaluation and treatment in Apert syndrome, *Clin Plast Surg* 18:291-307, 1991.

Gorlin RJ, Cohen MM Jr, Hennekam RCM: Apert syndrome (acrocephalosyndactyly). In *Syndromes of the head and neck*, ed 4, pp 654-658, New York, 2001, Oxford University Press.

Ibrahimi OA, Chiu ES, McCarthy JG et al: Understanding the molecular basis of Apert syndrome, *Plast Reconstr Surg* 115:264-270, 2005.

Katzen JT, McCarthy JG: Syndromes involving craniosynostosis and midface hypoplasia, *Otolaryngol Clin North Am* 33:1257-1284, 2000.

Kreiborg S, Cohen MM Jr: The oral manifestations of Apert syndrome, *J Craniofac Genet Dev Biol* 12:41-48, 1992.

Marsh JL, Galic M, Vannier MW: Surgical correction of the craniofacial dysmorphology of Apert syndrome, *Clin Plast Surg* 18:251-275, 1991.

Mulliken JB, Steinberger D, Kunze S et al: Molecular diagnosis of bilateral coronal synostosis, *Plast Reconstr Surg* 104:1603-1615, 1999.

Mandibulofacial Dysostosis

Fuente del Campo A, Martinez Elizondo M, Arnaud E: Treacher Collins syndrome (mandibulofacial dysostosis), *Clin Plast Surg* 21:613-623, 1994.

Gorlin RJ, Cohen MM Jr, Hennekam RCM: Mandibulofacial dysostosis (Treacher Collins syndrome, Franceschetti-Zwahlen-Klein syndrome). In *Syndromes of the head and neck*, ed 4, pp 799-802, New York, 2001, Oxford University Press.

Marszalek B, Wójcicki P, Kobus K et al: Clinical features, treatment and genetic background of Treacher Collins syndrome, *J Appl Genet* 43:223-233, 2002.

Posnick JC: Treacher Collins syndrome: perspectives in evaluation and treatment, *J Oral Maxillofac Surg* 55:1120-1133, 1997.

Posnick JC, Ruiz RL: Treacher Collins syndrome: current evaluation, treatment, and future directions, *Cleft Palate Craniofac J* 37:434, 2000.

2

Abnormalities of Teeth

CHAPTER OUTLINE

Environmental Alterations of Teeth

The abnormalities of the teeth can be divided into those that are influenced by environmental forces and those that are idiopathic and appear hereditary in nature. Later parts of this chapter delineate the idiopathic and hereditary alterations of teeth. Box 2-1 lists the major categories of tooth alteration that can be affected by environmental influences. In many cases the cause and effect are obvious; in others the primary nature of the problem is less distinct.

Box 2-1

Environmental Alterations of Teeth

- Developmental tooth defects
- Postdevelopmental structure loss
- Discolorations of teeth
- Localized disturbances in eruption

Box 2-2

Factors Associated with Enamel Defects

SYSTEMIC

- Birth-related trauma: Breech presentations, hypoxia, multiple births, premature birth, prolonged labor
- Chemicals: Antineoplastic chemotherapy, fluoride, lead, tetracycline, thalidomide, vitamin D
- Chromosomal abnormalities: Trisomy 21
- Infections: Chicken pox, cytomegalovirus (CMV), gastrointestinal infections, measles, pneumonia, respiratory infections, rubella, syphilis, tetanus
- Inherited diseases: Amelo-cerebro-hypohidrotic syndrome, amelo-onycho-hypohidrotic syndrome, epidermolysis bullosa, galactosemia, mucopolysaccharidosis IV, Nance-Horan syndrome, oculo-dento-osseous dysplasia, phenylketonuria, pseudohypoparathyroidism, tricho-dento-osseous syndrome, tuberous sclerosis, vitamin D-dependent rickets
- Malnutrition: Generalized malnutrition, vitamin-D deficiency, vitamin-A deficiency
- Metabolic disorders: Cardiac disease, celiac disease, gastrointestinal malabsorption, gastrointestinal lymphangiectasia, hepatobillary disease, hyperbilirubinemia, hypocalcemia, hypothyroidism, hypoparathyroidism, maternal diabetes, renal disease, toxemia of pregnancy
- Neurologic disorders: Cerebral palsy, mental retardation, sensorineural hearing defects

LOCAL

- Local acute mechanical trauma: Falls, gunshots, neonatal mechanical ventilation, ritual mutilation, surgery, vehicular accidents
- Electrical burn
- Irradiation
- Local infection: Acute neonatal maxillitis, periapical inflammatory disease

ENVIRONMENTAL EFFECTS ON TOOTH STRUCTURE DEVELOPMENT

The ameloblasts in the developing tooth germ are extremely sensitive to external stimuli, and many factors can result in abnormalities in the enamel (Box 2-2). The primary hereditary abnormalities of the enamel that are unrelated to other disorders are termed **amelogenesis imperfecta** (see page 99).

Dental enamel is unique in that remodeling does not occur after initial formation. Therefore, abnormalities in enamel formation are etched permanently on the tooth surface. The enamel develops in three major stages: (1) **matrix formation,** (2) **mineralization,** and (3) **maturation.** During matrix formation, the enamel proteins are laid down. In the next phase, minerals are deposited and the majority of the original proteins are removed. During the final maturation period, the enamel undergoes final mineralization and the remnants of the original proteins are removed. In the early stage of mineralization, the enamel is dull, white, and relatively soft. During the late stage of maturation, the final hard translucent enamel replaces this diffuse opaque enamel.

The timing of the ameloblastic damage has a great effect on the location and appearance of the defect in the enamel. The cause of the damage does not appear to be of major importance, because many different local and systemic stimuli can result in defects that have similar clinical appearances. The final enamel represents a record of all significant insults received during tooth development. Deciduous enamel contains a neonatal ring, and the rate of enamel apposition is estimated to be 0.023 mm/day. Using this knowledge, the clinician can accurately estimate the timing of an insult to the deciduous teeth to within 1 week. In the permanent dentition, the position of the enamel defects provides a rough estimate of the time of damage; however, available data on the chronology of tooth development are derived from a relatively small sample size, and the ranges of normal values are wide. In addition, gender and racial variations are not established thoroughly.

CLINICAL AND RADIOGRAPHIC FEATURES

Almost all visible environmental enamel defects can be classified into one of three patterns:

1. Hypoplasia
2. Diffuse opacities
3. Demarcated opacities

Subtle enamel defects can be masked by saliva, plaque, or poor illumination. When attempting to detect areas of altered enamel, the dentition should be cleaned thoroughly; then it should be dried with gauze. Dental operatory lights are an ideal light source (direct sunlight should be avoided). Plaque-disclosing solution can be used to highlight small defects. The altered enamel may be localized or present on numerous teeth,

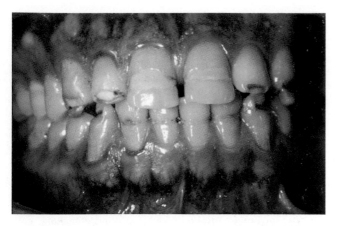

Fig. 2-1 Environmental enamel hypoplasia. Bilaterally symmetrical pattern of horizontal enamel hypoplasia of the anterior dentition. Maxillary central incisors have been restored previously. *(From Neville BW, Damm DD, White DK: Color atlas of clinical oral pathology, ed 2, Hamilton, 1999, BC Decker.)*

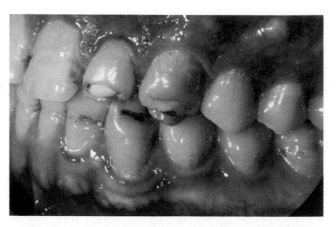

Fig. 2-2 Environmental enamel hypoplasia. Same patient as depicted in Fig. 2-1. Note the lack of enamel damage on bicuspids. *(From Neville BW, Damm DD, White DK: Color atlas of clinical oral pathology, ed 2, Hamilton, 1999, BC Decker.)*

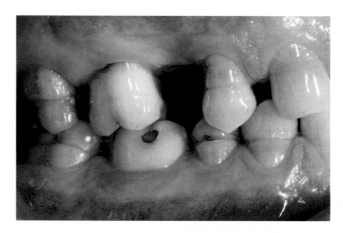

Fig. 2-3 Environmental enamel hypoplasia. Horizontal enamel hypoplasia of the bicuspids and second molars. Note sparing of the first molars. *(From Neville BW, Damm DD, White DK: Color atlas of clinical oral pathology, ed 2, Hamilton, 1999, BC Decker.)*

and all or part of the surfaces of each affected tooth may be involved. **Enamel hypoplasia** occurs in the form of pits, grooves, or larger areas of missing enamel. **Diffuse opacities of enamel** appear as variations in the translucency of the enamel. The affected enamel is of normal thickness; however, it has an increased white opacity with no clear boundary with the adjacent normal enamel. **Demarcated opacities** of enamel show areas of decreased translucence, increased opacity, and a sharp boundary with the adjacent enamel. The enamel is of normal thickness, and the affected opacity may be white, cream, yellow, or brown.

The crowns of the deciduous dentition begin to develop at approximately the fourteenth week of gestation and continue until the child is 12 months of age. Development of the crowns of the permanent dentition occurs from approximately 6 months to 15 years of age. The site of coronal damage correlates with the area of ameloblastic activity at the time of the injury; the affected enamel is restricted to the areas in which secretory activity or active maturation of the enamel matrix was occurring.

Environmental enamel abnormalities are extremely common. In a review of more than 1500 children from 12 to 15 years of age in an industrialized nation, the prevalence of enamel defects in the permanent dentition was 68.4%. Within this group, 67.2% demonstrated opacities, 14.6% revealed hypoplasia, and both patterns were seen in 13.4% of the children. The average number of affected teeth per individual was 3.6, with greater than 10% of the children having 10 or more teeth involved.

A common pattern is seen as a result of systemic influences, such as exanthematous fevers, that occur during the first 2 years of life. Horizontal rows of pits or diminished enamel are present on the anterior teeth and first molars (Figs. 2-1 and 2-2). The enamel loss is

bilaterally symmetric, and the location of the defects correlates well with the developmental stage of the affected teeth. A similar pattern of enamel defects can be seen in the cuspids, bicuspids, and second molars when the inciting event occurs around the age of 4 to 5 years (Fig. 2-3).

TURNER'S HYPOPLASIA

Another frequent pattern of enamel defects seen in permanent teeth is caused by periapical inflammatory disease of the overlying deciduous tooth. The altered tooth is called a **Turner's tooth** (after the clinician whose publications allowed this problem to be widely recognized). The appearance of the affected area varies according to the timing and severity of the insult. The enamel defects vary from focal areas of white, yellow, or brown discoloration to extensive hypoplasia, which can involve the entire crown. The process is noted most frequently in the permanent bicuspids because of their

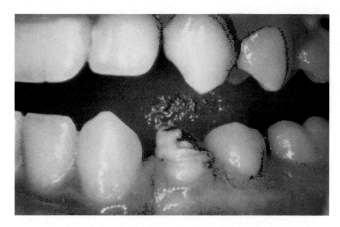

Fig. 2-4   Turner's hypoplasia. Extensive enamel hypoplasia of mandibular first bicuspid secondary to previous inflammatory process associated with overlying first deciduous molar. *(From Halstead CL, Blozis GG, Drinnan AJ et al: Physical evaluation of the dental patient, St Louis, 1982, Mosby.)*

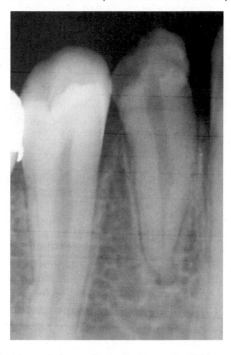

Fig. 2-5   Turner's hypoplasia. Radiograph of the same tooth depicted in Fig. 2-4. Note the lack of significant enamel and irregularity of the dentin surface. *(From Halstead CL, Blozis GG, Drinnan AJ et al: Physical evaluation of the dental patient, St Louis, 1982, Mosby.)*

relationship to the overlying deciduous molars (Figs. 2-4 and 2-5). Anterior teeth are involved less frequently because crown formation is usually complete before the development of any apical inflammatory disease in the relatively caries-resistant anterior deciduous dentition. Factors that determine the degree of damage to the permanent tooth by the overlying infection include the stage of tooth development, length of time the infection remains untreated, the virulence of the infective organisms, and the host resistance to the infection.

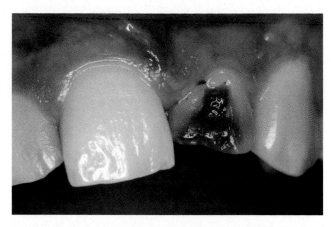

Fig. 2-6   Turner's hypoplasia. Extensive coronal hypoplasia of permanent maxillary left central incisor secondary to previous trauma to deciduous central incisor.

In addition to classic Turner's teeth, an increased prevalence of demarcated opacities has been reported in the permanent successors of carious primary teeth. In one report, if the primary tooth developed caries, the successor was twice as likely to demonstrate a circumscribed enamel defect. In addition, if the primary tooth was extracted for any reason other than trauma, then the prevalence of a demarcated enamel defect increased fivefold.

Traumatic injury to deciduous teeth also can cause significant alterations of the underlying dentition and the formation of Turner's teeth. This is not a rare occurrence; up to 45% of all children sustain injuries to their primary teeth. In a prospective study of 114 children with 255 traumatized primary teeth, 23% of the corresponding permanent teeth demonstrated developmental disturbances. The maxillary central incisors are affected in the majority of the cases; the maxillary lateral incisors are altered less frequently (Fig. 2-6). In several large reviews, the prevalence of involvement of the posterior teeth or mandibular incisors was less than 10% of all cases.

The frequency of traumatic damage of the anterior maxillary dentition is not surprising, considering the common occurrence of trauma to the deciduous dentition of the prominent anterior maxilla and the close anatomic relationship between the developing tooth bud and the apices of the overlying primary incisors. As would be expected, the clinical appearance of the alteration varies according to the timing and severity of the damage.

Because of the position of the primary apices relative to the tooth bud, the facial surface of the maxillary incisors is the location most frequently affected. Typically, the affected area appears as a zone of white or yellowish-brown discoloration with or without an area of horizontal enamel hypoplasia. The trauma also can cause displacement of the already formed hard-tooth substance in relation to the soft tissue of the remaining developing tooth. This results in a bend of the tooth known as **dilaceration** and can affect either the crown or the root of a tooth (see page 97). Severe trauma early in the development of the tooth can result in such disorganization of the bud that the resultant product may resemble a complex odontoma (see page 724). Similar levels of damage late in the formative process can lead to partial or total arrest in root formation.

MOLAR INCISOR HYPOMINERALIZATION

Over the last two to three decades, a number of publications have described a unique pattern of defective enamel that has been recognized most frequently in Northern Europe, although the pathosis is not limited to that geographic region. In the past this disorder most likely went undiagnosed because of the high prevalence of caries, but with the dramatic reduction in caries, these tooth changes have become more recognized.

Patients affected with **molar incisor hypomineralization** have enamel defects of one or more first permanent molars. The altered enamel may be white, yellow, or brown, with a sharp demarcation between the defective and surrounding normal enamel. Often, the involved enamel is soft and porous with a resemblance to discolored chalk or old Dutch cheese ("cheese molars"). Frequently, the incisors also are affected, but the defects generally are much less severe.

The enamel of the affected molars is very fragile and can chip easily. Often, affected molars are sensitive to cold, warm, or mechanical trauma. Toothbrushing is frequently painful, with a tendency for the children to avoid brushing these teeth. As would be expected, the lack of normal enamel and absence of appropriate hygiene lead to rapid development of caries. During attempts at dental therapy, these teeth often are highly sensitive and very difficult to anesthetize.

The cause of molar incisor hypomineralization is unknown, but many investigators believe the condition arises from a systemic influence during the first years of life, coinciding with the period of mineralization of the affected dentition. A number of prevalence studies have been performed with the results ranging from 3.6% to 25%.

HYPOPLASIA CAUSED BY ANTINEOPLASTIC THERAPY

As modern medicine increases the prevalence of successful therapy against childhood cancer, it has become evident that a number of developmental alterations arise secondary to use of therapeutic radiation or chemotherapy. As would be expected, developing teeth are affected most severely, with these therapies producing clinically obvious alterations most commonly in patients younger than 12 years and most extensively

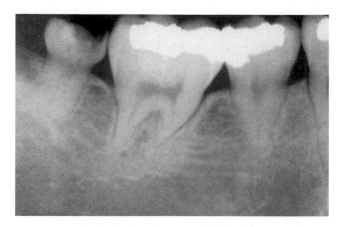

Fig. 2-7 Hypoplasia caused by antineoplastic therapy. Developmental radicular hypoplasia and microdontia caused by radiation therapy. *(From Neville BW, Damm DD, White DK: Color atlas of clinical oral pathology, ed 2, Hamilton, 1999, BC Decker.)*

in those younger than 5 years. The degree and severity of the developmental alterations are related to the patient's age at treatment, the form of therapy, and the dose and field of radiation, if used.

Although both chemotherapeutic agents and radiation therapy can be responsible for developmental abnormalities, the most severe alterations are associated with radiation. Doses as low as 0.72 Gy are associated with mild developmental defects in both enamel and dentin. As the dose escalates, so does the effect on the developing dentition and jaws. Frequently noted alterations include hypodontia, microdontia, radicular hypoplasia, and enamel hypoplasia (Fig. 2-7). In addition, mandibular hypoplasia and a reduction of the vertical development of the lower third of the face are not rare. The mandibular hypoplasia may be the direct effect of the radiation, reduced alveolar bone growth secondary to impaired root development, or (possibly) growth failure related to altered pituitary function caused by cranial radiation. Chemotherapy alone results in much less dramatic alterations but can produce an increased number of enamel hypoplasias and discolorations, slightly smaller tooth size, and occasional radicular hypoplasia that is less severe than that secondary to radiation.

DENTAL FLUOROSIS

The ingestion of excess amounts of fluoride also can result in significant enamel defects known as **dental fluorosis**. In 1901, Dr. Frederick S. McKay suggested the association between this altered enamel and an agent in the Colorado Springs, Colorado, water supply during investigation of the *Colorado brown stain* seen in the teeth of many of his patients. In 1909, Dr. F.L. Robertson noted a similar association in many of his patients in Bauxite, Arkansas (the home of bauxite mines for aluminum). In 1930, H.V. Churchill, a chemist in Bauxite who was employed by the Aluminum Company of America, discovered high concentrations of fluoride (13.7 ppm) in the water and contacted McKay for samples of the water in affected areas of Colorado. McKay's samples also demonstrated high levels of fluoride, and the final part of the puzzle was solved.

Although the fluoride produced an unusual and permanent dental stain, a resistance to caries also was noted. In 1931 the National Institutes of Health hired Dr. H. Trendley Dean to investigate the association between fluoride, the presence of dental fluorosis, and the prevalence of caries among children. Ultimately this led to the first water fluoridation clinical trial in Grand Rapids, Michigan. Because of the efforts of these pioneers and the simultaneous work of many others, it was discovered that fluoride in the water at 1.0 ppm reduced caries by 50% to 70%. Since 1962 fluoridation of drinking water is recommended, with the optimum range being 0.7 to 1.2 ppm. The lower concentration is recommended for warmer climates in which water consumption is thought to be higher, but this distinction has been questioned because of an evolving indoor lifestyle and the use of modern air-conditioning. In 1999 the United States Centers for Disease Control and Prevention designated fluoridation of drinking water as one of the ten great public health achievements of the twentieth century in the United States.

Initially, fluoride's ability to reduce caries was thought to be secondary to its incorporation into developing enamel, resulting in a stronger and more acid-resistant fluorapatite crystal. A number of more recent studies have suggested that the posteruptive effects of fluoride may be of equal or even greater importance. Researchers believe that continued exposure to topical fluoride contained in products such as toothpaste or fluoridated water inhibits demineralization, enhances remineralization, and exhibits antibacterial effects. In addition, they have suggested that preeruptive fluoride is most effective against pit and fissure caries, whereas smooth surface caries is affected most significantly by posteruptive exposure.

Consumption of optimally fluoridated water has been associated with a low prevalence of altered enamel, which usually is mild in degree. However, an increased prevalence of dental fluorosis has been noted in recent years. In addition, the relative caries reduction in fluoridated communities has improved between 8% and 37%. This has been attributed to the diffusion of fluoride to nonfluoridated areas through bottling and processing of foods and beverages with fluoridated water, as well as to the widespread use of fluoride toothpaste. Adult-strength fluoride toothpastes, fluoride supplements, infant foods, soft drinks, fruit juices, and industrial environmental emissions all represent potential sources of fluoride for children in their formative years. Infant formulas also used to contain significant amounts of fluoride; however, in 1979, U.S. manufacturers voluntarily agreed to dramatically limit fluoride in infant formulas. Despite this, some investigators have noted an increased prevalence of fluorosis continuing after 1979 in individuals who consumed powdered, concentrated formula that was reconstituted with optimally fluoridated water. To minimize the chance of fluorosis, the use of ready-to-feed formula or reconstitution with low-fluoride bottled water has been recommended.

Because of this dissemination of fluoride, the need for supplements in nonfluoridated areas is declining. In patients who use fluoride toothpastes, the anticariogenic benefit of supplements is very small or nonexistent and the risk of fluorosis at the community level becomes a certainty. Several investigators have recommended strongly that children younger than 7 years of age apply only a pea-sized amount of fluoride toothpaste on the toothbrush and avoid swallowing. Because young children tend to swallow almost all toothpaste placed on their brush, parents should be warned to avoid fluoridated toothpaste in children younger than 2 years of age and perform oral hygiene with only a toothbrush and water. In addition, fluoride supplements are recommended only in nonfluoridated areas for children who are at high risk for rampant caries. Finally, an effort is under way to alter the 1962 recommendation and lower the optimum level of fluoride in the public water supply to 0.7 ppm.

Fluoride appears to create its significant enamel defects through retention of the amelogenin proteins in the enamel structure, leading to the formation of hypomineralized enamel. These alterations create a permanent hypomaturation of the enamel in which an increased surface and subsurface porosity of the enamel is observed. This enamel structure alters the light reflection and creates the appearance of white, chalky areas. Most of the problems associated with dental fluorosis are aesthetic and concern the appearance of the anterior teeth. Therefore, the critical period for clinically significant dental fluorosis is during the second and third years of life, when these teeth are forming.

The severity of dental fluorosis is dose dependent, with higher intakes of fluoride during critical periods of tooth development being associated with more severe fluorosis. The affected teeth are caries resistant, and the altered tooth structure appears as areas of lusterless white opaque enamel that may have zones of yellow to dark-brown discoloration (Figs. 2-8 and 2-9). In the past, areas of moderate-to-severe enamel fluorosis were termed **mottled enamel.** True enamel hypoplasia is uncommon but can occur as deep, irregular, and brownish pits. Because other factors can result in

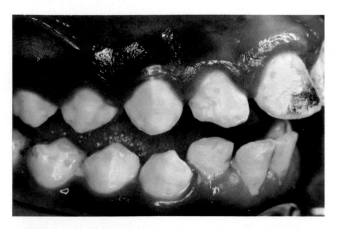

Fig. 2-8 Dental fluorosis. Dentition exhibiting lusterless, white, and opaque enamel.

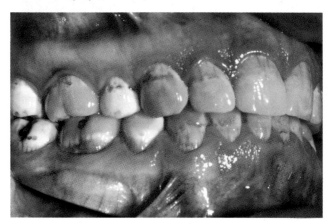

Fig. 2-9 Dental fluorosis. White opaque alteration of the bicuspids and second molars in a patient who also exhibits discoloration of the teeth secondary to tetracycline use. Patient moved to area of endemic fluorosis at 3 years of age.

a similar pattern of enamel damage, a definitive diagnosis requires that the defects be present in a bilaterally symmetric distribution, and evidence of prior excessive fluoride intake or elevated levels of fluoride in the enamel or other tissues should be found.

Recently, an increased prevalence of dental changes similar to dental fluorosis has been linked to amoxicillin use during early infancy. Commonly affected teeth include the permanent first molars and maxillary central incisors. The number of affected teeth appears to correlate with the duration of use. Although the mechanism of this alteration is unclear, the antibiotic may reduce gene expression of selected matrix proteins or reduce the activity of proteinases that hydrolyze matrix proteins. It also should be noted that one of the etiologic theories suggested for molar incisor hypomineralization (see page 58) is prior antibiotic therapy.

SYPHILITIC HYPOPLASIA

Congenital syphilis (see page 190) results in a pattern of enamel hypoplasia that is well known but currently so rare that lengthy discussion is not warranted. Anterior teeth altered by syphilis are termed **Hutchinson's incisors** and exhibit crowns that are shaped like straight-edge screwdrivers, with the greatest circumference present in the middle one third of the crown and a constricted incisal edge. The middle portion of the incisal edge often demonstrates a central hypoplastic notch. Altered posterior teeth are termed **mulberry molars** and demonstrate constricted occlusal tables with a disorganized surface anatomy that resembles the bumpy surface of a mulberry.

TREATMENT AND PROGNOSIS

Most defects in the enamel are cosmetic rather than functional dental problems. Those affected by dental fluorosis often benefit from surface microabrasion, which produces a dramatic and permanent improvement in the surface brown or yellow discoloration. Improvement in the white surface markings usually requires further restorative dentistry. Other types of environmental enamel hypoplasia have been associated with an increased prevalence of caries, with one study reporting more than twice the level in patients with such enamel defects. The decreased caries resistance is thought to be secondary to focal loss of enamel or because of imperfect enamel. The areas most frequently associated with an increased prevalence of caries demonstrate full-thickness enamel defects. Aesthetically or functionally defective teeth can be restored through a variety of cosmetically pleasing techniques, such as the following:
- Acid-etched composite resin restorations
- Labial veneers
- Full crowns

POSTDEVELOPMENTAL LOSS OF TOOTH STRUCTURE

Tooth structure can be lost after its formation by a variety of influences beyond the obvious cases related to caries or traumatic fractures. Destruction can begin on the enamel surface of the crown through abrasion, attrition, erosion, or abfraction. In addition, loss of tooth structure can begin on the dentin or cemental surfaces of the teeth by external or internal resorption.

TOOTH WEAR

Tooth wear, also termed *tooth surface loss,* is a normal physiologic process that occurs with aging but must be considered pathologic when the degree of destruction creates functional, aesthetic, or dental sensitivity problems. Although the four causes of tooth wear (i.e., **attrition, abrasion, erosion, abfraction**), often are discussed as independent pathoses, most of these types of tooth loss are the result of a combination of influences. Many cases of attrition are accelerated by the presence of abrasive materials in the mouth. Erosion or abrasion often further damages areas of dentin exposed by attrition or abfraction. Areas softened by erosion are more susceptible to attrition, abrasion, and abfraction. The clinician should appreciate that acquired environmental loss of tooth structure often is multifactorial.

Most researchers agree that the reported prevalence of tooth wear is increasing. This is explained partly by a greater awareness among clinicians and by the adult population retaining more natural teeth as they age. In addition, younger individuals appear to exhibit an increased tooth surface loss that many believe may be caused by a more acidic diet (e.g., acidic soft drinks, diet foods, fresh fruits).

Attrition is the loss of tooth structure caused by tooth-to-tooth contact during occlusion and mastication. The term comes from the Latin verb *attritum*, which refers to the action of rubbing against another surface. Some degree of attrition is physiologic, and the process becomes more noticeable with age. When the amount of tooth loss is extensive and begins to affect aesthetic appearance and function, the process must be considered pathologic.

The following factors can accelerate tooth destruction:
- Poor-quality or absent enamel (e.g., fluorosis, environmental or hereditary enamel hypoplasia, or dentinogenesis imperfecta)
- Premature contacts (edge-to-edge occlusion)
- Intraoral abrasives, erosion, and grinding habits

Abrasion is the pathologic wearing away of tooth structure or restoration secondary to the mechanical action of an external agent. The term arises from the Latin verb *abrasum*, which literally means *to scrape off* and implies wear or partial removal through a mechanical process. The most common cause of abrasion is toothbrushing that combines abrasive toothpaste with heavy pressure and a horizontal brushing stroke. Other items frequently associated with dental abrasion include pencils, toothpicks, pipe stems, and bobby pins (hair grips). Chewing tobacco, cracking nuts and seeds, biting fingernails or thread, and using dental floss inappropriately also can cause clinically significant abrasion. When tooth wear is accelerated by chewing an abrasive substance between opposing teeth, the process has been termed **demastication** and exhibits features of both attrition and abrasion.

Erosion is the loss of tooth structure caused by a nonbacterial chemical process. The term is derived from the Latin verb *erosum*, which literally means *to corrode* and implies gradual destruction of a surface by a chemical or electrolytic process. Some investigators have suggested that the term *dental corrosion* would be a more appropriate designation for this process, but review of modern dictionaries reveals both terms are acceptable, with little need for a disruption in the long-held nomenclature of tooth wear. Typically, the exposure to an acid is to blame, but chelating agents are occasionally the primary cause. Although saliva aids remineralization and contains bicarbonate with a significant buffering ability, this effect can be overwhelmed by xerostomia or excess acid. Causes for salivary gland hypofunction include salivary gland aplasia, dehydration, therapeutic radiation, medications and systemic conditions such as Sjögren syndrome, bulimia nervosa, and diabetes. The acidic source often is foods or drinks, but other causes include some medications (e.g., chewable vitamin C, aspirin tablets), swimming pools with poorly monitored pH, chronic involuntary regurgitation (e.g., hiatal hernia, esophagitis, chronic alcoholism, pregnancy), voluntary regurgitation (e.g., psychologic problems, bulimia, occupations that require low body weight), and industrial environmental exposure. Erosion from dental exposure to gastric secretions is termed **perimolysis**. Because saliva has the ability to remineralize tooth surfaces exposed to acid, it appears that areas of erosive damage must have some abrasive component that removes the softened enamel before remineralization.

Agreement on the prevalence of dental erosion does not exist. Some investigators believe erosion rarely is responsible solely for loss of tooth structure, although others list erosion as the leading cause of accelerated tooth wear.

Abfraction refers to the loss of tooth structure from occlusal stresses that create repeated tooth flexure with failure of enamel and dentin at a location away from the point of loading. The term is derived from the Latin words *ab* and *fractio*, which respectively translate into *away* and *breaking*. Dentin is able to withstand greater tensile stress than enamel. When occlusal forces are applied eccentrically to a tooth, the tensile stress is concentrated at the cervical fulcrum, leading to flexure that may produce disruption in the chemical bonds of the enamel crystals in the cervical areas. Once damaged, the cracked enamel can be lost or more easily removed by erosion or abrasion. Some investigators have suggested that the placement of occlusal restorations weakens the tooth's ability to resist the stresses of occlusion and predisposes to future abfractive lesions.

Like erosion, agreement on the prevalence of abfraction does not exist. Some propose that abfraction causes most cervical tooth loss; others believe that little evidence exists to indicate that this sequence of events actually occurs in the mouth. Some investigators have suggested that the engineering models used to justify abfraction have not taken into consideration the cushioning provided by the surrounding bone and periodontium, which may dissipate occlusal forces acting on a tooth. The pattern of cervical tooth loss tends to occur at sites with diminished serous salivary flow and could be explained by the initial loss of salivary protection rather than excess occlusal forces. Involvement by abfraction of the facial cervical areas of the anterior maxillary dentition is very puzzling, because the flexure during function would occur on the palatal surface of the tooth, not the facial surface. During function, investigators have found little evidence that strains in lingual enamel and dentin are any different from those that occur in facial sites; however, areas of focal cervical tooth loss occur almost exclusively on the facial surfaces. Finally, review of skulls from ancient Australian aborigines has revealed advanced tooth wear both occlusally and interproximally; and despite evidence of heavy occlusal loads, cervical defects were rare.

CLINICAL FEATURES

ATTRITION

Attrition can occur in both the deciduous and the permanent dentitions. As would be expected, the surfaces predominantly affected are those that contact the opposing dentition. Most frequently, the incisal and occlusal surfaces are involved, in addition to the lingual of the anterior maxillary teeth and the labial of the anterior mandibular teeth. Large, flat, smooth, and shiny wear facets are found in a relationship that corresponds to the pattern of occlusion. The interproximal contact points also are affected from the vertical movement of the teeth during function. Over time, this interproximal loss can result in a shortening of the arch length. Pulp exposure and dentin sensitivity are rare because of the slow loss of tooth structure and the apposition of reparative secondary dentin within the pulp chamber (Fig. 2-10).

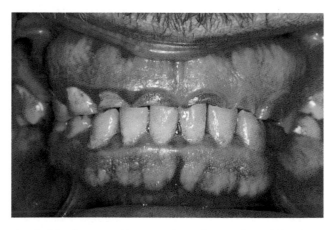

Fig. 2-10 Attrition. Extensive loss of coronal tooth height without pulp exposure in patient with anterior edge-to-edge occlusion.

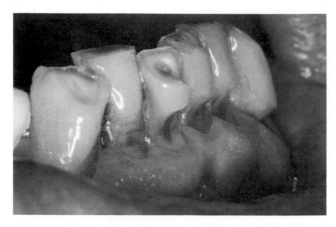

Fig. 2-11 Abrasion. Horizontal cervical notches on the anterior mandibular dentition. Note visible pulp canals that have been filled with tertiary dentin.

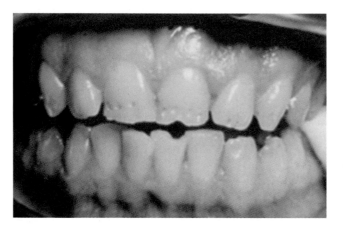

Fig. 2-12 Abrasion. Notching of the right central incisor caused by improper use of bobby pins. The patient also exhibits environmental enamel hypoplasia of the anterior dentition. *(Courtesy of Dr. Robert J. Gorlin.)*

ABRASION

Abrasion has a variety of patterns, depending on the cause. Toothbrush abrasion typically appears as horizontal cervical notches on the buccal surface of exposed radicular cementum and dentin (Fig. 2-11). The defects usually have sharply defined margins and a hard, smooth surface. If acid also is present, then the lesions will be more rounded and shallower. The degree of loss is greatest on prominent teeth (i.e., cuspids, bicuspids, teeth adjacent to edentulous areas) and occasionally is more advanced on the side of the arch opposite the dominant hand. Thread biting or the use of pipes or bobby pins usually produces rounded or V-shaped notches in the incisal edges of anterior teeth (Figs. 2-12 and 2-13). The inappropriate use of dental floss or toothpicks results in the loss of interproximal radicular cementum and dentin.

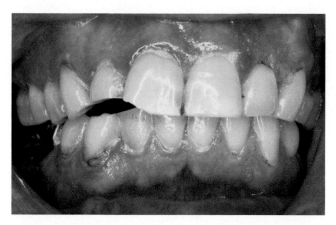

Fig. 2-13 **Abrasion.** Notching of the anterior dentition on the right side caused by long-term use of tobacco pipe.

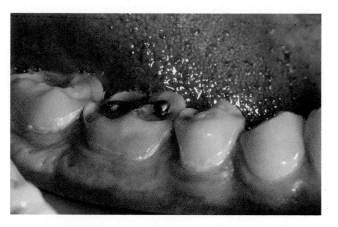

Fig. 2-15 **Erosion.** Extensive loss of buccal and occlusal tooth structure. Note that the amalgam margins are above the surface of the dentin.

A

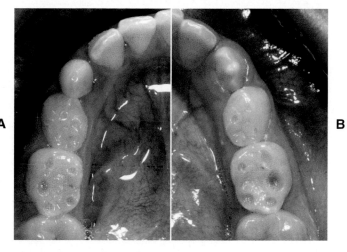

Fig. 2-14 **Erosion.** Multiple cupped-out depressions corresponding to the cusp tips.

B

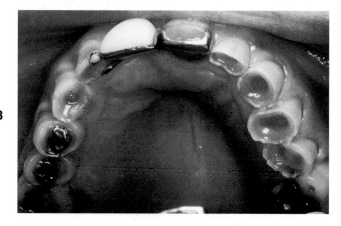

Fig. 2-16 **Erosion.** Occlusal view of the maxillary dentition exhibiting concave dentin depressions surrounded by elevated rims of enamel.

EROSION

In patients with **erosion,** the tooth loss does not correlate with functional wear patterns or with those typically associated with known abrasives. The predominant sites of tooth loss appear to correlate closely with those areas not protected by the serous secretions of the parotid and submandibular glands. The facial and palatal surfaces of the maxillary anterior teeth and the facial and occlusal surfaces of the mandibular posterior teeth are affected most frequently. Involvement of the lingual surfaces of the entire mandibular dentition is uncommon, possibly because of the protective buffering capacity of the submandibular serous saliva.

The classic pattern of dental erosion is the cupped lesion in which a central depression of dentin is surrounded by elevated enamel. Cupped areas are seen on the occlusal cusp tips, incisal edges, and marginal ridges (Fig. 2-14). In contrast to abrasion, erosion commonly affects the facial surfaces of the maxillary anteriors and appears as shallow spoon-shaped depressions

in the cervical portion of the crown. The posterior teeth frequently exhibit extensive loss of the occlusal surface, and the edges of metallic restorations subsequently may be above the level of the tooth structure (Fig. 2-15). After a portion of the cuspal enamel has been lost, the dentin is destroyed more rapidly than the remaining enamel, often resulting in a concave depression of the dentin surrounded by an elevated rim of enamel (Fig. 2-16). The more rapid dissolution of the dentin can lead to undermined enamel that often is lost easily by chipping. Occasionally, entire buccal cusps are lost and replaced by ski slope–like depressions that extend from the lingual cusp to the buccal cemento-enamel junction (Fig. 2-17). When palatal surfaces are affected, the exposed dentin has a concave surface and shows a peripheral white line of enamel (Fig. 2-18). Active erosion typically reveals a clean, unstained surface, whereas inactive sites become stained and discolored.

Focal facial tooth wear of the gingival portion has been given the nonspecific term, **noncarious cervical**

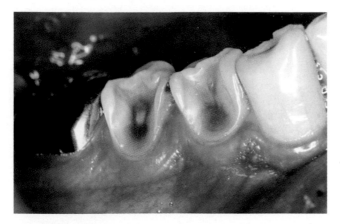

Fig. 2-17 Erosion. Extensive loss of enamel and dentin on the buccal surface of the maxillary bicuspids. The patient had sucked chronically on tamarinds (an acidic fruit).

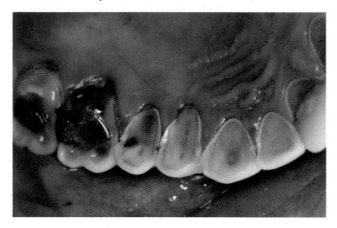

Fig. 2-18 Erosion. Palatal surfaces of the maxillary dentition in which the exposed dentin exhibits a concave surface and a peripheral white line of enamel. The patient had bulimia.

lesions, in an attempt to emphasize the multifactorial nature of the process. These cervical defects often are seen in association with loss of occlusal tooth structure, which has features of erosion, attrition, or both.

Erosion limited to the facial surfaces of the maxillary anterior dentition often is associated with dietary sources of acid. When the tooth loss is confined to the incisal portions of the anterior dentition of both arches, an external environmental source is suggested. When erosion is located on the palatal surfaces of the maxillary anterior teeth and the occlusal surfaces of the posterior teeth of both dentitions, regurgitation of gastric secretions is a probable cause. The location of the tooth structure loss may suggest the cause of the damage but is not completely reliable.

ABFRACTION

Abfraction appears as wedge-shaped defects limited to the cervical area of the teeth and may closely resemble cervical abrasion or erosion. Clues to the diagnosis include defects that are deep, narrow, and V-shaped

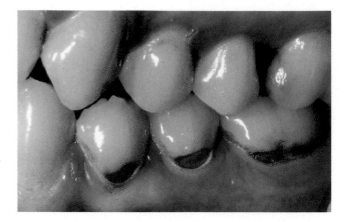

Fig. 2-19 Abfraction. Deep and narrow enamel cervical defects on the facial surface of the mandibular dentition. *(From Neville BW, Damm DD, White DK: Color atlas of clinical oral pathology, ed 2, Hamilton, 1999, BC Decker.)*

(which do not allow the toothbrush to contact the base of the defect) and often affect a single tooth with adjacent unaffected teeth (Fig. 2-19). In addition, occasional lesions are subgingival, a site typically protected from abrasion and erosion. The lesions predominantly affect bicuspids and molars, are seen almost exclusively on the facial surface, and exhibit a much greater prevalence in those with bruxism.

In all forms of tooth wear, the process typically proceeds at a slow rate that allows deposition of tertiary dentin and prevents pulp exposure, even when extensive loss of tooth structure is present (see Fig. 2-11). In some cases, and especially in the deciduous dentition, the tooth loss can proceed at a more accelerated rate that results in a near or frank exposure of the pulp. In a large review of 448 patients with tooth wear, 11.6% revealed near or direct pulp exposure. In addition, hypersensitivity was the presenting symptom in about one third of patients with tooth wear.

TREATMENT AND PROGNOSIS

Normal levels of attrition require no therapy, with intervention reserved for those cases that create a pathologic degree of tooth loss. The presence of advanced tooth wear in the deciduous dentition appears to correlate with subsequent tooth wear in adulthood, suggesting a continuation of the causative influences. Early diagnosis and intervention may assist in preserving the permanent dentition. Before any definitive action, the clinician must remember that tooth wear almost invariably has a multifactorial cause. Failure to recognize the interrelationships of these pathoses can lead to inappropriate therapy and failure of any attempted repair. Intervention should emphasize detailed diagnosis, preventive measures, and long-term monitoring. Immediate therapy should be directed toward resolution of tooth sensitivity and pain, but identifying the causes of tooth structure loss and protecting the remaining dentition also are important goals.

In patients affected by dental erosion, preventive interventions should attempt not only to reduce acid exposure but also to improve the oral cavity's ability to resist the effects of acid. Upon exposure to an acid, the saliva has the ability to achieve remineralization with time, but teeth are vulnerable to abrasion before completion of this action. Investigators have recommended a minimum 1-hour interval between acid exposure and toothbrushing in an attempt to minimize abrasion of the weakened enamel. Patients with erosion should limit toothbrushing to once a day in the morning because of the increased vulnerability of acid-etched enamel to abrasion and attrition. Low-abrasive toothpaste and professional guidance to prevent inappropriate, overzealous, or too frequent toothbrushing may assist in reducing associated abrasion. Consumption of buffering substances such as milk and cheese also is thought to be beneficial. Proper hydration is extremely important to maintain sufficient salivary flow. A suspected common cause of tooth loss is decreased salivary flow secondary to dehydration, often associated with strenuous work or athletic activities and possibly complicated by use of acidic soft drinks or sports beverages in the place of water. Chewing gum has been suggested as a method for decreasing dental erosion by increasing salivary flow after acid exposure, but others have demonstrated that enamel softened by acid can be damaged by the adjacent soft tissues during the movements of chewing in this time of vulnerability. Patients should be informed of the potential for loss of tooth structure associated with the overuse of acidic foods and drinks (e.g., wine, carbonated beverages, foods pickled in acetic acid, and citrate-containing fruits, fruit juices, and candies), chronic regurgitation, and improper oral hygiene techniques. Mouth guards and occlusal adjustment can be used to slow nocturnal attrition and to protect the teeth from frequent exposure to acid from regurgitation or industrial sources. Dental sensitivity can be reduced through the use of varnishes, mouthwashes, or toothpastes containing strontium chloride, stannous fluoride, or monofluorophosphate. If initially unsuccessful, these agents can be combined with iontophoresis.

Active restorative therapy is premature in the presence of ongoing tooth wear and should be postponed until the patient expresses strong aesthetic concerns, exhibits dental sensitivity that is nonresponsive to conservative interventions, or demonstrates progressive and uncontrollable wear. Once indicated, the minimum treatment necessary to solve the problem should be implemented. In lesions thought to represent abfraction, glass ionomer materials are recommended because of their greater resilience that allows the material to flex with the tooth. In areas of abrasion, a material with optimum resistance to the abrasive process should be chosen. In isolated teeth that continue to lose Class V restorations, continued abfraction is likely, and occlusal trauma should be eliminated. Replacement of lost posterior teeth and avoidance of edge-to-edge occlusion limit the effects of attrition. Lost tooth structure can be restored with composite resins, veneers, onlays, or full crowns. Restorative procedures that do not involve significant removal of remaining tooth structure are preferable in patients demonstrating extensive tooth wear.

The body may adapt to loss of tooth structure by continual eruption of the teeth, appositional alveolar bone deposition, and compensatory skeletal growth. If the process of tooth loss is slow, the vertical dimension often is maintained; in patients with rapid destruction, a loss of facial length occurs. Restoration of extensive loss of tooth structure is complex and should be performed only after a complete evaluation of the dentoalveolar complex.

INTERNAL AND EXTERNAL RESORPTION

In addition to loss of tooth structure that begins on the exposed coronal surfaces, destruction of teeth also can occur through resorption, which is accomplished by cells located in the dental pulp (i.e., **internal resorption**) or in the periodontal ligament (PDL) (i.e., **external resorption**). Internal resorption is a relatively rare occurrence, and most cases develop after injury to pulpal tissues, such as physical trauma or caries-related pulpitis. The resorption can continue as long as vital pulp tissue remains and may result in communication of the pulp with the PDL.

By contrast, external resorption is extremely common; with close examination, all patients are most likely to have root resorption on one or more teeth. In one radiographic review of 13,263 teeth, all patients showed evidence of root resorption, and 86.4% of the examined teeth demonstrated external resorption, with an average of 16 affected teeth per patient. Most areas of resorption are mild and of no clinical significance, but 10% of patients exhibit unusual amounts of external resorption.

The potential for resorption is inherent within the periodontal tissue of each patient, and this individual susceptibility to resorption is the most important factor in the degree of resorption that will occur after a stimulus. The factors reported to increase the severity of external resorption are delineated in Box 2-3. Many cases have been termed *idiopathic* because no factor could be found to explain the accelerated resorption. When pretreatment radiographs of a given patient exhibit a degree of resorption beyond that which is normally seen, the clinician should realize the potential risks involved in initiating procedures (e.g., ortho-

Factors Associated with External Resorption

- Cysts
- Dental trauma
- Excessive mechanical forces (e.g., orthodontic therapy)
- Excessive occlusal forces
- Grafting of alveolar clefts
- Hormonal imbalances
- Intracoronal bleaching of pulpless teeth
- Local involvement by herpes zoster
- Paget's disease of bone
- Periodontal treatment
- Periradicular inflammation
- Pressure from impacted teeth
- Reimplantation of teeth
- Tumors

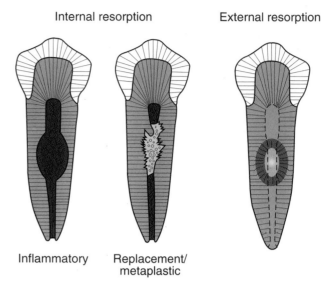

Internal resorption   External resorption

Inflammatory   Replacement/metaplastic

Fig. 2-20 Tooth resorption. Illustration contrasting the common patterns of internal and external tooth resorption. Internal resorption will result in a radiolucent enlargement of the pulp chamber or canal. In external resorption, the radiolucency is superimposed on the pulp canal, which should not be enlarged.

dontics) that are known to be associated with an increased risk of external resorption.

CLINICAL AND RADIOGRAPHIC FEATURES

Resorption of dentin or cementum can occur at any site that contacts vital soft tissue. Internal resorption is usually asymptomatic and discovered through routine radiographs. Pain may be reported if the process is associated with significant pulpal inflammation. Two main patterns are seen: (1) **inflammatory resorption** and (2) **replacement** or **metaplastic resorption** (Fig. 2-20). In inflammatory resorption, the resorbed dentin is replaced by inflamed granulation tissue. Although this pattern may involve any portion of the canal, the cervical zone is affected most frequently (and the pulpal inflammation is usually caused by bacterial invasion). The resorption continues as long as vital pulp remains; typically, the coronal pulp is necrotic, with the apical portion remaining vital. The results of pulp testing are variable. In this pattern the area of destruction usually appears as a uniform, well-circumscribed symmetric radiolucent enlargement of the pulp chamber or canal. When it affects the coronal pulp, the crown can display a pink discoloration (**pink tooth of Mummery**) as the vascular resorptive process approaches the surface (Fig. 2-21). When it occurs in the root, the original outline of the canal is lost and a balloonlike radiographic dilation of the canal is seen (Fig. 2-22). If the process continues, the destruction eventually can perforate the lateral root surface, which may be difficult to distinguish from external root resorption (Fig. 2-23). Although most cases are pro-

gressive, some cases are transient and usually arise in traumatized teeth or those that have recently undergone orthodontic or periodontal therapy.

The remaining pattern of internal resorption is termed *replacement* or *metaplastic resorption*. In this form, portions of the pulpal dentinal walls are resorbed and replaced with bone or cementum-like bone (see Fig. 2-20). Radiographically, replacement resorption appears as an enlargement of the canal, which is filled with a material that is less radiodense than the surrounding dentin. Because a central zone of the pulp is replaced with bone, the radiographic appearance often demonstrates partial obliteration of the canal. The outline of destruction is less defined than that seen in inflammatory resorption.

By contrast, external resorption typically appears as a "moth-eaten" loss of tooth structure in which the radiolucency is less well defined and demonstrates variations in density (Figs. 2-24 to 2-27). If the lesion overlies the pulp canal, then close examination demonstrates the retention of the unaltered canal through the area of the defect. Most cases involve the apical or midportions of the root. External resorption can create significant defects in the crowns of teeth before eruption (see Fig. 2-26). This pattern frequently is misdiagnosed as preeruptive caries and is thought by some investigators to be caused by defects in the enamel epithelium that allow connective tissue to come into direct contact with the enamel.

In reimplanted avulsed teeth, extensive external resorption of the root is extremely common without

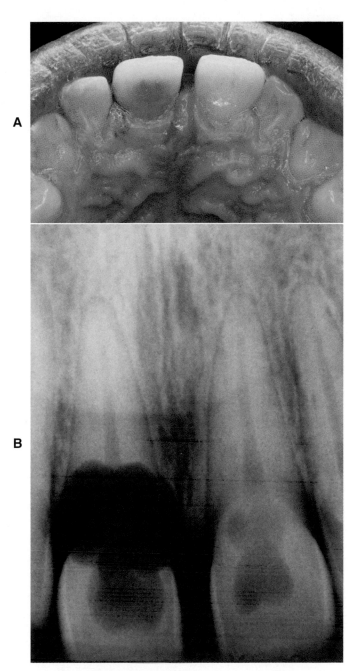

A

B

Fig. 2-21 **Internal resorption (pink tooth of Mummery).**
A, Pink discoloration of the maxillary central incisor.
B, Radiograph of same patient showing extensive resorption
of both maxillary central incisors.

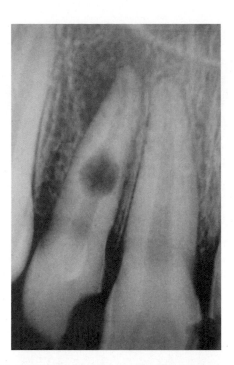

Fig. 2-22 **Internal resorption.** Balloonlike enlargement of
the root canal.

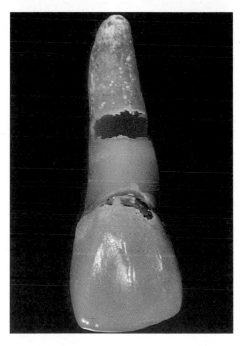

Fig. 2-23 **Internal resorption.** The destruction has resulted
in perforation of the lateral root surface.

rapid and appropriate intervention (see Fig. 2-25). If
the tooth remains outside of the socket without being
placed in a proper storage medium, then the PDL cells
will undergo necrosis. Without vital PDL cells, the surrounding bone will view the tooth as a foreign object
and initiate resorption and replacement by bone.

External resorption occurring during orthodontics
does not appear to be affected significantly by the
patient's sex or age, the severity of malocclusion, or the
type of mechanics used during therapy. Although the
patient's individual susceptibility has the strongest
influence, the single most important skeletodental predictor is the distance a tooth is moved during therapy.
The maxillary anterior teeth typically are the most
severely affected, particularly in patients who have
been treated with premolar extractions. Movement of

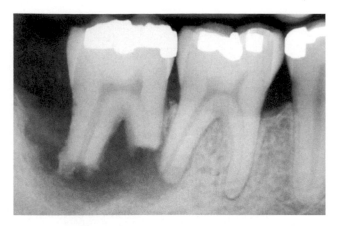

Fig. 2-24   External resorption. Extensive irregular destruction of both roots of the mandibular second molar associated with chronic periodontitis. *(Courtesy of Dr. Tommy Shimer.)*

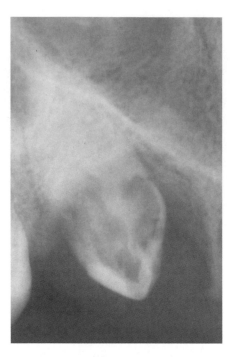

Fig. 2-26   External resorption. Extensive external resorption of the crown of the impacted right maxillary cuspid. Histopathologic examination revealed resorption without bacterial contamination or caries.

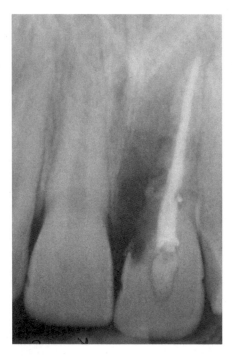

Fig. 2-25   External resorption. "Moth-eaten" radiolucent alteration of the maxillary left central incisor. The tooth had been reimplanted after traumatic avulsion. *(Courtesy of Dr. Harry Meyers.)*

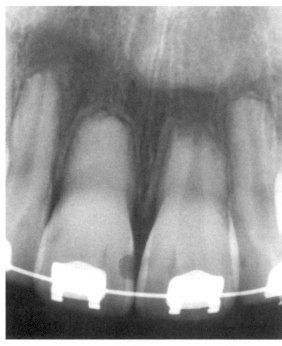

Fig. 2-27   External resorption. Diffuse external resorption of radicular dentin of maxillary dentition. This process arose after initiation of orthodontics.

teeth with an abnormal root shape such as dilaceration also has been associated with an increased severity of external resorption.

Occasionally, external resorption may begin in the cervical area and extend from a small opening to involve a large area of the dentin between the cementum and the pulp. The resorption can extend apically into the pulp or coronally under the enamel and simulate the pink tooth seen in internal resorption. The

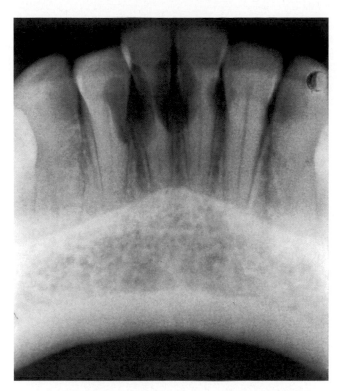

Fig. 2-28 Multiple idiopathic root resorption. Extensive invasive cervical resorption of several anterior mandibular teeth. *(Courtesy of Dr. Keith Lemmerman.)*

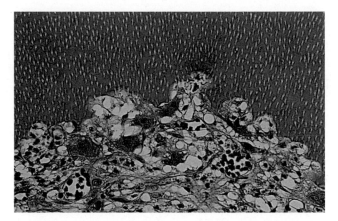

Fig. 2-29 Internal resorption. Resorption of the inner dentinal wall of the pulp. Note cellular and vascular fibrous connective tissue, which exhibits an adjacent inflammatory infiltrate and numerous dentinoclasts within resorptive lacunae.

source of radiation will shift distally). With this technique, the sites of external resorption appear to shift away from the pulp canal when the radiographs are compared. In addition, the radiographs can reveal which side of the root is affected in cases of external resorption.

HISTOPATHOLOGIC FEATURES

In patients with internal inflammatory resorption, the pulp tissue in the area of destruction is vascular and exhibits increased cellularity and collagenization. Immediately adjacent to the dentinal wall are numerous multinucleated dentinoclasts, which are histologically and functionally identical to osteoclasts (Fig. 2-29). An inflammatory infiltrate characterized by lymphocytes, histiocytes, and polymorphonuclear leukocytes is not uncommon. In replacement resorption, the normal pulp tissue is replaced by woven bone that fuses with the adjacent dentin. External resorption is similar in appearance, with numerous multinucleated dentinoclasts located in the areas of structure loss. Areas of resorption often are repaired through deposition of osteodentin. In large defects, external inflammatory resorption results in deposition of inflamed granulation tissue, and areas of replacement with woven bone may also be seen. Extensive bony replacement in areas of external resorption can lead to ankylosis.

TREATMENT AND PROGNOSIS

The treatment of internal and external resorption centers on the removal of all soft tissue from the sites of dental destruction. Internal resorption can be

cervical pattern of external resorption often is rapid and has been termed **invasive cervical resorption**. In some instances, several teeth may be involved, and an underlying cause for the accelerated destruction may not be obvious (**multiple idiopathic root resorption**) (Fig. 2-28). The exact cause of this pattern of resorption has been elusive, and it may result from a variety of inflammatory, traumatic, or bacterial stimuli affecting the clastic cells within the PDL. The process has been noted after orthodontic therapy, orthognathic surgery, other dentoalveolar surgery, root scaling or planing, internal bleaching of endodontically treated teeth, local trauma, bruxism, and tooth fracture. Other investigators believe this pattern of resorption can be triggered by periodontal pathogens and have seen good response to local mechanical débridement combined with systemic antibiotics.

In addition to invasive cervical resorption, generalized and progressive external resorption also can affect the apical portion of the roots. Although this pattern can occur secondary to an endocrine disturbance or one of a small number of systemic conditions, many of these cases are idiopathic and difficult to arrest.

If difficulty arises in distinguishing external from internal resorption, then the mesial-buccal-distal rule can be used through two radiographic exposures: one perpendicular and one mesial (objects closer to the stopped consistently if endodontic therapy successfully removes all vital pulp tissue before the process perforates into the PDL. Once perforation occurs, therapy becomes more difficult and the prognosis is poor. In such cases, initial placement of calcium hydroxide paste occasionally may result in remineralization of the site of perforation and stop the resorptive process. If remineralization of cervical sites of perforation is not successful, then surgical exposure and restoration of the defect may halt the process. Extraction often is necessary for radicular perforations that do not respond to therapy.

The first step in treating external resorption is the identification and elimination of any accelerating factor. Apically located sites cannot be approached without significant damage created by attempts at access. Those cases located in the cervical areas can be treated by surgical exposure, removal of all soft tissue from the defects, and restoration of the lost structure of the tooth. Because the cells responsible for the resorption are located within the PDL, endodontic therapy is not effective in stopping the process. In one report of generalized cervical resorption, therapy directed against local periodontal pathogens (débridement combined with systemic metronidazole and amoxicillin) stopped the resorption and was associated with an increased density of the adjacent crestal bone.

For avulsed teeth, the best way to prevent resorption is to maintain PDL vitality by immediate reimplantation or short-term use of a physiologic storage solution. Teeth reimplanted with an open apex should be monitored monthly; for teeth with a closed apex, endodontic therapy is necessary. Avulsed teeth with an open apex and nonvital PDL cells should not be implanted.

ENVIRONMENTAL DISCOLORATION OF TEETH

The color of normal teeth varies and depends on the shade, translucency, and thickness of the enamel. Abnormal colorations may be **extrinsic** or **intrinsic**. Extrinsic stains occur from surface accumulation of an exogenous pigment and typically can be removed with a surface treatment, whereas intrinsic discolorations arise from an endogenous material that is incorporated into the enamel or dentin and cannot be removed by prophylaxis with toothpaste or pumice. Box 2-4 lists the most frequently documented causes of tooth discolorations.

Dental fluorosis is discussed in the section on environmental effects on the structural development of the teeth (see page 58). The alterations associated with **amelogenesis imperfecta** (see page 99) and **dentinogenesis imperfecta** (see page 106) are presented later

---

Box 2-4

Tooth Discolorations

EXTRINSIC
- Bacterial stains
- Iron
- Tobacco
- Foods and beverages
- Gingival hemorrhage
- Restorative materials
- Medications

INTRINSIC
- Amelogenesis imperfecta
- Dentinogenesis imperfecta
- Dental fluorosis
- Erythropoietic porphyria
- Hyperbilirubinemia
- Ochronosis
- Trauma
- Localized red blood cell breakdown
- Medications

---

in this chapter in the text devoted to primary developmental alterations of the teeth.

CLINICAL FEATURES
EXTRINSIC STAINS

Bacterial stains are a common cause of surface staining of exposed enamel, dentin, and cementum. Chromogenic bacteria can produce colorations that vary from green or black-brown to orange. The discoloration occurs most frequently in children and is usually seen initially on the labial surface of the maxillary anterior teeth in the gingival one third. In contrast to most plaque-related discolorations, the black-brown stains most likely are not primarily of bacterial origin but are secondary to the formation of ferric sulfide from an interaction between bacterial hydrogen sulfide and iron in the saliva or gingival crevicular fluid.

Extensive use of **tobacco** products, **tea**, or **coffee** often results in significant brown discoloration of the surface enamel (Fig. 2-30). The tar within the tobacco dissolves in the saliva and easily penetrates the pits and fissures of the enamel. Smokers (of tobacco or marijuana) most frequently exhibit involvement of the lingual surface of the mandibular incisors; users of smokeless tobacco often demonstrate involvement of the enamel in the area of tobacco placement. Stains from beverages also often involve the lingual surface of the anterior teeth, but the stains are usually more widespread and less intense. In addition, foods that contain

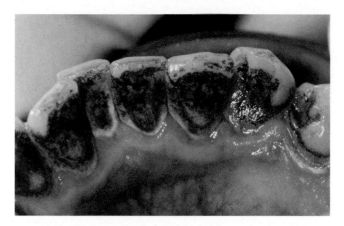

Fig. 2-30   Tobacco discoloration. Extrinsic brown stains of the enamel on the lingual surfaces of the anterior mandibular dentition secondary to long-term tobacco abuse.

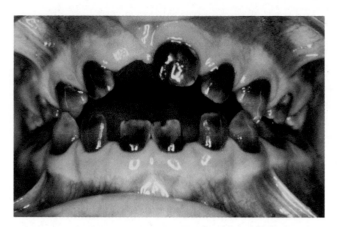

Fig. 2-31   Erythropoietic porphyria-related discoloration. Red-brown discoloration of the maxillary dentition.

abundant chlorophyll can produce a green discoloration of the enamel surface.

The green discoloration associated with chromogenic bacteria or the frequent consumption of chlorophyll-containing foods can resemble the pattern of green staining seen secondary to **gingival hemorrhage.** As would be expected, this pattern of discoloration occurs most frequently in patients with poor oral hygiene and erythematous, hemorrhagic, and enlarged gingiva. The color results from the breakdown of hemoglobin into green biliverdin.

A large number of **medications** may result in surface staining of the teeth. In the past, use of products containing high amounts of iron or iodine was associated with significant black pigmentation of the teeth. Exposure to sulfides, silver nitrate, or manganese can cause stains that vary from gray to yellow to brown to black. Copper or nickel may produce a green stain; cadmium, essential oils, and co-amoxiclav may be associated with a yellow to brown discoloration. Multiple recent reports have documented a yellow-brown staining of teeth associated with doxycycline, which can be removed by professional abrasive cleaning; the cause of this discoloration is unclear.

More recently, the most frequently reported culprits include **stannous fluoride** and **chlorhexidine.** Fluoride staining may be associated with the use of 8% stannous fluoride and is thought to be secondary to the combination of the stannous (tin) ion with bacterial sulfides. This black stain occurs predominantly in people with poor oral hygiene in areas of a tooth previously affected by early carious involvement. The labial surfaces of anterior teeth and the occlusal surfaces of posterior teeth are the most frequently affected. Chlorhexidine is associated with a yellow-brown stain that predominantly involves the interproximal surfaces near the gingival margins. The degree of staining varies with the concentration of the medication and the patient's susceptibility. Although an increased frequency has been associated with the use of tannin-containing beverages, such as tea and wine, effective brushing and flossing or frequent gum chewing can minimize staining. Chlorhexidine is not alone in its association with tooth staining; many oral antiseptics, such as Listerine and sanguinarine, also may produce similar changes.

INTRINSIC STAINS

Congenital erythropoietic porphyria (Günther disease) is an autosomal recessive disorder of porphyrin metabolism that results in the increased synthesis and excretion of porphyrins and their related precursors. Significant diffuse discoloration of the dentition is noted as a result of the deposition of porphyrin in the teeth (Fig. 2-31). Affected teeth demonstrate a marked red-brown coloration that exhibits a red fluorescence when exposed to a Wood's ultraviolet (UV) light. The deciduous teeth demonstrate a more intense coloration because porphyrin is present in the enamel and the dentin; in the permanent teeth, only the dentin is affected. Excess porphyrins also are present in the urine, which may reveal a similar fluorescence when exposed to a Wood's light.

Another autosomal recessive metabolic disorder, **alkaptonuria,** is associated with a blue-black discoloration termed *ochronosis* that occurs in connective tissue, tendons, and cartilage. On rare occasions, a blue discoloration of the dentition may be seen in patients who also are affected with Parkinson's disease.

Bilirubin is a breakdown product of red blood cells, and excess levels can be released into the blood in a number of conditions. The increased amount of bilirubin can accumulate in the interstitial fluid, mucosa, serosa, and skin, resulting in a yellow-green discoloration known as **jaundice** (see page 821). During periods of **hyperbilirubinemia,** developing teeth also may accumulate the pigment and become stained intrinsically. In most cases the deciduous teeth are affected as a result of hyperbilirubinemia during the neonatal period. The two most common causes are **erythroblastosis fetalis** and **biliary atresia.** Other diseases that less frequently display intrinsic staining of this type include the following:

- Premature birth
- ABO incompatibility
- Neonatal respiratory distress
- Significant internal hemorrhage
- Congenital hypothyroidism
- Biliary hypoplasia
- Metabolic diseases (tyrosinemia, α1-antitrypsin deficiency)
- Neonatal hepatitis

Erythroblastosis fetalis is a hemolytic anemia of newborns secondary to a blood incompatibility (usually Rh factor) between the mother and the fetus. Currently, this disorder is relatively uncommon because of the use of antiantigen gamma globulin at delivery in mothers with Rh-negative blood.

Biliary atresia is a sclerosing process of the biliary tree and is the leading cause of death from hepatic failure in children in North America. However, many affected children live after successful liver transplantation.

The extent of the dental changes correlates with the period of hyperbilirubinemia, and most patients exhibit involvement limited to the primary dentition. Occasionally, the cusps of the permanent first molars may be affected. In addition to enamel hypoplasia, the affected teeth frequently demonstrate a green discoloration **(chlorodontia).** The color is the result of the deposition of biliverdin (the breakdown product of bilirubin that causes jaundice) and may vary from yellow to deep shades of green (Fig. 2-32). The color of tooth structure formed after the resolution of the hyperbilirubinemia appears normal. The teeth often demonstrate a sharp dividing line, separating green portions (formed during hyperbilirubinemia) from normal-colored portions (formed after normal levels of bilirubin were restored).

Coronal discoloration is a frequent finding after **trauma,** especially in the deciduous dentition. Posttraumatic injuries may create pink, yellow, or dark-gray discoloration. Temporary pink discoloration that arises 1 to 3 weeks after trauma may represent localized vascular damage and often returns to normal in 1 to 3 weeks. In these instances, periapical radiographs are warranted to rule out internal resorption that may

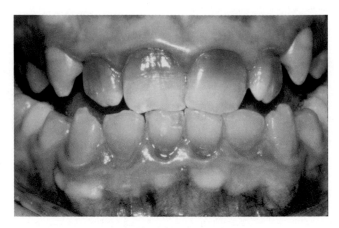

Fig. 2-32 Hyperbilirubinemia-related discoloration. Diffuse grayish-blue discoloration of the dentition. Cervical portions are stained most intensely. *(Courtesy of Dr. John Giunta.)*

produce a similar clinical presentation. A yellow discoloration is indicative of pulpal obliteration, termed **calcific metamorphosis,** and is discussed more fully in Chapter 3 (see page 123). The dark-gray discoloration is long-term and occurs in teeth with significant pulpal pathosis in which blood degradation products have diffused into the dentinal tubules. Endodontic therapy initiated before or shortly after the total death of the pulp often prevents the discoloration. The pulpal necrosis may be aseptic and not associated with significant tenderness to percussion, mobility, or associated periapical inflammatory disease. A related process secondary to **localized red blood cell destruction** also can result in discoloration of the teeth. Occasionally, during a postmortem examination, a pink discoloration of teeth is found. The crowns and necks of the teeth are affected most frequently, and the process is thought to arise from hemoglobin breakdown within the necrotic pulp tissue in patients in whom blood has accumulated in the head.

A similar pink or red discoloration of the maxillary incisors has been reported in living patients with **lepromatous leprosy** (see page 198). Although controversial, some investigators believe these teeth are involved selectively because of the decreased temperature preferred by the causative organism. This process is thought to be secondary to infection-related necrosis and the rupture of numerous small blood vessels within the pulp, with a secondary release of hemoglobin into the adjacent dentinal tubules.

Dental **restorative materials,** especially amalgam, can result in black-gray discolorations of teeth. This most frequently arises in younger patients who presumably have more open dentinal tubules. Large Class II proximal restorations of posterior teeth can produce discoloration of the overlying facial surface. In

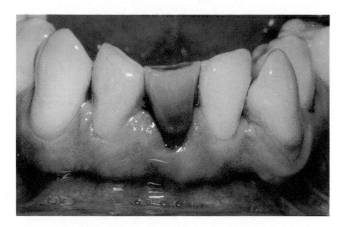

Fig. 2-33   Amalgam discoloration. Green-gray discoloration of mandibular central incisor, which had endodontic access preparation restored with amalgam.

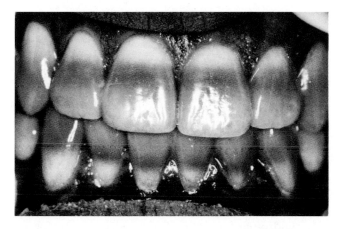

Fig. 2-34   Tetracycline-related discoloration. Diffuse brownish discoloration of the permanent dentition. *(Courtesy of Dr. John Fantasia.)*

addition, deep lingual metallic restorations on anterior incisors can significantly stain underlying dentin and produce visible grayish discoloration on the labial surface. To help reduce the possibility of discoloration, the clinician should not restore endodontically treated anterior teeth with amalgam (Fig. 2-33).

Several different **medications** can become incorporated into the developing tooth and result in clinically evident discoloration. The severity of the alterations is dependent on the time of administration, the dose, and the duration of the drug's use. The most infamous is **tetracycline,** with the affected teeth varying from bright yellow to dark brown and, in UV light, showing a bright-yellow fluorescence (Fig. 2-34). After chronic exposure to ambient light, the fluorescent yellow discoloration fades over months to years into a nonfluorescent brown discoloration. Often the facial surfaces of the anterior teeth will darken while the posterior dentition and lingual surfaces remain a fluorescent

yellow. The drug and its homologues can cross the placental barrier; therefore, administration should, if possible, be avoided during pregnancy and in children up to 8 years of age. All homologues of tetracycline are associated with discoloration and include chlortetracycline (gray-brown discoloration) and demethylchlortetracycline and oxytetracycline (yellow).

One semisynthetic derivative of tetracycline, **minocycline hydrochloride,** has been shown to produce significant discoloration of the dentition and also may affect teeth that are fully developed. Minocycline is a widely used medication for the treatment of acne and also is occasionally prescribed to treat rheumatoid arthritis. Its prevalence of use is increasing (and, presumably, so will the number of patients affected with discolored teeth and bone).

Although the mechanism is unknown, minocycline appears to bind preferentially to certain types of collagenous tissues (e.g., dental pulp, dentin, bone, dermis). Once in these tissues, oxidation occurs and may produce the distinctive discoloration. Some investigators believe supplementation with ascorbic acid (an antioxidant) can block formation of the discoloration. No matter the cause, once the pulp tissues are stained, the coloration can be seen through the overlying translucent dentin and enamel. The staining is not universal; only 3% to 6% of long-term users become affected. In those affected, the period of time before discoloration becomes evident can range from just 1 month to several years.

In susceptible individuals, minocycline creates discoloration in the skin, oral mucosa (see page 318), nails, sclera, conjunctiva, thyroid, bone, and teeth. Coloration of the bone occasionally results in a distinctive blue-gray appearance of the palate, mandibular tori, or anterior alveolar mucosa, which represents the black bone showing through the thin, translucent oral mucosa (see page 317). Several patterns of staining are noted in the dentition. Fully erupted teeth typically reveal a blue-gray discoloration of the incisal three fourths, with the middle one third being maximally involved. The exposed roots of erupted teeth demonstrate a dark-green discoloration, although the roots of developing teeth are stained dark black.

Another antibiotic, ciprofloxacin, is given intravenously to infants for *Klebsiella* spp. infections. Although less notable than tetracycline, this medication also has been associated with intrinsic tooth staining, usually a greenish discoloration.

TREATMENT AND PROGNOSIS

Careful polishing with fine pumice can remove most extrinsic stains on the teeth; typically, normal prophylaxis paste is insufficient. Stubborn stains often are resolved by mixing 3% hydrogen peroxide with the pumice or by using bicarbonated spray solutions. The use of jet prophylactic devices with a mild abrasive is the most effective. Recurrence of the stains is not uncommon unless the cause is reduced or eliminated. Improving the level of oral hygiene often minimizes the chance of recurrence.

Intrinsic discoloration is much more difficult to resolve because of the frequent extensive involvement of the dentin. Suggested aesthetic remedies include external bleaching of vital teeth, internal bleaching of nonvital teeth, bonded restorations, composite build-ups, laminate veneer crowns, and full crowns. The treatment must be individualized to fulfill the unique needs of each patient and his or her specific pattern of discoloration.

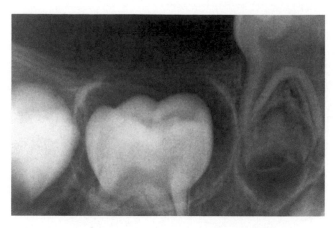

Fig. 2-35   Impaction of deciduous tooth. The right secondary primary molar demonstrates delayed eruption and enlarged pericoronal radiolucency. *(Courtesy of Dr. G. Thomas Kluemper.)*

LOCALIZED DISTURBANCES IN ERUPTION

IMPACTION

Eruption is the continuous process of movement of a tooth from its developmental location to its functional location. Teeth that cease to erupt before emergence are **impacted.** Some authors subdivide these non-erupted teeth into those that are obstructed by a physi-cal barrier (impacted) and those that appear to exhibit a lack of eruptive force (embedded). In many cases a tooth may appear to be embedded; however, on removal a previously undetected overlying odonto-genic hamartoma or neoplasm is discovered. There-fore, it appears appropriate to classify all these teeth as impacted.

CLINICAL AND RADIOGRAPHIC FEATURES

Impaction of deciduous teeth is extremely rare; when seen, it most commonly involves second molars (Fig. 2-35). Analysis of cases suggests that ankylosis plays a major role in the pathogenesis. In the permanent denti-tion, the most frequently impacted teeth are the man-dibular third molar, followed by maxillary third molars and maxillary cuspids. In decreasing order of fre-quency, impaction also may occur with mandibular premolars, mandibular canines, maxillary premolars, maxillary central incisors, maxillary lateral incisors, and mandibular second molars. First molars and max-illary second molars are rarely affected.

Lack of eruption most frequently is caused by crowd-ing and insufficient maxillofacial development. Proce-dures that create more space, such as removal of bicuspids for orthodontic purposes, are associated with

a decreased prevalence of third molar impaction. Impacted teeth are frequently diverted or angulated and eventually lose their potential to erupt (on comple-tion of root development). Other factors known to be associated with impaction include the following:

- Overlying cysts or tumors
- Trauma
- Reconstructive surgery
- Thickened overlying bone or soft tissue
- A host of systemic disorders, diseases, and syndromes

Impacted teeth may be partially erupted or com-pletely encased within the bone (i.e., full bony impac-tion). In addition, the impaction may be classified according to the angulation of the tooth in relationship to the remaining dentition: mesioangular, distoangular, vertical, horizontal, or inverted. On occasion, a small spicule of nonvital bone may be seen radiographically or clinically overlying the crown of partially erupted permanent posterior tooth (Fig. 2-36). The process is termed an **eruption sequestrum** and occurs when the osseous fragment becomes separated from the contigu-ous bone during eruption of the associated tooth. On occasion, mild sensitivity is noted in the area, espe-cially during eating.

TREATMENT AND PROGNOSIS

The choices of treatment for impacted teeth include the following:

- Long-term observation
- Orthodontically assisted eruption
- Transplantation
- Surgical removal

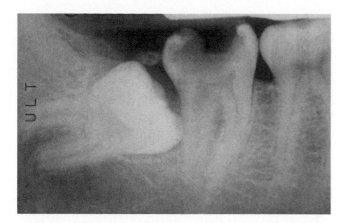

Fig. 2-36 Eruption sequestrum. A radiopaque fragment of sequestrating bone can be seen overlying an impacted third molar.

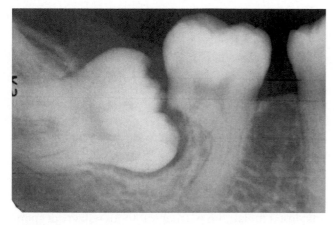

Fig. 2-37 Impaction-related tooth resorption. Mesioangular impaction of the right mandibular third molar associated with significant resorption of the distal root of the second molar. *(Courtesy of Dr. Richard Brock.)*

The presence of infection, nonrestorable carious lesions, cysts, tumors, or destruction of adjacent tooth and bone mandates extraction. Surgical removal of impacted teeth is the procedure performed most frequently by oral and maxillofacial surgeons. The choice of therapy in asymptomatic cases is an area of hot debate, and no immediate resolution is obvious. The risks associated with nonintervention include the following:

- Crowding of dentition
- Resorption, caries, and worsening of the periodontal status of adjacent teeth (Fig. 2-37)
- Development of pathologic conditions, such as infections, cysts, and tumors

The risks of intervention include the following:

- Transient or permanent sensory loss
- Alveolitis
- Trismus
- Infection
- Fracture
- Temporomandibular joint (TMJ) injury
- Periodontal injury
- Injury to adjacent teeth

Dental referral patterns provide a variety of perspectives of different dental practitioners. Many specialists (e.g., oral and maxillofacial surgeons, oral and maxillofacial pathologists) see a large percentage of significant pathologic conditions associated with impacted teeth compared with the experience of other clinicians. Although pathology rarely is associated with impacted teeth in children and young adults, numerous reports have documented an increased prevalence of problems in the later decades; therefore, any meaningful prospective studies must be lifelong rather than confined to just a few years. One review of 2646 pericoronal lesions submitted to an active oral pathology service revealed that 32.9% of cases had pathologically significant lesions, with strong relationship between increasing age and the prevalence of pericoronal pathosis. In this 6-year review were six primary squamous cell carcinomas arising from dentigerous cysts in addition to numerous odontogenic keratocysts and odontogenic tumors. Because of the frequent occurrence of significant pericoronal pathology, specialists often recommend extraction over close observation of impacted teeth.

The eruption sequestrum requires no therapy and usually undergoes spontaneous resorption or exfoliation.

ANKYLOSIS

Eruption continues after the emergence of the teeth to compensate for masticatory wear and the growth of the jaws. The cessation of eruption after emergence is termed **ankylosis** and occurs from an anatomic fusion of tooth cementum or dentin with the alveolar bone. Although the areas of union may be too subtle to be detected clinically and radiographically, histopathologic examination will demonstrate fusion between the affected tooth and the adjacent bone in almost all cases. Other terms for this process within the literature include **infraocclusion, secondary retention, submergence, reimpaction,** and **reinclusion.** *Secondary retention* is an acceptable term but may be confused with *retained primary teeth,* which maintain their emergence. *Submergence, reimpaction,* and *reinclusion* connote an active depression, and this is not the case.

The pathogenesis of ankylosis is unknown and may be secondary to one of many factors. Disturbances from changes in local metabolism, trauma, injury, chemical or thermal irritation, local failure of bone growth, and abnormal pressure from the tongue have been suggested. The periodontal ligament (PDL) might act as a barrier that prevents osteoblasts from applying bone directly onto cementum. Ankylosis could arise from a variety of factors that result in a deficiency of this natural barrier. Such loss could arise from trauma or a genetically decreased PDL gap. Other theories point to a disturbance between normal root resorption and hard tissue repair. Several investigators believe genetic predisposition has a significant influence and point to monozygotic twins who demonstrate strikingly similar patterns of ankylosis to support this hypothesis.

CLINICAL AND RADIOGRAPHIC FEATURES

Ankylosis may occur at any age; however, clinically the condition is most obvious if the fusion develops during the first two decades of life. Most patients reported in the literature with obvious alterations in occlusion are between the ages of 7 and 18 years, with a peak prevalence occurring in 8- to 9-year-old children. The reported prevalence of clinically detectable ankylosis in children varies from 1.3% to 8.9% and has been reported to be as high as 44% in siblings of those affected.

Although any tooth may be affected, the most commonly involved teeth in order of frequency are the mandibular primary first molar, the mandibular primary second molar, the maxillary primary first molar, and the maxillary primary second molar. Ankylosis of permanent teeth is uncommon. In the deciduous dentition, mandibular teeth are affected 10 times as often as the maxillary dentition. The occlusal plane of the involved tooth is below that of the adjacent dentition (infraocclusion) in a patient with a history of previous full occlusion (Fig. 2-38). A sharp, solid sound may

be noted on percussion of the involved tooth but can be detected only when more than 20% of the root is fused to the bone. Radiographically, absence of the PDL space may be noted; however, the area of fusion is often in the bifurcation and interradicular root surface, making radiographic detection most difficult (Fig. 2-39).

Ankylosed teeth that are allowed to remain in position can lead to a number of dental problems. The adjacent teeth often incline toward the affected tooth, frequently with the development of subsequent occlusal and periodontal problems. In addition, the opposing teeth often exhibit overeruption. Occasionally, the ankylosed tooth leads to a localized deficiency of the alveolar ridge or impaction of the underlying permanent tooth. An increased frequency of lateral open bite and crossbite is seen.

TREATMENT AND PROGNOSIS

Because they are fused to the adjacent bone, ankylosed teeth fail to respond to normal orthodontic forces, with attempts to move the ankylosed tooth occasionally resulting in intrusion of the anchor teeth. Recommended therapy for ankylosis of primary molars is variable and often is determined by the severity and timing of the process. When an underlying permanent successor is present, extraction of the ankylosed primary molar should not be performed until it becomes obvious that exfoliation is not proceeding normally or adverse occlusal changes are developing. After extraction of an ankylosed molar, the permanent tooth will erupt spontaneously in the majority of cases. In permanent teeth or primary teeth without underlying successors, prosthetic buildup can be placed to augment the occlusal height. Severe cases in primary teeth are treated best with extraction and space maintenance. Luxation of

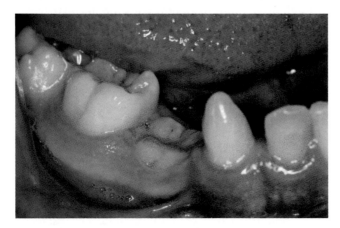

Fig. 2-38   Ankylosis. Deciduous molar well below the occlusal plane of the adjacent teeth.

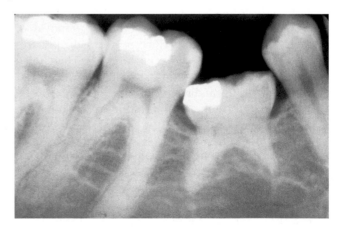

Fig. 2-39   Ankylosis. Radiograph of an ankylosed deciduous molar. Note the lack of periodontal ligament (PDL) space.

affected permanent teeth may be attempted with extraction forceps in an effort to break the ankylosis. It is hoped that the subsequent inflammatory reaction results in the formation of a new fibrous ligament in the area of previous fusion. In these cases, reevaluation in 6 months is mandatory. Finally, several reports have documented successful repositioning of an ankylosed permanent tooth with a combination of orthodontics, segmental osteotomy, and distraction osteogenesis.

Developmental Alterations of Teeth

Numerous developmental alterations of teeth can occur. Box 2-5 delineates the major reported alterations, and the following text pertains to these entities. These alterations may be primary or arise secondary to environmental influences (e.g., concrescence, hypercementosis, dilaceration). For the sake of convenience, both the primary and the environmental forms will be discussed together.

2-5

Developmental Alterations of Teeth

NUMBER
- Hypodontia
- Hyperdontia

SIZE
- Microdontia
- Macrodontia

SHAPE
- Gemination
- Fusion
- Concrescence
- Accessory cusps
- Dens invaginatus
- Ectopic enamel
- Taurodontism
- Hypercementosis
- Accessory roots
- Dilaceration

STRUCTURE
- Amelogenesis imperfecta
- Dentinogenesis imperfecta
- Dentin dysplasia type I
- Dentin dysplasia type II
- Regional odontodysplasia

DEVELOPMENTAL ALTERATIONS IN THE NUMBER OF TEETH

Variations in the number of teeth that develop are common. Several terms are useful in the discussion of the numeric variations of teeth. **Anodontia** refers to a total lack of tooth development. **Hypodontia** denotes the lack of development of one or more teeth; **oligodontia** (a subdivision of hypodontia) indicates the lack of development of six or more teeth. **Hyperdontia** is the development of an increased number of teeth, and the additional teeth are termed **supernumerary.** Terms such as *partial anodontia* are oxymorons and should be avoided. In addition, these terms pertain to teeth that failed to develop and should not be applied to teeth that developed but are impacted or have been removed.

Genetic control appears to exert a strong influence on the development of teeth. Hypodontia and hyperdontia have been noted in patients with a variety of syndromes (Boxes 2-6 and 2-7). In all of these syndromes, an increased prevalence of hypodontia or hyperdontia exists, but the strength of the association varies. Furthermore, the actual genetic contribution to the increased or decreased number of teeth may be unclear in some of these conditions. In addition to these syndromes, an increased prevalence of hypodontia is noted in patients with nonsyndromic cleft lip (CL) or cleft palate (CP).

Genetic influences still may affect nonsyndromic numeric alterations of teeth, because more than 200 genes are known to play a role in odontogenesis. Because of the complexity of the system, variations in tooth number arise in a wide variety of patterns. A large percentage of primary hypodontia cases appear to be inherited in an autosomal dominant fashion, with incomplete penetrance and variable expressivity, whereas a minority of examples present an autosomal recessive or sex-linked pattern. The environment is not without its influence, with occasional examples suggesting multifactorial inheritance. Several investigators have reported variable expression of hypodontia in monozygotic twins (confirmed by DNA fingerprinting). This discordance confirms the occasional multifactorial nature of the process. Overall, hypodontia most likely represents a variety of disorders caused by variable genetic and epigenetic factors.

Research has identified a gene mutation in only a small percentage of nonsyndromic hypodontia cases. Although this list will continue to lengthen over time, the currently implicated genes include the *PAX9* gene, the *MSX1* gene, the *AXIN2* gene, and He-Zhao deficiency, which is associated with an unknown gene that maps to chromosome 10q11.2. Although variable expressivity is common, most of these examples

Box 2-6

Syndromes Associated with Hypodontia

- Ankyloglossia superior
- Böök
- Cockayne
- Coffin-Lowry
- Cranio-oculo-dental
- Crouzon
- Down
- Ectodermal dysplasia
- Ectodermal dysplasia, cleft lip, cleft palate
- Ehlers-Danlos
- Ellis-van Creveld
- Focal dermal hypoplasia
- Freire-Maia
- Frontometaphyseal dysplasia
- Goldenhar
- Gorlin
- Gorlin-Chaudhry-Moss
- Hallermann-Streiff
- Hanhart
- Hurler
- Hypoglossia-hypodactylia
- Incontinentia pigmenti
- Johanson-Blizzard
- Lipoid proteinosis
- Marshall-White
- Melanoleukoderma
- Monilethrix-anodontia
- Oral-facial-digital type I
- Otodental dysplasia
- Palmoplantar keratosis, hypotrichosis, cysts of eyelid
- Progeria
- Rieger
- Robinson
- Rothmund-Thomson
- Sturge-Weber
- Tooth-and-nail
- Turner

Box 2-7

Syndromes Associated with Hyperdontia

- Apert
- Angio-osteohypertrophy
- Cleidocranial dysplasia
- Craniometaphyseal dysplasia
- Crouzon
- Curtius
- Down
- Ehlers-Danlos
- Ellis-van Creveld
- Fabry-Anderson
- Fucosidosis
- Gardner
- Hallermann-Streiff
- Incontinentia pigmenti
- Klippel-Trénaunay-Weber
- Laband
- Leopard
- Nance-Horan
- Oral-facial-digital types I and III
- Sturge-Weber
- Tricho-rhino-phalangeal

represent oligodontia and exhibit numerous missing teeth. Interestingly, the affected gene tends to correlate to the pattern of missing teeth. It must be stressed that these genes are involved in only a very small number of affected patients with hypodontia, and the genetic basis for the vast majority of hypodontia cases remains elusive.

Less information is available on the genetics of hyperdontia; however, like hypodontia, almost every possible pattern of inheritance has been suggested. In all likelihood, many cases are multifactorial and arise from a combination of genetics and environmental influences. In spite of this, studies on certain kindreds have suggested an autosomal dominant pattern of inheritance with incomplete penetrance, autosomal recessive inheritance with lesser penetrance in females, and X-linked inheritance.

Some investigators have implied that hypodontia is a normal variant, suggesting that humans are in an intermediate stage of dentitional evolution. A proposed future dentition would contain one incisor, one canine, one premolar, and two molars per quadrant. Conversely, others have suggested that hyperdontia represents atavism—the reappearance of an ancestral condition. The latter hypothesis is difficult to accept because some patients have had as many as four premolars in one quadrant, a situation that has never been reported in other mammals. The most widely accepted theory is that hyperdontia is the result of a localized and independent hyperactivity of dental lamina.

In contrast, hypodontia correlates with the absence of appropriate dental lamina. As discussed, the loss of the developing tooth buds in most instances appears to be genetically controlled. In spite of this, the environment most likely influences the final result or, in some cases, may be responsible completely for the lack of tooth formation. The dental lamina is extremely sensitive to external stimuli, and damage before tooth formation can result in hypodontia. Trauma, infection, radiation, chemotherapeutic medications, endocrine disturbances, and severe intrauterine disturbances have been associated with missing teeth.

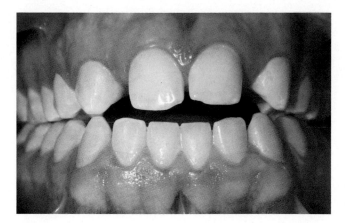

Fig. 2-40   Hypodontia. Developmentally missing maxillary lateral incisors. Radiographs revealed no underlying teeth, and there was no history of trauma or extraction.

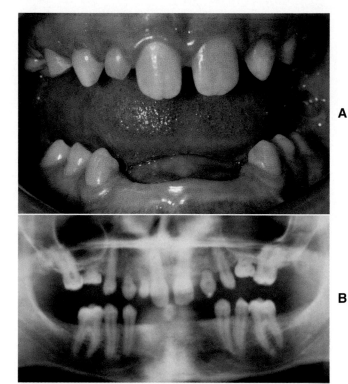

Fig. 2-41   Hypodontia. A, Multiple developmentally missing permanent teeth and several retained deciduous teeth in a female adult. **B,** The panoramic radiograph shows no unerupted teeth in either jaw.

CLINICAL FEATURES

HYPODONTIA

Failure of teeth to form is one of the most common dental developmental abnormalities, with a reported prevalence of 1.6% to 9.6% in permanent teeth when absence of third molars is excluded. The prevalence increases to 20% if third molars are considered. A female predominance of approximately 1.5:1 is reported. Anodontia is rare, and most cases occur in the presence of hereditary hypohidrotic ectodermal dysplasia (see page 741). Indeed, when the number of missing teeth is high or involves the most stable teeth (i.e., maxillary central incisors, first molars), the patient should be evaluated for ectodermal dysplasia. **Hypodontia** is uncommon in the deciduous dentition, with a prevalence that ranges from 0.5% to 0.9% and, when present, most frequently involves the lateral incisors. Absence of a deciduous tooth is associated strongly with an increased prevalence of a missing successor. Missing teeth in the permanent dentition are not rare, with third molars being the most commonly affected. After the molars, the second premolars and lateral incisors are absent most frequently (Fig. 2-40). Hypodontia is associated positively with microdontia (see page 83), reduced alveolar development, increased freeway space, and retained primary teeth (Fig. 2-41). In whites with missing teeth, approximately 80% will demonstrate loss of only one or two teeth.

Mutation of the *PAX9* gene creates an autosomal dominant pattern of oligodontia that can involve various teeth but most commonly affects most of the permanent molars. In severe cases, loss of the primary molars, second premolars, and permanent mandibular central incisors also may be seen. Mutation of the *MSX1* gene also is inherited as an autosomal dominant trait. Those affected with this mutation tend to demonstrate loss of the distal tooth of each type, with more severely affected individuals also revealing anterior progression of the agenesis. In these patients the most commonly missing teeth are the second premolars and third molars. In more severe cases, often the maxillary first premolars and maxillary lateral incisors also are missing. With the *MSX1* mutation, the degree of oligodontia is severe, with an average of approximately 12 missing teeth per patient. The He-Zhao deficiency arose in a large kindred from northwest China and includes a highly variable pattern of missing teeth that occurs only in the permanent dentition. The missing teeth may affect the entire dentition, but the condition most commonly involves the third molars, second premolars, and maxillary lateral incisors.

For dentists and their patients, the most critical discovery related to hypodontia revolves around the mutation of the *AXIN2* gene. This pattern of oligodontia is inherited as an autosomal dominant disorder, with the most commonly missing teeth being the permanent second and third molars, second premolars, lower incisors, and maxillary lateral incisors. The maxillary central incisors always are present and usually accompanied by the canines, first premolars, and first molars. However, the number and type of missing teeth are highly variable, a typical finding of inheritable oligodontia. Although the missing teeth can produce a significant oral problem, the presence of the *AXIN2* mutation in these kindreds also has been associated with development of adenomatous polyps of the colon and colorectal carcinoma. This suggests that patients with similar examples of oligodontia should be questioned closely for a family history of colon cancer, with further medical evaluation recommended for those possibly at risk.

Even in kindreds with an obviously inherited pattern of hypodontia or oligodontia, it must be stressed that, in the majority of the cases, the genes are yet to be discovered. The most common form of inherited hypodontia is an autosomal dominant pattern in which the average number of missing teeth is slightly more than two. Excluding the third molars, the most commonly missing teeth in these cases are the lower second premolars, upper second premolars, maxillary lateral incisors, and lower central incisors.

HYPERDONTIA

The prevalence of supernumerary permanent teeth in whites is between 0.1% and 3.8%, with a slightly higher rate seen in Asian populations. The frequency in the deciduous dentition is much lower and varies from 0.3% to 0.8%. Approximately 76% to 86% of cases represent single-tooth **hyperdontia,** with two supernumerary teeth noted in 12% to 23%, and three or more extra teeth noted in less than 1% of cases. Single-tooth hyperdontia occurs more frequently in the permanent dentition, and approximately 95% present in the maxilla, with a strong predilection for the anterior region. The most common site is the maxillary incisor region, followed by maxillary fourth molars and mandibular fourth molars, premolars, canines, and lateral incisors (Fig. 2-42). Supernumerary mandibular incisors are very rare. Although supernumerary teeth may be bilateral, most occur unilaterally (Figs. 2-43 and 2-44). In contrast to single-tooth hyperdontia, nonsyndromic multiple supernumerary teeth occur most frequently in the mandible. These multiple supernumerary teeth occur most often in the premolar region, followed by the molar and anterior regions, respectively (Fig. 2-45).

Although most supernumerary teeth occur in the jaws, examples have been reported in the gingiva, maxillary tuberosity, soft palate, maxillary sinus, sphenomaxillary fissure, nasal cavity, and between the orbit and the brain. The eruption of accessory teeth is

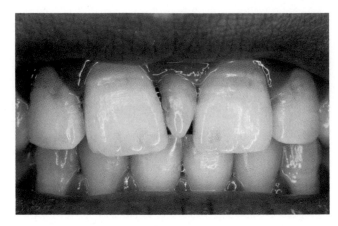

Fig. 2-42 Hyperdontia (mesiodens). Erupted supernumerary, rudimentary tooth of the anterior maxilla.

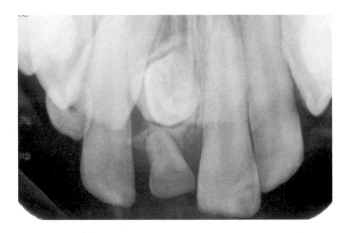

Fig. 2-43 Hyperdontia (mesiodens). Unilateral supernumerary tooth of the anterior maxilla, which has altered the eruption path of the maxillary right permanent central incisor.

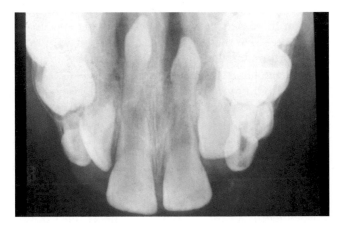

Fig. 2-44 Hyperdontia (mesiodens). Bilateral inverted supernumerary teeth of the anterior maxilla.

variable and dependent on the degree of space available; 75% of supernumerary teeth in the anterior maxilla fail to erupt. Unlike hypodontia, hyperdontia is positively correlated with macrodontia (see page 83) and exhibits a 2:1 male predominance. Although examples may be identified in older adults, most supernumerary teeth develop during the first two decades of life.

Several terms have been used to describe supernumerary teeth, depending on their location. A supernumerary tooth in the maxillary anterior incisor region is termed a **mesiodens** (see Fig. 2-42); an accessory fourth molar is often called a **distomolar** or **distodens.** A posterior supernumerary tooth situated lingually or buccally to a molar tooth is termed a **paramolar** (Fig. 2-46).

Supernumerary teeth are divided into **supplemental** (normal size and shape) or **rudimentary** (abnormal

shape and smaller size) types. Rudimentary supernumerary teeth are classified further into **conical** (small, peg-shaped), **tuberculate** (barrel-shaped anterior with more than one cusp), and **molariform** (small premolar-like or molarlike). Although odontomas are considered hamartomas and could be placed within this classification, these lesions traditionally are included in the list of odontogenic neoplasms and are discussed in Chapter 15 (page 724). The conical mesiodens represents one of the more common supernumerary teeth and can erupt spontaneously, whereas tuberculate examples are less frequent and rarely erupt.

Occasionally, normal teeth may erupt into an inappropriate position (e.g., a canine present between two premolars). This pattern of abnormal eruption is called **dental transposition.** Such misplaced teeth have been confused with supernumerary teeth; but in reality, patients exhibiting dental transposition have been reported to exhibit an increased prevalence of hypodontia, not hyperdontia. The teeth involved most frequently in transposition are the maxillary canines and first premolars. Crowding or malocclusion of these normal teeth may dictate reshaping, orthodontics, or extraction.

Accessory teeth may be present at or shortly after birth. Historically, teeth present in newborns have been called **natal teeth;** those arising within the first 30 days of life are designated **neonatal teeth.** This is an artificial distinction, and it appears appropriate to call all of these teeth *natal teeth* (Fig. 2-47). Although some authors have suggested that these teeth may represent predeciduous supernumerary teeth, most are prematurely erupted deciduous teeth (not supernumerary teeth). Approximately 85% of natal teeth are mandibular incisors, 11% are maxillary incisors, and 4% are posterior teeth.

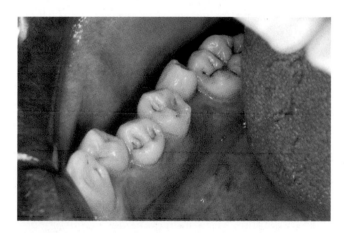

Fig. 2-45   Hyperdontia. Right mandibular dentition exhibiting four erupted bicuspids.

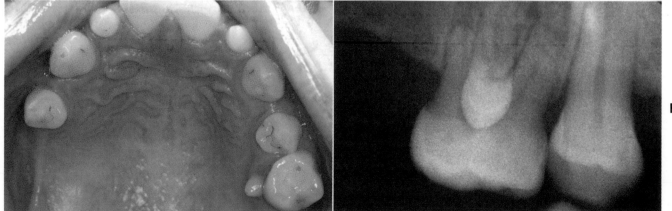

A   **B**

Fig. 2-46   Paramolar. A, Rudimentary tooth situated palatal to a maxillary molar in a patient who also exhibits hypodontia. **B,** Radiograph of the same patient showing a fully formed tooth overlying the crown of the adjacent molar.

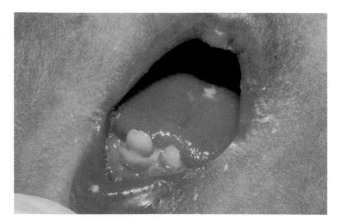

Fig. 2-47   Natal teeth. Mandibular central incisors that were erupted at birth.

TREATMENT AND PROGNOSIS

Sequelae associated with hypodontia include abnormal spacing of teeth, delayed tooth formation, delayed deciduous tooth exfoliation, late permanent tooth eruption, and altered dimension of the associated gnathic regions. The management of the patient with hypodontia depends on the severity of the case. No treatment may be required for a single missing tooth; prosthetic replacement often is needed when multiple teeth are absent. Therapeutic options include removable partial dentures, traditional fixed prosthodontics, resin-bonded bridges, or osseointegrated implants with associated prosthetic crowns. Use of fixed prosthodontics typically is not recommended for children because of the risk of pulp exposure during abutment preparation and because further growth can lead to infraocclusion and ankylosis of teeth held together by the prosthesis. Likewise, because implants act more like ankylosed teeth than erupting teeth, their use is not recommended before completion of skeletal growth except for patients with anodontia. For these reasons, a removable appliance or resin-bonded bridge often is appropriate in children and young adults while waiting for full dental and skeletal maturation.

In some cases of hypodontia, orthodontic therapy may improve the restorative treatment or even negate its need in selected patients. Patients with oligodontia exhibit an increased prevalence of orthodontics-associated external root resorption. This may be due to the altered root anatomy or to the extensive tooth movement that is required in some patients. Follow-up radiographs are recommended after 6 to 9 months of therapy to evaluate the root morphology for evidence of excessive resorption.

The presence of supernumerary teeth should be suspected if a significant delay is observed in the eruption of a localized portion of the dentition. Because of the decreased clarity in the anterior portion of a panoramic radiograph, this image should be combined with occlusal and periapical radiographs to fully visualize the area. Supernumerary teeth may develop long after eruption of the permanent dentition. Several publications have documented supernumerary bicuspids arising up to 11 years after completion of normal teeth development. In patients previously diagnosed with supernumerary teeth, or in those genetically predisposed, long-term monitoring for additional tooth development is warranted.

Early diagnosis and treatment often are crucial in minimizing the aesthetic and functional problems of the adjacent teeth. Because only 7% to 20% of supernumerary teeth exist without clinical complications, the standard of care is removal of the accessory tooth during the time of the early mixed dentition. Complications created by anterior supernumerary teeth tend to be more significant than those associated with extra teeth in the posterior regions. Reports have documented spontaneous eruption of the adjacent dentition in 75% of the cases if the supernumerary tooth is removed early. After removal of the supernumerary tooth, full eruption typically occurs within 18 months to 3 years. Impacted permanent teeth having closed apices or those associated with a tuberculate mesiodens may show a reduced tendency for spontaneous eruption. Permanent teeth that fail to erupt are treated best by surgical exposure with orthodontic eruption. Removal of unerupted deciduous teeth is not recommended, because most will erupt spontaneously.

A consequence of late therapy may include the delayed eruption, resorption of the adjacent teeth, displacement of the teeth with associated crowding, dilaceration, malocclusion, diastema formation, or eruption into the nasal cavity. Supernumerary teeth also predispose the area to subacute pericoronitis, gingivitis, periodontitis, abscess formation, and the development of any one of a large number of odontogenic cysts and tumors. In selected cases, clinical judgment may not dictate surgical removal, or patient resistance to therapy may be present. In these instances, regular monitoring is appropriate.

Natal teeth must be approached individually, with sound clinical judgment guiding appropriate therapy. As stated, the erupted teeth in most cases represent the deciduous dentition, and removal should not be performed hastily. If the teeth are mobile and at risk for aspiration, then removal is indicated. If mobility is not a problem and the teeth are stable, then they should be retained. Traumatic ulcerations of the adjacent soft tissue (**Riga-Fede disease**) (see page 287) may occur during breast-feeding but often can be resolved with appropriate measures.

DEVELOPMENTAL ALTERATIONS IN THE SIZE OF TEETH

Tooth size is variable among different races and between the sexes. The presence of unusually small teeth is termed **microdontia;** the presence of teeth larger than average is termed **macrodontia.** Although heredity is the major factor, both genetic and environmental influences affect the size of developing teeth. The deciduous dentition appears to be affected more by maternal intrauterine influences; the permanent teeth seem to be more affected by environment.

CLINICAL FEATURES

Although the size of teeth is variable, the two sides of the jaws are usually symmetrical. Despite this, when significant size variation is present, the entire dentition rarely is affected. Typically, only a few teeth are altered significantly in size. Differences in tooth sizes cannot be considered in isolation. Microdontia is associated strongly with hypodontia (see page 79); macrodontia often is seen in association with hyperdontia (see page 80). Females demonstrate a higher frequency of microdontia and hypodontia; males have a greater prevalence of macrodontia and hyperdontia.

MICRODONTIA

The term **microdontia** should be applied only when the teeth are physically smaller than usual. Normal-sized teeth may appear small when widely spaced within jaws that are larger than normal. This appearance has been historically termed **relative microdontia,** but it represents **macrognathia** (not microdontia). Diffuse true microdontia is uncommon but may occur as an isolated finding in Down syndrome, in pituitary dwarfism, and in association with a small number of rare hereditary disorders that exhibit multiple abnormalities of the dentition (Fig. 2-48).

Isolated microdontia within an otherwise normal dentition is not uncommon. The maxillary lateral incisor is affected most frequently and typically appears as a peg-shaped crown overlying a root that often is of normal length (Fig. 2-49). The mesiodistal diameter is reduced, and the proximal surfaces converge toward the incisal edge. The reported prevalence varies from 0.8% to 8.4% of the population, and the alteration appears to be autosomal dominant with incomplete penetrance. In addition, isolated microdontia often affects third molars. Interestingly, the maxillary lateral incisors and the third molars are among the most frequent teeth to be congenitally missing. When a peg-shaped tooth is present, the remaining permanent teeth often exhibit a slightly smaller mesiodistal size.

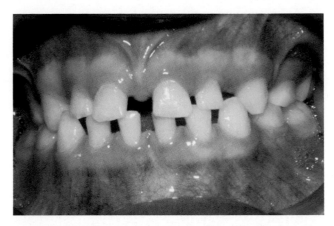

Fig. 2-48 **Diffuse microdontia.** Dentition in which the teeth are smaller than normal and widely spaced within the arch.

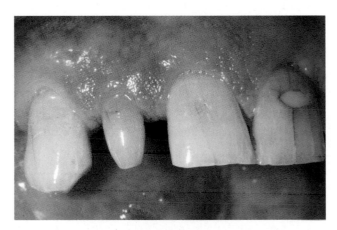

Fig. 2-49 **Isolated microdontia (peg lateral).** Small, cone-shaped right maxillary lateral incisor.

MACRODONTIA

Analogous to microdontia, the term **macrodontia (megalodontia, megadontia)** should be applied only when teeth are physically larger than usual and should not include normal-sized teeth crowded within a small jaw (previously termed **relative macrodontia**). In addition, the term *macrodontia* should not be used to describe teeth that have been altered by fusion or gemination. Diffuse involvement is rare, and typically only a few teeth are abnormally large. Diffuse macrodontia has been noted in association with pituitary gigantism (see page 831), otodental syndrome, XYY males, and pineal hyperplasia with hyperinsulinism. Macrodontia with unilateral premature eruption is not rare in hemifacial hyperplasia (see page 38). Authors have postulated that the unilateral bone growth resulting from this condition may also affect developing teeth on the altered side. Isolated macrodontia is reported to occur most frequently in incisors or canines but also has been seen in second premolars and third molars. In such situations, the alteration often occurs bilaterally.

TREATMENT AND PROGNOSIS

Treatment of the dentition is not necessary unless desired for aesthetic considerations. Maxillary peg laterals often are restored to full size by porcelain crowns.

DEVELOPMENTAL ALTERATIONS IN THE SHAPE OF TEETH

GEMINATION, FUSION, AND CONCRESCENCE

Double teeth (connated teeth, conjoined teeth) are two separate teeth exhibiting union by dentin and (perhaps) their pulps. The union may be the result of fusion of two adjacent tooth buds or the partial splitting of one into two. The development of isolated large or joined (i.e., double) teeth is not rare, but the literature is confusing when the appropriate terminology is presented. Historically, *gemination* was defined as an attempt of a single tooth bud to divide, with the resultant formation of a tooth with a bifid crown and, usually, a common root and root canal. Conversely, *fusion* was considered the union of two normally separated tooth buds with the resultant formation of a joined tooth with confluence of dentin. Finally, *concrescence* was the union of two teeth by cementum without confluence of the dentin.

Many investigators have found these definitions confusing and open to debate. A double tooth found in the place of a maxillary permanent central incisor is a good example of the controversy. If the joined tooth is counted as one and the tooth number is correct, then the anomaly could result from the division of a single tooth bud or the fusion of the permanent tooth bud with the bud of an adjacent mesiodens. Some have suggested that the terms *gemination, fusion,* and *concrescence* should be discontinued, and all of these anomalies should be termed *twinning.* This also is confusing because other investigators use *twinning* to refer to the development of two separate teeth that arose from the complete separation of one tooth bud (this also is arguable).

Because of this confusion in terminology, the use of the term *twinning* cannot be recommended. Extra teeth are termed **supernumerary,** and another name is not necessary. Even though the exact pathogenesis may be questionable in some cases (whether caused by fusion of adjacent buds or partial split of one bud), the terms

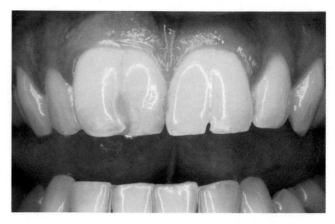

Fig. 2-50 Bilateral gemination. Two double teeth. The tooth count was normal when each anomalous tooth was counted as one.

gemination, fusion, and *concrescence* serve a useful purpose because they are the most descriptive of the clinical presentation. **Gemination** is defined as a single enlarged tooth or joined (i.e., double) tooth in which the tooth count is normal when the anomalous tooth is counted as one. **Fusion** is defined as a single enlarged tooth or joined (i.e., double) tooth in which the tooth count reveals a missing tooth when the anomalous tooth is counted as one. **Concrescence** is union of two adjacent teeth by cementum alone, without confluence of the underlying dentin. Unlike fusion and gemination, concrescence may be developmental or postinflammatory. When two teeth develop in close proximity, developmental union by cementum is possible. In addition, areas of inflammatory damage to the roots of teeth are repaired by cementum once the inciting process resolves. Concrescence of adjacent teeth may arise in initially separated teeth in which cementum deposition extends between two closely approximated roots in a previous area of damage.

CLINICAL FEATURES
GEMINATION AND FUSION

Double teeth (**gemination** and **fusion**) occur in both the primary and the permanent dentitions, with a higher frequency in the anterior and maxillary regions (Figs. 2-50 to 2-54). In the permanent dentition, the prevalence of double teeth in whites is approximately 0.3% to 0.5%, whereas the frequency in deciduous teeth is greater, with a reported prevalence from 0.5% to 2.5%. Asian populations tend to demonstrate a higher occurrence that exceeds 5% in some studies. In both dentitions, incisors and canines are the most commonly affected teeth. Involvement of posterior primary teeth, premolars, and permanent molars also can occur.

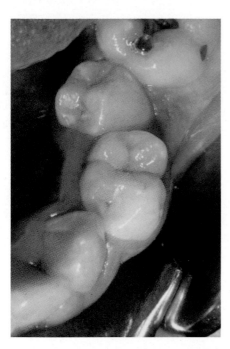

Fig. 2-51   Gemination. Mandibular bicuspid exhibiting bifid crown.

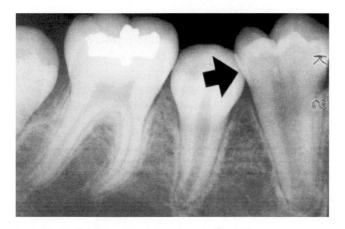

Fig. 2-52   Gemination. Same patient as depicted in Fig. 2-51. Note the bifid crown and shared root canal.

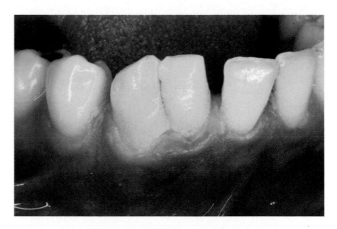

Fig. 2-53   Fusion. Double tooth in the place of the mandibular right lateral incisor and cuspid.

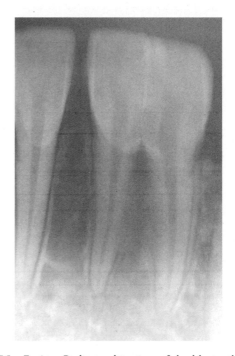

Fig. 2-54   Fusion. Radiographic view of double tooth in the place of the mandibular central and lateral incisors. Note separate root canals.

Gemination is more common in the maxilla, whereas fusion tends to occur more frequently in the mandible. Bilateral cases are uncommon (Fig. 2-55).

Gemination and fusion appear similar and may be differentiated by assessing the number of teeth in the dentition. Some authors have suggested that gemination demonstrates a single root canal. Separate canals are present in fusion, but this does not hold true in all cases (Fig. 2-56). A variety of appearances are noted with both fusion and gemination. The processes may result in an otherwise anatomically correct tooth that is greatly enlarged. A bifid crown may be seen overly-ing two completely separated roots, or the joined crowns may blend into one enlarged root with a single canal.

CONCRESCENCE

Concrescence is two fully formed teeth, joined along the root surfaces by cementum. The process is noted more frequently in the posterior and maxillary regions. The developmental pattern often involves a second molar tooth in which its roots closely approximate the adjacent impacted third molar (Fig. 2-57). The postinflammatory pattern frequently involves carious molars

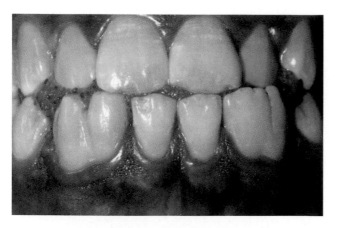

Fig. 2-55 Fusion. Bilateral double teeth in the place of the mandibular lateral incisors and cuspids.

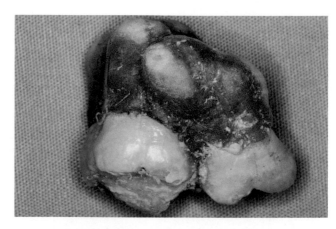

Fig. 2-57 Concrescence. Union by cementum of adjacent maxillary molars.

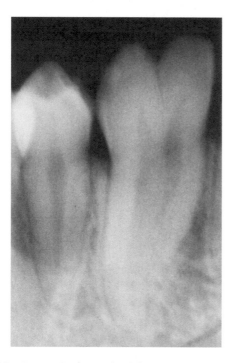

Fig. 2-56 Fusion. Radiograph of the same patient depicted in Fig. 2-55. Note the bifid crown overlying the single root canal; the contralateral radiograph revealed a similar pattern.

in which the apices overlie the roots of horizontally or distally angulated third molars. This latter pattern most frequently arises in a carious tooth that exhibits large coronal tooth loss. The resultant large pulpal exposure often permits pulpal drainage, leading to a resolution of a portion of the intrabony pathosis. Cemental repair then occurs (Figs. 2-58 and 2-59).

TREATMENT AND PROGNOSIS

The presence of double teeth (i.e., gemination or fusion) in the deciduous dentition can result in crowding, abnormal spacing, and delayed or ectopic eruption of the underlying permanent teeth. When detected, the progression of eruption of the permanent teeth should be monitored closely by careful clinical and radiographic observation. When appropriate, extraction may be necessary to prevent an abnormality in eruption. Occasionally, fusion in the primary dentition is associated with absence of the underlying permanent successor.

Several approaches are available for the treatment of joined teeth in the permanent dentition, and the treatment of choice is determined by the patient's particular needs. Rare reports of successful surgical division have been documented. In most cases of surgical division, endodontic therapy was performed. Selected shaping with or without placement of full crowns has been used in many cases. Other patients exhibit pulpal or coronal anatomic features that are resistant to reshaping and require surgical removal with prosthetic replacement. Double teeth often will demonstrate a pronounced labial or lingual groove that may be prone to develop caries. In such cases, placement of a fissure sealant or composite restoration is appropriate if the tooth is to be retained.

Patients with concrescence often require no therapy unless the union interferes with eruption; then surgical removal may be warranted. Postinflammatory concrescence must be kept in mind whenever extraction is planned for nonvital teeth with apices that overlie the roots of an adjacent tooth. Significant extraction difficulties can be experienced on attempted removal of a tooth that is unexpectedly joined to its neighbor. Surgical separation often is required to complete the procedure without loss of a significant portion of the surrounding bone.

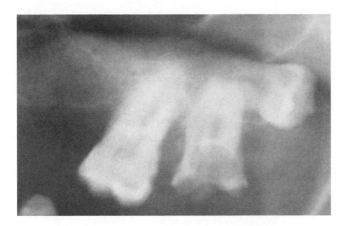

Fig. 2-58   Concrescence. Union by cementum of maxillary second and third molars. Note the large carious defect of the second molar.

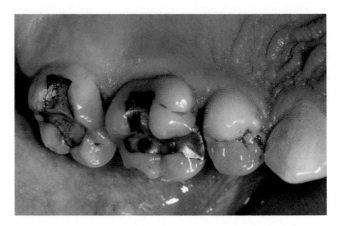

Fig. 2-60   Cusp of Carabelli. Accessory cusp on the mesiolingual surface of the maxillary first molar.

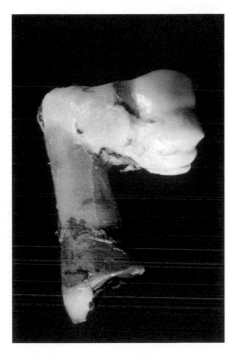

Fig. 2-59   Concrescence. Gross photograph of the same teeth depicted in Fig. 2-58. Histopathologic examination revealed that union occurred in the area of cemental repair previously damaged by a periapical inflammatory lesion.

ACCESSORY CUSPS

The cuspal morphology of teeth exhibits minor variations among different populations; of these, three distinctive patterns deserve further discussion: (1) **cusp of Carabelli,** (2) **talon cusp,** and (3) **dens evaginatus.** When an accessory cusp is present, the other permanent teeth often exhibit a slightly increased tooth size.

CLINICAL AND RADIOGRAPHIC FEATURES

CUSP OF CARABELLI

The **cusp of Carabelli** is an accessory cusp located on the palatal surface of the mesiolingual cusp of a maxillary molar (Fig. 2-60). The cusp may be seen in the permanent or deciduous dentitions and varies from a definite cusp to a small indented pit or fissure. When present, the cusp is most pronounced on the first molar and is increasingly less obvious on the second and third molars. When a cusp of Carabelli is present, the remaining permanent teeth often are larger than normal mesiodistally, but a similar association in deciduous tooth size is typically not noted. A significant variation exists among different populations, with the prevalence reported to be as high as 90% in whites and rare in Asians. An analogous accessory cusp is seen occasionally on the mesiobuccal cusp of a mandibular permanent or deciduous molar and is termed a *protostylid*.

TALON CUSP

A **talon cusp** is a well-delineated additional cusp that is located on the surface of an anterior tooth and extends at least half the distance from the cemento-enamel junction to the incisal edge. A talon cusp is thought to represent the end of a continuum that extends from a normal cingulum, to an enlarged cingulum, to a small accessory cusp, and, finally, to a full-formed talon cusp. Investigators have muddied the literature associated with this spectrum by categorizing all enlarged cingula as talon cusps and developing a classification system for the degree of enlargement. These classification systems make prevalence data difficult to evaluate and should be discouraged.

Three fourths of all reported talon cusps are located in the permanent dentition. The cusps predominantly

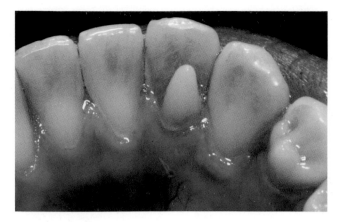

Fig. 2-61   Talon cusp. Accessory cusp present on the lingual surface of a mandibular lateral incisor.

occur on permanent maxillary lateral (55%) or central (33%) incisors but have been seen less frequently on mandibular incisors (6%) and maxillary canines (4%) (Fig. 2-61). Their occurrence in the deciduous dentition is very rare, with the vast majority noted on maxillary central incisors. In almost all cases the accessory cusp projects from the lingual surface of the affected tooth and forms a three-pronged pattern that resembles an eagle's talon. On rare occasions, the cusp may project from the facial surface or from both surfaces of a single tooth. A deep developmental groove may be present where the cusp fuses with the underlying surface of the affected tooth. Most, but not all, talon cusps contain a pulpal extension. Radiographically, the cusp is seen overlying the central portion of the crown and includes enamel and dentin (Fig. 2-62). Only a few cases demonstrate visible pulpal extensions on dental radiographs.

Extensive prevalence studies have not been performed, but estimates suggest the frequency of talon cusp in the population ranges from less than 1% to 8%. Variations among different population groups and inconsistent definitions of a talon cusp make a definitive calculation difficult. The process does appear to occur more frequently in Asians, Native Americans, the Inuit, and those of Arab descent. Both sexes may be affected, and the occurrence may be unilateral or bilateral. The accessory cusp has been seen in association with other dental anomalies (e.g., supernumerary teeth, odontomas, impacted teeth, peg-shaped lateral incisors, dens invaginatus, posterior dens evaginatus).

In isolated cases, genetic influences appear to have an effect, because identical talon cusps occasionally have been documented in twins. Talon cusps also have been seen in patients with Rubinstein-Taybi syndrome, Mohr syndrome, Ellis-van Creveld syndrome, incontinentia pigmenti achromians, and Sturge-Weber angiomatosis. Although the strength of association between

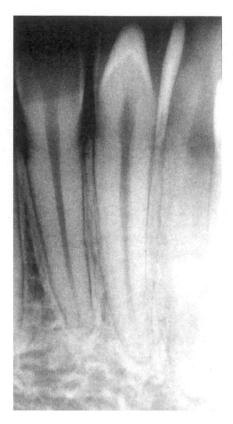

Fig. 2-62   Talon cusp. Radiograph of same patient shown in Fig. 2-61. Note the enamel and dentin layers within the accessory cusp.

the presence of talon cusps and these syndromes generally is not clear, Rubinstein-Taybi syndrome is strongly correlated as demonstrated by a study of 45 affected patients in which 92% demonstrated talon cusps. Other characteristic features of this syndrome include growth and mental retardation, broad thumbs and great toes, and a number of other orodental features (thin upper lip, retrognathia, micrognathia, narrow high-arched palate, submucous cleft palate, and cleft palate [rarely]).

DENS EVAGINATUS

Dens evaginatus (central tubercle, tuberculated cusp, accessory tubercle, occlusal pearl, evaginated odontome, Leong premolar, tuberculated premolar) is a cusplike elevation of enamel located in the central groove or lingual ridge of the buccal cusp of premolar or molar teeth (Fig. 2-63). Although this pattern of accessory cusps has been reported on molars, dens evaginatus typically occurs on premolar teeth, is usually bilateral, and demonstrates a marked mandibular predominance. Deciduous molars are affected infrequently. The accessory cusp normally consists of enamel and dentin, with pulp present in about half of the cases. Although the prevalence is variable, most

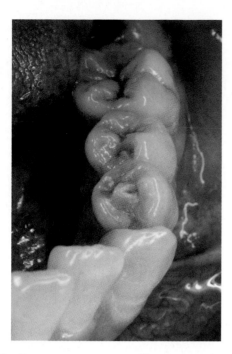

Fig. 2-63 **Dens evaginatus.** Cusplike elevation located in the central groove of mandibular first bicuspid.

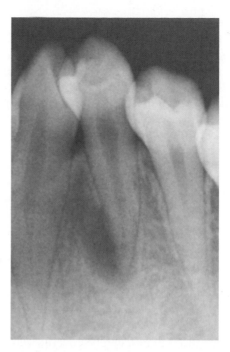

Fig. 2-64 **Dens evaginatus.** Radiograph of teeth depicted in Fig. 2-63. Note the tuberculated occlusal anatomy. Attrition on the accessory cusp led to pulpal necrosis and periapical inflammatory disease.

reviews suggest a frequency between 1% and 4%. The anomaly is encountered most frequently in Asians, the Inuit, and Native Americans but is rare in whites. Researchers expect an increased prevalence of this anomaly in the United States secondary to immigration by Asians and by Hispanics of mestizo heritage (i.e., those of mixed European and Native American ancestry). Radiographically, the occlusal surface exhibits a tuberculated appearance, and often a pulpal extension is seen in the cusp (Fig. 2-64). The accessory cusp frequently creates occlusal interferences that are associated with significant clinical problems. In one large study, more than 80% of the tubercles were worn or fractured, with pulpal pathosis noted in more than 25% of patients. Pulpal necrosis is common and may occur through a direct exposure or invasion of patent, immature dentinal tubules. In addition to abnormal wear and pulpal pathosis, the accessory cusp also may result in dilaceration, displacement, tilting, or rotation of the tooth.

Frequently, dens evaginatus is seen in association with another variation of coronal anatomy, **shovel-shaped incisors**. This alteration also occurs predominantly in Asians, with a prevalence of approximately 15% in whites but close to 100% in Native Americans and the Inuit. Affected incisors demonstrate prominent lateral margins, creating a hollowed lingual surface that resembles the scoop of a shovel (Fig. 2-65). Typically, the thickened marginal ridges converge at

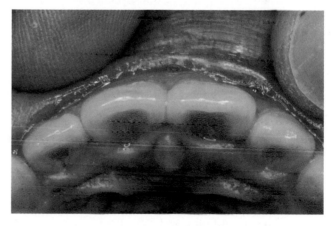

Fig. 2-65 **Shovel-shaped incisors.** Chinese patient exhibiting maxillary incisors with prominent lateral margins, which create a hollowed lingual surface.

the cingulum; not uncommonly, a deep pit, fissure, or dens invaginatus is found at this junction. Maxillary lateral and central incisors most frequently are affected, with mandibular incisors and canines less commonly reported.

TREATMENT AND PROGNOSIS

Patients with cusps of Carabelli require no therapy unless a deep groove is present between the accessory cusp and the surface of the mesiolingual cusp of the molar. These deep grooves should be sealed to prevent carious involvement.

Patients with talon cusps on mandibular teeth often require no therapy; talon cusps on maxillary teeth frequently interfere with occlusion and should be removed. Other complications include compromised aesthetics, displacement of teeth, caries, periodontal problems, and irritation of the adjacent soft tissue (e.g., tongue or labial mucosa). Because many of these cusps contain pulp, rapid removal often results in pulpal exposure. Removal without the loss of vitality may be accomplished through periodic grinding of the cusp, with time allowed for tertiary dentin deposition and pulpal recession. At the end of each grinding session, the exposed dentin should be coated with a desensitizing agent such as fluoride varnish, which also may speed the rate of pulpal recession. Even with slow reduction and no direct pulp exposure, loss of vitality is possible when large numbers of immature dentin tubules are exposed. After successful removal of the cusp, the exposed dentin can be covered with calcium hydroxide, the peripheral enamel etched, and a composite resin placed.

On eruption, the affected tooth should be inspected for the presence of a deep fissure at the junction between the talon cusp and the surface of the tooth. If a fissure is present, it should be restored to avoid early carious extension into the nearby dental pulp. Reports also have documented the continuation of this fissure down the surface of the root, with subsequent development of lateral radicular inflammatory lesions secondary to the access provided to oral flora by the deep groove. In these latter cases, further surgery is required to expose the groove for appropriate cleansing.

Dens evaginatus typically results in occlusal problems and often leads to pulpal death. In affected teeth, removal of the cusp often is indicated, but attempts to maintain vitality have met with only partial success. Slow, periodic grinding of the cusp exposes immature patent dentinal tubules and may lead to irreversible pulpitis without direct exposure. To reduce the chance of pulpal pathosis, elimination of opposing occlusal interferences combined with removal of minimal dentin and treatment of the area with stannous fluoride has been recommended. More rapid cuspal removal with indirect or direct pulp capping also has proven beneficial in some patients. Other investigators support removal of occlusal interferences, protection of the cusp from fracture by the placement of surrounding resin reinforcement, and delaying cuspal removal until evidence of significant dentinal maturation, pulpal recession, and apical root closure are present.

Shovel-shaped incisors should be inspected for surface defects at the point where the marginal ridges

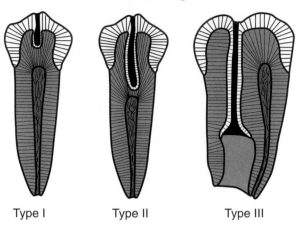

Coronal dens invaginatus

Type I   Type II   Type III

Fig. 2-66 Dens invaginatus. Illustration depicting the three types of coronal dens invaginatus.

converge. Any deep fissures or invaginations should be restored shortly after eruption to prevent carious exposure of the adjacent pulp.

DENS INVAGINATUS (DENS IN DENTE)

Dens invaginatus is a deep surface invagination of the crown or root that is lined by enamel. Oehlers described this condition thoroughly in three classic articles published from 1957 to 1958. Two forms, coronal and radicular, are recognized.

CLINICAL AND RADIOGRAPHIC FEATURES

By a great margin, **coronal dens invaginatus** is seen more frequently; the reported prevalence varies from 0.04% to 10% of all patients. In order of decreasing frequency, the teeth affected most often include the permanent lateral incisors, central incisors, premolars, canines, and molars. Involvement of deciduous teeth has been reported but is uncommon. A strong maxillary predominance is seen.

The depth of the invagination varies from a slight enlargement of the cingulum pit to a deep infolding that extends to the apex. As would be expected, before eruption the lumen of the invagination is filled with soft tissue similar to the dental follicle (i.e., reduced enamel epithelium with a fibrous connective tissue wall). On eruption, this soft tissue loses its vascular supply and becomes necrotic.

Historically, coronal dens invaginatus has been classified into three major types (Fig. 2-66). Type I exhibits an invagination that is confined to the crown. The invagination in type II extends below the cemento-

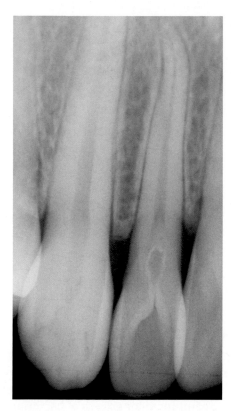

Fig. 2-67   Coronal dens invaginatus type II. Maxillary lateral incisor exhibiting invagination of the surface enamel that extends below the cementoenamel junction.

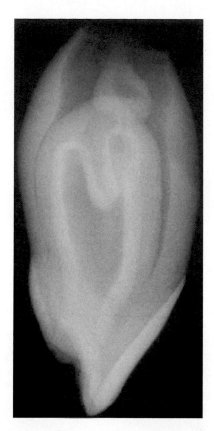

Fig. 2-68   Coronal dens invaginatus type II. Bulbous maxillary cuspid exhibiting a dilated invagination lined by enamel.

enamel junction and ends in a blind sac that may or may not communicate with the adjacent dental pulp (Figs. 2-67 and 2-68). Large invaginations may become dilated and contain dystrophic enamel in the base of the dilatation (Fig. 2-69). Type III extends through the root and perforates in the apical or lateral radicular area without any immediate communication with the pulp. In this latter type, the enamel that lines the invagination is often replaced by cementum close to the radicular perforation. This perforation provides direct communication from the oral cavity to the intraosseous periradicular tissues and often produces inflammatory lesions in the presence of a vital pulp (Figs. 2-70 and 2-71).

Occasionally, the invagination may be rather large and resemble a tooth within a tooth, hence the term **dens in dente.** In other cases the invagination may be dilated and disturb the formation of the tooth, resulting in anomalous tooth development termed **dilated odontome.** Involvement may be singular, multiple, or bilateral.

Radicular dens invaginatus is rare and thought to arise secondary to a proliferation of Hertwig's root sheath, with the formation of a strip of enamel that extends along the surface of the root. This pattern of

A

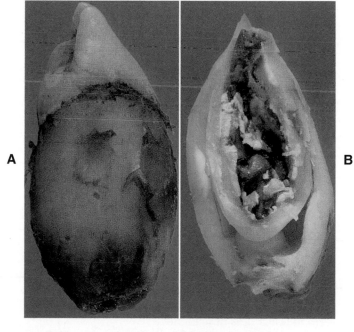

B

Fig. 2-69   Coronal dens invaginatus type II. Gross photograph of a sectioned tooth. Note the dilated invagination with apical accumulation of dystrophic enamel.

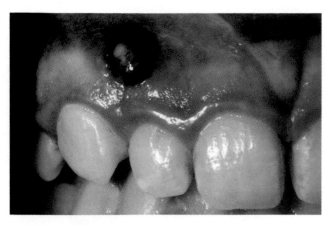

Fig. 2-70 Coronal dens invaginatus type III. Parulis overlying vital maxillary cuspid and lateral incisor. The cuspid contained a dens invaginatus that perforated the mesial surface of its root.

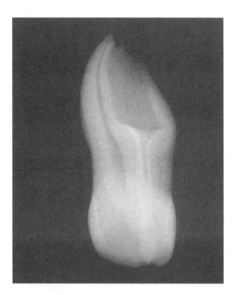

Fig. 2-71 Coronal dens invaginatus type III. Maxillary cuspid exhibiting an enamel invagination that parallels the pulp canal and perforates the lateral root surface. (*Courtesy of Dr. Brian Blocher.*)

enamel deposition is similar to that frequently seen in association with radicular **enamel pearls** (see Ectopic Enamel). Rather than protrude from the surface (as seen in an enamel pearl), the altered enamel forms a surface invagination into the dental papilla (Fig. 2-72). Cementum-lined invaginations of the root have been reported, but these represent a simple variation of root morphology and should not be included under the term *radicular dens invaginatus.*

Radiographically, the affected tooth demonstrates an enlargement of the root. Close examination often reveals a dilated invagination lined by enamel, with the

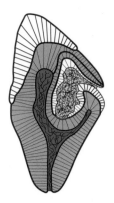

Fig. 2-72 Radicular dens invaginatus. Illustration depicting the radicular form of dens invaginatus.

opening of the invagination situated along the lateral aspect of the root.

TREATMENT AND PROGNOSIS

On eruption, the invagination of the affected tooth communicates with the oral cavity, and the soft tissue within the lumen undergoes necrosis (providing an excellent environment for growth of bacteria). In small type I invaginations, the opening of the invagination should be restored after eruption in an attempt to prevent carious involvement and subsequent pulpal inflammation. If the invagination is not detected quickly, then pulpal necrosis frequently results. With larger invaginations the contents of the lumen and any carious dentin must be removed; then a calcium hydroxide base may be placed to help treat any possible microcommunications with the adjacent pulp. In cases with obvious pulpal communication or signs of pulpal pathosis, both the invagination and the adjacent pulp canal require endodontic therapy. In teeth with open apices, apexification with calcium hydroxide or mineral trioxide aggregate often is successful, followed by final obturation.

Type III invaginations associated with periradicular inflammatory lesions require endodontic-like therapy of the perforating invagination. Once again, before final obturation with gutta-percha, temporary placement of calcium hydroxide helps to build dentinal bridges and maintain vitality of the adjacent pulp. If vitality is lost, endodontic therapy of the parallel root canal also becomes necessary. Some cases do not respond to conservative endodontic therapy and require periapical surgery and retrofill. Large and extremely dilated invaginations often have abnormal crowns and need to be extracted.

If the invagination does not significantly disrupt the morphologic appearance of the tooth, then complications of radicular dens invaginatus are rare unless the radicular opening is exposed to the oral cavity. After exposure occurs, carious involvement often leads to pulpal necrosis. Openings close to the anatomic neck of the tooth should be exposed and restored to minimize damage to the tooth and surrounding structures.

ECTOPIC ENAMEL

Ectopic enamel refers to the presence of enamel in unusual locations, mainly the tooth root. The most widely known are **enamel pearls.** These are hemispheric structures that may consist entirely of enamel or contain underlying dentin and pulp tissue. Most enamel pearls project from the surface of the root and are thought to arise from a localized bulging of the odontoblastic layer. This bulge may provide prolonged contact between Hertwig's root sheath and the developing dentin, triggering induction of enamel formation. Similar internal projections of enamel into the underlying dentin rarely have been reported in the crowns of teeth.

In addition to enamel pearls, **cervical enamel extensions** also occur along the surface of dental roots. These extensions represent a dipping of the enamel from the cementoenamel junction toward the bifurcation of molar teeth. This pattern of ectopic enamel forms a triangular extension of the coronal enamel that develops on the buccal surface of molar teeth directly overlying the bifurcation. The base of the triangle is continuous with the inferior portion of the coronal enamel; the leading point of the triangle extends directly toward the bifurcation of the tooth. These areas of ectopic enamel have been called *cervical enamel projections,* but this terminology is confusing because no significant exophytic projections are seen.

CLINICAL AND RADIOGRAPHIC FEATURES

ENAMEL PEARLS

Enamel pearls are found most frequently on the roots of maxillary molars (mandibular molars are the second most frequent site). It is uncommon for maxillary premolars and incisors to be affected. Involvement of deciduous molars is not rare. The prevalence of enamel pearls varies (1.1% to 9.7% of all patients) according to the population studied and is highest in Asians. In most cases, one pearl is found, but as many as four pearls have been documented on a single tooth. The majority occur on the roots at the furcation area or near the cementoenamel junction (Fig. 2-73). Radiographically, pearls appear as well-defined, radiopaque nodules along the root's surface (Fig. 2-74). Mature internal enamel pearls appear as well-defined circular areas of

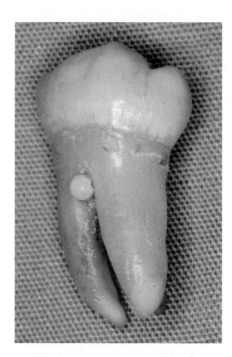

Fig. 2-73   Enamel pearl. Mass of ectopic enamel located in the furcation area of a molar tooth. *(Courtesy of Dr. Joseph Beard.)*

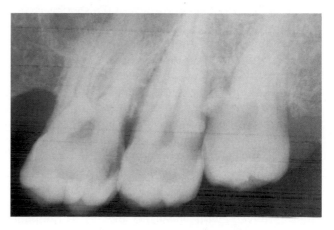

Fig. 2-74   Enamel pearl. Radiopaque nodule on the mesial surface of the root of the maxillary third molar. Another less distinct enamel pearl is present on the distal root of the second molar.

radiodensity extending from the dentinoenamel junction into the underlying coronal dentin.

The enamel surface of pearls precludes normal periodontal attachment with connective tissue, and a hemidesmosomal junction probably exists. This junction is less resistant to breakdown; once separation occurs, rapid loss of attachment is likely. In addition, the exophytic nature of the pearl is conducive to plaque retention and inadequate cleansing.

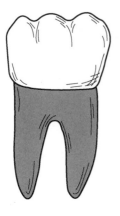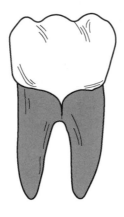

Normal cervical enamel   Cervical enamel extension

Fig. 2-75 Cervical enamel extension. Illustration of a normal molar adjacent to a molar exhibiting V-shaped elongation of enamel extending toward the bifurcation.

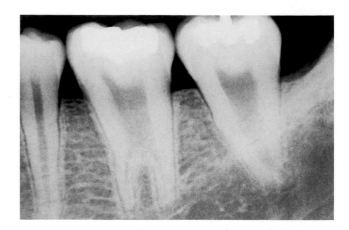

Fig. 2-76 Taurodontism. Mandibular molar teeth exhibiting increased pulpal apicoocclusal height with apically positioned pulpal floor and bifurcation. *(Courtesy of Dr. Michael Kahn.)*

CERVICAL ENAMEL EXTENSIONS

As mentioned previously, **cervical enamel extensions** are located on the buccal surface of the root overlying the bifurcation (Fig. 2-75). Mandibular molars are affected slightly more frequently than maxillary molars. In reviews of extracted teeth in the lower 48 United States, the prevalence is surprisingly high, with approximately 20% of molars being affected. Similar studies demonstrate an even greater prevalence in other locations such as Japan, China, and Alaska, with cervical enamel extensions discovered in 50% to 78% of extracted molars. Cervical enamel extensions may occur on any molar, but they are seen less frequently on third molars. Because connective tissue cannot attach to enamel, these extensions have been correlated positively with localized loss of periodontal attachment with furcation involvement. On review of a large number of dentitions with periodontal furcation involvement, a significantly higher frequency of cervical enamel extensions was found compared with dentitions without furcation involvement. In addition, the greater the degree of cervical extension, the higher the frequency of furcation involvement.

In addition to periodontal furcation involvement, cervical enamel extensions (in some cases) have been associated with the development of inflammatory cysts that are histopathologically identical to inflammatory periapical cysts. The cysts develop along the buccal surface over the bifurcation and most appropriately are called **buccal bifurcation cysts** (see page 698). The association between cervical enamel extensions and this unique inflammatory cyst is controversial.

TREATMENT AND PROGNOSIS

When enamel pearls are detected radiographically, the area should be viewed as a weak point of periodontal attachment. Meticulous oral hygiene should be maintained in an effort to prevent localized loss of periodontal support. If removal of the lesion is contemplated, then the clinician must remember that enamel pearls occasionally contain vital pulp tissue.

For teeth with cervical enamel extensions and associated periodontal furcation involvement, therapy is directed at achieving a more durable attachment and providing access to the area for appropriate cleaning. Reports have suggested that flattening or removing the enamel in combination with an excisional new attachment procedure and furcation plasty may accomplish this.

TAURODONTISM

Taurodontism is an enlargement of the body and pulp chamber of a multirooted tooth, with apical displacement of the pulpal floor and bifurcation of the roots. This pattern of molar formation has been found in ancient Neanderthals, and the overall shape of the taurodont resembles that of the molar teeth of cud-chewing animals (*tauro* = bull; *dont* = tooth).

CLINICAL AND RADIOGRAPHIC FEATURES

Affected teeth tend to be rectangular and exhibit pulp chambers with a dramatically increased apicoocclusal height and a bifurcation close to the apex (Fig. 2-76). The diagnosis usually is made subjectively from the radiographic appearance. The degree of taurodontism

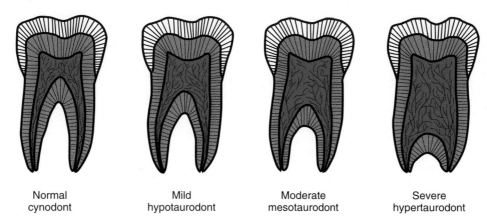

| Normal cynodont | Mild hypotaurodont | Moderate mesotaurodont | Severe hypertaurodont |

Fig. 2-77   Taurodontism. Illustration exhibiting the classification of taurodontism according to the degree of apical displacement of the pulpal floor.

has been classified into *mild* (**hypotaurodontism**), *moderate* (**mesotaurodontism**), and *severe* (**hypertaurodontism**), according to the degree of apical displacement of the pulpal floor (Fig. 2-77). Witkop and colleagues and Shifman and Chanannel presented useful biometric criteria for the determination of taurodontism. These reports contain information that is useful in epidemiologic studies of the process.

Some investigators include examples of taurodontism in premolar teeth; others argue that taurodontism is not shown by premolars. This argument is academic because the presence of taurodontism in premolars cannot be documented *in situ*. Investigations of taurodontism in premolar teeth require the examination of extracted teeth, because the necessary radiographs depict the tooth in a mesiodistal orientation.

Taurodontism may be unilateral or bilateral and affects permanent teeth more frequently than deciduous teeth. There is no sex predilection. The reported prevalence is highly variable (0.5% to 46%) and most likely is related to different diagnostic criteria and racial variations. In the United States most reports indicate a prevalence of 2.5% to 3.2% of the population. Some investigators believe the alteration is more of a variation of normal rather than a definitive pathologic anomaly. The process often demonstrates a field effect, with the involvement of all molars. When this occurs, the first molar is usually affected least, with increasing severity noted in the second and third molars, respectively.

Taurodontism may occur as an isolated trait or as a component of a specific syndrome (Box 2-8). An increased frequency of taurodontism has been reported in patients with hypodontia, cleft lip, and cleft palate. Investigations have shown that taurodontism may develop in the presence of any one of a large

---

Box 2-8

Syndromes Associated with Taurodontism

- Amelogenesis imperfecta, hypoplastic type IE
- Amelogenesis imperfecta-taurodontism type IV
- Cranioectodermal
- Ectodermal dysplasia
- Hyperphosphatasia-oligophrenia-taurodontism
- Hypophosphatasia
- Klinefelter
- Lowe
- Microdontia-taurodontia-dens invaginatus
- Microcephalic dwarfism-taurodontism
- Oculo-dento-digital dysplasia
- Oral-facial-digital type II
- Rapp-Hodgkin
- Scanty hair-oligodontia-taurodontia
- Sex chromosomal aberrations (e.g., XXX, XYY)
- Down
- Tricho-dento-osseous types I, II, and III
- Tricho-onycho-dental
- Wolf-Hirschhorn

---

number of different genetic alterations. These findings suggest that chromosomal abnormalities may disrupt the development of the tooth's form and that taurodontism is not the result of a specific genetic abnormality.

TREATMENT AND PROGNOSIS

Patients with taurodontism require no specific therapy. Coronal extension of the pulp is not seen; therefore, the process does not interfere with routine restorative procedures. Some investigators have suggested the taurodontic shape may exhibit decreased stability and

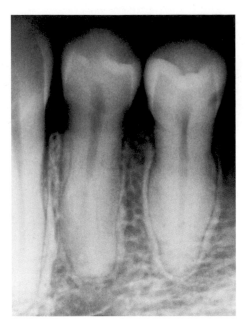

Fig. 2-78   Hypercementosis. Mandibular bicuspids exhibiting thickening and blunting of the roots.

Box 2-9

Factors Associated with Hypercementosis

LOCAL FACTORS
- Abnormal occlusal trauma
- Adjacent inflammation (e.g., pulpal, periapical, periodontal)
- Unopposed teeth (e.g., impacted, embedded, without antagonist)
- Repair of vital root fracture

SYSTEMIC FACTORS
- Acromegaly and pituitary gigantism
- Arthritis
- Calcinosis
- Paget disease of bone
- Rheumatic fever
- Thyroid goiter
- Gardner syndrome
- Vitamin A deficiency (possibly)

strength as an abutment tooth in prosthetic procedures, but this hypothesis has not been verified. If endodontic therapy is required, then the shape of the pulp chamber frequently increases the difficulty of locating, instrumenting, and obturating the pulp canals. One bit of good news is that patients have to demonstrate significant periodontal destruction before bifurcation involvement occurs.

HYPERCEMENTOSIS

Hypercementosis (cemental hyperplasia) is a non-neoplastic deposition of excessive cementum that is continuous with the normal radicular cementum.

CLINICAL AND RADIOGRAPHIC FEATURES

Radiographically, affected teeth demonstrate a thickening or blunting of the root, but the exact amount of increased cementum often is difficult to ascertain because cementum and dentin demonstrate similar radiodensities (Fig. 2-78). The enlarged root is surrounded by the radiolucent PDL space and the adjacent intact lamina dura. On occasion, the enlargement may be significant enough to suggest the possibility of a cementoblastoma (see page 655). However, the cementoblastoma usually can be distinguished on the basis of associated pain, cortical expansion, and continued enlargement.

Hypercementosis may be isolated, involve multiple teeth, or appear as a generalized process. In a study of more than 22,000 affected teeth, the mandibular molars were affected most frequently, followed by the mandibular and maxillary second premolars and mandibular first premolars. In this study, a 2.5:1 mandibular predominance was noted.

Hypercementosis occurs predominantly in adulthood, and the frequency increases with age, most likely secondary to cumulative exposure to causative influences. Its occurrence has been reported in younger patients, and many of these cases demonstrate a familial clustering, suggesting hereditary influence.

Box 2-9 lists several local and systemic factors that have been associated with an increased frequency of the cemental deposition. All of the listed systemic factors exhibit a weak association with hypercementosis except for **Paget's disease of bone** (see page 623). Numerous authors have reported significant hypercementosis in patients with Paget's disease, and this disorder should be considered whenever generalized hypercementosis is discovered in a patient of the appropriate age. In spite of the association with a number of disorders, most localized cases of hypercementosis are not related to any systemic disturbance.

HISTOPATHOLOGIC FEATURES

The periphery of the root exhibits deposition of an excessive amount of cementum over the original layer of primary cementum. The excessive cementum may be hypocellular or exhibit areas of cellular cementum

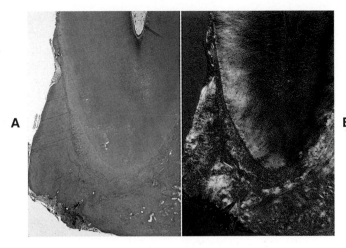

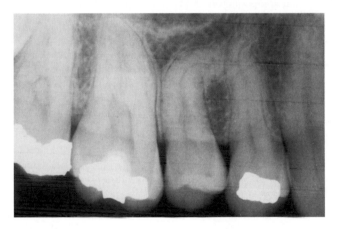

Fig. 2-79   Hypercementosis. A, Dental root exhibiting excessive deposition of cellular and acellular cementum. The dividing line between dentin and cementum is indistinct. **B,** Polarized light demonstrating the sharp dividing line between the tubular dentin and osteocementum.

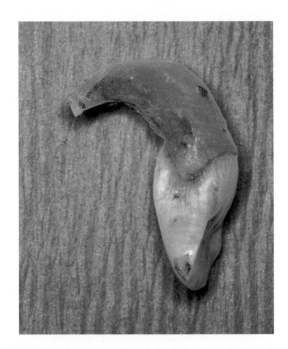

Fig. 2-80   Dilaceration. Sharp curvature of the root of a maxillary central incisor.

that resemble bone (osteocementum). Often the material is arranged in concentric layers and may be applied over the entire root or be limited to the apical portion. On routine light microscopy, distinguishing between dentin and cementum often is difficult, but viewing the section with polarized light helps to discriminate between the two different layers (Fig. 2-79).

TREATMENT AND PROGNOSIS

Patients with hypercementosis require no treatment. Because of a thickened root, occasional problems have been reported during the extraction of an affected tooth. Sectioning of the tooth may be necessary in certain cases to aid in removal.

DILACERATION

Dilaceration is an abnormal angulation or bend in the root or, less frequently, the crown of a tooth (Figs. 2-80 and 2-81). Although most examples are idiopathic, a number of teeth with dilaceration appear to arise after an injury that displaces the calcified portion of the tooth germ, and the remainder of the tooth is formed at an abnormal angle. The damage frequently follows avulsion or intrusion of the overlying primary predecessor, an event that usually occurs before 4 years of age. Injury-related dilaceration more frequently affects the anterior dentition and often creates both a functional and a cosmetic dental problem. Less frequently the bend develops secondary to the presence of an adjacent cyst, tumor, or odontogenic hamartoma (e.g., odontoma, supernumerary tooth) (Fig. 2-82).

Fig. 2-81   Dilaceration. Maxillary second bicuspid exhibiting mesial inclination of the root. The patient reported no history of injury to this area. *(Courtesy of Dr. Lawrence Bean.)*

CLINICAL AND RADIOGRAPHIC FEATURES

In one review of 1166 randomly selected patients, 176 dilacerated teeth were identified. Of these teeth, the most commonly affected were the mandibular third molars, followed by the maxillary second premolars and mandibular second molars. The maxillary and mandibular incisors were the least frequently affected, representing approximately 1% of the series. This contrasts with other authors who have reported a high frequency of dilaceration involving anterior teeth. In reality the molars most likely demonstrate the highest

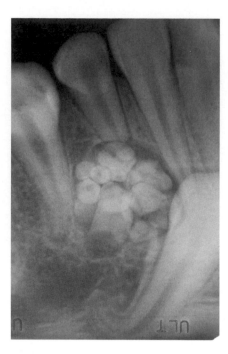

Fig. 2-82 Dilaceration. Root angulation of a mandibular cuspid. Development has been altered by the presence of an adjacent compound odontoma. *(Courtesy of Dr. Brent Bernard.)*

prevalence of dilaceration but are not highlighted because of a lack of associated clinical problems in most instances. Occasionally, involvement of the deciduous teeth is reported, and some have been associated with prior trauma secondary to neonatal laryngoscopy and endotracheal intubation. The age of the patient and the direction and degree of force appear to determine the extent of the tooth's malformation. The abnormal angulation may be present anywhere along the length of the tooth.

Altered maxillary anterior teeth frequently demonstrate the bend in the crown or the coronal half of the root; failure of eruption is often seen. Affected mandibular incisors also exhibit involvement of the crown or the superficial portion of the root, but more frequently they erupt into full occlusion. Those that achieve eruption often follow an altered path and present in a labial or lingual position. Many of the affected teeth, especially anterior mandibular teeth, are nonvital and associated with periapical inflammatory lesions. Typically, altered posterior teeth demonstrate involvement of the apical half of the root and frequently do not exhibit delayed eruption.

TREATMENT AND PROGNOSIS

The treatment and prognosis vary according to the severity of the deformity. Altered deciduous teeth often demonstrate inappropriate resorption and result in delayed eruption of the permanent teeth. Extraction is indicated when necessary for the normal eruption of the succedaneous teeth. Patients with minor dilaceration of permanent teeth frequently require no therapy. Those teeth that exhibit delayed or abnormal eruption may be exposed and orthodontically moved into position. In some cases with extensive deformation of the affected tooth, perforation of the buccal alveolar ridge by the malpositioned root may occur on repositioning. In such cases, amputation of the root apex with subsequent endodontic therapy may be necessary. Grossly deformed teeth require surgical removal. The extraction of affected teeth may be difficult and result in root fracture on removal. When attempting to perform endodontic procedures, the clinician must use great care to avoid root perforation of teeth with significant dilaceration.

Root dilaceration concentrates stress if the affected tooth is used as an abutment for a dental prosthetic appliance. This increased stress may affect the stability and longevity of the abutment tooth. Splinting of the dilacerated tooth to an adjacent tooth results in a multirooted abutment and overcomes the stress-related problems.

SUPERNUMERARY ROOTS

The term **supernumerary roots** refers to the development of an increased number of roots on a tooth compared with that classically described in dental anatomy.

CLINICAL AND RADIOGRAPHIC FEATURES

Any tooth may develop accessory roots, and involvement has been reported in both the deciduous and the permanent dentitions. Data on the frequency of supernumerary roots are sparse, but the prevalence appears to vary significantly among different races. The most frequently affected teeth are the permanent molars (especially third molars) from either arch and mandibular cuspids and premolars (Fig. 2-83). In some instances the supernumerary root is divergent and seen easily on radiographs; in other cases the additional root is small, superimposed over other roots, and difficult to ascertain.

TREATMENT AND PROGNOSIS

No treatment is required for supernumerary roots, but the detection of the accessory root is of critical importance when endodontic therapy or exodontia is undertaken. Extracted teeth always should be examined closely to ensure that all roots have been removed successfully, because accessory roots may not be obvious on the presurgical radiographs. Just as important is the

Table **2-1**   **Classification of Amelogenesis Imperfecta**

Type	Pattern	Specific Features	Inheritance
IA	Hypoplastic	Generalized pitted	Autosomal dominant
IB	Hypoplastic	Localized pitted	Autosomal dominant
IC	Hypoplastic	Localized pitted	Autosomal recessive
ID	Hypoplastic	Diffuse smooth	Autosomal dominant
IE	Hypoplastic	Diffuse smooth	X-linked dominant
IF	Hypoplastic	Diffuse rough	Autosomal dominant
IG	Hypoplastic	Enamel agenesis	Autosomal recessive
IIA	Hypomaturation	Diffuse pigmented	Autosomal recessive
IIB	Hypomaturation	Diffuse	X-linked recessive
IIC	Hypomaturation	Snow-capped	X-linked
IID	Hypomaturation	Snow-capped	Autosomal dominant?
IIIA	Hypocalcified	Diffuse	Autosomal dominant
IIIB	Hypocalcified	Diffuse	Autosomal recessive
IVA	Hypomaturation-hypoplastic	Taurodontism present	Autosomal dominant
IVB	Hypoplastic-hypomaturation	Taurodontism present	Autosomal dominant

Modified from Witkop CJ Jr: Amelogenesis imperfecta, dentinogenesis imperfecta and dentin dysplasia revisited: problems in classification, *J Oral Pathol* 17:547-553, 1988.

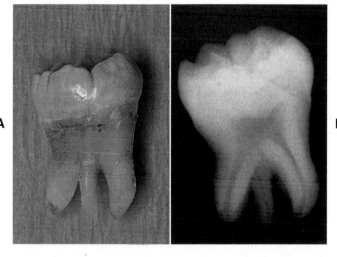

A **B**

Fig. 2-83   Supernumerary root. A, Gross photograph showing a mandibular molar with a supernumerary root. **B,** Periapical radiograph of the extracted tooth.

search for accessory canals during endodontic access procedures, because failure to discover these additional openings often results in a lack of resolution of the associated inflammatory process.

DEVELOPMENTAL ALTERATIONS IN THE STRUCTURE OF TEETH

AMELOGENESIS IMPERFECTA

Amelogenesis imperfecta encompasses a complicated group of conditions that demonstrate developmental alterations in the structure of the enamel in the absence of a systemic disorder. Box 2-2 (see page 55) lists several systemic diseases associated with enamel disorders that are not considered isolated amelogenesis imperfecta.

At least 14 different hereditary subtypes of amelogenesis imperfecta exist, with numerous patterns of inheritance and a wide variety of clinical manifestations. As proof of the complicated nature of the process, several different classification systems exist. The most widely accepted is that developed by Witkop (Table 2-1), and this part of the text adheres to this classification. The dissertation by Witkop and Sauk (and Witkop's 1988 review) are works of art, and they should be used if the clinician desires more information.

An ideal classification system for amelogenesis imperfecta has not been established yet. Witkop's classification relies on the phenotype and pedigree (i.e., clinical appearance and apparent pattern of inheritance). Classification by clinical appearance is problematic, because different phenotypes have been noted within a single affected family. In addition, similar phenotypes may be seen in individuals with very different molecular patterns of disease. One example of the potential confusion occurs in kindreds affected with certain variants of autosomal dominant amelogenesis imperfecta in which homozygotes exhibit generalized thin hypoplasia, whereas heterozygotes exhibit localized enamel pitting. Using the current nomenclature, different individuals within this kindred would be placed into multiple categories (e.g., types IB, ID, IF).

Although the molecular basis underlying the majority of amelogenesis imperfecta remains poorly defined, the genetics associated with several variations of amelo-

Table **2-2**   **Modified Classification of Amelogenesis Imperfecta**

Inheritance	Phenotype	Related Genes
Autosomal dominant	Generalized pitted	
Autosomal dominant	Localized hypoplastic	ENAM
Autosomal dominant	Generalized thin	ENAM
Autosomal dominant	Hypocalcification	
Autosomal dominant	With taurodontism	DLX3
Autosomal recessive	Localized hypoplastic	
Autosomal recessive	Generalized thin	
Autosomal recessive	Pigmented hypomaturation	MMP20, KLK4
Autosomal recessive	Hypocalcification	
X-linked	Generalized thin	AMELX
X-linked	Diffuse hypomaturation	AMELX
X-linked	Snow-capped hypomaturation	

genesis imperfecta has been clarified. This has led investigators to suggest a future classification system based primarily on the mode of inheritance with secondary discriminators that include the phenotype and molecular basis (site of chromosomal mutation, when known). Although the push for a new classification system is not new, the progress in defining the molecular genetics of amelogenesis imperfecta has been slow and currently prevents complete agreement on a transition to a genetics-directed system of classification. As the molecular basis of the disease becomes better clarified, the move to a new pattern of classification seems inevitable.

Investigations into the genetics are ongoing and producing results that are not only interesting but also directly applicable to patient care. To date, mutations in five genes have been associated with amelogenesis imperfecta. Each gene can be mutated in a variety of ways, often creating diverse and distinct phenotypic patterns.

The **AMELX gene** is associated with the enamel protein **amelogenin,** which constitutes up to 90% of enamel matrix. AMELX-associated variants of amelogenesis imperfecta are X-linked with 14 different mutations currently known. Because of the effect of lyonization, the male and female phenotypes are variable but often associated with the genotype. The male phenotypes include both the diffuse smooth hypoplastic and the hypomaturation variants.

The **ENAM gene** is associated with another enamel protein, **enamelin,** which represents approximately 1% to 5% of enamel matrix. Mutations of the ENAM gene have been correlated with some autosomal dominant and recessive patterns of hypoplastic amelogenesis imperfecta, ranging from minor pitting to diffuse generalized thin enamel.

The **MMP-20 gene** codes for a proteinase named **enamelysin;** mutation of this gene has been associated with the autosomal recessive, pigmented hypomaturation variant of amelogenesis imperfecta.

The protease, **kallikrein-4**, is associated with the **KLK4 gene**, the mutation of which has been shown to be involved with some forms of hypomaturation amelogenesis imperfecta. Both enamelysin and kallikrein-4 are thought necessary for the removal of enamel matrix proteins during the maturation stage of enamel development.

The **DLX3 gene** is in a group of genes that code for a number of proteins that are critical for craniofacial, tooth, hair, brain, and neural development; mutation of this gene has been associated with the hypoplastic-hypomaturation variants of amelogenesis imperfecta with taurodontism.

Another strong candidate is the **AMBN gene** that codes for the protein **ameloblastin,** which constitutes about 5% of enamel matrix. Although not proven to be associated with amelogenesis imperfecta, this gene locus is a strong candidate for some of the autosomal dominant patterns.

Although no one has compiled a complete list of amelogenesis imperfecta types using the proposed new classification, Table 2-2 provides a rough idea of how this might be organized. Despite these exciting molecular genetic discoveries, it must be stressed how little is known and how much remains to be investigated. When studying large numbers of kindreds affected by amelogenesis imperfecta, only rare families will demonstrate mutation of one of the currently known genes.

The formation of enamel is a multistep process, and problems may arise in any one of the steps. In general, the development of enamel can be divided into three major stages:
1. Elaboration of the organic matrix
2. Mineralization of the matrix
3. Maturation of the enamel

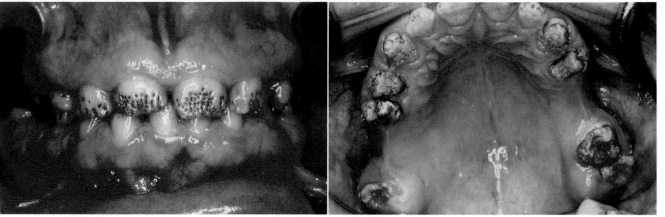

Fig. 2-84 **Hypoplastic amelogenesis imperfecta, generalized pitted pattern. A,** Note the numerous pinpoint pits scattered across the surface of the teeth. The enamel between the pits is of normal thickness, hardness, and coloration. **B,** Occlusal view of same patient showing diffuse involvement of all maxillary teeth, which would be inconsistent with environmental damage. *(A from Stewart RE, Prescott GH: Oral facial genetics, St Louis, 1976, Mosby;* **B** *courtesy of Dr. Joseph S. Giansanti.)*

The hereditary defects of the formation of enamel also are divided along these lines: hypoplastic, hypocalcified, and hypomaturation.

CLINICAL AND RADIOGRAPHIC FEATURES

Amelogenesis imperfecta may be inherited as an autosomal dominant, autosomal recessive, or X-linked disorder, with an estimated frequency between 1:718 and 1:14,000 of the population. As in any hereditary condition, clustering of affected patients in certain geographic areas may occur (resulting in an increased prevalence of the disorder in those areas). Additionally, the stringency of the diagnostic criteria may influence the reported prevalence in any given study. In general, both the deciduous and the permanent dentitions are diffusely involved.

HYPOPLASTIC AMELOGENESIS IMPERFECTA

In patients with hypoplastic amelogenesis imperfecta, the basic alteration centers on inadequate deposition of enamel matrix. Any matrix present is mineralized appropriately and radiographically contrasts well with the underlying dentin. In the **generalized pattern,** pinpoint-to-pinhead–sized pits are scattered across the surface of the teeth and do not correlate with a pattern of environmental damage (Fig. 2-84). The buccal surfaces of the teeth are affected more severely, and the pits may be arranged in rows or columns. Staining of the pits may occur. Variable expressivity is seen within groups of affected patients. The enamel between the pits is of normal thickness, hardness, and coloration.

In the **localized pattern,** the affected teeth demonstrate horizontal rows of pits, a linear depression, or one large area of hypoplastic enamel surrounded by a zone of hypocalcification. Typically, the altered area is located in the middle third of the buccal surfaces of the teeth. The incisal edge or occlusal surface usually is not affected. Both dentitions (or only the primary teeth) may be affected. All the teeth may be altered, or only scattered teeth may be affected. When the involvement is not diffuse, the pattern of affected teeth does not correlate with a specific time in development. The autosomal recessive type (type IC) is more severe and typically demonstrates involvement of all teeth in both dentitions.

In the **autosomal dominant smooth pattern,** the enamel of all teeth exhibits a smooth surface and is thin, hard, and glossy (Fig. 2-85). The absence of appropriate enamel thickness results in teeth that are shaped like crown preparations and demonstrate open contact points. The color of the teeth varies from opaque white to translucent brown. Anterior open bite is not rare. Radiographically, the teeth exhibit a thin peripheral outline of radiopaque enamel. Often, unerupted teeth exhibiting resorption are seen.

The **X-linked smooth pattern** has been stated to arise from an X-linked dominant mutation and is a lesson in the lyonization effect. On approximately the sixteenth day of embryonic life in all individuals with two X chromosomes, one member of the pair is inactivated in each cell. As a result of this event, females are mosaics, with a mixture of cells, some with active maternal X chromosomes and others with active paternal X chromosomes. Usually the mix is of

the coronal enamel is removed, except for the cervical portion that is occasionally calcified better. Unerupted teeth and anterior open bite are not rare. Both patterns are similar, but the autosomal recessive examples are generally more severe than the autosomal dominant cases. Radiographically, the density of the enamel and dentin are similar. Before eruption the teeth are normal in shape; however, after a period of function much of the cuspal enamel is lost, with the occlusal surface becoming the most irregular.

AMELOGENESIS IMPERFECTA WITH TAURODONTISM (HYPOMATURATION/ HYPOPLASTIC AMELOGENESIS IMPERFECTA)

This type of amelogenesis imperfecta exhibits enamel hypoplasia in combination with hypomaturation. The deciduous and the permanent dentitions are diffusely involved. Historically, two patterns have been recognized that are similar but differentiated by the thickness of the enamel and the overall tooth size. When studying a single kindred, phenotypic variation is seen that would place members of the same family in both

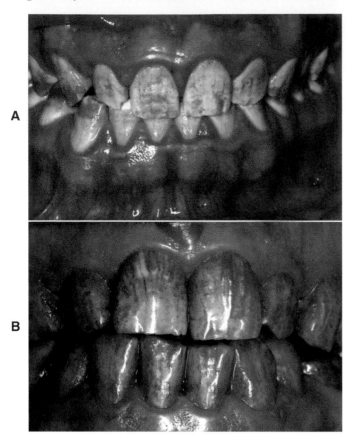

Fig. 2-87   Hypomaturation amelogenesis imperfecta, X-linked. A, Male patient exhibiting diffuse yellow-white dentition. **B,** The patient's mother exhibits vertical bands of white, opaque enamel and translucent enamel. *(Courtesy of Dr. Carlos Salinas.)*

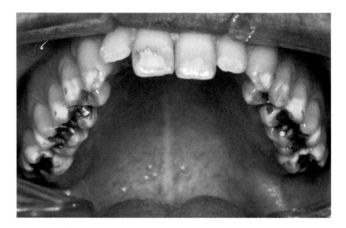

Fig. 2-88   Hypomaturation amelogenesis imperfecta, snow-capped pattern. Dentition exhibiting zone of white opaque enamel in the incisal and occlusal one fourth of the enamel surface. *(Courtesy of Dr. Heddie O. Sedano.)*

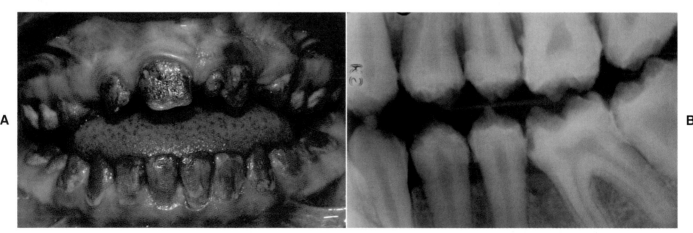

Fig. 2-89   Hypocalcified amelogenesis imperfecta. A, Dentition exhibiting diffuse yellow-brown discoloration. Note numerous teeth with loss of coronal enamel except for the cervical portion. **B,** Radiograph of the same patient. Note the extensive loss of coronal enamel and the similar density of enamel and dentin.

divisions; therefore, many believe these divisions should be joined into one phenotype termed merely **amelogenesis imperfecta with taurodontism.**

In the presentation known as the **hypomaturation-hypoplastic pattern,** the predominant defect is one of enamel hypomaturation in which the enamel appears as mottled yellow-white to yellow-brown. Pits are seen frequently on the buccal surfaces of the teeth. Radiographically, the enamel appears similar to dentin in density, and large pulp chambers may be seen in single-rooted teeth in addition to varying degrees of taurodontism.

In the **hypoplastic-hypomaturation pattern,** the predominant defect is one of enamel hypoplasia in which the enamel is thin but also hypomature. Except for the decrease in the thickness of the enamel, this pattern is radiographically similar to the hypomaturation-hypoplastic variant.

A pattern of teeth alteration similar to amelogenesis imperfecta with taurodontism is seen in the systemic disorder, **tricho-dento-osseous syndrome.** This autosomal dominant disorder is mentioned here because the diagnosis may not be readily apparent without a high index of suspicion (Fig. 2-90). In addition to the dental findings, the predominant systemic changes are present variably and include kinky hair, osteosclerosis, and brittle nails. The kinky hair is present at birth but may straighten with age. The osteosclerosis primarily affects the base of the skull and the mastoid process. The mandible often exhibits a shortened ramus and an obtuse angle.

Some authors have suggested that amelogenesis imperfecta with taurodontism may represent partial expression of the tricho-dento-osseous syndrome. Recent studies have identified distinctly different gene mutations that are responsible for tricho-dento-osseous syndrome and amelogenesis imperfecta with taurodontism. However, other investigators dispute this fact, showing evidence that some examples of this pattern of amelogenesis imperfecta appear allelic (different mutation on the same gene) to the syndrome. If only dental changes are seen in the absence of hair or bone changes, either in the individual or within the family, then the diagnosis of amelogenesis imperfecta appears appropriate.

HISTOPATHOLOGIC FEATURES

The histopathologic alterations present in amelogenesis imperfecta are not evident in routine preparations. Because decalcification of the teeth is necessary before processing to allow sectioning of paraffin-embedded specimens, all the enamel is lost. To examine the enamel structure of altered teeth, ground sections of nondecalcified specimens are prepared. The alterations discovered are highly diverse and vary with each clinical type of amelogenesis imperfecta. Detailed descriptions of such alterations were provided by Witkop and Sauk.

TREATMENT AND PROGNOSIS

The clinical implications of amelogenesis imperfecta vary according to the subtype and its severity, but the main problems are aesthetics, dental sensitivity, and loss of vertical dimension. In addition, in some types of amelogenesis imperfecta there is an increased prevalence of caries, anterior open bite, delayed eruption, tooth impaction, or associated gingival inflammation.

A 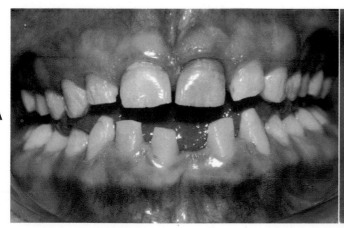 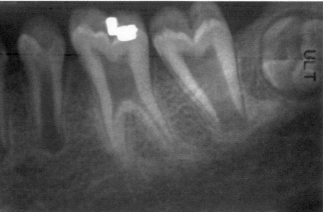 **B**

Fig. 2-90   Tricho-dento-osseous syndrome. A, Dentition exhibiting diffuse enamel hypoplasia and hypomaturation. At birth, the patient exhibited a kinky "steel wool" texture to her hair; with time, the hair straightened. A high index of suspicion was required to arrive at the diagnosis. **B,** Radiograph of the same patient showing significant taurodontism of the first molar and thin enamel, which is similar in density to the dentin.

Table **2-3** **Dentinogenesis Imperfecta**

Shields	Clinical Presentation	Witkop
Dentinogenesis imperfecta I	Osteogenesis imperfecta with opalescent teeth	Dentinogenesis imperfecta
Dentinogenesis imperfecta II	Isolated opalescent teeth	Hereditary opalescent teeth
Dentinogenesis imperfecta III	Isolated opalescent teeth	Brandywine isolate

Data from Shields ED: A new classification of heritable human enamel defects and a discussion of dentin defects. In Jorgenson RJ, Paul NW: *Dentition: genetic effects (birth defects original article series)*, vol 19, no. 1, pp 107-127, New York, 1983, Alan R Liss; Witkop CJ Jr: Amelogenesis imperfecta, dentinogenesis imperfecta and dentin dysplasia revisited: problems in classification, *J Oral Pathol* 17:547-553, 1988.

Patients with generalized thin enamel hypoplasia demonstrate minimal normal enamel associated with rapid attrition. These variants require full coverage as soon as is practical; if the treatment is delayed, a loss of usable crown length occurs. In those patients without sufficient crown lengths, full dentures (overdentures in some cases) often become the only satisfactory approach.

The other types of amelogenesis imperfecta demonstrate less rapid tooth loss, and the aesthetic appearance often is the prime consideration. Many less severe cases can be improved by the placement of full crowns or facial veneers on clinically objectionable teeth. In some cases a lack of good enamel bonding of veneers occurs and does not result in a durable restoration. The use of glass ionomer cements with dentinal adhesives often overcomes this weakness.

DENTINOGENESIS IMPERFECTA (HEREDITARY OPALESCENT DENTIN; CAPDEPONT'S TEETH)

Dentinogenesis imperfecta is a hereditary developmental disturbance of the dentin in the absence of any systemic disorder. Similar dental changes may be seen in conjunction with the systemic hereditary disorder of bone, **osteogenesis imperfecta** (see page 613). Dentin defects associated with this bone disease are termed **osteogenesis imperfecta with opalescent teeth.** Extensive pedigrees of individuals with dentinogenesis imperfecta have been studied, and none have exhibited other changes suggestive of osteogenesis imperfecta. Genetic research has confirmed that osteogenesis imperfecta with opalescent teeth clearly is a separate disease from dentinogenesis imperfecta.

The various types of osteogenesis imperfecta have been associated with mutation of the **COL1A1** or **COL1A2 gene** that encodes production of type I collagen; in contrast, dentinogenesis imperfecta is associated with mutation of the **DSPP** (dentin sialophosphoprotein) **gene.** Currently, eight mutations of the DSPP gene are known; seven are associated with dentinogenesis imperfecta, with the eighth known to create dentin dysplasia type II.

Like amelogenesis imperfecta, the classification of the disorders of dentin is gradually evolving as the result of these recent molecular genetic findings. Two systems, one by Witkop and the other by Shields, historically were well accepted but not totally satisfactory (Table 2-3). Dentinogenesis imperfecta formerly was divided into *hereditary opalescent dentin* (Shields type II) and the *Brandywine isolate* (Shields type III).

The defining phenotypic feature of the Brandywine isolate was the presence of unusual pulpal enlargement known as *shell teeth.* Current evidence strongly suggests that the Brandywine isolate represents nothing more than variable expressivity of the gene for dentinogenesis imperfecta. The original review of the isolate revealed only 8% of the kindred with shell teeth. Investigators have documented enlarged pulps in affected individuals whose parents and children have classic dentinogenesis imperfecta. Finally, identical patterns of expression have been seen in other large kindreds with no connection to the Brandywine isolate. Subsequently, a single mutation of the *DSPP* gene has been shown to cause both phenotypic patterns, strongly supporting the assumption that the phenotypes previously termed *dentinogenesis imperfecta type II* and *dentinogenesis imperfecta type III* represent a single disease with variable expressions. A modified classification of dentin disorders therefore seems warranted (Table 2-4), and continued use of the Shields or Witkop nomenclature does not appear justified.

CLINICAL AND RADIOGRAPHIC FEATURES

The prevalence of dentinogenesis imperfecta is not randomly distributed throughout the United States and Europe. Most cases can be traced to whites (people of English or French ancestry) from communities close to the English Channel. The disorder is autosomal dominant and occurs in about 1:8000 whites in the United States.

The dental alterations in dentinogenesis imperfecta and osteogenesis imperfecta with opalescent teeth are similar clinically, radiographically, and histopathologically. All teeth in both dentitions are affected. The

Table **2-4**   **Modified Classification of Hereditary Disorders Affecting Dentin**

Disorder	Inheritance	Involved Gene or Genes
Osteogenesis imperfecta with opalescent teeth	Autosomal dominant or recessive	*COL1A1, COL1A2*
Dentinogenesis imperfecta	Autosomal dominant	*DSPP*
Dentin dysplasia type I	Autosomal dominant	
Dentin dysplasia type II	Autosomal dominant	*DSPP*

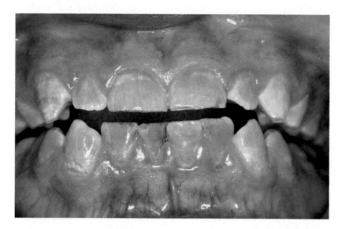

Fig. 2-91   Dentinogenesis imperfecta. Dentition exhibiting diffuse brownish discoloration and slight translucence.

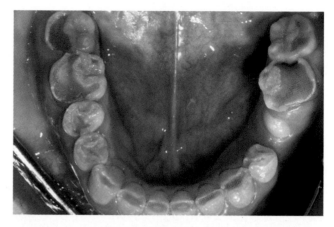

Fig. 2-92   Dentinogenesis imperfecta. Dentition exhibiting grayish discoloration with significant enamel loss and attrition.

severity of the dental alterations varies with the age at which the tooth developed. Deciduous teeth are affected most severely, followed by the permanent incisors and first molars, with the second and third molars being least altered.

The dentitions have a blue-to-brown discoloration, often with a distinctive translucence (Fig. 2-91). The enamel frequently separates easily from the underlying defective dentin. Once exposed, the dentin often demonstrates significantly accelerated attrition (Fig. 2-92). Radiographically, the teeth have bulbous crowns, cervical constriction, thin roots, and early obliteration of the root canals and pulp chambers (Fig. 2-93).

The trait exhibits close to 100% penetrance but variable expressivity. Significant, clinically obvious enamel hypoplasia is noted in some patients (Fig. 2-94). Researchers believe that the enamel abnormality is a secondary defect and not a direct expression of the dentinogenesis imperfecta gene. Although the pulps are usually obliterated by excess dentin production, some teeth may show normal-sized pulps or pulpal enlargement (shell teeth).

Shell teeth demonstrate normal-thickness enamel in association with extremely thin dentin and dramatically enlarged pulps (Fig. 2-95). The thin dentin may involve the entire tooth or be isolated to the root. This

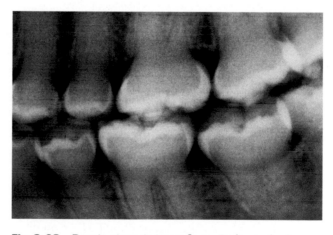

Fig. 2-93   Dentinogenesis imperfecta. Radiograph of dentition exhibiting bulbous crowns, cervical constriction, and obliterated pulp canals and chambers.

rare abnormality has been seen most frequently in deciduous teeth in the presence of dentinogenesis imperfecta. The alteration may be unassociated with dentinogenesis imperfecta as an isolated finding in both dentitions and demonstrate normal tooth shape and coloration, a negative family history, and diffuse involvement. In the isolated variant, slow but progressive root resorption occurs.

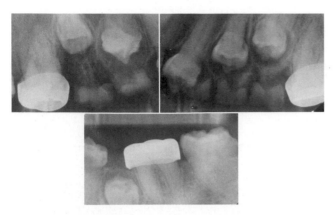

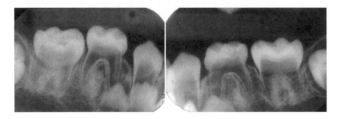

Fig. 2-94 Dentinogenesis imperfecta. Radiograph of dentition exhibiting bulbous crowns, early obliteration of the pulp, and enamel hypoplasia. *(From Levin LS, Leaf SH, Jelmine RJ et al: Dentinogenesis imperfecta in the Brandywine isolate (DI type III): clinical, radiologic, and scanning electron microscopic studies of the dentition, Oral Surg Oral Med Oral Pathol 56:267-274, 1983.)*

Fig. 2-95 Shell teeth. Dentition exhibiting normal thickness enamel, extremely thin dentin, and dramatically enlarged pulps.

Several kindreds affected with dentinogenesis imperfecta also have been shown to demonstrate progressive, sensorineural, high-frequency hearing loss. Jaw position has been shown to affect the anatomy of the inner ear, and premature tooth loss has been associated with hearing deficits. At this time, it is unclear if the hearing loss is correlated with the *DSPP* mutation or an alteration secondary to the primary gnathic changes. Investigators wonder if dental restoration may prevent the hearing loss or if the *DSPP* gene may directly affect bone formation and the structure of the inner ear.

HISTOPATHOLOGIC FEATURES

As expected, affected teeth demonstrate altered dentin. The dentin adjacent to the enamel junction appears similar to normal dentin, but the remainder is distinctly abnormal. Short misshapen tubules course through an atypical granular dentin matrix, which often demonstrates interglobular calcification (Fig. 2-96). Scanty atypical odontoblasts line the pulp surface, and cells

Fig. 2-96 Dentinogenesis imperfecta. Coronal dentin exhibiting short misshapen tubules within atypical granular dentin matrix.

can be seen entrapped within the defective dentin. In ground sections the enamel is normal in most patients; however, about one third of the patients have hypoplastic or hypocalcified defects.

TREATMENT AND PROGNOSIS

The entire dentition is at risk because of numerous problems. The root canals become threadlike and may develop microexposures, resulting in periapical inflammatory lesions. In spite of the risk of enamel loss and significant attrition, the teeth are not good candidates for full crowns because of cervical fracture. The success of full coverage is best in teeth with crowns and roots that exhibit close to a normal shape and size. Overlay dentures placed on teeth that are covered with fluoride-releasing glass ionomer cement have been used with success in some cases.

Additional therapeutic approaches have been used, but long-term follow-up is incomplete. In patients with extensive attrition, the vertical dimension has been rebuilt by placing nonprecious metal castings with adhesive luting agents on teeth that have received no preparation and are not subject to significant occlusal stress. The newer composites combined with a dentin-bonding agent have been used in areas subject to occlusal wear. When large kindreds have been followed over a long term, most of those affected are candidates for full dentures or implants by 30 years of age in spite of the numerous interventions. Newer materials and interventions may alter this outlook.

DENTIN DYSPLASIA

Dentin dysplasia was initially categorized in 1939. Two major patterns exist: type I and type II. By definition, dentin dysplasia should have no correlation with sys-

Systemic Diseases Correlated with Dentin Dysplasia-like Alterations

- Calcinosis universalis
- Rheumatoid arthritis and vitaminosis D
- Sclerotic bone and skeletal anomalies
- Tumoral calcinosis

temic disease or dentinogenesis imperfecta. An unusual combination of type I and type II dentin dysplasia has been reported, but these cases represent variable pulpal anatomy that has been documented well in dentin dysplasia type I. Systemic diseases reported to be associated with similar dentin changes are listed in Box 2-10.

As evidenced by the clinical and radiographic descriptions that follow, dentin dysplasia type II is closely related to dentinogenesis imperfecta. In addition, genetic evaluation has shown that dentin dysplasia type II arises from mutation of the *DSPP* gene (see Dentinogenesis Imperfecta) and is allelic (different mutation of the same gene) to dentinogenesis imperfecta. The phenotypic and genotypic findings are so close that some might choose to classify dentin dysplasia type II as a variation of dentinogenesis imperfecta rather than grouping it with dentin dysplasia type I. Indeed, before the current era of molecular genetics, Witkop remarked on the close similarities of these two diseases and mentioned the possibility of reclassification.

CLINICAL AND RADIOGRAPHIC FEATURES

DENTIN DYSPLASIA TYPE I

Dentin dysplasia type I (radicular dentin dysplasia), has been referred to as **rootless teeth,** because the loss of organization of the root dentin often leads to a shortened root length. The process exhibits an autosomal dominant pattern of inheritance and an approximate prevalence of 1:100,000. The enamel and coronal dentin are normal clinically and well formed (Fig. 2-97), but the radicular dentin loses all organization and subsequently is shortened dramatically (Fig. 2-98). Wide variation in root formation is produced because dentinal disorganization may occur during different stages of tooth development. If the dentin organization is lost early in tooth development, markedly deficient roots are formed; later disorganization results in minimal root malformation. The variability is most pronounced in permanent teeth and

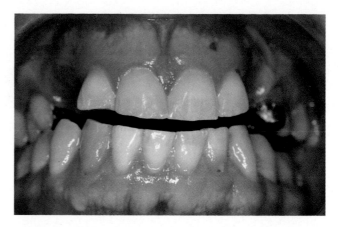

Fig. 2-97 Dentin dysplasia type I. Dentition exhibiting attrition but otherwise normal coronal coloration and morphology.

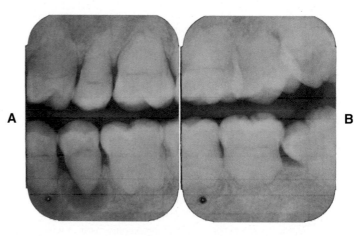

Fig. 2-98 Dentin dysplasia type I. Posterior dentition exhibiting dramatically shortened roots, absence of pulp canals, and small, crescent-shaped pulp chambers. Note radiolucency at apex of mandibular bicuspid. *(Courtesy of Dr. Michael Quinn.)*

may vary not only from patient to patient but also from tooth to tooth in a single patient. Because of the shortened roots, the initial clinical signs are extreme tooth mobility and premature exfoliation, spontaneously or secondary to minor trauma. Less frequently, delayed eruption is the presenting symptom. The strength of the radicular dentin is reduced, with the teeth being predisposed to fracture during extractions.

Radiographically, the deciduous teeth often are affected severely, with little or no detectable pulp, and roots that are markedly short or absent. The permanent teeth vary according to the proportion of organized versus disorganized dentin (Fig. 2-99). Several years ago, a subclassification of dentin dysplasia type I was proposed and has become widely accepted (Box 2-11).

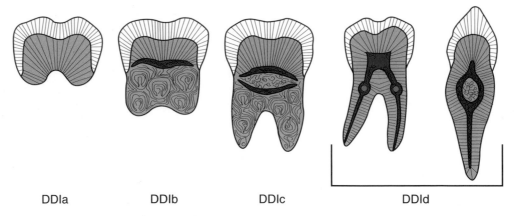

DDIa   DDIb   DDIc   DDId

Fig. 2-99   Dentin dysplasia type I. Illustration demonstrating the variability of the radiographic appearance according to the degree of dentin disorganization within the root.

Subclassification of Dentin Dysplasia Type I

- DDIa: No pulp chambers, no root formation, and frequent periapical radiolucencies
- DDIb: A single small horizontally oriented and crescent-shaped pulp, roots only a few millimeters in length, and frequent periapical radiolucencies
- DDIc: Two horizontally oriented and crescent-shaped pulpal remnants surrounding a central island of dentin, significant but shortened root length, and variable periapical radiolucencies
- DDId: Visible pulp chambers and canals, near normal root length, enlarged pulp stones that are located in the coronal portion of the canal and create a localized bulging of the canal and root, constriction of the pulp canal apical to the stone, and few periapical radiolucencies

---

In general, the teeth without root canals are those that frequently develop periapical radiolucencies without obvious cause (see Fig. 2-98). The radiolucencies represent periapical inflammatory disease and appear secondary to caries or spontaneous coronal exposure of microscopic threads of pulpal remnants present within the defective dentin. The subclassification system has proven to be beneficial, because it assists in highlighting the mild DDId variant that often is not quickly recognized as dentin dysplasia and can be confused with dentin dysplasia type II. On occasion, reports have demonstrated patients with classic DDId-like involvement of the anteriors and bicuspids but without affected molars.

A similar but unrelated disorder is **fibrous dysplasia of dentin.** This autosomal dominant disorder exhibits teeth that are normal clinically. Radiographically the teeth are normal in shape but demonstrate a radiodense product filling the pulp chambers and canals. In contrast to dentinogenesis imperfecta, small foci of radiolucency can be seen in the pulp. In contrast to dentin dysplasia type I, no crescent pulp chambers and no decrease in root length are seen. The radiodense intrapulpal material consists of fibrotic dentin.

DENTIN DYSPLASIA TYPE II

Dentin dysplasia type II (coronal dentin dysplasia) is inherited as an autosomal dominant hereditary disorder that exhibits numerous features of dentinogenesis imperfecta. In contrast to dentin dysplasia type I, the root length is normal in both dentitions. The deciduous teeth closely resemble those of dentinogenesis imperfecta. Clinically, the teeth demonstrate a blue-to-amber-to-brown translucence. Radiographically, the dental changes include bulbous crowns, cervical constriction, thin roots, and early obliteration of the pulp. The permanent teeth demonstrate normal clinical coloration; however, radiographically, the pulp chambers exhibit significant enlargement and apical extension. This altered pulpal anatomy has been described as *thistle tube-shaped* or *flame-shaped* (Figs. 2-100 and 2-101). Pulp stones develop in the enlarged pulp chambers.

A similar but unrelated disorder is **pulpal dysplasia.** This process develops in teeth that are normal clinically. Radiographically, both dentitions exhibit thistle tube–shaped pulp chambers and multiple pulp stones.

HISTOPATHOLOGIC FEATURES

In patients with dentin dysplasia type I, the coronal enamel and dentin are normal. Apical to the point of disorganization, the central portion of the root forms

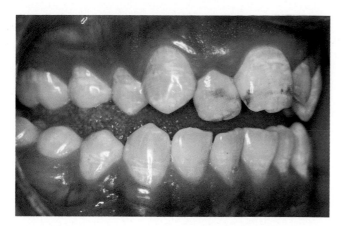

Fig. 2-100 **Dentin dysplasia type II.** Permanent dentition that does not exhibit translucence, as noted in the deciduous teeth. The patient also exhibits mild fluorosis of the enamel.

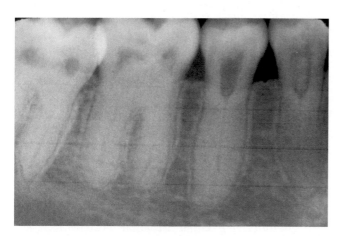

Fig. 2-101 **Dentin dysplasia type II.** Radiographic appearance of the dentition depicted in Fig. 2-100. Note thistle tube-shaped enlargements of the pulp chambers and numerous pulp stones.

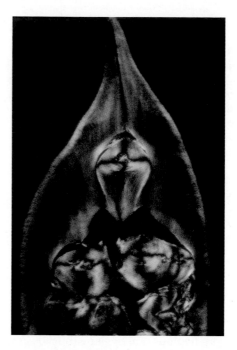

Fig. 2-102 **Dentin dysplasia type I.** Polarized light view of affected tooth demonstrating a classic "stream flowing around boulders" appearance.

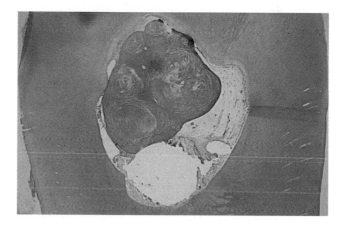

Fig. 2-103 **Dentin dysplasia type II.** Affected tooth exhibiting large pulp stone within the pulp chamber.

whorls of tubular dentin and atypical osteodentin. These whorls exhibit a peripheral layer of normal dentin, giving the root the appearance of a "stream flowing around boulders" (Fig. 2-102).

In patients with dentin dysplasia type II, the deciduous teeth demonstrate the pattern described in dentinogenesis imperfecta. The permanent teeth exhibit normal enamel and coronal dentin. Adjacent to the pulp, numerous areas of interglobular dentin are seen. The radicular dentin is atubular, amorphous, and hypertrophic. Pulp stones develop in any portion of the chamber (Fig. 2-103).

TREATMENT AND PROGNOSIS

In patients with dentin dysplasia type I, preventive care is of foremost importance. Perhaps as a result of short-

ened roots, early loss from periodontitis is frequent. In addition, pulp vascular channels extend close to the dentinoenamel junction; therefore, even shallow occlusal restorations can result in pulpal necrosis. Meticulous oral hygiene must be established and maintained.

If periapical inflammatory lesions develop, the root length guides the therapeutic choice. Conventional endodontic therapy requires mechanical creation of canal paths and has been successful in teeth without extremely short roots. Teeth with short roots demonstrate pulpal ramifications that eliminate conventional

Box 2-12

Pathoses Noted in Association with Regional Odontodysplasia

- Ectodermal dysplasia
- Epidermal nevi
- Hypophosphatasia
- Hydrocephalus
- Ipsilateral facial hypoplasia
- Neurofibromatosis
- Orbital coloboma
- Rh factor incompatibility
- Vascular nevi

Box 2-13

Proposed Causations for Regional Odontodysplasia

- Abnormal migration of neural crest cells
- Latent virus
- Local circulatory deficiency
- Local trauma or infection
- Hyperpyrexia
- Malnutrition
- Medication used during pregnancy
- Radiation therapy
- Somatic mutation

endodontic treatment as an appropriate therapeutic option. Periapical curettage and retrograde amalgam seals have demonstrated short-term success.

Dentin dysplasia type II demonstrates similar problems, and meticulous oral hygiene must be established. The deciduous teeth can be approached in a manner similar to that used for dentinogenesis imperfecta. In the permanent teeth, an increased risk of periapical inflammatory lesions is also seen. Because the pulp canals are not usually obliterated completely, endodontic therapy is accomplished more readily.

REGIONAL ODONTODYSPLASIA (GHOST TEETH)

Regional odontodysplasia is a localized, nonhereditary developmental abnormality of teeth with extensive adverse effects on the formation of enamel, dentin, and pulp. Most cases are idiopathic, but a number have been related to various syndromes, growth abnormalities, neural disorders, and vascular malformations (Box 2-12). A number of causes have been proposed (Box 2-13), but the most popular theory revolves around an alteration in the vascular supply. Several cases have occurred in patients with vascular nevi of the head and neck; in addition, similar changes have been induced in animals by restricting the vascular flow to an area of the jaws.

CLINICAL AND RADIOGRAPHIC FEATURES

Regional odontodysplasia is an uncommon finding that occurs in both dentitions and exhibits no racial predilection and a slight female predominance. A review of the age at the time of diagnosis reveals a bimodal peak that correlates with the normal time of eruption of the deciduous (2 to 4 years) and permanent (7 to 11 years) dentitions. Typically, the process affects a focal area of

the dentition, with involvement of several contiguous teeth. A maxillary predominance exists with a predilection for the anterior teeth. Occasionally, an unaffected tooth may be intermixed within a row of altered teeth. Ipsilateral involvement of both arches and bilateral changes in the same jaw have been reported. Although rare generalized involvement has been documented, the presence of regional odontodysplasia in more than two quadrants is rare. Involvement of the deciduous dentition is typically followed by similarly affected permanent teeth. In the area of altered teeth, the surrounding bone often exhibits a lower density; in addition, hyperplasia of the soft tissue may be noted overlying affected teeth that are impacted.

Many of the affected teeth fail to erupt. Erupted teeth demonstrate small irregular crowns that are yellow to brown, often with a very rough surface. Caries and associated periapical inflammatory lesions are fairly common. Because of dentinal clefts and very long pulp horns, pulpal necrosis is common (often in the absence of an obvious cause). Radiographically, the altered teeth demonstrate extremely thin enamel and dentin surrounding an enlarged radiolucent pulp, resulting in a pale wispy image of a tooth; hence the term **ghost teeth** (Fig. 2-104). A lack of contrast is seen between the dentin and the enamel, with an indistinct or "fuzzy" appearance of the coronal silhouette. Short roots and open apices may be seen. The enlarged pulps frequently demonstrate one or more prominent pulp stones. The most common presenting signs and symptoms include delayed or failure of eruption, early exfoliation, abscess formation, malformed teeth, and noninflammatory gingival enlargement.

HISTOPATHOLOGIC FEATURES

In ground sections the thickness of the enamel varies, resulting in an irregular surface. The prism structure of the enamel is irregular or lacking with a laminated

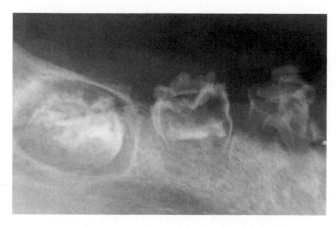

Fig. 2-104 Regional odontodysplasia (ghost teeth).
Posterior mandibular dentition exhibiting enlarged pulps and
extremely thin enamel and dentin. *(Courtesy of Dr. John B. Perry.)*

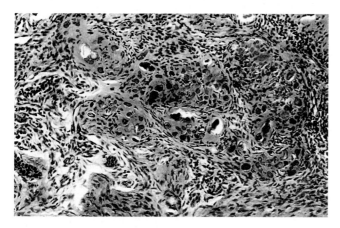

Fig. 2-105 Regional odontodysplasia. Follicular tissue
contains scattered collections of enameloid conglomerates
and islands of odontogenic epithelium.

appearance. The dentin contains clefts scattered
through a mixture of interglobular dentin and amorphous material. Globular areas of poorly organized
tubular dentin and scattered cellular inclusions often
are seen. The pulp tissue contains free or attached
stones that may exhibit tubules or consist of laminated
calcification. The follicular tissue surrounding the
crown may be enlarged and typically exhibits focal collections of basophilic enamel-like calcifications called
enameloid conglomerates (Fig. 2-105). This pattern
of calcification is not specific for regional odontodysplasia and has been seen in other processes with
disturbed enamel formation, such as amelogenesis
imperfecta. Scattered islands of odontogenic epithelium and other patterns of intramural calcification also
are seen.

TREATMENT AND PROGNOSIS

The basic approach to therapy of regional odontodysplasia is directed toward retention of the altered teeth,
whenever possible, to allow for appropriate development and preservation of the surrounding alveolar
ridge. Endodontic therapy on nonvital teeth that have
sufficient hard tissue to allow restoration has been performed successfully. Unerupted teeth should remain
untouched, restoring function with a removable partial
prosthesis until the skeletal growth period has passed.
Erupted teeth can be covered with etched-retained restorations or stainless steel crowns until final restorations can be placed after the completion of growth.
Because of the fragile nature of the coronal hard tissue
and the ease of pulp exposure, tooth preparation is
contraindicated. Severely affected and infected teeth
often are not salvageable and need to be removed.
Although ankylosis has been seen with autotrans-
planted teeth, normal bicuspids have been autotrans-
planted into the extraction sites of the abnormal
dentition. This approach can successfully restore masticatory function, allowing appropriate facial development, and preventing ridge atrophy and supereruption
of the opposing dentition. Osseointegrated implants
have been placed in growing children with hypodontia
and could be used in the setting of regional odontodysplasia. Because implants essentially become ankylosed,
they have the potential to become embedded upon
continued gnathic growth in a child. For this reason,
implants generally should be reserved for patients who
have completed pubertal growth.

Although vitality of the abnormal dentition often is
difficult to maintain, such efforts may bring significant
rewards. Several investigators have shown continued
dentinal development of teeth affected by regional
odontodysplasia. In cases monitored for many years,
the teeth lost their ghostly appearance and revealed a
resultant decrease in pulp size, a significant increase in
dentin thickness, and ultimate relative normalization
of the radicular anatomy. In contrast, the enamel
remained hypoplastic. The surrounding bone became
well developed and lost its diminished density. Only a
few reports of this phenomenon exist, however, most
likely because the prior treatment of choice has been
extraction.

BIBLIOGRAPHY

General References
Gorlin RJ, Cohen MM, Hennekam RCM: *Syndromes of the head
and neck*, ed 4, New York, 2001, Oxford University Press.
Stewart RE, Prescott GH: *Oral facial genetics*, St Louis, 1976,
Mosby.

Witkop CJ: Clinical aspects of dental anomalies, *Int Dent J* 26:378-390, 1976.

Witkop CJ, Rao S: Inherited defects in tooth structure. In Bergsma D: *Birth defects. Original article series*, vol 7, no 7, pp 153-184, Baltimore, 1971, Williams & Wilkins.

Environmental Effects on Tooth Structure Development

Andreasen JO, Sundström B, Ravn JJ: The effect of traumatic injuries to primary teeth on their permanent successors. 1. A clinical and histologic study of 117 injured permanent teeth, *Scand J Dent Res* 79:219-283, 1971.

Bentley EM, Ellwood RP, Davies RM: Fluoride ingestion from toothpaste by young children, *Br Dent J* 186:460-462, 1999.

Broadbent JM, Thomson WM, Williams SM: Does caries in primary teeth predict enamel defects in permanent teeth? A longitudinal study, *J Dent Res* 84:260-264, 2005.

Brook AH, Smith JM: Environmental causes of enamel defects, *Ciba Found Symp* 205:212-225, 1997.

Browne D, Whelton H, O'Mullane D: Fluoride metabolism and fluorosis, *J Dent* 33:177-186, 2005.

Centers for Disease Control and Prevention: Ten great public health achievements—United States, 1990-1999, *MMWR Morb Mortal Wkly Rep* 48:241-243, 1999.

Centers for Disease Control and Prevention: Recommendations for using fluoride to prevent and control dental caries in the United States, *MMWR Recomm Rep* 50(RR-14):1-42, 2001.

Churchill HV: Occurrence of fluorides in some waters of the United States, *J Ind Eng Chem* 23:996-998, 1931.

Croll TP: Esthetic correction for teeth with fluorosis and fluorosis-like enamel dysmineralization, *J Esthet Dent* 10:21-29, 1998.

Dean HT: Endemic fluorosis and its relation to dental caries, *Public Health Rep* 53:1443-1452, 1938.

Fayle SA: Molar incisor hypomineralisation: restorative management, *Eur J Paediatr Dent* 4:121-126, 2003.

Groeneveld A, Van Eck AAMJ, Backer Dirks O: Fluoride in caries prevention: is the effect pre- or post-eruptive? *J Dent Res* 69(spec iss):751-755, 1990.

Holtta P, Alaluusua S, Saarinen-Pinkala UM et al: Long-term adverse effects on dentition in children with poor-risk and autologous stem cell transplantation with or without total body irradiation, *Bone Marrow Transplant* 29:121-127, 2002.

Hong L, Levy SM, Warren JJ et al: Association of amoxicillin use during early childhood with developmental tooth enamel defects, *Arch Pediatr Adolesc Med* 159:943-948, 2005.

Kaste SC, Hopkins KP, Bowman LC: Dental abnormalities in long-term survivors of head and neck rhabdomyosarcoma, *Med Pediatr Oncol* 25:96-101, 1995.

Marec-Berard P, Azzi D, Chaux-Bodard AG et al: Long-term effects of chemotherapy on dental status in children treated for nephroblastoma, *Pediatr Hematol Oncol* 22:581-588, 2005.

Marshall TA, Levy SM, Warren JJ et al: Association between intakes of fluoride from beverages during infancy and dental fluorosis of primary teeth, *J Am Col Nutr* 23:108-116, 2004.

McKay FS, Black GV: An investigation of mottled teeth: an endemic developmental imperfection of the enamel and teeth, heretofore unknown in the literature of dentistry, *Dent Cosmos* 58:477-484, 1916.

Montero MJ, Douglass JM, Mathieu GM: Prevalence of dental caries and enamel defects in children in Connecticut Head Start children, *Pediatr Dent* 25:235-239, 2003.

Pajari U, Lanning M: Developmental defects of teeth in survivors of childhood ALL are related to the therapy and age at diagnosis, *Med Pediatr Oncol* 24:310-314, 1995.

Pendrys DG: Risk of enamel fluorosis in nonfluoridated and optimally fluoridated populations: considerations for the dental professional, *J Am Dent Assoc* 131:746-755, 2000.

Pendrys DG, Katz RV: Risk factors for enamel fluorosis in optimally fluoridated children born after the US manufacturer's decision to reduce the fluoride concentration of infant formula, *Am J Epidemiol* 148:967-974, 1998.

Peterson J: Solving the mystery of the Colorado brown stain, *J Hist Dent* 45:57-61, 1997.

Pourghadiri M, Longhurst P, Watson TF: A new technique for the controlled removal of mottled enamel: measurement of enamel loss, *Br Dent J* 184:239-241, 1998.

Price RBT, Loney RW, Doyle MG et al: An evaluation of a technique to remove stains from teeth using microabrasion, *J Am Dent Assoc* 134:1066-1071, 2003.

Riordan PJ: The place of fluoride supplements in caries prevention today, *Aust Dent J* 41:335-342, 1996.

Riordan PJ: Fluoride supplements for young children; analysis of the literature focusing on benefits and risks, *Community Dent Oral Epidemiol* 27:72-83, 1999.

Rodd HD, Davidson LE: The aesthetic management of severe dental fluorosis in the young patient, *Dent Update* 24:408-411 1997.

Seow WK: Clinical diagnosis of enamel defects: pitfalls and practical guidelines, *Int Dent J* 47:173-182, 1997.

Suckling GW: Developmental defects of enamel—historical and present day perspective of their pathogenesis, *Adv Dent Res* 3:87-94, 1989.

Turner JG: Injury to the teeth of succession by abscess of the temporary teeth, *Brit Dent J* 30:1233-1237, 1909.

von Arx T: Developmental disturbances of permanent teeth following trauma to the primary dentition, *Aust Dent J* 38:1-10, 1993.

Weerheijm KL: Molar incisor hypomineralisation (MIH), *Eur J Paediatr Dent* 4:114-120, 2003.

Weerheijm KL: Molar incisor hypomineralisation (MIH): clinical presentation, aetiology and management, *Dent Update* 31:9-12, 2004.

Weerheijm KL, Groen HJ, Beentjes VEVM et al: Prevalence of cheese molars in eleven-year-old Dutch children, *J Dent Child* 68:259-262, 2001.

Postdevelopmental Loss of Tooth Structure

Amaechi BT, Higham SM, Edgar WM: Influence of abrasion in clinical manifestation of human dental erosion, *J Oral Rehabil* 30:407-413, 2003.

Bakland LK: Root resorption, *Dent Clin North Am* 36:491-507, 1992.

Beertsen W, Piscaer M, Van Winkelhoff AF et al: Generalized cervical root resorption associated with periodontal disease, *J Clin Periodontol* 28:1067-1073, 2001.

Caliskan MK, Türkün M: Prognosis of permanent teeth with internal resorption: a clinical review, *Endod Dent Traumatol* 13:75-81, 1997.

Eccles JD: Tooth surface loss from abrasion, attrition and erosion, *Dent Update* 7:373-381, 1982.

Fuss Z, Tsesis I, Lin S: Root resorption—diagnosis, classification and treatment choices based on stimulation factors, *Dent Traumatol* 19:175-182, 2003.

Gartner AH, Mack T, Somerlott RG et al: Differential diagnosis of internal and external resorption, *J Endod* 2:329-334, 1976.

Goultschin J, Nitzan D, Azaz B: Root resorption. Review and discussion, *Oral Surg Oral Med Oral Pathol* 54:586-590, 1982.

Grippo JO: Abfractions: a new classification of hard tissue lesions of teeth, *J Esthet Dent* 3:14-19, 1991.

Grippo JO, Simring M: Dental "erosions" revisited, *J Am Dent Assoc* 126:619-630, 1995.

Grippo JO, Simring M, Schreiner S: Attrition, abrasion, corrosion and abfraction revisited. A new perspective on tooth surface lesions, *J Am Dent Assoc* 135:1109-1118, 2004.

Harris EF, Boggan BW, Wheeler DA: Apical root resorption in patients treated with comprehensive orthodontics, *J Tenn Dent Assoc* 81:30-33, 2001.

Heithersay GS: Clinical, radiologic, and histopathologic features of invasive cervical resorption, *Quintessence Int* 30:27-37, 1999.

House RC, Grisius R, Bliziotes MM et al: Perimolysis: unveiling the surreptitious vomiter, *Oral Surg Oral Med Oral Pathol* 51:152-155, 1981.

Kelleher M, Bishop K: The aetiology and clinical appearance of tooth wear, *Eur J Prosthodont Restor Dent* 5:157-160, 1997.

Kelleher M, Bishop K: Tooth surface loss: an overview, *Br Dent J* 186:61-66, 1999.

Khan F, Young WG, Daley TJ: Dental erosion and bruxism. A tooth wear analysis from South East Queensland, *Aust Dent J* 43:117-127, 1998.

Kofod T, Würtz V, Melsen B: Treatment of an anklosed central incisor by single tooth dento-osseous osteotomy and a simple distraction device, *Am J Orthod Dentofacial Orthop* 127:72-80, 2005.

Krasner P: Advances in the treatment of avulsed teeth, *Dent Today* 22:84-87, 2003.

Lambrechts P, van Meerbeek B, Perdigão J et al: Restorative therapy for erosive lesions, *Eur J Oral Sci* 104:229-240, 1996.

Lee WC, Eakle WS: Possible role of tensile stress in the etiology of cervical erosive lesions of teeth, *J Prosthet Dent* 52:374-379, 1984.

Lee WC, Eakle WS: Stress-induced cervical lesions: review of advances in the past 10 years, *J Prosthet Dent* 75:487-494, 1996.

Levitch LC, Bader JD, Shugars DA et al: Non-carious cervical lesions, *J Dent* 22:195-207, 1994.

Litonjua LA, Andreana S, Bush PJ et al: Tooth wear: attrition, erosion, and abrasion, *Quintessence Int* 34:435-446, 2003.

Litonjua LA, Andreana S, Patra AK et al: An assessment of stress analyses in the theory of abfraction, *Biomed Mater Eng* 14:311-321, 2004.

Litonjua LA, Bush PJ, Andreana S et al: Effects of occlusal load in cervical lesions, *J Oral Rehabil* 31:225-232, 2004.

Massler M, Malone AJ: Root resorption in human permanent teeth: a roentgenographic study, *Am J Orthod* 40:619-633, 1954.

Milosevic A: Toothwear: aetiology and presentation, *Dent Update* 25:6-11, 1998.

Milosevic A: Toothwear: management, *Dent Update* 25:50-55, 1998.

Moody GH, Muir KF: Multiple idiopathic root resorption. A case report and discussion of pathogenesis, *J Clin Periodontol* 18:577-580, 1991.

Mummery JH: The pathology of "pink spots" on teeth, *Br Dent J* 41:301-311, 1920.

Ne RF, Witherspoon DE, Gutmann JL: Tooth resorption, *Quintessence Int* 30:9-25, 1999.

Newman WG: Possible etiologic factors in external root resorption, *Am J Orthod* 67:522-539, 1975.

Rabinowitch BZ: Internal resorption, *Oral Surg Oral Med Oral Pathol* 33:263-282, 1972.

Ram D, Cohenca N: Therapeutic protocols for avulsed permanent teeth: review and clinical update, *Pediatr Dent* 26:251-255, 2004.

Rees JS: The role of cuspal flexure in the development of abfraction lesions: a finite element study, *Eur J Oral Sci* 106:1028-1032, 1998.

Sameshima GT, Sinclair PM: Predicting and preventing root resorption: I. Diagnostic factors, *Am J Orthod Dentofacial Orthop* 119:505-510, 2001.

Schätzle M, Tanner SD, Bosshardt DD: Progressive, generalized, apical idiopathic root resorption and hypercementosis, *J Periodontol* 76:2002-2011, 2005.

Sivasithamparam K, Harbrow D, Vinczer E et al: Endodontic sequelae of dental erosion, *Aust Dent J* 48:97-101, 2003.

Smith BGN, Bartlett DW, Robb ND: The prevalence, etiology and management of tooth wear in the United Kingdom, *J Prosthet Dent* 78:367-372, 1997.

Tronstad L: Root resorption-etiology, terminology and clinical manifestations, *Endod Dent Traumatol* 4:241-252, 1988.

Yap AUJ, Neo JCL: Non-carious cervical tooth loss: part 1, *Dent Update* 22:315-318, 1995.

Yap AUJ, Neo JCL: Non-carious cervical tooth loss: part 2, management, *Dent Update* 22:364-368, 1995.

Young WG: The oral medicine of tooth wear, *Aust Dent J* 46:236-250, 2001.

Young WG: Tooth wear: diet analysis and advice, *Int Dent J* 55:68-72, 2005.

Young WG, Khan F: Sites of dental erosion are saliva-dependent, *J Oral Rehabil* 29:35-43, 2002.

Discolorations of Teeth

Alto LAM, Pomarico L, Souza IPR et al: Green pigmentation of deciduous teeth: report of two cases, *J Dent Child* 71:179-182, 2004.

Ayaslioglu E, Erkek E, Oba AA et al: Doxycycline-induced staining of permanent adult dentition, *Aust Dent J* 50:273-275, 2005.

Bowles WH: Protection against minocycline pigment formation by ascorbic acid (vitamin C), *J Esthet Dent* 10:182-186, 1998.

Cabrerizo-Merino CC, Garcia-Ballesta C, Onate-Sanchez RE et al: Stomatological manifestations of Günther's disease, *J Pedod* 14:113-116, 1990.

Cheek CC, Heymann HO: Dental and oral discoloration associated with minocycline and other tetracycline analogs, *J Esthet Dent* 11:43-48, 1999.

Dayan D, Heifferman A, Gorski M et al: Tooth discoloration—extrinsic and intrinsic factors, *Quintessence Int* 14:195-199, 1983.

Eisenberg E, Bernick SM: Anomalies of the teeth with stains and discolorations, *J Prev Dent* 2:7-20, 1975.

Friedman S: Internal bleaching: long-term outcomes and complications, *J Am Dent Assoc* 128:51S-55S, 1997.

Giunta JL, Tsamtsouris A: Stains and discolorations of teeth: review and case reports, *J Pedod* 2:175-182, 1978.

Holan G, Fuks AB: The diagnostic value of coronal dark-gray discoloration in primary teeth following traumatic injuries, *Pediatr Dent* 18:224-227, 1996.

Link J: Discoloration of the teeth in alkaptonuria (ochronosis) and parkinsonism, *Chronicle* 36:130, 1973.

Morisaki I, Abe K, Tong LS et al: Dental findings of children with biliary atresia: report of seven cases, *J Dent Child* 57:220-223, 1990.

Nelson R, Parker SRS: Doxycycline-induced staining of adult teeth: the first reported case, *Arch Dermatol* 142:1081-1082, 2006.

Rendall JR, McDougall AC: Reddening of the upper central incisors associated with periapical granuloma in lepromatous leprosy, *Br J Oral Surg* 13:271-277, 1976.

Sainio P, Syrjanen S, Keijala JP et al: Postmortem pink teeth phenomenon: an experimental study and a survey of the literature, *Proc Finn Dent Soc* 86:29-35, 1990.

Sánchez AR, Rogers RS III, Sheridan PJ: Tetracycline and other tetracycline-derivative staining of the teeth and oral cavity, *Int J Dermatol* 43:709-715, 2004.

Siekert RG, Gibilisco JA: Discoloration of the teeth in alkaptonuria (ochronosis) and parkinsonism, *Oral Surg Oral Med Oral Pathol* 29:197-199, 1970.

Tredwin CJ, Scully C, Bagan-Sebastian JV: Drug-induced disorders of teeth, *J Dent Res* 84:596-602, 2005.

van der Bijl P, Pitigoi-Aron G: Tetracycline and calcified tissues, *Ann Dent* 54:69-72, 1995.

Watanabe K, Shibata T, Kurosawa T et al: Bilirubin pigmentation of human teeth caused by hyperbilirubinemia, *J Oral Pathol Med* 28:128-130, 1999.

Westbury LW, Najera A: Minocycline-induced intraoral pharmacogenic pigmentation: case reports and review of the literature, *J Periodontol* 68:84-91, 1997.

Wray A, Welbury R: Treatment of intrinsic discoloration in permanent anterior teeth in children and adolescents, *Int J Paediatr Dent* 11:309-315, 2001.

Localized Disturbances in Eruption

Alling CC III, Catone GA: Management of impacted teeth, *J Oral Maxillofac Surg* 51(suppl 1):3-6, 1993.

Bianchi SD, Roccuzzo M: Primary impaction of primary teeth: a review and report of three cases, *J Clin Pediatr Dent* 15:165-168, 1991.

Chu FCS, Li TKL, Lui VKB et al: Prevalence of impacted teeth and associated pathologies—a radiographic study of Hong Kong Chinese population, *Hong Kong Med J* 9:158-163, 2003.

Curran AE, Damm DD, Drummond JF: Pathologically significant pericoronal lesions in adults: histopathologic evaluation, *J Oral Maxillofac Surg* 60:613-617, 2002.

Dewhurst SN, Harris JC, Bedi R: Infraocclusion of primary molars in monozygotic twins: report of two cases, *Int J Paediatr Dent* 7:25-30, 1997.

Douglass J, Tinanoff N: The etiology, prevalence, and sequelae of infraocclusion of primary molars, *J Dent Child* 58:481-483, 1991.

Ekim SL, Hatibovic-Kofman S: A treatment decision-making model for infraoccluded primary molars, *Int J Paediatr Dent* 11:340-346, 2001.

Kim T-W, Årtun J, Behbehani F et al: Prevalence of third molar impaction in orthodontic patients treated nonextraction and with extraction of 4 premolars, *Am J Orthod Dentofacial Orthop* 123:138-145, 2003.

Frank CA: Treatment options for impacted teeth, *J Am Dent Assoc* 131:623-632, 2000.

Mercier P, Precious D: Risks and benefits of removal of impacted third molars, *J Oral Maxillofac Surg* 21:17-27, 1993.

Peterson LJ: Rationale for removing impacted teeth: when to extract or not to extract, *J Am Dent Assoc* 123:198-204, 1992.

Qunitero E, Giunta ME, Cahuana A et al: Primary molars in severe infraocclusion: a retrospective study, *Eur J Paediatr Dent* 4:78-83, 2003.

Razdolsky Y, El-Biaky TH, Dessner S et al: Movement of ankylosed permanent teeth with a distraction device, *J Clin Orthod* 38:612-620, 2004.

Developmental Alterations in Number of Teeth

Bodin I, Julin P, Thomsson M: Hyperdontia. I. Frequency and distribution of supernumerary teeth among 21,609 patients, *Dentomaxillofac Radiol* 7:15-17, 1978.

Carter NE, Gillgrass TJ, Hobson RS et al: The interdisciplinary management of hypodontia: orthodontics, *Br Dent J* 194:361-366, 2003.

Foley J: Surgical removal of supernumerary teeth and the fate of incisor eruption, *Eur J Paediatr Dent* 5:35-40, 2004.

Frazier-Bowers SA, Guo DC, Cavender A et al: A novel mutation in human PAX9 causes molar oligodontia, *J Dent Res* 81:129-133, 2002.

Itro A, Difalco P, Urcicuolo V et al: The aesthetic and functional restoration in the case of partial edentulism in young patients, *Minerva Stomatol* 54:281-292, 2005.

Kates GA, Needleman HL, Holmes LB: Natal and neonatal teeth: a clinical study, *J Am Dent Assoc* 109:441-443, 1984.

Kindelan JD, Rysiecki G, Childs WP: Hypodontia: genotype or environment? A case report of monozygotic twins, *Br J Orthod* 25:175-178, 1998.

Kolens-Fuśe FJ: Tooth agenesis: in search of mutation behind failed dental development, *Med Oral Patol Oral Cir Bucal* 9:385-395, 2004.

Lammi L, Arte S, Somer M et al: Mutations in AXIN2 cause familial tooth agenesis and predispose to colorectal cancer, *Am J Hum Genet* 74:1043-1050, 2004.

Lamour CJ, Mossey PA, Thind BS et al: Hypodontia—a retrospective review of prevalence and etiology. Part 1, *Quintessence Int* 36:263-270, 2005.

Lidral AC, Reising BC: The role of MSX1 in human tooth agenesis, *J Dent Res* 81:274-278, 2002.

Longtin R: Chew on this: mutation may be responsible for tooth loss, colon cancer, *J Natl Cancer Inst* 96:987-989, 2004.

Peck S, Peck L: Classification of maxillary tooth transposition, *Am J Orthod Dentofac Orthop* 107:505-517, 1995.

Rajab LD, Hamdan MAM: Supernumerary teeth: review of the literature and a survey of 152 cases, *Int J Paediatr Dent* 12:244-254, 2002.

Rao PP, Chidzonga MM: Supernumerary teeth: literature review, *Cent Afr J Med* 47:22-26, 2001.

Russell KA, Flowarczna MA: Mesiodens—diagnosis and management of a common supernumerary tooth, *J Can Dent Assoc* 69:362-366, 2003.

Salcido-Gárcia JF, Ledesma-Montes C, Hernández-Flores F et al: Frequency of supernumerary teeth in Mexican population, *Med Oral Patol Oral Cir Bucal* 9:403-409, 2004.

Shapira Y, Kuftinec MM: Tooth transposition—a review of the literature and treatment considerations, *Angle Orthod* 59:271-276, 1989.

Spouge JD, Feasby WH: Erupted teeth in the newborn, *Oral Surg Oral Med Oral Pathol* 22:198-208, 1966.

Yusof WZ: Non-syndrome multiple supernumerary teeth: literature review, *J Can Dent Assoc* 56:147-149, 1990.

Developmental Alterations in Size of Teeth

Bailit HL: Dental variation among populations. An anthropologic view, *Dent Clin North Am* 19:125-139, 1975.

Brook AH: A unifying aetiological explanation for anomalies of human tooth number and size, *Arch Oral Biol* 29:373-378, 1984.

Dugmore CR: Bilateral macrodontia of mandibular second premolars: a case report, *Int J Paediatr Dent* 11:69-73, 2001.

Rootkin-Gray VFAI, Sheehy EC: Macrodontia of a mandibular second premolar: a case report, *J Dent Child* 68:347-349, 2001.

Rushton MA: Partial gigantism of face and teeth, *Br Dent J* 62:572-578, 1937.

Townsend GC: Hereditability of deciduous tooth size in Australian aboriginals, *Am J Phys Anthropol* 53:297-300, 1980.

Townsend GC, Brown T: Hereditability of permanent tooth size, *Am J Phys Anthropol* 49:497-504, 1978.

Gemination, Fusion, Concrescence

Alpöz AR, Munanoğlu D, Oncag O: Mandibular bilateral fusion in primary dentition: case report, *J Dent Child* 70:74-76, 2003.

Brook AH, Winter GB: Double teeth: a retrospective study of "geminated" and "fused" teeth in children, *Br Dent J* 129:123-130, 1970.

Duncan WK, Helpin ML: Bilateral fusion and gemination: a literature analysis and case report, *Oral Surg Oral Med Oral Pathol* 64:82-87, 1987.

Hamasha AA, Al-Khateeb T: Prevalence of fused and geminated teeth in Jordanian adults, *Quintessence Int* 35:556-559, 2004.

Levitas TC: Gemination, fusion, twinning and concrescence, *J Dent Child* 32:93-100, 1965.

Romito LM: Concrescence: report of a rare case, *Oral Surg Oral Med Oral Pathol Oral Radiol Endod* 97:325-327, 2004.

Ruprecht A, Batniji S, El-Neweihi E: Double teeth: the incidence of gemination and fusion, *J Pedod* 9:332-337, 1985.

Tasa GL, Lukacs JR: The prevalence and expression of primary double teeth in western India, *J Dent Child* 68:196-200, 2001.

Yuen SWH, Chan JCY, Wei SHY: Double primary teeth and their relationship with the permanent successors: a radiographic study of 376 cases, *Pediatr Dent* 9:42-48, 1987.

Accessory Cusps

Bailit HL: Dental variation among populations. An anthropologic view, *Dent Clin North Am* 19:125-139, 1975.

Bloch-Zupan A, Stachtou J, Emmanouil D et al: Oro-dental features as useful diagnostic tool in Rubinstein-Taybi syndrome, *Am J Med Genet A* 143A:570-573, 2007.

Dankner E, Harari D, Rotstein I: Dens evaginatus of anterior teeth. Literature review and radiographic survey of 15,000 teeth, *Oral Surg Oral Med Oral Pathol Oral Radiol Endod* 81:472-476, 1996.

Falomo OO: The cusp of Carabelli: frequency, distribution, size and clinical significance in Nigeria, *West Afr J Med* 21:322-324, 2002.

Gaynor WN: Dens evaginatus—how does it present and how should it be managed? *N Z Dent J* 98:104-107, 2002.

Geist JR: Dens evaginatus: case report and review of the literature, *Oral Surg Oral Med Oral Pathol* 67:628-631, 1989.

Glavina D, Škrinjarić T: Labial talon cusp on maxillary central incisors: a rare development dental anomaly, *Coll Antropol* 29:227-231, 2005.

Hattab FN, Yassin OM, Al-Nimri KS: Talon cusp in permanent dentition associated with other dental anomalies: review of literature and reports of seven cases, *J Dent Child* 63:368-376, 1996.

Jeevarathan J, Deepti A, Muthu MS et al: Labial and lingual talon cusps of a primary lateral incisor: a case report, *Pediatr Dent* 27:303-306, 2005.

Levitan ME, Himel VT: Dens evaginatus: literature review, pathophysiology, and comprehensive treatment regimen, *J Endod* 32:1-9, 2006.

Liu JF, Chen LR: Talon cusp affecting the primary maxillary central incisors in two sets of female twins: report of two cases, *Pediatr Dent* 17:362-364, 1995.

McCulloch KJ, Mills CM, Greenfeld RS et al: Dens evaginatus: review of the literature and report of several clinical cases, *J Can Dent Assoc* 64:104-106, 110-113, 1998.

Mellor JK, Ripa LW: Talon cusp: a clinically significant anomaly, *Oral Surg Oral Med Oral Pathol* 29:225-228, 1970.

Ooshima T, Ishida R, Mishima K et al: The prevalence of developmental anomalies of teeth and their association with tooth size in the primary and permanent dentitions of 1650 children, *Int J Paediat Dent* 6:87-94, 1996.

Saini TS, Kharat DU, Mokeem S: Prevalence of shovel-shaped incisors in Saudi Arabian dental patients, *Oral Surg Oral Med Oral Pathol* 70:540-544, 1990.

Segura-Egea JJ, Jiménez-Rubio A, Ríos-Santos JV et al: Dens evaginatus of anterior teeth (talon cusp): report of five cases, *Quintessence Int* 34:272-277, 2003.

Dens Invaginatus

Hülsmann M: Dens invaginatus: aetiology, classification, prevalence, diagnosis, and treatment considerations, *Int Endod J* 30:79-90, 1997.

Jaramillo A, Fernández R, Villa P: Endodontic treatment of dens invaginatus: a 5-year follow-up, *Oral Surg Oral Med Oral Pathol Oral Radiol Endod* 101:E15-E21, 2006.

Nallapati S: Clinical management of a maxillary lateral incisor with vital pulp and type 3 dens invaginatus: a case report, *J Endod* 30:726-731, 2004.

Oehlers FAC: Dens invaginatus (dilated composite odontome). I. Variations of the invagination process and associated anterior crown forms, *Oral Surg Oral Med Oral Pathol* 10:1204-1218, 1957.

Oehlers FAC: Dens invaginatus (dilated composite odontome). II. Associated posterior crown forms and pathogenesis, *Oral Surg Oral Med Oral Pathol* 10:1302-1316, 1957.

Oehlers FAC: The radicular variety of dens invaginatus, *Oral Surg Oral Med Oral Pathol* 11:1251-1260, 1958.

Payne M, Craig GT: A radicular dens invaginatus, *Br Dent J* 169:94-95, 1990.

Ridell K, Mejàre I, Matsson L: Dens invaginatus: a retrospective study of prophylactic invagination treatment, *Int J Paediatr Dent* 11:92-97, 2001.

Ectopic Enamel

Cavanha AO: Enamel pearls, *Oral Surg Oral Med Oral Pathol* 19:373-382, 1965.

Craig GT: The paradental cyst, a specific inflammatory odontogenic cyst, *Br Dent J* 141:9-14, 1976.

Fowler CB, Brannon RB: The paradental cyst: a clinicopathologic study of six new cases and review of the literature, *J Oral Maxillofac Surg* 47:243-348, 1989.

Goldstein AR: Enamel pearls as a contributing factor in periodontal breakdown, *J Am Dent Assoc* 99:210-211, 1979.

Hou G-L, Tsai C-C: Relationship between periodontal furcation involvement and molar cervical enamel projections, *J Periodontol* 58:715-721, 1987.

Kaugars GE: Internal enamel pearls: report of case, *J Am Dent Assoc* 107:941-943, 1983.

Matthews DC, Tabesh M: Detection of localized tooth-related factors that predispose to periodontal infections, *Periodontol 2000* 34:136-150, 2004.

Moskow BS, Canut PM: Studies on root enamel: (2) enamel pearls—a review of their morphology, localization, nomenclature, occurrence, classification, histogenesis and incidence, *J Clin Periodontol* 17:275-281, 1990.

Pompura JR, Sándor GKB, Stoneman DW: The buccal bifurcation cyst: a prospective study of treatment outcomes in 44 sites, *Oral Surg Oral Med Oral Pathol Oral Radiol Endod* 83:215-221, 1997.

Risnes S: The prevalence, location, and size of enamel pearls on human molars, *Scand J Dent Res* 82:403-412, 1974.

Zee K-Y, Bratthall G: Prevalence of cervical enamel projection and its correlation with furcation involvement in Eskimos' dry skulls, *Swed Dent J* 27:43-48, 2003.

Taurodontism

Durr DP, Campos CA, Ayers CS: Clinical significance of taurodontism, *J Am Dent Assoc* 100:378-381, 1980.

Llamas R, Jimenez-Planas A: Taurodontism in premolars, *Oral Surg Oral Med Oral Pathol* 75:501-505, 1993.

Ruprecht A, Batniji S, El-Neweihi E: The incidence of taurodontism in dental patients, *Oral Surg Oral Med Oral Pathol* 63:743-747, 1987.

Shaw JCM: Taurodont teeth in South African races, *J Anat* 62:476-498, 1928.

Shifman A, Chanannel I: Prevalence of taurodontism found in radiographic dental examination of 1,200 young adult Israeli patients, *Community Dent Oral Epidemiol* 6:200-203, 1978.

Tsesis I, Shifman A, Kaufman AY: Taurodontism: an endodontic challenge. Report of a case, *J Endod* 29:353-355, 2003.

Witkop CJ, Keenan KM, Cervenka J et al: Taurodontism: an anomaly of teeth reflecting disruptive developmental homeostasis, *Am J Med Genet* 4(suppl):85-97, 1988.

Hypercementosis

Fox L: Paget's disease (osteitis deformans) and its effect on maxillary bones and teeth, *J Am Dent Assoc* 20:1823-1829, 1933.

Gardner BS, Goldstein H: The significance of hypercementosis, *Dent Cosmos* 73:1065-1069, 1931.

Leider AS, Garbarino VE: Generalized hypercementosis, *Oral Surg Oral Med Oral Pathol* 63:375-380, 1987.

Napier-Souza L, Monteiro-Lima-Junio S, Garcia-Santos-Pimenta FJ: Atypical hypercementosis versus cementoblastoma, *Dentomaxillofac Radiol* 33:267-270, 2004.

Rao VM, Karasick D: Hypercementosis—an important clue to Paget disease of the maxilla, *Skeletal Radiol* 9:126-128, 1982.

See R, Nixon PP: Generalised hypercementosis: a case report, *Prim Dent Care* 11:119-122, 2004.

Weinberger A: The clinical significance of hypercementosis, *Oral Surg Oral Med Oral Pathol* 7:79-87, 1954.

Dilaceration

Celik E, Aydinlik E: Effect of a dilacerated root in stress distribution to the tooth and supporting tissues, *J Prosthet Dent* 65:771-777, 1991.

Chew MT, Ong M M-A: Orthodontic-surgical management of an impacted dilacerated maxillary central incisor: a clinical case report, *Pediatr Dent* 26:341-344, 2004.

Ligh RQ: Coronal dilaceration, *Oral Surg Oral Med Oral Pathol* 51:567, 1981.

Hamasha AA, Al-Khateeb T, Darwazeh A: Prevalence of dilaceration in Jordanian adults, *Int Endod J* 35:910-912, 2002.

Seow WK, Perham S, Young WG et al: Dilaceration of a primary maxillary incisor associated with neonatal laryngoscopy, *Pediatr Dent* 12:321-324, 1990.

Stewart DJ: Dilacerate unerupted maxillary central incisors, *Br Dent J* 145:229-233, 1978.

van Gool AV: Injury to the permanent tooth germ after trauma to the deciduous predecessor, *Oral Surg Oral Med Oral Pathol* 35:2-12, 1973.

Supernumerary Roots

Badger GR: Three-rooted mandibular first primary molar, *Oral Surg Oral Med Oral Pathol* 53:547, 1982.

Kannan SK, Suganya, Santharam H et al: Supernumerary roots, *Indian J Dent Res* 13:116-119, 2002.

Krolls SO, Donahue AH: Double-rooted maxillary primary canines, *Oral Surg Oral Med Oral Pathol* 49:379, 1980.

Younes SA, Al-Shammery AR, El-Angbawi MF: Three-rooted permanent mandibular first molars of Asian and black groups in the Middle East, *Oral Surg Oral Med Oral Pathol* 69:102-105, 1990.

Amelogenesis Imperfecta

Aldred MJ, Crawford PJM: Amelogenesis imperfecta—toward a new classification, *Oral Dis* 1:2-5, 1995.

Aldred MJ, Crawford PJM: Molecular biology of hereditary enamel defects, *Ciba Found Symp* 205:200-209, 1997.

Aldred MJ, Crawford PJM, Savarirayan R et al: It's only teeth—are there limits to genetic testing? *Clin Genet* 63:333-339, 2003.

Aldred MJ, Savarirayan R, Crawford PJM: Amelogenesis imperfecta: a classification and catalogue for the 21st century, *Oral Dis* 9:19-23, 2003.

Aldred MJ, Savarirayan R, Lamande SR et al: Clinical and radiographic features of a family with autosomal dominant amelogenesis imperfecta with taurodontism, *Oral Dis* 8:62-68, 2002.

Crawford PJM, Aldred MJ: Amelogenesis imperfecta with taurodontism and the tricho-dento-osseous syndrome: separate conditions or a spectrum of disease? *Clin Genet* 38:44-50, 1990.

Dong J, Amor D, Aldreds MJ et al: DLX3 mutation associated with autosomal dominant amelogenesis imperfecta with taurodontism, *Am J Med Genet A* 133A:138-141, 2005.

Kim J-W, Seymen F, Lin BP-J et al: ENAM mutations in autosomal-dominant amelogenesis imperfecta, *J Dent Res* 84:278-282, 2005.

Nusier M, Yassin O, Hart TC et al: Phenotypic diversity and revision of the nomenclature for autosomal recessive amelogenesis imperfecta, *Oral Surg Oral Med Oral Pathol Oral Radiol Endod* 97:220-230, 2004.

Ozdemir D, Hart PS, Ryu OH et al: MMP20 active-site mutation in hypomaturation amelogenesis imperfecta, *J Dent Res* 84:1031-1035, 2005.

Price JA, Wright JT, Walker SJ et al: Tricho-dento-osseous syndrome and amelogenesis imperfecta with taurodontism are genetically distinct conditions, *Clin Genet* 56:35-40, 1999.

Seow WK: Clinical diagnosis and management strategies of amelogenesis imperfecta variants, *Pediatr Dent* 15:384-393, 1993.

Seow WK: Taurodontism of the mandibular first permanent molar distinguishes between the tricho-dento-osseous (TDO) syndrome and amelogenesis imperfecta, *Clin Genet* 43:240-246, 1993.

Shields ED: A new classification of heritable human enamel defects and a discussion of dentin defects. In Jorgenson RJ, Paul NW: *Dentition: genetic effects, birth defects.* Original article series, vol 19, no 1, pp 107-127, New York, 1983, Alan R. Liss.

Stephanopoulos G, Garefalaki M-E: Genes and related proteins involved in amelogenesis imperfecta, *J Dent Res* 84:1117-1126, 2005.

Sundell S, Koch G: Hereditary amelogenesis imperfecta. I. Epidemiology and clinical classification in a Swedish child population, *Swed Dent J* 9:157-169, 1985.

Witkop CJ Jr: Amelogenesis imperfecta, dentinogenesis imperfecta and dentin dysplasia revisited: problems in classification, *J Oral Pathol* 17:547-553, 1988.

Witkop CJ Jr, Sauk JJ Jr: Heritable defects of enamel. In Stewart RE, Prescott GH: *Oral facial genetics*, pp 151-226, St Louis, 1976, Mosby.

Wright JT, Hart PS, Aldred MJ et al: Relationship of phenotype and genotype in X-linked amelogenesis imperfecta, *Connect Tissue Res* 44(suppl 1):72-78, 2003.

Dentinogenesis Imperfecta

Hursey RJ, Witkop CJ Jr, Miklashek D et al: Dentinogenesis imperfecta in a racial isolate with multiple hereditary defects, *Oral Surg Oral Med Oral Pathol* 9:641-658, 1956.

Joshi N, Parkash H: Oral rehabilitation in dentinogenesis imperfecta with overdentures: case report, *J Clin Pediatr Dent* 22:99-102, 1998.

Kim J-W, Hu J C-C, Lee J-I et al: Mutational hot spot in the DSPP gene causing dentinogenesis imperfecta type II, *Hum Genet* 116:186-191, 2005.

Kim J-W, Nam S-H, Jang K-T et al: A novel splice acceptor mutation in the DSPP gene causing dentinogenesis imperfecta type II, *Hum Genet* 115:248-254, 2004.

Levin LS: The dentition in the osteogenesis imperfecta syndrome, *Clin Orthop* 159:64-74, 1981.

Levin LS, Leaf SH, Jelmini RJ et al: Dentinogenesis imperfecta in the Brandywine isolate (DI type III): clinical, radiologic, and scanning electron microscopic studies of the dentition, *Oral Surg Oral Med Oral Pathol* 56:267-274, 1983.

Ranta H, Lukinmaa P-L, Waltimo J: Heritable dentin defects: nosology, pathology, and treatment, *Am J Med Genet* 45:193-200, 1993.

Rushton MA: A new form of dentinal dysplasia: shell teeth, *Oral Surg Oral Med Oral Pathol* 7:543-549, 1954.

Shields ED, Bixler D, El-Kafrawy AM: A proposed classification for heritable human dentine defects with a description of a new entity, *Arch Oral Biol* 18:543-553, 1973.

Witkop CJ Jr: Amelogenesis imperfecta, dentinogenesis imperfecta and dentin dysplasia revisited: problems in classification, *J Oral Pathol* 17:547-553, 1988.

Witkop CJ Jr: Hereditary defects of dentin, *Dent Clin North Am* 19:25-45, 1975.

Witkop CJ Jr, MacLean CJ, Schmidt PJ et al: Medical and dental findings in the Brandywine isolate, *Ala J Med Sci* 3:382-403, 1966.

Dentin Dysplasia

Bixler D: Heritable disorders affecting dentin. In Stewart RE, Prescott GH: *Oral facial genetics*, pp 227-262, St Louis, 1976.

Comer TL, Gound TG: Hereditary pattern for dentinal dysplasia type Id: a case report, *Oral Surg Oral Med Oral Pathol Oral Radiol Endod* 94:51-53, 2002.

Duncan WK, Perkins TM, O'Carroll MK: Type I dentin dysplasia: report of two cases, *Ann Dent* 50:18-21, 1991.

O'Carroll MK, Duncan WK, Perkins TM: Dentin dysplasia: review of the literature and a proposed subclassification based on radiographic findings, *Oral Surg Oral Med Oral Pathol* 72:119-125, 1991.

Parekh S, Kyriazidou A, Bloch-Zupan A et al: Multiple pulp stones and shortened roots of unknown etiology, *Oral Surg Oral Med Oral Pathol, Oral Radiol Endod* 101:e139-142, 2006.

Rajpar MH, Koch MJ, Davies RM et al: Mutation of the signal peptide region of the bicistronic gene DSPP affects translocation to the endoplasmic reticulum and results in defective dentine biomineralization, *Hum Mol Genet* 11:2559-2565, 2002.

Ranta H, Lukinmaa P-L, Waltimo J: Heritable dentin defects: nosology, pathology, and treatment, *Am J Med Genet* 45:193-200, 1993.

Rao SR, Witkop CJ Jr, Yamane GM: Pulpal dysplasia, *Oral Surg Oral Med Oral Pathol* 30:682-689, 1970.

Rosenberg LR, Phelan JA: Dentin dysplasia type II: review of the literature and report of a family, *J Dent Child* 50:372-375, 1983.

Rushton MA: A case of dentinal dysplasia, *Guys Hosp Rep* 89:369-373, 1939.

Scola SM, Watts PG: Dentinal dysplasia type I. A subclassification, *Br J Orthod* 14:175-179, 1987.

Shields ED, Bixler D, El-Kafrawy AM: A proposed classification for heritable human dentine defects with a description of a new entity, *Arch Oral Biol* 18:543-553, 1973.

Steidler NE, Radden BG, Reade PC: Dentinal dysplasia: a clinicopathologic study of eight cases and review of the literature, *Br J Oral Maxillofac Surg* 22:274-286, 1984.

Tidwell E, Cunningham CJ: Dentinal dysplasia: endodontic treatment, with case report, *J Endod* 5:372-376, 1979.

Van Dis ML, Allen CM: Dentinal dysplasia type I: a report of four cases, *Dentomaxillofac Radiol* 18:128-131, 1989.

Wesley RK, Wysocki GP, Mintz SM et al: Dentin dysplasia type I. Clinical, morphologic, and genetic studies of a case, *Oral Surg Oral Med Oral Pathol* 41:516-524, 1976.

Witkop CJ Jr: Manifestations of genetic diseases in the human pulp, *Oral Surg Oral Med Oral Pathol* 32:278-316, 1971.

Witkop CJ Jr: Hereditary defects of dentin, *Dent Clin North Am* 19:25-45, 1975.

Witkop CJ Jr: Amelogenesis imperfecta, dentinogenesis imperfecta and dentin dysplasia revisited: problems in classification, *J Oral Pathol* 17:547-553, 1988.

Regional Odontodysplasia

Cahuana A, González Y, Palma C: Clinical management of regional odontodysplasia, *Pediatr Dent* 27:34-39, 2005.

Crawford PJM, Aldred MJ: Regional odontodysplasia: a bibliography, *J Oral Pathol Med* 18:251-263, 1989.

Gardner DG: The dentinal changes in regional odontodysplasia, *Oral Surg Oral Med Oral Pathol* 38:887-897, 1974.

Hamdan MA, Sawair FA, Rajab LD et al: Regional odontodysplasia: a review of the literature and report of a case, *Int J Paediatr Dent* 14:363-370, 2004.

Kahn MA, Hinson RL: Regional odontodysplasia. Case report with etiologic and treatment considerations, *Oral Surg Oral Med Oral Pathol* 72:462-467, 1991.

Kerebel L-M, Kerebel B: Soft-tissue calcifications of the dental follicle in regional odontodysplasia: a structural and ultrastructural study, *Oral Surg Oral Med Oral Pathol* 56:396-404, 1983.

Lowe O, Duperon DF: Generalized odontodysplasia, *J Pedod* 9:232-243, 1985.

Sadeghi EM, Ashrafi MH: Regional odontodysplasia: clinical, pathologic and therapeutic considerations, *J Am Dent Assoc* 102:336-339, 1981.

Tervonon SA, Stratmann U, Mokrys K et al: Regional odontodysplasia: a review of the literature and report of four cases, *Clin Oral Invest* 8:45-51, 2004.

von Arx T: Autotransplantation for treatment of regional odontodysplasia. Case report with 6-year follow-up, *Oral Surg Oral Med Oral Pathol Oral Radiol Endod* 85:304-307, 1998.

Walton JL, Witkop CJ Jr, Walker PO: Odontodysplasia. Report of three cases with vascular nevi overlying the adjacent skin of the face, *Oral Surg Oral Med Oral Pathol* 46:676-684, 1978.

Zegarelli EV, Kutscher AH, Applebaum E et al: Odontodysplasia, *Oral Surg Oral Med Oral Pathol* 16:187-193, 1963.

3

Pulpal and Periapical Disease

CHAPTER OUTLINE

PULPITIS

The initial response of the dental pulp to injury is not significantly different from that seen in other tissues. However, the final result can be different because of the rigid dentinal walls of the pulp chamber. When external stimuli reach a noxious level, degranulation of mast cells, decreased nutrient flow, and cellular damage occur. Numerous inflammatory mediators (e.g., histamine, bradykinin, neurokinins, neuropeptides, prostaglandins) are released. These mediators cause vasodilation, increased blood inflow, and vascular leakage with edema. In normal tissue, increased blood flow promotes healing through removal of inflammatory mediators, and swelling of the injured tissue usually occurs. However, the dental pulp exists in a very confined area.

Pulpal response to noxious stimuli is meant to eliminate any invading organisms, remove cellular debris, and limit tissue damage. Paradoxically, the inflammatory reaction can lead to increased pulpal injury or even death of the pulp. Previous theories have suggested that the associated increased vascular pulpal pressures could compress venous return and lead to "self-strangulation" and pulpal necrosis. Today researchers recognize that the increased fluid pressure usually is localized to the area of inflamed pulp immediately adjacent to the affected dentin. Increased interstitial pressure in areas of inflammation leads to increased flow of fluid back into capillaries of adjacent unin-

flamed tissue and increased drainage. In this manner, the increased fluid pressure from inflammation is counteracted and typically does not lead to a generalized increase in pulpal fluid pressure, effectively preventing "self-strangulation." Although many consider the dental pulp very fragile, the defense mechanisms work well the vast majority of time and rarely result in widespread necrosis. Localized pulpal abscesses often are able to heal after formation of reparative dentin and cessation of the noxious stimulus. In spite of numerous defense mechanisms, severe localized pulpal damage can overwhelm the system and spread progressively to the apical portion of the pulp, potentially producing widespread pulpal necrosis. In caries, whenever bacteria reach the tertiary dentin, the defense barriers have been breached, the degree of **pulpitis** will be severe, and the chance for pulpal recovery is minimal.

Four main types of noxious stimuli are common causes of pulpal inflammation:
1. *Mechanical damage.* Mechanical sources of injury include traumatic accidents, iatrogenic damage from dental procedures, attrition, abrasion, and barometric changes.
2. *Thermal injury.* Severe thermal stimuli can be transmitted through large uninsulated metallic restorations or may occur from such dental procedures as cavity preparation, polishing, and exothermic chemical reactions of dental materials.

3. *Chemical irritation.* Chemical-related damage can arise from erosion or from the inappropriate use of acidic dental materials.
4. *Bacterial effects.* Bacteria can damage the pulp through toxins or directly after extension from caries or transportation via the vasculature.

Pulpitis can be classified as the following:
- Acute or chronic
- Subtotal or generalized
- Infected or sterile

The best classification system is one that guides the appropriate treatment. *Reversible pulpitis* denotes a level of pulpal inflammation in which the tissue is capable of returning to a normal state of health if the noxious stimuli are removed. *Irreversible pulpitis* implies that a higher level of inflammation has developed in which the dental pulp has been damaged beyond the point of recovery. Often, frank invasion by bacteria is the crossover point from reversible to irreversible pulpitis.

CLINICAL FEATURES
REVERSIBLE PULPITIS

When exposed to temperature extremes, teeth with **reversible pulpitis** exhibit a sudden mild-to-moderate pain **(pulpalgia)** of short duration. Although heat may initiate pain, the affected tooth responds most to cold stimuli (e.g., ice, beverages, cold air). Contact with sweet or sour foods and beverages also may cause pain. The pain does not occur without stimulation and subsides within seconds after the stimulus is removed. Typically, the tooth responds to electric pulp testing at lower levels of current than an appropriate control tooth. Mobility and sensitivity to percussion are absent. If the pulpitis is allowed to progress, then the duration of the pain on stimulation can become longer and the pulp may become affected irreversibly.

IRREVERSIBLE PULPITIS

Patients with early **irreversible pulpitis** generally have sharp, severe pain on thermal stimulation, and the pain continues after the stimulus is removed. Cold is especially uncomfortable, although heat or sweet and acidic foods also can elicit pain. In addition, the pain may be spontaneous or continuous and may be exacerbated when the patient lies down. The tooth responds to electric pulp testing at lower levels of current.

In the early stages of irreversible pulpitis, the pain often can be localized easily to the individual offending tooth; with increasing discomfort, however, the patient is unable to identify the offending tooth within a quadrant.

In the later stages of irreversible pulpitis, the pain increases in intensity and is experienced as a throbbing pressure that can keep patients awake at night. At this point, heat increases the pain; however, cold may produce relief. The tooth responds to electric pulp testing at higher levels of current or demonstrates no response. Mobility and sensitivity to percussion are usually absent because significant inflammation has not spread yet to the apical area. If pulpal drainage occurs (e.g., crown fracture, fistula formation), then the symptoms may resolve—only to return if the drainage ceases.

The dramatic and painful cases of acute pulpitis are the ones that are recalled most easily by both patients and clinicians. In spite of this, the process may take years, the pattern of symptomatology is highly variable, and often the patient may have no symptoms. A number of large retrospective studies of patients presenting for endodontic therapy of teeth with radiographic evidence of periapical inflammatory disease have shown that in approximately half of these cases the associated pulpitis and necrosis were asymptomatic. Severe pulpitis with abscess formation and necrosis may be asymptomatic, whereas mild pulpitis may cause excruciating pain.

CHRONIC HYPERPLASTIC PULPITIS

One unique pattern of pulpal inflammation is **chronic hyperplastic pulpitis (pulp polyp)**. This condition occurs in children and young adults who have large exposures of the pulp in which the entire dentinal roof often is missing. The most frequently involved teeth are the deciduous or succedaneous molars, which have large pulp chambers in these age groups. Mechanical irritation and bacterial invasion result in a level of chronic inflammation that produces hyperplastic granulation tissue that extrudes from the chamber and often fills the associated dentinal defect (Figs. 3-1 to 3-3). The apex may be open and reduces the chance of pulpal necrosis secondary to venous compression. The tooth is asymptomatic except for a possible feeling of pressure when it is placed into masticatory function.

Typically, the diagnosis of pulpitis is straightforward and easily correlated with a diseased tooth that can be stimulated to produce the associated symptoms. If such a correlation is not obvious, then it should raise suspicion that the symptoms may not be pulpally related. The tooth that is the source of pulpal pain may be difficult to identify in some instances. Although pulpal pain never crosses the midline, it can be referred from arch to arch, making pulp testing of both arches a necessity in difficult cases. Numerous disorders such as myofascial pain, trigeminal neuralgia, atypical facial neuralgia, migraine headaches, cluster headaches, nasal or sinus pathoses, and angina pectoris have been reported to mimic pulpalgia in some patients. If these conditions are not recognized as causing pain, then

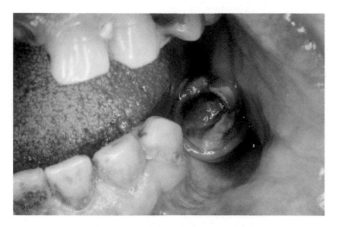

Fig. 3-1   Chronic hyperplastic pulpitis. Erythematous granulation tissue extruding from the pulp chamber of the mandibular first molar.

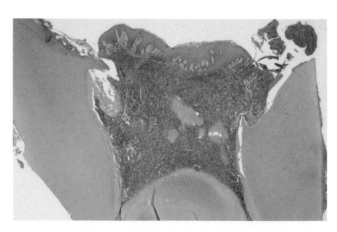

Fig. 3-3   Chronic hyperplastic pulpitis. Same tooth as depicted in Fig. 3-2. Chronically inflamed granulation tissue fills the coronal defect. Note surface stratified squamous epithelium.

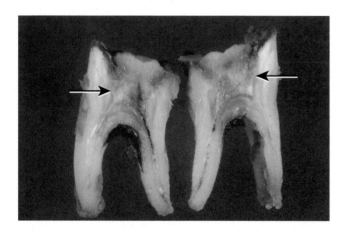

Fig. 3-2   Chronic hyperplastic pulpitis. Gross photograph demonstrating hyperplastic pulp tissue filling a large coronal carious defect. Arrows delineate the previous roof of the pulp chamber.

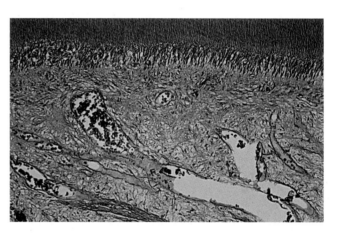

Fig. 3-4   Reversible pulpitis. Dental pulp exhibiting hyperemia and edema. The adjacent dentin was cut recently during placement of a dental restoration.

sequential extractions or endodontic procedures may be performed inappropriately.

The diagnosis of pulpalgia is made from a combination of the clinical presentation and the response of the teeth to percussion, thermal stimuli, and electric pulp testing. The predictive value of these tests is sometimes less than optimal. When the procedures demonstrate that the pulp is disease free, results are highly reliable. However, when a pulp appears to test positively for irreversible pulpitis, histopathologic examination may demonstrate no obvious evidence of pulpal disease. The practitioner should use all available tests, clinical information, and personal judgment in an attempt to arrive at an appropriate diagnosis. Future improvements in diagnostic methods, such as laser Doppler

flowmetry and pulse oximetry devices, may help to increase accuracy.

HISTOPATHOLOGIC FEATURES

Basically, the histopathology is primarily of academic interest and does not usually affect treatment significantly. Numerous investigations have shown a surprising lack of correlation between histopathologic findings and the clinical symptoms in the majority of pulps examined.

In patients with reversible pulpitis, the pulp usually shows hyperemia, edema, and a few inflammatory cells underlying the area of affected dentinal tubules (Fig. 3-4). Tertiary dentin may be noted in the adjacent

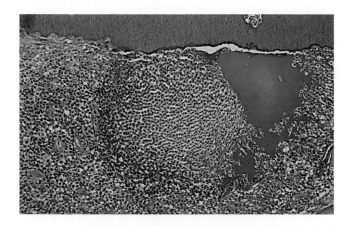

Fig. 3-5 Irreversible pulpitis. Dental pulp exhibiting acute inflammatory infiltrate consisting predominantly of polymorphonuclear leukocytes.

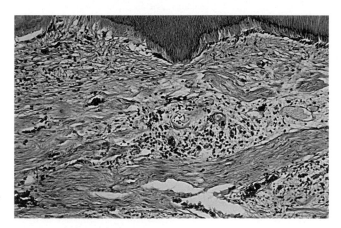

Fig. 3-6 Irreversible pulpitis. Same tooth as depicted in Fig. 3-5. The dental pulp exhibits an area of fibrosis and chronic inflammation peripheral to the zone of abscess formation.

dentinal wall, and scattered acute inflammatory cells are found occasionally.

Irreversible pulpitis often demonstrates congestion of the venules that results in focal necrosis. This necrotic zone contains polymorphonuclear leukocytes and histiocytes (Fig. 3-5). The surrounding pulp tissue usually exhibits fibrosis and a mixture of plasma cells, lymphocytes, and histiocytes (Fig. 3-6).

Chronic hyperplastic pulpitis demonstrates a cap of subacutely inflamed granulation tissue that fills the entire space of the original pulp chamber and histopathologically resembles a pyogenic granuloma (see page 518). The surface of the polyp may or may not be covered with stratified squamous epithelium, which migrates from the adjacent gingiva or arises from sloughed epithelium within the oral fluids (see Fig. 3-3). The deeper pulp tissue within the canals typically

demonstrates fibrosis and a chronic inflammatory infiltrate. Pulpal calcifications are common in both the radicular and coronal portions. Often the apical portion of the pulp tissue is normal, with minimal inflammation or fibrosis.

TREATMENT AND PROGNOSIS

Reversible pulpitis is treated by removal of the local irritant. On occasion, analgesic medications sometimes are desirable. The prognosis of reversible pulpitis is good if action is taken early enough. The tooth should be tested for vitality after the symptoms have subsided to ensure that irreversible damage has not occurred.

Irreversible and chronic hyperplastic pulpitis are treated by extraction of the tooth or by root canal therapy.

SECONDARY AND TERTIARY DENTIN

Formation of dentin proceeds throughout life. The dentin formed before completion of the crown is called **primary dentin.** This process is followed by the formation of **secondary dentin.** The same odontoblasts that formed the primary dentin remain functional and produce secondary dentin. With advancing age, deposition of secondary dentin leads to smaller pulp chambers and canal systems. The deposition of dentin is slow and gradual but does increase after the age of 35 to 40 years. Forensic scientists have shown that the formation of secondary dentin occurs so consistently that the width ratio of the dentin taken at three different root levels correlates very closely with age. Early widespread formation of secondary dentin has been seen in association with **progeria,** a condition associated with accelerated aging. On occasion, significant traumatic injury can lead to early obliteration of the pulp chamber and canal (**calcific metamorphosis**) in the affected tooth.

In functioning teeth, deposition begins in the coronal portions of the tooth and proceeds to the apical areas. Many investigators believe that this type of dentin, termed **physiologic secondary dentin,** occurs as a result of aging. A significantly decreased amount of secondary dentin has been described in impacted teeth, suggesting that functional forces of occlusion promote the deposition. Interestingly, the deposition in impacted teeth appears to begin in the apical areas and spreads coronally.

Although production of physiologic secondary dentin and a resultant decrease in pulpal size are related most strongly to aging, the process is more advanced in males and has been associated positively with calcification-related diseases (e.g., arthritis, gout, kidney stones, gall stones, atherosclerosis, hypertension). Deposition within the pulp chamber often is not totally uniform. In posterior teeth, the greatest deposition is seen on the pulpal floor, to a lesser extent on the roof, and least on the sidewalls. Therefore, with age, pulp chambers decrease significantly in height but not extensively in width.

Localized new dentin also is laid down in areas of focal injury. This dentin is more haphazardly organized and is termed **tertiary (reactionary, reparative, irregular, or irritation) dentin.** This localized dentin formation may occur in response to the following:

- Attrition
- Fracture
- Erosion
- Abrasion
- Caries
- Periodontal disease
- Mechanical injury from dental procedures
- Irritation from dental materials

Injury of the peripheral odontoblastic processes is all that is required to initiate tertiary dentin formation. If the stimulus is mild to moderate, then the tertiary dentin typically is produced by surviving odontoblasts and is termed *reactionary dentin.* This type of tertiary dentin is more regular in appearance and continuous with the tubules of the primary and secondary dentin. If the stimulus is more severe and leads to the death of the primary odontoblasts, then a new generation of odontoblasts may arise from undifferentiated cells within the pulp and continue to form tertiary dentin that is termed *reparative dentin.* Researchers believe that these new odontoblasts arise from subodontoblastic cells or pericytes. During primary dentin formation, the odontoblasts incorporate a number of growth factors, such as transforming growth factor-β (TGF-β), into the intertubular matrix. Investigators have suggested that these growth factors may be released secondary to dentinal injury or cavity restoration and may be involved in the signaling for differentiation of the secondary generation of odontoblasts. Demineralization of dentin during caries also releases significant amounts of calcium and phosphates. These minerals often diffuse toward the pulp and assist in sclerosis of the tubules as calcium phosphate. In many ways, dentin not only acts as the backbone of the tooth but also as a storehouse of bioactive materials awaiting release during critical times of injury.

The initial layer of reparative dentin is atubular and known as *interface dentin (fibrodentin).* This thin band may be acellular or exhibit scattered nuclear inclusions. After deposition of the interface dentin, the remainder of the reparative dentin is tubular but not continuous with the primary, secondary, or reactionary dentin. This lack of communication further assists in protecting the pulp from the external stimulus. When

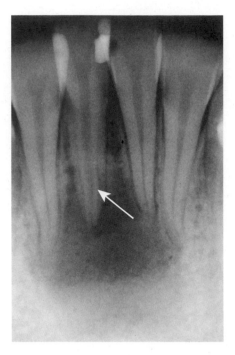

Fig. 3-7   Physiologic secondary dentin. Periapical abscess with all four teeth nonresponsive to electric pulp testing. Decreased deposition of physiologic secondary dentin on the right central incisor (*arrow*) delineated the origin of the infection; endodontic treatment of this tooth resolved the lesion.

the primary odontoblasts die, their dentinal tubules are filled with degenerated odontoblastic processes and are termed *dead tracts.* These tubules usually are sealed off from the pulp by the reparative dentin.

CLINICAL AND RADIOGRAPHIC FEATURES

As noted on periapical radiographs, the deposition of secondary dentin results in diminishing size of pulp chambers and canals. In addition to being used as an estimate of age, secondary dentin appears to reduce sensitivity of the affected teeth, susceptibility to dentinal caries, and the trauma of dental procedures. Although production of secondary dentin makes pulp exposure during operative procedures less likely, it also increases the difficulty of locating the pulp chamber and canals during endodontic therapy. On occasion, large inflammatory lesions may involve more than one apex; the size of the canals can be used to help determine the original focus of infection because the canal may be larger in the tooth that became nonvital earlier (Fig. 3-7). Teeth affected by calcific metamorphosis often are discovered clinically by a yellow discoloration of the crown; radiographically, the affected teeth exhibit an accelerated closure of the pulp chamber and

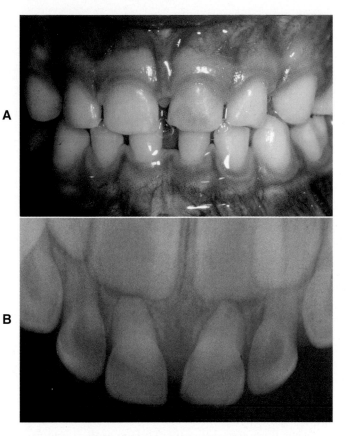

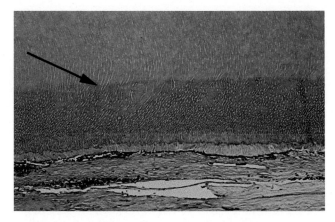

Fig. 3-9 Physiologic secondary dentin. A distinct line of demarcation (*arrow*) separates the primary dentin and physiologic secondary dentin.

Fig. 3-8 Calcific metamorphosis. A, Left deciduous maxillary central incisor exhibiting yellow discoloration. **B,** Radiograph of the same patient showing total calcification of the pulp chambers and canals of the deciduous maxillary incisors. (*Courtesy of Dr. Jackie L. Banahan.*)

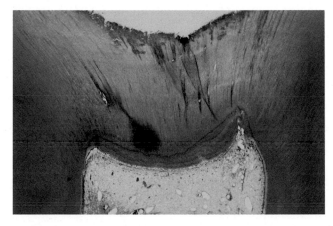

Fig. 3-10 Reparative secondary dentin. Localized deposition of secondary dentin (*bottom*) at the pulpal end of the dentinal tubules affected by the carious process.

canal when compared with adjacent or contralateral teeth (Fig. 3-8). In such cases the pulpal space may appear to be obliterated completely or reduced dramatically. This alteration usually follows trauma to the tooth and may be seen as early as 3 months after the traumatic episode; however, usually the condition is not detected for about 1 year.

HISTOPATHOLOGIC FEATURES

Physiologic secondary dentin consists of regular tubular dentin that is applied onto the primary dentin. These two layers of dentin can be separated by a line of demarcation, often indicated by a bending of the tubules (Fig. 3-9). With advancing age, as the odontoblasts undergo degenerative changes, the physiologic secondary dentin becomes more irregular with fewer tubules.

The quality and appearance of tertiary dentin depend on the severity of the noxious stimulus that promoted its formation. Tertiary dentin is localized to

the pulpal end of the odontoblastic processes that were affected (Fig. 3-10). With a mild stimulus, such as abrasion or attrition, reactionary dentin exhibits slow deposition characterized by tubules that are continuous with the secondary dentin and only slightly irregular. With more severe damage (e.g., a rapidly progressing carious lesion), reparative dentin is formed, a process that occurs more rapidly and consists of a thin layer of interface dentin on which is deposited irregular dentin with widely scattered, disorganized tubules.

TREATMENT AND PROGNOSIS

In studies of teeth exhibiting calcific metamorphosis, the vast majority of affected teeth never develop clinical or radiographic features suggestive of periapical inflammatory disease; therefore, endodontic therapy should be performed only if periapical pathosis or negative vitality testing is present. Even if a canal space cannot be identified radiographically, conventional root canal therapy usually can locate and negotiate the pulp canal. Because of the dramatically reduced canal space, location of the pulp canal can be difficult, and care must be exercised during access preparation to prevent perforation. If endodontic therapy is unsuccessful, then periapical surgery can be performed in those cases with evidence of periapical inflammatory disease. If vitality testing is positive, then periodic reevaluation appears prudent. To improve dental aesthetics, full coverage is recommended for discolored anterior teeth with large restorations. Otherwise, bleaching often effectively resolves the discoloration.

PULPAL CALCIFICATIONS

Calcifications within the dental pulp are not rare, but the frequency is difficult to determine. Reported rates vary from 8% to 90%, but several investigators have documented a prevalence of approximately 20% in individual teeth reviewed radiographically. Because radiographically detectable pulp stones typically exceed 200 μm in diameter, the prevalence in a histopathologic review would be expected to be much higher. There appears to be a strong association between long-standing chronic pulpitis and the presence of pulpal calcification; in addition, the prevalence of pulpal calcifications increases with age. However, some examples appear to be developmental with a familial tendency.

The three types of pulpal calcifications are:
1. Denticles
2. Pulp stones
3. Diffuse linear calcifications

All pulpal calcifications start out as free bodies within the pulp tissue, but many may become attached or embedded in the dentinal walls of the pulp.

Denticles are believed to form as a result of an epitheliomesenchymal interaction within the developing pulp. Epithelial strands originating from the root sheath, or cervical extensions into the pulp chamber adjacent to furcations, induce odontoblastic differentiation of the surrounding mesenchyme of the dental papilla, forming the core of the denticle. Odontoblasts deposit tubular dentin as they move away from the central epithelium and produce thimble-shaped structures surrounding the epithelium. Denticles form during the period of root development and occur in the root canal and the pulp chamber adjacent to the furcation areas of multirooted teeth. Because denticle development typically precedes completion of the primary dentin, most denticles become attached to or embedded in the dentin.

Pulp stones are believed to develop around a central nidus of pulp tissue (e.g., collagen fibril, ground substance, necrotic cell remnants). Initial calcification begins around the central nidus and extends outward in a concentric or radial pattern of regular calcified material. Pulp stones are formed within the coronal portions of the pulp and may arise as a part of age-related or local pathologic changes. Most pulp stones develop after tooth formation is completed and are usually free or attached. In rare instances, stones may become embedded.

Diffuse linear calcifications do not demonstrate the lamellar organization of pulp stones; they exhibit areas of fine, fibrillar, irregular calcification that often parallel the vasculature. These calcifications may be present in the pulp chamber or canals, and the frequency increases with age.

CLINICAL AND RADIOGRAPHIC FEATURES

Denticles and pulp stones can reach sufficient size to be detected on intraoral radiographs as radiopaque enlargements within the pulp chamber or canal (Fig. 3-11). Diffuse calcifications are not detectable radiographically.

Other than rare difficulties during endodontic procedures, pulpal calcifications are typically of little clinical significance. Some investigators associate the calcifications with dental neuralgias, but the high frequency of these lesions in the absence of clinical symptoms argues against this relationship. On occasion, the pulpal calcifications may become very large and may interfere with root formation, possibly leading to early periodontal destruction and tooth loss. Prominent pulpal calcifications have been noted in association with certain disease processes, such as the following:

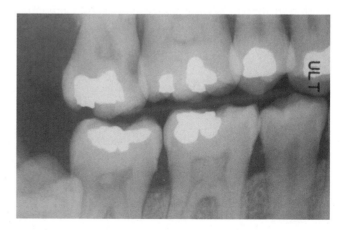

Fig. 3-11 Pulp stones. Multiple teeth demonstrating radiographically obvious calcifications within the pulp chambers.

- Dentin dysplasia type Id (see page 108)
- Dentin dysplasia type II (see page 108)
- Pulpal dysplasia (see page 110)
- Tumoral calcinosis
- Calcinosis universalis
- Ehlers-Danlos syndrome (see page 755)

If all of the patient's teeth have enlarged pulp chambers containing calcifications, the possibility of dentin dysplasia type II should be investigated. If the stones are located in the coronal portion of root canals that exhibit enlargement and bulging, then dentin dysplasia type 1d should be considered. Both of these rare conditions are associated with abnormally shaped pulp chambers or canals; therefore, such a diagnosis should not be considered when pulp stones are noted in the absence of pulpal changes.

HISTOPATHOLOGIC FEATURES

Denticles consist of tubular dentin surrounding a central nest of epithelium. With time, the central epithelium degenerates and the tubules undergo sclerosis, making their detection difficult. Most denticles are attached or embedded. Those that remain free in the pulp occasionally develop outer layers of irregular fibrillar calcification or lamellated layers of calcification similar to those seen in pulp stones.

Pulp stones demonstrate a central amorphous mass of irregular calcification surrounded by concentric lamellar rings of regular calcified material (Fig. 3-12). Occasionally, a peripheral layer of tubular dentin may be applied by odontoblasts, which arise from the surrounding pulp tissue in response to the presence of the pulp stone. In addition, fibrillar irregular calcified material also may be evident on the periphery of pulp stones.

Diffuse linear calcifications consist entirely of fine, fibrillar, and irregular calcifications that develop in the pulp chambers and canals (Fig. 3-13). This material often is deposited in a linear fashion along the course of a blood vessel or nerve.

TREATMENT AND PROGNOSIS

No treatment is required. Most pulpal calcifications are not associated with any significant clinical alterations.

PERIAPICAL GRANULOMA (CHRONIC APICAL PERIODONTITIS)

The term **periapical granuloma** refers to a mass of chronically or subacutely inflamed granulation tissue at the apex of a nonvital tooth. This commonly used name is not totally accurate because the lesion does not show true granulomatous inflammation microscopically. Although the term **apical periodontitis** may be more appropriate, it may prove confusing to the clinician. Formation of apical inflammatory lesions represents a defensive reaction secondary to the presence of microbial infection in the root canal with spread of related toxic products into the apical zone. Initially, the defense reaction eliminates noxious substances that exit the canals. With time, however, the host reaction becomes less effective with microbial invasion or spread of toxins into the apical area. Although the infection typically is bacterial in origin, the presence of yeasts occasionally is demonstrated. Although controversial, an increased prevalence of human cytomegalovirus and, to a lesser extent, Epstein-Barr virus has been documented in symptomatic periapical inflammatory disease; some clinicians believe this to be more than a secondary infestation.

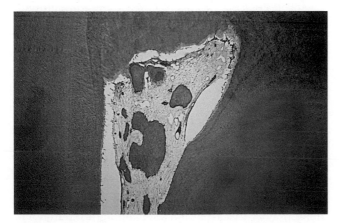

Fig. 3-12   Pulp stones. Multiple stones within the pulp chamber.

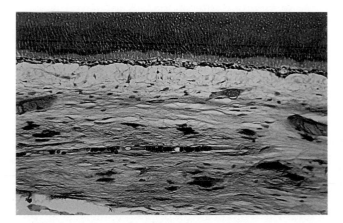

Fig. 3-13   Diffuse linear pulpal calcifications. Fine, fibrillar calcifications parallel the course of the neurovascular channels within the pulp canal.

In the early stages of infection, neutrophils predominate and radiographic alterations are not present; this phase of periapical inflammatory disease is termed *acute apical periodontitis*. The involved inflammatory cells are primarily neutrophils and release prostaglandins, which activate osteoclasts to resorb the surrounding bone, leading to a detectable periapical radiolucency. Researchers believe that this bone destruction is an attempt to prevent the spread of the infection and provide space for the arrival of defense cells specialized against the infectious process. With time, chronic inflammatory cells begin to dominate the host response. Mediators released by lymphocytes reduce further osteoclastic activity while also stimulating fibroblasts and the microvasculature. Because of these actions, chronic lesions often are asymptomatic and demonstrate little additional change radiographically.

Periapical granulomas may arise after quiescence of a **periapical abscess** or may develop as the initial periapical pathosis. These lesions are not necessarily static. In addition to possible **periapical cyst** formation, a worsening of the pulpal infection can lead to a reappearance of inflammation, redevelopment of symptoms, and possible enlargement of the associated radiolucency. Secondary acute inflammatory changes within a periapical granuloma have been termed a *phoenix abscess*, after the mythical bird that would die, only to arise again from its own ashes. In progressive periapical granulomas, the enlargement often is not continuous but occurs in spurts associated with periodic acute exacerbations.

CLINICAL AND RADIOGRAPHIC FEATURES

The initial phase of periapical inflammatory disease—acute periapical periodontitis—creates a constant dull, throbbing pain. The associated tooth responds negatively to vitality testing or reveals a delayed positive result. Typically, pain on biting or percussion is present, and no obvious radiographic alterations are noted. If the acute inflammatory process evolves into a chronic pattern, then the associated symptoms diminish. In many instances, chronic periapical inflammatory disease is detected without any previous recollection of a prior acute phase.

Most periapical granulomas are asymptomatic, but pain and sensitivity can develop if acute exacerbation occurs. Typically, the involved tooth does not demonstrate mobility or significant sensitivity to percussion. The soft tissue overlying the apex may or may not be tender. The tooth does not respond to thermal or electric pulp tests unless the pulpal necrosis is limited to a single canal in a multirooted tooth. Periapical granulomas represent approximately 75% of apical inflammatory lesions and 50% of those that have failed to respond to conservative endodontic measures.

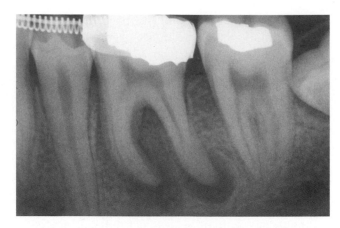

Fig. 3-14   Periapical granulomas. Discrete periapical radiolucencies associated with the apices of the mandibular first molar. *(Courtesy of Dr. Garth Bobrowski.)*

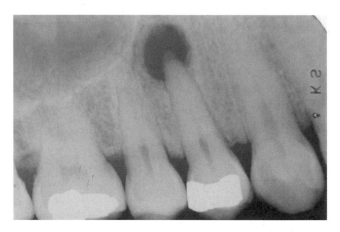

Fig. 3-15   Periapical granuloma. Well-defined radiolucency associated with the apex of the maxillary first bicuspid. *(Courtesy of Dr. Frank Beylotte.)*

Most lesions are discovered on routine radiographic examination. The associated radiolucencies are variable, ranging from small, barely perceptible lesions to lucencies exceeding 2 cm in diameter (Figs. 3-14 to 3-16). Affected teeth typically reveal loss of the apical lamina dura. The lesion may be circumscribed or ill-defined and may or may not demonstrate a surrounding radiopaque rim. Root resorption is not uncommon (Fig. 3-17). Although lesions greater than 200 mm^2 often represent periapical cysts, numerous investigators have been unable to distinguish periapical granulomas from periapical cysts simply on the basis of size and radiographic appearance. Because periapical inflammatory disease is not static and granulomas can transform into cysts or abscesses (and vice versa) without significant radiographic change, it is not

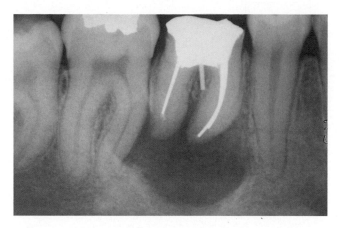

Fig. 3-16 Periapical granuloma. Large, well-defined radiolucency associated with the apices of the mandibular first molar. *(Courtesy of Dr. Robert E. Loy.)*

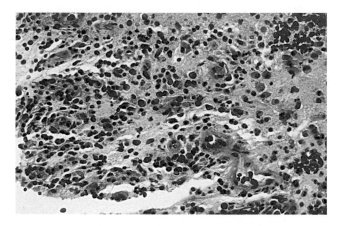

Fig. 3-18 Periapical granuloma. Granulation tissue exhibits mixed inflammatory infiltrate consisting of lymphocytes, plasma cells, and histiocytes.

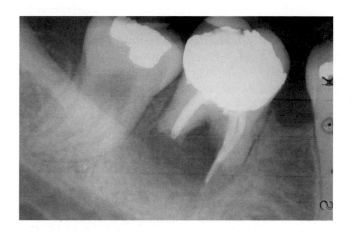

Fig. 3-17 Periapical granuloma. Ill-defined radiolucency associated with the mandibular first molar, which exhibits significant root resorption.

surprising that the radiographic features are not diagnostic.

HISTOPATHOLOGIC FEATURES

Periapical granulomas consist of inflamed granulation tissue surrounded by a fibrous connective tissue wall. The granulation tissue demonstrates a variably dense lymphocytic infiltrate that is intermixed frequently with neutrophils, plasma cells, histiocytes, and, less frequently, mast cells and eosinophils (Fig. 3-18). When numerous plasma cells are present, scattered eosinophilic globules of gamma globulin **(Russell bodies)** may be seen. In addition, clusters of lightly basophilic particles **(pyronine bodies)** also may be present in association with the plasmacytic infiltrate. Both of these plasma cell products are not specific for the periapical granuloma and may be found within any accumulation of plasma cells. Epithelial rests of Malassez may be identified within the granulation tissue. Collections of cholesterol clefts, with associated multinucleated giant cells and areas of red blood cell extravasation with hemosiderin pigmentation, may be present. Although the source of the cholesterol is unclear, this material often is noted in areas of long-term inflammation and may accumulate from dying inflammatory cells, disintegrating red blood cells, or degenerating cystic epithelium. The cholesterol attracts macrophages and foreign body giant cells, which are unable to degrade the material but release inflammatory and bone resorptive mediators. Significant cholesterol accumulation can continue the inflammatory process in the absence of active microbial infection. Small foci of acute inflammation with focal abscess formation may be seen but do not warrant the diagnosis of periapical abscess.

TREATMENT AND PROGNOSIS

Apical inflammatory lesions result from the presence of microorganisms or their toxic products in the root canal, the apical tissues, or both. Successful treatment depends on the reduction and control of the offending organisms. Because of the anatomic complexity of the root canal systems, some investigators believe absolute eradication of all microorganisms is unlikely; the goal of endodontics is to reduce the microbial load to a level that is insufficient to maintain periapical inflammation. If the tooth can be maintained, then root canal therapy can be performed. Nonrestorable teeth must be extracted, followed by curettage of all apical soft tissue. In symptomatic cases, nonsteroidal antiinflammatory drugs (NSAIDs) are beneficial; use of systemic antibiotic medications is not recommended unless associated swelling or systemic changes are present.

Teeth treated endodontically should be evaluated at 1- and 2-year intervals (at a minimum) to rule out possible lesional enlargement and to ensure appropriate healing. In addition, many clinicians believe that evaluations at 1, 3, and 6 months are appropriate. Strong emphasis should be placed on the importance of the recall appointments.

Lesions may fail to heal for several reasons:
- Cyst formation
- Persistent pulpal infection (e.g., poor access design, missed canals, perforated canals, vertical root fractures, inadequate aseptic technique or instrumentation, leaking fillings)
- Extraradicular infection (usually localized periapical actinomycotic colonization)
- Accumulation of endogenous debris (e.g., cholesterol crystals)
- Periapical foreign material
- Associated periodontal disease
- Penetration of the adjacent maxillary sinus
- Fibrous scar formation (see following)

If initial conventional therapy is unsuccessful, endodontic retreatment represents the best approach for minimizing the bacterial contamination and should be considered before periapical surgery. Periapical surgery remains an important tool for resolution of periapical inflammatory disease, but often it is reserved for lesions larger than 2 cm or those associated with teeth that are not appropriate for conventional endodontic therapy. Periapical surgery should include thorough curettage of all periradicular soft tissue, amputation of the apical portion of the root, and sealing the foramen of the canal.

All soft tissue removed during periapical surgical procedures should be submitted for histopathologic examination. These surgical sites represent areas that have failed to respond to appropriate therapy; as such, histopathologic examination and diagnostic confirmation are mandatory. The primary motivation for this examination is not to discover whether the lesion represents a periapical granuloma or cyst; the examination is conducted to eliminate the possibility of a more serious process unrelated to periapical inflammatory disease. In an active oral and maxillofacial pathology service, discovery of unexpected neoplasms within specimens removed during periapical surgery is not rare.

On occasion, the defect created by periapical inflammatory lesions may fill with dense collagenous tissue rather than normal bone (Fig. 3-19). These **fibrous (periapical) scars** occur most frequently when both the facial and lingual cortical plates have been lost (Fig.

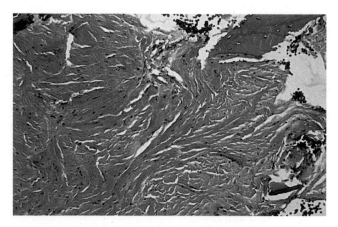

Fig. 3-19 Periapical fibrous scar. Dense, fibrous connective tissue with vital bone and no significant inflammatory infiltrate.

3-20); however, they occasionally arise in areas with intact cortical plates. If during surgery both plates are discovered to be missing, then the patient should be informed of the possibility of scar formation. The development of a periapical scar is not an indication for future surgery.

PERIAPICAL CYST (RADICULAR CYST; APICAL PERIODONTAL CYST)

Epithelium at the apex of a nonvital tooth presumably can be stimulated by inflammation to form a true epithelium-lined cyst, or **periapical cyst.** The inflammatory response appears to increase the production of keratinocyte growth factor by periodontal stroma cells, leading to increased proliferation of normally quiescent epithelium in the area. The source of the epithelium is usually a rest of Malassez but also may be traced to crevicular epithelium, sinus lining, or epithelial lining of fistulous tracts. Cyst development is common; the reported frequency varies from 7% to 54% of periapical radiolucencies.

The wide disparity of prevalence most likely is related to the stringency of the diagnostic criteria used in a particular study. Several investigators believe the diagnosis of a periapical cyst can be made only after a lesion has been examined entirely with serial or step sectioning of the specimen. Review of random sections of a fragmented and epithelialized periapical granuloma could appear to be an epithelium-lined cavity that did not exist in reality. When strict criteria are used, the prevalence of periapical cysts appears to be approximately 15%. When the cyst and root are removed totally, two variations of periapical cyst have been described. **Periapical pocket cysts** are characterized by an incomplete epithelial lining because of extension

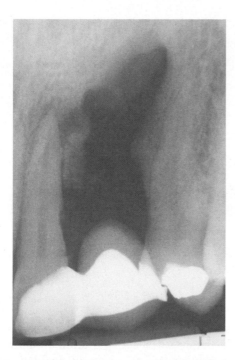

Fig. 3-20 Periapical fibrous scar. Periapical radiolucency of maxilla at the previous site of extraction in which both cortical plates were lost. The site was filled with dense collagenous tissue. *(Courtesy of Dr. James Tankersley.)*

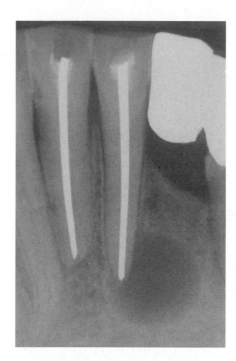

Fig. 3-21 Periapical cyst. Well-circumscribed radiolucency intimately associated with the apex of the mandibular central incisor. Note the loss of lamina dura in the area of the lesion.

of the apical portion of the tooth into the cyst lumen. **Periapical true cysts** form a complete epithelium-lined baglike structure that is adjacent to, but separated from, the tooth apex. Because distinguishing between an epithelialized periapical granuloma, a "pocket" cyst, or a "true" cyst has little postsurgical implications, laborious histopathologic examination and subclassification are impractical.

Periapical cysts represent a fibrous connective tissue wall lined by epithelium with a lumen containing fluid and cellular debris. Theoretically, as the epithelium desquamates into the lumen, the protein content is increased. Fluid enters the lumen in an attempt to equalize the osmotic pressure, and slow enlargement occurs. Most periapical cysts grow slowly and do not attain a large size.

On occasion, a similar cyst, best termed a **lateral radicular cyst,** may appear along the lateral aspect of the root. Like the periapical cyst, this lesion also usually arises from rests of Malassez, and the source of inflammation may be periodontal disease or pulpal necrosis with spread through a lateral foramen. Radiographically, these cysts mimic developmental **lateral periodontal cysts** (see page 692). Histopathologically, however, they are consistent with cysts of inflammatory origin.

Periapical inflammatory tissue that is not curetted at the time of tooth removal may give rise to an inflam-

matory cyst called a **residual periapical cyst.** With time, many of these cysts exhibit an overall reduction in size, and spontaneous resolution can occur from a lack of continued inflammatory stimulus.

CLINICAL AND RADIOGRAPHIC FEATURES

PERIAPICAL CYST

Typically, patients with periapical cysts have no symptoms unless there is an acute inflammatory exacerbation. In addition, if the cyst reaches a large size, then swelling and mild sensitivity may be noted. Movement and mobility of adjacent teeth are possible as the cyst enlarges. The tooth from which the cyst originated does not respond to thermal and electric pulp testing.

The radiographic pattern is identical to that of a periapical granuloma. Cysts may develop even in small periapical radiolucencies, and the radiographic size cannot be used for the definitive diagnosis. A loss of the lamina dura is seen along the adjacent root, and a rounded radiolucency encircles the affected tooth apex (Fig. 3-21). Root resorption is common (Fig. 3-22). With enlargement, the radiolucency often flattens out as it approaches adjacent teeth. Significant growth is possible, and lesions occupying an entire quadrant have been noted (Fig. 3-23). Although periapical cysts more frequently achieve greater size than periapical

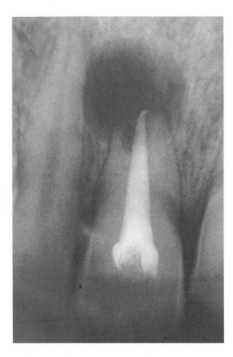

Fig. 3-22   Periapical cyst. Radiolucency associated with the maxillary central incisor, which exhibits significant root resorption.

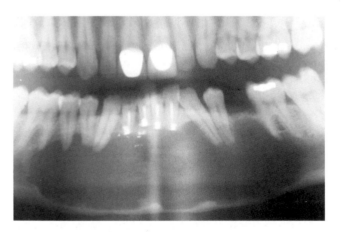

Fig. 3-23   Periapical cyst. Large unilocular radiolucency extending from the mandibular first molar to the contralateral first molar. *(Courtesy of Dr. John R. Cramer.)*

granulomas, neither the size nor the shape of the lesion can be considered a definitive diagnostic criterion. Periapical cysts also are known to involve deciduous teeth. These are most frequently associated with molar teeth and appear as a radiolucent zone that surrounds the roots and fills the interradicular space at the bifurcation (Fig. 3-24).

LATERAL RADICULAR CYST

Lateral radicular cysts appear as discrete radiolucencies along the lateral aspect of the root (Fig. 3-25). Loss of lamina dura and an obvious source of inflam-

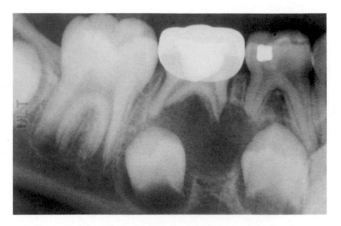

Fig. 3-24   Periapical cyst. Radiolucency involving the bifurcation and apices of the deciduous right mandibular second molar.

mation may not be detected without a high index of suspicion. Before surgical exploration of laterally positioned radiolucencies, a thorough evaluation of the periodontal status and vitality of adjacent teeth should be performed. Many examples of the so-called globulomaxillary cyst (see page 28) prove to be of inflammatory origin and represent lateral radicular cysts (Fig. 3-26).

RESIDUAL PERIAPICAL CYST

The residual periapical cyst appears as a round-to-oval radiolucency of variable size within the alveolar ridge at the site of a previous tooth extraction (Figs. 3-27 and 3-28). As the cyst ages, degeneration of the cellular contents within the lumen occasionally leads to dystrophic calcification and central luminal radiopacity (Fig. 3-29).

HISTOPATHOLOGIC FEATURES

The histopathologic features of all three types of inflammatory cysts are similar. The cyst is lined by stratified squamous epithelium, which may demonstrate exocytosis, spongiosis, or hyperplasia (Fig. 3-30). As seen in dentigerous cysts, scattered mucous cells or areas of ciliated pseudostratified columnar epithelium may be noted in periapical cysts (Fig. 3-31). Although some maxillary periapical cysts lined by pseudostratified columnar epithelium may have originated from the adjacent sinus lining, the presence of mucous cells or respiratory-like epithelium also can be observed in mandibular cysts. The ability of odontogenic epithelium to demonstrate such specialized differentiation represents an example of *prosoplasia* (forward metaplasia) and highlights the diverse potential of odontogenic epithelium. The cyst lumen may be filled with fluid and

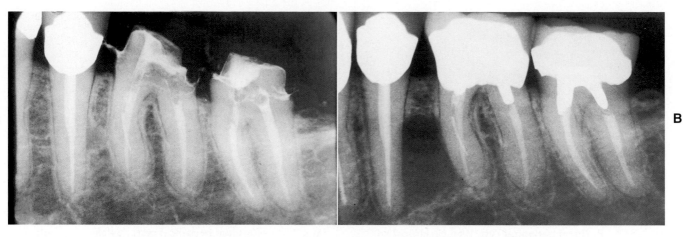

Fig. 3-25   Lateral radicular cyst. A, Periapical radiograph of the left side of the posterior mandible taken at time of completion of endodontic therapy of the bicuspid and molars. **B,** Subsequent radiograph taken 27 months later. Note radiolucency between bicuspid and first molar extending laterally from the mesial root of the first molar. *(Courtesy of Dr. Carroll Gallagher.)*

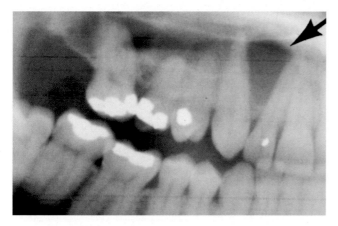

Fig. 3-26   Lateral radicular cyst. Inverted pear-shaped radiolucency between the maxillary lateral incisor and cuspid *(arrow).* The lateral incisor ultimately proved to be nonvital.

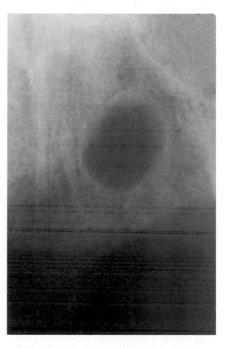

Fig. 3-27   Residual periapical cyst. Persistent radiolucency of the mandibular body at the site of previous tooth extraction.

cellular debris. On occasion, the lining epithelium may demonstrate linear or arch-shaped calcifications known as *Rushton bodies* (Fig. 3-32). Dystrophic calcification, cholesterol clefts with multinucleated giant cells, red blood cells, and areas of hemosiderin pigmentation may be present in the lumen, wall, or both. The wall of the cyst consists of dense fibrous connective tissue, often with an inflammatory infiltrate containing lymphocytes variably intermixed with neutrophils, plasma cells, histiocytes, and (rarely) mast cells and eosinophils.

Occasionally, the walls of inflammatory cysts will contain scattered **hyaline bodies (pulse granuloma, giant-cell hyaline angiopathy).** These bodies appear as small circumscribed pools of eosinophilic material

that exhibits a corrugated periphery of condensed collagen often surrounded by lymphocytes and multinucleated giant cells (Fig. 3-33). The eosinophilic material may be uniform or contain a variable mixture of lymphocytes, plasma cells, multinucleated giant cells, neutrophils, necrotic debris, and dystrophic calcification. Initially, these foci were thought to be a vascular degenerative process or a foreign body reaction to machinery oil or vegetable matter. Subsequently, these bodies

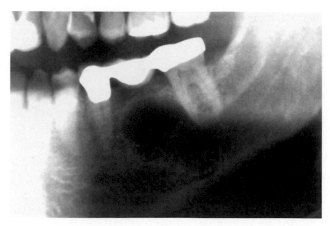

Fig. 3-28   Residual periapical cyst. Well-circumscribed radiolucency in the extraction site of the left mandibular first molar.

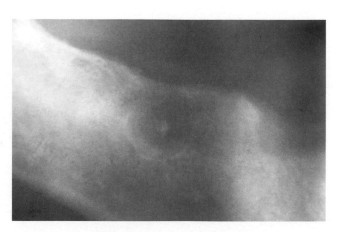

Fig. 3-29   Residual periapical cyst. Radiolucency with central radiopacity of the right mandibular body.

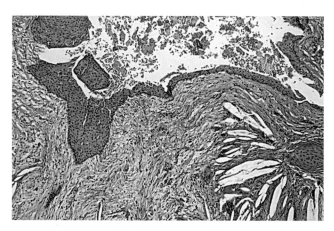

Fig. 3-30   Periapical cyst. Cyst lined by stratified squamous epithelium. Note connective tissue wall, which contains a chronic inflammatory infiltrate and numerous cholesterol clefts.

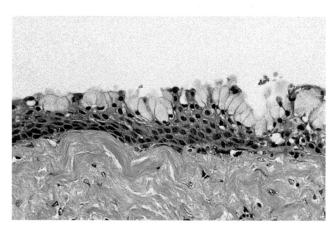

Fig. 3-31   Periapical cyst. Stratified squamous epithelial lining containing numerous mucous cells.

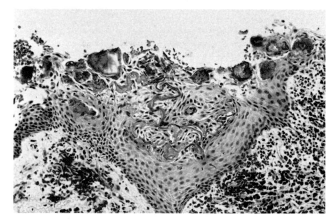

Fig. 3-32   Periapical cyst. Squamous epithelial cyst lining exhibiting numerous irregular and curvilinear Rushton bodies.

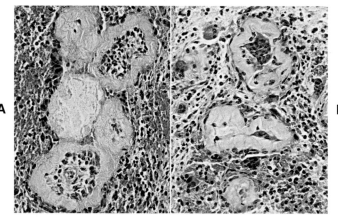

Fig. 3-33   Hyaline bodies. A, Multiple hyaline bodies appearing as corrugated collagenous rings surrounding lymphocytes and plasma cells; note early hyaline body filled with serum. **B,** Multiple hyaline bodies with numerous multinucleated giant cells within and around the corrugated collagenous rings.

have been shown to represent pools of inflammatory exudate (i.e., extravasated serum) that ultimately undergoes fibrosis and occasionally dystrophic calcification. The multinucleated giant cells are drawn to the site for removal of insoluble hemosiderin granules. Hyaline bodies may be found in any area of chronic intraosseous inflammation, especially periapical inflammatory disease.

TREATMENT AND PROGNOSIS

A periapical cyst is treated in the same manner as a periapical granuloma. When clinical and radiographic features indicate a periapical inflammatory lesion, extraction or conservative nonsurgical endodontic therapy is performed. Although some authors believe that large cystic lesions cannot be resolved with conventional endodontics, experienced clinicians have successfully used nonsurgical root canal therapy for large areas of periapical inflammatory disease that approach 2 cm in diameter. Larger lesions associated with restorable teeth have been treated successfully with conservative endodontic therapy when combined with biopsy and marsupialization, decompression, or fenestration. As with any periapical inflammatory lesion, minimal follow-up at 1 and 2 years is advised strongly.

If the radiolucency fails to resolve, then the lesion often can be managed successfully by nonsurgical endodontic retreatment. As previously mentioned, periapical surgery typically is performed for lesions exceeding 2 cm and those associated with teeth that are not suitable for conventional endodontics. Biopsy is indicated to rule out other possible pathologic processes.

Because any number of odontogenic and nonodontogenic cysts and tumors can mimic the appearance of a residual periapical cyst, all of these cysts should be excised surgically. All inflammatory foci in the area of a lateral radicular cyst should be eliminated and the patient observed in a manner similar to that described for the periapical cyst. In some instances, lateral radicular cysts are removed before tooth vitality testing or periodontal evaluation for an adjacent focus of infection. If this diagnosis is made, then a thorough evaluation for an inflammatory source is mandatory.

Cysts of inflammatory origin do not recur after appropriate management. Fibrous scars are possible, especially when both cortical plates have been lost; once diagnosed, no further therapy for fibrous scars is indicated. In rare instances, development of squamous cell carcinoma has been reported within periapical cysts; therefore, even in the absence of symptoms, treatment is required for all persistent intrabony pathoses that have not been diagnosed definitively by histopathologic examination.

PERIAPICAL ABSCESS

The accumulation of acute inflammatory cells at the apex of a nonvital tooth is termed a **periapical abscess.** Acute inflammatory lesions with abscess formation may arise as the initial periapical pathosis or from an acute exacerbation of a chronic periapical inflammatory lesion (see discussion of phoenix abscess, page 128). Frequently, the source of the infection is obvious. On occasion, however, pulpal death may be trauma related, and the tooth may contain neither a cavity nor a restoration.

In the earliest stage of all forms of periapical inflammatory disease, the periapical periodontal ligament (PDL) fibers may exhibit acute inflammation but no frank abscess formation. This localized alteration, best termed **acute apical periodontitis,** may or may not proceed to abscess formation. Although this process often occurs in association with a nonvital tooth, acute apical periodontitis may be found in vital teeth secondary to trauma, high occlusal contacts, or wedging by a foreign object. The clinical presentation often closely resembles that of a periapical abscess and must be considered in the differential diagnosis.

CLINICAL AND RADIOGRAPHIC FEATURES

Many investigators subdivide periapical abscesses into **acute** and **chronic** types. However, these are misnomers because both types represent acute inflammatory reactions. Periapical abscesses should be designated as **symptomatic** or **asymptomatic** on the basis of their clinical presentations.

Periapical abscesses become symptomatic as the purulent material accumulates within the alveolus. The initial stages produce tenderness of the affected tooth that often is relieved by direct application of pressure. With progression, the pain becomes more intense, often with extreme sensitivity to percussion, extrusion of the tooth, and swelling of the tissues. The offending tooth does not respond to cold or electric pulp testing. Headache, malaise, fever, and chills may be present.

Radiographically, abscesses may demonstrate a thickening of the apical periodontal ligament, an ill-defined radiolucency, or both; however, often no appreciable alterations can be detected because insufficient time has occurred for significant bone destruction. Phoenix abscesses demonstrate the outline of the original chronic lesion, with or without an associated ill-defined bone loss.

With progression, the abscess spreads along the path of least resistance. The purulence may extend through the medullary spaces away from the apical area, resulting in **osteomyelitis,** or it may perforate the

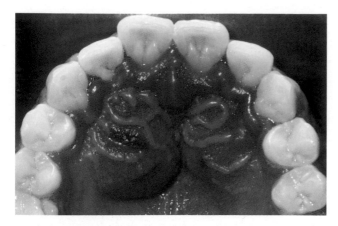

Fig. 3-34 **Periapical abscess.** Bilateral soft tissue swelling of the anterior palate.

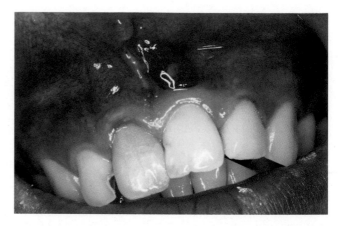

Fig. 3-36 **Parulis.** Erythematous mass of granulation tissue overlying the left maxillary central incisor. Note discoloration of the maxillary right central incisor.

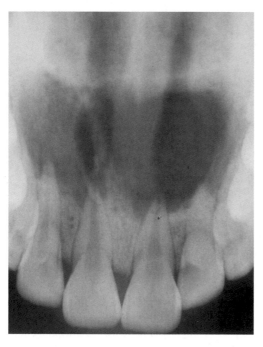

Fig. 3-35 **Periapical abscess.** Same patient as depicted in Fig. 3-34. Multiple, overlapping radiolucencies of the anterior maxilla are present. All four maxillary incisors exhibit pulpal necrosis.

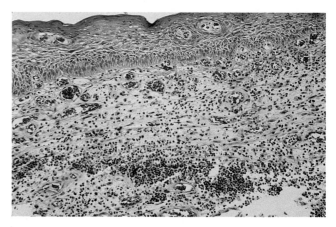

Fig. 3-37 **Parulis.** Normal connective tissue has been replaced by acutely inflamed granulation tissue, which exhibits focal areas of neutrophilic abscess formation. Note the central sinus tract, which courses from the base of the specimen toward the surface epithelium.

cortex and spread diffusely through the overlying soft tissue (as **cellulitis**). Each of these occurrences is described later in the chapter.

Once an abscess is in soft tissue, it can cause cellulitis or may channelize through the overlying soft tissue. The cortical plate may be perforated in a location that permits entrance into the oral cavity. The purulent material can accumulate in the connective tissue overlying the bone and can create a sessile swelling or perforate through the surface epithelium and drain through an intraoral sinus (Figs. 3-34 and 3-35). At the intraoral opening of a sinus tract, a mass of subacutely inflamed granulation tissue often is found, known as a **parulis (gum boil)** (Figs. 3-36 and 3-37). Occasionally, the nonvital tooth associated with the parulis may be difficult to determine, and insertion of a gutta-percha point into the tract can aid in detection of the offending tooth during radiographic examination (Fig. 3-38). Dental abscesses also may channelize through the overlying skin and drain via a **cutaneous sinus** (Fig. 3-39).

Most dental-related abscesses perforate buccally because the bone is thinner on the buccal surface. However, infections associated with maxillary lateral incisors, the palatal roots of maxillary molars, and mandibular second and third molars typically drain through the lingual cortical plate.

If a chronic path of drainage is achieved, a periapical abscess typically becomes asymptomatic because of

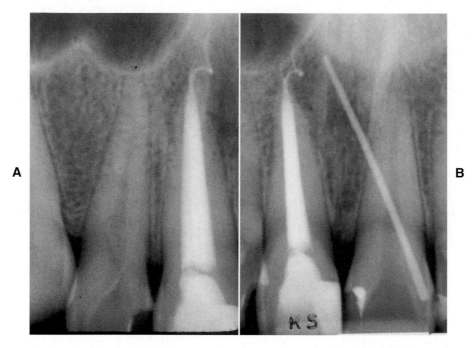

Fig. 3-38   Periapical abscess. A, Same patient as depicted in Fig. 3-36. None of the incisors demonstrates an obvious periapical radiolucency. (The large radiolucency at the top is the anterior portion of the maxillary sinus.) **B,** Gutta-percha point revealed that the right maxillary incisor was the source of the infection.

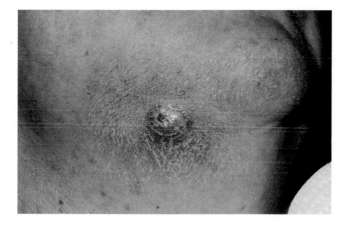

Fig. 3-39   Cutaneous sinus. Erythematous, firm, and sensitive enlargement of the skin inferior to the right body of the mandible.

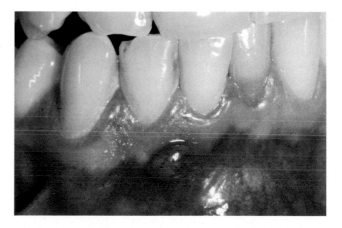

Fig. 3-40   Parulis. Asymptomatic yellow-red nodule of the anterior mandibular alveolar mucosa. The adjacent teeth were asymptomatic and appeared clinically normal.

a lack of accumulation of purulent material within the alveolus. Occasionally, such infections are discovered during a routine oral examination after detection of a parulis or drainage through a large carious defect (Figs. 3-40 and 3-41). If the drainage site becomes blocked, then signs and symptoms of the abscess frequently become evident in a short time. On occasion, periapical infections can spread through the bloodstream and result in systemic symptoms such as fever, lymphade-

nopathy, and malaise. The risk of dissemination appears to be less for periapical abscesses that drain freely.

HISTOPATHOLOGIC FEATURES

Biopsy specimens from pure abscesses are uncommon because the material is in liquid form. Abscesses consist of a sea of polymorphonuclear leukocytes often intermixed with inflammatory exudate, cellular debris,

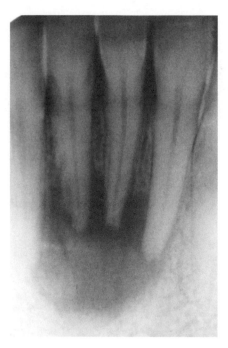

Fig. 3-41 Periapical abscess. Same patient as depicted in Fig. 3-40. Periapical radiolucency associated with the nonvital mandibular lateral incisor.

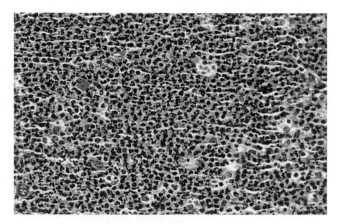

Fig. 3-42 Periapical abscess. Sheet of polymorphonuclear leukocytes intermixed with scattered histiocytes.

necrotic material, bacterial colonies, or histiocytes (Fig. 3-42). Phoenix abscesses can maintain a soft tissue component; they present as subacutely inflamed periapical granulomas or cysts intermixed with areas of significant abscess formation. In these cases the pathologist typically diagnoses the primary lesion but comments about the abscess formation.

TREATMENT AND PROGNOSIS

Treatment of the patient with a periapical abscess consists of drainage and elimination of the focus of infection. Those abscesses associated with a patent fistulous tract may be asymptomatic but, nevertheless, should be treated. With localized periapical abscesses, the signs and symptoms typically diminish significantly within 48 hours of initiation of appropriate drainage. When the abscess causes clinical expansion of the bone or soft tissue adjacent to the apex of the affected tooth, incisional drainage of the swelling should be considered because this technique appears to be associated with more rapid resolution of the inflammatory process when compared with drainage through the root canal. If the affected tooth is extruded, then reduction of the occlusion is recommended because chronic occlusal trauma has been shown to delay resolution of the inflammatory process. Unless contraindicated, treatment with NSAIDs usually is appropriate preoperatively, immediately postoperatively, and for subsequent

pain control. Typically, use of antibiotic medications for a well-localized and easily drained periapical abscess in a healthy patient is unnecessary. Antibiotic coverage should be reserved for the medically compromised and patients with significant cellulitis or clinical evidence of dissemination (i.e., fever, lymphadenopathy, malaise). Medical conditions that favor more widespread infection include diabetes mellitus, neutropenia, malignancy, immunosuppression, or use of therapeutic corticosteroid medications or cytotoxic drugs. Patients with significant cellulitis must be treated aggressively and monitored closely. Complications, such as cavernous sinus thrombosis, mediastinitis, cervical necrotizing fasciitis, and cerebral abscess, can be life threatening. Once the infection has been resolved by extraction or appropriate endodontic therapy, the affected bone typically heals.

Usually, a sinus tract resolves spontaneously after the offending tooth is extracted or endodontically treated. Sinus tracts that persist are thought to contain sufficient infectious material along the fistulous tract to maintain the surface granulation tissue, and surgical removal with curettage of the tract is required for resolution.

CELLULITIS

If an abscess is not able to establish drainage through the surface of the skin or into the oral cavity, it may spread diffusely through fascial planes of the soft tissue. This acute and edematous spread of an acute inflammatory process is termed **cellulitis**. Although numerous patterns of cellulitis can be seen from the spread of dental infections, two especially dangerous forms warrant further discussion: (1) **Ludwig's angina** and (2) **cavernous sinus thrombosis.**

Ludwig's angina, named after the German physician who described the seriousness of the disorder in 1836, refers to cellulitis of the submandibular region. Angina comes from the Latin word *angere*, which means *to strangle* (an apt term, considering the clinical features described in the following section). In approximately 70% of cases, Ludwig's angina develops from spread of an acute infection from the lower molar teeth. Other situations associated with this clinical presentation are peritonsillar or parapharyngeal abscesses, oral lacerations, fractures of the mandible, or submandibular sialadenitis. Although the process may occur in otherwise healthy individuals, there is an increased prevalence in patients who are immunocompromised secondary to disorders such as diabetes mellitus, organ transplantation, acquired immunodeficiency syndrome (AIDS), and aplastic anemia.

The cavernous sinus is a major dural sinus that is encased between the meningeal and periosteal layers of the dura. The meningeal layer contains the trochlear and oculomotor nerves and the maxillary and ophthalmic branches of the trigeminal nerve. In addition, the internal carotid artery and abducens nerve travel within the sinus. The sinus receives venous drainage from the orbit via the superior and inferior ophthalmic veins. Infection of the sinus can produce a variety of clinical symptoms related to the numerous anatomic structures that course through this site.

Cavernous sinus thrombosis can occur via an anterior or posterior pathway. Infection from the maxillary anterior teeth can perforate the facial maxillary bone and spread to the canine space. A septic thrombus develops in the valveless facial veins coursing through this space, propagating in a retrograde fashion from the angular vein to the inferior ophthalmic vein through the inferior orbital fissure into the cavernous sinus. The posterior pathway is followed by infections originating from maxillary premolar or molar teeth, which demonstrate buccal or infratemporal space involvement that may spread via the emissary veins from the pterygoid venous plexus to the inferior petrosal sinus and into the cavernous sinus. Overall, cavernous sinus thrombosis is relatively uncommon, and orodental infections are responsible in approximately 10% of the cases.

CLINICAL FEATURES
LUDWIG'S ANGINA

Ludwig's angina is an aggressive and rapidly spreading cellulitis that involves the sublingual, submandibular, and submental spaces. Once the infection enters the submandibular space, it may extend to the lateral pharyngeal space and then to the retropharyngeal space. This extension may result in spread to the mediastinum, with several serious consequences.

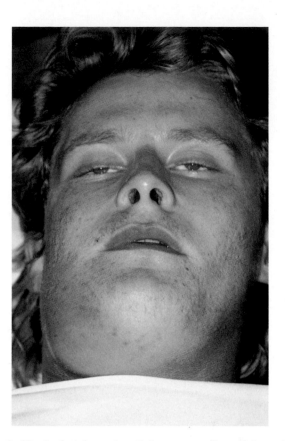

Fig. 3-43   Ludwig's angina. Soft tissue swelling of the right submandibular region. (*Courtesy of Dr. Brian Blocher.*)

Ludwig's angina creates massive swelling of the neck that often extends close to the clavicles (Fig. 3-43). Involvement of the sublingual space results in elevation, posterior enlargement, and protrusion of the tongue **(woody tongue)**, which can compromise the airway. Submandibular space spread causes enlargement and tenderness of the neck above the level of the hyoid bone **(bull neck)**. Although initially unilateral, spread to the contralateral neck typically occurs. Pain in the neck and floor of mouth may be seen in addition to restricted neck movement, dysphagia, dysphonia, dysarthria, drooling, and sore throat. Involvement of the lateral pharyngeal space can cause respiratory obstruction secondary to laryngeal edema. Tachypnea, dyspnea, tachycardia, stridor, restlessness, and the patient's need to maintain an erect position suggest airway obstruction. Fever, chills, leukocytosis, and an elevated sedimentation rate may be seen. Classically, obvious collections of pus are not present.

CAVERNOUS SINUS THROMBOSIS

Cavernous sinus thrombosis appears as an edematous periorbital enlargement with involvement of the eyelids and conjunctiva. In cases involving the canine space, swelling is also typically present along the lateral border

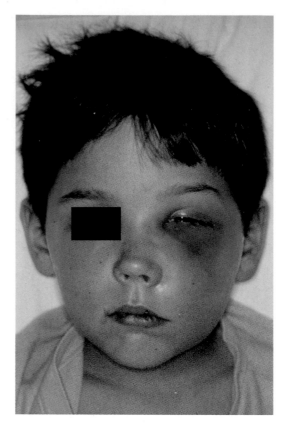

Fig. 3-44   Cellulitis involving canine space. Erythematous and edematous enlargement of the left side of the face with involvement of the eyelids and conjunctiva. Patients with odontogenic infections involving the canine space are at risk for cavernous sinus thrombosis. *(Courtesy of Dr. Richard Ziegler.)*

of the nose and may extend up to the medial aspect of the eye and periorbital area (Fig. 3-44). Protrusion and fixation of the eyeball often are evident, in addition to induration and swelling of the adjacent forehead and nose. Pupil dilation, lacrimation, photophobia, and loss of vision may occur. Pain over the eye and along the distribution of the ophthalmic and maxillary branches of the trigeminal nerve often are present. Proptosis, chemosis, and ptosis are noted in greater than 90% of affected patients. The cavernous sinuses freely communicate via the intercavernous sinus. Although many cases are initially unilateral, without appropriate therapy, the infection may spread to the contralateral side.

Fever, chills, headache, sweating, tachycardia, nausea, and vomiting can occur. With progression, signs of central nervous system (CNS) involvement develop. Meningitis, tachycardia, tachypnea, irregular breathing, stiffening of the neck, and deepening stupor with or without delirium indicate advanced toxemia

and meningeal involvement. Occasionally, brain abscesses may result.

TREATMENT AND PROGNOSIS
LUDWIG'S ANGINA

Treatment of Ludwig's angina centers around four activities:
1. Maintenance of the airway
2. Incision and drainage
3. Antibiotic therapy
4. Elimination of original focus of infection

Of primary importance is management of an intact airway. On initial observation, many clinicians administer systemic corticosteroid medications, such as intravenous (IV) dexamethasone, in an attempt to reduce the cellulitis. This procedure often protects the airway and allows more rapid penetration of antibiotic medications in the infected fascial spaces. Such therapy significantly reduces the need for an artificial airway; in the majority of the cases, tracheotomy or intubation is not required.

If signs or symptoms of impending airway obstruction develop, fiber-optic nasotracheal intubation or tracheostomy should be performed. Orotracheal intubation often is very difficult because of the presence of trismus and swollen soft tissues. Because intubation is difficult in patients with such massive neck enlargement and may cause laryngospasm or discharge of pus into the bronchial tree, tracheostomy is preferred if there is any chance of significant intubation complications. On occasion, cricothyroidotomy is performed instead of a tracheostomy because of a perceived lower risk of spreading the infection to the mediastinum.

High-dose penicillin is the antibiotic of choice. Aminoglycoside therapy is given for resistant organisms, and clindamycin or chloramphenicol is used in penicillin-sensitive patients. The antibiotic medication is adjusted according to the patient's response and culture results from aspirates of fluid from the enlargements.

Although large accumulations of purulent material are rare, decompression of the sublingual, submental, and submandibular spaces should be performed when fluctuance is present. If the infection remains diffuse, indurated, and brawny, then surgical intervention is at the discretion of the clinician and often is governed by the patient's response to noninvasive therapy. Computed tomography (CT) of the neck and chest is recommended for patients with extensive cervical infection to rule out spread into the mediastinum.

Before the use of modern antibiotic medications, the mortality from Ludwig's angina often exceeded 50%. Although this rate has been reduced to less than 10%, deaths still occur as the result of complications such as pericarditis, pneumonia, mediastinitis, sepsis, empyema, and respiratory obstruction.

CAVERNOUS SINUS THROMBOSIS

The therapeutic cornerstones for cavernous sinus thrombosis secondary to dental infections are surgical drainage combined with high-dose antibiotic medications similar to those administered for patients with Ludwig's angina. The offending tooth should be extracted, and drainage is required if fluctuance is present. Administration of systemic corticosteroid drugs is indicated only in patients who have developed pituitary insufficiency in advanced cases of cavernous sinus thrombosis. Some investigators also prescribe anticoagulant medications to prevent thrombosis and septic emboli; conversely, others believe that thrombosis limits the infection and that the use of anticoagulant drugs may promote hemorrhagic lesions in the orbit and brain.

In older series the mortality rate approached 75%. Even with current medical advances and modern antibiotic medications, the mortality rate remains at approximately 30%, with fewer than 40% of patients achieving full recovery.

OSTEOMYELITIS

Osteomyelitis is an acute or chronic inflammatory process in the medullary spaces or cortical surfaces of bone that extends away from the initial site of involvement. The term *osteomyelitis* has been used to encompass a wide variety of pathoses. This section describes the classic pattern of osteomyelitis. The vast majority of osteomyelitis cases are caused by bacterial infections and result in an expanding lytic destruction of the involved bone, with suppuration and sequestra formation. Many believe that this condition is more appropriately termed *suppurative osteomyelitis, bacterial osteomyelitis,* or *secondary osteomyelitis.* This pattern of osseous pathosis is in contrast to an ill-defined group of idiopathic inflammatory disorders of bone that do not respond consistently to antibacterial medications and typically demonstrate ultimate sclerosis of bone without suppuration or sequestra formation. This second pattern of inflammatory bone disease is most appropriately termed *primary chronic osteomyelitis* but often is included under the term *diffuse sclerosing osteomyelitis.* This disorder and several other patterns of inflammatory bone disease (e.g., focal sclerosing osteomyelitis, proliferative periostitis, alveolar osteitis) are unique and are covered separately later in the chapter. Osteoradionecrosis is excluded from this discussion because this is primarily a problem of hypoxia, hypocellularity, and hypovascularity in which the presence of bacteria represents a secondary colonization of non-

healing bone rather than a primary bacterial infection (see page 296). In addition, bisphosphonate-associated osteonecrosis represents another unique pattern that is discussed in a later chapter and appears more strongly related to altered bone metabolism (see page 299).

Suppurative osteomyelitis of the jaws is uncommon in developed countries, but it continues to be a source of significant difficulty in developing nations. In Europe and North America, most cases arise after odontogenic infections or traumatic fracture of the jaws. In addition, many cases reported in Africa occur in the presence of acute necrotizing ulcerative gingivitis (ANUG) or noma.

Chronic systemic diseases, immunocompromised status, and disorders associated with decreased vascularity of bone appear to predispose people to osteomyelitis. Tobacco use, alcohol abuse, IV drug abuse, diabetes mellitus, exanthematous fevers, malaria, sickle cell anemia, malnutrition, malignancy, collagen vascular diseases, and AIDS have been associated with an increased frequency of osteomyelitis. In addition to radiation, several diseases (e.g., osteopetrosis, dysosteosclerosis, late Paget's disease, end-stage cemento-osseous dysplasia) may result in hypovascularized bone that is predisposed to necrosis and inflammation.

Acute suppurative osteomyelitis exists when an acute inflammatory process spreads through the medullary spaces of the bone and insufficient time has passed for the body to react to the presence of the inflammatory infiltrate. **Chronic suppurative osteomyelitis** exists when the defensive response leads to the production of granulation tissue, which subsequently forms dense scar tissue in an attempt to wall off the infected area. The encircled dead space acts as a reservoir for bacteria, and antibiotic medications have great difficulty reaching the site. This pattern begins to evolve about 1 month after the spread of the initial acute infection and results in a smoldering process that is difficult to manage unless the problem is approached aggressively.

CLINICAL AND RADIOGRAPHIC FEATURES

Patients of all ages can be affected by osteomyelitis. There is a strong male predominance, approaching 75% in some reviews. Most cases involve the mandible. Maxillary disease becomes important primarily in pediatric patients and in cases that arise from ANUG or noma (in African populations).

ACUTE SUPPURATIVE OSTEOMYELITIS

Patients with acute osteomyelitis have signs and symptoms of an acute inflammatory process that has typically been less than 1 month in duration. Fever,

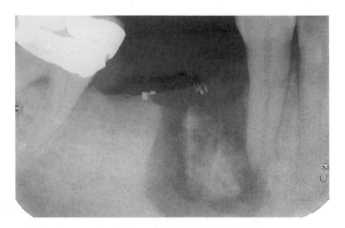

Fig. 3-45   Acute osteomyelitis. Ill-defined area of radiolucency of the right body of the mandible.

Fig. 3-46   Acute osteomyelitis with sequestrum. Radiolucency of the right body of the mandible with central radiopaque mass of necrotic bone. *(Courtesy of Dr. Michael Meyrowitz.)*

A 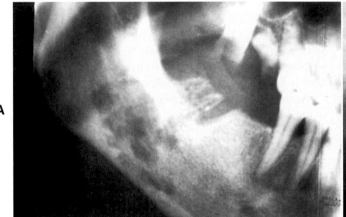   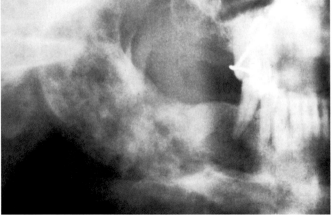 **B**

Fig. 3-47   Chronic osteomyelitis. A, Ill-defined area of radiolucency of the right body of the mandible adjacent to a recent extraction site. **B,** After the initial intervention, the patient failed to return for follow-up because of lack of significant pain. An enlarged, ill-defined radiolucency of the right body of the mandible was discovered 2 years after the initial surgery. *(Courtesy of Dr. Charles Waldron.)*

leukocytosis, lymphadenopathy, significant sensitivity, and soft tissue swelling of the affected area may be present. The radiographs may be unremarkable or may demonstrate an ill-defined radiolucency (Fig. 3-45). Periosteal new bone formation also may be seen in response to subperiosteal spread of the infection. This proliferation is more common in young patients and presents as a single-layered linear radiopaque line separated from the normal cortex by an intervening radiolucent band. On occasion, paresthesia of the lower lip, drainage, or exfoliation of fragments of necrotic bone may be discovered. A fragment of necrotic bone that has separated from the adjacent vital bone is termed a **sequestrum.** Sequestra often exhibit spontaneous exfoliation (Fig. 3-46). On occasion, fragments of

necrotic bone may become surrounded by new vital bone, known as an **involucrum.**

CHRONIC SUPPURATIVE OSTEOMYELITIS

If acute osteomyelitis is not resolved expeditiously, the entrenchment of **chronic osteomyelitis** occurs, or the process may arise primarily without a previous acute episode. Swelling, pain, sinus formation, purulent discharge, sequestrum formation, tooth loss, or pathologic fracture may occur. Patients may experience acute exacerbations or periods of decreased pain associated with chronic smoldering progression (Fig. 3-47).

Radiographs reveal a patchy, ragged, and ill-defined radiolucency that often contains central radiopaque sequestra. On CT scan, the osteolytic change is contin-

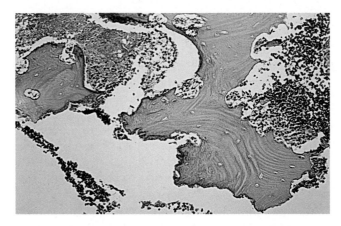

Fig. 3-48 Acute osteomyelitis. Nonvital bone exhibits loss of the osteocytes from the lacunae. Peripheral resorption, bacterial colonization, and surrounding inflammatory response also can be seen.

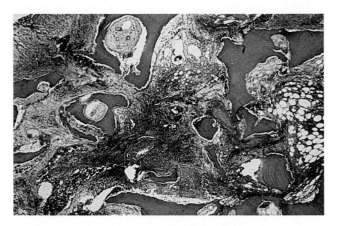

Fig. 3-49 Chronic osteomyelitis. Chronically inflamed and reactive fibrous connective tissue filling the intertrabecular spaces.

uous and may exhibit spread to the periosteum by direct extension. This is in contrast to primary chronic osteomyelitis, in which multifocal and separate areas of osteolysis are present within zones of sclerosis. Occasionally, the surrounding bone may exhibit an increased radiodensity, and the cortical surface can demonstrate significant osteogenic periosteal hyperplasia. In spite of the potential for peripheral sclerosis, the main radiographic feature of suppurative osteomyelitis is one of an expanding radiolucent osteolytic change.

Because of an anatomic peculiarity, large portions of each jawbone receive their blood supply through multiple arterial loops originating from a single vessel. Involvement of this single feeder vessel can lead to necrosis of a large portion of the affected bone. Sequestration that has involved an entire quadrant of the jaw has been reported in long-standing cases of chronic osteomyelitis.

HISTOPATHOLOGIC FEATURES
ACUTE SUPPURATIVE OSTEOMYELITIS

Generation of biopsy material from patients with acute osteomyelitis is not common because of the predominantly liquid content and lack of a soft tissue component. When submitted, the material consists predominantly of necrotic bone. The bone shows a loss of the osteocytes from their lacunae, peripheral resorption, and bacterial colonization (Fig. 3-48). The periphery of the bone and the haversian canals contain necrotic debris and an acute inflammatory infiltrate consisting of polymorphonuclear leukocytes. The submitted material will be diagnosed as a sequestrum unless a good clinicopathologic correlation points to the appropriate diagnosis of acute osteomyelitis.

CHRONIC SUPPURATIVE OSTEOMYELITIS

Biopsy material from patients with chronic osteomyelitis demonstrates a significant soft tissue component that consists of chronically or subacutely inflamed fibrous connective tissue filling the intertrabecular areas of the bone (Fig. 3-49). Scattered sequestra and pockets of abscess formation are common.

TREATMENT AND PROGNOSIS
ACUTE SUPPURATIVE OSTEOMYELITIS

If obvious abscess formation is noted, the treatment of acute osteomyelitis consists of antibiotic medications and drainage. Microbiologic study of the infectious material typically reveals a polymicrobial infection of organisms normally present in the oral cavity. The antibiotic medications most frequently selected include penicillin, clindamycin, cephalexin, cefotaxime, tobramycin, and gentamicin.

In most patients a sufficient and appropriate antibiotic regimen aborts the infection and averts the need for surgical intervention. In patients receiving appropriate antibiotic medications, investigators have suggested that nonvital bone fragments could be allowed to remain in place as scaffolding for the future development of new bone.

CHRONIC SUPPURATIVE OSTEOMYELITIS

Chronic osteomyelitis is difficult to manage medically, presumably because pockets of dead bone and organisms are protected from antibiotic drugs by the surrounding wall of fibrous connective tissue. Surgical intervention is mandatory. The antibiotic medications are similar to those used in the acute form but must be given intravenously in high doses.

The extent of the surgical intervention depends on the spread of the process; removal of all infected material down to good bleeding bone is mandatory in all cases. For small lesions, curettage, removal of necrotic bone, and saucerization are sufficient. In patients with more extensive osteomyelitis, decortication or saucerization often is combined with transplantation of cancellous bone chips. In cases of persisting osteomyelitis, resection of the diseased bone followed by immediate reconstruction with an autologous graft is required. Weakened jawbones must be immobilized.

The goal of surgery is removal of all infected tissue. Persistence of chronic osteomyelitis is typically the result of incomplete removal of diseased tissue. On successful elimination of all infected material, resolution is expected. Adjunctive procedures (e.g., hyperbaric oxygen) are rarely necessary if thorough surgical curettage and sequestrectomy have been accomplished. In an attempt to remove all areas of necrotic bone thoroughly, tetracycline has been administered 48 hours in advance of surgery and used as a fluorescent marker of vital bone. At the time of surgery, necrotic bone will not fluoresce under the ultraviolet (UV) light of a Wood's lamp, indicating that it should be removed.

Management of persistent cases of chronic osteomyelitis often requires use of more sophisticated techniques. Scintigraphic techniques with technetium 99m (^{99m}Tc-labeled phosphorus compounds) can be used to evaluate the therapeutic response and progress of treatment. Hyperbaric oxygen is recommended primarily for the rare patient who does not respond to standard therapy or for disease arising in hypovascularized bone (e.g., osteoradionecrosis, osteopetrosis, Paget's disease, cemento-osseous dysplasia).

DIFFUSE SCLEROSING OSTEOMYELITIS

Diffuse sclerosing osteomyelitis is an ill-defined, highly controversial, evolving area of dental medicine. This diagnosis encompasses a group of presentations that are characterized by pain, inflammation, and varying degrees of gnathic periosteal hyperplasia, sclerosis, and lucency. On occasion, diffuse sclerosing osteomyelitis can be confused with secondarily inflamed intraosseous pathoses (florid cemento-osseous dysplasia) (see page 641) or Paget's disease of bone (see page 623). In spite of the clinical and radiographic similarities, these processes can be separated from diffuse sclerosing osteomyelitis because of various clinical, radiographic, and histopathologic differences.

The remaining pathoses can be grouped under three categories:
1. Diffuse sclerosing osteomyelitis
2. Primary chronic osteomyelitis
3. Chronic tendoperiostitis

Although the concepts regarding the nature of these conditions continue to be clarified, many believe chronic tendoperiostitis may represent a subset of primary chronic osteomyelitis, whereas two other disorders, **synovitis-acne-pustulosis hyperostosis-osteomyelitis** (SAPHO) **syndrome** and **chronic recurrent multifocal osteomyelitis** (CRMO), constitute primary chronic osteomyelitis with additional extragnathic manifestations. Whether these represent variations of a single disorder or different pathologic processes is highly debated with no clear answer at this time. It appears prudent for clinicians to consider all possibilities in an effort to ensure the most appropriate care for patients affected by these conditions.

In the purist's view, **diffuse sclerosing osteomyelitis** is different from primary chronic osteomyelitis and all its variants. This term should be used only when an obvious infectious process directly is responsible for sclerosis of bone. In these cases, chronic intraosseous bacterial infection creates a smoldering mass of chronically inflamed granulation tissue that incites sclerosis of the surrounding bone.

Primary chronic osteomyelitis often is confused with, but must be distinguished from, chronic suppurative osteomyelitis (secondary chronic osteomyelitis). In contrast to suppurative osteomyelitis, an association with a bacterial infection is not obvious, and suppuration and sequestration characteristically are absent. A number of causes have been proposed, such as an altered immune response to an organism of low virulence, but no single theory has received widespread acceptance. In contrast to suppurative osteomyelitis, a primary infectious cause cannot be proven, because many studies have been unable to culture organisms and the condition does not respond to long-term antibiotic therapy.

Although initially thought to be an obscure infectious process, the clinical presentation of **chronic tendoperiostitis** is similar to that of primary chronic osteomyelitis; today many clinicians believe it represents a reactive alteration of bone that is initiated and exacerbated by chronic overuse of the masticatory muscles, predominantly the masseter and digastric. In a large series of patients, parafunctional muscle habits (e.g., bruxism, clenching, nail biting, co-contraction, inability to relax jaw musculature) were known or became evident during follow-up. In neurophysiologic studies, masseter inhibitory reflexes were abnormal in the vast majority of patients studied. The cause of chronic tendoperiostitis is controversial, and some investigators believe this disorder may represent a variation of primary chronic osteomyelitis, in which parafunctional muscle habits exacerbate the process but are not the initial cause.

On occasion, gnathic lesions presenting as primary chronic osteomyelitis occur in patients with other significant systemic manifestations. As the name implies, CRMO includes involvement of multiple bones that is thought by many to represent a widespread variant of primary chronic osteomyelitis. As previously discussed, SAPHO syndrome is an acronym for a complex clinical presentation that includes synovitis, acne, pustulosis, hyperostosis, and osteitis in which the osseous lesions mirror those of primary chronic osteomyelitis and CRMO. The cause of SAPHO is unknown, but it is thought to arise in genetically predisposed individuals who develop an autoimmune disturbance secondary to exposure to dermatologic bacteria. Although not found consistently, an increased prevalence of histocompatibility antigen 27 (HLA 27) in patients with SAPHO has been noted by several investigators. Researchers theorize that an abnormal immune response to the microorganism cross-reacts with normal bone or joint structures, leading to the variety of clinical manifestations. Other immunologic factors have been suggested to cause chronic osteomyelitis and CRMO, but again this theory currently is unproven.

CLINICAL AND RADIOGRAPHIC FEATURES

DIFFUSE SCLEROSING OSTEOMYELITIS

Diffuse sclerosing osteomyelitis is similar to the localized variant (condensing osteitis; see page 147); however, the disorder is also very different. It arises almost exclusively in adulthood, does not exhibit a sex predominance, and primarily occurs in the mandible. An increased radiodensity develops around sites of chronic infection (e.g., periodontitis, pericoronitis, apical inflammatory disease) in a manner very similar to the increased radiodensity that may be seen surrounding areas of chronic suppurative osteomyelitis. Typically, the altered area is restricted to a single site but may be multifocal or extend to fill an entire quadrant.

The sclerosis centers on the crestal portions of the tooth-bearing alveolar ridge and does not appear to originate in the areas of attachment of the masseter or digastric muscle (Fig. 3-50). The radiodensities do not develop from previously radiolucent fibro-osseous lesions and do not exhibit the predilection for black females, as is found in those patients with florid cemento-osseous dysplasia. Pain and swelling are not typical.

PRIMARY CHRONIC OSTEOMYELITIS

Primary chronic osteomyelitis is most commonly discovered as an isolated process that typically is localized to the mandible. Extragnathic evidence of SAPHO syndrome or CRMO is seen much less frequently. The

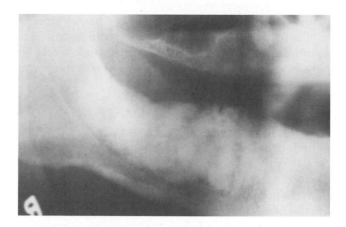

Fig. 3-50   Diffuse sclerosing osteomyelitis. Diffuse area of increased radiodensity of the right body of the mandible in the tooth-bearing area. No other quadrants were involved. *(Courtesy of Dr. Louis M. Beto.)*

onset of symptoms tends to demonstrate two peaks, one in adolescence and the other in adults after the fifth decade of life. Affected patients have recurrent episodes of pain, swelling, local induration, and limited mouth opening that is not associated with any obvious dental infection. During periods of disease activity, regional lymphadenopathy and reduced sensation in the distribution of the inferior alveolar nerve may be present. Absence of fever, purulence, sequestration, and sinus formation are characteristic. The lack of an obvious association with an odontogenic infection and the nonsuppurative presentation clearly separate this condition from chronic suppurative osteomyelitis.

In the early stages of primary chronic osteomyelitis, radiographs tend to demonstrate a mixed pattern, with areas of radiolucent osteolysis intermingled with zones of sclerosis. In contrast to the pattern noted in CT images of suppurative osteomyelitis, the osteolytic areas are not continuous and alternate with zones of sclerosis. The affected area of the bone typically is thickened and demonstrates a periosteal proliferation that is more solid than the typical laminated proliferative periostitis of inflammatory origin. Facial asymmetry is not uncommon and often takes years to resolve secondary to slow remodeling. Over time, the affected area becomes predominantly sclerotic, but during subsequent periods of disease activity, new foci of osteolysis and cortical bone destruction appear. These newly affected areas subsequently undergo sclerosis, awaiting the next cycle of disease activity. With disease progression, the clinical symptoms typically diminish and the affected bone demonstrates progressive sclerosis and a reduction in the volume. Radiolucent osteolytic areas may remain, but they tend to be relatively small and widely scattered. Overall, the predominant radiographic alteration of primary chronic osteomyelitis is medullary sclerosis, a pattern that is noted invariably in affected patients. Skeletal scintigraphy demonstrates significant uptake in the affected areas and should be performed in all patients in an effort to rule out extra-gnathic involvement.

CHRONIC TENDOPERIOSTITIS

Although the mean age of occurrence is 40 years, chronic tendoperiostitis may occur in people of all ages. There is no sex predilection. Recurrent pain, swelling of the cheek, and trismus are classic symptoms. Suppuration and an associated infectious cause are not found. Microbiologic cultures are typically negative, with the lesions failing to respond to appropriate antibiotic medications. Uncommon spontaneous resolution with development of radiographic normalcy has been noted.

In most instances, the sclerosis is limited to a single quadrant and centers on the anterior region of the mandibular angle and posterior portion of the mandibular body (i.e., attachment of the masseter muscle). Occasionally, the cuspid and premolar region and the anterior mandible (i.e., attachment of the digastric muscle) may be involved. Relatively radiolucent zones are apparent within the areas of radiodensity, but histopathologic examination reveals only dense bone, formation of reactive bone, and relatively few signs of inflammation. The inferior border of the mandibular body is typically affected, and significant erosion of the inferior border appears just anterior to the angle of the mandible.

SAPHO SYNDROME

Patients with SAPHO syndrome are usually younger than 60 years old and have chronic multifocal osteomyelitis that is typically associated with negative microbiologic cultures and is nonresponsive to antibiotic therapy. In contrast to bacterial osteomyelitis, the osteolytic areas are scattered randomly within areas of sclerotic bone. Periosteal new bone formation is common but not related to cortical bone perforation. Investigation of the entire skeleton by bone scintigraphy classically reveals involvement of multiple sites. The most frequently involved location is the anterior chest wall, with the sternum, clavicles, and ribs being affected individually or together. Other bones occasionally involved include the spine, pelvis, and long bones.

In early gnathic lesions, diffuse osteolytic zones are more prominent than sclerosis; the affected bone is enlarged because of significant production of periosteal new bone. With time, the bone becomes more sclerotic and decreases in size because of diminished periosteal apposition, while the osteolytic zones become smaller and fewer. External bone resorption and deformity of the mandible are characteristic in older lesions.

In some instances, multiple bone lesions are present without associated skin involvement. In these cases the osseous abnormalities have been termed **CRMO.** Scintigraphy and radiographs will demonstrate synchronous or metachronous involvement of multiple bones such as the clavicle, humerus, radius, femur, or tibia. Mandibular involvement in CRMO occurs in less than 10% of reported cases. Dermatologic involvement may be absent, appear after some delay, or be so subtle as to escape detection. The interval between initial recognition of bone lesions and ultimate development of skin alterations has been as long as 20 years. Commonly associated skin lesions include palmoplantar pustulosis, pustular or plain psoriasis, acne conglobata or ulcerans, and hidradenitis suppurativa.

HISTOPATHOLOGIC FEATURES
DIFFUSE SCLEROSING OSTEOMYELITIS

Diffuse sclerosing osteomyelitis demonstrates sclerosis and remodeling of bone. The haversian canals are scattered widely and little marrow tissue can be found. Although the sclerosis occurs adjacent to areas of inflammation, the bone is not typically intermixed with a significant inflammatory soft tissue component. If the adjacent inflammatory process extends into the sclerotic bone, then necrosis often occurs. The necrotic bone separates from the adjacent vital tissue and becomes surrounded by subacutely inflamed granulation tissue. Secondary bacterial colonization often is visible.

PRIMARY CHRONIC OSTEOMYELITIS

Similar histopathologic features are seen in primary chronic osteomyelitis, SAPHO syndrome, and CRMO. In the areas of sclerosis, numerous irregular trabeculae of pagetoid bone are present and demonstrate extensive evidence of remodeling with prominent reversal lines, osteoblastic rimming, and focal areas of osteoclastic activity (Fig. 3-51). Intertrabecular fibrosis is present, with scattered lymphocytes and plasma cells. Present in many, but not all examples, are foci of microabscess formation, hyalinization around small blood vessels, and subperiosteal bone formation. The microabscesses have been correlated with the osteolytic foci noted during active phases of the disease. In obvious contrast to chronic suppurative osteomyelitis, bone necrosis, bacterial colonization, and frank purulence are absent.

CHRONIC TENDOPERIOSTITIS

Chronic tendoperiostitis demonstrates sclerosis and remodeling of the cortical and subcortical bone with a resultant increase in bone volume. If chronic inflam-

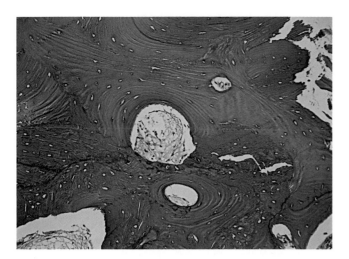

Fig. 3-51 Primary chronic osteomyelitis. Trabeculae of sclerotic, pagetoid bone showing numerous resting and reversal lines.

matory cells are present, then they are located in cortical resorption defects and the subcortical bone adjacent to sites of muscle insertion.

TREATMENT AND PROGNOSIS
DIFFUSE SCLEROSING OSTEOMYELITIS

Diffuse sclerosing osteomyelitis is treated best through resolution of the adjacent foci of chronic infection. After resolution of the infection, the sclerosis remodels in some patients but remains in others. The persistent sclerotic bone is hypovascular, does not exhibit typical remodeling, and is very sensitive to inflammation. The patient and the clinician should work together to avoid future problems with periodontitis or apical inflammatory disease. With long-term alveolar resorption after denture placement, the altered bone does not exhibit typical resorption and exposure with secondary osteomyelitis can develop. These secondary lesions can be treated in the same way as a primary acute or chronic osteomyelitis (see page 143).

PRIMARY CHRONIC OSTEOMYELITIS

Even with significant surgical and medical intervention, the disease course is characterized by flares separated by partial remissions. Most treatments directed toward elimination of infection have been proven ineffective. Long-term antibiotic treatment with or without hyperbaric oxygen therapy has not produced consistent long-term success. Surgical decortication has decreased the intensity and frequency of symptoms but has failed to resolve the process totally. Because of inconsistent results from surgical intervention, extensive surgery is contraindicated, especially in young,

growing patients. Corticosteroid medications, NSAIDs, and calcitonin have been reported to relieve symptoms but usually are associated with incomplete resolution. In a limited number of publications, IV administration of bisphosphonates has shown significant therapeutic benefits. Of the bisphosphonates that have been evaluated (alendronate, disodium clodronate, and pamidronate), a single infusion of alendronate produced the most remarkable response, resulting in complete disappearance of pain within 24 hours, dramatic suppression of bone turnover as confirmed by skeletal scintigraphy, and long-term remission.

CHRONIC TENDOPERIOSTITIS

Treatment of chronic tendoperiostitis as a form of osteomyelitis has been most unsatisfactory. Large series of patients have been treated with antibiotic medications, explorations, intraoral decortication, implantation of gentamicin beads, hyperbaric oxygen, and corticosteroid drugs with no significant effect. Treatment directed toward resolution of muscle overuse has resulted in significantly decreased symptoms in most patients and total resolution in a minority. Therapeutic approaches include the following:
- Muscular relaxation instructions (soft diet, avoidance of parafunctional habits)
- Rotation exercises
- Occlusal splint therapy
- Myofeedback
- Muscle relaxant drugs (e.g., diazepam, mefenoxalon)

CONDENSING OSTEITIS (FOCAL SCLEROSING OSTEOMYELITIS)

Localized areas of bone sclerosis associated with the apices of teeth with pulpitis (from large carious lesions or deep coronal restorations) or pulpal necrosis are termed **condensing osteitis**. The association with an area of inflammation is critical, because these lesions can resemble several other intrabony processes that produce a somewhat similar pattern.

CLINICAL AND RADIOGRAPHIC FEATURES

This secondary sclerosis of bone is seen most frequently in children and young adults but also can occur in older adults. The classic alteration consists of a localized, usually uniform zone of increased radiodensity adjacent to the apex of a tooth that exhibits a thickened periodontal ligament space or an apical inflammatory lesion (Fig. 3-52). Clinical expansion should not be present. Most cases occur in the premolar and molar areas of the mandible, and the dental pulp of the

4

Periodontal Diseases

CHAPTER OUTLINE

In this textbook of oral and maxillofacial pathology, the discussion of periodontal diseases is limited appropriately in scope. However, several fine textbooks are available on periodontology and can provide the reader with more information on the background, microbiology, clinical presentations, diagnostic procedures, and current therapies used to treat these diseases.

GINGIVITIS

Gingivitis refers to inflammation limited to the soft tissues that surround the teeth. It does not include the inflammatory processes that may extend into the underlying alveolar ridge, periodontal ligament, or cementum. The primary types of gingivitis are listed in Box 4-1. This part of the text concentrates on the plaque-related types. **Necrotizing ulcerative gingivitis** (NUG), **medication-influenced gingivitis,** and a specific type of allergic gingivitis **(plasma cell gingivitis)** are presented later in this chapter. Additional forms of allergic gingivitis are discussed in Chapter 9. The gingivitis associated with specific infections (e.g., herpes simplex, human immunodeficiency virus [HIV]) is discussed in Chapters 5 and 7. The gingiva is a frequent site of involvement in several of the dermatologic vesiculoerosive diseases; these are well described in Chapter 16.

CLINICAL FEATURES

Most cases of gingivitis occur from lack of proper oral hygiene, which leads to the accumulation of dental plaque and calculus; however, many other factors can affect the gingiva's susceptibility to the oral flora. The frequency of gingivitis is high in all age groups, but its true prevalence is difficult to determine because of the lack of a standardized method of measurement. Clinically detectable inflammatory changes of the gingiva begin in childhood and increase with age. With similar amounts of dental plaque, the severity of gingivitis is greater in adults than in prepubertal children. Around the time of puberty, there is a period of increased susceptibility to gingivitis **(puberty gingivitis),** with the peak prevalence of involvement occurring between the ages of 9 and 14 years (Fig. 4-1). Between the ages of 11 and 17 years, the frequency declines; then a slow increase is seen until the prevalence approaches 100% in the sixth decade of life.

In most age groups, females demonstrate a lower frequency of gingivitis than do males (although females have periods of increased susceptibility). This may be due more to better oral hygiene in females than to a physiologic difference between the sexes. In addition to the years of puberty, females exhibit a greater susceptibility to gingivitis when they are exposed to the high levels of progesterone associated with pregnancy

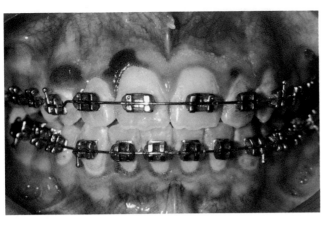

Fig. 4-1 Puberty gingivitis. Erythematous gingivitis that arose at time of initial menses and was slow to respond to local therapy.

Box 4-1

Types of Gingivitis

- Plaque-related gingivitis
- Necrotizing ulcerative gingivitis (NUG)
- Medication-influenced gingivitis
- Allergic gingivitis
- Specific infection-related gingivitis
- Dermatosis-related gingivitis

Box 4-2

Systemic Factors Associated with Gingivitis

1. Hormonal changes
   - Puberty
   - Pregnancy
   - Oral contraceptive use
2. Stress
3. Substance abuse
4. Poor nutrition
   - Ascorbate (vitamin C) deficiency (see page 826)
5. Certain medications (see page 163)
   - Phenytoin
   - Calcium channel blockers
   - Cyclosporine
6. Diabetes mellitus (see page 842)
7. Down syndrome
8. Immune dysfunction
9. Heavy-metal poisoning (see page 313)

Box 4-3

Local Factors Associated with Gingivitis

1. Local trauma
2. Tooth crowding with overlapping
3. Dental anomalies
   - Enamel pearls (see page 93)
   - Enamel and radicular grooves
4. Tooth fracture
5. Dental caries
6. Gingival recession
7. High frenum attachments
8. Iatrogenic factors
   - Overhanging restorations
   - Removable prostheses
   - Orthodontic appliances
9. Inadequate lip closure
10. Mouth breathing

---

or some forms of oral contraceptives. Progesterone appears to increase the permeability of gingival blood vessels, thereby rendering the area more sensitive to bacterial, physical, and chemical irritants.

A number of other systemic factors have been shown to increase the frequency of gingivitis and are listed in Box 4-2. In contrast, smoking and use of many antibiotic drugs, corticosteroid medications, and nonsteroidal antiinflammatory drugs (NSAIDs) have been correlated with a reduced gingival response to plaque. Various local factors that can be related to gingivitis are shown in Box 4-3.

Injury to the gingiva from mastication, oral hygiene techniques, or other habits may result in a breach of the oral mucosa, with secondary infection from the local flora. Most such injuries result in transient areas of erythema. However, if the trauma follows a chronic pattern, then areas of persistently swollen, erythematous gingiva may result. Patients who are mouth breathers or demonstrate incomplete lip closure can display a unique pattern of gingivitis in which the anterior facial gingiva is smooth, swollen, and red (Fig. 4-2).

In a large group of patients that was controlled for the local and systemic factors, a variety of severity in gingivitis was seen. Susceptibility to plaque-related gingivitis appears to vary within the population, and the individual traits seem to determine the severity of gingivitis, independent of the degree of plaque accumulation. Even after removal of the causative plaque and resolution of the associated gingivitis, individuals identified as being susceptible to gingivitis exhibit measurable differences in gingival crevicular fluid volume from patients who have demonstrated resistance to plaque-related gingivitis. In addition, evidence suggests that susceptibility to gingivitis appears linked to susceptibility to future development of periodontitis. In the future, such research may allow identification of patients who are susceptible to gingivitis and ultimately periodontitis, and appropriate interventions could be instituted.

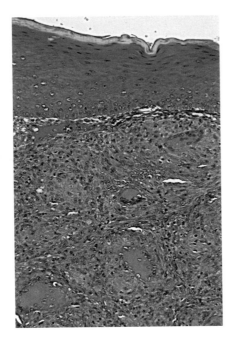

Fig. 4-14 Granulomatous gingivitis. Focal collection of histiocytes, lymphocytes, and multinucleated giant cells within the superficial lamina propria of the gingiva.

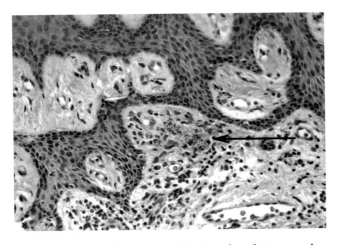

Fig. 4-15 Foreign body gingivitis. Particles of pigmented foreign material (*arrow*) intermixed with lymphocytes and plasma cells. This biopsy was obtained from the patient depicted in Fig. 4-13.

lamina propria. Because the immune reaction in lichen planus tends to be composed primarily of lymphocytes, the presence of significant numbers of plasma cells, histiocytes, or neutrophils in the absence of plaque-related gingivitis should suggest a thorough search for subtle foreign material.

In the majority of cases, the foreign material appears as black or brown-black granules. In many cases, colorless, translucent crystal structures are noted and may be intermixed with black granules. These crystals often are difficult to detect unless viewed under polarized light. To ensure that any foreign material is not an artifact introduced during processing, it should be present in multiple sections.

TREATMENT AND PROGNOSIS

When all the histopathologic and clinical investigations have been performed, the final differential diagnosis of granulomatous gingivitis is usually narrowed down to a localized form of orofacial granulomatosis (see page 341) or a foreign body reaction. Without definitive demonstration of foreign material, a complete physical evaluation for diseases known to be associated with orofacial granulomatosis is mandatory. On occasion, patients with orofacial granulomatosis initially have gingival lesions but eventually develop more widespread manifestations such as cheilitis granulomatosa, cobblestone buccal mucosa, or vestibular linear hyperplastic folds.

Surgical excision of the affected tissue is the therapy of choice for those cases related to foreign material. In persistently atrophic or erosive areas of foreign body gingivitis, overlaying the damaged area with a graft from a healthy gingival donor site may be a better option than complete excision. In an attempt to prevent future introduction of iatrogenic foreign material, it appears appropriate to follow certain guidelines:
- The clinician should use extreme care when trimming restorations or using abrasive instruments close to gingival margins.
- Air abrasion (i.e., sandblasting) should be used cautiously.
- Dental prophylaxis should be delayed for 2 days after scaling, root planing, and curettage procedures.

Patients who do not respond to surgical removal and have recurrences of granulomatous gingivitis despite cautious dental care probably should be classified as having orofacial granulomatosis and managed accordingly.

DESQUAMATIVE GINGIVITIS

Most clinicians use the term **desquamative gingivitis** to describe gingival epithelium that spontaneously sloughs or can be removed with minor manipulation. The process most likely represents a manifestation of one of several different vesiculoerosive diseases. Histopathologic and immunologic investigations of this condition reveal that most patients exhibit features that are diagnostic of pemphigoid or lichen planus. Other diagnoses that are made less frequently include linear IgA disease, pemphigus vulgaris, epidermolysis bullosa acquisita, systemic lupus erythematosus (SLE), chronic ulcerative stomatitis, and paraneoplastic pemphigus. The gingival manifestations of these mucosal and dermatologic diseases are described in greater detail in Chapter 16, so further discussion here is not warranted.

DRUG-RELATED GINGIVAL HYPERPLASIA (DRUG-RELATED GINGIVAL OVERGROWTH)

Drug-related gingival hyperplasia refers to an abnormal growth of the gingival tissues secondary to use of a systemic medication. The term is a misnomer because neither the epithelium nor the cells within the connective tissue exhibit either hyperplasia or hypertrophy. The increased gingival size is due to an increased amount of extracellular matrix, predominantly collagen. Therefore, several authors designate the alteration as **medication-associated gingival enlargement** or **gingival overgrowth**. These designations are further supported by investigators who have suggested the gingival changes arise from interference with normal intracellular collagen degradation. It is known that gingival collagen constantly undergoes physiologic remodeling, and the process must be tightly controlled to maintain a constant volume of the gingival tissues. Investigators have suggested that cyclosporine, phenytoin, and nifedipine are all associated with calcium deregulation, which disrupts the normal collagen phagocytosis and remodeling process. If this is true, then the increased collagen does not occur from hyperplasia but from impaired collagen degradation and remodeling.

A list of medications reported to be associated with gingival hyperplasia is provided in Box 4-4. Of these medications, a strong association has been noted only with cyclosporine (Fig. 4-16), phenytoin, and nifedipine (Fig. 4-17). In the remainder, the prevalence is much lower or the association is weak or anecdotal. As new drugs have been developed, the list of offending medications has grown. When cyclosporine and nifedipine are used concurrently, the severity of the associated hyperplasia often is increased (Fig. 4-18).

Box 4-4

Medications Reported to be Associated with Gingival Hyperplasia

Anticonvulsants
- Carbamazepine
- Ethosuximide
- Ethotoin
- Felbamate
- Mephenytoin
- Methsuximide
- Phenobarbital
- Phensuximide
- Phenytoin
- Primidone
- Sodium valproate
- Vigabatrin

Calcium channel blockers
- Amlodipine
- Bepridil
- Diltiazem
- Felodipine
- Nicardipine
- Nifedipine
- Nimodipine
- Nitrendipine
- Verapamil

Cyclosporine
Erythromycin
Oral contraceptives

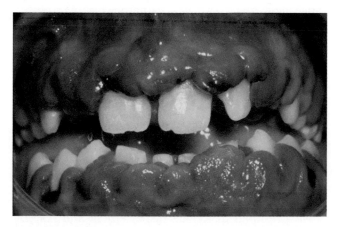

Fig. 4-16   Cyclosporine-related gingival hyperplasia. Diffuse, erythematous, and fibrotic gingival hyperplasia.

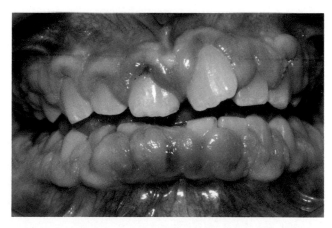

Fig. 4-17   Nifedipine-related gingival hyperplasia. Diffuse, fibrotic gingival hyperplasia after 1 month of intensive oral hygiene. Significant erythema, edema, and increased enlargement were present before intervention.

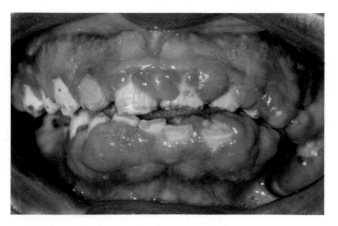

Fig. 4-18 Cyclosporine- and nifedipine-related gingival hyperplasia. Dramatic gingival hyperplasia in a patient using two drugs associated with gingival enlargement.

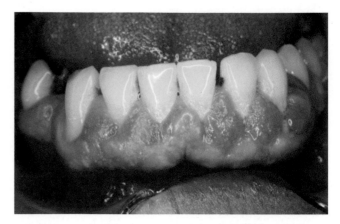

Fig. 4-19 Mild phenytoin-related gingival hyperplasia. Gingival enlargement present predominantly in the interdental papillae.

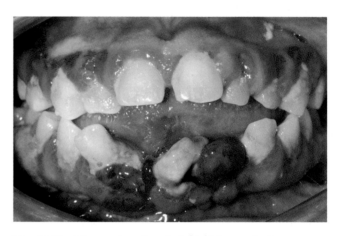

Fig. 4-20 Phenytoin-related gingival hyperplasia. Significant erythematous gingival hyperplasia is covering portions of the crowns of numerous teeth.

The prevalence of these hyperplasias varies widely; however, as reported in one critical review of the literature, the prevalence related to use of phenytoin is approximately 50%. Cyclosporine and nifedipine each produce significant changes in about 25% of patients treated. Whether there is a relationship between the particular dose and the risk or severity of the hyperplasia is a controversial issue. Investigators have suggested that susceptibility to cyclosporine gingival hyperplasia is associated with certain histocompatibility antigen (HLA) types, whereas other HLA types appear to protect against hyperplasia. Whether similar correlations exist for the other forms of medication-associated gingival hyperplasia is unknown.

The degree of gingival enlargement appears to be related significantly to the patient's susceptibility and the level of oral hygiene. In observations of patients with excellent oral hygiene, gingival overgrowth (as ascertained by pseudopocket formation) is reduced dramatically or not present. Even with good oral hygiene, however, some degree of gingival enlargement can be discovered in susceptible individuals, although in many cases the changes are difficult to detect. Rigorous oral hygiene often can limit the severity to clinically insignificant levels. Of the medications discussed, cyclosporine appears to be the least responsive to the institution of a rigorous program of oral hygiene; even with this medication, however, the elimination of gingival inflammation results in noticeable clinical improvement. In addition, the degree of drug-associated gingival hyperplasia appears to be markedly higher in smokers.

CLINICAL FEATURES

Because young patients use phenytoin most often, the gingival hyperplasia it induces is primarily a problem in people younger than age 25. Cases related to the calcium channel blockers occur mainly in middle-aged or older adults. Cyclosporine is used over a broad age range, and this correlates with the age of reported hyperplasia. A greater risk for gingival hyperplasia occurs when the drug is used in children, especially adolescents. No sex or race predilection is present.

After 1 to 3 months of drug use, the enlargements originate in the interdental papillae and spread across the tooth surfaces (Fig. 4-19). The anterior and facial segments are the most frequently involved areas. In extensive cases, the hyperplastic gingiva can cover a portion (or all) of the crowns of many of the involved teeth (Figs. 4-20 and 4-21). Extension lingually and occlusally can interfere with speech and mastication. In one report, significant lingual expansion of the gingiva resulted in tongue displacement and respiratory distress. Edentulous areas are generally not affected, but significant hyperplasia under poorly

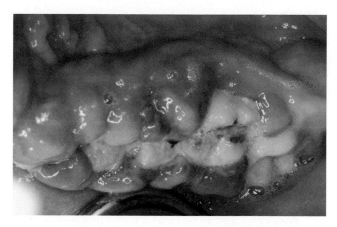

Fig. 4-21   Phenytoin-related gingival hyperplasia.
Significant gingival hyperplasia almost totally covers the crowns of the posterior maxillary dentition. *(Courtesy of Dr. Ann Drummond and Dr. Timothy Johnson.)*

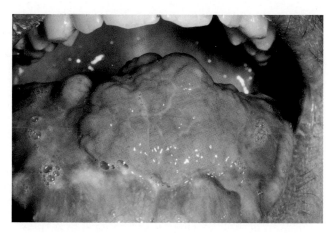

Fig. 4-23   Nongingival cyclosporine hyperplasia. Exophytic and granulomatous-appearing mass of the dorsal surface of the tongue that arose in a bone marrow transplant patient who was receiving cyclosporine for graft-versus-host disease (GVHD).

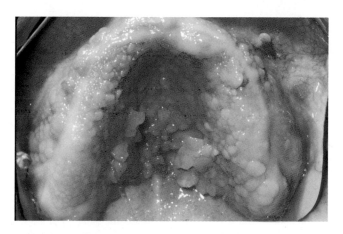

Fig. 4-22   Phenytoin-related palatal hyperplasia. Extensive hyperplasia of palatal mucosa in an edentulous patient with poor denture hygiene.

maintained dentures and around implants has been noted (Fig. 4-22).

Nongingival soft tissue growths that resemble pyogenic granulomas have been reported in allogenic bone marrow transplant recipients who are receiving cyclosporine for graft-versus-host disease (GVHD) (Fig. 4-23). It is thought that cyclosporine triggers the proliferations in areas chronically inflamed by GVHD.

In the absence of inflammation, the enlarged gingiva is normal in color and firm, with a surface that may be smooth, stippled, or granular. With inflammation, the affected gingiva often becomes dark red and edematous, with a surface that is friable, bleeds easily, and occasionally is ulcerated. Pyogenic granuloma-like enlargements occasionally are seen in the presence of heavy inflammation.

HISTOPATHOLOGIC FEATURES

The exact histopathologic changes that occur in people with drug-induced gingival hyperplasia are difficult to ascertain because of variations in the techniques of investigation. In spite of this, most controlled microscopic examinations of hyperplastic gingival tissues removed from lesions caused by phenytoin or the dihydropyridines reveal redundant tissue of apparently normal composition. Those cases related to cyclosporine use demonstrate an increased amount of collagen per unit volume, with a normal density of fibroblasts.

The overlying surface epithelium may demonstrate elongation of the rete ridges, with long extensions into the underlying lamina propria. In patients with secondary inflammation, there is increased vascularity and a chronic inflammatory cellular infiltrate that most frequently consists of lymphocytes and plasma cells. In patients with pyogenic granuloma-like overgrowths, the proliferations often demonstrate an increased vascularity and significant subacute inflammation.

TREATMENT AND PROGNOSIS

Discontinuation of the offending medication by the attending physician often results in cessation, and possibly some regression, of the gingival enlargement; even substitution of one medication for another may be beneficial. If the patient's response allows drug substitution, then cyclosporine can be replaced with tacrolimus; phenytoin with carbamazepine, lamotrigine, gabapentin, sulthiame, topiramate, or valproic acid; and nifedipine with isradipine or atenolol. Often the response to medication substitution is not immediate.

Unless the degree of hyperplasia dramatically affects aesthetics and function, allowing at least 6 to 12 months between discontinuation of the offending medication and the decision whether to proceed with surgical therapy is recommended. If the drug use is mandatory, then professional cleaning, frequent reevaluations, and home plaque control are important. Antiplaque agents, such as chlorhexidine, have been beneficial in the prevention of plaque buildup and the associated gingival hyperplasia.

Systemic or topical folic acid has been shown to ameliorate the gingival hyperplasia in some cases. In addition, several authors have documented significant resolution of cyclosporine-related gingival hyperplasia after a short course of metronidazole or azithromycin. Although the mechanism is not clear, it appears these antibiotic medications can inhibit proliferation of collagen fibers along with their antimicrobial abilities. Azithromycin also may be beneficial in resolving gingival hyperplasia related to nifedipine and phenytoin.

Although gingival hyperplasia is associated with increased probing depths, some investigators do not believe this necessarily leads to exaggerated attachment loss or an increased loss of teeth. Therefore, some clinicians exercise watchful waiting and do not perform invasive therapy without evidence of attachment loss, inappropriate aesthetics, or disruption of speech or mastication. When objectionable alterations are noted and all other interventions fail to achieve significant resolution, eradication of the excess gingival tissues remains the treatment of choice. This can be achieved by surgical removal, by chemosurgical techniques, by means of electrosurgery, or by use of a carbon dioxide laser. Histopathologic examination of all excised tissue is mandatory to confirm the diagnosis. Recurrence is not uncommon, especially in patients with inadequate oral hygiene. Although recurrences may arise in as little as 3 months, most surgical results are maintained for at least 12 months.

GINGIVAL FIBROMATOSIS (FIBROMATOSIS GINGIVAE; ELEPHANTIASIS GINGIVAE)

Gingival fibromatosis is a slowly progressive gingival enlargement caused by a collagenous overgrowth of the gingival fibrous connective tissue. In spite of the name, this disorder bears no relationship to the hypercellular and neoplastic fibromatoses that can occur in soft tissue and bone (see pages 515 and 658).

Gingival fibromatosis may be familial or idiopathic. Other findings sometimes seen in conjunction with gingival fibromatosis include hypertrichosis (Fig. 4-24), generalized aggressive periodontitis, epilepsy, mental retardation, sensorineural deafness, hypothy-

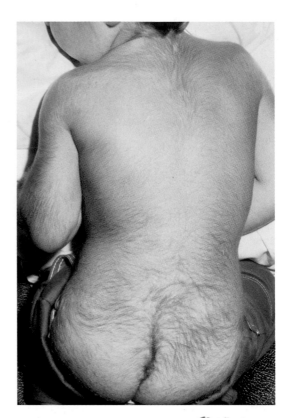

Fig. 4-24 Hypertrichosis in association with gingival fibromatosis. Dramatically increased body hair of the back and buttocks in a patient with gingival fibromatosis. *(Courtesy of Dr. George Blozis.)*

roidism, chondrodystrophia, and growth hormone deficiency. The familial variations may occur as an isolated finding or in association with one of several hereditary syndromes (e.g., **Zimmermann-Laband, Murray-Puretic-Drescher, Rutherfurd, multiple hamartoma** [see page 760], **Cross, Ramon, Jones, prune belly**).

In most cases of isolated gingival fibromatosis, an autosomal dominant pattern of inheritance is seen; however, autosomal recessive examples also have been noted. Incomplete penetrance and variable expressivity are seen. Even in cases with similar patterns of inheritance, genetic heterogeneity of gingival fibromatosis has been noted and confirms that this alteration represents a group of clinically similar disorders. In the autosomal dominant pattern of isolated gingival fibromatosis, one of three different mutations, *GINGF* (*HGF1*), *GINGF2* (*HGF2*), and *GINGF3* (*HGF3*), have been documented and correlates respectively to chromosomes 2p21, 5q13-q22, and 2p22.3-p23.3. Of the three defined loci, only the SOS1 (son of sevenless-1) gene associated with the GINGF locus has been identified. In studies of another kindred with hereditary gingival fibromatosis and hypertrichosis, this presentation

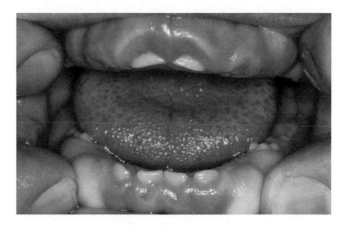

Fig. 4-25   Gingival fibromatosis. A young child with cheeks retracted by the parent. Note erythematous gingival hyperplasia arising in association with erupting deciduous dentition. *(Courtesy of Dr. George Blozis.)*

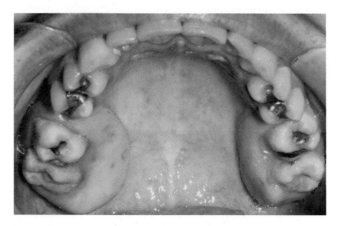

Fig. 4-27   Localized gingival fibromatosis. Bilateral and symmetrical fibrotic enlargements of the palatal surfaces of the posterior maxillary alveolar ridges.

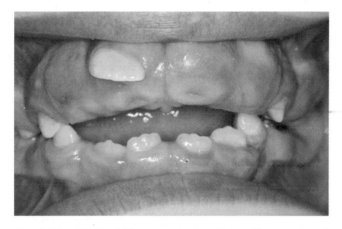

Fig. 4-26   Gingival fibromatosis. Significant fibrotic gingival hyperplasia with resultant delayed eruption of numerous teeth. *(From Neville BW, Damm DD, White DK, Waldron CA: Color atlas of clinical oral pathology, Philadelphia, 1991, Lea & Febiger.)*

was not linked to either mutation known at that time (*GINGF* or *GINGF1*), further confirming the genetic heterogeneity in this hereditary gingival fibromatosis.

CLINICAL FEATURES

In most instances, the enlargement begins before age 20 and often is correlated with the eruption of the deciduous or permanent teeth (Fig. 4-25). Most investigators believe that the presence of teeth probably is necessary for the condition to occur. After the process has begun, it can overgrow the associated teeth and even interfere with lip closure. Failure or delay in eruption of subsequent teeth may be evident (Fig. 4-26). In some instances, a tooth may have erupted into a normal position, but the fibrous connective tissue continues to cover the crown and prevent visualization.

The gingival changes may be generalized or localized to one or more quadrants. Either jaw may be involved, but the maxilla is affected more frequently and demonstrates a greater degree of enlargement. Palatal surfaces are typically increased in thickness more than the buccal side. Typically, extension past the alveolar mucosal junction into the mucobuccal fold is not seen, but palatal extensions can cause significant distortion of the contour of the palate and, at times, almost can meet in the midline.

In localized cases, the hyperplasia may involve a group of teeth and remain stable or, at a later date, may extend to other segments of one or both jaws. One distinctive and not uncommon pattern involves the posterior maxillary alveolar ridge. In this pattern, the hyperplastic tissue forms bilaterally symmetrical enlargements that extend posteriorly and palatally from the posterior alveolar ridges (Fig. 4-27). Less commonly, the overgrowth also may be isolated to the facial gingiva of the lower molars.

The gingiva is firm, normal in color, and covered by a surface that is smooth or finely stippled. In older patients, the surface may develop numerous papillary projections. The frenular attachments may appear to divide the gingival tissues of the alveolar ridge into lobules. Associated clinical problems include poor aesthetics, prolonged retention of deciduous teeth, abnormal occlusion, inadequate lip closure, and difficulty in eating and speaking.

HISTOPATHOLOGIC FEATURES

The enlargements of gingival fibromatosis consist of dense hypocellular, hypovascular collagenous tissue, which forms numerous interlacing bundles that appear to run in all directions. The surface epithelium often

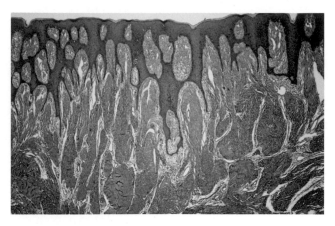

Fig. 4-28   Gingival fibromatosis. Surface stratified squamous epithelium exhibiting long, thin rete ridges and underlying dense, fibrous connective tissue.

exhibits long, thin rete ridges that extend deeply into the underlying fibrous connective tissue (Fig. 4-28). Inflammation is absent to mild. On occasion, scattered islands of odontogenic epithelium, foci of dystrophic calcification, or areas of osseous metaplasia may be seen. Electron microscopic examination demonstrates a mixture of both fibroblasts and myofibroblast-like cells.

TREATMENT AND PROGNOSIS

Conservative treatment consists of gingivectomy in conjunction with a rigorous program of oral hygiene. Follow-up is recommended because there is a tendency for recurrence within a few years. Investigators have suggested that the frequency of recurrence is less if gingivectomy is delayed until after full eruption of the permanent dentition. In severe cases, selective extraction of teeth (and gingivectomy) often is required to achieve a normal gingival morphology.

PERIODONTITIS

Periodontitis refers to an inflammation of the gingival tissues in association with some loss of both the attachment of the periodontal ligament and bony support. With progressive loss of attachment, significant destruction of the periodontal ligament and adjacent alveolar bone can occur. Apical migration of the crevicular epithelium along the root surface results in the formation of periodontal pockets. Loosening and eventual loss of teeth are possible.

For more than a century, the presence of the disease has been correlated with the accumulation of dental plaque on the tooth and under the gingiva. Despite this, current evidence suggests that dental plaque is part of the natural human microflora. In some patients with extensive dental plaque, destructive lesions of the periodontium do not develop. Many investigators now believe that periodontitis occurs not from the mere presence of dental plaque but as a result of shifts in the proportions of bacterial species in the plaque, possibly related to changes in the dentogingival environment (e.g., a soft diet or a highly fermentable carbohydrate content diet).

Dramatic differences exist in the content of dental plaque in areas of healthy and diseased periodontium. Healthy sites are colonized primarily by facultative gram-positive organisms, such as actinomycetes and streptococci; plaque within areas of active periodontitis contains anaerobic and microaerophilic gram-negative flora. Of the more than 500 types of bacteria that may reside in the oral cavity, only a few have been related to periodontitis, and the specific types often correlate with the clinical patterns of periodontitis. Chronic periodontitis is associated strongly with *Actinobacillus actinomycetemcomitans, Tannerella forsythensis* (formerly *Bacteroides forsythus*), and *Porphyromonas gingivalis.* Additional organisms frequently thought to be involved include *Prevotella intermedia, Campylobacter rectus, Treponema denticola,* and *Fusobacterium nucleatum.* Although controversial, some investigators also have suggested that human cytomegalovirus and other herpesviruses could play a contributing role.

The pathogenic organisms exist in an organized community termed a **biofilm.** Bacteria growing in biofilms are relatively protected from normal host defenses and exhibit an increased resistance to locally or systemically administered antibiotic medications. Lipopolysaccharides released from the biofilms are thought to trigger release of catabolic inflammatory mediators that lead to the loss of attachment. Mechanical disruption of this organized bacterial biofilm may be an important factor associated with successful treatment of periodontitis.

The presence of pathogenic bacteria is essential but insufficient to produce periodontitis. Although mild-to-moderate periodontitis is present in the majority of adults, only 10% to 15% of the population develops severe, generalized disease. The variation of susceptibility to periodontitis appears related to genetic influences on host response, with 50% of the risk for chronic periodontitis attributed to heredity, 20% to tobacco abuse, and another 20% to colonization by specific pathogenic bacteria.

The classification of periodontitis, as delineated by the American Academy of Periodontology, is listed in Box 4-5. In 1999 this classification underwent significant revision, with consolidation of many previously distinct disorders. The concept of "early-onset periodontitis" and all of its subdivisions has been reclassi-

Box 4-5

Classification of Periodontitis

1. Chronic periodontitis
   - Localized
   - Generalized
2. Aggressive periodontitis
   - Localized
   - Generalized
3. Periodontitis as a manifestation of systemic diseases
   - Associated with hematologic disorders
   - Associated with genetic disorders
   - Not otherwise specified
4. Necrotizing periodontal diseases
   - Necrotizing ulcerative gingivitis (NUG)
   - Necrotizing ulcerative periodontitis (NUP)
5. Abscesses of the periodontium
   - Gingival abscess
   - Periodontal abscess
   - Pericoronal abscess (in association with pericoronitis)
6. Periodontitis associated with endodontic lesions

Box 4-6

Systemic Disorders with Premature Attachment Loss

1. Acatalasia
2. Acrodynia
3. Acquired immunodeficiency syndrome (AIDS)
4. Blood dyscrasias
   - Leukemia
   - Agranulocytosis
   - Cyclic neutropenia
5. Chédiak-Higashi syndrome
6. Cohen syndrome
7. Crohn's disease
8. Diabetes mellitus
9. Dyskeratosis congenita
10. Ehlers-Danlos syndrome, types IV and VIII
11. Glycogen storage disease
12. Haim-Munk syndrome
13. Hemochromatosis
14. Hypophosphatasia
15. Kindler syndrome
16. Langerhans cell disease
17. Leukocyte dysfunctions with associated extraoral infections
18. Oxalosis
19. Papillon-Lefèvre syndrome
20. Sarcoidosis
21. Trisomy 21

fied as **aggressive periodontitis**. The following text concentrates on the chronic form of periodontitis; a later section discusses the aggressive forms of periodontitis. From this list it should be clear that periodontitis represents a heterogeneous group of disorders.

Periodontitis associated with systemic disease is not rare, and Box 4-6 lists many of the disorders that may be associated with a premature loss of periodontal attachment. **Necrotizing ulcerative periodontitis** (NUP) represents the loss of attachment that often occurs in association with necrotizing ulcerative gingivitis (NUG) (see page 157). This form has been correlated with aggressive invasion by a number of spirochetes and *Prevotella intermedia*.

CLINICAL AND RADIOGRAPHIC FEATURES

CHRONIC PERIODONTITIS

With the decline in caries, **chronic periodontitis** has become the primary cause of tooth loss in patients older than 35 years of age. A national survey found that 44% of adults in the United States had attachment loss of 3 mm or more in at least one site. The disorder demonstrates an increased prevalence in males, although researchers believe that much of this effect is related to poorer oral hygiene and dental-visit behavior. In addition, an increased prevalence of chronic periodontitis is associated with the following:

- Advancing age
- Smoking
- Diabetes mellitus
- Osteoporosis
- HIV infection
- Lower socioeconomic level

Local factors also may predispose patients to isolated periodontal defects; these include tooth shape and alignment, presence and quality of dental restorations, poor interdental contact, calculus formation, subgingival dental caries, traumatic occlusion, and abnormal alveolar bone or gingival anatomy.

Conversely, it appears that the presence of significant periodontitis may place patients at risk for an increased prevalence or greater severity of certain medical disorders. Although controversial, increasing evidence links periodontitis with an elevated risk for coronary artery disease, stroke, progressive diabetes mellitus, respiratory diseases, and delivery of low–birth weight babies. If true, then it is unclear if these associations are due to dissemination of triggering host inflammatory mediators or the spread of bacteria or their related toxins. Although strong direct associations have been documented, the epidemiology is difficult to

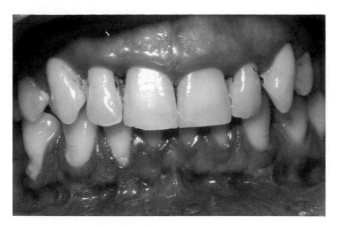

Fig. 4-29   Adult periodontitis. Diffuse gingival erythema with blunting and apical positioning of the gingival margins. *(Courtesy of Dr. Samuel Jasper.)*

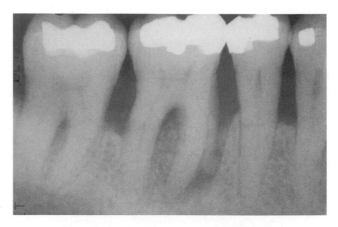

Fig. 4-30   Advanced adult periodontitis. Generalized horizontal bone loss with an isolated vertical defect involving the mesial root of the first molar.

interpret because of the additional risk factors associated with both conditions. For example, cardiovascular disease has been related to periodontitis, but the nature of this association is cloudy because both are strongly associated with smoking. Numerous interventional studies are ongoing to investigate the possible reduction in these medical disorders secondary to elimination and control of periodontitis.

In chronic periodontitis, no abnormalities of the immune system are found. Periodontitis begins in youth and early adulthood, takes years to decades to progress, and includes cyclic patterns of exacerbation and remission. The assumption that periodontitis is a disease of aging has been challenged, and most believe the increased periodontal destruction observed in older adults reflects a lifetime of disease accumulation rather than an age-specific disease.

In patients with periodontitis, gingivitis is present and precedes the development of significant periodontal lesions. Although many sites may demonstrate gingivitis and few progress to attachment loss, lifelong local measures directed against sites of gingivitis represent an effective approach for prevention of chronic periodontitis. As loss of attachment occurs, blunting and apical positioning of the gingival margins typically are present (Fig. 4-29). Periodontal disease is present when a loss of attachment can be demonstrated through the use of a periodontal probe. In the absence of significant gingival hyperplasia, a measurement of pocket depths greater than 3 to 4 mm indicates destruction of the periodontal ligament and resorption of adjacent alveolar bone; however, clinical attachment loss is the best measurement of accumulated periodontal destruction and represents the diagnostic gold standard. High-quality dental radiographs exhibit a decreased vertical height of the bone surrounding the affected teeth (Fig.

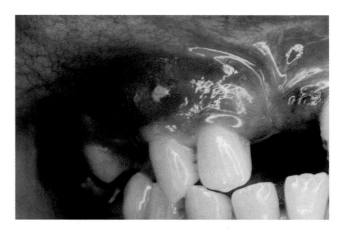

Fig. 4-31   Periodontal abscess. Localized erythematous gingival enlargement with central purulent drainage.

4-30). With advanced bone loss, tooth mobility is present.

NECROTIZING ULCERATIVE PERIODONTITIS

NUP presents similarly to NUG (see page 157), but it also demonstrates loss of clinical attachment and alveolar bone. This destructive form of periodontitis may arise within a zone of preexisting periodontitis, or it may represent a sequela of a single or multiple episodes of NUG. Many believe that NUG and NUP represent different stages of the same infection. Patients affected with this pattern frequently are younger than most patients affected with chronic periodontitis and often demonstrate immunosuppression or malnutrition.

PERIODONTAL ABSCESS

A **periodontal abscess** (Figs. 4-31 and 4-32) is a localized purulent infection of the gingiva with involvement of the adjacent periodontal attachment and alveolar

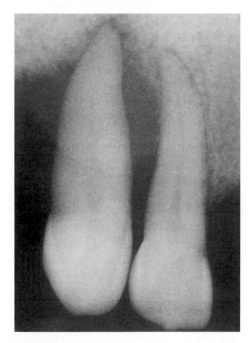

Fig. 4-32   Periodontal abscess. Same patient as depicted in Fig. 4-31. Note extensive loss of bone support associated with the maxillary cuspid.

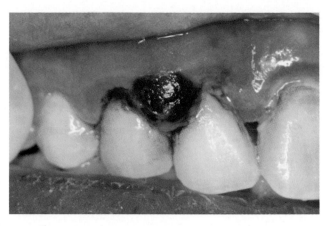

Fig. 4-33   Periodontal abscess. Dark-red and hemorrhagic enlargement of the interdental papilla between the maxillary right lateral incisor and cuspid.

bone. On occasion, an abscess may be localized to the marginal or interdental gingiva without involvement of the adjacent periodontal ligament or alveolar bone. This lesion is termed a **gingival abscess** and often is secondary to plaque or foreign material that has become entrapped in the gingival sulcus.

A periodontal abscess often arises in a preexisting periodontal lesion and usually is precipitated by alterations in the subgingival flora, host resistance, or both. Factors frequently associated with abscess formation are closure of the entrance into a periodontal pocket, furcation involvement, or diabetes. Many cases arise in patients actively undergoing periodontal therapy, perhaps because of incomplete removal of deep calculus with microbial penetration of the soft tissue surrounding the pocket or premature sealing of the coronal opening to the pocket. Other factors involved less frequently are trauma and anatomic dental anomalies, such as enamel pearls (see page 93) and dens invaginatus (see page 90). Most cases arise in adults; periodontal abscesses in children are rare and most frequently the result of a foreign body that has been introduced into previously healthy periodontal tissues.

A periodontal abscess appears as a zone of gingival enlargement along the lateral aspect of a tooth. The involved gingiva may be erythematous and edematous, with a slick, red surface, or it may be hemorrhagic, with a dark-red coloration (Fig. 4-33). Common symptoms include the following:

- Throbbing pain
- Extreme sensitivity to palpation of the affected gingiva
- Sensitivity, mobility, or extrusion of the adjacent tooth
- Foul taste
- Lymphadenopathy
- Fever, leukocytosis, and malaise (occasionally)

Probing or gentle pressure on the affected gingiva often results in the expression of pus from the sulcus. The abscess may drain through an overlying sinus tract. With drainage, the abscess becomes asymptomatic but can demonstrate acute exacerbations if the mucosa heals over and the pressure builds again. Radiographs often demonstrate bone loss associated with the previous periodontal defect or additional radiolucency secondary to the current acute process. In some cases, the infection can spread into the periapical region and create a combined periodontal-endodontic lesion.

PERICORONITIS

Pericoronitis is an inflammatory process that arises within the tissues surrounding the crown of a partially erupted tooth. The inflammatory reaction often arises when food debris and bacteria are present beneath the gingival flap overlying the crown. Other predisposing factors include stress and upper respiratory infections, especially tonsillitis or pharyngitis.

These gingival flaps can exhibit long periods of chronic inflammation without symptoms. If the debris and bacteria become entrapped deep within the gingival flap, then abscess formation develops. Abscess development is seen most frequently in association with the mandibular third molars, and the predominant symptoms are extreme pain in the area, a foul taste, and inability to close the jaws. The pain may

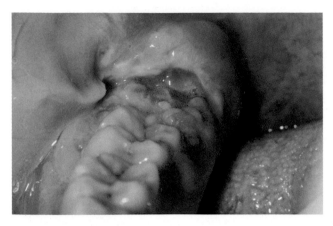

Fig. 4-34   Pericoronitis. Painful erythematous enlargement of the soft tissues overlying the crown of the partially erupted right mandibular third molar.

radiate to the throat, ear, or floor of the mouth. The affected area is erythematous and edematous, and the patient often has lymphadenopathy, fever, leukocytosis, and malaise (Fig. 4-34). NUG-like necrosis may develop in areas of persistent pericoronitis.

HISTOPATHOLOGIC FEATURES

When soft tissue from areas of periodontitis is examined microscopically, gingivitis is present and the crevicular epithelium lining the pocket is hyperplastic, with extensive exocytosis of acute inflammatory cells. The adjacent connective tissue exhibits an increased vascularity and contains an inflammatory cellular infiltrate consisting predominantly of lymphocytes and plasma cells, but with a variable number of polymorphonuclear leukocytes. Frequently, large colonies of microorganisms, representing plaque and calculus, are noted.

TREATMENT AND PROGNOSIS

PERIODONTITIS

Initial attention must be directed toward elimination of any existing risk factors. Even with appropriate treatment and improved oral hygiene, many patients fail to respond to therapy unless certain factors (e.g., smoking, inadequately controlled diabetes) are eliminated. Once these influences have been managed, the treatment of periodontitis is directed toward stopping the loss of attachment. The foremost goal of this process is the elimination of the pathogenic bacterial plaque. Scaling, root planing, and curettage can be used to treat early periodontal lesions. In deeper pockets, a surgical flap may be required to gain access to the tooth for neces-

sary débridement. At this time, the underlying bone may be recontoured (if necessary) to aid in the resolution of the periodontal pocket.

In some bony defects, regeneration of the attachment can be attempted through interdental denudation or the placement of autogenous bone grafts, allografts, or alloplastic materials. Often these grafts are used in conjunction with materials such as polytetrafluoroethylene in an attempt to achieve guided tissue regeneration in moderate-to-advanced periodontal defects.

Because of the chronic nature of periodontitis, antibiotic medications are not generally used except in patients who do not respond to conventional therapy. Inappropriate use of antibiotic agents can lead to overgrowth of potentially pathogenic organisms and development of bacterial drug resistance. When required, tetracycline or metronidazole are used most frequently. The choice of antibiotic medication always should be guided by microbiologic analysis with susceptibility testing. Several studies also suggest that NSAIDs may help slow the progression of bone loss in some cases of destructive periodontitis.

Several forms of local antibiotic delivery have been developed. The antibiotic drugs are placed directly into sites of refractory periodontitis and consist of gels, ointments, nonresorbable fibers, and resorbable polymers. These antibiotic agents represent an adjunct to scaling and root planing and should be limited to sites that are resistant to conventional therapy alone. Although short-term benefits have been demonstrated, many investigations have revealed limited long-term positive effects when compared with scaling and root planing without antibiotic medications.

In many cases the prognosis for chronic periodontitis correlates directly with the patient's desire to maintain oral health. Long-term studies show that periodontal health can be maintained after appropriate periodontal therapy if a program of rigorous oral hygiene and professional care is established. Professional scaling and root planing modify the composition of the plaque microflora so that pathogenic plaques are converted to those with bacterial types normally found in healthy mouths. Bacterial morphotypes return to pretreatment levels 42 days after professional prophylaxis, but pathogenic complexes capable of inducing attachment loss require approximately 3 months to be reestablished functionally. In patients with less-than-optimal oral hygiene or with isolated defects that cannot be self-cleaned, a loss of attachment can be prevented if professional scaling and root planing are performed at 3-month intervals.

Many clinicians believe that the average individual is neither motivated nor sufficiently effective in maintaining the level of plaque control necessary to prevent periodontal disease. In these cases, supplementing normal hygiene techniques with regular professional cleaning and interventions such as counterrotational electric toothbrushes with automatic timers, antimicrobial mouth rinses (e.g., essential oils, chlorhexidine), and toothpastes containing triclosan with 2% Gantrez copolymer may prove beneficial. Other interventions occasionally recommended include medications to temper the host response (e.g., NSAIDs, doxycycline at subantimicrobial dose).

Destructive periodontal disease that is nonresponsive to normal therapy in compliant patients is termed **refractory periodontitis.** In such cases the patient should be reevaluated closely for any predisposing risk factors (such as smoking) or systemic diseases known to be associated with an increased prevalence of periodontitis. Subgingival microbial cultures can be obtained to assist in selection of an appropriate antibiotic intervention. Antimicrobial therapy may be combined with more frequent periodontal maintenance therapy and stronger reinforcement of the patient's oral hygiene techniques.

Investigators are beginning to discover genetic markers for those patients who are at risk for developing severe, progressive periodontitis. Many envision a future in which patients are evaluated for the presence of these markers, with susceptible individuals monitored closely for early colonization by periodontal pathogens. If colonization is detected, then it could be eliminated easily and inexpensively. Attempts at vaccine development have been hindered by the multifactorial nature of periodontitis combined with the complexity of the bacterial biofilms.

NECROTIZING ULCERATIVE PERIODONTITIS

Once any underlying influence (e.g., immunosuppression, malnutrition) has been resolved, NUP often responds well to irrigation, débridement of the necrotic areas, effective oral hygiene measures, and administration of systemic antibiotic medications. Failure to respond to standard therapy mandates a thorough physical evaluation to rule out the possibility of an underlying disease.

PERIODONTAL ABSCESS

A gingival or periodontal abscess is treated by drainage through the sulcus or by an incision through the overlying mucosa. Thorough cleansing of the area with removal of all foreign material, plaque, and calculus should be performed. Penicillin or other antibiotic drugs are prescribed when a fever is present. Analgesic agents are prescribed, and the patient receives a soft diet, is told to use warm saltwater rinses, and is instructed to return each day until the symptoms have resolved. After the acute phase has passed, the patient

is treated for any underlying chronic pathologic periodontal condition.

PERICORONITIS

Acute pericoronitis is treated with gentle antiseptic lavage under the gingival flap to remove gross food debris and bacteria. Systemic antibiotic agents are used if a fever or general symptoms are noted. The patient is instructed to use warm saltwater rinses and to return in 24 hours. Once the acute phase has subsided, the tooth can be extracted if long-term maintenance is contraindicated. If tooth retention is desirable, then the overlying gingival flap is removed surgically, followed by elimination of all food debris and bacterial colonies by thorough curettage.

AGGRESSIVE PERIODONTITIS

Although periodontitis is much more frequent in older adults, it also can be a significant problem in children and young adults. Before the 1999 reclassification by the American Academy of Periodontology, destructive periodontal disease in younger patients was termed **early-onset periodontitis** and subdivided into **prepubertal**, **localized juvenile**, **generalized juvenile**, and **rapidly progressing** forms of periodontitis. The "early-onset" designation was discontinued during the 1999 workshop because the term was deemed too restrictive. Many argued that this pattern of periodontitis can occur at any age and is not restricted to patients younger than 35 years old. It was agreed that an appropriate classification system should not be based on age but should consider primarily the clinical, radiographic, historical, and laboratory findings.

The 1999 workshop concluded that the most logical classification system should not be age dependent or require knowledge of rates of progression. In general, the new designation of **localized aggressive periodontitis** replaces the older term, **localized juvenile periodontitis,** whereas **generalized aggressive periodontitis** supersedes **generalized juvenile periodontitis.** The pattern previously designated as **prepubertal periodontitis** has been associated with a systemic leukocyte dysfunction termed *leukocyte adhesion syndrome.* This disease currently is classified as one of the forms of periodontitis presenting as a manifestation of a systemic disease.

By definition, aggressive periodontitis occurs in otherwise healthy people; there should be no association with a systemic disease process. In keeping with this definition, the diagnosis is one of exclusion, and all systemic disorders known to be related to premature loss of attachment (see Box 4-6) should be ruled out before the definitive diagnosis is made.

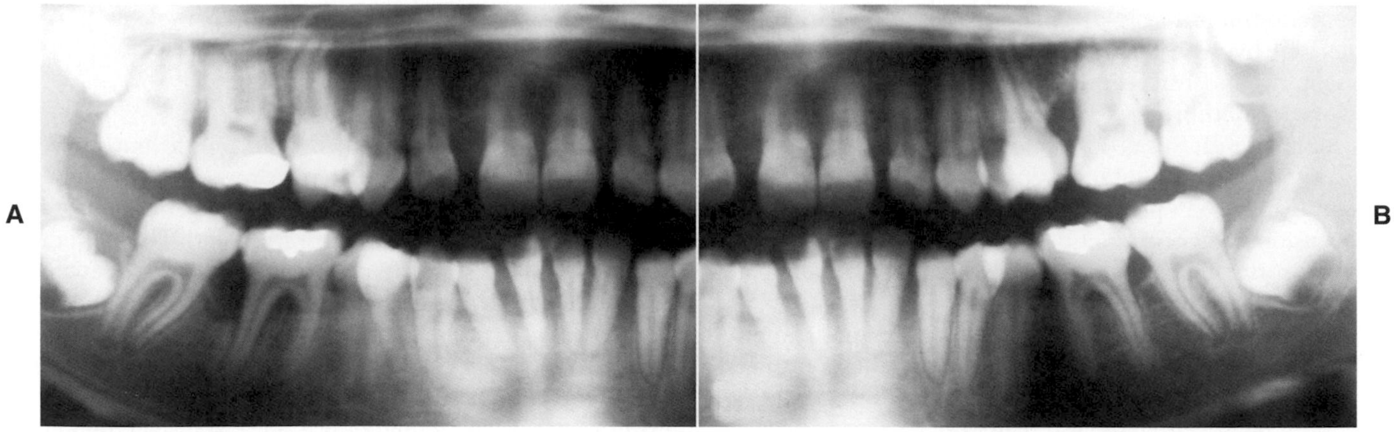

Fig. 4-35   Localized aggressive periodontitis. A, Loss of bone support in the area of the first molars and incisors of both maxillary and mandibular right quadrants in a 14-year-old patient. **B,** Left quadrants of the same patient depicted in **A.** Note the similar pattern of bone loss in the area of the first molars and incisors.

In contrast to chronic disease, aggressive periodontitis appears to be correlated with one or more deficiencies in the immune response, rather than with inappropriate accumulations of plaque and calculus. Researchers believe that aggressive periodontitis represents a number of different pathoses that have been grouped together because of similar clinical presentations. Suspected pathogens that are commonly found in these diseases include *Actinobacillus actinomycetemcomitans, Prevotella intermedia, Porphyromonas gingivalis,* and a variety of other less common organisms. The response to therapy often hinges on the successful elimination of these organisms. As mentioned in the discussion of periodontitis (see page 168), an association with a number of viruses has been suggested but disputed by others.

The majority of patients with aggressive periodontitis have a demonstrable neutrophil dysfunction but without systemic manifestations. In the localized variant, a number of affected patients demonstrate a specific defect of bactericidal activity toward *A. actinomycetemcomitans.* Although this is a controversial topic, several investigators have suggested that aggressive periodontitis requires specific bacterial flora and the presence of a selective immune dysfunction that allows these pathogens to flourish. This unique pattern of immune alteration may explain the failure to defend appropriately against certain periodontal pathogens without exhibiting systemic signs of immunodeficiency.

Familial aggregation of patients with aggressive periodontitis is noted and suggests an underlying genetic foundation, which may be transmitted in some families as an autosomal dominant trait with reduced penetrance (some patients can harbor mutation without clinical evidence of disease). In all likelihood, aggressive periodontitis is genetically heterogeneous, meaning the mutation of any one of several different gene loci can result in the disease; however, only one of these causative mutations is identified within a kindred. With this knowledge, it would not be surprising to encounter variations in inheritance patterns in different geographic locations and ethnic groups.

CLINICAL AND RADIOGRAPHIC FEATURES

LOCALIZED AGGRESSIVE PERIODONTITIS

As previously stated, aggressive periodontitis can be localized or generalized. One large study of children aged 5 to 17 years in the United States demonstrated a prevalence of 0.53% for the localized form and 0.13% for the generalized variant. **Localized aggressive periodontitis** typically begins around the ages of 11 to 13 years and has a strong familial tendency. The following specific features have been delineated by the American Academy of Periodontology:

- Circumpubertal onset
- Robust serum antibody response to infecting agents
- Attachment loss localized to the first molars and incisors, with involvement of no more than two teeth other than the first molars and incisors

This form may appear to localize around the first molars and the incisors, possibly because these teeth have been erupted for the longest duration (Fig. 4-35). In numerous clinical studies, minimal supragingival plaque or calculus has been documented; however, this finding has been disputed. The rate of bone destruction is three to five times faster than that seen in chronic periodontitis.

In the first molar regions, radiographs reveal vertical bone resorption that often is bilateral and symmetrical. In classic cases an arc-shaped zone of bone loss extends from the distal aspect of the second bicuspid to the mesial aspect of the second molar. Similar involvement is apparent around the anterior teeth. Tooth migration and mobility are common. If untreated, then the process often continues until the teeth are exfoliated. In about one third of patients affected with localized aggressive periodontitis, progression to more generalized disease occurs.

Of all the pathogens in dental plaque, A. *actinomycetemcomitans* appears to be predominant in localized aggressive periodontitis. This bacterium is present in disease sites in more than 90% of cases. Its ability to invade gingival tissue has created difficulties in mechanical eradication. Knowledge of its importance to the disease process has led to remarkable advances in therapy.

GENERALIZED AGGRESSIVE PERIODONTITIS

Generalized aggressive periodontitis may not represent a distinct disease entity but, rather, may occur in a collection of young adults with advanced periodontal disease. Many cases may represent localized aggressive periodontitis that has become more generalized with time; other cases initially demonstrate generalized disease. As with the localized variant, a significant percentage of cases demonstrate neutrophil dysfunction. The American Academy of Periodontology recognizes the following features:

- Usually diagnosed in patients younger than 30 years old but may occur at any age
- Poor serum antibody response to infecting agents
- Pronounced episodic destruction of periodontal attachment and alveolar bone
- Generalized loss of attachment that must affect at least three teeth other than the first molars and incisors

Most affected patients are between the ages of 12 and 32. In contrast to many examples of the localized variant, heavy plaque, calculus, and marked gingival inflammation may be present. Compared with the localized variant, more teeth are affected and the bone loss is not restricted to specific areas of the jaws.

Although the localized pattern is associated primarily with A. *actinomycetemcomitans*, the pathogens active in the generalized variant are more complex, more closely aligned to chronic periodontitis, and also involve organisms such as *Prevotella intermedia*, *Porphyromonas gingivalis*, *Tannerella forsythensis*, *Fusobacterium nuclea-*

tum, *Campylobacter rectus*, and various spirochetes. In patients whose disease progresses from the localized to generalized pattern, the associated periodontal pathogens often become more diverse as the patient ages and the disease becomes more widespread.

HISTOPATHOLOGIC FEATURES

The microscopic examination of granulation tissue removed from sites of aggressive periodontitis does not differ dramatically from that seen in chronic periodontitis. In spite of this, initial histopathologic examination of the material removed from active sites of disease is mandatory to rule out the possibility of other disease processes, such as Langerhans cell disease (see page 590). Even when the attachment loss presents in a classic localized pattern, systemic disease cannot be eliminated without an examination of tissue. The definitive diagnosis centers on the clinical, radiographic, histopathologic, and microbiologic findings, combined with the family history and leukocyte function tests.

TREATMENT AND PROGNOSIS

Unlike the treatment used for patients with chronic periodontitis, scaling and root planing alone do not stop progression of aggressive periodontitis. The defects in leukocyte function, in addition to the invasive capabilities of the involved pathogenic organisms, mandate the use of antibiotics in combination with mechanical removal of subgingival plaque and inflamed periodontal tissues. Although tetracycline, amoxicillin and clavulanate potassium, minocycline, and erythromycin can be used in selected patients, the combination of high-dose (500 mg three times per day) amoxicillin and metronidazole has been shown to be most effective in controlling the involved periodontal pathogens, especially A. *actinomycetemcomitans*. Therapy often is predicated on microbiologic testing to ensure selection of the most appropriate antimicrobial agent. Some investigators have claimed better results if the scaling and root planing are completed within a 24-hour period, rather than treating a quadrant at a time over an extended period. Reinfection of previously cleaned areas by organisms from untreated sites is thought to worsen the response to therapy.

A reevaluation with professional prophylaxis is performed once a month for 6 months and then every 3 months thereafter. Specimens for anaerobic cultures are obtained at each 3-month recall. Patients with refractory disease or significant colonization by pathogenic organisms receive additional courses of appropriate antibiotics. Long-term follow-up is mandatory because of the possibility of reinfection or incomplete elimination of the organisms. The presence of deep residual pockets is associated with disease progression. In such circumstances, periodontal surgery often is performed to eliminate these defects. This intervention is directed at any pocket consistently deeper than 5 mm and typically is performed after 2 to 6 months of nonsurgical therapy.

Dental practitioners should alert proband patients with aggressive periodontitis of the possible genetic transmission of the disease process. In general, patients diagnosed with localized aggressive periodontitis typically exhibit relatively stable disease, whereas those initially diagnosed with generalized involvement often continue to lose periodontal attachment and teeth. Patients who smoke and those who present for therapy with advanced clinical attachment loss tend to demonstrate a worse prognosis and respond less reliably to therapy.

PAPILLON-LEFÈVRE SYNDROME

In 1924, Papillon and Lefèvre initially described the syndrome that bears their names. This autosomal recessive disorder predominantly demonstrates oral and dermatologic manifestations; similar dermatologic changes can be seen in the absence of oral findings (**keratoderma palmoplantar of Unna-Thost syndrome** and **Meleda disease**). Because of the autosomal recessive inheritance pattern, the parents typically are not affected; consanguinity is noted in approximately one third of cases. The predominant oral finding is accelerated periodontitis that appears to be caused by defects in neutrophil function and multiple immune-mediated mechanisms.

Genetic studies of patients with Papillon-Lefèvre syndrome have mapped the major gene locus to chromosome 11q14-q21 and revealed mutation and loss of function of the cathepsin C gene. This gene is important in the structural growth and development of the skin and is critical for appropriate immune response of myeloid and lymphoid cells. Researchers believe that the loss of appropriate function of the cathepsin C gene results in an altered immune response to infection. In addition, the altered gene may affect the integrity of the junctional epithelium surrounding the tooth.

A closely related disease, **Haim-Munk syndrome,** also exhibits palmoplantar keratosis, progressive periodontal disease, recurrent skin infections, and several skeletal malformations. In this syndrome, the skin manifestations are more severe and the periodontal disease is milder. Studies have demonstrated that Haim-Munk syndrome and many examples of prepubertal periodontitis also exhibit mutation of the cathepsin C gene and represent allelic variants of the mutated gene responsible for Papillon-Lefèvre syndrome.

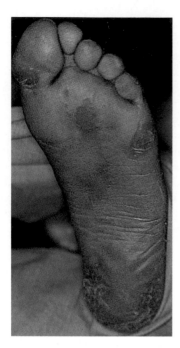

Fig. 4-36   Papillon-Lefèvre syndrome. Plantar keratosis of the foot.

CLINICAL AND RADIOGRAPHIC FEATURES

Papillon-Lefèvre syndrome exhibits a prevalence of one to four per million people in the population, and carriers are thought to be present in two to four per thousand persons. In most cases, the dermatologic manifestations become clinically evident in the first 3 years of life. Diffuse transgredient (first occurs on the palms and soles and then spreads to the dorsa of the hands and feet) palmar-plantar keratosis develops, with occasional reports of diffuse follicular hyperkeratosis, nail dystrophy, hyperhidrosis, and keratosis on the elbows and knees (Fig. 4-36). Other less common sites of involvement include the legs, thighs, dorsal surface of the fingers and toes, and (rarely) the trunk. Although the appearance of the dermatologic manifestations is variable, the lesions typically present as white, light-yellow, brown, or red plaques and patches that develop crusts, cracks, or deep fissures. Some patients describe worsening in the winter, and others describe keratotic desquamation, which may be confused with psoriasis.

The oral manifestations consist of dramatically advanced periodontitis that is seen in both the deciduous and the permanent dentitions and develops soon after the eruption of the teeth. Extensive hyperplastic and hemorrhagic gingivitis is seen (Fig. 4-37). A rapid loss of attachment occurs, with the teeth soon lacking osseous support and radiographically appearing to

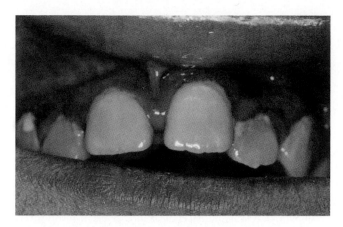

Fig. 4-37   Papillon-Lefèvre syndrome. Generalized erythematous gingivitis.

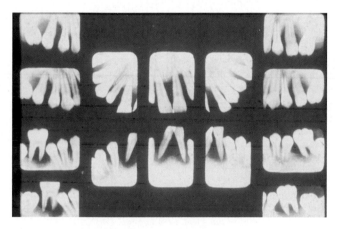

Fig. 4-38   Papillon-Lefèvre syndrome. Multifocal sites of bone loss in all four quadrants. *(From Giansanti JS, Hrabak RP, Waldron CA: Palmoplantar hyperkeratosis and concomitant periodontal destruction [Papillon-Lefèvre syndrome], Oral Surg Oral Med Oral Pathol 36:40, 1973.)*

float in the soft tissue (Fig. 4-38). Without aggressive therapy, the loss of the dentition is inevitable. Mobility and migration of the teeth are observed consistently, and mastication often is painful because of the lack of support. The teeth spontaneously exfoliate or are removed because of sensitivity during function. This process prematurely eliminates the deciduous dentition; with eruption of the permanent teeth, the destructive pattern is duplicated. When the teeth are absent, the alveolar mucosa is normal in appearance.

Although other pathogenic bacteria have been isolated from sites of active disease, *Actinobacillus actinomycetemcomitans* has been related directly to the periodontal destruction. Although a hereditary component exists and leukocyte dysfunction can be demonstrated, it appears that an infection with a specific, potent bacterium, such as *A. actinomycetemcomitans*,

must be present for the periodontal component to develop. Interestingly, one investigation documented the development of appropriate peripheral leukocyte function after successful resolution of the pathogenic organisms responsible for the periodontitis. This indicates that the leukocyte dysfunction may be induced by infection with *A. actinomycetemcomitans* (possibly secondary to generated leukotoxins).

In addition to the dermatologic and oral manifestations, numerous investigators have documented less frequent findings. Retardation of somatic development and ectopic calcifications of the falx cerebri and choroid plexus have been reported, in addition to an increased susceptibility to infections beyond the oral cavity. Pyoderma, furunculosis, pneumonia, hepatic abscesses, and other infections have been documented.

HISTOPATHOLOGIC FEATURES

Once again, the histopathologic features of Papillon-Lefèvre syndrome resemble those seen in chronic periodontitis and are not specific. Submitted tissue often contains hyperplastic crevicular epithelium with exocytosis. The underlying connective tissue exhibits increased vascularity and a mixed inflammatory cellular infiltrate consisting predominantly of polymorphonuclear leukocytes, lymphocytes, histiocytes, and plasma cells. Initially, histopathologic examination is recommended to rule out other pathologic causes of the periodontal destruction.

TREATMENT AND PROGNOSIS

The most successful treatment of the skin lesions has been retinoid (e.g., etretinate) administration, which has resulted in remarkable improvement with complete clearance in the majority of patients. Surprisingly, a few authors have reported improvement of the associated periodontal disease during periods of retinoid use, but others have disputed this claim. Possible adverse reactions caused by retinoid administration include angular cheilitis, dry lips, hair loss, arthralgia, tendinous and ligamentous calcifications, and teratogenicity. In an attempt to avoid these drug-related adverse reactions, patients with mild dermatologic manifestations often are treated with topical lubricants, keratolytic agents (salicylic or lactic acid), corticosteroid agents, or antibiotics medications.

Attempts at resolution of the periodontal disease often have been frustrating. In spite of extensive periodontal therapy and antibiotic agents, in many patients the disease progresses until all teeth are lost. However, several investigators have reported a cessation of attachment loss, and two different treatment approaches have been used.

Despite the use of numerous antibiotic medications, several reports document a difficulty in resolution of the infection associated with teeth that already exhibit attachment loss. In some of the cases, all of the periodontally involved deciduous teeth were extracted, followed by a period of edentulousness with antibiotic treatment in an attempt to remove the causative pathogens. Tetracycline was successful in preventing the redevelopment of periodontitis in the permanent teeth after the extractions, as well as in the resolution of the infection in the deciduous dentition. However, penicillin, erythromycin, metronidazole, and tetracycline were all unsuccessful in resolving active sites of periodontitis.

The second approach revolves around direct attack against *A. actinomycetemcomitans*. In numerous studies of patients with destructive periodontitis associated with *A. actinomycetemcomitans*, therapy with high-dose amoxicillin and metronidazole has proven effective when combined with high patient compliance and strong supportive periodontal therapy. A variety of other regimens have been used with variable success in different geographic regions, suggesting the possibility of inconsistent effectiveness related to local patterns of antibiotic resistance. It appears clear that elimination of *A. actinomycetemcomitans* and continued control of plaque and calculus are mandatory, but the antibiotic agent best suited for this task can vary.

Through the use of mechanical plaque control and appropriate antibiotic medications directed toward *A. actinomycetemcomitans*, the course of the disease might be altered. The progression of attachment loss is slowed dramatically, and the teeth that erupt after the initiation of therapy do not develop periodontal destruction. Rigorous oral hygiene, chlorhexidine mouth rinses, frequent professional prophylaxis, and periodic appropriate antibiotic therapy are necessary for long-term maintenance.

BIBLIOGRAPHY

General Reference
Newman MG, Takei H, Carranza FA et al: *Clinical periodontology*, ed 10, Philadelphia, 2006, WB Saunders.

Gingivitis
American Academy of Periodontology: Parameter on plaque-induced gingivitis, *J Periodontol* 71(suppl):851-852, 2000.
American Academy of Periodontology: Treatment of plaque-induced gingivitis, chronic periodontitis, and other clinical conditions, *J Periodontol* 72:1790-1800, 2001.
Fransson C, Berglundh T, Lindhe J: The effects of age on the development of gingivitis. Clinical, microbiological and histological findings, *J Clin Periodontol* 23:379-385, 1996.
Gunsolley JC: A meta-analysis of six-month studies of antiplaque and antigingivitis agents, *J Am Dent Assoc* 137:1649-1657, 2006.

Löe H, Theilade E, Jensen SB: Experimental gingivitis in man, *J Periodontol* 36:177-187, 1965.
Löe H, Theilade E, Jensen SB et al: Experimental gingivitis in man. 3. Influence of antibiotics on gingival plaque development, *J Periodontol Res* 2:282-289, 1967.
Moskow BS, Polson AM: Histologic studies on the extension of the inflammatory infiltrate in human periodontitis, *J Clin Periodontol* 18:534-542, 1991.
Schätzle M, Löe H, Lang NP et al: The clinical course of chronic periodontitis. IV. Gingival inflammation as a risk factor in tooth mortality, *J Clin Periodontol* 31:1122-1127, 2004.
Tatakis DN, Trombelli L: Modulation of clinical expression of plaque-induced gingivitis. I. Background review and rationale, *J Clin Periodontol* 31:229-238, 2004.
Theilade E, Wright WH, Jensen SB et al: Experimental gingivitis in man. II. A longitudinal clinical and bacteriologically investigation, *J Periodontol Res* 1:1-13, 1966.
Trombelli L: Susceptibility to gingivitis: a way to predict periodontal disease? *Oral Health Prev Dent* 2(suppl 1):265-269, 2004.
Trombelli L, Scapoli C, Orlandini E et al: Modualtion of clinical expression of plaque-induced gingivitis. III. Response of "high responders" and "low responders" to therapy, *J Clin Periodontol* 31:253-259, 2004.

Necrotizing Ulcerative Gingivitis
American Academy of Periodontology: Parameter on acute periodontal diseases, *J Periodontol* 71(suppl):863-866, 2000.
Arendorf TM, Bredekamp B, Cloete C-A: Seasonal variation of acute necrotising ulcerative gingivitis in South Africans, *Oral Dis* 7:150-154, 2001.
Contreras A, Falkler Jr WA, Enwonwu C et al: Human *herpesviridae* in acute necrotizing ulcerative gingivitis in children in Nigeria, *Oral Microbiol Immuol* 12:259-265, 1997.
Hartnett AC, Shiloah J: The treatment of acute necrotizing ulcerative gingivitis, *Quintessence Int* 22:95-100, 1991.
Horning GM: Necrotizing gingivostomatitis-NUG to noma, *Compend Contin Educ Dent* 17:951-962, 1996.
Horning GM, Cohen ME: Necrotizing ulcerative gingivitis, periodontitis, and stomatitis: clinical staging and predisposing factors, *J Periodontol* 66:990-998, 1995.
Jiménez LM, Duque FL, Baer PN et al: Necrotizing ulcerative periodontal diseases in children and young adults in Medellín, Columbia, 1965-2000, *J Int Acad Periodontol* 7:55-63, 2005.
Johnson BD, Engel D: Acute necrotizing ulcerative gingivitis: a review of diagnosis, etiology and treatment, *J Periodontol* 57:141-150, 1986.
Rowland RW: Necrotizing ulcerative gingivitis, *Ann Periodontol* 4:65-73, 1999.
Wade DN, Kerns DG: Acute necrotizing ulcerative gingivitis-periodontitis: a literature review, *Mil Med* 5:337-342, 1998.

Plasma Cell Gingivitis
Kerr DA, McClatchey KD, Regezi JA: Allergic gingivostomatitis (due to gum chewing), *J Periodontol* 42:709-712, 1971.
Kerr DA, McClatchey KD, Regezi JA: Idiopathic gingivostomatitis: cheilitis, glossitis, gingivitis syndrome: atypical gingivostomatitis plasma-cell gingivitis, plasmacytosis of gingiva, *Oral Surg Oral Med Oral Pathol* 32:402-423, 1971.
Lubow RM, Cooley RL, Hartman KS et al: Plasma-cell gingivostomatitis: report of a case, *J Periodontol* 55:235-241, 1984.
MacLeod RL, Ellis JE: Plasma cell gingivitis related to the use of herbal toothpaste, *Br Dent J* 166:375-376, 1989.
Mahler V, Hornstein OP: Plasma cell gingivitis: treatment with 2% fusidic acid, *J Am Acad Dermatol* 34:145-146, 1996.

Marker P, Krogdahl A: Plasma cell gingivitis apparently related to the use of khat: report of a case, *Br Dent J* 192:311-313, 2002.

Owings JR: An atypical gingivostomatitis: report of four cases, *J Periodontol* 40:538-542, 1969.

Perry HO, Deffner NF, Sheridan PJ: Atypical gingivostomatitis: nineteen cases, *Arch Dermatol* 107:872-878, 1973.

Serio FG, Siegel MA: Plasma cell gingivitis of unusual origin: report of a case, *J Periodontol* 62:390-393, 1991.

Silverman S Jr, Lozada F: An epilogue to plasma-cell gingivostomatitis (allergic gingivostomatitis), *Oral Surg Oral Med Oral Pathol* 43:211-217, 1977.

Sollecito TP, Greenberg MS: Plasma cell gingivitis: report of two cases, *Oral Surg Oral Med Oral Pathol* 73:690-693, 1992.

Timms MS, Sloan P: Association of supraglottic and gingival idiopathic plasmacytosis, *Oral Surg Oral Med Oral Pathol* 71:451-453, 1991.

Granulomatous Gingivitis

Daley TD, Wysocki GP: Foreign body gingivitis: an iatrogenic disease? *Oral Surg Oral Med Oral Pathol* 69:708-712, 1990.

Gordon SC, Daley TD: Foreign body gingivitis: clinical and microscopic features of 61 cases, *Oral Surg Oral Med Oral Pathol Oral Radiol Endod* 83:562-570, 1997.

Gordon SC, Daley TD: Foreign body gingivitis: identification of the foreign material by energy-dispersive x-ray microanalysis, *Oral Surg Oral Med Oral Pathol Oral Radiol Endod* 83:571-576, 1997.

Gravitis K, Daley TD, Lochhead MA: Management of patients with foreign body gingivitis: report of 2 cases with histologic findings, *J Can Dent Assoc* 71:105-109, 2005.

Koppang HS, Roushan A, Srafilzadeh A et al: Foreign body gingival lesions: distribution, morphology, identification by x-ray energy dispersive analysis and possible origin of foreign material, *J Oral Pathol Med* 36:161-172, 2007.

Lombardi T, Kuffer R, Dubrez B: Polishing-paste-induced silica granuloma of the gingiva, *Dermatology* 203:177-179, 2001.

Mignogna MD, Fedele S, LoRusso L et al: Orofacial granulomatosis with gingival onset, *J Clin Periodontol* 28:692-696, 2001.

Drug-Related Gingival Hyperplasia

American Academy of Periodontology: Informational paper. Drug-associated gingival enlargement, *J Periodontol* 75:1424-1431, 2004.

Botha PJ: Drug-induced gingival hyperplasia and its management—a literature review, *J Dent Assoc S Afr* 52:659-664, 1997.

Brunet L, Miranda J, Farré M et al: Gingival enlargement induced by drugs, *Drug Saf* 15:219-231, 1996.

Butler RT, Kalkwarf KL, Kaldahl WB: Drug-induced gingival hyperplasia: phenytoin, cyclosporine, and nifedipine, *J Am Dent Assoc* 114:56-60, 1987.

Camargo PM, Melnick PR, Pirih FQM et al: Treatment of drug-induced gingival enlargement: aesthetic and functional considerations, *Periodontol 2000* 27:131-138, 2001.

Desai P, Silver JG: Drug-induced gingival enlargements, *J Can Dent Assoc* 64:263-268, 1998.

Dongari A, McDonnell HT, Langlais RP: Drug-induced gingival overgrowth, *Oral Surg Oral Med Oral Pathol* 76:543-548, 1993.

Eggerath J, English H, Leichter JW: Drug-associated gingival enlargement: case report and review of aetiology, management and evidenced-based outcomes of treatment, *J N Z Soc Periodontol* 88:7-14, 2005.

Hall EE: Prevention and treatment considerations in patients with drug-induced gingival enlargement, *Curr Opin Periodontol* 4:59-63, 1997.

Hassell TM, Hefti AF: Drug-induced gingival overgrowth: old problem, new problem, *Crit Rev Oral Biol Med* 2:103-137, 1991.

McCulloch CA: Drug-induced fibrosis: interference with intracellular collagen degradation pathway, *Curr Opin Drug Discov Devel* 7:720-724, 2004.

Meisel P, Schwahn C, John U et al: Calcium antagonists and deep gingival pockets in the population-based SHIP study, *Br J Clin Pharmacol* 60:552-559, 2005.

Woo S-B, Allen CM, Orden A et al: Non-gingival soft tissue overgrowths after allogeneic marrow transplantation, *Bone Marrow Transplant* 17:1127-1132, 1996.

Gingival Fibromatosis

Coletta RD, Graner E: Hereditary gingival fibromatosis: a systematic review, *J Periodontol* 77:753-764, 2006.

Hart TC, Zhang Y, Gorry MC et al: A mutation in the SOS1 gene causes hereditary gingival fibromatosis type 1, *Am J Hum Genet* 70:943-954, 2002.

Jorgenson RJ, Cocker ME: Variation in the inheritance and expression of gingival fibromatosis, *J Periodontol* 45:472-477, 1974.

Mangino M, Pizzuti A, Dallapiccola B et al: Hereditary gingival fibromatosis (HGF) with hypertrichosis is unlinked to the HGF1 and HGF2 loci, *Am J Med Genet* 116A:312-314, 2003.

Rushton MA: Hereditary or idiopathic hyperplasia of the gums, *Dent Pract Dent Rec* 7:136-146, 1957.

Shashi V, Pallos D, Pettenati MJ et al: Genetic heterogeneity of gingival fibromatosis on chromosome 2p, *J Med Genet* 36:683-686, 1999.

Takagi M, Yamamoto H, Mega H et al: Heterogeneity in the gingival fibromatoses, *Cancer* 68:2202-2212, 1991.

Xiao S, Bu L, Zhu L et al: A new locus for hereditary gingival fibromatosis (GINGF2) maps to 5q13-q22, *Genomics* 74:180-185, 2001.

Ye X, Shi L, Cheng Y et al: A novel locus for autosomal dominant hereditary gingival fibromatosis, GINGF3, maps to chromosome 2q22.3-p23.3, *Clin Genet* 68:239-244, 2005.

Periodontitis

Albandar JM: Global risk factors and risk indicators for periodontal diseases, *Periodontol 2000* 29:177-206, 2002.

American Academy of Periodontology: Position paper. Supportive periodontal therapy (SPT), *J Periodontol* 69:502-506, 1998.

American Academy of Periodontology: Parameter on acute periodontal diseases, *J Periodontol* 71:863-866, 2000.

American Academy of Periodontology: Parameter on "refractory" periodontitis, *J Periodontol* 71:859-860, 2000.

American Academy of Periodontology: Informational paper. Modulation of the host response in periodontal therapy, *J Periodontol* 73:460-470, 2003.

American Academy of Periodontology: Position paper. Diagnosis of periodontal diseases, *J Periodontol* 74:1237-1247, 2003.

American Academy of Periodontology: Informational paper. Implications of genetic technology for the management of periodontal diseases, *J Periodontol* 76:850-857, 2005.

American Academy of Periodontology: Position paper. Epidemiology of periodontal diseases, *J Periodontol* 76:1406-1419, 2005.

Armitage G: Development of a classification system for periodontal diseases and conditions, *Ann Periodontol* 4:1-6, 1999.

Bataineh AB, Al Qudah MA: The predisposing factors of pericoronitis of mandibular third molars in a Jordanian population, *Quintessence Int* 34:227-231, 2003.

Cappuyns I, Gugerli P, Mombelli A: Viruses in periodontal disease—a review, *Oral Dis* 11:219-229, 2005.

Corbet EF: Diagnosis of acute periodontal lesions, *Periodontol 2000* 34:204-216, 2004.

Gaggl AJ, Rainer H, Grund E et al: Local oxygen therapy for treating acute necrotizing periodontal disease in smokers, *J Periodontol* 77:31-38, 2006.

Greenstein G: Periodontal response to mechanical non-surgical therapy: a review, *J Periodontol* 63:118-130, 1992.

Dentino AR, Kassab MW, Renner EJ: Prevention of periodontal diseases, *Dent Clin North Am* 49:573-594, 2005.

Ismail AI, Morrison EC, Burt BA et al: Natural history of periodontal disease in adults: findings from the Tecumseh periodontal disease study, 1959-87, *J Dent Res* 69:430-435, 1990.

Kinane DF, Hart TC: Genes and genetic polymorphisms associated with periodontal disease, *Crit Rev Oral Biol Med* 14:430-449, 2003.

Lindhe J, Nyman S: Long-term maintenance of patients treated for advanced periodontal disease, *J Clin Periodontol* 11:504-514, 1984.

Loos BG, John RP, Laine ML: Identification of genetic risk factors for periodontitis and possible mechanisms of action, *J Clin Periodontol* 32(suppl 6):159-179, 2005.

Meng HX: Periodontal abscess, *Ann Periodontol* 4:79-82, 1999.

Minsk L: Diagnosis and treatment of acute periodontal conditions, *Compend Contin Educ Dent* 27:8-11, 2006.

Newman HN: Plaque and chronic inflammatory periodontal disease: a question of ecology, *J Clin Periodontol* 17:533-541, 1990.

Novak MJ: Necrotizing ulcerative periodontitis, *Ann Periodontol* 4:74-77, 1999.

Preshaw PM, Seymour RA, Heasman PA: Current concepts in periodontal pathogenesis, *Dent Update* 21:570-578, 2004.

Rees JS, Midda M: Update on periodontology: 1. Current concepts in the histopathology of periodontal disease, *Dent Update* 18:418-422, 1991.

Scannapieco FA: Systemic effects of periodontal diseases, *Den Clin North Am* 49:533-550, 2005.

Slots J: Herpesviruses in periodontal diseases, *Periodontol 2000* 38:33-62, 2005.

Tatakis DN, Kumar PS: Etiology and pathogenesis of periodontal diseases, *Dent Clin North Am* 49:491-516, 2005.

Tonetti MS, D'Aiuto F, Nibali L et al: Treatment of periodontitis and endothelial function, *N Engl J Med* 35:911-920, 2007.

Aggressive Periodontitis

Albandar JM, Brown LJ, Genco RJ et al: Clinical classification of periodontitis in adolescents and young adults, *J Periodontol* 68:545-555, 1997.

American Academy of Periodontology: Parameter on aggressive periodontitis, *J Periodontol* 71:867-869, 2000.

American Academy of Periodontology: Position paper. Periodontal diseases of children and adolescents, *J Periodontol* 74:1696-1704, 2003.

Armitage GC: Development of a classification system for periodontal diseases and conditions, *Ann Periodontol* 4:1-6, 1999.

Donly KJ, Ashkenazi M: Juvenile periodontitis: a review of pathogenesis, diagnosis and treatment, *J Clin Pediatr Dent* 16:73-78, 1992.

Guerrero A, Griffiths GS, Nibali L et al: Adjunctive benefits of systemic amoxicillin and metronidazole in non-surgical treatment of generalized aggressive periodontitis: a randomized placebo-controlled clinical trial, *J Clin Periodontol* 32:1096-1107, 2005.

Hughes FJ, Syed M, Koshy B et al: Prognostic factors in the treatment of generalized aggressive periodontitis: I. Clinical features and initial outcome, *J Clin Periodontol* 33:663-670, 2006.

Kamma JJ, Slots J: Herpesviral-bacterial interactions in aggressive periodontitis, *J Clin Periodontol* 30:420-426, 2003.

Kinane DF, Hart TC: Genes and genetic polymorphisms associated with periodontal disease, *Crit Rev Oral Biol Med* 14:430-449, 2003.

Lindhe J, Liljenberg B: Treatment of localized juvenile periodontitis: results after 5 years, *J Clin Periodontol* 11:399-410, 1984.

Löe H, Brown LJ: Early onset periodontitis in the United States of America, *J Periodontol* 62:608-616, 1991.

Mongardini C, van Steenberghe D, Dekeyser C et al: One stage full- versus partial-mouth disinfection in the treatment of chronic adult or generalized early-onset periodontitis. I. Long-term clinical observations, *J Periodontol* 70:632-645, 1999.

Novak MJ, Novak KF: Early-onset periodontitis, *Curr Opin Periodontol* 3:45-58, 1996.

Tonetti MS, Mombelli A: Early-onset periodontitis, *Ann Periodontol* 4:39-52, 1999.

Xajigeorgiou C, Sakellari D, Slini T et al: Clinical and microbiological effects of different antimicrobials on generalized aggressive periodontitis, *J Clin Periodontol* 33:254-264, 2006.

Papillon-Lefèvre Syndrome

Ahuja V, Shin RH, Mudgil A et al: Papillon-Lefèvre syndrome: a successful outcome, *J Periodontol* 76:1996-2001, 2005.

Gorlin RJ, Sedano H, Anderson VE: The syndrome of palmar-plantar hyperkeratosis and premature destruction of the teeth: a clinical and genetic analysis of the Papillon-Lefèvre syndrome, *J Pediatr* 65:895-908, 1964.

Hart TC, Hart PS, Bowden DW et al: Mutations of the cathepsin C gene are responsible for Papillon-Lefèvre syndrome, *J Med Genet* 36:881-887, 1999.

Hart TC, Hart PS, Michalec M et al: Haim-Munk syndrome and Papillon-Lefèvre syndrome are allelic mutations in cathepsin C, *J Med Genet* 37:88-94, 2000.

Hattab FN, Amin WM: Papillon-Lefèvre syndrome with albinism: a review of the literature and report of 2 brothers, *Oral Surg Oral Med Oral Pathol Oral Radiol Endod* 100:709-716, 2005.

Hewitt C, McCormick D, Linden G: The role of cathepsin C in Papillon-Lefèvre syndrome, prepubertal periodontitis, and aggressive periodontitis, *Hum Mutat* 23:222-228, 2004.

Lundgren T, Crossner C-G, Twetman S et al: Systemic retinoid medication and periodontal health in patients with Papillon-Lefèvre syndrome, *J Clin Periodontol* 23:176-179, 1996.

Noack B, Görgens H, Hoffmann TH et al: Novel mutations in the *cathepsin C* gene in patients with pre-pubertal aggressive periodontitis and Papillon-Lefèvre syndrome, *J Dent Res* 83:368-370, 2004.

Pacheco JJ, Coelho C, Salazar F et al: Treatment of Papillon-Lefèvre syndrome periodontitis, *J Clin Periodontol* 29:370-374, 2002.

Wiebe CB, Häkkinen L, Putnins EE et al: Successful periodontal maintenance of a case with Papillon-Lefèvre syndrome: 12-year follow-up and review of the literature, *J Periodontol* 72:824-830, 2001.

5

Bacterial Infections

CHAPTER OUTLINE

IMPETIGO

Impetigo is a superficial infection of the skin that is caused by *Streptococcus pyogenes* (group A streptococcus) and *Staphylococcus aureus,* either separately or together. The term *impetigo* is derived from a Latin word meaning "attack," because of its common presentation as a scabbing eruption. Two clinically distinctive patterns are seen, **nonbullous impetigo** and **bullous impetigo.** Intact epithelium is normally protective against infection; therefore, many cases arise in damaged skin such as preexisting dermatitis, cuts, abrasions, or insect bites. Secondary involvement of an area of dermatitis has been termed **impetiginized dermatitis.** An increased prevalence is associated with debilitating systemic conditions such as human immunodeficiency virus (HIV) infection, type 2 diabetes mellitus, or dialysis.

CLINICAL FEATURES

Nonbullous impetigo (impetigo contagiosa) is the more prevalent pattern and occurs most frequently on the legs, with less common involvement noted on the trunk, scalp, or face. The facial lesions usually develop around the nose and mouth. In many patients with facial involvement, the pathogenic bacteria are harbored in the nose and spread onto the skin into previ-

ously damaged sites such as scratches or abrasions. Often, facial lesions will have a linear pattern that corresponds to previous fingernail scratches. The infection is more prevalent in school-aged children but also may be seen in adults. The peak occurrence is during the summer or early fall in hot, moist climates. Impetigo is contagious and easily spread in crowded or unsanitary living conditions.

Nonbullous impetigo initially appears as red macules or papules, with the subsequent development of fragile vesicles. These vesicles quickly rupture and become covered with a thick, amber crust (Fig. 5-1). The crusts are adherent and have been described as "cornflakes glued to the surface." Some cases may be confused with exfoliative cheilitis (see page 304) or recurrent herpes simplex (see page 243). Pruritus is common, and scratching often causes the lesions to spread (Fig. 5-2). Lymphangitis, cellulitis, fever, anorexia, and malaise are uncommon, although leukocytosis occurs in about half of affected patients.

Bullous impetigo usually is caused by *S. aureus* and also has been termed **staphylococcal impetigo.** Like the nonbullous form, it most frequently affects the extremities, trunk, and face. Infants and newborns are infected most commonly, but the disease also may occur in children and adults. The lesions are characterized by superficial vesicles that rapidly enlarge to form larger flaccid bullae. Initially, the bullae are filled with

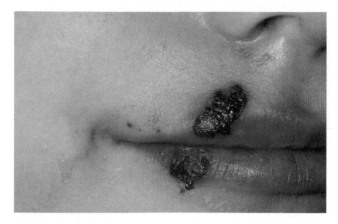

Fig. 5-1   Impetigo. Amber crusts of the skin and vermilion border of the lips.

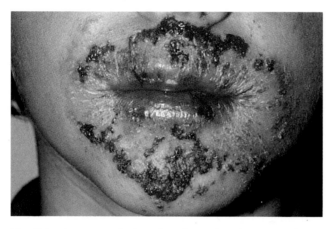

Fig. 5-2   Impetigo. Scaly and amber-colored crusts of the perioral skin.

clear serous fluid, but the contents of the bullae quickly become more turbid and eventually purulent. Although the bullae may remain intact, they usually rupture and develop a thin brown crust that some describe as "lacquer." Weakness, fever, and diarrhea may be seen. Lymphadenopathy and cellulitis are unusual complications. Meningitis and pneumonia are very rare but may lead to serious complications, even death.

DIAGNOSIS

A strong presumptive diagnosis can normally be made from the clinical presentation. When the diagnosis is not obvious clinically or the infection fails to respond to standard therapy within 7 days, the definitive diagnosis requires isolation of *S. pyogenes* or *S. aureus* from cultures of involved skin.

TREATMENT AND PROGNOSIS

For patients with nonbullous impetigo involving only a small area with few lesions, topical mupirocin has been shown to be effective. Fusidic acid (available in Europe, not in the United States) also has been very effective; however, increasing reports of resistance are diminishing its use. Removal of the crusts with a clean cloth soaked in warm soapy water is recommended before application of topical therapy, rather than placing the medication on inert, dried, exfoliating skin. For bullous or more extensive lesions, topical antibiotic drugs often are insufficient; the treatment of choice is a 1-week course of a systemic oral antibiotic. The best antibiotic is one that is effective against both *S. pyogenes* and penicillin-resistant *S. aureus*. Cephalexin, trimethoprim-sulfamethoxazole, dicloxacillin, flucloxacillin, and amoxicillin-clavulanic acid represent good current choices. Erythromycin or clindamycin can be used in patients sensitive to penicillin, but resistance by *S. aureus* to erythromycin has become an increasing problem. If left untreated, then the lesions often enlarge slowly and spread. Serious complications, such as acute glomerulonephritis, are rare but possible in prolonged cases. Inappropriate diagnosis and treatment with topical corticosteroids may produce resolution of the surface crusts, but infectious, red, raw lesions remain.

ERYSIPELAS

Erysipelas is a superficial skin infection most commonly associated with β-hemolytic streptococci (usually group A, such as *Streptococcus pyogenes*, but occasionally other groups such as group C, B, or G). Other less common causative organisms include *Staphylococcus aureus*, *Streptococcus pneumoniae* (i.e., pneumococcus), *Klebsiella pneumoniae*, *Yersinia enterocolitica*, and *Haemophilus influenzae*. The infection rapidly spreads through the lymphatic channels, which become filled with fibrin, leukocytes, and streptococci. Although also associated with ergotism, the term *Saint Anthony's fire* has been used to describe erysipelas. Because the French House of St. Anthony, an eleventh-century hospital, had fiery red walls similar to the color of erysipelas, the term *Saint Anthony's fire* was used to describe this disease. Today, classical facial erysipelas is a rare and often forgotten diagnosis. At times, the appropriate diagnosis has been delayed because of confusion with facial cellulitis from dental infections.

CLINICAL FEATURES

Erysipelas tends to occur primarily in young and older adult patients or in those who are debilitated, diabetic, immunosuppressed, obese, or alcoholic. Patients who

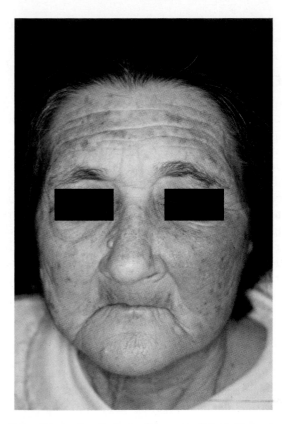

Fig. 5-3 **Erysipelas.** Red, swollen area of the left cheek. (*Courtesy Dr. Arthur Gonty*).

have areas of chronic lymphedema or large surgical scars (such as postmastectomy or saphenous venectomy) also are susceptible to this disease. The infection may occur anywhere on the skin, especially in areas of previous trauma. The most commonly affected site is the leg in areas affected by tinea pedis (athlete's foot). The face, arm, and upper thigh also frequently are infected. In facial erysipelas, an increased prevalence is noted in the winter and spring months, whereas summer is the peak period of involvement of the lower extremities.

When lesions occur on the face, they normally appear on the cheeks, eyelids, and bridge of the nose, at times producing a butterfly-shaped lesion that may resemble lupus erythematosus (see page 794). If the eyelids are involved, then they may become edematous and shut, thereby resembling angioedema (see page 356). The affected area is painful, bright red, well circumscribed, swollen, indurated, and warm to the touch (Fig. 5-3). Often the affected skin will demonstrate a surface texture that resembles an orange peel (*peau d'orange*). High fever and lymphadenopathy often are present. Lymphangitis, leukocytosis, nausea, and vomiting occur infrequently. Diagnostic confirmation is difficult because cultures usually are not beneficial.

TREATMENT AND PROGNOSIS

The treatment of choice is penicillin. Alternative antibiotic drugs include macrolides such as erythromycin, cephalosporins such as cephalexin, and fluoroquinolones such as ciprofloxacin. On initiation of therapy, the area of skin involvement often enlarges, probably secondary to the release of toxins from the dying streptococci. A rapid resolution is noted within 48 hours. Without appropriate therapy, possible complications include abscess formation, gangrene, necrotizing fasciitis, toxic shock syndrome with possible multiple organ failure, thrombophlebitis, acute glomerulonephritis, septicemia, endocarditis, and death. Recurrences may develop in the same area, most likely in a previous zone of damaged lymphatics or untreated athlete's foot. With repeated recurrences, permanent and disfiguring enlargements may result. In cases with multiple recurrences, prophylaxis with oral penicillin has been used.

STREPTOCOCCAL TONSILLITIS AND PHARYNGITIS

Tonsillitis and **pharyngitis** are extremely common and may be caused by many different organisms. The most common causes are group A, β-hemolytic streptococci, adenoviruses, enteroviruses, influenza, parainfluenza, and Epstein-Barr virus. Although a virus causes the majority of pharyngitis cases, infection with group A streptococci is responsible for 15% to 30% of acute pharyngitis cases in children and 5% to 10% of cases in adults. Adults who are parents of school-aged children or work in close association with children are at increased risk for developing this infection. Spread is typically by person-to-person contact through respiratory droplets or oral secretions, with a short incubation period of 2 to 5 days. Uncommonly, outbreaks of streptococcal pharyngitis have been associated with contaminated food, often inappropriately handled cold salads containing foodstuffs such as eggs, mayonnaise, tuna, potatoes, or cheese.

CLINICAL FEATURES

Although the infection can occur at any age, the greatest prevalence occurs in children 5 to 15 years old, with most cases in temperate climates arising in the winter or early spring. The signs and symptoms of **tonsillitis** and **pharyngitis** vary from mild to intense. Common findings include sudden onset of sore throat, temperature of 101° to 104° F, dysphagia, tonsillar hyperplasia, redness of the oropharynx and tonsils, palatal petechiae, cervical lymphadenopathy, and a yellowish tonsillar exudate that may be patchy or

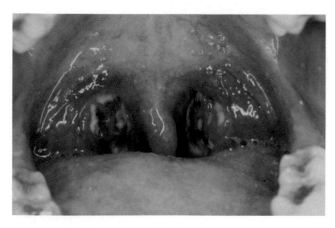

Fig. 5-4   Tonsillitis. Hyperplastic pharyngeal tonsils, with yellowish exudate of crypts.

confluent (Fig. 5-4). Other occasional findings include a "beefy" red and swollen uvula, excoriated nares, and a scarlatiniform rash (see next topic). Systemic symptoms, such as headache, malaise, anorexia, abdominal pain, and vomiting, may be noted, especially in younger children. Conjunctivitis, coryza (rhinorrhea), cough, hoarseness, discrete ulcerative lesions, anterior stomatitis, absence of fever, a viral exanthem, and diarrhea typically are associated with the viral infections and normally are not present in streptococcal pharyngotonsillitis.

DIAGNOSIS

Although the vast majority of pharyngitis cases are caused by a viral infection, reviews have shown that about 70% of adults in the United States receive antibiotic therapy. In an attempt to minimize overuse, antibiotics should not be prescribed without confirmation of bacterial infection. Except for very rare infections such as *Corynebacterium diphtheriae* (see page 186) and *Neisseria gonorrhoeae* (see page 193), antibiotics are of no benefit for acute pharyngitis except for those related to group A streptococci.

Patients exhibiting features strongly suggestive of a viral infection (see previous section) should not receive antibiotic therapy or microbiologic testing for streptococcal infection. Because the clinical features of streptococcal pharyngitis overlap those of viral origin, the diagnosis cannot be based solely on clinical features; however, laboratory testing of all patients with sore throat cannot be justified. Diagnostic testing is recommended only for those patients with clinical and epidemiologic findings that suggest streptococcal infection or for those in close contact with a well-documented case. Although less sensitive than throat culture, rapid antigen detection testing provides quick results and exhibits good sensitivity and specificity. If negative

results are obtained in children, then confirmatory throat cultures should be performed.

TREATMENT AND PROGNOSIS

Streptococcal pharyngitis usually is self-limited and resolves spontaneously within 3 to 4 days after onset of symptoms. In addition to reducing the localized morbidity of the infection, the main goals of therapy are to prevent development of acute rheumatic fever and complications such as peritonsillar or retropharyngeal abscess, deep tissue cellulitis, toxic shock–like syndrome, bacteremia, arthralgia, and acute glomerulonephritis. Initiation of appropriate therapy within the first 9 days after development of the pharyngitis will prevent rheumatic fever. Patients are considered noncontagious 24 hours after initiation of appropriate antibiotic therapy.

Group A streptococci are uniformly sensitive to penicillin. Although oral penicillin remains the therapy of choice, amoxicillin and cephalosporin drugs such as cephalexin, cefadroxil, cefuroxime, and cefprozil also are effective. Erythromycin is used in patients who have a known sensitivity to penicillin. Newer macrolides (e.g., clarithromycin, azithromycin) have similar effectiveness but cause less gastrointestinal distress when compared with erythromycin.

No single regimen eliminates pharyngeal pathogenic streptococci in 100% of treated patients. Posttherapeutic laboratory testing is recommended in patients with a family history of rheumatic fever, during outbreaks of acute rheumatic fever or streptococcal glomerulonephritis, during outbreaks of streptococcal pharyngitis in semiclosed communities, and when "ping pong" spread is occurring within a family. In these cases, clindamycin or amoxicillin-clavulanic acid often is able to clear the organism in patients who continue to demonstrate positive culture after penicillin therapy.

SCARLET FEVER (SCARLATINA)

Scarlet fever is a systemic infection produced by group A, β-hemolytic streptococci. The disease begins as a streptococcal tonsillitis with pharyngitis in which the organisms elaborate an erythrogenic toxin that attacks the blood vessels and produces the characteristic skin rash. The condition occurs in susceptible patients who do not have antitoxin antibodies. The incubation period ranges from 1 to 7 days, and the significant clinical findings include fever, enanthem, and exanthem.

CLINICAL FEATURES

Scarlet fever is most common in children from the ages of 3 to 12 years. The enanthem of the oral mucosa involves the tonsils, pharynx, soft palate, and tongue

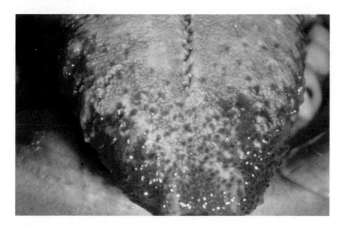

Fig. 5-5   Scarlet fever. Dorsal surface of the tongue exhibiting white coating in association with numerous enlarged and erythematous fungiform papillae (white strawberry tongue).

(see discussion of streptococcal pharyngotonsillitis in previous section). The tonsils, soft palate, and pharynx become erythematous and edematous, and the tonsillar crypts may be filled with a yellowish exudate. In severe cases, the exudates may become confluent and can resemble diphtheria (see page 186).

Scattered petechiae may be seen on the soft palate. During the first 2 days, the dorsal surface of the tongue demonstrates a white coating through which only the fungiform papillae can be seen; this has been called **white strawberry tongue** (Fig. 5-5). By the fourth or fifth day, **red strawberry tongue** develops when the white coating desquamates to reveal an erythematous dorsal surface with hyperplastic fungiform papillae.

Classically, in untreated cases, fever develops abruptly around the second day. The patient's temperature peaks at approximately 103° F and returns to normal within 6 days. The exanthematous rash develops within the first 2 days and becomes widespread within 24 hours. The classic rash of scarlet fever is distinctive and often is described as "a sunburn with goose pimples." Pinhead punctate areas that are normal in color project through the erythema, giving the skin of the trunk and extremities a sandpaper texture. The rash is more intense in areas of pressure and skin folds. Often, transverse red streaks, known as **Pastia's lines,** occur in the skin folds secondary to the capillary fragility in these zones of stress. In contrast, the skin of the face usually is spared or may demonstrate erythematous cheeks with circumoral pallor.

The rash usually clears within 1 week, and then a period of desquamation of the skin occurs. This scaling begins on the face at the end of the first week and spreads to the rest of the skin by the third week, with the extremities being the last affected. The desquamation of the face produces small flakes; the skin of the

trunk comes off in thicker, larger flakes. This period of desquamation may last from 3 to 8 weeks.

DIAGNOSIS

A culture of throat secretions may be used to confirm the diagnosis of streptococcal infection, but this has been replaced by several methods of rapid detection of antigens that are specific for group A, β-hemolytic streptococci. Failure to respond to appropriate antibiotics should alert the clinician that the detected streptococci may represent an intercurrent carrier state, and other causes of infection should be investigated.

TREATMENT AND PROGNOSIS

Treatment of scarlet fever and the associated streptococcal pharyngitis is necessary to prevent the possibility of complications, such as peritonsillar or retropharyngeal abscess, sinusitis, or pneumonia. Late complications are rare and include otitis media, acute rheumatic fever, glomerulonephritis, arthralgia, meningitis, and hepatitis. The treatment of choice is oral penicillin, with erythromycin reserved for patients who are allergic to penicillin. Ibuprofen can be used to reduce the fever and relieve the associated discomfort. The fever and symptoms show dramatic improvement within 48 hours after the initiation of treatment. With appropriate therapy, the prognosis is excellent.

TONSILLAR CONCRETIONS AND TONSILLOLITHIASIS

Anatomically, the pharyngeal tonsils demonstrate numerous deep, twisted, and epithelial-lined invaginations. These tonsillar crypts function to increase the surface area for interaction between the immune cells within the lymphoid tissue and the oral environment. These convoluted crypts commonly are filled with desquamated keratin and foreign material and secondarily become colonized with bacteria, usually *Actinomyces* spp. The contents of the invaginations often become compacted and form a mass of foul-smelling material known as a **tonsillar concretion.** Occasionally, the condensed necrotic debris and bacteria undergo dystrophic calcification and form a **tonsillolith.** Recurrent tonsillar inflammation may promote the development of these tonsillar concretions.

CLINICAL AND RADIOGRAPHIC FEATURES

Although tonsillar concretions and tonsilloliths are not uncommon, published reports are rare, often documenting unusually large examples. The affected

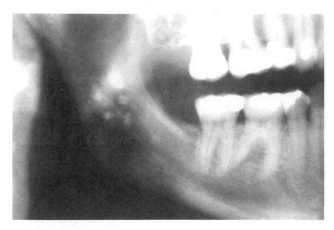

Fig. 5-6 Tonsilloliths. Cluster of radiopacities in the midportion of the ascending ramus.

tonsil will demonstrate one or more enlarged crypts filled with yellow debris that varies in consistency from soft to friable to fully calcified. In contrast to acute tonsillitis, the surrounding tonsillar tissue is not acutely painful, dramatically inflamed, or significantly edematous. Tonsilloliths can develop over a wide age range, from childhood to old age, with a mean patient age in the early 40s. Men are affected twice as frequently as women. These calcifications vary from small clinically insignificant lesions to massive calcifications more than 14 cm in length. Tonsilloliths may be single or multiple, and bilateral cases have been reported.

Many tonsillar concretions and tonsilloliths, especially the smaller examples, are asymptomatic. However, these calcifications can promote recurrent tonsillar infections and may lead to pain, abscess formation, ulceration, dysphagia, chronic sore throat, irritable cough, otalgia, or halitosis. Occasionally, patients will report a dull ache or a sensation of a foreign object in the throat that is relieved on removal of the tonsillar plug. In patients with large stones, clinical examination often reveals a hard, yellow submucosal mass of the affected tonsil. In older adult patients, large tonsilloliths can be aspirated and produce significant secondary pulmonary complications. Most frequently, tonsilloliths are discovered on panoramic radiographs as radiopaque objects superimposed on the midportion of the mandibular ramus (Fig. 5-6). On occasion, calcifications initially thought to be bilateral are proven to be unilateral with a panoramic ghost image present on the contralateral side.

DIAGNOSIS

A strong presumptive diagnosis can be made through a combination of the clinical and radiographic features. After detection on a panoramic radiograph, if further diagnostic confirmation of tonsilloliths is deemed necessary, then their presence can be confirmed with computed tomography (CT), magnetic resonance imaging (MRI), or the demonstration of the calculi on removal of the affected tonsil.

TREATMENT AND PROGNOSIS

Tonsilloliths discovered incidentally during evaluation of a panoramic radiograph often are not treated unless associated with significant tonsillar hyperplasia or clinical symptoms. Affected individuals occasionally try to remove tonsillar concretions with instruments such as straws, toothpicks, and dental instruments. Such therapy has the potential to damage the surrounding tonsillar tissue and should be discouraged. Patients should be educated to attempt removal by gargling warm salt water or using pulsating jets of water.

Superficial calculi can be enucleated or curetted; deeper tonsilloliths require local excision. Redevelopment of removed concretions is common. One group successfully used laser cryptolysis to reduce the extent of the tonsillar invaginations and stop the redevelopment of the concretions. If evidence of associated chronic tonsillitis is seen, then tonsillectomy provides definitive therapy.

DIPHTHERIA

Diphtheria is a life-threatening infection produced by *Corynebacterium diphtheriae*. The disease was first described in 1826, and *C. diphtheriae* (also termed *Klebs-Löffler bacillus*) was discovered initially by Klebs in 1883 and isolated in pure culture by Löffler in 1884. Humans are the sole reservoir, and the infection is acquired through contact with an infected person or carrier. The bacterium produces a lethal exotoxin that causes tissue necrosis, thereby providing nutrients for further growth and leading to peripheral spread. However, an effective antitoxin has been available since 1913, and immunization has been widespread in North America since 1922.

In the first edition of this textbook, it was stated that diphtheria was included mainly for historical interest because the world was on the threshold of virtual eradication of this infection in developed countries. However, a relatively recent epidemic in Russia reveals how rapidly such advances can be reversed in the absence of an effective immunization program. The epidemic began in Moscow and spread to involve all of the newly independent states of the former Soviet Union. During this outbreak, more than 150,000 cases were reported with approximately 4500 deaths. This one epidemic represented more than 90% of all cases reported between 1990 and 1995. The process was finally controlled by administration of vaccine to all children, adolescents, and adults (regardless of immunization histories).

In addition to this epidemic, infections may occur in people who are immunosuppressed or who have failed to receive booster injections as required. Isolated outbreaks still are reported in the urban poor and Native American populations of North America. Occasional reports from industrialized nations continue to document individuals who have returned home after contracting the infection while visiting a developing country.

CLINICAL FEATURES

The signs and symptoms of diphtheria arise 1 to 5 days after exposure to the organism. The initial systemic symptoms, which include low-grade fever, headache, malaise, anorexia, sore throat, and vomiting, arise gradually and may be mild. Although skin wounds may be involved, the infection predominantly affects mucosal surfaces and may produce exudates of the nasal, tonsillar, pharyngeal, laryngotracheal, conjunctival, or genital areas. Involvement of the nasal cavity is often accompanied with prolonged mucoid or hemorrhagic discharge. The oropharyngeal exudate begins on one or both tonsils as a patchy, yellow-white, thin film that thickens to form an adherent gray covering. With time, the membrane may develop patches of green or black necrosis. The superficial epithelium is an integral portion of this exudate, and attempts at removal are difficult and may result in bleeding. The covering may continue to involve the entire soft palate, uvula, larynx, or trachea, resulting in stridor and respiratory difficulties. Palatal perforation has rarely been reported.

During the Russian epidemic, patients with lesions isolated to the oral cavity were documented. In these patients, scattered areas of necrosis were noted on the buccal mucosa, upper and lower lips, hard and soft palate, or tongue. Such localization is rare and makes diagnosis more difficult.

The severity of the infection correlates with the spread of the membrane. Local obstruction of the airway can be lethal. Involvement of the tonsils leads to significant cervical lymphadenopathy, which often is associated with an edematous neck enlargement known as *bull neck*. Toxin-related paralysis may affect oculomotor, facial, pharyngeal, diaphragmatic, and intercostal muscles. The soft palatal paralysis can lead to nasal regurgitation during swallowing. Oral or nasal involvement has been reported to spread to the adjacent skin of the face and lips.

Cutaneous diphtheria can occur anywhere on the body and is characterized by chronic skin ulcers that frequently are associated with infected insect bites and also may harbor other pathogens such as *Staphylococcus aureus* or *Streptococcus pyogenes*. These skin lesions can arise even in vaccinated patients and typically are not associated with systemic toxic manifestations. When contracted by travelers from developed nations, the diagnosis often is delayed because of the nonspecific clinical presentation and a low index of suspicion. The cutaneous lesions represent an important reservoir of infection and can lead to more typical and lethal diphtheria in unprotected contacts.

Although bacteremia is rare, circulating toxin can result in systemic complications. Myocarditis and neurologic difficulties are seen most frequently and are usually discovered in patients with severe nasopharyngeal diphtheria. Myocarditis may exhibit as progressive weakness and dyspnea or lead to acute congestive heart failure. Neuropathy is not uncommon in patients with severe diphtheria, and palatal paralysis is the most commonly seen manifestation. A peripheral polyneuritis resembling Guillain-Barré syndrome also may occur.

DIAGNOSIS

Although the clinical presentation can be distinctive in severe cases, laboratory confirmation should be sought in all instances. The specimen for culture should be obtained from underneath the diphtheric membrane, if possible, or from the surface of the membrane. Culture material also should be obtained from the nasal mucosa. Diphtheria also must be kept in mind for any patient who has traveled to a disease-endemic area and has chronic skin ulcerations. In these cases, wound swab specimens should be examined for *C. diphtheriae*.

TREATMENT AND PROGNOSIS

Treatment of the patient with diphtheria should be initiated at the time of the clinical diagnosis and should not be delayed until the results of the culture are received. Antitoxin should be administered in combination with antibiotics to prevent further toxin production, to stop the local infection, and to prevent transmission. Erythromycin, procaine penicillin, or intravenous (IV) penicillin may be used. Most patients are no longer infectious after 4 days of antibiotic therapy, but some may retain vital organisms. The patient is not considered to be cured until three consecutive negative culture specimens are obtained.

Before the development of the antitoxin, the mortality rate approached 50%, usually from cardiac or neurologic complications. The current mortality rate is less than 5%, but the outcome is unpredictable. Development of myocarditis is an important predictor of mortality.

Deaths still occur in the United States because of delays in therapy secondary to lack of suspicion. With worldwide travel and visitors from across the globe, prevention is paramount. Even in those vaccinated as children, it must be remembered that a booster inoculation is required every 10 years.

SYPHILIS (LUES)

Syphilis is a worldwide chronic infection produced by *Treponema pallidum*. The organism is extremely vulnerable to drying; therefore, the primary modes of transmission are sexual contact or from mother to fetus. Although the risk of infection from blood transfusion is negligible because of serologic testing of donors, transmission through exposure to infected blood is theoretically possible because the organism may survive up to 5 days in refrigerated blood. Humans are the only proven natural host for syphilis.

After the advent of penicillin therapy in the 1940s, the incidence of syphilis slowly decreased for many years but often demonstrated peaks and troughs in approximately 10-year cycles. In 2000 the United States had the fewest reported cases of primary and secondary syphilis since reporting began in 1941. From 2001 to 2004, the rate increased primarily as a result of increases among men who have sex with men (MSM). In 2004, 84% of reported cases occurred in men, and the Centers for Disease Control and Prevention (CDC) estimates 64% of the total number was among MSM. In women, the prevalence decreased each year from 2000 to 2003 but leveled off and remained stable in 2004. In 2004, men were affected 5.9 times more frequently than women.

Although the data vary from year to year, a significant and prolonged increased prevalence has been seen in blacks, with the rate in 2004 being 5.6 times greater than that among whites. Most of the recent increases have been found in black men. Because of the recent trends in the surveillance data, current national health policy is stressing enhanced prevention measures directed toward blacks and MSM.

Oral sex is thought to have played an increasingly important contribution to the recent surge in a number of sexually transmitted diseases in MSM. Because the risk of HIV transmission through oral sex is lower than the rate associated with vaginal or anal sex, many falsely believed that unprotected oral sex was a safe or no-risk sexual practice and represented a good replacement for other higher-risk behaviors.

In patients with syphilis, the infection undergoes a characteristic evolution that classically proceeds through three stages. A syphilitic patient is highly infectious only during the first two stages, but pregnant women also may transmit the infection to the fetus during the latent stage. Maternal transmission during the first two stages of infection almost always results in miscarriage, stillbirth, or an infant with congenital malformations. The longer the mother has had the infection, the less the chance of fetal infection. Infection of the fetus may occur at any time during pregnancy, but the stigmata do not begin to develop until after the fourth month of gestation. The clinical changes secondary to the fetal infection are known as **congenital syphilis**. Between 1997 and 2002, a 63% reduction in the prevalence of congenital syphilis was noted, a figure that correlates closely with decreases in primary and secondary syphilis rates among women during that time. Continued national interventions attempt to ensure that all pregnant women receive prenatal care, including screening for syphilis early in the pregnancy.

Oral syphilitic lesions are uncommon but may occur in any stage. Many of the changes are secondary to obliterative endarteritis, which occurs in areas of infection.

CLINICAL FEATURES

PRIMARY SYPHILIS

Primary syphilis is characterized by the **chancre** that develops at the site of inoculation, becoming clinically evident 3 to 90 days after the initial exposure. The majority of chancres are solitary, although multiple lesions may be seen occasionally. The external genitalia and anus are the most common sites, and the affected area begins as a papular lesion, which develops a central ulceration. Less than 2% of chancres occur in other locations, but the oral cavity is the most common extragenital site. Oral lesions are seen most commonly on the lip, but other sites include the tongue, palate, gingiva, and tonsils (Fig. 5-7). The upper lip is affected more frequently in males, whereas lower lip involvement is predominant in females. Some believe this selective labial distribution may reflect the surfaces most actively involved during fellatio and cunnilingus. The oral lesion appears as a painless, clean-based ulceration or, rarely, as a vascular proliferation resembling a pyogenic granuloma. Regional lymphadenopathy, which may be bilateral, is seen in most patients. At this time the organism is spreading systemically through the lymphatic channels, setting the stage for future progression. If untreated, then the initial lesion heals within 3 to 8 weeks.

SECONDARY SYPHILIS

The next stage is known as *secondary* (disseminated) *syphilis* and is discovered clinically 4 to 10 weeks after the initial infection. The lesions of secondary syphilis may arise before the primary lesion has resolved com-

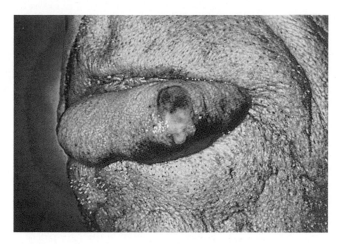

Fig. 5-7   Chancre of primary syphilis. Ulceration of the
dorsal surface of the tongue on the left side. *(From Neville BW,
Damm DD, White DK: Color atlas of clinical oral pathology, ed 2,
Hamilton, 1999, BC Decker.)*

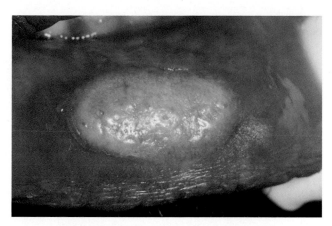

Fig. 5-9   Mucous patch of secondary syphilis.
Circumscribed white plaque on the lower labial mucosa.
(Courtesy of Dr. Pete Edmonds.)

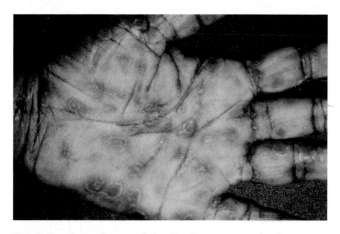

Fig. 5-8   Secondary syphilis. Erythematous rash of
secondary syphilis affecting the palms of the hands. *(Courtesy of
Dr. John Maize.)*

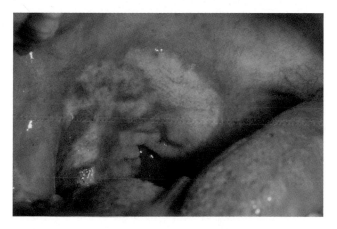

Fig. 5-10   Mucous patch of secondary syphilis. Irregular
thickened white plaque of the right soft palate.

pletely. During secondary syphilis, systemic symptoms
often arise. The most common are painless lymphadenopathy, sore throat, malaise, headache, weight loss,
fever, and musculoskeletal pain. A consistent sign is
a diffuse, painless, maculopapular cutaneous rash,
which is widespread and can even affect the palmar
and plantar areas (Fig. 5-8). The rash also may involve
the oral cavity and appear as red, maculopapular
areas. Although the skin rash may result in areas of
scarring and hyperpigmentation or hypopigmentation,
it heals without scarring in the vast majority of
patients.

In addition, roughly 30% of patients have focal areas
of intense exocytosis and spongiosis of the oral mucosa,
leading to zones of sensitive whitish mucosa known as
mucous patches (Figs. 5-9 and 5-10). Occasionally,
several adjacent patches can fuse and form a serpen-

tine or snailtrack pattern. Subsequently, superficial
epithelial necrosis may occur, leading to sloughing and
exposure of the underlying raw connective tissue.
These may appear on any mucosal surface but are
found commonly on the tongue, lip, buccal mucosa,
and palate. Elevated mucous patches also may be centered over the crease of the oral commissure and have
been termed **split papules.** Occasionally, papillary
lesions that may resemble viral papillomas arise during
this time and are known as **condylomata lata.**
Although these lesions typically occur in the genital or
anal regions, rare oral examples occur (Fig. 5-11). In
contrast to the isolated chancre noted in the primary
stage, multiple lesions are typical of secondary syphilis.
Spontaneous resolution usually occurs within 3 to 12
weeks; however, relapses may occur during the next
year.

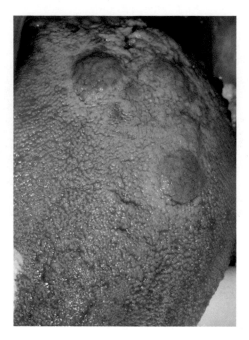

Fig. 5-11 **Condyloma lata.** Multiple indurated and slightly papillary nodules on the dorsal tongue. *(Courtesy of Dr. Karen Novak.)*

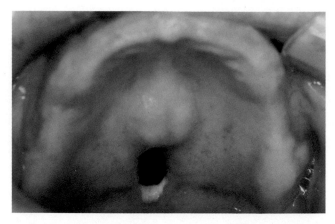

Fig. 5-12 **Tertiary syphilis.** Perforation of the hard palate. *(Courtesy of Dr. George Blozis.)*

On occasion, especially in the presence of a compromised immune system, secondary syphilis can exhibit an explosive and widespread form known as **lues maligna**. This form has prodromal symptoms of fever, headache, and myalgia, followed by the formation of necrotic ulcerations, which commonly involve the face and scalp. Oral lesions are present in more than 30% of affected patients. Malaise, pain, and arthralgia are seen occasionally. Several cases of lues maligna have been reported in patients with acquired immunodeficiency syndrome (AIDS) (see page 264), and this possibility should be kept in mind whenever HIV-infected patients have atypical ulcerations of the skin or oral mucosa.

TERTIARY SYPHILIS

After the second stage, patients enter a period in which they are free of lesions and symptoms, known as **latent syphilis**. This period of latency may last from 1 to 30 years; then (in approximately 30% of patients) the third stage, which is known as *tertiary syphilis,* develops. The third stage of syphilis includes the most serious of all complications. The vascular system can be affected significantly through the effects of the earlier arteritis. Aneurysm of the ascending aorta, left ventricular hypertrophy, aortic regurgitation, and congestive heart failure may occur. Involvement of the central nervous system (CNS) may result in tabes dorsalis, general paralysis, psychosis, dementia, paresis, and death.

Ocular lesions such as iritis, choroidoretinitis, and Argyll Robertson pupil (fails to react to light but responds to accommodation) may occur. Less significant, but more characteristic, are scattered foci of granulomatous inflammation, which may affect the skin, mucosa, soft tissue, bones, and internal organs. This active site of granulomatous inflammation, known as a **gumma,** appears as an indurated, nodular, or ulcerated lesion that may produce extensive tissue destruction. Intraoral lesions usually affect the palate or tongue. When the palate is involved, the ulceration frequently perforates through to the nasal cavity (Fig. 5-12). The tongue may be involved diffusely with gummata and appear large, lobulated, and irregularly shaped. This lobulated pattern is termed **interstitial glossitis** and is thought to be the result of contracture of the lingual musculature after healing of gummas. Diffuse atrophy and loss of the dorsal tongue papillae produce a condition called **luetic glossitis** (Fig. 5-13). In the past, this form of atrophic glossitis was thought to be precancerous, but several more recent publications dispute this concept.

CONGENITAL SYPHILIS

In 1858, Sir Jonathan Hutchinson described the changes found in congenital syphilis and defined the following three pathognomonic diagnostic features, known as **Hutchinson's triad:**
- Hutchinson's teeth
- Ocular interstitial keratitis
- Eighth nerve deafness

Like many diagnostic triads, few patients exhibit all three features.

Infants infected with syphilis can display signs within 2 to 3 weeks of birth. These early findings include growth retardation, fever, jaundice, anemia, hepatosplenomegaly, rhinitis, rhagades (circumoral

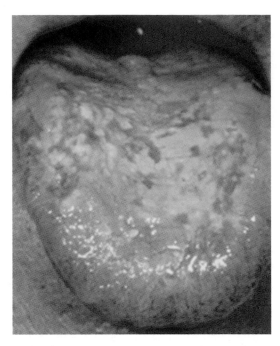

Fig. 5-13   Atrophic glossitis of tertiary syphilis. Dorsal surface of the tongue exhibiting loss of filiform papillae and areas of epithelial atrophy and hyperkeratosis. *(Courtesy of Dr. Robert J. Gorlin.)*

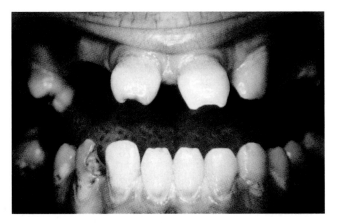

Fig. 5-14   Hutchinson's incisors of congenital syphilis. Dentition exhibiting crowns tapering toward the incisal edges. *(From Halstead CL, Blozis GG, Drinnan AJ et al: Physical evaluation of the dental patient, St Louis, 1982, Mosby.)*

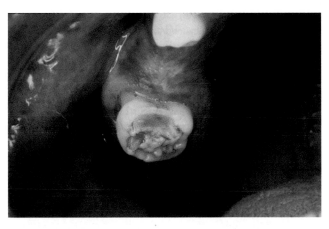

Fig. 5-15   Mulberry molar of congenital syphilis. Maxillary molar demonstrating occlusal surface with numerous globular projections.

radial skin fissures), and desquamative maculopapular, ulcerative, or vesiculobullous skin eruptions. Untreated infants who survive often develop tertiary syphilis with damage to the bones, teeth, eyes, ears, and brain. It is these findings that were described well by Hutchinson. The infection alters the formation of both the anterior teeth (**Hutchinson's incisors**) and the posterior dentition (**mulberry molars, Fournier's molars, Moon's molars**). Hutchinson's incisors exhibit their greatest mesiodistal width in the middle third of the crown. The incisal third tapers to the incisal edge, and the resulting tooth resembles a straightedge screwdriver (Fig. 5-14). The incisal edge often exhibits a central hypoplastic notch. Mulberry molars taper toward the occlusal surface with a constricted grinding surface. The occlusal anatomy is abnormal, with numerous disorganized globular projections that resemble the surface of a mulberry (Fig. 5-15).

Interstitial keratitis of the eyes is not present at birth but usually develops between the ages of 5 and 25 years. The affected eye has an opacified corneal surface, with a resultant loss of vision. In addition to Hutchinson's triad, a number of other alterations such as saddle-nose deformity, high-arched palate, frontal bossing, hydrocephalus, mental retardation, gummas, and neurosyphilis may be seen. Table 5-1 delineates the prevalence rates of the stigmata of congenital syphilis in a cohort of affected patients.

HISTOPATHOLOGIC FEATURES

The histopathologic picture of the oral lesions in the syphilitic patient is not specific. During the first two stages, the pattern is similar. The surface epithelium is ulcerated in primary lesions and may be ulcerated or hyperplastic in the secondary stage. The underlying lamina propria may demonstrate an increase in the number of vascular channels, and an intense chronic inflammatory reaction is present. The infiltrate is composed predominantly of lymphocytes and plasma cells and often demonstrates a perivascular pattern (Fig. 5-16). Although the presence of plasma cells within the infiltrate may suggest the diagnosis of syphilis on the skin, their presence in areas of oral ulceration is commonplace and therefore not necessarily of diagnostic significance. In secondary syphilis, ulceration may not be present and the surface epithelium often

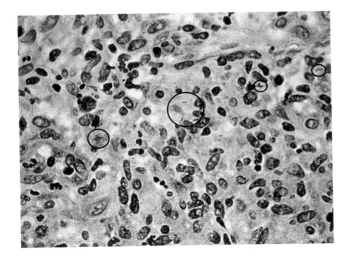

Fig. 5-25   Tuberculosis. Acid-fast stain of specimen depicted in Fig. 5-24 exhibiting scattered mycobacterial organisms presenting as small red rods.

Ziehl-Neelsen or other acid-fast stains, are required to demonstrate the mycobacteria (Fig. 5-25). Because of the relative scarcity of the organisms within tissue, the special stains successfully demonstrate the organism in only 27% to 60% of cases. Therefore, a negative result does not completely rule out the possibility of TB.

DIAGNOSIS

Approximately 2 to 4 weeks after initial exposure, a cell-mediated hypersensitivity reaction to tubercular antigens develops. This reaction is the basis for the purified protein derivative (PPD) skin test (i.e., tuberculin skin test), which uses a filtered precipitate of heat-sterilized broth cultures of *M. tuberculosis*. Positivity runs as high as 80% in developing nations; only 5% to 10% of the population in the United States is positive. A positive tuberculin skin test result indicates exposure to the organism and does not distinguish infection from active disease. A negative tuberculin skin test result does not totally rule out the possibility of TB. False-negative reactions have been documented in older adults; the immunocompromised; patients with sarcoidosis, measles, or Hodgkin's lymphoma; and when the antigen was placed intradermally. The false-negative rate may be as high as 66% in patients with AIDS.

Special mycobacterial stains and culture of infected sputum or tissue must be used to confirm the diagnosis of active disease. Even if detected with special stains, identification of the organism by culture is appropriate. This identification is important because some forms of nontuberculous mycobacteria have a high level of resistance to traditional antituberculous therapy and frequently require surgical excision. Because 4 to 6 weeks may be required to identify the organism in

culture, antituberculous therapy often is initiated before definitive classification. Polymerase chain reaction (PCR) is also used to identify *M. tuberculosis* DNA and speeds the diagnosis without the need to await culture results.

TREATMENT AND PROGNOSIS

M. tuberculosis can mutate and develop resistance to single-agent medications. To combat this ability, multiagent therapy is the treatment of choice for an active infection, and treatment usually involves two or more active drugs for several months to years. A frequently used protocol consists of an 8-week course of isoniazid, rifampin, and pyrazinamide, followed by a 16-week course of isoniazid and rifampin. Other first-line medications include ethambutol and streptomycin. Relapse rates of approximately 1.5% are seen. With an alteration of doses and the administration schedule, the response to therapy in patients with AIDS has been good, but relapses and progression of infection have been seen.

A different protocol termed *chemoprophylaxis* is used for patients who have a positive PPD skin test but no signs or symptoms of active disease. Although this situation does not mandate therapy, several investigators have demonstrated the value of therapy, especially in young individuals. **Bacillus Calmette-Guérin (BCG) vaccine** for TB is available to approximately 85% of the global population, but its use is restricted in the United States because of a controversy related to its effectiveness.

LEPROSY (HANSEN DISEASE)

Leprosy is a chronic infectious disease produced by *Mycobacterium leprae*. Because of worldwide efforts coordinated by the World Health Organization (WHO), a dramatic decrease in the prevalence of leprosy has been seen over the past 15 years. Since the mid-1980s, the number of estimated cases of active leprosy has dropped from between 10 and 12 million to 1.15 million, with the number of officially registered cases falling 85%. However, leprosy remains a public health problem in many areas of the world. Approximately 82% of all currently reported cases are noted in five countries: Brazil, India, Indonesia, Myanmar, and Nigeria.

The organism has a low infectivity, and exposure rarely results in clinical disease. Small endemic areas of infection are present in Louisiana and Texas, but most patients in the United States have been infected abroad. Many believe that the organism requires a cool host body temperature for survival. Although the exact route of transmission is not known, the high number of organisms in nasal secretions suggests that in some cases the initial site of infection may be the nasal or oropharyngeal mucosa. Although humans are considered the major host, other animals (e.g., armadillo, chimpanzee, mangabey monkey) may be additional possible reservoirs of infection. The nine-banded armadillo is relatively unique because of its low body core temperature, and it is naturally susceptible to the infection. Infected armadillos have been discovered in Louisiana.

For decades, leprologists have believed the bacillus is highly temperature dependent and produces lesions primarily in cooler parts of the body, such as the skin, nasal cavity, and palate. This concept has been questioned because the organism may be seen in significant numbers at sites of core body temperature, such as the liver and spleen. Recently, one investigator mapped common sites of oral involvement and compared this pattern to a map of the local temperature. This comparison demonstrated that the oral lesions tend to occur more frequently in the areas of the mouth with a lower surface temperature. The temperature-dependent theory of leprosy infection remains an area of interest and controversy.

Historically, two main clinical presentations are noted, and these are related to the immune reaction to the organism. The first, called **tuberculoid leprosy,** develops in patients with a high immune reaction. Typically, the organisms are not found in skin biopsy specimens, skin test results to heat-killed organisms (lepromin) are positive, and the disease is usually localized. The second form, **lepromatous leprosy,** is seen in patients who demonstrate a reduced cell-mediated immune response. These patients exhibit numerous organisms in the tissue, do not respond to lepromin skin tests, and exhibit diffuse disease. Borderline and less common variations exist. Active disease progresses through stages of invasion, proliferation, ulceration, and resolution with fibrosis. The incubation period is prolonged, with an average of 2 to 5 years for the tuberculoid type and 8 to 12 years for the lepromatous variant.

CLINICAL FEATURES

Currently, leprosy is classified into two separate categories, **paucibacillary** and **multibacillary,** with the distinction influencing the recommended form of therapy. Because laboratory services such as skin smears often are not available, patients are increasingly being classified on clinical grounds using the number of lesions (primarily skin) and the number of body areas affected.

Paucibacillary leprosy corresponds closely to the tuberculoid pattern of leprosy and exhibits a small

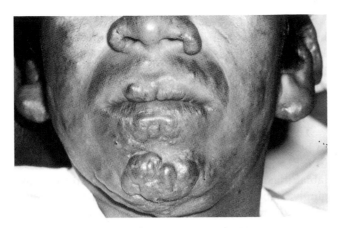

Fig. 5-26   Multibacillary (lepromatous) leprosy. Numerous thickened facial nodules.

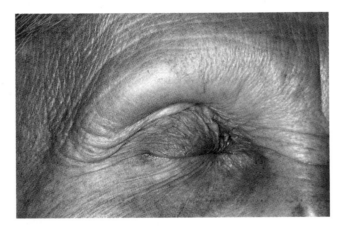

Fig. 5-27   Multibacillary (lepromatous) leprosy. Loss of eyebrows and eyelashes.

number of well-circumscribed, hypopigmented skin lesions. Nerve involvement usually results in anesthesia of the affected skin, often accompanied by a loss of sweating. Oral lesions are rare in this variant.

Multibacillary leprosy corresponds well to the lepromatous pattern of leprosy and begins slowly with numerous, ill-defined, hypopigmented macules or papules on the skin that, with time, become thickened (Fig. 5-26). The face is a common site of involvement, and the skin enlargements can lead to a distorted facial appearance **(leonine facies).** Hair, including the eyebrows and lashes, often is lost (Fig. 5-27). Nerve involvement leads to a loss of sweating and decreased light touch, pain, and temperature sensors. This sensory loss begins in the extremities and spreads to most of the body. Nasal involvement results in nosebleeds, stuffiness, and a loss of the sense of smell. The hard tissue of the floor, septum, and bridge of the nose may be affected. Collapse of the bridge of the nose is considered pathognomonic.

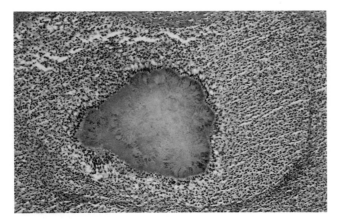

Fig. 5-34 Actinomycosis. Colony of actinomycotic organisms surrounded by polymorphonuclear leukocytes.

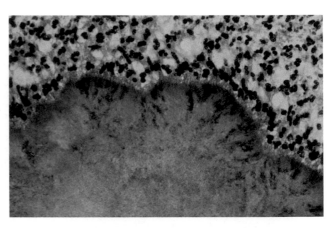

Fig. 5-35 Actinomycosis. Actinomycotic colony exhibiting club-shaped filaments arranged in a radiating rosette pattern.

the primary change is one of variable hyperplasia. Tonsillar hyperplasia thought to be secondary to actinomycotic infestation of the crypts does not appear responsive to antibiotics, probably because of the superficial location of the bacterial colonies. Tonsillectomy is generally the most effective treatment for this situation.

Salivary gland involvement also is not unusual. Intraductal colonization by the organism may lead to infections in both the submandibular and parotid glands, resulting in abscess formation in the submandibular and masseter spaces, respectively. In addition, more localized infections occur in minor salivary gland ducts, which also may demonstrate mucous plugs or sialoliths.

Actinomycotic osteomyelitis of the mandible and maxilla has been reported. Trauma, periodontal infections, nonvital teeth, and extraction sites have all provided access. Ill-defined areas of radiolucency, often surrounded by radiopacity, may be found with or without involvement of the overlying soft tissue.

Intrabony colonization of dentigerous cysts without other significant clinical or radiographic spread has been reported. Periapical inflammatory lesions involved by the bacteria can result in lesions that are difficult to resolve with standard endodontic treatment, but such lesions typically remain localized and do not evolve into invasive cervicofacial actinomycosis.

HISTOPATHOLOGIC FEATURES

The tissue removed from areas of active infection demonstrates a peripheral band of fibrosis encasing a zone of chronically inflamed granulation tissue surrounding large collections of polymorphonuclear leukocytes and, with luck, colonies of organisms (Fig. 5-34). The colonies consist of club-shaped filaments that form a

radiating rosette pattern (Fig. 5-35). With hematoxylin and eosin (H&E) stains, the central core stains basophilic and the peripheral portion is eosinophilic. Methenamine silver stains demonstrate the organisms well. If the colonies of actinomycetes become displaced from the exudate, then a rim of neutrophils typically clings to the periphery of the organisms.

DIAGNOSIS

The diagnosis of actinomycosis is achieved ideally by culture, but less than 50% of cases are positive because of the overgrowth of associated bacteria, prior antibiotic therapy, or improper anaerobic media conditions. Lacking positive culture results, a strong presumptive diagnosis can be obtained through a demonstration of the typical colonies in lesional biopsy material. The material for culture and histopathologic examination is typically obtained during surgical exploration, with fine-needle aspiration being a satisfactory substitute in many cases. Sulfur granules in infections other than actinomycosis are so rare that their demonstration strongly supports the diagnosis. If desired, then fluorescein-conjugated antiserum can be used on the granules to specifically identify the *Actinomyces* species.

TREATMENT AND PROGNOSIS

The treatment of choice for actinomycosis in chronic fibrosing cases is prolonged high doses of antibiotics in association with abscess drainage and excision of the sinus tracts. A high antibiotic concentration is required to penetrate larger areas of suppuration and fibrosis. Although penicillin remains the standard of care with no documented *in vivo* resistance, some clinicians believe amoxicillin represents a better first-choice antibiotic. Other investigators have demonstrated *in vitro* resistance to penicillin and recommend tetracycline, which is as effective as penicillin and is the drug of choice for patients with a known allergy to penicillin. Early cervicofacial actinomycosis typically responds to a 5- to 6-week course of penicillin; patients with deep-seated infections may require up to 12 months.

In cases of osteomyelitis caused by actinomycetes, antibiotic therapy alone often is associated with persistent disease. Adequate débridement appears to be the cornerstone of therapy and ultimately determines the success of the subsequent antibiotic treatment. When combined with appropriate surgery, a 3-month course of penicillin usually is curative. In resistant cases, repeated débridement should be combined with cultures to direct future antibiotic therapy. Care should be taken to ensure that colonization of bony sequestra by actinomycotic colonies is not mistaken for invasive actinomycotic osteomyelitis.

Several authors have indicated that localized acute actinomycotic infections may be treated more conservatively than the deep, chronic cases of actinomycosis. Localized periapical and pericoronal actinomycosis, tongue abscesses, and focal subacute sialadenitis with intraductal involvement frequently respond well to surgical removal of infected tissue. In these cases it appears best to reserve antibiotics for patients in whom local surgical excision fails.

CAT-SCRATCH DISEASE

Cat-scratch disease is an infectious disorder that begins in the skin but classically spreads to the adjacent lymph nodes. This infection is the most common cause of chronic regional lymphadenopathy in children, with an estimated 22,000 cases occurring annually in the United States. This disease has been recognized since 1931, but the definitive cause was not determined until the 1980s. Isolation and culture of the organism were finally achieved in 1988. The causative organism was initially named *Rochalimaea henselae* but was reclassified as *Bartonella henselae*. On very rare occasions, cat-scratch disease is caused by related species, *Bartonella quintana* or *Bartonella clarridgeiae*.

Almost all cases arise after contact with a cat, usually a kitten. Cat fleas appear to be involved in the transmission of the causative organism among cats, but the role of fleas in the transmission from cats to humans is unclear. Most human infections appear to follow scratches, licks, or bites from domestic cats. Infection from other sources is highly unlikely, but the disease rarely has been described via dogs, monkeys, porcupine quills, and thorns. Person-to-person transmission has not been documented.

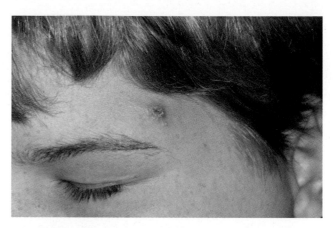

Fig. 5-36   Cat-scratch disease. Papule that developed at initial site of injury.

CLINICAL FEATURES

Eighty percent of the cases occur in patients younger than 21 years of age. Cat-scratch disease begins as a papule or pustule that develops in 3 to 14 days along the initial scratch line (Fig. 5-36). The lymph node changes develop in approximately 3 weeks and often may be accompanied by fever or malaise (Fig. 5-37). Scratches on the face typically lead to submandibular lymphadenopathy, and the patient may be referred to dental practitioners to rule out an odontogenic infection. Often the primary site of trauma may have resolved by the time that the symptomatic lymphadenopathy is diagnosed. Therefore, cat-scratch disease must be considered strongly in the differential diagnosis of patients with unexplained symptomatic lymphadenopathy. In about half of the cases, a single node is involved. Multiple regional nodes are affected in about 20%, and nodal enlargement is discovered in multiple sites in about 33%. Suppuration is noted in approximately 10% of affected patients.

A few patients with cat-scratch disease demonstrate unusual presentations. The infection can appear as an intraoral mass in the buccal mucosa when lymphoid aggregates become involved from an adjacent cutaneous primary site. Scratches in the preauricular area may localize in parotid lymphoid tissue and can cause significant parotid pain or even temporary facial paralysis. Other less common problems include granulomatous osteomyelitis, arthralgias, encephalopathy, erythematous and maculopapular rashes, splenomegaly, hepatic lesions, thrombocytopenia, pneumonia, anemia, pleural effusions, and recurrent bacterial infections.

Primary lesions adjacent to the eye can result in a conjunctival granuloma that is associated with preauricular lymphadenopathy (**oculoglandular syndrome**

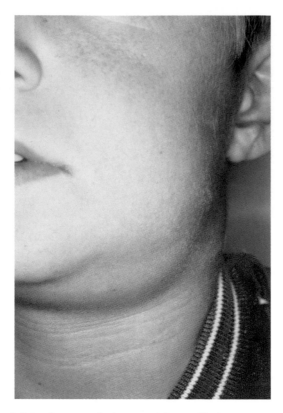

Fig. 5-37   Cat-scratch disease. Submandibular lymphadenopathy has developed after initial trivial injury to skin. (*Courtesy of Dr. George Blozis.*)

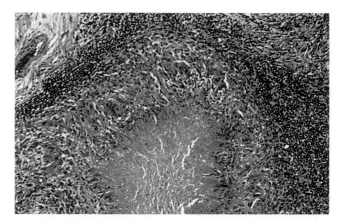

Fig. 5-38   Cat-scratch disease. Intranodal area of necrosis surrounded by a band of epithelioid histiocytes and lymphocytes.

HISTOPATHOLOGIC FEATURES

The involved lymph nodes are enlarged as a result of significant cortical hyperplasia, which classically contains areas of stellate suppurative necrosis surrounded by a band of histiocytes and neutrophils (Fig. 5-38). In some cases, significant necrosis is absent, but areas of karyorrhexis are present around proliferations of plump vascular channels that often exhibit thickened eosinophilic walls. On staining with the Warthin-Starry method, cat-scratch bacilli are usually found in areas without significant necrosis. As the disease progresses and necrosis increases, the organisms become more difficult to identify. In addition, the Brown-Hopps method of gram staining may be used to highlight the bacilli. Recently, a commercially available monoclonal antibody against *B. henselae* has been used to demonstrate the organisms via immunoperoxidase techniques on paraffin-embedded material. Upon immunostaining, the organisms are highlighted dramatically, an important advance over the previous special stains. One downside is the failure of this specific antibody to react with the organisms in the exceptional cases of cat-scratch disease caused by *B. quintana* or *B. clarridgeiae*.

Bacillary angiomatosis reveals lobular proliferations of small blood vessels in an edematous to fibrotic stroma. The supporting connective tissue typically demonstrates a significant number of neutrophils and leukocytoclasis, important clues to the diagnosis. Also present are variably sized amphophilic and granular aggregates that upon Warthin-Starry staining prove to be masses of the causative bacteria.

DIAGNOSIS

Today the diagnosis of cat-scratch disease usually is established via serologic tests that demonstrate a high degree of sensitivity and specificity. The most widely

of Parinaud); this pattern is thought to occur when an individual touches fur moistened with the cat's saliva during grooming. When the individual rubs their eye, the organism is transmitted to the conjunctiva.

During the past 2 decades, an unusual subcutaneous vascular proliferation, histopathologically similar to histiocytoid hemangioma, has been recognized in patients with AIDS. This proliferation has been termed **bacillary angiomatosis,** with most cases being definitively associated with *Bartonella henselae*. In a minority of the cases, bacillary angiomatosis is caused by a related organism, *B. quintana*. The affected areas often resemble Kaposi's sarcoma (see page 270) and appear as variable numbers of red-to-purple skin lesions. These may be macular, papular, or pedunculated and exhibit a widespread distribution on the skin. Pain and tenderness are common. The larger lesions are friable and bleed easily.

Oral lesions have been seen in bacillary angiomatosis and also may resemble Kaposi's sarcoma. The affected areas may exhibit zones of alveolar bone loss or may be within the soft tissue and appear as a proliferative vascular lesion.

used is an indirect fluorescent antibody assay for detecting antibodies to *B. henselae.* Another commercially available method is an enzyme-linked immunosorbent assay (ELISA) for IgM antibodies to the organism. Polymerase chain reaction (PCR) techniques also are available but are not widely used.

TREATMENT AND PROGNOSIS

Cat-scratch disease is a self-limiting condition and normally resolves within 4 months. The use of local heat, analgesics, and aspiration of the node on suppuration is the typical pattern of therapy. If persistent discomfort makes nodal aspiration necessary, then drainage should be achieved with a needle that is tunneled into the node laterally through normal skin 1 to 2 cm away from the lesion. Incision directly into the node could result in a chronic draining sinus.

Although the organism has demonstrated sensitivity to a number of antibiotics in culture, the results in immunocompetent patients have been inconsistent and difficult to evaluate because the disease is self-limited in most cases. Antibiotics typically are reserved for those cases that demonstrate a prolonged course or severe involvement. Use of antibiotic drugs in patients with AIDS and bacillary angiomatosis has produced dramatic resolution within 2 days. Although a number of medications have been used successfully, the primary antibiotics used for cat-scratch disease or bacillary angiomatosis are azithromycin, erythromycin, doxycycline, rifampin, ciprofloxacin, and gentamicin.

SINUSITIS

Sinusitis is one of the most common health complaints in the United States. To understand the problem, the clinician must first have some knowledge of sinus anatomy. Adults have bilateral maxillary, frontal, sphenoid, ethmoid, and mastoid sinuses. Except for the mastoid sinuses, these cavities drain into the nose through openings called **ostia**. The frontal, sphenoid, and maxillary sinuses must drain through the middle meatus. In addition, the ethmoids are located bilaterally in this area of the nose and present as a labyrinth of 3 to 15 small sinuses, which drain through smaller ostia. The ostiomeatal complex, with its numerous narrow openings (Fig. 5-39), is the key to sinus disease because it is the primary nasal site for the deposition of foreign matter from inspired air.

Normal sinuses are lined by pseudostratified columnar epithelium with cilia. The cilia are necessary to move the sinus secretions toward the ostia. Gravity also is beneficial in removing the secretions, except in the maxillary sinus where there is a superior location of the

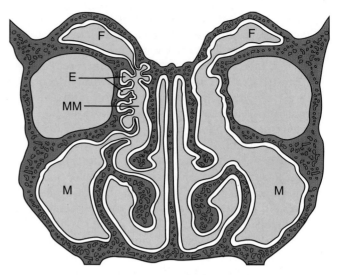

Fig. 5-39   The paranasal sinuses. Illustration demonstrating the ostiomeatal complex and its importance to appropriate sinus drainage. The left side demonstrates the typical narrow middle meatus through which all sinus drainage must pass. The right side reveals enlargement of the middle meatus, such as that achieved through corrective endoscopic surgery. *M,* Maxillary sinus; *F,* frontal sinus; *E,* ethmoid sinuses; *MM,* middle meatus.

ostial opening and, therefore, the ciliary apparatus becomes even more important. Normal function of the paranasal sinuses depends on the following:
- Patency of the ostial openings
- Proper function of the ciliary apparatus
- Quality of the nasal secretions

Disruption of this balance leads to sinusitis. For a long time, researchers believed that primary inflammation of the lining of the maxillary antrum was the major cause of sinusitis; however, advances have demonstrated that most sinus disease begins from a blockage of the ostiomeatal complex that disrupts normal drainage, decreases ventilation, and precipitates disease. Less common localized sinus infections can occur from focal areas of inflammation within a single sinus, such as a dental infection affecting the maxillary sinus.

Approximately 10% of maxillary sinusitis cases arise from an odontogenic source such as infection from the maxillary teeth, dental trauma, noninflammatory odontogenic pathoses, or iatrogenic causes such as dental extractions, maxillary osteotomies, or placement of dental implants. In such cases, therapy requires resolution of the odontogenic pathosis in addition to management of the sinus infection.

All of the sinuses contain bacteria. In a person with sinusitis, infection is present initially or as the disease evolves. With bacteria already present in the sinuses, changes as minor as a slight mucosal thickening in the ostiomeatal complex can lead to improper sinus drainage and infection. The most common predisposing factors are a recent upper respiratory viral infection or allergic rhinitis. Other less common causes include cystic fibrosis, immotile cilia syndrome, bronchiectasis, developmental abnormalities, and immunodeficiency (including AIDS).

In otherwise healthy patients, the most common organisms responsible for acute sinusitis are *Streptococcus pneumoniae*, *Haemophilus influenzae*, and *Moraxella catarrhalis*. If not corrected, some cases of acute sinusitis may become chronic. *Chronic sinusitis* is defined as recurring episodes of acute sinusitis or symptomatic sinus disease lasting longer than 3 months. In these cases the bacteria tend to be anaerobes and are most frequently *Streptococcus*, *Bacteroides*, or *Veillonella* spp. When sinusitis arises secondary to an odontogenic infection, the causative organisms are usually those that predominate in periodontal or endodontic infections and include bacteria such as *Peptostreptococcus* spp., *Fusobacterium* spp., *Prevotella* spp., *Bacteroides* spp., and *Porphyromonas* spp.

Infrequently, in an environment of chronic sinusitis, an area of dystrophic calcification (**antrolith**) may develop and be detected radiographically. The nidus for this calcification may be endogenous from materials such as inflamed mucus, pus, or clots. In other cases the source may be exogenous from tooth roots or foreign bodies, such as dental materials, vegetable matter, paper, glass, and stone. Focal antral calcification also has been seen in sinuses filled with a fungal ball of *Aspergillus fumigatus* (noninvasive mycetoma) (see page 234). A sinus that is unresponsive to therapy and exhibits focal antrolith formation within a diffuse soft tissue opacification is highly suggestive of noninvasive aspergillosis.

CLINICAL AND RADIOGRAPHIC FEATURES

Presenting symptoms of acute sinusitis in adults include headache, fever, and facial pain over the affected sinus. Anorexia, photophobia, and malaise also may be seen. Anterior nasal or posterior pharyngeal discharge is present; it may be thick or thin in consistency and appear clear, mucoid, or purulent. Children, with their less complex sinuses, typically have only persistent cough, fever, and purulent rhinorrhea. Localized involvement of the maxillary sinus can occur as pain over the cheekbone, toothache, periorbital pain, or temporal headache. Maxillary sinusitis is associated with increased pain when the head is held upright and less discomfort when the patient is supine.

Chronic sinusitis is less diagnostic, and radiographic imaging becomes more important. Frequent complaints include facial pressure, pain, or a sensation of obstruction. In some cases, nonspecific symptoms, such as headache, sore throat, lightheadedness, or generalized fatigue, also may be present or even dominate. Radiographically, the involved sinus has a cloudy, increased density (Fig. 5-40).

At times, sinusitis can be confused with an odontogenic infection. In such cases, close examination of periapical radiographs, a thorough periodontal examination, and assessment of tooth vitality often will rule out or point to an odontogenic infection. A sinus infection should be strongly considered when patients complain of pain from several teeth, demonstrate tenderness over one or both of the maxillary sinuses, exhibit nasal congestion, or have a nasal discharge accompanied by a foul odor, fever, and headache.

In addition to the patient's symptoms, the diagnosis in the past often was made by procedures such as transillumination and by plain radiographs, such as the Waters, Caldwell-Luc, lateral, and submental vertex views. Today, when the diagnosis is in question, many clinicians use nasal endoscopy and computed tomography (CT). Areas of infection and sites of improper drainage will be found. These techniques not only confirm the diagnosis but also pinpoint the primary pathologic alteration that led to the obstructive sinusitis.

An antrolith appears radiographically as a radiodense focus within the sinus. The calcification often is seen in association with a thickening of the antral lining or diffuse clouding of the affected sinus.

TREATMENT AND PROGNOSIS

Although acute sinusitis is usually a self-limiting disease, antibiotics are frequently prescribed. Few placebo-controlled, double-blind, randomized clinical trials have been published, and the results are inconsistent. Although the supporting evidence is weak, the few well-performed trials suggest that patients with more severe signs and symptoms may benefit from an antibiotic, whereas those with less severe manifestations do not require antibiotic therapy.

If antibiotics are used, the first-line therapy for acute sinusitis in otherwise healthy patients is amoxicillin. Because of drug resistance, additional medications are used if the patient does not respond to the initial antibiotic. Amoxicillin-clavulanate, trimethoprim-sulfamethoxazole, or cefaclor are good antibiotic drugs for resistant cases. Although topical decongestants shrink nasal membranes and improve ostial drainage, they are not recommended because of the resultant decreased ciliary function and decreased mucosal

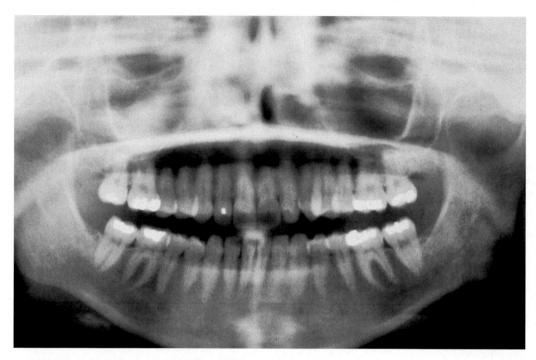

Fig. 5-40   Sinusitis. Cloudy right maxillary antrum.

blood flow, which leads to impaired antibiotic delivery. The effect of systemic antihistamine and decongestant medications on sinusitis has not been studied adequately.

In otherwise healthy adult patients, chronic sinusitis that is not responsive to typical medical management often is corrected surgically. In the past, radical stripping of the diseased sinus mucosa was the therapy of choice. Today, nasal endoscopy has shown that sinusitis is a disease of obstruction and that mucosal inflammation is usually a secondary development. Functional endoscopic sinus surgery enlarges the ostial openings and corrects blockages in the ostiomeatal complex, often with a rapid resolution of the signs and symptoms (see Fig. 5-35). The surgery is delicate because it extends close to the orbit and the central nervous system. Each patient's unique anatomy should be evaluated carefully by CT and nasal endoscopy before surgery.

Although endoscopic surgery is considered by many to be the current standard of care for chronic sinusitis, a few investigators still use the more invasive Caldwell-Luc procedure in selected patients. Although the Caldwell-Luc procedure is associated with a higher prevalence of significant complications, it also is associated with a lower number of reoperations when compared with the less invasive endoscopic procedure. Therefore, some clinicians continue to use the old technique in patients who demonstrate recurrent disease limited to the maxillary sinus and prefer a single major operation rather than multiple, less invasive procedures.

When the infection is isolated to a single maxillary sinus and associated with a odontogenic cause, the dental pathosis must be resolved in addition to treating the diseased sinus. Although the Caldwell-Luc procedure continues to be used, endoscopic shaver-assisted techniques are becoming more popular to perform an antrostomy and accomplish removal of pathoses, such as irreversibly diseased antral lining, polyps, tooth fragments, and foreign material. When the sinus disease is caused by an oroantral communication, defects less than 5 mm typically close spontaneously. With small openings, the defect can be covered and protected during the early stages of healing with a resorbable barrier such as an absorbable gelatin sponge. Oroantral fistulae larger that 5 mm should be closed primarily, but this should be done only after resolution of any associated acute infection within the associated sinus.

In children, continued medical management is the therapy of choice for uncomplicated acute or recurrent acute sinusitis. The anatomy in the child, with the decreased distance between the orbit and brain, increases the difficulty of any surgical procedure. Surgical management is indicated in only a small number of childhood sinusitis cases. Suppurative sinusitis extending into surrounding tissues or true chronic sinusitis caused by serious underlying systemic disease are examples of indications for the surgical management of sinus disease in a child.

BIBLIOGRAPHY

General References

Gorbach SL, Bartlett JG, Blacklow NR: *Infectious diseases*, ed 2, Philadelphia, 1998, WB Saunders.

Holmes KK: *Sexually transmitted diseases*, ed 3, New York, 1999, McGraw-Hill.

Katz SL, Gershon AA, Hotez PJ et al: *Krugman's infectious diseases of children*, ed 10, St Louis, 1999, Mosby.

Streptococcal Infections (Impetigo; Erysipelas; Streptococcal Pharyngitis and Tonsillitis; Scarlet Fever)

Bialecki C, Feder HM, Grant-Kels JM: The six classic childhood exanthems: a review and update, *J Am Acad Dermatol* 21:891-903, 1989.

Bisno AL, Gerber MA, Gwaltney Jr JM et al: Practice guidelines for the diagnosis and management of group A streptococcal pharyngitis, *Clin Infect Dis* 35:113-125, 2002.

Bonnetblanc J-M, Bédane C: Erysipelas. Recognition and management, *Am J Clin Dermatol* 4:157-163, 2003.

Bratton RL, Neese RE: St. Anthony's fire: diagnosis and management of erysipelas, *Am Fam Physician* 51:401-404, 1995.

Gerber MA: Diagnosis and treatment of pharyngitis in children, *Pediatr Clin North Am* 52:729-747, 2005.

Giunta JL: Comparison of erysipelas and odontogenic cellulitis, *J Endod* 13:291-294, 1987.

Hirschmann JV: Impetigo: etiology and therapy, *Curr Clin Top Infect Dis* 22:42-51, 2002.

Jaggi P, Shulman ST: Group A streptococcal infections, *Pediatr Rev* 27:99-105, 2006.

Katzenell U, Shemer J, Bar-Dayan Y: Streptococcal contamination of food: an unusual cause of epidemic pharyngitis, *Epidemiol Infect* 127:179-184, 2001.

Kolokotronis A, Doumas S, Lambroudi M et al: Facial and perioral primary impetigo: a clinical study, *J Clin Pediatr Dent* 29:341-346, 2005.

Koning S, Verhagen AP, van Suijlekom-Smit LW et al: Interventions for impetigo, *Cochrane Database Syst Rev* 2:CD003261, 2004.

Ochs MW, Dolwick MF: Facial erysipelas: report of a case and review of the literature, *J Oral Maxillofac Surg* 49:1116-1120, 1991.

Österlund A, Kahlmeter G, Hæggman S et al: *Staphylococcus aureus* resistance to fusidic acid among Swedish children: a follow-up study, *Scand J Infect Dis* 38:332-334, 2006.

Pavlotsky F, Amrani S, Trau H: Recurrent erysipelas: risk factors, *J Dtsch Dermatol Ges* 2:89-95, 2004.

Pichichero M, Casy J: Comparison of European and U.S. results for cephalosporin versus penicillin treatment of group A streptococcal tonsillopharyngitis, *Eur J Clin Microbiol Infect Dis* 25:354-364, 2006.

Török L: Uncommon manifestations of erysipelas, *Clin Dermatol* 23:515-518, 2005.

Watkins P: Impetigo: aetiology, complications and treatment options, *Nurs Stand* 19:50-54, 2005.

Tonsillar Concretions and Tonsillolithiasis

Cooper MM, Steinberg JJ, Lastra M et al: Tonsillar calculi: report of a case and review of the literature, *Oral Surg Oral Med Oral Pathol* 55:239-243, 1983.

Finkelstein Y, Talmi YP, Ophir D et al: Laser cryptolysis for the treatment of halitosis, *Otolaryngol Head Neck Surg* 131:372-377, 2004.

Özcan E, Ural A, Öktemer TK et al: Bilateral tonsillolithiasis: a case report, *Oral Surg Oral Med Oral Pathol Oral Radiol Endod* 102:e17-18, 2006.

Myers NE, Compliment JM, Post JC et al: Tonsilloliths a common finding in pediatric patients, *Nurse Pract* 31:53-54, 2006.

Ram S, Siar CH, Ismail SM et al: Pseudo bilateral tonsilloliths: a case report and review of the literature, *Oral Surg Oral Med Oral Pathol Oral Radiol Endod* 98:110-114, 2004.

Sezer B, Tugsel Z, Bilgen C: An unusual tonsillolith, *Oral Surg Oral Med Oral Pathol Oral Radiol Endod* 95:471-473, 2003.

Verghese A, Fernando C, Roberson D et al: The foul-smelling, removable tonsillar concretion: a poorly appreciated manifestation of colonization with *Actinomyces*, *J Tenn Med Assoc* 83:71-73, 1990.

Diphtheria

Centers for Disease Control and Prevention: Fatal respiratory diphtheria in a U.S. traveler to Haiti–Pennsylvania, 2003, *MMWR Morb Mortal Wkly Rep* 52:1285-1286, 2004.

deBenoist A-C, White JM, Efstratiou et al: Imported cutaneous diphtheria, United Kingdom, *Emerg Infect Dis* 10:511-513, 2004.

Galazka A: Implications of the diphtheria epidemic in the former Soviet Union for immunization programs, *J Infect Dis* 181(suppl 1):S244-248, 2000.

Galazka A: The changing epidemiology of diphtheria in the vaccine era, *J Infect Dis* 181(suppl 1):S2-9, 2000.

Hadfield TL, McEvoy P, Polotsky Y et al: The pathology of diphtheria, *J Infect Dis* 181(suppl 1):S116-120, 2000.

Jayashree M, Shruthi N, Singhi S: Predictors of outcome in patients with diphtheria receiving intensive care, *Indian Pediatr* 43:155-160, 2006.

Nikolaeva IN, Astafeva NV, Barer GM et al: Diphtheria of the oral mucosa, *Stomatologiia (Mosk)* 74:26-28, 1995.

Syphilis

Barrett AW, Dorrego MV, Hodgson TA et al: The histopathology of syphilis of the oral mucosa, *J Oral Pathol Med* 33:286-291, 2004.

Centers for Disease Control and Prevention: Congenital syphilis–United States, 2002, *MMWR Morb Mortal Wkly Rep* 53:716-719, 2004.

Centers for Disease Control and Prevention: Primary and secondary syphilis–United States, 2003-2004, *MMWR Morb Mortal Wkly Rep* 55:2659-2673, 2006.

Centers for Disease Control and Prevention: Transmission of primary and secondary syphilis by oral sex–Chicago, Illinois, 1998-2002, *MMWR Morb Mortal Wkly Rep* 53:966-968, 2004.

Fiumara NJ, Lessel S: Manifestations of late congenital syphilis: an analysis of 271 patients, *Arch Dermatol* 102:78-83, 1970.

Leão JC, Gueiros LA, Porter SR: Oral manifestations of syphilis, *Clinics* 61:161-166, 2006.

Little JW: Syphilis: an update, *Oral Surg Oral Med Oral Pathol Oral Radiol Endod* 100:3-9, 2005.

Meyer I, Abbey LM: The relationship of syphilis to primary carcinoma of the tongue, *Oral Surg Oral Med Oral Pathol* 30:678-681, 1970.

Meyer I, Shklar G: The oral manifestations of acquired syphilis: a study of eighty-one cases, *Oral Surg Oral Med Oral Pathol* 23:45-61, 1967.

Gonorrhea

Centers for Disease Control and Prevention: Increases in fluoroquinolone-resistant *Neisseria gonorrhoeae* among men who have sex with men–United States, 2003, and revised recommendations for gonorrhea treatment, 2004, *MMWR Morb Mortal Wkly Rep* 53:335-338, 2004.

Centers for Disease Control and Prevention: Screening tests to detect *Chlamydia trachomatis* and *Neisseria gonorrhoeae* infection–2002, *MMWR Morb Mortal Wkly Rep* 51(RR-15):1-38, 2002.

Giunta JL, Fiumara NJ: Facts about gonorrhea and dentistry, *Oral Surg Oral Med Oral Pathol* 62:529-531, 1986.

Janier M, Lassau F, Casin I et al: Pharyngeal gonorrhoea: the forgotten reservoir, *Sex Transm Infect* 79:345, 2003.

Little JW: Gonorrhea: update, *Oral Surg Oral Med Oral Pathol Oral Radiol Endod* 101:137-143, 2006.

Miller KE: Diagnosis and treatment of *Neisseria gonorrhoeae* infections, *Am Fam Physician* 73:1779-1184, 2006.

Siegel MA: Syphilis and gonorrhea, *Dent Clin North Am* 40:369-383, 1996.

Williams LN: The risks of oral-genital contact: a case report, *Gen Dent* 50:282-284, 2002.

Tuberculosis

Centers for Disease Control and Prevention: Emergence of *Mycobacterium tuberculosis* with extensive resistance to second-line drugs–worldwide, 2000-2004, *MMWR Morb Mortal Wkly Rep* 55:301-305, 2006.

Centers for Disease Control and Prevention: Trends in tuberculosis incidence–United States, 2006, *MMWR Morb Mortal Wkly Rep* 56:245-250, 2007.

Darlington CC, Salman I: Oral tuberculous lesions, *Am Rev Tuberc* 35:147-179, 1937.

Eng H-L, Lu S-Y, Yang C-H et al: Oral tuberculosis, *Oral Surg Oral Med Oral Pathol Oral Radiol Endod* 81:415-420, 1996.

Kolokotronis A, Avramidou E, Zaraboukas T et al: Oral tuberculosis associated with a treatment with anti-rheumatic drugs, *J Oral Pathol Med* 35:123-125, 2006.

Mandel L: Tuberculous cervical node calcifications mimicking sialolithiasis: a case report, *J Oral Maxollofac Surg* 64:1439-1442, 2006.

Phelan JA, Jimenez V, Tompkins DC: Tuberculosis, *Dent Clin North Am* 40:327-341, 1996.

Rinaggio J: Tuberculosis, *Dent Clin North Am* 47:449-465, 2003.

Samaranayake LP: Re-emergence of tuberculosis and its variants: implications for dentistry, *Int Dent J* 52:330-336, 2002.

Yepes JF, Sullivan J, Pinto A: Tuberculosis: medical management update, *Oral Surg Oral Med Oral Pathol Oral Radiol Endod* 98:267-273, 2004.

Leprosy

Brand PW: Temperature variations and leprosy deformity, *Int J Lepr* 27:1-7, 1959.

Girdhar BK, Desikan KV: A clinical study of the mouth in untreated lepromatous patients, *Lepr Rev* 50:25-35, 1979.

Handa S, Saraswat A, Radotra BD et al: Chronic macrocheilia: a clinico-pathologic study of 28 patients, *Clin Exp Dermatol* 28:245-250, 2003.

Prabhu SR, Daftary DK: Clinical evaluation of oro-facial lesions of leprosy, *Odontostomatol Trop* 4:83-95, 1981.

Reichart P: Facial and oral manifestations in leprosy: an evaluation of seventy cases, *Oral Surg Oral Med Oral Pathol* 41:385-399, 1976.

Rendall JR, McDougall AC: Reddening of the upper central incisors associated with periapical granuloma in lepromatous leprosy, *Br J Oral Surg* 13:271-277, 1976.

Ramos-e-Silva M: Facial and oral aspects of some venereal and tropical diseases, *Acta Dermatovenerol Croat* 12:173-180, 2004.

Scheepers A: Correlation of oral surface temperature and the lesions of leprosy, *Int J Lepr* 66:214-217, 1998.

Scheepers A, Lemmer J, Lownie JF: Oral manifestations of leprosy, *Lepr Rev* 64:37-43, 1993.

Scollard DM, Skinsnes OK: Oropharyngeal leprosy in art, history, and medicine, *Oral Surg Oral Med Oral Pathol Oral Radiol Endod* 87:463-470, 1999.

World Health Organization: WHO expert committee on leprosy, *World Health Organ Tech Rep Ser* 874:1-43, 1998.

Noma

Adekeye EO, Ord RA: Cancrum oris: principles of management and reconstructive surgery, *J Maxillofac Surg* 11:160-170, 1983.

Baratti-Mayer D, Pittet B, Montandon D et al: Noma: an "infectious" disease of unknown aetiology, *Lancet Infect Dis* 3:419-431, 2003.

Berthold P: Noma: a forgotten disease, *Dent Clin North Am* 47:559-574, 2003.

Bourgeois DM, Leclercq MH: The World Health Organization initiative on noma, *Oral Dis* 5:172-174, 1999.

Enwonwu CO: Noma–the ulcer of extreme poverty, *N Engl J Med* 354:221-224, 2006.

Enwonwu CO, Falkler WA Jr, Phillips RS: Noma (cancrum oris), *Lancet* 368:147-156, 2006.

Uohara GI, Knapp MJ: Oral fusospirochetosis and associated lesions, *Oral Surg Oral Med Oral Pathol* 24:113-123, 1967.

Actinomycosis

Bhargava D, Bhusnurmath B, Sundaram KR et al: Tonsillar actinomycosis: a clinicopathologic study, *Acta Tropica* 80:163-168, 2001.

Bennhoff DF: Actinomycosis: diagnostic and therapeutic considerations and a review of 32 cases, *Laryngoscope* 94:1198-1217, 1984.

Miller M, Haddad AJ: Cervicofacial actinomycosis, *Oral Surg Oral Med Oral Pathol Oral Radiol Endod* 85:496-508, 1998.

Nagler R, Peled M, Laufer D: Cervicofacial actinomycosis. A diagnostic challenge, *Oral Surg Oral Med Oral Pathol Oral Radiol Endod* 83:652-656, 1997.

Robinson JL, Vaudry WL, Dobrovolsky W: Actinomycosis presenting as osteomyelitis in the pediatric population, *Pediatr Infect Dis J* 24:365-369, 2005.

Rush JR, Sulte HR, Cohen DM et al: Course of infection and case outcome in individuals diagnosed with microbial colonies morphologically consistent with *Actinomyces* species, *J Endod* 28:613-618, 2002.

Sakellariou PL: Periapical actinomycosis: report of a case and review of the literature, *Endod Dent Traumatol* 12:151-154, 1996.

Sprague WG, Shafer WG: Presence of actinomyces in dentigerous cyst: report of two cases, *J Oral Surg* 21:243-245, 1963.

Cat-Scratch Disease

Centers for Disease Control: Cat-scratch disease in children–Texas, September 2000–August 2001, *MMWR Morb Mortal Wkly Rep* 51:212-214, 2002.

Cheuk W, Chan AK, Wong MC et al: Confirmation of diagnosis of cat scratch disease by immunohistochemistry, *Am J Surg Pathol* 30:274-275, 2006.

English CK, Wear DJ, Margileth AM et al: Cat-scratch disease: isolation and culture of the bacterial agent, *JAMA* 259:1347-1352, 1988.

English R: Cat-scratch disease, *Pediatr Rev* 27:123-128, 2006.

Lamps LW, Scott MA: Cat-scratch disease. Historic, clinical, and pathologic perspectives, *Am J Clin Pathol* 121(suppl 1):S71-80, 2004.

Margileth AM, Wear DJ, English CK: Systemic cat scratch disease: report of 23 patients with prolonged or recurrent severe bacterial infection, *J Infect Dis* 155:390-402, 1987.

Wear DJ, Margileth AM, Hadfield TL et al: Cat scratch disease: a bacterial infection, *Science* 221:1403-1405, 1983.

Windsor JJ: Cat-scratch disease: epidemiology, aetiology and treatment, *Br J Biomed Sci* 58:101-110, 2001.

Sinusitis

Boork I: Sinusitis of odontogenic origin, *Otolaryngol Head Neck Surg* 135:349-355, 2006.

Jacobsen PL, Casagrande AM: Sinusitis as a source of dental pain, *Dent Today* 22:110-113, 2003.

Kennedy DW: First-line management of sinusitis: a national problem? Overview, *Otolaryngol Head Neck Surg* 103(suppl):847-854, 1990.

Kennedy DW: First-line management of sinusitis: a national problem? Surgical update, *Otolaryngol Head Neck Surg* 103(suppl):884-886, 1990.

Lopatin AS, Sysolyatin SP, Sysolyatin PG et al: Chronic maxillary sinusitis of dental origin: is external surgical approach mandatory? *Laryngoscope* 112:1056-1059, 2002.

Mehra P, Murad H: Maxillary sinus disease of odontogenic origin, *Otolaryngol Clin North Am* 37:347-364, 2004.

Närkiö-Mäkelä M, Qvarnberg Y: Endoscopic sinus surgery or Caldwell-Luc operation in the treatment of chronic and recurrent maxillary sinusitis, *Acta Otolaryngol Suppl* 529:177-180, 1997.

Ogata Y, Okinaka Y, Takahashi M: Antrolith associated with aspergillosis of the maxillary sinus: report of a case, *J Oral Maxillofac Surg* 55:1339-1341, 1997.

Richtsmeier WJ: Medical and surgical management of sinusitis in adults, *Ann Otol Rhinol Laryngol* 101(suppl 155):46-50, 1992.

6

Fungal and Protozoal Diseases

CHAPTER OUTLINE

CANDIDIASIS

Infection with the yeastlike fungal organism *Candida albicans* is termed **candidiasis** or, as the British prefer, **candidosis.** An older name for this disease is *moniliasis;* the use of this term should be discouraged because it is derived from the archaic designation *Monilia albicans.* Other members of the *Candida* genus, such as *C. tropicalis, C. krusei, C. parapsilosis,* and *C. guilliermondii,* may also be found intraorally, but they rarely cause disease.

Like many other pathogenic fungi, *C. albicans* may exist in two forms—a trait known as **dimorphism.** The yeast form of the organism is believed to be relatively innocuous, but the hyphal form is usually associated with invasion of host tissue.

Candidiasis is by far the most common oral fungal infection in humans and has a variety of clinical manifestations, making the diagnosis difficult at times. In fact, *C. albicans* may be a component of the normal oral microflora, with as many as 30% to 50% of people simply carrying the organism in their mouths without clinical evidence of infection. This rate of carriage has been shown to increase with age, and *C. albicans* can be recovered from the mouths of nearly 60% of dentate patients older than 60 years who have no sign of oral mucosal lesions. At least three general factors may determine whether clinical evidence of infection exists:
1. The immune status of the host
2. The oral mucosal environment
3. The strain of *C. albicans*

In the past, candidiasis was considered to be only an opportunistic infection, affecting individuals who were debilitated by another disease. Certainly, such patients make up a large percentage of those with candidal infections today. However, now clinicians recognize that oral candidiasis may develop in people who are otherwise healthy. As a result of this complex host and organism interaction, candidal infection may range from mild, superficial mucosal involvement seen in most patients to fatal, disseminated disease in severely immunocompromised patients. This chapter focuses on those clinical presentations of candidiasis that affect the oral mucosa.

CLINICAL FEATURES

Candidiasis of the oral mucosa may exhibit a variety of clinical patterns, which are summarized in Table 6-1. Many patients will display a single pattern, although some individuals will exhibit more than one clinical form of oral candidiasis.

PSEUDOMEMBRANOUS CANDIDIASIS

The best recognized form of candidal infection is **pseudomembranous candidiasis.** Also known as *thrush,* pseudomembranous candidiasis is characterized by the presence of adherent white plaques that resemble cottage cheese or curdled milk on the oral mucosa (Figs. 6-1 and 6-2). The white plaques are composed of tangled masses of hyphae, yeasts, desquamated epithe-

Table **6-1**   **Clinical Forms of Oral Candidiasis**

Clinical Type	Appearance and Symptoms	Common Sites	Associated Factors and Comments
Pseudomembranous (thrush)	Creamy-white plaques, removable; burning sensation, foul taste	Buccal mucosa, tongue, palate	Antibiotic therapy, immunosuppression
Erythematous	Red macules, burning sensation	Posterior hard palate, buccal mucosa, dorsal tongue	Antibiotic therapy, xerostomia, immunosuppression, idiopathic
Central papillary atrophy (median rhomboid glossitis)	Red, atrophic mucosal areas; asymptomatic	Midline posterior dorsal tongue	Idiopathic, immunosuppression
Chronic multifocal	Red areas, often with removable white plaques; burning sensation, asymptomatic	Posterior palate, posterior dorsal tongue, angles of mouth	Immunosuppression, idiopathic
Angular cheilitis	Red, fissured lesions; irritated, raw feeling	Angles of mouth	Idiopathic, immunosuppression, loss of vertical dimension
Denture stomatitis (chronic atrophic candidiasis, denture sore mouth)	Red, asymptomatic	Confined to palatal denture-bearing mucosa	Probably not true infection; denture often is positive on culture but mucosa is not
Hyperplastic (candidal leukoplakia)	White plaques that are not removable; asymptomatic	Anterior buccal mucosa	Idiopathic, immunosuppression; care must be taken not to confuse this with other keratotic lesions with superimposed candidiasis
Mucocutaneous	White plaques, some of which may be removable; red areas	Tongue, buccal mucosa, palate	Rare; inherited or sporadic idiopathic immune dysfunction
Endocrine-candidiasis syndromes	White plaques, most of which are not removable	Tongue, buccal mucosa, palate	Rare; endocrine disorder develops after candidiasis

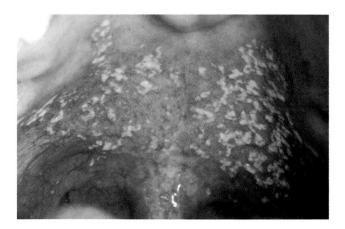

Fig. 6-1 Pseudomembranous candidiasis. Multiple white plaques on the soft palate.

lial cells, and debris. Scraping them with a tongue blade or rubbing them with a dry gauze sponge can remove these plaques. The underlying mucosa may appear normal or erythematous. If bleeding occurs, then the mucosa has probably also been affected by another process, such as lichen planus or cancer chemotherapy.

Pseudomembranous candidiasis may be initiated by exposure of the patient to broad-spectrum antibiotics (thus eliminating competing bacteria) or by impairment of the patient's immune system. The immune dysfunctions seen in leukemic patients (see page 587) or those infected with human immunodeficiency virus (HIV) (see page 264) are often associated with pseudomembranous candidiasis. Infants may also be affected, ostensibly because of their underdeveloped immune systems. Antibiotic exposure is typically responsible for an acute (rapid) expression of the condition; immunologic problems usually produce a chronic (slow-

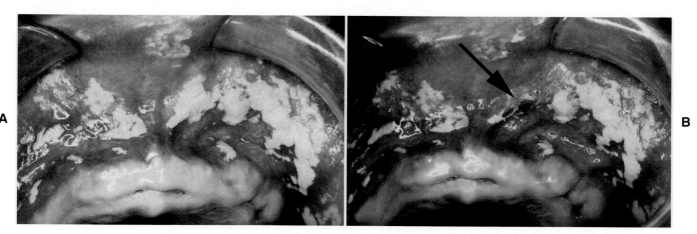

Fig. 6-2 Pseudomembranous candidiasis. A, Classic "curdled milk" appearance of the oral lesions of pseudomembranous candidiasis. This patient had no apparent risk factors for candidiasis development. **B,** Removal of one of the pseudomembranous plaques (*arrow*) reveals a mildly erythematous mucosal surface. *(From Allen CM, Blozis GG: Oral mucosal lesions. In Cummings CW, Fredrickson JM, Harker LA et al, editors:* Otolaryngology: head and neck surgery, *ed 3, St Louis, 1998, Mosby.)*

onset, long-standing) form of pseudomembranous candidiasis.

Symptoms, if present at all, are usually relatively mild, consisting of a burning sensation of the oral mucosa or an unpleasant taste in the mouth, variably described as salty or bitter. Sometimes patients complain of "blisters," when in fact they feel the elevated plaques rather than true vesicles. The plaques are characteristically distributed on the buccal mucosa, palate, and dorsal tongue.

ERYTHEMATOUS CANDIDIASIS

In contrast to the pseudomembranous form, patients with erythematous candidiasis either do not show white flecks, or a white component is not a prominent feature. Erythematous candidiasis is undoubtedly more common than pseudomembranous candidiasis, although it is often overlooked clinically. Several clinical presentations may be seen. **Acute atrophic candidiasis** or "antibiotic sore mouth," typically follows a course of broad-spectrum antibiotic therapy. Patients often complain that the mouth feels as if a hot beverage had scalded it. This burning sensation is usually accompanied by a diffuse loss of the filiform papillae of the dorsal tongue, resulting in a reddened, "bald" appearance of the tongue (Fig. 6-3). Burning mouth syndrome (see page 873) frequently manifests with a scalded sensation of the tongue; however, the tongue appears normal in that condition. Patients who suffer from xerostomia for any reason (e.g., pharmacologic, postradiation therapy, Sjögren syndrome) have an increased prevalence of erythematous candidiasis that is commonly symptomatic as well.

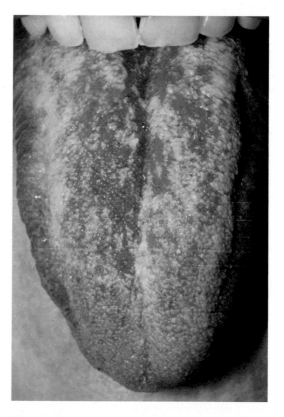

Fig. 6-3 Erythematous candidiasis. The patchy, denuded areas (not the white areas) of the dorsal tongue represent erythematous candidiasis. The patient had received a broad-spectrum antibiotic.

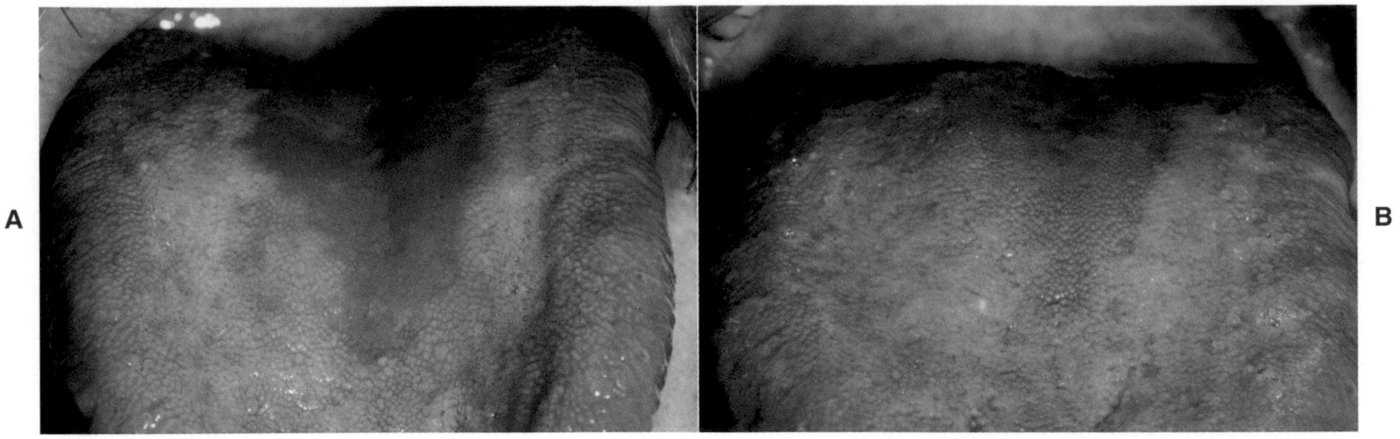

Fig. 6-4 **Erythematous candidiasis. A,** Severe presentation of central papillary atrophy. In this patient the lesion was asymptomatic. **B,** Marked regeneration of the dorsal tongue papillae occurred 2 weeks after antifungal therapy with fluconazole.

Other forms of erythematous candidiasis are usually asymptomatic and chronic. Included in this category is the condition known as **central papillary atrophy** of the tongue, or **median rhomboid glossitis.** In the past, this was thought to be a developmental defect of the tongue, occurring in 0.01% to 1.00% of adults. The lesion was supposed to have resulted from a failure of the embryologic tuberculum impar to be covered by the lateral processes of the tongue. Theoretically, the prevalence of central papillary atrophy in children should be identical to that seen in adults; however, in one study in which 10,000 children were examined, not a single lesion was detected. Other investigators have noted a consistent relationship between the lesion and *C. albicans,* and similar lesions have been induced experimentally on the dorsal tongues of rats.

Clinically, central papillary atrophy appears as a well-demarcated erythematous zone that affects the midline, posterior dorsal tongue and often is asymptomatic (Fig. 6-4). The erythema is due in part to the loss of the filiform papillae in this area. The lesion is usually symmetrical, and its surface may range from smooth to lobulated. Often the mucosal alteration resolves with antifungal therapy, although occasionally only partial resolution can be achieved.

Some patients with central papillary atrophy may also exhibit signs of oral mucosal candidal infection at other sites. This presentation of erythematous candidiasis has been termed **chronic multifocal candidiasis.** In addition to the dorsal tongue, the sites that show involvement include the junction of the hard and soft palate and the angles of the mouth. The palatal lesion appears as an erythematous area that, when the tongue is at rest, contacts the dorsal tongue lesion, resulting in what is called a "kissing lesion" because of the intimate proximity of the involved areas (Fig. 6-5).

The involvement of the angles of the mouth **(angular cheilitis, perlèche)** is characterized by erythema, fissuring, and scaling (Fig. 6-6). Sometimes this condition is seen as a component of chronic multifocal candidiasis, but it often occurs alone, typically in an older person with reduced vertical dimension of occlusion and accentuated folds at the corners of the mouth. Saliva tends to pool in these areas, keeping them moist and thus favoring a yeast infection. Patients often indicate that the severity of the lesions waxes and wanes. Microbiologic studies have indicated that 20% of these cases are caused by *C. albicans* alone, 60% are due to a combined infection with *C. albicans* and *Staphylococcus aureus,* and 20% are associated with *S. aureus* alone. Infrequently, the candidal infection more extensively involves the perioral skin, usually secondary to actions that keep the skin moist (e.g., chronic lip licking, thumb sucking), creating a clinical pattern known as **cheilocandidiasis** (Fig. 6-7). Other causes of exfoliative cheilitis often must be considered in the differential diagnosis (see page 304).

Denture stomatitis should be mentioned because it is often classified as a form of erythematous candidiasis, and some authors may use the term *chronic atrophic candidiasis* synonymously. This condition is characterized by varying degrees of erythema, sometimes accompanied by petechial hemorrhage, localized to the denture-bearing areas of a maxillary removable dental prosthesis (Figs. 6-8 and 6-9). Although the clinical appearance can be striking, the process is rarely symptomatic. Usually the patient admits to wearing the denture continuously, removing it only periodically to

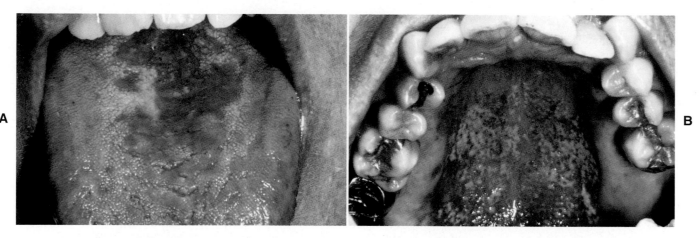

Fig. 6-5 **Candidiasis. A,** Multifocal oral candidiasis characterized by central papillary atrophy of the tongue and other areas of involvement. **B,** Same patient showing a "kissing" lesion of oral candidiasis on the hard palate.

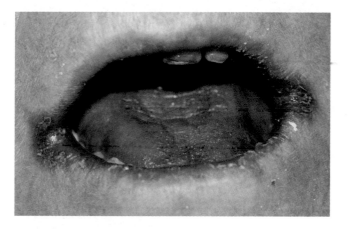

Fig. 6-6 **Angular cheilitis.** Characteristic lesions appear as fissured, erythematous alterations of the skin at the corners of the mouth.

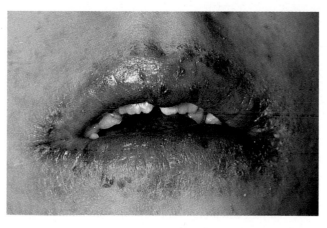

Fig. 6-7 **Cheilocandidiasis.** The exfoliative lesions of the vermilion zone and perioral skin are due to superficial candidal infection.

clean it. Whether this represents actual infection by *C. albicans* or is simply a tissue response by the host to the various microorganisms living beneath the denture remains controversial. The clinician should also rule out the possibility that this reaction could be caused by improper design of the denture (which could cause unusual pressure on the mucosa), allergy to the denture base, or inadequate curing of the denture acrylic.

Although *C. albicans* is often associated with this condition, biopsy specimens of denture stomatitis seldom show candidal hyphae actually penetrating the keratin layer of the host epithelium. Therefore, this lesion does not meet one of the main defining criteria for the diagnosis of infection—host tissue invasion by the organism. Furthermore, if the palatal mucosa and tissue-contacting surface of the denture are swabbed and separately

streaked onto a Sabouraud's agar slant, then the denture typically shows much heavier colonization by yeast (Fig. 6-10).

CHRONIC HYPERPLASTIC CANDIDIASIS (CANDIDAL LEUKOPLAKIA)

In some patients with oral candidiasis, there may be a white patch that cannot be removed by scraping; in this case the term *chronic hyperplastic candidiasis* is appropriate. This form of candidiasis is the least common and is also somewhat controversial. Some investigators believe that this condition simply represents candidiasis that is superimposed on a preexisting leukoplakic lesion, a situation that may certainly exist at times. In some instances, however, the candidal organism alone may be capable of inducing a hyperkeratotic lesion.

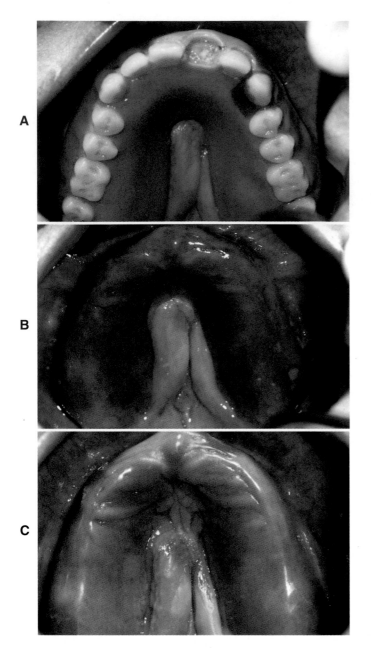

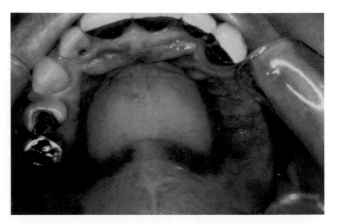

Fig. 6-9   Denture stomatitis. Denture stomatitis, not associated with *Candida albicans*, confined to the denture-bearing mucosa of a maxillary partial denture framework.

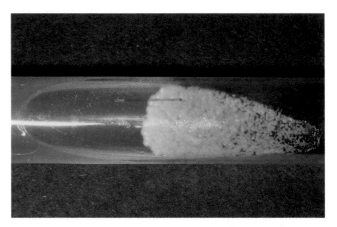

Fig. 6-10   Denture stomatitis. This Sabouraud's agar slant has been streaked with swabs obtained from erythematous palatal mucosa (*left side of the slant*) and the tissue-bearing surface of the denture (*right side of the slant*). Extensive colonization of the denture is demonstrated, whereas little evidence of yeast associated with the mucosa is noted.

Fig. 6-8   Denture stomatitis. A, Maxillary denture with incomplete palatal vault associated with midline tissue hyperplasia. **B,** Mucositis corresponds to the outline of the prosthesis. **C,** Resolution of mucositis after antifungal therapy and appropriate denture cleansing.

Such lesions are usually located on the anterior buccal mucosa and cannot clinically be distinguished from a routine leukoplakia (Fig. 6-11). Often the leukoplakic lesion associated with candidal infection has a fine intermingling of red and white areas, resulting in a speckled leukoplakia (see page 392). Such lesions may have an increased frequency of epithelial dysplasia histopathologically.

The diagnosis is confirmed by the presence of candidal hyphae associated with the lesion and by complete resolution of the lesion after antifungal therapy (Fig. 6-12).

MUCOCUTANEOUS CANDIDIASIS

Severe oral candidiasis may also be seen as a component of a relatively rare group of immunologic disorders known as *mucocutaneous candidiasis*. Several distinct immunologic dysfunctions have been identified, and the severity of the candidal infection correlates with the severity of the immunologic defect. Most cases are sporadic, although an autosomal recessive pattern of inheritance has been identified in some families. The immune problem usually becomes evident during the first few years of life, when the patient begins to have candidal infections of the mouth, nails, skin, and other mucosal surfaces. The oral lesions are usually described as thick, white plaques that typically do not rub off (essentially chronic hyperplastic candidiasis), although the other clinical forms of candidiasis may also be seen.

In some patients with mucocutaneous candidiasis, mutations in the autoimmune regulator (AIRE) gene have been documented, with the resultant formation of autoantibodies directed against the person's own tissues (Fig. 6-13). In most instances the immunologic attack is directed against the endocrine glands; however, the reasons for this tissue specificity are

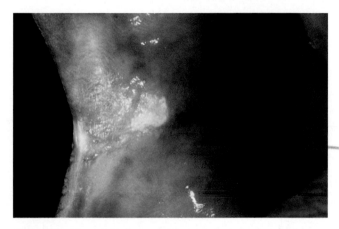

Fig. 6-11 **Hyperplastic candidiasis.** This lesion of the anterior buccal mucosa clinically resembles a leukoplakia because it is a white plaque that cannot be removed by rubbing. With antifungal therapy, such a lesion should resolve completely.

currently unclear. Young patients with mucocutaneous candidiasis should be evaluated periodically because any one of a variety of endocrine abnormalities (i.e., **endocrine-candidiasis syndrome**, **autoimmune polyendocrinopathy-candidiasis-ectodermal dystrophy [APECED] syndrome**), as well as iron-deficiency anemia, may develop in addition to the candidiasis. These endocrine disturbances include hypothyroidism, hypoparathyroidism, hypoadrenocorticism (Addison's disease), and diabetes mellitus. Typically, the endocrine abnormality develops months or even years after the onset of the candidal infection. One recent study has documented increased prevalence of oral and esophageal carcinoma in this condition, with these malignancies affecting approximately 10% of adults with APECED syndrome. This finding represents another justification for periodic reevaluation of these individuals.

Interestingly, the candidal infection remains relatively superficial rather than disseminating throughout the body. Both the oral lesions and any cutaneous involvement (usually presenting as roughened, foul-smelling cutaneous plaques and nodules) can be controlled with continuous use of relatively safe systemic antifungal drugs.

HISTOPATHOLOGIC FEATURES

The candidal organism can be seen microscopically in either an exfoliative cytologic preparation or in tissue sections obtained from a biopsy specimen. On staining with the periodic acid-Schiff (PAS) method, the candidal hyphae and yeasts can be readily identified (Fig.

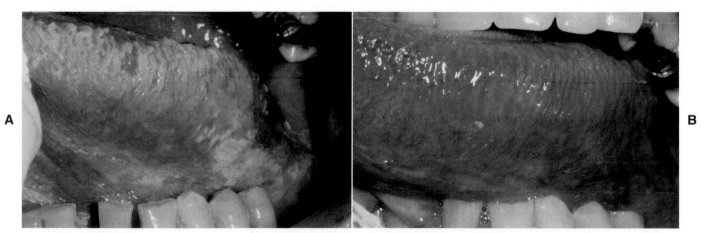

Fig. 6-12 **Hyperplastic candidiasis. A,** These diffuse white plaques clinically appear as leukoplakia, but they actually represent an unusual presentation of hyperplastic candidiasis. **B,** Treatment with clotrimazole oral troches shows complete resolution of the white lesions within 2 weeks, essentially confirming the diagnosis of hyperplastic candidiasis. If any white mucosal alteration had persisted, a biopsy of that area would have been mandatory.

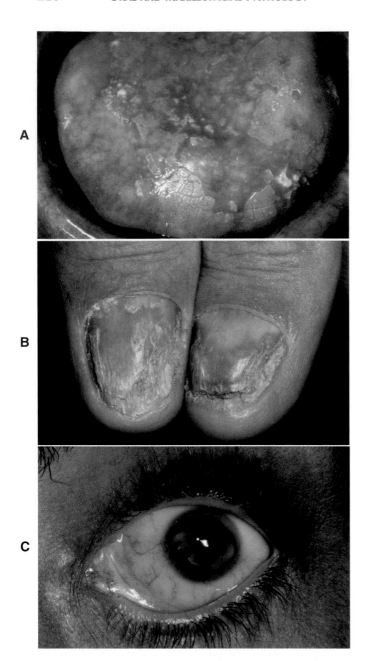

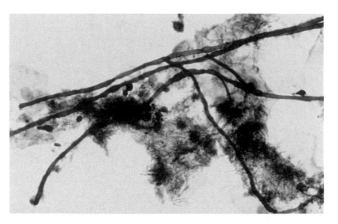

Fig. 6-14   Candidiasis. This cytologic preparation demonstrates tubular-appearing fungal hyphae and ovoid yeasts of *Candida albicans.* (PAS stain.)

Fig. 6-13   Autoimmune polyendocrinopathy-candidiasis-ectodermal dystrophy (APECED) syndrome.
A, Erythematous candidiasis diffusely involving the dorsal tongue of a 32-year-old man. **B,** Same patient showing nail dystrophy. **C,** Corneal keratopathy is also noted. Patient had a history of the onset of hypoparathyroidism and hypoadrenocorticism, both diagnosed in the second decade of life.

6-14). The PAS method stains carbohydrates, contained in abundance by fungal cell walls; the organisms are easily identified by the bright-magenta color imparted by the stain. To make a diagnosis of candidiasis, one must be able to see hyphae or pseudohyphae (which are essentially elongated yeast cells). These hyphae are approximately 2 μm in diameter, vary in their length, and may show branching. Often the hyphae are accompanied by variable numbers of yeasts, squamous epithelial cells, and inflammatory cells.

A 10% to 20% potassium hydroxide (KOH) preparation may also be used to rapidly evaluate specimens for the presence of fungal organisms. With this technique, the KOH lyses the background of epithelial cells, allowing the more resistant yeasts and hyphae to be visualized.

The disadvantages of the KOH preparation include the following:

- Lack of a permanent record
- Greater difficulty in identifying the fungal organisms, compared with PAS staining
- Inability to assess the nature of the epithelial cell population with respect to other conditions, such as epithelial dysplasia or pemphigus vulgaris

The histopathologic pattern of oral candidiasis may vary slightly, depending on which clinical form of the infection has been submitted for biopsy. The features that are found in common include an increased thickness of parakeratin on the surface of the lesion in conjunction with elongation of the epithelial rete ridges (Fig. 6-15). Typically, a chronic inflammatory cell infiltrate can be seen in the connective tissue immediately subjacent to the infected epithelium, and small collections of neutrophils (microabscesses) are often identified in the parakeratin layer and the superficial spinous cell layer near the organisms (Fig. 6-16). The candidal hyphae are embedded in the parakeratin layer and rarely penetrate into the viable cell layers of the epithelium unless the patient is extremely immunocompromised.

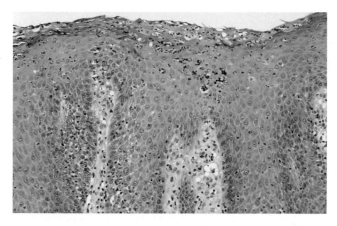

Fig. 6-15   Candidiasis. This medium-power photomicrograph shows a characteristic pattern of parakeratosis, neutrophilic microabscesses, a thickened spinous layer, and chronic inflammation of the underlying connective tissue associated with long-standing candidal infection of the oral mucosa.

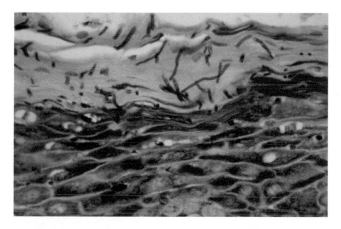

Fig. 6-16   Candidiasis. This high-power photomicrograph shows the tubular hyphae of *Candida albicans* embedded in the parakeratin layer. (PAS stain.)

DIAGNOSIS

The diagnosis of candidiasis is usually established by the clinical signs in conjunction with exfoliative cytologic examination. Although a culture can definitively identify the organism as *C. albicans,* this process may not be practical in most office settings. The cytologic findings should demonstrate the hyphal phase of the organism, and antifungal therapy can then be instituted. If the lesion is clinically suggestive of chronic hyperplastic candidiasis but does not respond to antifungal therapy, then a biopsy should be performed to rule out the possibility of *C. albicans* superimposed on epithelial dysplasia, squamous cell carcinoma, or lichen planus.

The definitive identification of the organism can be made by means of culture. A specimen for culture is obtained by rubbing a sterile cotton swab over the lesion and then streaking the swab on the surface of a Sabouraud's agar slant. *C. albicans* will grow as creamy, smooth-surfaced colonies after 2 to 3 days of incubation at room temperature.

TREATMENT AND PROGNOSIS

Several antifungal medications have been developed for managing oral candidiasis, each with its advantages and disadvantages (Table 6-2).

POLYENE AGENTS
NYSTATIN

In the 1950s the polyene antibiotic nystatin was the first effective treatment for oral candidiasis. Nystatin is formulated for oral use as a suspension or pastille (lozenge). Many patients report that nystatin has a very bitter taste, which may reduce patient compliance; therefore, the taste has to be disguised with sucrose and flavoring agents. If the candidiasis is due to xerostomia, the sucrose content of the nystatin preparation may contribute to xerostomia-related caries in these patients. The gastrointestinal tract poorly absorbs nystatin and the other polyene antibiotic, amphotericin; therefore, their effectiveness depends on direct contact with the candidal organisms. This necessitates multiple daily doses so that the yeasts are adequately exposed to the drug. Nystatin combined with triamcinolone acetonide cream or ointment can be applied topically and is effective for angular cheilitis that does not have a bacterial component.

AMPHOTERICIN B

For many years in the United States, the use of amphotericin B was restricted to intravenous (IV) treatment of life-threatening systemic fungal infections. This medication subsequently became available as an oral suspension for the management of oral candidiasis. Unfortunately, the interest in this formulation of the drug was scant, and it is no longer marketed in the United States.

IMIDAZOLE AGENTS

The imidazole-derived antifungal agents were developed during the 1970s and represented a major step forward in the management of candidiasis. The two drugs of this group that are used most frequently are clotrimazole and ketoconazole.

CLOTRIMAZOLE

Like nystatin, clotrimazole is not well absorbed and must be administered several times each day. It is formulated as a pleasant-tasting troche (lozenge) and

Table **6-2**   **Antifungal Medications**

Generic Name	Trade Name	Indications	Dosage
Nystatin	Mycostatin pastilles Mycostatin oral suspension	Oral candidiasis	One or two pastilles (200,000-400,000 units) dissolved slowly in the mouth 4-5 times daily for 10-14 days
Clotrimazole	Mycelex oral troches	Oral candidiasis	Dissolve 1 troche (10 mg) slowly in the mouth, 5 times daily for 10-14 days
Ketoconazole	Nizoral tablets	Oral candidiasis	Not to be used as initial therapy for oral candidiasis
		Blastomycosis	One tablet (200 mg) daily for 1-2 weeks for candidiasis
		Coccidioidomycosis Histoplasmosis Paracoccidioidomycosis	Minimum treatment period for systemic mycoses is 6 months
Fluconazole	Diflucan tablets	Oral candidiasis Cryptococcal meningitis	For oral candidiasis: 2 tablets (200 mg) on day 1 and then 1 tablet (100 mg) daily for 1-2 weeks
Itraconazole	Sporanox capsules	Blastomycosis Histoplasmosis	For blastomycosis and histoplasmosis: two capsules (200 mg) daily, increasing by 100-mg increments up to 400 mg daily in divided doses if no clinical response is noted
		Aspergillosis refractory to amphotericin B therapy	For aspergillosis: 200-400 mg daily For life-threatening situations: loading dose of 200 mg TID for first 3 days, then dose can be reduced Treatment should continue for at least 3 months for all of the above
Itraconazole	Sporanox oral solution	Oral candidiasis	10 mL (100 mg) vigorously swished in the mouth and swallowed, twice daily for 1-2 weeks
Amphotericin B	Fungizone oral suspension	Oral candidiasis	1 mL (100 mg) rinse and hold in the mouth for as long as possible, QID, PC and HS for 2 weeks

TID, Three times a day; *QID*, four times a day; *PC*, after meals; *HS*, at bedtime.

produces few side effects. The efficacy of this agent in treating oral candidiasis can be seen in Fig. 6-12. Clotrimazole cream is also effective treatment for angular cheilitis, because this drug has antibacterial and antifungal properties.

KETOCONAZOLE

Ketoconazole was the first antifungal drug that could be absorbed across the gastrointestinal tract, thereby providing systemic therapy by an oral route of administration. The single daily dose was much easier for patients to use; however, several disadvantages have been noted. Patients must not take antacids or H$_2$-blocking agents because an acidic environment is required for proper absorption. If a patient is to take ketoconazole for more than 2 weeks, then liver function studies are recommended because approximately 1 in 10,000 individuals will experience idiosyncratic liver toxicity from the agent. For this reason, the U.S. Food and Drug Administration has stated that ketoconazole should not be used as initial therapy for routine oral candidiasis. Furthermore, ketoconazole has been

Side Effects/Adverse Reactions	Drug Interactions
Nausea, diarrhea, vomiting with large doses	None known
Mild elevations of liver enzymes in 15% of patients	No significant drug interactions
Periodic assessment of liver function in patients with hepatic impairment	
Nausea, vomiting	
Serious hepatotoxicity in 1:10,000 patients	Serious and/or life-threatening interactions with terfenadine, astemizole, or cisapride
Monitoring of liver function is indicated for patients with preexisting hepatic problems, patients who develop symptoms of hepatic failure, or patients treated for >28 days	Metabolism of cyclosporine, tacrolimus, methylprednisolone, midazolam, triazolam, coumarin-like drugs, phenytoin, and rifampin may be altered
Serum testosterone is lowered	
Nausea, vomiting	
Anaphylaxis	
Rare cases of hepatotoxicity, ranging from mild transient elevation of liver enzymes to hepatic failure	
Headache, nausea, vomiting, abdominal pain, diarrhea	Clinically or potentially significant side effects have been noted with the following medications: oral hypoglycemic agents, coumarin-like drugs, phenytoin, cyclosporine, rifampin, theophylline, terfenadine, cisapride, astemizole, rifabutin, and tacrolimus
Rare cases of hepatoxicity	Serious and/or life-threatening interactions with terfenadine, astemizole, pimozide, quinidine, oral triazolam, oral midazolam, and cisapride
Liver function should be monitored in patients with preexisting hepatic problems on therapy for more than 1 month	Lovastatin and simvastatin should be discontinued
Nausea, diarrhea, vomiting	Increased plasma concentrations may be seen with warfarin, ritonavir, indinavir, vinca alkaloid agents, diazepam, cyclosporine, dihydropyridine medications, tacrolimus, digoxin, and methylprednisolone
Rare cases of hepatotoxicity	Serious and/or life-threatening interactions with terfenadine, astemizole, oral triazolam, oral midazolam, and cisapride
Liver function should be monitored in patients with preexisting hepatic problems on therapy for more than 1 month	Lovastatin and simvastatin should be discontinued
Nausea, diarrhea, vomiting	
Rash, gastrointestinal symptoms	No significant drug interactions

implicated in drug interactions with macrolide antibiotics (e.g., erythromycin), the gastrointestinal motility-enhancing agent cisapride, and the antihistamine astemizole, all of which may produce potentially life-threatening cardiac arrhythmias.

TRIAZOLES

The triazoles are the newest group of antifungal drugs. Both fluconazole and itraconazole have been approved for treating candidiasis in the United States.

FLUCONAZOLE

Fluconazole appears to be more effective than ketoconazole; it is well absorbed systemically, and an acidic environment is not required for absorption. A relatively long half-life allows for once-daily dosing, and liver toxicity is rare at the doses used to treat oral candidiasis. Some reports have suggested that fluconazole may not be appropriate for long-term preventive therapy because resistance to the drug seems to develop in some instances. Known drug interactions include a potentiation of the effects of phenytoin (Dilantin), an antiseizure medication; warfarin compounds (anticoagulants); and sulfonylureas (oral hypoglycemic agents). Other drugs that may interact with fluconazole are summarized in Table 6-2.

ITRACONAZOLE

Itraconazole has proven efficacy against a variety of fungal diseases, including histoplasmosis, blastomycosis, and fungal conditions of the nails. Recently, itraconazole solution was approved for management of oropharyngeal candidiasis, and this appears to have an efficacy equivalent to clotrimazole and fluconazole. As with fluconazole, significant drug interactions are possible, and itraconazole is contraindicated for patients taking astemizole, triazolam, midazolam, and cisapride. (See Table 6-2 for other potential drug interactions.)

POSACONAZOLE

This new triazole compound has been shown to be effective in the management of oropharyngeal candidiasis in patients with HIV infection. Given the cost of this drug and the proven effectiveness of other, less expensive, oral antifungal agents, the use of this medication for treatment of routine oral candidiasis would be difficult to justify.

ECHINOCANDINS

This new class of antifungal drugs acts by interfering with candidal cell wall synthesis. The formation of β-1,3-glucan, which is a principal component of the candidal cell wall, is disrupted and results in permeability of the cell wall with subsequent demise of the candidal organism. These medications are not well absorbed; consequently they must be administered intravenously and are reserved for more life-threatening candidal infections. Examples include caspofungin, micafungin, and anidulafungin.

OTHER ANTIFUNGAL AGENTS
IODOQUINOL

Although not strictly an antifungal drug, iodoquinol has antifungal and antibacterial properties. When compounded in a cream base with a corticosteroid, this material is very effective as topical therapy for angular cheilitis.

In most cases, oral candidiasis is an annoying superficial infection that is easily resolved by antifungal therapy. If infection should recur after treatment, then a thorough investigation of potential factors that could predispose to candidiasis, including immunosuppression, may be necessary. In only the most severely com-

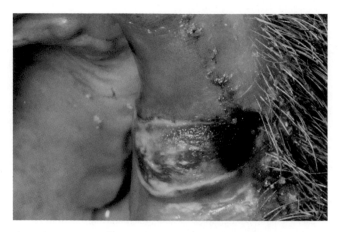

Fig. 6-17   Candidiasis. This necrotic lesion of the upper lip developed in a man with uncontrolled type I diabetes mellitus. Biopsy and culture showed a rare example of invasive oral infection by *Candida albicans*.

promised patient will candidiasis cause deeply invasive disease (Fig. 6-17).

HISTOPLASMOSIS

Histoplasmosis, the most common systemic fungal infection in the United States, is caused by the organism *Histoplasma capsulatum*. Like several other pathogenic fungi, *H. capsulatum* is dimorphic, growing as a yeast at body temperature in the human host and as a mold in its natural environment. Humid areas with soil enriched by bird or bat excrement are especially suited to the growth of this organism. This habitat preference explains why histoplasmosis is seen endemically in fertile river valleys, such as the region drained by the Ohio and Mississippi Rivers in the United States. Airborne spores of the organism are inhaled, pass into the terminal passages of the lungs, and germinate.

Approximately 500,000 new cases of histoplasmosis are thought to develop annually in the United States. Other parts of the world, such as Central and South America, Europe, and Asia, also report numerous cases. Epidemiologic studies in endemic areas of the United States suggest that 80% to 90% of the population in these regions has been infected.

CLINICAL AND RADIOGRAPHIC FEATURES

Most cases of histoplasmosis produce either no symptoms or such mild symptoms that the patient does not seek medical treatment. The expression of disease depends on the quantity of spores inhaled, the immune status of the host, and perhaps the strain of *H. capsula-*

tum. Most individuals who become exposed to the organism are relatively healthy and do not inhale a large number of spores; therefore, they have either no symptoms or they have a mild, flulike illness for 1 to 2 weeks. The inhaled spores are ingested by macrophages within 24 to 48 hours, and specific T-lymphocyte immunity develops in 2 to 3 weeks. Antibodies directed against the organism usually appear several weeks later. With these defense mechanisms, the host is usually able to destroy the invading organism, although sometimes the macrophages simply surround and confine the fungus so that viable organisms can be recovered years later. Thus patients who formerly lived in an endemic area may have acquired the organism and later express the disease at some other geographic site if they become immunocompromised.

Acute histoplasmosis is a self-limited pulmonary infection that probably develops in only about 1% of people who are exposed to a low number of spores. With a high concentration of spores, as many as 50% to 100% of individuals may experience acute symptoms. These symptoms (e.g., fever, headache, myalgia, nonproductive cough, anorexia) result in a clinical picture similar to that of influenza. Patients are usually ill for 2 weeks, although calcification of the hilar lymph nodes may be detected as an incidental finding on chest radiographs years later.

Chronic histoplasmosis also primarily affects the lungs, although it is much less common than acute histoplasmosis. The chronic form usually affects older, emphysematous, white men or immunosuppressed patients. Clinically, it appears similar to tuberculosis. Patients typically exhibit cough, weight loss, fever, dyspnea, chest pain, hemoptysis, weakness, and fatigue. Chest roentgenograms show upper-lobe infiltrates and cavitation.

Disseminated histoplasmosis is even less common than the acute and chronic types. It occurs in 1 of 2000 to 5000 patients who have acute symptoms. This condition is characterized by the progressive spread of the infection to extrapulmonary sites. It usually occurs in either older, debilitated, or immunosuppressed patients. In some areas of the United States, 2% to 10% of patients with **acquired immunodeficiency syndrome** (AIDS) (see page 277) develop disseminated histoplasmosis. Tissues that may be affected include the spleen, adrenal glands, liver, lymph nodes, gastrointestinal tract, central nervous system (CNS), kidneys, and oral mucosa. Adrenal involvement may produce hypoadrenocorticism (**Addison's disease**) (see page 841).

Most oral lesions of histoplasmosis occur with the disseminated form of the disease. The most commonly affected sites are the tongue, palate, and buccal mucosa.

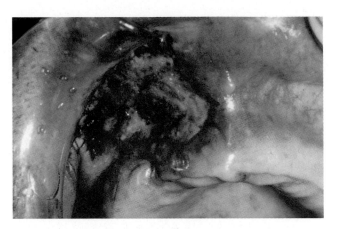

Fig. 6-18 Histoplasmosis. This ulcerated granular lesion involves the maxillary buccal vestibule and is easily mistaken clinically for carcinoma. Biopsy established the diagnosis. *(From Allen CM, Blozis GG: Oral mucosal lesions. In Cummings CW, Fredrickson JM, Harker LA et al, editors: Otolaryngology: head and neck surgery, ed 3, St Louis, 1998, Mosby.)*

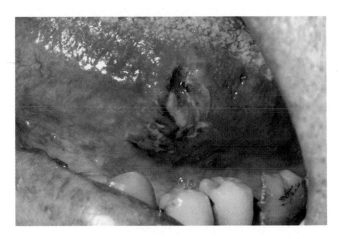

Fig. 6-19 Histoplasmosis. This chronic ulceration of the ventral and lateral tongue represents an oral lesion of histoplasmosis that had disseminated from the lungs. The lesion clinically resembles carcinoma; because of this high-risk site, biopsy is mandatory.

The condition usually appears as a solitary, variably painful ulceration of several weeks' duration; however, some lesions may appear erythematous or white with an irregular surface (Fig. 6-18). The ulcerated lesions have firm, rolled margins, and they may be indistinguishable clinically from a malignancy (Fig. 6-19).

HISTOPATHOLOGIC FEATURES

Microscopic examination of lesional tissue shows either a diffuse infiltrate of macrophages or, more commonly, collections of macrophages organized into granulomas (Fig. 6-20). Multinucleated giant cells are usually seen

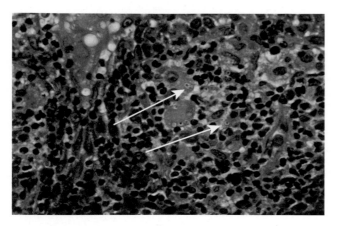

Fig. 6-20   Histoplasmosis. This medium-power photomicrograph shows scattered epithelioid macrophages admixed with lymphocytes and plasma cells. Some macrophages contain organisms of *Histoplasma capsulatum* *(arrows)*.

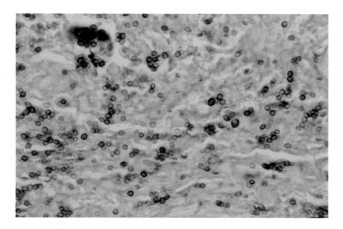

Fig. 6-21   Histoplasmosis. This high-power photomicrograph of a tissue section readily demonstrates the small yeasts of *Histoplasma capsulatum*. (Grocott-Gomori methenamine silver stain.)

in association with the granulomatous inflammation. The causative organism can be identified with some difficulty in the routine hematoxylin and eosin (H&E)-stained section; however, special stains, such as the PAS and Grocott-Gomori methenamine silver methods, readily demonstrate the characteristic 1- to 2-μm yeasts of *H. capsulatum* (Fig. 6-21).

DIAGNOSIS

The diagnosis of histoplasmosis can be made by histopathologic identification of the organism in tissue sections or by culture. Other helpful diagnostic studies include serologic testing in which antibodies directed against *H. capsulatum* are demonstrated and antigen produced by the yeast is identified.

TREATMENT AND PROGNOSIS

Acute histoplasmosis, because it is a self-limited process, generally warrants no specific treatment other than supportive care with analgesic and antipyretic agents. Often the disease is not treated because the symptoms are so nonspecific and the diagnosis is not readily evident.

Patients with chronic histoplasmosis require treatment, despite the fact that up to half of them may recover spontaneously. Often the pulmonary damage is progressive if it remains untreated, and death may result in up to 20% of these cases. The treatment of choice is intravenous amphotericin B, particularly in severe cases. However, significant kidney damage can result from this therapy; therefore, itraconazole may be used in nonimmunosuppressed patients because it is associated with fewer side effects, but this medication requires daily dosing for at least 3 months. Although ketoconazole and fluconazole have been used for treatment of histoplasmosis, these agents appear to be less effective than itraconazole and less likely to produce a desired therapeutic response.

Disseminated histoplasmosis is a very serious condition that results in death in 80% to 90% of patients if they remain untreated. Amphotericin B is usually indicated for such patients; once the life-threatening phase of the disease is under control, daily itraconazole is necessary for 6 to 18 months. Despite therapy, however, a mortality rate of 7% to 23% is observed. Itraconazole alone may be used if the patient is nonimmunocompromised and has relatively mild to moderate disease; however, the response rate is slower than for patients receiving amphotericin B, and the relapse rate may be higher.

BLASTOMYCOSIS

Blastomycosis is a relatively uncommon disease caused by the dimorphic fungus known as *Blastomyces dermatitidis*. Although the organism is rarely isolated from its natural habitat, it seems to prefer rich, moist soil, where it grows as a mold. Much of the region in which it grows overlaps the territory associated with *H. capsulatum* (affecting the eastern half of the United States). The range of blastomycosis extends farther north, however, including Wisconsin, Minnesota, and the Canadian provinces surrounding the Great Lakes. Sporadic cases have also been reported in Africa, India, Europe, and South America. By way of comparison, histoplasmosis appears to be at least ten times more common than blastomycosis. In several series of cases, a prominent adult male predilection has been noted, often with a male-to-female ratio as high as 9:1. Researchers have attributed this to the greater degree of outdoor activity (e.g., hunting, fishing) by men in areas where the organism grows. The occurrence of blastomycosis in immunocompromised patients is relatively rare.

CLINICAL AND RADIOGRAPHIC FEATURES

Blastomycosis is almost always acquired by inhalation of spores, particularly after a rain. The spores reach the alveoli of the lungs, where they begin to grow as yeasts at body temperature. In most patients, the infection is probably halted and contained in the lungs, but it may become hematogenously disseminated in a few instances. In order of decreasing frequency, the sites of dissemination include skin, bone, prostate, meninges, oropharyngeal mucosa, and abdominal organs.

Although most cases of blastomycosis are either asymptomatic or produce only very mild symptoms, patients who do experience symptoms usually have pulmonary complaints. **Acute blastomycosis** resembles pneumonia, characterized by high fever, chest pain, malaise, night sweats, and productive cough with mucopurulent sputum. Rarely, the infection may precipitate life-threatening adult respiratory distress syndrome.

Chronic blastomycosis is more common than the acute form, and it may mimic tuberculosis; both conditions are often characterized by low-grade fever, night sweats, weight loss, and productive cough. Chest radiographs may appear normal, or they may demonstrate diffuse infiltrates or one or more pulmonary or hilar masses. Unlike the situation with tuberculosis and histoplasmosis, calcification is not typically present. Cutaneous lesions usually represent the spread of infection from the lungs, although occasionally they are the only sign of disease. Such lesions begin as erythematous nodules that enlarge, becoming verrucous or ulcerated (Figs. 6-22 and 6-23).

Oral lesions of blastomycosis may result from either extrapulmonary dissemination or local inoculation with the organism. These lesions may have an irregular, erythematous or white intact surface, or they may appear as ulcerations with irregular rolled borders and varying degrees of pain (Figs. 6-24 and 6-25). Clinically, because the lesions resemble squamous cell carcinoma, biopsy and histopathologic examination are required.

HISTOPATHOLOGIC FEATURES

Histopathologic examination of lesional tissue typically shows a mixture of acute inflammation and granulomatous inflammation surrounding variable numbers of yeasts. These organisms are 8 to 20 μm in diameter.

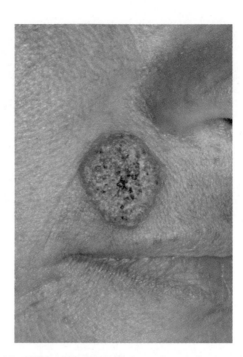

Fig. 6-22 Blastomycosis. This granular erythematous plaque of cutaneous blastomycosis has affected the facial skin. *(Courtesy of Dr. William Welton.)*

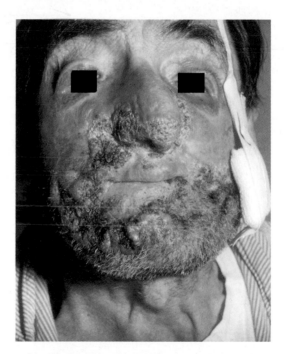

Fig. 6-23 Blastomycosis. Severe cutaneous infection by *Blastomyces dermatitidis.* *(Courtesy of Dr. Emmitt Costich.)*

They are characterized by a doubly refractile cell wall (Fig. 6-26) and a broad attachment between the budding daughter cell and the parent cell. Like many other fungal organisms, *B. dermatitidis* can be detected more easily using special stains, such as the Grocott-Gomori methenamine silver and PAS methods. Iden-

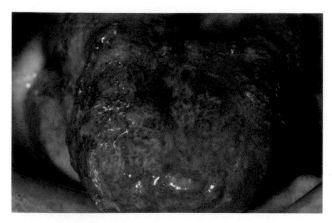

Fig. 6-24   Blastomycosis. These irregular ulcerations of the tongue represent blastomycosis. Direct inoculation was thought to have occurred from the patient's habit of chewing dried horse manure ("Kentucky field candy"), in which the organism was probably growing.

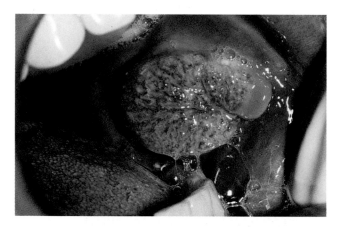

Fig. 6-25   Blastomycosis. Granular exophytic and indurated mass on the buccal mucosa.

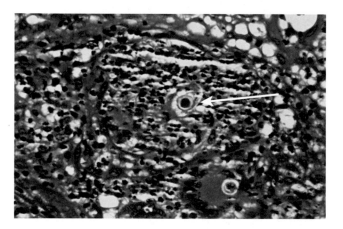

Fig. 6-26   Blastomycosis. This high-power photomicrograph shows the large yeasts of *Blastomyces dermatitidis* (*arrow*) and a pronounced host inflammatory response to the organism.

tification of these organisms is especially important because this infection often induces a benign reaction of the overlying epithelium in mucosal or skin lesions called **pseudoepitheliomatous (pseudocarcinomatous) hyperplasia.** Because this benign elongation of the epithelial rete ridges may look like squamous cell carcinoma at first glance under the microscope, careful inspection of the underlying inflamed lesional tissue is mandatory.

DIAGNOSIS

Rapid diagnosis of blastomycosis can be performed by microscopic examination of either histopathologic sections or an alcohol-fixed cytologic preparation. The most rapid means of diagnosis, however, is the KOH preparation, which may be used for examining scrapings from a suspected lesion. The most accurate method of identifying *B. dermatitidis* is by obtaining a culture specimen from sputum or fresh biopsy material and growing the organism on Sabouraud's agar. This is a slow technique, however, sometimes taking as long as 3 to 4 weeks for the characteristic mycelium-to-yeast conversion to take place. A specific DNA probe has been developed, allowing immediate identification of the mycelial phase that usually appears by 5 to 7 days in culture. Serologic studies and skin testing are usually not helpful because of lack of reactivity and specificity.

TREATMENT AND PROGNOSIS

As stated previously, most patients with blastomycosis require no treatment. Even in the case of symptomatic acute blastomycosis, administration of systemic amphotericin B is indicated only if one or more of the following is noted:

- Patient is seriously ill (AIDS, organ transplant recipient, other immune suppression disorder)
- Patient is not improving clinically
- Patient is ill for more than 2 or 3 weeks

Patients with chronic blastomycosis or extrapulmonary lesions need treatment. Itraconazole is generally recommended, particularly if the infection is mild or moderate. Although ketoconazole and fluconazole are active against *B. dermatitidis*, these drugs have been shown to be less effective than itraconazole. Amphotericin B is reserved for patients who are severely ill or show no response to itraconazole.

Disseminated blastomycosis occurs in only a small percentage of infected patients and, with proper treatment, the outlook for the patient is reasonably good. Still, mortality rates ranging from 4% to 22% have been described over the past 20 years, with men, blacks, and patients with HIV infection tending to have less favorable outcomes.

PARACOCCIDIOIDOMYCOSIS (SOUTH AMERICAN BLASTOMYCOSIS)

Paracoccidioidomycosis is a deep fungal infection that is caused by *Paracoccidioides brasiliensis*. The condition is seen most frequently in patients who live in either South America (primarily Brazil, Colombia, Venezuela, Uruguay, and Argentina) or Central America. However, immigrants from those regions and visitors to those areas can acquire the infection. Within some endemic areas, the nine-banded armadillo has been shown to harbor *P. brasiliensis* (similar to the situation seen with leprosy) (see page 198). Although there is no evidence that the armadillo directly infects humans, it may be responsible for the spread of the organism in the environment.

Paracoccidioidomycosis has a distinct predilection for males, with a 15:1 male-to-female ratio typically reported. This striking difference is thought to be attributable to a protective effect of female hormones (because β-estradiol inhibits the transformation of the hyphal form of the organism to the pathogenic yeast form). This theory is supported by the finding of an equal number of men and women who have antibodies directed against the yeast.

CLINICAL FEATURES

Patients with paracoccidioidomycosis are typically middle-aged at the time of diagnosis, and most are employed in agriculture. Most cases of paracoccidioidomycosis are thought to appear initially as pulmonary infections after exposure to the spores of the organism. Although infections are generally self-limiting, *P. brasiliensis* may spread by a hematogenous or lymphatic route to a variety of tissues, including lymph nodes, skin, and adrenal glands. Adrenal involvement often results in hypoadrenocorticism (**Addison's disease**) (see page 841).

Oral lesions appear as mulberry-like ulcerations that most commonly affect the alveolar mucosa, gingiva, and palate (Fig. 6-27). The lips, tongue, oropharynx, and buccal mucosa are also involved in a significant percentage of cases. In most patients with oral lesions, more than one oral mucosal site is affected.

HISTOPATHOLOGIC FEATURES

Microscopic evaluation of tissue obtained from an oral lesion may reveal pseudoepitheliomatous hyperplasia in addition to ulceration of the overlying surface epithelium. *P. brasiliensis* elicits a granulomatous inflammatory host response that is characterized by collections of epithelioid macrophages and multinucleated giant cells (Fig. 6-28). Scattered, large (up to 30 μm in diam-

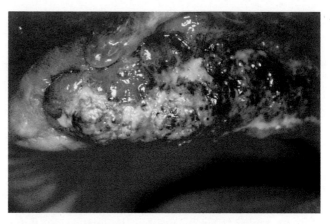

Fig. 6-27 Paracoccidioidomycosis. This granular, erythematous, and ulcerated lesion of the maxillary alveolus represents infection by *Paracoccidioides brasiliensis*. (*Courtesy of Dr. Ricardo Santiago Gomez.*)

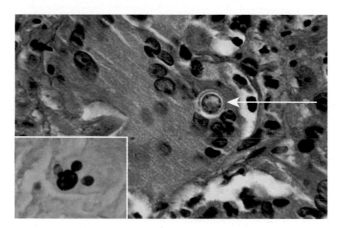

Fig. 6-28 Paracoccidioidomycosis. This high-power photomicrograph shows a large yeast of *Paracoccidioides brasiliensis* (*arrow*) within the cytoplasm of a multinucleated giant cell. A section stained with the Grocott-Gomori methenamine silver method (*inset*) illustrates the characteristic "Mickey Mouse ears" appearance of the budding yeasts. (*Courtesy of Dr. Ricardo Santiago Gomez.*)

eter) yeasts are readily identified after staining of the tissue sections with the Grocott-Gomori methenamine silver or PAS method. The organisms often show multiple daughter buds on the parent cell, resulting in an appearance that has been described as resembling "Mickey Mouse ears" or the spokes of a ship's steering wheel ("mariner's wheel").

DIAGNOSIS

Demonstration of the characteristic multiple budding yeasts in the appropriate clinical setting is usually adequate to establish a diagnosis of paracoccidioidomycosis. Specimens for culture can be obtained, but *P. brasiliensis* grows quite slowly.

TREATMENT AND PROGNOSIS

The method of management of patients with paracoccidioidomycosis depends on the severity of the disease presentation. Sulfonamide derivatives have been used since the 1940s to treat this infection. These drugs are still used today in many instances to treat mild-to-moderate cases, particularly in developing countries with limited access to the newer, more expensive antifungal agents. For severe involvement, intravenous amphotericin B is usually indicated. Cases that are not life threatening are best managed by oral itraconazole, although therapy may be needed for several months. Ketoconazole can also be used, although the side effects are typically greater than those associated with itraconazole.

COCCIDIOIDOMYCOSIS (SAN JOAQUIN VALLEY FEVER; VALLEY FEVER; COCCI)

Coccidioides immitis is the fungal organism responsible for **coccidioidomycosis**. *C. immitis* grows saprophytically in the alkaline, semiarid, desert soil of the southwestern United States and Mexico, with isolated regions also noted in Central and South America. As with several other pathogenic fungi, *C. immitis* is a dimorphic organism, appearing as a mold in its natural environment of the soil and as a yeast in tissues of the infected host. Arthrospores produced by the mold become airborne and can be inhaled into the lungs of the human host, producing infection.

Coccidioidomycosis is confined to the Western hemisphere and is endemic throughout the desert regions of southwestern United States and Mexico; however, with modern travel taking many visitors to and from the Sunbelt, this disease can be encountered virtually anywhere in the world. It is estimated that 100,000 people are infected annually in the United States, although 60% of this group are asymptomatic.

CLINICAL FEATURES

Most infections with *C. immitis* are asymptomatic, although approximately 40% of infected patients experience a flulike illness and pulmonary symptoms within 1 to 3 weeks after inhaling the arthrospores. Fatigue, cough, chest pain, myalgias, and headache are commonly reported, lasting several weeks with spontaneous resolution in most cases. Occasionally, the immune response may trigger a hypersensitivity reaction that causes the development of an erythema multiforme-like cutaneous eruption (see page 776) or erythema nodosum. Erythema nodosum is a condition that usually affects the skin of the legs and is characterized by the appearance of multiple painful erythematous inflammatory nodules in the subcutaneous connective tissue. This hypersensitivity reaction occurring in conjunction with coccidioidomycosis is termed **valley fever**, and it resolves as the host cell-mediated immune response controls the pulmonary infection.

Chronic progressive pulmonary coccidioidomycosis is relatively rare. It mimics tuberculosis, with its clinical presentation of persistent cough, hemoptysis, chest pain, low-grade fever, and weight loss.

Disseminated coccidioidomycosis occurs when the organism spreads hematogenously to extrapulmonary sites. This occurs in less than 1% of cases, but it is a more serious problem. The most commonly involved areas include skin, lymph nodes (including cervical lymph nodes), bone and joints, and the meninges. Immunosuppression greatly increases the risk of dissemination. The following groups are particularly susceptible:

- Patients taking large doses of systemic corticosteroids (organ transplant recipients)
- Patients who are being treated with cancer chemotherapy
- Patients in the end stages of HIV infection
- Patients who are pregnant

Infants and older adult patients, both of whom may have suboptimally functioning immune systems, also may be at increased risk for disseminated disease. Persons of color (e.g., blacks, Filipinos, Native Americans) also seem to have an increased risk, but it is unclear whether their susceptibility is due to genetic causes or socioeconomic factors, such as poor nutrition.

The cutaneous lesions may appear as papules, subcutaneous abscesses, verrucous plaques, and granulomatous nodules. Of prime significance to the clinician is the predilection for these lesions to develop in the area of the central face, especially the nasolabial fold. Oral lesions are distinctly uncommon, and these have been described as ulcerated granulomatous nodules.

HISTOPATHOLOGIC FEATURES

Biopsy material shows large (20 to 60 μm), round spherules that may contain numerous endospores. The host response may be variable, ranging from a suppurative, neutrophilic infiltrate to a granulomatous inflammatory response. In some cases the two patterns of inflammation are seen concurrently. Special stains, such as the PAS and Grocott-Gomori methenamine silver methods, enable the pathologist to identify the organism more readily.

DIAGNOSIS

The diagnosis of coccidioidomycosis can be confirmed by culture or identification of characteristic organisms in biopsy material. If the organisms do not have a classic microscopic appearance, then *in situ* hybridization studies using specific complementary DNA probes for *C. immitis* can be performed to definitively identify the fungus. Cytologic preparations from bronchial swabbings or sputum samples may also reveal the organisms.

Serologic studies are helpful in supporting the diagnosis, and they may be performed at the same time as skin testing. Skin testing by itself may be of limited value in determining the diagnosis because many patients in endemic areas have already been exposed to the organism and have positive test findings.

TREATMENT

The decision whether or not to treat a particular patient affected by coccidioidomycosis depends on the severity and extent of the infection and the patient's immune status. Relatively mild symptoms in an immunocompetent person do not warrant treatment. Amphotericin B is administered for the following groups:

- Immunosuppressed patients
- Patients with severe pulmonary infection
- Patients who have disseminated disease
- Patients who are pregnant
- Patients who appear to be in a life-threatening situation concerning the infection

For many cases of coccidioidomycosis, fluconazole or itraconazole is the drug of choice, usually given in high doses for an extended period of time. Although the response of the disease to these oral azole medications may be somewhat slower than that of amphotericin B, the side effects and complications of therapy are far fewer. Ketoconazole also may be used as an alternative treatment for mild-to-moderate cases of coccidioidomycosis.

CRYPTOCOCCOSIS

Cryptococcosis is a relatively uncommon fungal disease caused by the yeast *Cryptococcus neoformans.* This organism normally causes no problem in immunocompetent people, but it can be devastating to the immunocompromised patient. The incidence of cryptococcosis increased dramatically during the 1990s, primarily because of the AIDS epidemic. At that time, this was the most common life-threatening fungal infection in these patients. However, with the advent of highly active anti-retroviral therapy (HAART) (see page 280), this complication has become less of a problem in the United States. In countries where the population cannot afford HAART, cryptococcosis remains a significant cause of death for AIDS patients. The disease has a worldwide distribution because of its association with the pigeon (with the organism living in the deposits of excreta left by the birds). Unlike many other pathogenic fungi, *C. neoformans* grows as a yeast both in the soil and in infected tissue. The organism usually produces a prominent mucopolysaccharide capsule that appears to protect it from host immune defenses.

The disease is acquired by inhalation of *C. neoformans* spores into the lungs, resulting in an immediate influx of neutrophils, which destroys most of the yeasts. Macrophages soon follow, although resolution of infection in the immunocompetent host ultimately depends on an intact cell-mediated immune system.

CLINICAL FEATURES

Primary cryptococcal infection of the lungs is often asymptomatic; however, a mild flulike illness may develop. Patients complain of productive cough, chest pain, fever, and malaise. Most patients with a diagnosis of cryptococcosis have a significant underlying medical problem related to immune suppression (e.g., systemic corticosteroid therapy, cancer chemotherapy, malignancy, AIDS). It is estimated that 5% to 10% of AIDS patients acquire this infection (see page 264).

Dissemination of the infection is common in these immunocompromised patients, and the most frequent site of involvement is the meninges, followed by skin, bone, and the prostate gland.

Cryptococcal meningitis is characterized by headache, fever, vomiting, and neck stiffness. In many instances, this is the initial sign of the disease.

Cutaneous lesions develop in 10% to 15% of patients with disseminated disease. These are of particular importance to the clinician, because the skin of the head and neck is often involved. The lesions appear as erythematous papules or pustules that may ulcerate, discharging a puslike material rich in cryptococcal organisms (Fig. 6-29).

Although oral lesions are relatively rare, they have been described either as craterlike, nonhealing ulcers that are tender on palpation or as friable papillary erythematous plaques. Dissemination to salivary gland tissue also has been reported rarely.

HISTOPATHOLOGIC FEATURES

Microscopic sections of a cryptococcal lesion generally show a granulomatous inflammatory response to the organism. The extent of the response may vary, however, depending on the host's immune status and the strain of the organism. The yeast appears as a round-to-ovoid structure, 4 to 6 μm in diameter, surrounded by a clear halo that represents the capsule. Staining with the PAS or Grocott-Gomori methenamine silver method readily identifies the fungus;

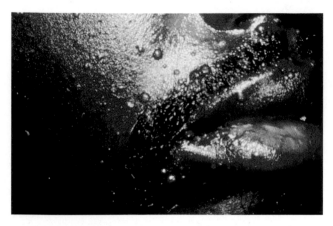

Fig. 6-29   Cryptococcosis. These papules of the facial skin represent disseminated cryptococcal infection in a patient infected with human immunodeficiency virus (HIV). *(Courtesy of Dr. Catherine Flaitz.)*

moreover, a mucicarmine stain uniquely demonstrates its mucopolysaccharide capsule.

DIAGNOSIS

The diagnosis of cryptococcosis can be made by several methods, including biopsy and culture. Detection of cryptococcal polysaccharide antigen in the serum or cerebrospinal fluid is also useful as a diagnostic procedure.

TREATMENT AND PROGNOSIS

Management of cryptococcal infections can be very difficult because most of the affected patients have an underlying medical problem. Before amphotericin B was developed, cryptococcosis was almost uniformly fatal. For cryptococcal meningitis, a combination of systemic amphotericin B and another antifungal drug (flucytosine) is used initially for 2 weeks in most cases to treat this disease. Then, either fluconazole or itraconazole is given for an additional minimal period of 10 weeks. For relatively mild cases of pulmonary cryptococcosis, only fluconazole or itraconazole may be used. These drugs produce far fewer side effects than do amphotericin B and flucytosine, and they have proven to be important therapeutic tools for managing this type of infection.

ZYGOMYCOSIS (MUCORMYCOSIS; PHYCOMYCOSIS)

Zygomycosis is an opportunistic, frequently fulminant, fungal infection that is caused by normally saprobic organisms of the class Zygomycetes, including such genera as *Absidia*, *Mucor*, *Rhizomucor*, and *Rhizopus*.

These organisms are found throughout the world, growing in their natural state on a variety of decaying organic materials. Numerous spores may be liberated into the air and inhaled by the human host.

Zygomycosis may involve any one of several areas of the body, but the rhinocerebral form is most relevant to the oral health care provider. Zygomycosis is noted especially in insulin-dependent diabetics who have uncontrolled diabetes and are ketoacidotic; ketoacidosis inhibits the binding of iron to transferrin, allowing serum iron levels to rise. The growth of these fungi is enhanced by iron, and patients who are taking deferoxamine (an iron-chelating agent used in the treatment of diseases such as thalassemia) are also at increased risk for developing zygomycosis. As with many other fungal diseases, this infection affects immunocompromised patients as well, including bone marrow transplant recipients, patients with AIDS, and those receiving systemic corticosteroid therapy. Only rarely has zygomycosis been reported in apparently healthy individuals.

CLINICAL AND RADIOGRAPHIC FEATURES

The presenting symptoms of rhinocerebral zygomycosis may be exhibited in several ways. Patients may experience nasal obstruction, bloody nasal discharge, facial pain or headache, facial swelling or cellulitis, and visual disturbances with concurrent proptosis. Symptoms related to cranial nerve involvement (e.g., facial paralysis) are often present. With progression of disease into the cranial vault, blindness, lethargy, and seizures may develop, followed by death.

If the maxillary sinus is involved, the initial presentation may be seen as intraoral swelling of the maxillary alveolar process, the palate, or both. If the condition remains untreated, palatal ulceration may evolve, with the surface of the ulcer typically appearing black and necrotic. Massive tissue destruction may result if the condition is not treated (Figs. 6-30 and 6-31).

Radiographically, opacification of the sinuses may be observed in conjunction with patchy effacement of the bony walls of the sinuses (Fig. 6-32). Such a picture may be difficult to distinguish from that of a malignancy affecting the sinus area.

HISTOPATHOLOGIC FEATURES

Histopathologic examination of lesional tissue shows extensive necrosis with numerous large (6 to 30 μm in diameter), branching, nonseptate hyphae at the periphery (Fig. 6-33). The hyphae tend to branch at 90-degree angles. The extensive tissue destruction and necrosis associated with this disease are undoubtedly attribut-

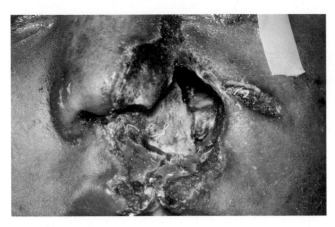

Fig. 6-30   Zygomycosis. Diffuse tissue destruction involving the nasal and maxillary structures caused by a *Mucor* species. *(Courtesy of Dr. Sadru Kabani.)*

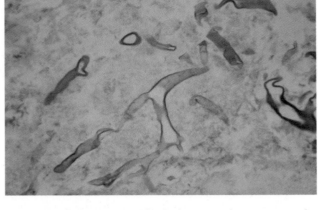

Fig. 6-33   Zygomycosis. This high-power photomicrograph shows the large, nonseptate fungal hyphae characteristic of the zygomycotic organisms.

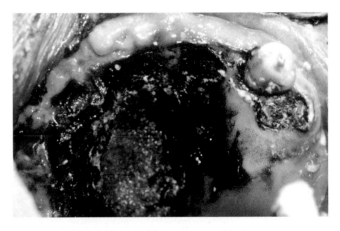

Fig. 6-31   Zygomycosis. The extensive black, necrotic lesion of the palate represents zygomycotic infection that extended from the maxillary sinus in a patient with poorly controlled type I diabetes mellitus. *(Courtesy of Dr. Michael Tabor.)*

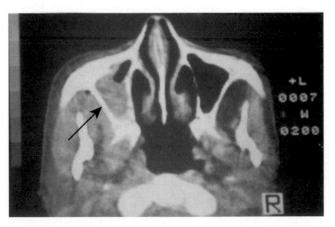

Fig. 6-32   Zygomycosis. This computed tomography (CT) scan demonstrates the opacification of the left maxillary sinus *(arrow)*.

able to the preference of the fungi for invasion of small blood vessels. This disrupts normal blood flow to the tissue, resulting in infarction and necrosis. A neutrophilic infiltrate usually predominates in the viable tissue, but the host inflammatory cell response to the infection may be minimal, particularly if the patient is immunosuppressed.

DIAGNOSIS

Diagnosis of zygomycosis is usually based on the histopathologic findings. Because of the grave nature of this infection, appropriate therapy must be instituted in a timely manner (often without the benefit of definitive culture results).

TREATMENT AND PROGNOSIS

Successful treatment of zygomycosis consists of rapid accurate diagnosis of the condition, followed by radical surgical débridement of the infected, necrotic tissue and systemic administration of high doses of one of the lipid formulations of amphotericin B. Magnetic resonance imaging (MRI) of the head may be useful in determining the extent of disease involvement so that surgical margins can be planned. In addition, control of the patient's underlying disease (e.g., diabetic ketoacidosis) must be attempted. Despite such therapy, the prognosis is usually poor, with approximately 60% of patients who develop rhinocerebral zygomycosis dying of their disease. Should the patient survive, the massive tissue destruction that remains presents a challenge both functionally and aesthetically. Prosthetic obturation of palatal defects may be necessary.

ASPERGILLOSIS

Aspergillosis is a fungal disease that is characterized by noninvasive and invasive forms. Noninvasive aspergillosis usually affects a normal host, appearing either as an allergic reaction or a cluster of fungal hyphae. Localized invasive infection of damaged tissue may be seen in a normal host, but a more extensive invasive infection is often evident in the immunocompromised patient. With the advent of intensive chemotherapeutic regimens, the AIDS epidemic, and both solid-organ and bone marrow transplantation, the prevalence of invasive aspergillosis has increased dramatically in the past 20 years. Patients with uncontrolled diabetes mellitus are also susceptible to *Aspergillus* spp. infections. Rarely, invasive aspergillosis has been reported to affect the paranasal sinuses of apparently normal immunocompetent individuals.

Normally, the various species of the *Aspergillus* genus reside worldwide as saprobic organisms in soil, water, or decaying organic debris. Resistant spores are released into the air and inhaled by the human host, resulting in opportunistic fungal infection second in frequency only to candidiasis. Interestingly, most species of *Aspergillus* cannot grow at 37° C; only the pathogenic species have the ability to replicate at body temperature.

The two most commonly encountered species of *Aspergillus* in the medical setting are A. *flavus* and A. *fumigatus*, with A. *fumigatus* being responsible for 90% of the cases of aspergillosis. The patient may acquire such infections in the hospital (**"nosocomial"** infection), especially if remodeling or building construction is being performed in the immediate area. Such activity often stirs up the spores, which are then inhaled by the patient.

CLINICAL FEATURES

The clinical manifestations of aspergillosis vary, depending on the host immune status and the presence or absence of tissue damage. In the normal host, the disease may appear as an allergy affecting either the sinuses (**allergic fungal sinusitis**) or the bronchopulmonary tract. An asthma attack may be triggered by inhalation of spores by a susceptible person. Sometimes a low-grade infection becomes established in the maxillary sinus, resulting in a mass of fungal hyphae called an **aspergilloma.** Occasionally, the mass will undergo dystrophic calcification, producing a radiopaque body called an **antrolith** within the sinus.

Another presentation that may be encountered by the oral health care provider is aspergillosis after tooth extraction or endodontic treatment, especially in the maxillary posterior segments. Presumably, tissue

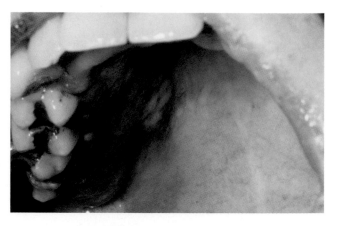

Fig. 6-34   Aspergillosis. This young woman developed a painful purplish swelling of her hard palate after induction chemotherapy for leukemia.

damage predisposes the sinus to infection, resulting in symptoms of localized pain and tenderness accompanied by nasal discharge. Immunocompromised patients are particularly susceptible to oral aspergillosis, and some investigators have suggested that the portal of entry may be the marginal gingiva and gingival sulcus. Painful gingival ulcerations are initially noted, and peripherally the mucosa and soft tissue develops diffuse swelling with a gray or violaceous hue (Fig. 6-34). If the disease is not treated, extensive necrosis, seen clinically as a yellow or black ulcer, and facial swelling evolve.

Disseminated aspergillosis occurs principally in immunocompromised patients, particularly in those who have leukemia or who are taking high daily doses of corticosteroids. Such patients usually exhibit symptoms related to the primary site of inoculation: the lungs. The patient typically has chest pain, cough, and fever, but such symptoms are vague. Therefore, obtaining an early, accurate diagnosis may be difficult. Once the fungal organism obtains access to the bloodstream, infection can spread to such sites as the CNS, eye, skin, liver, gastrointestinal tract, bone, and thyroid gland.

HISTOPATHOLOGIC FEATURES

Tissue sections of invasive *Aspergillus* spp. lesions show varying numbers of branching, septate hyphae, 3 to 4 μm in diameter (Figs. 6-35 and 6-36). These hyphae show a tendency to branch at an acute angle and to invade adjacent small blood vessels. Occlusion of the vessels often results in the characteristic pattern of necrosis associated with this disease. In the immunocompetent host, a granulomatous inflammatory response—in addition to necrosis—can be expected. In the immunocompromised patient, however, the inflam-

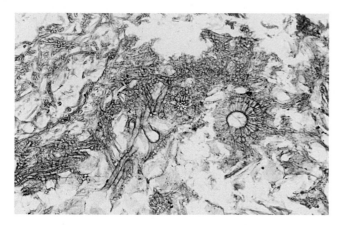

Fig. 6-35   Aspergillosis. This photomicrograph reveals fungal hyphae and a fruiting body of an *Aspergillus* species.

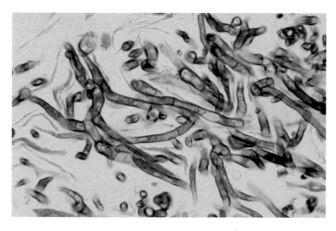

Fig. 6-36   Aspergillosis. This high-power photomicrograph shows the characteristic septate hyphae of *Aspergillus* species. (Grocott-Gomori methenamine silver stain.)

matory response is often weak or absent, leading to extensive tissue destruction.

Noninvasive forms of aspergillosis have histopathologic features that differ from invasive aspergillosis, however. The aspergilloma, for example, is characterized by a tangled mass of hyphae with no evidence of tissue invasion. Allergic fungal sinusitis, on the other hand, histopathologically exhibits large pools of eosinophilic inspissated mucin with interspersed sheetlike collections of lymphocytes and eosinophils. Relatively few fungal hyphae are identified, and then only with careful examination after methenamine silver staining.

DIAGNOSIS

Although the diagnosis of fungal infection can be established by identification of hyphae within tissue sections, this finding is only suggestive of aspergillosis because other fungal organisms may appear similar microscopically. Ideally, the diagnosis should be supported by culture of the organism from the lesion; however, from a practical standpoint, treatment may need to be initiated immediately to prevent the patient's demise. Culture specimens of sputum and blood are of limited value because they are often negative despite disseminated disease.

TREATMENT AND PROGNOSIS

Treatment depends on the clinical presentation of aspergillosis. For immunocompetent patients with a noninvasive aspergilloma, surgical débridement may be all that is necessary. Patients who have allergic fungal sinusitis are treated with débridement and corticosteroid drugs. For localized invasive aspergillosis in the immunocompetent host, débridement followed by antifungal medication is indicated. Although systemic amphotericin B therapy was considered appropriate in the past, recent studies have shown that voriconazole, a triazole antifungal agent, is more effective for treating these patients. In one large series of patients with invasive aspergillosis, 71% of those treated with voriconazole were alive after 12 weeks of therapy, compared with 58% survival in the group who received standard amphotericin B treatment. Itraconazole has also been approved as an alternative therapy. Immunocompromised patients who have invasive aspergillosis should be treated by aggressive débridement of necrotic tissue, combined with systemic antifungal therapy as described previously.

The prognosis for immunocompromised patients is much worse compared with immunocompetent individuals, particularly if the infection is disseminated. Even with appropriate therapy, only about one third of these patients survive. Because aspergillosis in the immunocompromised patient usually develops while the individual is hospitalized, particular attention should be given to the ventilation system in the hospital to prevent patient exposure to the airborne spores of *Aspergillus* spp.

TOXOPLASMOSIS

Toxoplasmosis is a relatively common disease caused by the obligate intracellular protozoal organism *Toxoplasma gondii*. For normal, healthy adults, the organism poses no problems, and an estimated 16% to 23% of adults in the United States may have had asymptomatic infection, based on an epidemiologic study that examined serologic samples from more than 4000 randomized individuals. However, the prevalence of infection has considerable geographic variation around the world. Unfortunately, the disease can be devastating for the developing fetus or the immunocompromised patient. Other mammals, particularly members of the cat family, are vulnerable to infection, and cats are considered to be the definitive host. *T. gondii* multiplies in the intestinal tract of the cat by means of a sexual life cycle, discharging numerous oocysts in the cat feces. Another animal or human can ingest these oocysts, resulting in the production of disease.

CLINICAL FEATURES

In the normal, immunocompetent individual, infection with *T. gondii* is often asymptomatic. If symptoms develop, they are usually mild and resemble infectious mononucleosis; patients may have a low-grade fever, cervical lymphadenopathy, fatigue, and muscle or joint pain. These symptoms may last from a few weeks to a few months, although the host typically recovers without therapy. Sometimes the lymphadenopathy involves one or more of the lymph nodes in the para-oral region, such as the buccal or submental lymph node. In such instances, the oral health care provider may discover the disease.

In immunosuppressed patients, toxoplasmosis may represent a new, primary infection or, more frequently, reactivation of previously encysted organisms. The principal groups at risk include the following:
- AIDS patients
- Transplant recipients
- Cancer patients

Manifestations of infection can include necrotizing encephalitis, pneumonia, and myositis or myocarditis. In the United States, it is estimated that from 3% to 10% of AIDS patients (see page 264) will experience CNS involvement. CNS infection is very serious. Clinically, the patient may complain of headache, lethargy, disorientation, and hemiparesis.

Congenital toxoplasmosis occurs when a nonimmune mother contracts the disease during her pregnancy and the organism crosses the placental barrier, infecting the developing fetus. The potential effects of blindness, mental retardation, and delayed psychomotor development are most severe if the infection occurs during the first trimester of pregnancy.

HISTOPATHOLOGIC FEATURES

Histopathologic examination of a lymph node obtained from a patient with active toxoplasmosis shows characteristic reactive germinal centers exhibiting an accumulation of eosinophilic macrophages. The macrophages encroach on the germinal centers and accumulate within the subcapsular and sinusoidal regions of the node (Fig. 6-37).

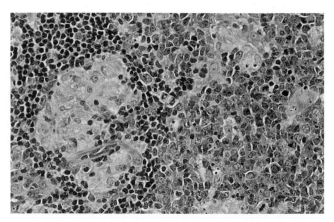

Fig. 6-37 Toxoplasmosis. This high-power photomicrograph shows an accumulation of eosinophilic macrophages within a lymph node. *(Courtesy of Dr. John Kalmar.)*

DIAGNOSIS

The diagnosis of toxoplasmosis is usually established by identification of rising serum antibody titers to *T. gondii* within 10 to 14 days after infection. Immunocompromised patients, however, may not be able to generate an antibody response; therefore, the diagnosis may rest on the clinical findings and the response of the patient to therapy.

Biopsy of an involved lymph node may suggest the diagnosis, and the causative organisms can sometimes be detected immunohistochemically using antibodies directed against *T. gondii*–specific antigens (Fig. 6-38). The diagnosis should also be confirmed by serologic studies, if possible.

TREATMENT AND PROGNOSIS

Most healthy adults with toxoplasmosis require no specific treatment because of the mild symptoms and self-limiting course. Perhaps more importantly, pregnant women should avoid situations that place them at risk for the disease. Handling or eating raw meat or cleaning a cat litter box should be avoided until after delivery. If exposure during pregnancy is suspected, treatment with a combination of sulfadiazine and pyrimethamine often prevents transmission of *T. gondii* to the fetus. Because these drugs act by inhibiting folate metabolism of the protozoan, folinic acid is given concurrently to help prevent hematologic complications in the patient. A similar drug regimen is used to treat immunosuppressed individuals with toxoplasmosis, although clindamycin may be substituted for sulfadiazine in managing patients who are allergic to sulfa drugs. Because most cases of toxoplasmosis in AIDS patients represent reactivation of encysted organisms, prophylactic administration of trimethoprim and sul-

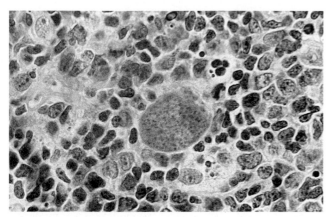

Fig. 6-38   Toxoplasmosis. In this high-power photomicrograph, an encysted organism of toxoplasmosis is highlighted by an immunohistochemical study. *(Courtesy of Dr. John Kalmar.)*

famethoxazole is generally recommended, particularly if the patient's CD4+ T-lymphocyte count is less than 100 cells/μL.

BIBLIOGRAPHY

Candidiasis

Akpan A, Morgan R: Oral candidiasis, *Postgrad Med J* 78:455-459, 2002.

Allen CM: Diagnosing and managing oral candidiasis, *J Am Dent Assoc* 123:77-82, 1992.

Arendoff TM, Walker DM: The prevalence and intra-oral distribution of *Candida albicans* in man, *Arch Oral Biol* 25:1-10, 1980.

Barbeau J, Séguin J, Goulet JP et al: Reassessing the presence of *Candida albicans* in denture-related stomatitis, *Oral Surg Oral Med Oral Pathol Oral Radiol Endod* 95:51-59, 2003.

Baughman RA: Median rhomboid glossitis: a developmental anomaly? *Oral Surg Oral Med Oral Pathol* 31:56-65, 1971.

Bennett JE: Echinocandins for candidemia in adults without neutropenia, *N Engl J Med* 355:1154-1159, 2006.

Bergendal T, Isacsson G: A combined clinical, mycological and histological study of denture stomatitis, *Acta Odontol Scand* 41:33-44, 1983.

Blomgren J, Berggren U, Jontell M: Fluconazole versus nystatin in the treatment of oral candidiasis, *Acta Odontol Scand* 56:202-205, 1998.

Eisenbarth GS, Gottlieb PA: Autoimmune polyendocrine syndromes, *N Engl J Med* 350:2068-2079, 2004.

Fotos PG, Vincent SD, Hellstein JW: Oral candidosis: clinical, historical and therapeutic features of 100 cases, *Oral Surg Oral Med Oral Pathol* 74:41-49, 1992.

Heimdahl A, Nord CE: Oral yeast infections in immunocompromised and seriously diseased patients, *Acta Odontol Scand* 48:77-84, 1990.

Holmstrup P, Axéll T: Classification and clinical manifestations of oral yeast infections, *Acta Odontol Scand* 48:57-59, 1990.

Kleinegger CL, Lockhart SR, Vargas K et al: Frequency, intensity, species, and strains of oral *Candida* vary as a function of host age, *J Clin Microbiol* 34:2246-2254, 1996.

Lehner T: Oral thrush, or acute pseudomembranous candidiasis: a clinicopathologic study of forty-four cases, *Oral Surg Oral Med Oral Pathol* 18:27-37, 1964.

Monaco JG, Pickett AB: The role of *Candida* in inflammatory papillary hyperplasia, *J Prosthet Dent* 45:470-471, 1981.

Odds FC, Arai T, Disalvo AF et al: Nomenclature of fungal diseases: a report and recommendations from a sub-committee of the International Society for Human and Animal Mycology (ISHAM), *J Med Vet Mycol* 30:1-10, 1992.

Öhman S-C, Dahlen G, Moller A et al: Angular cheilitis: a clinical and microbial study, *J Oral Pathol* 15:213-217, 1986.

Peterson P, Pitkänen J, Sillanpää N et al: Autoimmune polyendocrinopathy candidiasis ectodermal dystrophy (APECED): a model disease to study molecular aspects of endocrine autoimmunity, *Clin Exp Immunol* 135:348-357, 2004.

Rautemaa R, Hietanen J, Niissalo S et al: Oral and oesophageal squamous cell carcinoma—a complication or component of autoimmune polyendocrinopathy-candidiasis-ectodermal dystrophy (APECED, APS-I), *Oral Oncol* 43:607-613, 2007.

Rodu B, Griffin IL, Gockerman JP: Oral candidiasis in cancer patients, *South Med J* 77:312-314, 1984.

Samaranayake LP, Cheung LK, Samaranayake YH: Candidiasis and other fungal diseases of the mouth, *Dermatol Ther* 15:251-269, 2002.

Sanguineti A, Carmichael JK, Campbell K: Fluconazole-resistant *Candida albicans* after long-term suppressive therapy, *Arch Intern Med* 153:1122-1124, 1993.

Sitheeque MAM, Samaranayake LP: Chronic hyperplastic candidosis/candidiasis (candidal leukoplakia), *Crit Rev Oral Biol Med* 14:253-267, 2003.

Terai H, Shimahara M: Atrophic tongue associated with *Candida*, *J Oral Pathol Med* 34:397-400, 2005.

Terrell CL: Antifungal agents. II. The azoles, *Mayo Clin Proc* 74:78-100, 1999.

Vazquez JA, Skiest DJ, Nieto L et al: A multicenter randomized trial evaluation posaconazole versus fluconazole for the treatment of oropharyngeal candidiasis in subjects with HIV/AIDS, *Clin Infect Dis* 42:1179-1186, 2006.

Histoplasmosis

Bradsher RW: Histoplasmosis and blastomycosis, *Clin Infect Dis* 22(suppl 2):S102-111, 1996.

Couppié P, Clyti E, Nacher M et al: Acquired immunodeficiency syndrome-related oral and/or cutaneous histoplasmosis: a descriptive and comparative study of 21 cases in French Guiana, *Int J Dermatol* 41:571-576, 2002.

Leal-Alcure M, Di Hipólito-Júnior O, Paes de Almeida O et al: Oral histoplasmosis in an HIV-negative patient, *Oral Surg Oral Med Oral Pathol Oral Radiol Endod* 101:E33-36, 2006.

Lortholary O, Denning DW, Dupont B: Endemic mycoses: a treatment update, *J Antimicrob Chemother* 43:321-331, 1999.

Motta ACF, Galo R, Grupioni-Lourenço A et al: Unusual orofacial manifestations of histoplasmosis in renal transplanted patient, *Mycopathologia* 161:161-165, 2006.

Myskowski PL, White MH, Ahkami R: Fungal disease in the immunocompromised host, *Dermatol Clin* 15:295-305, 1997.

Samaranayake LP: Oral mycoses in HIV infection, *Oral Surg Oral Med Oral Pathol* 73:171-180, 1992.

Sarosi GA, Johnson PC: Disseminated histoplasmosis in patients infected with human immunodeficiency virus, *Clin Infect Dis* 14(suppl 1):S60-67, 1992.

Sharma OP: Histoplasmosis: a masquerader of sarcoidosis, *Sarcoidosis* 8:10-13, 1991.

Wheat LJ, Kauffman CA: Histoplasmosis, *Infect Dis Clin North Am* 17:1-19, 2003.

Blastomycosis

Areno JP, Campbell GD, George RB: Diagnosis of blastomycosis, *Semin Respir Infect* 12:252-262, 1997.

Assaly RA, Hammersley JR, Olson DE et al: Disseminated blastomycosis, *J Am Acad Dermatol* 48:123-127, 2003.

Bradsher RW: Clinical features of blastomycosis, *Semin Respir Infect* 12:229-234, 1997.

Bradsher RW, Chapman SW, Pappas PG: Blastomycosis, *Infect Dis Clin North Am* 17:21-40, 2003.

Davies SF, Sarosi GA: Epidemiological and clinical features of pulmonary blastomycosis, *Semin Resp Infect* 12:206-218, 1997.

Dworkin MS, Duckro AN, Proia L et al: The epidemiology of blastomycosis in Illinois and factors associated with death, *Clin Infect Dis* 41:e107-111, 2005.

Greenberg SB: Serious waterborne and wilderness infections, *Crit Care Clin* 15:387-414, 1999.

Klein BS, Vergeront JM, Weeks RJ et al: Isolation of *Blastomyces dermatitidis* in soil associated with a large outbreak of blastomycosis in Wisconsin, *N Engl J Med* 314:529-534, 1986.

Lemos LB, Baliga M, Guo M: Blastomycosis: the great pretender can also be an opportunist—initial clinical diagnosis and underlying diseases in 123 patients, *Ann Diagn Pathol* 6:194-203, 2002.

Meyer KC, McManus F-J, Maki DG: Overwhelming pulmonary blastomycosis associated with the adult respiratory distress syndrome, *N Engl J Med* 329:1231-1236, 1993.

Reder PA, Neel B: Blastomycosis in otolaryngology: review of a large series, *Laryngoscope* 103:53-58, 1993.

Rose HD, Gingrass DJ: Localized oral blastomycosis mimicking actinomycosis, *Oral Surg Oral Med Oral Pathol* 54:12-14, 1982.

Paracoccidioidomycosis

Bagagli E, Franco M, Bosco S et al: High frequency of *Paracoccidioides brasiliensis* infection in armadillos (*Dasypus novemcinctus*): an ecological study, *Med Mycol* 41:217-223, 2003.

Bethlem EP, Capone D, Maranhao B et al: Paracoccidioidomycosis, *Curr Opin Pulm Med* 5:319-325, 1999.

Bruinmet E, Castaneda E, Restrepo A: Paracoccidioidomycosis: an update, *Clin Microbiol Rev* 6:89-117, 1993.

Godoy H, Reichart PA: Oral manifestations of paracoccidioidomycosis. Report of 21 cases from Argentina, *Mycoses* 46:412-417, 2003.

Gorete dos Santos-Nogueira M, Queiroz-Andrade GM, Tonelli E: Clinical evolution of paracoccidioidomycosis in 38 children and teenagers, *Mycopathologia* 161:73-81, 2006.

Paes de Almeida O, Jorge J, Scully C: Paracoccidioidomycosis of the mouth: an emerging deep mycosis, *Crit Rev Oral Biol Med* 14:268-274, 2003.

San-Blas G: Paracoccidioidomycosis and its etiologic agent *Paracoccidioides brasiliensis*, *J Med Vet Mycol* 31:99-113, 1993.

San-Blas G, Restrepo A, Clemons K et al: Paracoccidioidomycosis, *J Med Vet Mycol* 30(suppl 1):59-71, 1992.

Sposto MR, Mendes-Giannini MJ, Moraes RA et al: Paracoccidioidomycosis manifesting as oral lesions: clinical, cytological and serological investigation, *J Oral Pathol Med* 23:85-87, 1994.

Sposto MR, Scully C, Paes de Almeida O et al: Oral paracoccidioidomycosis: a study of 36 South American patients, *Oral Surg Oral Med Oral Pathol* 75:461-465, 1993.

Coccidioidomycosis

Ampel NM, Dols CL, Galgiani JN: Coccidioidomycosis during human immunodeficiency virus infection: results of a prospective study in a coccidioidal endemic area, *Am J Med* 94:235-240, 1993.

Arnold MG, Arnold JC, Bloom DC et al: Head and neck manifestations of disseminated coccidioidomycosis, *Laryngoscope* 114:747-752, 2004.

Biller JA, Scheuller MC, Eisele DW: Coccidioidomycosis causing massive cervical lymphadenopathy, *Laryngoscope* 114:1892-1894, 2004.

Chiller TM, Galgiani JN, Stevens DA: Coccidioidomycosis, *Infect Dis Clin North Am* 17:41-57, 2003.

Crum NF, Ballon-Landa G: Coccidioidomycosis in pregnancy: case report and review of the literature, *Am J Med* 119:993.e11-993.e17, 2006.

DiCaudo DJ: Coccidioidomycosis: a review and update, *J Am Acad Dermatol* 55:929-942, 2006.

Galgiani JN, Ampel NM, Blair JE et al: Coccidioidomycosis, *Clin Infect Dis* 41:1217-1223, 2005.

Galgiani JN, Catanzaro A, Cloud GA et al: Comparison of oral fluconazole and itraconazole for progressive, nonmeningeal coccidioidomycosis, *Ann Intern Med* 133:676-686, 2000.

Kim A, Parker SS: Coccidioidomycosis: case report and update on diagnosis and management, *J Am Acad Dermatol* 46:743-747, 2002.

Rodriguez RA, Konia T: Coccidioidomycosis of the tongue, *Arch Pathol Lab Med* 129:e4-e6, 2005.

Schneider E, Hajjeh RA, Spiegel RA et al: A coccidioidomycosis outbreak following the Northridge, Calif, earthquake, *J Am Med Assoc* 277:904-908, 1997.

Cryptococcosis

Christianson JC, Engber W, Andes D: Primary cutaneous cryptococcosis in immunocompetent and immunocompromised hosts, *Med Mycol* 41:177-188, 2003.

Leggiadro RJ, Barrett FF, Hughes WT: Extrapulmonary cryptococcosis in immunocompromised infants and children, *Pediatr Infect Dis J* 11:43-47, 1992.

Levitz SM: The ecology of *Cryptococcus neoformans* and the epidemiology of cryptococcosis, *Rev Infect Dis* 13:1163-1169, 1991.

Mehrabi M, Bagheri S, Leonard MK et al: Mucocutaneous manifestation of cryptococcal infection: report of a case and review of the literature, *J Oral Maxillofac Surg* 63:1543-1549, 2005.

Monteil RA, Hofman P, Michiels JF et al: Oral cryptococcosis: case report of salivary gland involvement in an AIDS patient, *J Oral Pathol Med* 26:53-56, 1997.

Namiq AL, Tollefson T, Fan F: Cryptococcal parotitis presenting as a cystic parotid mass: report of a case diagnosed by fine-needle aspiration cytology, *Diagn Cytopathol* 33:36-38, 2005.

Nosanchuk JD, Shoham S, Fries BC et al: Evidence of zoonotic transmission of *Cryptococcus neoformans* from a pet cockatoo to an immunocompromised patient, *Ann Intern Med* 132:205-208, 2000.

Patz EF, Goodman PC: Pulmonary cryptococcosis, *J Thorac Imaging* 7:51-55, 1992.

Perfect JR, Casadevall A: Cryptococcosis, *Infect Dis Clin North Am* 16:837-874, 2002.

Ruhnke M: Mucosal and systemic fungal infections in patients with AIDS, *Drugs* 64:1163-1180, 2004.

Schmidt-Westhausen A, Grunewald T, Reichart PA et al: Oral cryptococcosis in a patient with AIDS. A case report, *Oral Dis* 1:77-79, 1995.

Scully C, Paes De Almeida O: Orofacial manifestations of the systemic mycoses, *J Oral Pathol Med* 21:289-294, 1992.

Subramanian S, Mathai D: Clinical manifestations and management of cryptococcal infection, *J Postgrad Med* 51(suppl 1):S21-S26, 2005.

Yao Z, Liao W, Chen R: Management of cryptococcosis in non-HIV-related patients, *Med Mycol* 43:245-251, 2005.

Zygomycosis

Chayakulkeeree M, Ghannoum MA, Perfect JR: Zygomycosis: the re-emerging fungal infection, *Eur J Clin Microbiol Infect Dis* 25:215-229, 2006.

Gonzalez CE, Rinaldi MG, Sugar AM: Zygomycosis, *Infect Dis Clin North Am* 16:895-914, 2002.

Greenberg RN, Mullane K, van Burik J-AH et al: Posaconazole as salvage therapy for zygomycosis, *Antimicrob Agents Chemother* 50:126-133, 2006.

Huang J-S, Kok S-H, Lee J-J et al: Extensive maxillary sequestration resulting from mucormycosis, *Br J Oral Maxillofac Surg* 43:532-534, 2005.

Jayasuriya NSS, Tilakaratne WM, Amaratunga EAPD et al: An unusual presentation of rhinofacial zygomycosis due to *Cunninghamella* sp. in an immunocompetent patient: a case report and literature review, *Oral Dis* 12:67-69, 2006.

Kyrmizakis DE, Doxas PG, Hajiioannou JK et al: Palate ulcer due to mucormycosis, *J Laryngol Otol* 116:146-147, 2002.

Jones AC, Bentsen TY, Freedman PD: Mucormycosis of the oral cavity, *Oral Surg Oral Med Oral Pathol* 75:455-460, 1993.

Lador N, Polacheck I, Gural A et al: A trifungal infection of the mandible: case report and literature review, *Oral Surg Oral Med Oral Pathol Oral Radiol Endod* 101:451-456, 2006.

Leitner C, Hoffmann J, Zerfowski M et al: Mucormycosis: necrotizing soft tissue lesion of the face, *J Oral Maxillofac Surg* 61:1354-1358, 2003.

O'Neill BM, Alessi AS, George EB et al: Disseminated rhinocerebral mucormycosis: a case report and review of the literature, *J Oral Maxillofac Surg* 64:326-333, 2006.

Roden MM, Zaoutis TE, Buchanan WL et al: Epidemiology and outcome of zygomycosis: a review of 929 reported cases, *Clin Infect Dis* 41:634-653, 2005.

Schütz P, Behbhani JH, Khan ZU et al: Fatal rhino-orbito-cerebral zygomycosis caused by *Apophysomyces elegans* in a healthy patient, *J Oral Maxillofac Surg* 64:1795-1802, 2006.

Spellberg B, Edwards J, Ibrahim A: Novel perspectives on mucormycosis: pathophysiology, presentation and management, *Clin Microbiol Rev* 18:556-569, 2005.

Aspergillosis

Clancy CJ, Nguyen MH: Invasive sinus aspergillosis in apparently immunocompetent hosts, *J Infect* 37:229-240, 1998.

Correa MEP, Soares AB, de Souza CA et al: Primary aspergillosis affecting the tongue of a leukemic patient, *Oral Dis* 9:49-53, 2003.

Falworth MS, Herold J: Aspergillosis of the paranasal sinuses. A case report and radiographic review, *Oral Surg Oral Med Oral Pathol Oral Radiol Endod* 81:255-260, 1996.

Karabulut AB, Kabakas F, Berköz Ö et al: Hard palate perforation due to invasive aspergillosis in a patient with acute lymphoblastic leukemia, *Int J Pediatr Otorhinolaryngol* 69:1395-1398, 2005.

Manuel RJ, Kibbler CC: The epidemiology and prevention of invasive aspergillosis, *J Hosp Infect* 39:95-109, 1998.

Marr KA, Patterson T, Denning D: Aspergillosis: pathogenesis, clinical manifestations, and therapy, *Infect Dis Clin North Am* 16:875-894, 2002.

Myoken Y, Sugata T, Fujita Y et al: Early diagnosis and successful management of atypical invasive *Aspergillus* sinusitis in a hematopoietic cell transplant patient: a case report, *J Oral Maxillofac Surg* 64:860-863, 2006.

Myoken Y, Sugata T, Kyo T-I et al: Pathologic features of invasive oral aspergillosis in patients with hematologic malignancies, *J Oral Maxillofac Surg* 54:263-270, 1996.

Ogata Y, Okinaka Y, Takahashi M: Antrolith associated with aspergillosis of the maxillary sinus: report of a case, *J Oral Maxillofac Surg* 55:1339-1341, 1997.

Rhodes JC, Jensen HE, Nilius AM et al: Aspergillus and aspergillosis, *J Med Vet Mycol* 30(suppl 1):51-57, 1992.

Schubert MS: Allergic fungal sinusitis, *Clin Rev Allergy Immunol* 30:205-216, 2006.

Segal BH, Walsh TJ: Current approaches to diagnosis and treatment of invasive aspergillosis, *Am J Respir Crit Care Med* 173:707-717, 2006.

Toxoplasmosis

Azaz B, Milhem I, Hasson O: Acquired toxoplasmosis of a submandibular lymph node in a 13-year-old boy: case report, *Pediatr Dent* 16:378-380, 1994.

Beasley DM, Egerman RS: Toxoplasmosis, *Semin Perinatol* 22:332-338, 1998.

García-Pola M-J, González-García M, García-Martín JM et al: Submaxillary adenopathy as sole manifestation of toxoplasmosis: case report and literature review, *J Otolaryngol* 31:122-125, 2002.

Luft BJ, Hafner R, Korzun AH et al: Toxoplasmic encephalitis in patients with the acquired immunodeficiency syndrome, *N Engl J Med* 329:995-1000, 1993.

Mamidi A, DeSimone JA, Pomerantz RJ: Central nervous system infections in individuals with HIV-1 infection, *J Neurovirol* 8:158-167, 2002.

Montoya JG, Rosso F: Diagnosis and management of toxoplasmosis, *Clin Perinatol* 32:705-726, 2005.

Moran WJ, Tom DWK, King D et al: Toxoplasmosis lymphadenitis occurring in a parotid gland, *Otolaryngol Head Neck Surg* 94:237-240, 1986.

Rorman E, Zamir CS, Rilkis I et al: Congenital toxoplasmosis—prenatal aspects of *Toxoplasma gondii* infection, *Reprod Toxicol* 21:458-472, 2006.

7

Viral Infections

CHAPTER OUTLINE

HUMAN HERPES VIRUSES

The term **herpes** comes from the ancient Greek word meaning *to creep or crawl*. The human herpesvirus (HHV) family is officially known as **Herpetoviridae**, and its best-known member is **herpes simplex virus (HSV)**, a DNA virus. Two types of HSV are known to exist: type I (HSV-1 or HHV-1) and type 2 (HSV-2 or HHV-2). Other members of the HHV family include **varicella-zoster virus** (VZV or HHV-3), **Epstein-Barr virus** (EBV or HHV-4), **cytomegalovirus** (CMV or HHV-5), and several more recently discovered members, HHV-6, HHV-7, and HHV-8.

Humans are the only natural reservoir for these viruses, which are endemic worldwide and share many features. All eight types cause a primary infection and remain latent within specific cell types for the life of the individual. On reactivation, these viruses are associated with recurrent infections that may be symptomatic or asymptomatic. The viruses are shed in the saliva or genital secretions, providing an avenue for infection of new hosts. Each type is known to transform cells in tissue culture, with several strongly associated with specific malignancies. Of the various types, the following sections will concentrate on the herpes simplex viruses, varicella-zoster virus, cytomegalovirus, and Epstein-Barr virus. Much less is known about herpesvirus types 6, 7, and 8.

Human herpesviruses 6 and **7 (HHV-6, HHV-7)** are closely related, commonly isolated from saliva, usually transmitted by respiratory droplets, and exhibit a prevalence rate of infection close to 90% by age 5 in the United States. Both viruses are associated with a primary infection that usually is asymptomatic but can exhibit an erythematous macular eruption that may demonstrate intermixed slightly elevated papules. The cutaneous manifestation of HHV-6 creates a specific pattern, **roseola (exanthema subitum),** whereas HHV-7 may cause a similar roseola-like cutaneous eruption. The primary latency resides in CD4 T lymphocytes, and reactivation occurs most frequently in immunocompromised patients. Recurrences can result in widespread multiorgan infection, including encephalitis, pneumonitis, bone-marrow suppression, and hepatitis.

Human herpesvirus 8 (HHV-8) appears to be involved in the pathogenesis of **Kaposi's sarcoma (KS)** (see page 557) and has been termed **Kaposi's sarcoma herpesvirus (KSHV).** In patients with normal immune systems, primary infection usually is asymptomatic, with sexual contact (especially male homosexual) being the most common pattern of transmission. The virus has been found without difficulty in saliva, suggesting another possible pattern of transmission. Associated symptoms such as transient fever, lymphadenopathy, and arthralgias are rarely reported.

Circulating B lymphocytes appear to be the major cell of latency. In addition to Kaposi's sarcoma, HHV-8 also has been associated with a small variety of lymphomas and Castleman's disease.

HERPES SIMPLEX VIRUS

The two herpes simplex viruses are similar structurally but different antigenically. In addition, the two exhibit epidemiologic variations.

HSV-1 is spread predominantly through infected saliva or active perioral lesions. HSV-1 is adapted best and performs more efficiently in the oral, facial, and ocular areas. The pharynx, intraoral sites, lips, eyes, and skin above the waist are involved most frequently.

HSV-2 is adapted best to the genital zones, is transmitted predominantly through sexual contact, and typically involves the genitalia and skin below the waist. Exceptions to these rules do occur, and HSV-1 can be seen in a pattern similar to that of HSV-2 and vice versa. The clinical lesions produced by both types are identical, and both produce the same changes in tissue. The viruses are so similar that antibodies directed against one cross-react against the other. Antibodies to one of the types decrease the chance of infection with the other type; if infection does occur, the manifestations often are less severe.

Clinically evident infections with HSV-1 exhibit two patterns. The initial exposure to an individual without antibodies to the virus is called the **primary infection.** This typically occurs at a young age, often is asymptomatic, and usually does not cause significant morbidity. At this point, the virus is taken up by the sensory nerves and transported to the associated sensory or, less frequently, the autonomic ganglia where the virus remains in a latent state. With HSV-1 infection, the most frequent site of latency is the trigeminal ganglion, but other possible sites include the nodose ganglion of the vagus nerve, dorsal root ganglia, and the brain. The virus uses the axons of the sensory neurons to travel back and forth to the peripheral skin or mucosa.

Secondary, recurrent, or **recrudescent HSV-1 infection** occurs with reactivation of the virus, although many patients may show only asymptomatic viral shedding in the saliva. Symptomatic recurrences are fairly common and affect the epithelium supplied by the sensory ganglion. Spread to an uninfected host can occur easily during periods of asymptomatic viral shedding or from symptomatic active lesions. When repeatedly tested, approximately one third of individuals with HSV-1 antibodies occasionally shed infectious viral particles, even without active lesions being present. In addition, the virus may spread to other sites in the same host to establish residency at the sensory ganglion of the new location. Numerous conditions such

as old age, ultraviolet light, physical or emotional stress, fatigue, heat, cold, pregnancy, allergy, trauma, dental therapy, respiratory illnesses, fever, menstruation, systemic diseases, or malignancy have been associated with reactivation of the virus, but only ultraviolet light exposure has been demonstrated unequivocally to induce lesions experimentally. More than 80% of the primary infections are purported to be asymptomatic, and reactivation with asymptomatic viral shedding greatly exceeds clinically evident recurrences.

HSV does not survive long in the external environment, and almost all primary infections occur from contact with an infected person who is releasing the virus. The usual incubation period is 3 to 9 days. Because HSV-1 usually is acquired from contact with contaminated saliva or active perioral lesions, crowding and poor hygiene promote exposure. Lower socioeconomic status correlates with earlier exposure. In developing countries, more than 50% of the population is exposed by 5 years of age, 95% by 15 years of age, and almost universal exposure by 30 years of age. On the other hand, upper socioeconomic groups in developed nations exhibit less than 20% exposure at 5 years of age and only 50% to 60% in adulthood. Regardless of the socioeconomic group, prevalence tends to increase with age, and many investigators report a frequency of prior infection that approaches 90% of the population by age 60. The low childhood exposure rate in the privileged groups is followed by a second peak during the college years of life. The age of initial infection also affects the clinical presentation of the symptomatic primary infections. In symptomatic cases, individuals exposed to HSV-1 at an early age tend to exhibit gingivostomatitis; those initially exposed later in life often demonstrate pharyngotonsillitis.

As mentioned previously, antibodies to HSV-1 decrease the chance of infection with HSV-2 or lessen the severity of the clinical manifestations. The dramatic increase recently seen in HSV-2 is due partly to lack of prior exposure to HSV-1, increased sexual activity, and lack of barrier contraception. HSV-2 exposure correlates directly with sexual activity. Exposure of those younger than age 14 is close to zero, and most initial infections occur between the ages of 15 and 35. The prevalence varies from near zero in celibate adults to more than 80% in prostitutes. Because many of those infected with HSV-2 refrain from sexual activity when active lesions are present, many investigators believe that at least 70% of primary infections are contracted from individuals during asymptomatic viral shedding.

In addition to clinically evident infections, HSV has been implicated in a number of noninfectious processes. More than 15% of cases of **erythema multiforme** are preceded by a symptomatic recurrence of HSV 3 to 10 days earlier (see page 776), and some investigators believe that up to 60% of mucosal erythema multiforme may be triggered by HSV. In some instances, the attacks of erythema multiforme are frequent enough to warrant antiviral prophylaxis. An association with cluster headaches and a number of cranial neuropathies has been proposed, but definitive proof is lacking.

On rare occasions, asymptomatic release of HSV will coincide with attacks of aphthous ulcerations. The ulcerations are not infected with the virus. In these rare cases, the virus may be responsible for the initiation of the autoimmune destruction; conversely, the immune dysregulation that produces aphthae may have allowed the release of the virions. In support of the lack of association between HSV and aphthae in the general population of patients with aphthous ulcerations, prophylactic oral acyclovir does not decrease the recurrence rate of the aphthous ulcerations. Although the association between HSV and recurrent aphthous ulcerations is weak, it may be important in small subsets of patients (see page 331).

HSV also has been associated with oral carcinomas, but much of the evidence is circumstantial. The DNA from HSV has been extracted from the tissues of some tumors but not from others. HSV may aid carcinogenesis through the promotion of mutations, but the oncogenic role, if any, is uncertain.

CLINICAL FEATURES

Acute herpetic gingivostomatitis (primary herpes) is the most common pattern of symptomatic primary HSV infection, and more than 90% are the result of HSV-1. In a study of more than 4000 children with antibodies to HSV-1, Juretić found that only 12% of those infected had clinical symptoms and signs severe enough to be remembered by the affected children or their parents. Some health care practitioners suspect that the percentage of primary infections that exhibit clinical symptoms is much higher, whereas others believe the prevalence is lower. Many primary infections may manifest as pharyngitis that mimics the pattern seen in common colds. Further studies are needed to fully answer this question.

Most cases of acute herpetic gingivostomatitis arise between the ages of 6 months and 5 years, with the peak prevalence occurring between 2 and 3 years of age. In spite of these statistics, occasional cases have been reported in patients over 60 years of age. Development before 6 months of age is rare because of protection by maternal anti-HSV antibodies. The onset is abrupt and often accompanied by anterior cervical lymphadenopathy, chills, fever (103° to 105° F), nausea, anorexia, irritability, and sore mouth lesions. The manifestations vary from mild to severely debilitating.

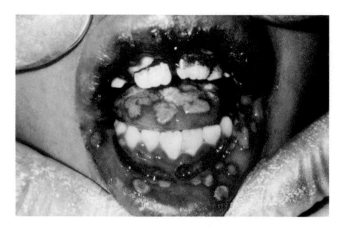

Fig. 7-1   Acute herpetic gingivostomatitis. Widespread yellowish mucosal ulcerations. *(Courtesy of Dr. David Johnsen.)*

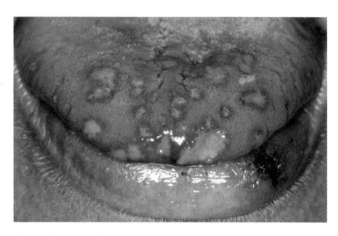

Fig. 7-2   Acute herpetic gingivostomatitis. Numerous coalescing, irregular, and yellowish ulcerations of the dorsal surface of the tongue.

Initially the affected mucosa develops numerous pinhead vesicles, which rapidly collapse to form numerous small, red lesions. These initial lesions enlarge slightly and develop central areas of ulceration, which are covered by yellow fibrin (Fig. 7-1). Adjacent ulcerations may coalesce to form larger, shallow, irregular ulcerations (Fig. 7-2). Both the movable and attached oral mucosa can be affected, and the number of lesions is highly variable. In all cases the gingiva is enlarged, painful, and extremely erythematous (Fig. 7-3). In addition, the affected gingiva often exhibits distinctive punched-out erosions along the midfacial free gingival margins (Fig. 7-4). It is not unusual for the involvement of the labial mucosa to extend past the wet line to include the adjacent vermilion border of the lips. Satellite vesicles of the perioral skin are fairly common. Self-inoculation of the fingers, eyes, and genital areas can occur. Mild cases usually resolve within 5 to 7 days; severe cases may extend to 2 weeks. Rare complications include keratoconjunctivitis, esophagitis, pneumonitis, meningitis, and encephalitis.

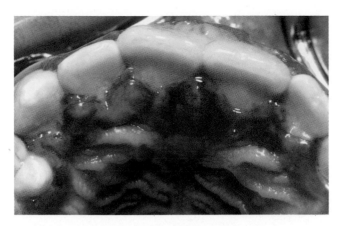

Fig. 7-3   Acute herpetic gingivostomatitis. Painful, enlarged, and erythematous palatal gingiva.

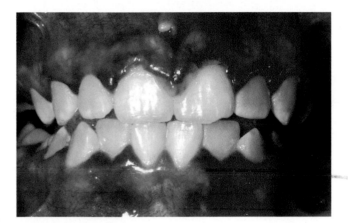

Fig. 7-4   Acute herpetic gingivostomatitis. Painful, enlarged, and erythematous facial gingiva. Note erosions of the free gingival margin.

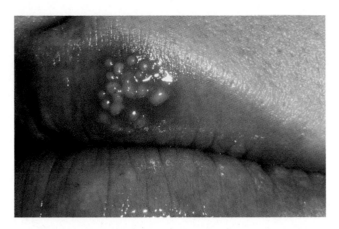

Fig. 7-5   Herpes labialis. Multiple fluid-filled vesicles on the lip vermilion.

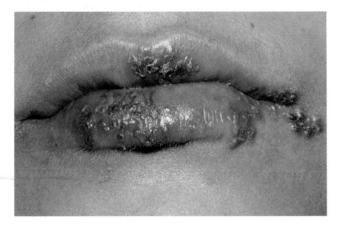

Fig. 7-6   Herpes labialis. Multiple sites of recurrent herpetic infection secondary to spread of viral fluid over cracked lips.

As mentioned previously, when the primary infection occurs in adults, some symptomatic cases exhibit **pharyngotonsillitis.** Sore throat, fever, malaise, and headache are the initial symptoms. Numerous small vesicles develop on the tonsils and posterior pharynx. The vesicles rapidly rupture to form numerous shallow ulcerations, which often coalesce with one another. A diffuse, gray-yellow exudate forms over the ulcers in many cases. Involvement of the oral mucosa anterior to Waldeyer's ring occurs in less than 10% of these cases. HSV appears to be a significant cause of pharyngotonsillitis in young adults who are from the higher socioeconomic groups with previously negative test findings for HSV antibodies. Most of these infections are HSV-1, but increasing proportions are HSV-2. The clinical presentation closely resembles pharyngitis secondary to streptococci or infectious mononucleosis, making the true frequency difficult to determine.

Recurrent herpes simplex infections (secondary herpes, recrudescent herpes) may occur either at the site of primary inoculation or in adjacent areas of surface epithelium supplied by the involved ganglion. The most common site of recurrence for HSV-1 is the vermilion border and adjacent skin of the lips. This is known as **herpes labialis** ("cold sore" or "fever blister"). Prevalence studies suggest that from 15% to 45% of the United States population have a history of herpes labialis. In some patients, ultraviolet light or trauma can trigger recurrences. Prodromal signs and symptoms (e.g., pain, burning, itching, tingling, localized warmth, erythema of the involved epithelium) arise 6 to 24 hours before the lesions develop. Multiple small, erythematous papules develop and form clusters of fluid-filled vesicles (Fig. 7-5). The vesicles rupture and crust within 2 days. Healing usually occurs within 7 to 10 days. Symptoms are most severe in the first 8 hours, and most active viral replication is complete within 48 hours. Mechanical rupture of intact vesicles and the release of the virus-filled fluid may result in the spreading of the lesions on lips previously cracked from sun exposure (Fig. 7-6). Recurrences are observed less commonly on the skin of the nose, chin, or cheek. The

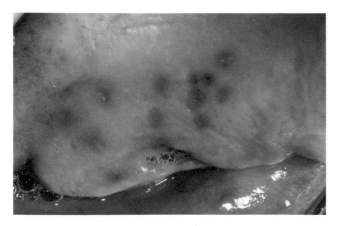

Fig. 7-7   Intraoral recurrent herpetic infection. Early lesions exhibiting as multiple erythematous macules on the hard palate. Lesions appeared a few days after extraction of a tooth.

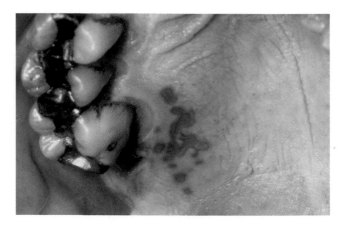

Fig. 7-8   Intraoral recurrent herpetic infection. Multiple coalescing ulcerations on the hard palate.

majority of those affected experience approximately 2 recurrences annually, but a small percentage may experience outbreaks that occur monthly or even more frequently.

On occasion, some lesions arise almost immediately after a known trigger and appear without any preceding prodromal symptoms. These rapidly developing recurrences tend to respond less favorably to treatment.

Recurrences also can affect the oral mucosa. In the immunocompetent patient, involvement is limited almost always to keratinized mucosa that is bound to bone (attached gingiva and hard palate). These sites often exhibit subtle changes, and the symptoms are less intense. The lesions begin as 1- to 3-mm vesicles that rapidly collapse to form a cluster of erythematous macules that may coalesce or slightly enlarge (Figs. 7-7 and 7-8). The damaged epithelium is lost, and a central yellowish area of ulceration develops. Healing takes place within 7 to 10 days.

Less common presentations of HSV-1 do occur. Infection of the thumbs or fingers is known as **herpetic whitlow (herpetic paronychia),** which may occur as a result of self-inoculation in children with orofacial herpes (Fig. 7-9). Before the uniform use of gloves, medical and dental personnel could infect their digits from contact with infected patients, and they were the most likely group affected by this form of HSV-I infection. Recurrences on the digits are not unusual and may result in paresthesia and permanent scarring.

Cutaneous herpetic infections also can arise in areas of previous epithelial damage. Parents kissing areas of dermatologic injury in children represent one vector. Wrestlers and rugby players also may contaminate areas of abrasion, a lesion called **herpes gladiato-**

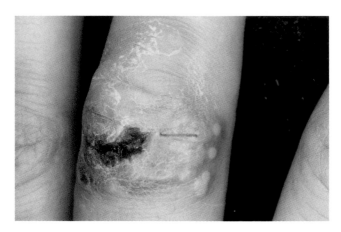

Fig. 7-9   Herpetic whitlow. Recurrent herpetic infection of the finger.

rum or **scrumpox.** On occasion, herpes simplex has been spread over the bearded region of the face into the minor injuries created by daily shaving, leading to a condition known as **herpes barbae** (*barbae* is Latin for "of the beard"). Ocular involvement may occur in children, often resulting from self-inoculation. Patients with diffuse chronic skin diseases, such as eczema, pemphigus, and Darier's disease, may develop diffuse life-threatening HSV infection, known as **eczema herpeticum (Kaposi's varicelliform eruption).** Newborns may become infected after delivery through a birth canal contaminated with HSV, usually HSV-2. Without treatment, there is greater than a 50% mortality rate.

HSV recurrence in immunocompromised hosts can be significant. Without proper immune function, recurrent herpes can persist and spread until the infection is treated with antiviral drugs, until immune status returns, or until the patient dies. On the skin, the lesions

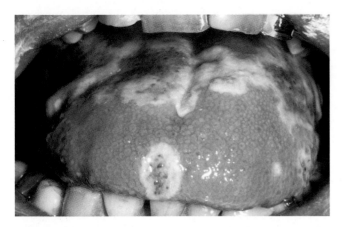

Fig. 7-10 Chronic herpetic infection. Numerous mucosal erosions, each of which is surrounded by a slightly raised, yellow-white border, in a patient with acute myelogenous leukemia.

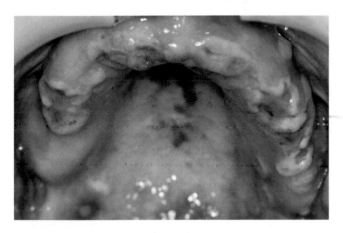

Fig. 7-11 Chronic herpetic infection. Numerous shallow herpetic erosions with raised, yellow and circinate borders on the maxillary alveolar ridge in an immunocompromised patient.

continue to enlarge peripherally, with the formation of an increasing zone of superficial cutaneous erosion. Oral mucosa also can be affected and usually is present in conjunction with herpes labialis. Although most oral mucosal involvement begins on the bound mucosa, it often is not confined to these areas. The involved sites begin as areas of necrotic epithelium that are brownish and raised above the surface of the adjacent intact epithelium. Typically, these areas are much larger than the usual pinhead lesions found in immunocompetent patients. With time, the area of involvement spreads laterally. The enlarging lesion is a zone of superficial necrosis or erosion, often with a distinctive circinate, raised, yellow border (Figs. 7-10 and 7-11). This border represents the advancing margin of active viral destruction. Microscopic demonstration of HSV infection in a chronic ulceration on the movable oral mucosa is

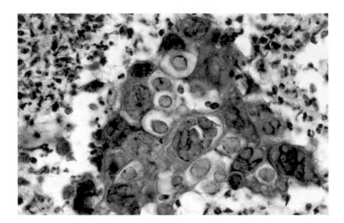

Fig. 7-12 Herpes simplex. Altered epithelial cells exhibiting ballooning degeneration, margination of chromatin, and multinucleation.

ominous, and all such patients should be evaluated thoroughly for possible immune dysfunction or underlying occult disease processes.

Although a yellow curvilinear border often is present in many chronic herpetic ulcerations noted in immunocompromised patients, this distinctive feature might be missing. Several authors have reported persistent oral ulcerations in patients with **acquired immunodeficiency syndrome** (AIDS) that lack the distinctive periphery, often are nonspecific clinically, and may mimic aphthous ulcerations, necrotizing stomatitis, or ulcerative periodontal disease. Biopsy of persistent ulcerations in patients with AIDS is mandatory and may reveal any one of a number of infectious or neoplastic processes. These ulcers may reveal histopathologic evidence of herpesvirus, often combined with diagnostic features of CMV (HHV-5) coinfection (see page 255).

HISTOPATHOLOGIC FEATURES

The virus exerts its main effects on the epithelial cells. Infected epithelial cells exhibit acantholysis, nuclear clearing, and nuclear enlargement, which has been termed **ballooning degeneration** (Fig. 7-12). The acantholytic epithelial cells are termed **Tzanck cells** (not specific for herpes; refers to a free-floating epithelial cell in any intraepithelial vesicle). Nucleolar fragmentation occurs with a condensation of chromatin around the periphery of the nucleus. Multinucleated, infected epithelial cells are formed when fusion occurs between adjacent cells (see Fig. 7-12). Intercellular edema develops and leads to the formation of an intraepithelial vesicle (Fig. 7-13). Mucosal vesicles rupture rapidly; those on the skin persist and develop secondary infiltration by inflammatory cells. Once they have ruptured, the mucosal lesions demonstrate a

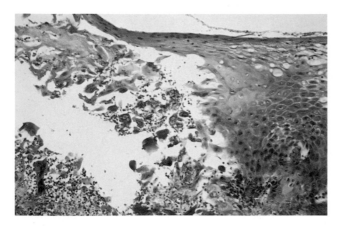

Fig. 7-13   Herpes simplex. Intraepithelial vesicle demonstrating acantholytic and virally altered epithelial cells.

surface fibrinopurulent membrane. Often at the edge of the ulceration or mixed within the fibrinous exudate are the scattered Tzanck or multinucleated epithelial cells.

DIAGNOSIS

With a thorough knowledge of the clinical presentations, the clinician can make a strong presumptive diagnosis of HSV infection. On occasion, HSV infections can be confused with other diseases, and laboratory confirmation is desirable. Viral isolation from tissue culture inoculated with the fluid of intact vesicles is the most definitive diagnostic procedure. The problem with this technique in primary infections is that up to 2 weeks can be required for a definitive result. Laboratory tests to detect HSV antigens by direct fluorescent assay or viral DNA by polymerase chain reaction (PCR) of specimens of active lesions also are available. Serologic tests for HSV antibodies are positive 4 to 8 days after the initial exposure. Confirmation of primary infection by serology requires a specimen obtained within 3 days of the presentation and a second sample approximately 4 weeks later. In such cases the initial specimen should be negative, with antibodies discovered only in the convalescent sample. These antibody titers are useful in documenting past exposure and are used primarily in epidemiologic studies.

Intact vesicles are rare intraorally. Therefore, using intraoral viral culture as the sole means of diagnostic confirmation of HSV infection is inappropriate. Research has shown that asymptomatic oral HSV shedding occurs in up to 9% of the general population. During periods of mental or physical stress, asymptomatic viral shedding rises to approximately one third of those previously exposed to the virus. In immunocompromised patients, the prevalence rises to 38%; this percentage is low and most likely would double if the investigation were restricted to those previously exposed to the virus. Therefore, culture of lesions contaminated with saliva that might contain coincidentally released HSV is meaningless unless supplemented by additional diagnostic procedures.

Two of the most commonly used diagnostic procedures are the cytologic smear and tissue biopsy, with cytologic study being the least invasive and most cost-effective. The virus produces distinctive histopathologic alterations within the infected epithelium. Only VZV produces similar changes, but these two infections usually can be differentiated on a clinical basis. Fluorescent monoclonal antibody typing can be performed on the direct smears or on infected cells obtained from tissue culture.

If diagnostic features of herpesvirus are discovered in a biopsy of a persistent ulceration in an immunocompromised patient, immunocytochemical studies for CMV also should be performed to rule out coinfection. The histopathologic features of CMV can be missed easily, resulting in patients not receiving the most appropriate therapy.

TREATMENT AND PROGNOSIS

In the past, primary herpetic gingivostomatitis was treated best symptomatically; however, if the infection is diagnosed early, antiviral medications can have a significant influence. Patients should be instructed to restrict contact with active lesions to prevent the spread to other sites and people. As mentioned previously, autoinoculation of the eyes can result in ocular involvement with the possibility of recurrence. Repeated ocular reinfection can produce permanent damage and blindness. HSV is the leading infectious cause of blindness in the United States.

When acyclovir suspension is initiated during the first 3 symptomatic days in a rinse-and-swallow technique five times daily for 5 days (children: 15 mg/kg up to the adult dose of 200 mg), significant acceleration in clinical resolution is seen. Once therapy is initiated, development of new lesions ceases. In addition, the associated eating and drinking difficulties, pain, healing time, duration of fever, and viral shedding are shortened dramatically. The use of a topical spray with 0.5% or 1.0% dyclonine hydrochloride also dramatically, but temporarily, decreases the mucosal discomfort. Compounding pharmacists also can provide tetracaine lollipops that can be used for rapid and profound numbing of the affected mucosa. Viscous lidocaine and topical benzocaine should be avoided in pediatric patients because of reports of lidocaine-induced seizures in children and an association between topical benzocaine and methemoglobinemia.

Nonsteroidal antiinflammatory drugs (NSAIDs), such as ibuprofen, also help alleviate the discomfort. Use of antiviral medications in capsule or tablet form is much less effective because of the increased time these formulations require to exert a significant effect.

Recurrent herpes labialis has been treated with everything from ether to voodoo; nothing has solved the problem for all patients. Of the antiherpetic medications, acyclovir ointment in polyethylene glycol was the initial formulation available for topical therapy. Acyclovir ointment has been of limited benefit for herpes labialis in immunocompetent patients, because its base is thought to prevent significant absorption. Subsequently, penciclovir cream became available in a base that allows increased absorption through the vermilion border. Use of this formulation has resulted in a statistically significant, although clinically minimal, reduction in healing time and pain (duration decreased approximately 1 day). Although the best results are obtained if use of penciclovir cream is initiated during the prodrome, late application has produced a measurable clinical benefit. Other current choices are acyclovir cream and an over-the-counter formulation of 10% n-docosanol cream. Although acyclovir cream does appear more effective than n-docosanol, both of these therapeutic choices are associated with statistically significant, but clinically minimal, reduction in healing time and pain, but at a lesser degree than that associated with penciclovir cream.

Systemic acyclovir and the two newer related medications, valacyclovir and famciclovir, appear to demonstrate similar effectiveness against HSV. However, valacyclovir and famciclovir exhibit improved bioavailability and more convenient oral dosing schedules. Of the three medications, a dosing schedule with valacyclovir, consisting of an initial 2 g taken on recognition of prodromal symptoms followed by another 2 g 12 hours later, has been most successful in minimizing the recurrences. The effects of this treatment are reduced significantly if it is not initiated during the prodrome. Although much less convenient, 400 mg of acyclovir taken five times daily for 5 days appears to produce similar results. For patients whose recurrences appear to be associated with dental procedures, a regimen of 2 g of valacyclovir taken twice on the day of the procedure and 1 g taken twice the next day may suppress or minimize any associated attack. In individuals with a known trigger that extends over a period of time (e.g., skiing, beach vacation), prophylactic short-term use of one of the antivirals (acyclovir, 400 mg twice a day [b.i.d.]; valacyclovir 1 g daily; or famciclovir 250 mg b.i.d.) has been shown to reduce the prevalence and severity of any associated recurrence.

Most cases of recurrent herpes labialis are infrequent; therefore, rarely can regular use of systemic antiviral medications be justified in immunocompetent individuals. Long-term suppression of recurrences with an antiviral medication is reserved by many for patients with more than six recurrences per year, those suffering from HSV-triggered erythema multiforme, and the immunocompromised. In recent years the emergence of acyclovir-resistant HSV has been seen with increasing frequency. Such resistance has arisen almost exclusively in immunocompromised patients receiving intermittent therapy, and the use of prophylactic therapy does not appear to be associated with emergence of resistant strains. In immunocompromised patients, the viral load tends to be high and replication is not suppressed completely by antiviral therapy, creating the environment for generating drug-resistant mutants. Although resistance is seen primarily in immunocompromised patients, cavalier use of antiviral medications for mild cases of recurrent herpes infection probably is inappropriate.

The pain associated with intraoral secondary herpes usually is not intense, and many patients do not require treatment. Some studies have shown chlorhexidine to exert antiviral effects *in vivo* and *in vitro*. In addition, acyclovir appears to function synergistically with chlorhexidine. Extensive clinical trials have not been performed, but chlorhexidine alone or in combination with acyclovir suspension may be beneficial in patients who desire or require therapy of intraoral lesions.

Immunocompromised hosts with HSV infections often require intravenous (IV) antiviral medications to control the problem. Furthermore, severely immunosuppressed individuals, such as bone marrow transplant patients and those with AIDS, often need prophylactic doses of oral acyclovir, valacyclovir, or famciclovir. On occasion, viral resistance develops, resulting in the onset of significant herpetic lesions. Any herpes lesions that do not respond to appropriate therapy within 5 to 10 days most likely are the result of resistant strains. At this point the initial antiviral therapy should be repeated at an elevated dose. If this intervention fails, IV trisodium phosphonoformate hexahydrate (foscarnet) is administered. If the infection persists, IV cidofovir is recommended. Another antiviral, adenine arabinoside (vidarabine), is reserved for patients in whom all of the previously described medications have failed. In resistant cases that have been treated successfully, it appears that only the peripheral virus mutates, because future recurrences often are once again sensitive to the first-line antivirals. Ulcerations that reveal coinfection with HSV and CMV respond well to ganciclovir, with foscarnet used in refractory cases.

Although a successful live-virus vaccine has been available for the closely related varicella virus for over 25 years, similar approaches against HSV have produced less satisfactory results. Significant research for a potential vaccine is ongoing and offers hope for the future.

VARICELLA (CHICKENPOX)

The **varicella-zoster virus** (VZV, HHV-3) is similar to herpes simplex virus (HSV) in many respects. **Chickenpox** represents the primary infection with the VZV; latency ensues, and recurrence is possible as **herpes zoster,** often after many decades. The virus is presumed to be spread through air droplets or direct contact with active lesions. Most cases of chickenpox arise between the ages of 5 and 9, with greater than 90% of the U.S. population being infected by 15 years of age. In contrast to infection with HSV, most cases are symptomatic. The incubation period is 10 to 21 days, with an average of 15 days.

CLINICAL FEATURES

The symptomatic phase of VZV infection usually begins with malaise, pharyngitis, and rhinitis. In older children and adults, additional symptoms (e.g., headache, myalgia, nausea, anorexia, vomiting) occasionally are seen. This is followed by a characteristic, intensely pruritic exanthem. The rash begins on the face and trunk, followed by involvement of the extremities. Each lesion rapidly progresses through stages of erythema, vesicle, pustule, and hardened crust (Figs. 7-14 and 7-15). The early vesicular stage is the classic presentation. The centrally located vesicle is surrounded by a zone of erythema and has been described as "a dewdrop on a rose petal." In contrast to herpes simplex, the lesions typically continue to erupt for 4 days; in some cases the exanthem's arrival may extend to 7 or more days. Old crusted lesions intermixed with newly formed and intact vesicles are commonplace. Affected individuals are contagious from 2 days before the exanthem until all the lesions crust. Fever usually is present during the active phase of the exanthem. The severity of the cutaneous involvement is variable and often more severe in adults and in household members secondarily infected by the initial patient.

Perioral and oral manifestations are fairly common and may precede the skin lesions. The vermilion border of the lips and the palate are the most common sites of involvement, followed by the buccal mucosa. Occasionally, gingival lesions resemble those noted in primary HSV infections, but distinguishing between the two is not difficult because the lesions of varicella tend to be relatively painless. The lesions begin as 3- to 4-mm, white, opaque vesicles that rupture to form 1- to 3-mm ulcerations (Fig. 7-16). The prevalence and number of the oral lesions correlate with the severity of

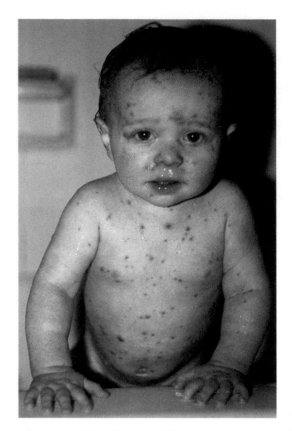

Fig. 7-14   Varicella. Infant with diffuse erythematous and vesicular rash. *(Courtesy of Dr. Sherry Parlanti.)*

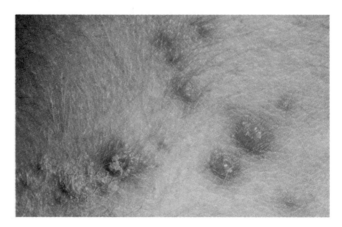

Fig. 7-15   Varicella. Numerous vesicles with surrounding erythema and early crusting.

the extraoral infection. In mild cases, oral lesions are present in about one third of affected individuals. Often only 1 or 2 oral ulcers are evident, and typically these heal within 1 to 3 days. In contrast, patients with severe infections almost always have oral ulcerations, often numbering up to 30 lesions and persisting for 5 to 10 days. In severe cases of chickenpox, old ruptured lesions will often become intermixed with fresh vesicles.

Complications can occur, with the need for hospitalization in children approximating 1 in 600 in the

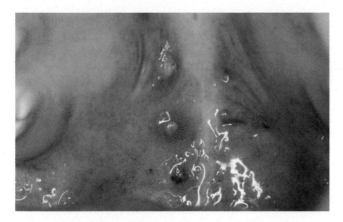

Fig. 7-16   Varicella. White opaque vesicles on the hard palate. (*Courtesy of Tristan Neville.*)

prevaccine era. Possible complications include Reye's syndrome, secondary skin infections, encephalitis, cerebellar ataxia, pneumonia, gastrointestinal disturbances (e.g., vomiting, diarrhea, associated dehydration), and hematologic events (i.e., thrombocytopenia, pancytopenia, hemolytic anemia, sickle cell crisis).

In childhood the most frequent complications are secondary skin infections, followed by encephalitis and pneumonia. With enhanced public education and decreased use of aspirin in children, the prevalence of Reye's syndrome is decreasing. Although associated bacterial infections had decreased after the introduction of antibiotics, an increased prevalence of significant complications related to secondary infections caused by group A, β-hemolytic streptococci was seen during the 1990s. These organisms have created life-threatening infections and areas of highly destructive necrotizing fasciitis.

The prevalence of complications in adults exceeds that noted in children. The most common and serious complication is varicella pneumonitis, which features dry cough, tachypnea, dyspnea, hemoptysis, chest pain, and cyanosis. Encephalitis and clinically significant pneumonia are diagnosed in 1 in 375 affected adults older than 20 years of age. The central nervous system (CNS) involvement typically produces ataxia but may result in headaches, drowsiness, convulsions, or coma. The risk of death is reported to be 15 times greater in adults compared with children, mostly because of an increased prevalence of encephalitis.

Infection during pregnancy can produce congenital or neonatal chickenpox. Involvement early in the pregnancy can result in spontaneous abortion or congenital defects. Although complications can occur in newborns, the effects of maternal varicella infection appear minimal. A multicenter prospective study of live births associated with maternal varicella infection revealed only a 1.2% prevalence of embryopathy. However, infection of the mother close to delivery can result in a severe fetal infection caused by a lack of maternal antibodies.

Infection in immunocompromised patients also can be most severe. The cutaneous involvement typically is extensive and may be associated with high fever, hepatitis, pneumonitis, pancreatitis, gastrointestinal obstruction, and encephalitis. Before effective antiviral therapy, the mortality rate in immunocompromised individuals was approximately 7%. Secondary bacterial infections often complicate the process.

HISTOPATHOLOGIC FEATURES

The cytologic alterations are virtually identical to those described for HSV. The virus causes acantholysis, with formation of numerous free-floating Tzanck cells, which exhibit nuclear margination of chromatin and occasional multinucleation.

DIAGNOSIS

The diagnosis of chickenpox usually can be made from a history of exposure to VZV within the last 3 weeks and the presence of the typical exanthem. Confirmation can be obtained through a demonstration of viral cytopathologic effects present within the epithelial cells harvested from the vesicular fluid. These cytologic changes are identical to those found in herpes simplex, and further confirmation sometimes is desired. Viral isolation in cell culture or rapid diagnosis from fluorescein-conjugated VZV monoclonal antibodies can be performed. Finally, serum samples can be obtained during the acute stage and 14 to 28 days later. The later sample should demonstrate a significant (fourfold) increase in antibody titers to VZV.

TREATMENT AND PROGNOSIS

Before the current antiviral medications became available, the treatment of varicella primarily was symptomatic. Warm baths with soap or baking soda, application of calamine lotion, and systemic diphenhydramine still are used to relieve pruritus. VZV has a lipid envelope that is destroyed rapidly by soap and other detergents. Lotions with diphenhydramine are not recommended because of reports of toxicity secondary to percutaneous absorption of the medication. Antipyretics other than aspirin should be given to reduce fever.

Use of peroral antiviral medications such as acyclovir, valacyclovir, and famciclovir has been shown to reduce the duration and severity of the infection if it is administered within the first 24 hours of the rash. Routine use of these antiviral medications is not recommended in immunocompetent children with uncomplicated chickenpox. Typically, such therapy is reserved for patients at risk for more severe disease, such as those over 13 years of age and individuals who contract the disease from a family member. Intravenous formulations are used in immunosuppressed patients or those exhibiting a progressive, severe infection. Treatment with one of the available antiviral medications does not alter the antibody response to VZV or reduce immunity later in life.

In patients without evidence of immunity who become exposed to VZV and are at high risk for severe disease or complications, purified varicella-zoster immune globulin can be given to modify the clinical manifestations of the infection. Individuals at risk include immunocompromised patients, pregnant women, premature infants, and neonates whose mothers do not have evidence of immunity. The U.S.-licensed manufacturer of the immune globulin marketed the material under the name VZIG but discontinued production in October 2004. At the time of this writing, the immune globulin is being made by a Canadian company and is known as *VariZIG*. This product has not completed full U.S. Food and Drug Administration (FDA) approval and is currently classified as an investigational new drug (IND). In an attempt to improve access during this critical period of transition, an expanded access protocol has been approved by a central institutional review board (IRB), with the FDA not requiring additional local IRB approval at the treatment site. VariZIG is most effective if administered within 96 hours of initial exposure. In most instances the material can be delivered from the distributor to the treatment site within 24 hours.

A live attenuated varicella vaccine has been available since 1974 and has been used extensively outside the United States, especially in Japan. In 1995 the vaccine was approved for use in the United States. Before that time, the annual incidence of infection in the United States was approximately 4 million, with an associated 11,000 hospitalizations and 100 deaths. Vaccination is recommended for children between 12 and 18 months of age, as well as for all susceptible individuals over the age of 13. Although the vaccination rates vary by state, the national coverage is approximately 85% and has led to a reduction of reported infection rates that also is around 85%.

During the first year after vaccination, the efficacy appears to be 100% but drops to 95% after 7 years. When breakthrough infections do occur, they usually are very mild. Because of continued exposure to wild virus, previously vaccinated patients have not required boosters to maintain immunity. As the prevalence of the wild virus diminishes, booster vaccines may be required to maintain lifelong immunity. Extensive

follow-up of vaccinated groups is ongoing; if antibody levels wane with time, booster immunizations will be recommended. It should be remembered that the vaccine is a live virus that can be spread to individuals in close contact. Vaccine recipients who develop a rash should avoid contact with those at risk, such as immunocompromised or pregnant individuals.

The national health objectives for 2010 included a goal to obtain and maintain ≥95% vaccination coverage among first graders for hepatitis B, diphtheria, tetanus, pertussis, poliovirus, measles, mumps, rubella, and varicella. The measles, mumps, and rubella (MMR) vaccine currently has achieved a 93% vaccination rate, whereas the frequency for the varicella vaccine remains below 90%. Use of a combined measles, mumps, rubella, and varicella (MMRV) vaccine has demonstrated comparable effectiveness and safety. This approach would provide protection via a single injection and have the potential to increase the vaccination rate for varicella more rapidly.

HERPES ZOSTER (SHINGLES)

After the initial infection with VZV (chickenpox), the virus is transported up the sensory nerves and presumably establishes latency in the dorsal spinal ganglia. Clinically evident **herpes zoster** occurs after reactivation of the virus, with the involvement of the distribution of the affected sensory nerve. Zoster occurs during the lifetime of 10% to 20% of individuals, and the prevalence of attacks increases with age. With the increasing average age of the population, an increased prevalence of herpes zoster is expected. Unlike herpes simplex virus (HSV), single rather than multiple recurrences are the rule. Immunosuppression, HIV-infection, treatment with cytotoxic or immunosuppressive drugs, radiation, presence of malignancies, old age, alcohol abuse, stress (emotional or physical), and dental manipulation are predisposing factors for reactivation.

CLINICAL FEATURES

The clinical features of herpes zoster can be grouped into three phases: (1) prodrome, (2) acute, and (3) chronic. During initial viral replication, active ganglionitis develops with resultant neuronal necrosis and severe neuralgia. This inflammatory reaction is responsible for the prodromal symptoms of intense pain that precedes the rash in more than 90% of the cases. As the virus travels down the nerve, the pain intensifies and has been described as burning, tingling, itching, boring, prickly, or knifelike. The pain develops in the area of epithelium innervated by the affected sensory nerve (dermatome). Typically, one dermatome is affected, but involvement of two or more can occur. The tho-

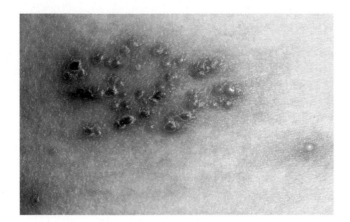

Fig. 7-17   Herpes zoster. Cluster of vesicles with surrounding erythema of the skin.

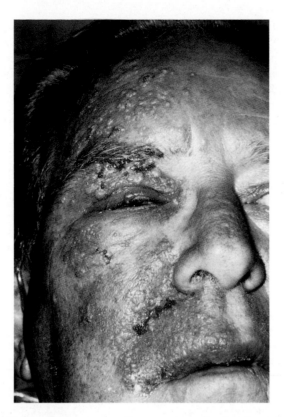

Fig. 7-18   Herpes zoster. Numerous crusting facial vesicles that extend to the midline.

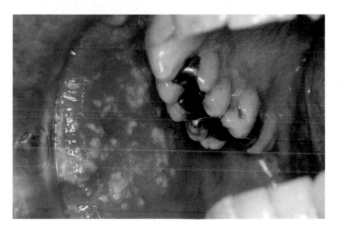

Fig. 7-19   Herpes zoster. Numerous white opaque vesicles on the right buccal mucosa of the same patient depicted in Fig. 7-18.

racic dermatomes are affected in about two thirds of cases. This prodromal pain, which may be accompanied by fever, malaise, and headache, normally is present 1 to 4 days before the development of the cutaneous or mucosal lesions. During this period (before the exanthem) the pain may masquerade as sensitive teeth, otitis media, migraine headache, myocardial infarction, or appendicitis, depending on which dermatome is affected.

Approximately 10% of affected individuals will exhibit no prodromal pain. Conversely, on occasion there may be recurrence in the absence of vesiculation of the skin or mucosa. This pattern is called **zoster sine herpete** (zoster without rash), and affected patients have severe pain of abrupt onset and hyperesthesia over a specific dermatome. Fever, headache, myalgia, and lymphadenopathy may or may not accompany the recurrence.

The acute phase begins as the involved skin develops clusters of vesicles set on an erythematous base (Fig. 7-17). Within 3 to 4 days, the vesicles become pustular and ulcerate, with crusts developing after 7 to 10 days. The lesions tend to follow the path of the affected nerve and terminate at the midline (Fig. 7-18). The exanthem typically resolves within 2 to 3 weeks in otherwise healthy individuals. On healing, scarring with hypopigmentation or hyperpigmentation is not unusual.

Oral lesions occur with trigeminal nerve involvement and may be present on the movable or bound mucosa. The lesions often extend to the midline and frequently are present in conjunction with involvement of the skin overlying the affected quadrant. Like varicella, the individual lesions manifest as 1- to 4-mm, white, opaque vesicles that rupture to form shallow ulcerations (Fig. 7-19). Involvement of the maxilla may be associated with devitalization of the teeth in the affected area.

Several reports have documented significant bone necrosis with loss of teeth in areas involved with herpes zoster. Because of the close anatomic relationship between nerves and blood vessels within neurovascular bundles, inflammatory processes within nerves have the potential to extend to adjacent vessels. It is postulated that the gnathic osteonecrosis may be secondary to damage of the blood vessels supplying the alveolar ridges and teeth, leading to focal ischemic necrosis. Of the reported cases, there is almost an equal distribution between the maxilla and mandible, with both sexes affected similarly. Although the average patient age is approximately 55, a wide range has been seen from the second to late eighth decade. The average interval between the appearance of the exanthem and the osteonecrosis is 21 days, but it has been reported as late as 42 days.

Ocular involvement is not unusual and can be the source of significant morbidity, including permanent blindness. The ocular manifestations are highly variable and may arise from direct viral-mediated epithelial damage, neuropathy, immune-mediated damage, or secondary vasculopathy. If the tip of the nose is involved, this is a sign that the nasociliary branch of the fifth cranial nerve is involved, suggesting the potential for ocular infection. In these cases, referral to an ophthalmologist is mandatory.

Facial paralysis has been seen in association with herpes zoster of the face or external auditory canal. **Ramsay Hunt syndrome** is the combination of cutaneous lesions of the external auditory canal and involvement of the ipsilateral facial and auditory nerves. The syndrome causes facial paralysis, hearing deficits, vertigo, and a number of other auditory and vestibular symptoms. In multiple studies of patients thought to have Bell's palsy (see page 859), evidenced of active VZV infection was detected in approximately 30% of patients by polymerase chain reaction (PCR) or via demonstration of appropriate antibody titers, suggesting an underlying viral cause for many cases of "idiopathic" facial paralysis. Similar associations also have been demonstrated with HSV and EBV.

Approximately 15% of affected patients progress to the chronic phase of herpes zoster, which is characterized by pain **(postherpetic neuralgia)** that persists longer than 3 months after the initial presentation of the acute rash. Postherpetic neuralgia is uncommon in individuals under the age of 50 but affects at least 50% of patients older than 60 years of age. The pain is described as burning, throbbing, aching, itching, or stabbing, often with flares caused by light stroking of the area or from contact with adjacent clothing. Most of these neuralgias resolve within 1 year, with half of the patients experiencing resolution after 2 months. Rare cases may last up to 20 years, and patients have been known to commit suicide as a result of the severe, lancinating quality of the pain. Although the cause is unknown, some investigators believe chronic VZV ganglionitis is responsible. Clearance of the pain has been reported within days after initiation of long-term famciclovir, with recurrence of the pain if the medication is stopped. Additional double-blind, placebo-controlled studies will need to be performed to confirm this observation.

HISTOPATHOLOGIC FEATURES

The active vesicles of herpes zoster are identical microscopically to those seen in the primary infection, varicella. For more information, refer to the previous portions of the chapter on the histopathologic presentation of varicella and herpes simplex.

DIAGNOSIS

The diagnosis of herpes zoster often can be made from the clinical presentation, but other procedures may be necessary in atypical cases. Viral culture can confirm the clinical impression but takes at least 24 hours. Cytologic smears demonstrate viral cytopathologic effects, as seen in varicella and HSV. In most cases the clinical presentation allows the clinician to differentiate zoster from HSV, but cases of zosteriform recurrent HSV infection, although uncommon, do exist. A rapid diagnosis can be obtained through the use of direct staining of cytologic smears with fluorescent monoclonal antibodies for VZV. This technique gives positive results in almost 80% of the cases. Molecular techniques such as dot-blot hybridization and PCR also can be used to detect VZV.

TREATMENT AND PROGNOSIS

Before the development of the current antiviral medications, therapy for herpes zoster was directed toward supportive and symptomatic measures. Fever should be treated with antipyretics that do not contain aspirin. Antipruritics, such as diphenhydramine, can be administered to decrease itching. Skin lesions should be kept dry and clean to prevent secondary infection; antibiotics may be administered to treat such secondary infections.

Early therapy with appropriate antiviral medications such as acyclovir, valacyclovir, and famciclovir has been found to accelerate healing of the cutaneous and mucosal lesions, reduce the duration of the acute pain, and decrease the duration of postherpetic neuralgia. These medications are most effective if initiated within 72 hours after development of the first vesicle. The newer generation of antiviral drugs, famciclovir and valacyclovir, may be more successful than acyclovir in reducing the prevalence of postherpetic neuralgia.

Once the skin lesions have healed, the neuralgia may become the worst aspect of the disease and often is the most difficult to resolve successfully. This intense pain has been treated with variable results by a variety of methods, including analgesics, narcotics, tricyclic antidepressants, anticonvulsants, gabapentin, percutaneous electric nerve stimulation, biofeedback, nerve blocks, and topical anesthetics. As mentioned previously, postherpetic neuralgia may be related to chronic VZV ganglionitis and respond to long-term famciclovir. In those who do not respond to famciclovir, IV acyclovir often leads to clinical improvement.

One topical treatment, capsaicin, has had significant success, with almost 80% of patients experiencing some pain relief; however, the medication's effect often does not occur until 2 weeks or more of therapy. Capsaicin is derived from red peppers and is not recommended for placement on mucosa or open cutaneous lesions. Capsaicin has been associated with significant burning, stinging, and redness in 40% to 70% of patients, with up to 30% discontinuing therapy because of this side effect. After use, patients must be warned to wash their hands and avoid contact with mucosal surfaces.

Corticosteroid therapy has been used in the hope it might decrease the neural inflammation and associated chronic pain. Although conflicting research has been published, studies have shown no long-term benefit when corticosteroids are added to an acyclovir regimen. In addition, an increased prevalence of side effects was noted in groups treated with corticosteroids.

A live attenuated VZV vaccine has been approved for use in adults 60 years of age or older. The vaccine, Zostavax, is 14 times more potent than Varivax, the vaccine for chickenpox. In a study of more than 38,000 adults, Zostavax markedly decreased the prevalence of herpes zoster, as well as the morbidity and frequency of postherpetic neuralgia in those who did develop the infection. In an October 2006 press release, the Advisory Committee on Immunization Practices of the Centers for Disease Control and Prevention (CDC) recommended that the vaccine be given to all people 60 years of age and older. This recommendation is being reviewed and becomes official only when published in the CDC's *Morbidity and Mortality Weekly Report.*

INFECTIOUS MONONUCLEOSIS (MONO; GLANDULAR FEVER; "KISSING DISEASE")

Infectious mononucleosis is a symptomatic disease resulting from exposure to Epstein-Barr virus (EBV, HHV-4). The infection usually occurs by intimate contact. Intrafamilial spread is common, and once a person is exposed, EBV remains in the host for life. Children usually become infected through contaminated saliva on fingers, toys, or other objects. Adults usually contract the virus through direct salivary transfer, such as shared straws or kissing, hence, the nickname "kissing disease." Exposure during childhood usually is asymptomatic, and most symptomatic infec-

tions arise in young adults. In developing nations, exposure usually occurs by age 3 and is universal by adolescence. In the United States, introduction to the virus often is delayed, with close to 50% of college students lacking previous exposure. These unexposed adults become infected at a rate of 10% to 15% per year while in college. Infection in adulthood is associated with a higher risk (i.e., 30% to 50%) for symptomatic disease.

Besides infectious mononucleosis, EBV has been demonstrated in the lesions of **oral hairy leukoplakia** (OHL) (see page 268) and has been associated with a number of lymphoproliferative disorders, a variety of lymphomas (most notably African Burkitt's lymphoma) (see page 600), nasopharyngeal carcinoma (see page 428), some gastric carcinomas, possibly breast and hepatocellular carcinomas, salivary lymphoepithelial carcinomas, and occasional smooth muscle tumors. However, direct proof of a cause-and-effect relationship is lacking.

CLINICAL FEATURES

Most EBV infections in children are asymptomatic. In children younger than 4 years of age with symptoms, most have fever, lymphadenopathy, pharyngitis, hepatosplenomegaly, and rhinitis or cough. Children older than 4 years of age are affected similarly but exhibit a much lower prevalence of hepatosplenomegaly, rhinitis, and cough.

Most young adults experience fever, lymphadenopathy, pharyngitis, and tonsillitis. Hepatosplenomegaly and rash are seen less frequently. In adults older than 40 years of age, fever and pharyngitis are the predominant findings, with less than 30% demonstrating lymphadenopathy. Less frequent signs and symptoms in this group include hepatosplenomegaly, rash, and rhinitis or cough. Possible significant complications include splenic rupture, thrombocytopenia, autoimmune hemolytic anemia, aplastic anemia, and neurologic problems with seizures. These complications are uncommon at any age but more frequently develop in children.

In classic infectious mononucleosis in a young adult, prodromal fatigue, malaise, and anorexia occur up to 2 weeks before the development of pyrexia. The body temperature may reach 104° F and lasts from 2 to 14 days. Prominent lymphadenopathy is noted in more than 90% of the cases and typically appears as enlarged, symmetrical, and tender nodes, frequently with involvement of the posterior and anterior cervical chains. Enlargement of parotid lymphoid tissue rarely has been reported and can be associated with facial nerve palsy. More than 80% of affected young adults have oropharyngeal tonsillar enlargement, sometimes with diffuse surface exudates and secondary tonsillar

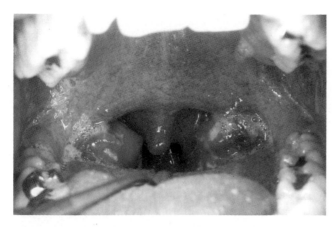

Fig. 7-20   Infectious mononucleosis. Hyperplastic pharyngeal tonsils with yellowish crypt exudates. *(Courtesy of Dr. George Blozis.)*

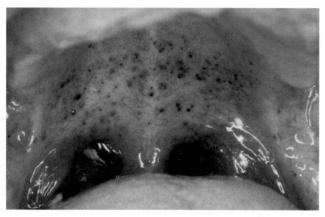

Fig. 7-21   Infectious mononucleosis. Numerous petechiae of the soft palate. *(Courtesy of Dr. George Blozis.)*

abscesses (Fig. 7-20). The lingual tonsils, which are located on the base of the tongue and extend from the circumvallate papilla to the epiglottis, can become hyperplastic and compromise the airway. Rare fatalities have been reported from respiratory difficulties secondary to the combined effects of hyperplasia of the lingual and palatine tonsils, arytenoid hypertrophy, pharyngeal edema, uvular edema, and epiglottal swelling.

Oral lesions other than lymphoid enlargement also may be seen. Petechiae on the hard or soft palate are present in about 25% of patients (Fig. 7-21). The petechiae are transient and usually disappear within 24 to 48 hours. **Necrotizing ulcerative gingivitis (NUG)** (see page 157) also is fairly common. NUG-like pericoronitis (see page 171) and necrotizing ulcerative mucositis (see page 158) occur less frequently. Cases of NUG that are refractory to normal therapy should be evaluated to rule out the possibility of EBV.

A controversial symptom complex called **chronic fatigue syndrome** has been described, and several investigators have tried to associate EBV with this problem. Patients complain of rather nonspecific symptoms of chronic fatigue, fever, pharyngitis, myalgias, headaches, arthralgias, paresthesias, depression, and cognitive defects. These patients often demonstrate elevations in EBV antibody titers, but this finding alone is insufficient to prove a definite cause-and-effect relationship. Several studies have cast serious doubt on a relationship between EBV and the chronic fatigue syndrome.

DIAGNOSIS

The diagnosis of infectious mononucleosis is suggested by the clinical presentation and should be confirmed through laboratory procedures. The white blood cell (WBC) count is increased, with the differential count showing relative lymphocytosis that can become as high as 70% to 90% during the second week. Atypical lymphocytes usually are present in the peripheral blood. The classic serologic finding in mononucleosis is the presence of Paul-Bunnell heterophil antibodies (immunoglobulins that agglutinate sheep erythrocytes). A rapid test for these antibodies is available and inexpensive. More than 90% of infected young adults have positive findings for the heterophil antibody, but infected children younger than age 4 frequently have negative results. Indirect immunofluorescent testing to detect EBV-specific antibodies should be used in those suspected of having an EBV infection but whose findings were negative on the Paul-Bunnell test. Enzyme-linked immunosorbent assays (ELISA) and recombinant DNA-derived antigens also may be used in place of the indirect immunofluorescent test.

TREATMENT AND PROGNOSIS

In most cases, infectious mononucleosis resolves within 4 to 6 weeks. Non–aspirin-containing antipyretics and NSAIDs can be used to minimize the most common symptoms. Infrequent complications include splenic rupture, EBV-related hepatitis, and Bell's palsy. Patients with significant enlargement of the spleen should avoid contact sports to prevent the rare possibility of splenic rupture. On occasion, the fatigue may become chronic. In immunocompromised patients, a polyclonal B-lymphocyte proliferation may occur and possibly lead to death.

The tonsillar involvement may, on occasion, resemble streptococcal pharyngitis or tonsillitis (see page 183). However, treatment with ampicillin and penicillin should be avoided because the use of these antibiotics in infectious mononucleosis has been associated with a higher than normal prevalence of allergic morbilliform skin rashes.

Corticosteroid use is the recommended therapy in many textbooks. Such drugs, however, should not be used indiscriminately because the person's immune response appears to be the most important factor in fighting the infection and preventing a potentially fatal polyclonal B-lymphocyte proliferation. In addition, an increased prevalence of encephalitis and myocarditis has been noted in patients who have infectious mononucleosis and are treated with steroids. Corticosteroid use produces a shortened duration of fever and shrinkage of enlarged lymphoid tissues, but its use should be restricted to life-threatening cases (e.g., those with upper-airway obstruction because of massive lymphadenopathy, tonsillar hyperplasia, and oropharyngeal edema). If corticosteroid therapy fails to resolve the airway obstruction, acute tonsillectomy and tracheostomy may be necessary.

Although antiviral medications such as acyclovir, valacyclovir, and famciclovir have been used successfully for temporary resolution of oral hairy leukoplakia, these medications do not demonstrate clinically obvious benefit for patients with infectious mononucleosis. Although the medications most likely have an effect on viral replication, the main clinical manifestations appear to be secondary to the immune response to EBV-infected activated B lymphocytes and are not altered by the medical intervention.

CYTOMEGALOVIRUS

Cytomegalovirus (CMV, HHV-5) is similar to the other human herpes viruses (i.e., after the initial infection, latency is established and reactivation is possible under conditions favorable to the virus). CMV can reside latently in salivary gland cells, endothelium, macrophages, and lymphocytes. Most clinically evident disease is found in neonates or in immunosuppressed adults. In infants, the virus is contracted through the placenta, during delivery, or during breast-feeding. The next peak of transmission occurs during adolescence, predominantly from the exchange of bodily fluids as this group begins sexual activity. Transmission also has been documented from blood transfusion and organ transplantation. The prevalence of neonatal CMV infection varies from 0.5% to 2.5%. By the age of 30, almost 40% of the population is infected; by age 60, 80% to 100% are infected. Screening of healthy middle-aged adult blood donors reveals that approximately 50% have been exposed to CMV.

CLINICAL FEATURES

At any age, almost 90% of CMV infections are asymptomatic. In clinically evident neonatal infection, the infant appears ill within a few days. Typical features include hepatosplenomegaly, extramedullary cutaneous erythropoiesis, and thrombocytopenia (often with

associated petechial hemorrhages). Significant encephalitis frequently leads to severe mental and motor retardation.

Although the majority of acute CMV infections are asymptomatic, less than 10% may include a nonspecific pattern of symptoms that ranges from an influenza-like presentation to lethal multiorgan involvement. In a review of 115 hospitalized immunocompetent adults with CMV infection, the most common symptoms (in order) include fever, joint and muscle pain, shivering, abdominal pain, nonproductive cough, cutaneous eruption (maculopapular rash), and diarrhea. Associated signs include hepatomegaly, splenomegaly, adenopathy, pharyngitis, jaundice, and evidence of meningeal irritation. The authors stress that symptomatic CMV infection should not be dismissed in immunocompetent patients and should be considered in any patient with unexplained persistent fever.

In contrast to patients with infectious mononucleosis, only about one third of patients with CMV infection demonstrate pharyngitis and lymphadenopathy. Rarely, immunocompetent patients may show signs of an acute sialadenitis that diffusely involves all of the major and minor salivary glands. In such cases, xerostomia often is noted and the affected glands are painful. Involvement of the major glands usually results in clinically obvious enlargements of the parotid and submandibular glands. Unusual complications of primary CMV infection include myocarditis, pneumonitis, and septic meningitis.

Evident CMV involvement is not unusual in immunocompromised transplant patients. In some cases a temporary mild fever is the only evidence; in others, the infection becomes aggressive and is characterized by significant hepatitis, leukopenia, pneumonitis, gastroenteritis, and, more rarely, a progressive wasting syndrome.

CMV disease is common in patients with AIDS (see page 264). CMV chorioretinitis affects almost one third of patients with AIDS and tends to progress rapidly, often resulting in blindness. Bloody diarrhea from CMV colitis is fairly common but may respond to appropriate antiviral medications.

Although oral lesions from CMV infection have been documented in a number of immunosuppressive conditions, reports of oral involvement by CMV have been increasing since the advent of the AIDS epidemic. Most affected patients have chronic mucosal ulcerations, and CMV changes are found on biopsy. Occasionally, chronic oral ulcerations in immunocompromised patients will demonstrate coinfection (usually CMV combined with HSV).

Neonatal CMV infection also can produce developmental tooth defects. Examination of 118 people with a history of neonatal CMV infection revealed tooth

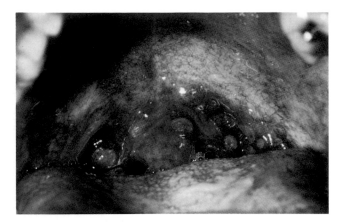

Fig. 7-23   Herpangina. Numerous aphthouslike ulcerations of the soft palate.

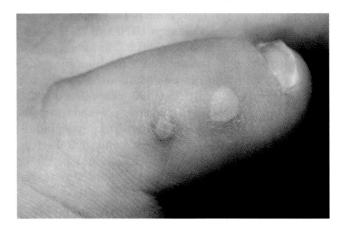

Fig. 7-24   Hand-foot-and-mouth disease. Multiple vesicles of the skin of the toe. *(Courtesy of Dr. Samuel J. Jasper.)*

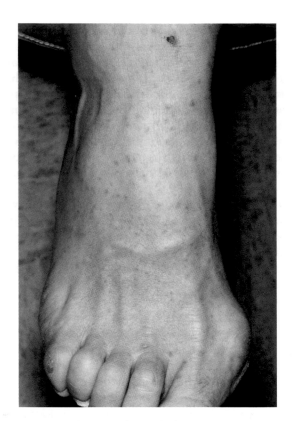

Fig. 7-25   Hand-foot-and-mouth disease. Numerous erythematous macules of the foot.

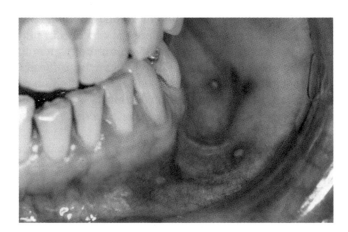

Fig. 7-26   Hand-foot-and-mouth disease. Multiple aphthouslike ulcerations of the mucobuccal fold.

ally accompanied by cough, rhinorrhea, anorexia, vomiting, diarrhea, myalgia, and headache.

The name fairly well describes the location of the lesions. Oral lesions and those on the hands almost always are present; involvement of other cutaneous sites is more variable. The oral lesions arise without prodromal symptoms and precede the development of the cutaneous lesions. Sore throat and mild fever are present. The cutaneous lesions range from a few to dozens and primarily affect the borders of the palms and soles and the ventral surfaces and sides of the fingers and toes (Fig. 7-24). Rarely other sites, especially the buttocks, external genitals, and legs, may be involved. The individual cutaneous lesions begin as erythematous macules that develop central vesicles and heal without crusting (Fig. 7-25).

The oral lesions resemble those of herpangina but may be more numerous and are not confined to the posterior areas of the mouth. The number of lesions ranges from 1 to 30. The buccal mucosa, labial mucosa, and tongue are the most common sites to be affected, but any area of the oral mucosa may be involved (Fig.

7-26). The individual vesicular lesions rapidly ulcerate and are typically 2 to 7 mm in diameter but may be larger than 1 cm. Most of these ulcerations resolve within 1 week.

ACUTE LYMPHONODULAR PHARYNGITIS

Acute lymphonodular pharyngitis is characterized by sore throat, fever, and mild headache, which may last from 4 to 14 days. Low numbers (one to five) of yellow to dark-pink nodules develop on the soft palate or ton-

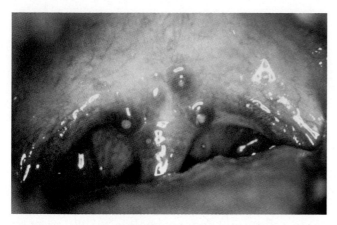

Fig. 7-27 Acute lymphonodular pharyngitis. Numerous dark-pink and yellow lymphoid aggregates. *(Courtesy of Dr. George Blozis.)*

sillar pillars (Fig. 7-27). The nodules represent hyperplastic lymphoid aggregates and resolve within 10 days without vesiculation or ulceration. Few cases have been described, and whether this represents a distinct clinical entity is as yet unresolved. The possibility that the sore throat and palatal lymphoid hyperplasia represent features of herpangina or some other infection cannot be excluded without further documentation of additional cases.

HISTOPATHOLOGIC FEATURES

In patients with herpangina and hand-foot-and-mouth disease, the areas of affected epithelium exhibit intracellular and intercellular edema, which leads to extensive spongiosis and the formation of an intraepithelial vesicle. The vesicle enlarges and ruptures through the epithelial basal cell layer, with the resultant formation of a subepithelial vesicle. Epithelial necrosis and ulceration soon follow. Inclusion bodies and multinucleated epithelial cells are absent.

DIAGNOSIS

The diagnoses of herpangina, hand-foot-and-mouth disease, and acute lymphonodular pharyngitis usually are made from the distinctive clinical manifestations. In patients with atypical presentations, laboratory confirmation appears prudent. Viral isolation from culture can be performed, and analysis of stool specimens is the best technique in patients with only mucosal lesions. Throat culture findings tend to be positive predominantly during the early acute stage. The culture of cutaneous lesions is best for the diagnosis of hand-foot-and-mouth disease. A serologic demonstration of rising enteroviral antibody titers between the acute and convalescent stages can be used to confirm the diagnosis in questionable cases. Polymerase chain reaction (PCR)

assay is increasingly available and replacing viral culture in many diagnostic laboratories.

TREATMENT AND PROGNOSIS

In most instances, the infection is self-limiting and without significant complications. Therapy for patients with an enterovirus infection is directed toward symptomatic relief. Nonaspirin antipyretics and topical anesthetics, such as dyclonine hydrochloride, often are beneficial.

Occasionally, certain strains produce infections with a more aggressive clinical course. During the 1998 epidemic in Taiwan, a large group of physicians reported 405 patients with severe disease and 78 deaths. Patients with more significant complications demonstrated higher body temperature (>102° F), fever for longer than 3 days, more serious vomiting, and greater lethargy. When these findings are present, the physician must monitor the patient more closely for the development of more serious complications.

RUBEOLA (MEASLES)

Rubeola is an infection produced by a virus in the family Paramyxovirus, genus *Morbillivirus,* and exhibits a variable prevalence that is correlated to the degree of vaccine use. Measles vaccine has been in wide use in the United States since 1963 and is 95% effective, resulting in a 98% reduction in the prevalence of this infection. Before 1963, virtually all children acquired measles, but the vaccine produced a continued and significant decline until the late 1980s. From 1989 to 1991, a major resurgence occurred with an increasing proportion of cases among unvaccinated preschool-aged children, particularly minority residents of densely populated urban areas. In addition, a smaller number of cases appeared to be associated with vaccine failure.

CLINICAL FEATURES

Most cases of measles arise in the winter and are spread through respiratory droplets. The incubation period is from 10 to 12 days, and affected individuals are infectious from 2 days before becoming symptomatic until 4 days after appearance of the associated rash. The virus is associated with significant lymphoid hyperplasia that often involves sites such as the lymph nodes, tonsils, adenoids, and Peyer's patches. Giant cell infiltration is noted in various tissues along with a vasculitis that is responsible for the characteristic skin rash.

There are three stages of the infection, with each stage lasting 3 days and justifying the designation *nineday measles.* The first 3 days are dominated by the three

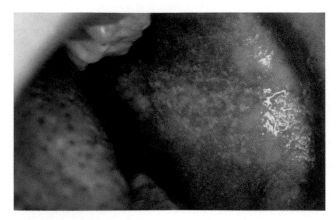

Fig. 7-28   Rubeola. Numerous blue-white Koplik's spots of buccal mucosa. *(Courtesy of Dr. Robert J. Achterberg.)*

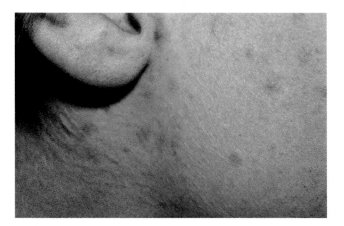

Fig. 7-29   Rubeola. Erythematous maculopapular rash of the face. *(Courtesy of Dr. Robert J. Achterberg.)*

Cs: **C**oryza (runny nose), **C**ough (typically brassy and uncomfortable), and **C**onjunctivitis (red, watery, and photophobic eyes). Fever typically accompanies these symptoms. During this initial stage, the most distinctive oral manifestation, **Koplik's spots,** is seen. Multiple areas of mucosal erythema are visible on the buccal and labial mucosa, and less often on the soft palate; within these areas are numerous small, blue-white macules (Fig. 7-28). In addition, similar spots rarely are noted on the inner conjunctival folds of the eye or the vaginal mucosa. These pathognomonic spots represent foci of epithelial necrosis and have been described as "grains of salt" on a red background.

As the second stage begins, the fever continues, the Koplik's spots fade, and a maculopapular and erythematous (morbilliform) rash begins. The face is involved first, with eventual downward spread to the trunk and extremities. Ultimately, a diffuse erythematous maculopapular eruption is formed, which tends to blanch on pressure (Fig. 7-29). Abdominal pain secondary to lymphatic involvement is not rare.

In the third stage, the fever ends. The rash begins to fade and demonstrates a similar downward progression with replacement by a brown pigmentary staining. Ultimately, desquamation of the skin is noted in the areas previously affected by the rash.

Common complications in young children are otitis media, pneumonia, persistent bronchitis, and diarrhea. Acute appendicitis occasionally is seen secondary to vascular obstruction created by the swelling of Peyer's patches. Encephalitis develops in approximately 1 in 1000 cases, often resulting in death or permanent brain damage and mental retardation. In about 1 in 100,000 cases, a delayed complication termed **subacute sclerosing panencephalitis** (SSPE) arises as late as 11 years after the initial infection. This degenerative disorder of the CNS leads to personality changes, seizures, coma, and death. Widespread vaccine use has virtually eliminated SSPE in developed nations. In the United States, one to two deaths occur for every 1000 reported cases of measles. In developing countries, the infection often is more severe, and the case-to-fatality rate can be as high as 25%. The most common causes of death are pneumonia and acute encephalitis.

Measles in immunocompromised patients can be serious, with a high risk of complications and death. Most of these patients exhibit either an atypical rash or no exanthem. Pneumonitis is the primary complication. The fatality rate of measles in patients with a malignancy is greater than 50%; AIDS-associated measles results in the death of more than one third of affected patients.

Koplik's spots are not the only oral manifestation that may be associated with measles. Candidiasis, necrotizing ulcerative gingivitis (NUG), and necrotizing stomatitis may occur if significant malnutrition also is present. Severe measles in early childhood can affect odontogenesis and result in pitted enamel hypoplasia of the developing permanent teeth. Enlargement of accessory lymphoid tissues such as the lingual and pharyngeal tonsils also may be noted.

HISTOPATHOLOGIC FEATURES

Because of the reduced prevalence of measles and the transient nature of Koplik's spots, few oral and maxillofacial pathologists have had the opportunity to view these lesions microscopically. Initially, Koplik's spots represent areas of focal hyperparakeratosis in which the underlying epithelium exhibits spongiosis, intercellular edema, dyskeratosis, and epithelial syncytial giant cells. The number of nuclei within these giant cells ranges from three to more than 25. Close examination of the epithelial cells often reveals pink-staining inclusions in the nuclei or, less commonly, in the cytoplasm.

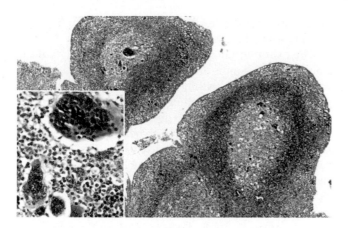

Fig. 7-30   Rubeola. Histopathologic section of pharyngeal tonsil demonstrating lymphoid hyperplasia with scattered multinucleated giant cells. *Inset* reveals high-power magnification of Warthin-Finkeldey giant cells.

On electron microscopy, the inclusions have been shown to represent microtubular aggregates characteristic of the causative paramyxovirus. As the spot ages, the epithelium exhibits heavy exocytosis by neutrophils leading to microabscess formation, epithelial necrosis, and, ultimately, ulceration. Frequently, examination of the epithelium adjacent to the ulceration will reveal the suggestive syncytial giant cells.

Examination of hyperplastic lymphoid tissue during the prodromal stage of measles often reveals a similar alteration. In 1931, Warthin and Finkeldey, in two separate publications, reported an unusual finding in patients who had their tonsils removed within 1 to 5 days of the clinical appearance of measles. Within the hyperplastic lymphoid tissue, there were numerous multinucleated giant lymphocytes (Fig. 7-30). These multinucleated cells subsequently have been termed **Warthin-Finkeldey giant cells** and were thought for a time to be specific for measles. Since that time, however, similar-appearing cells have been noted in a variety of lymphoproliferative conditions such as lymphoma, Kimura's disease, AIDS-related lymphoproliferative disease, and lupus erythematosus.

DIAGNOSIS

The diagnosis of typical measles in an epidemic setting usually is straightforward and based on the clinical features and history. Laboratory confirmation can be of value in isolated or atypical cases. Viral isolation or rapid detection of viral antigens is possible, but confirmation usually is established through a demonstration of rising serologic antibody titers. The antibodies appear within 1 to 3 days after the beginning of the exanthem and peak in about 3 to 4 weeks.

TREATMENT AND PROGNOSIS

With a complication rate of 21%, the best treatment for measles is a good vaccination program; rubeola is part of the widely used MMR vaccine. In an attempt to stop the resurgence of measles that began in 1989, the vaccination schedule was altered and the pockets of young, unvaccinated children were targeted. This action brought the transmission of indigenous measles to record lows. Although the number is variable from year to year, since 1993 the annual incidence of reported cases in the United States typically is well below 500. Total eradication of the infection is technically feasible with existing vaccines but will require universal cooperation and enthusiasm from across the globe. Renewed emphasis in the noncompliant sections of society must be stressed. In addition, a new two-dose vaccination schedule has been adopted in an attempt to decrease the vaccine failures. Currently, routine vaccination is recommended for all children between the ages of 12 and 15 months, with a second dose administered between the ages of 4 and 6 years.

In otherwise healthy patients with measles, fluids and nonaspirin antipyretics are recommended for symptomatic relief. Immunocompromised patients also may be treated with one of a number of medications that have shown promise but definitively have not been proven to be efficacious. The most promising is ribavirin; however, immunoglobulin, interferon, and vitamin A also are being used.

RUBELLA (GERMAN MEASLES)

Rubella is a mild viral illness that is produced by a virus in the family Togavirus, genus *Rubivirus*. The greatest importance of this infection lies not in its effects on those who contract the acute illness, but in its capacity to induce birth defects in the developing fetus. The infection occurs primarily in the winter and spring, is contracted through respiratory droplets, and it is transmitted to nearly 100% of individuals in close living conditions. The incubation time is from 14 to 21 days, and infected patients are contagious from 1 week before the exanthem to about 5 days after the development of the rash. Infants with a congenital infection may release virus for up to 1 year.

In the past, this infection occurred in cycles, with localized epidemics every 6 to 9 years and pandemics every 10 to 30 years. The last pandemic occurred from 1962 to 1964. In 1964 and 1965, the United States alone had more than 12.5 million cases, which resulted in more than 10,000 fetal deaths (direct effects or secondary to therapeutic abortions) and 20,000 infants born with **congenital rubella syndrome** (CRS).

An effective vaccine, first released in 1969, is used widely and has dramatically affected the epidemiology of the infection and broken the cycle of occurrences. The vaccine is contraindicated in the following groups:

- Pregnant women
- Immunodeficient patients
- Patients with acute febrile illnesses
- Patients with a known allergy to components of the vaccine

Researchers postulated that the protection of children also would eliminate the risk of exposure to women in the childbearing years. A 99% decrease in the infection was seen between 1969 and 1988, but young adults remain susceptible. Like rubeola, 1989 and 1990 demonstrated a slight resurgence of rubella, which was the result of a lack of vaccination diligence. More than 70% of the current cases occur in patients older than 15 years of age, and 10% to 25% of young adults remain susceptible. Of course, this should change when the previously vaccinated children grow into adults. For the present, the vaccination of postpubertal females must be stressed. Persons are presumed to be immune if they have received at least one dose of the MMR or were born before 1957. For pregnant females who have not received the vaccine, their immunity should be confirmed by demonstration of serum rubella IgG.

Initially, a single dose of the vaccine was thought to be sufficient to confer permanent immunity. Continued immunity appears to be permanent only if exposure to the virus occurs periodically, essentially serving as "booster doses." With almost total vaccination coverage throughout the population of the United States, reexposures are not occurring and immunity is waning. To combat this loss of immunity in a highly vaccinated population, additional boosters may become necessary. Already, two doses of MMR vaccine are recommended, the first at 12 to 15 months of age and the second at the age of 4 to 6 years. Some believe a third dose may become necessary in the future.

CLINICAL FEATURES

A large percentage of infections are asymptomatic; the frequency of symptoms is greater in adolescents and adults. Prodromal symptoms may be seen 1 to 5 days before the exanthem and include fever, headache, malaise, anorexia, myalgia, mild conjunctivitis, coryza, pharyngitis, cough, and lymphadenopathy. The lymphadenopathy may persist for weeks and is noted primarily in the suboccipital, postauricular, and cervical chains. The most common complication is arthritis, which increases in frequency with age and usually

arises subsequent to the rash. Rare complications include encephalitis and thrombocytopenia.

The exanthematous rash is often the first sign of the infection and begins on the face and neck, with spread to the entire body within 1 to 3 days. The rash forms discrete pink macules, then papules, and finally fades with flaky desquamation. The rash fades as it spreads and often exhibits facial clearing before the completion of its spread into the lower body areas. Generally, the rash is resolved completely by day 3, giving rise to the designation *three-day measles*.

Oral lesions, known as **Forchheimer's sign,** have been reported to be present in about 20% of the cases. These consist of small, discrete, dark-red papules that develop on the soft palate and may extend onto the hard palate. This enanthem arises simultaneously with the rash, becoming evident in about 6 hours after the first symptoms and not lasting longer than 12 to 14 hours. Palatal petechiae also may occur.

The risk of CRS correlates with the time of infection. The frequency of transmission from an infected mother is greater than 80% during the first 12 weeks of pregnancy, with the risk of fetal damage decreasing dramatically at 8 weeks and becoming rare after 20 weeks of gestation. The classic triad of CRS consists of deafness, heart disease, and cataracts. Deafness is the most common manifestation, affecting more than 80% of patients. This hearing loss may not become evident until 2 years of age and usually is bilateral. Less common, late emerging complications include encephalopathy, mental retardation, diabetes mellitus, and thyroid disorders.

DIAGNOSIS

The diagnosis of rubella is contingent on laboratory tests because the clinical presentation of the acquired infection is typically subclinical, mild, or nonspecific. Although viral culture is possible, serologic analysis is the mainstay of diagnosis.

TREATMENT AND PROGNOSIS

Rubella is mild, and therapy usually is not required. Nonaspirin antipyretics and antipruritics may be useful in patients with significant fever or symptomatic cutaneous involvement. Passive immunity may be provided by the administration of human rubella immunoglobulin. If immunoglobulin is given within a few days of exposure, it decreases the severity of the infection. This therapy typically is reserved for pregnant patients who decline abortion.

During the 1962 to 1965 worldwide rubella epidemic, the estimated number of infections in the United States was 12.5 million. These infections were associated with 20,000 infants born with CRS, 11,250 fetal deaths, and 2100 neonatal deaths. Because of the two-dose vaccination schedule with the MMR and at least 95% vaccination coverage among school-aged children, in 2004, rubella was declared no longer to be endemic in the United States. The annual reported incidence of rubella was 23 in 2001, 18 in 2002, 7 in 2003, and 9 in 2004. Approximately half of these infections occurred in individuals born outside the United States. Likewise, from 2001 to 2004, only four cases of CRS were reported, and three of the mothers of these infants were not born in the United States.

MUMPS (EPIDEMIC PAROTITIS)

Mumps is an infection caused by a virus in the family Paramyxovirus, genus *Rubulavirus,* which causes a diffuse disease of exocrine glands. Although the salivary glands are the best known sites of involvement, the pancreas, choroid plexus, and mature ovaries and testes also frequently are involved. The involved glands exhibit edema and lymphocytic infiltration. As with measles and rubella, the epidemiology has been affected dramatically by the MMR vaccine. Before the advent of widespread vaccination, epidemics were seen every 2 to 5 years; nearly everyone was exposed with 90% of the infections occurring before age 15. The vaccine directed against mumps was released in 1967, but its use was not accepted nationally until 1977. At that time, vaccination became the norm for children 12 to 15 months of age. The vaccine has a success rate of 75% to 95%. Most individuals born before 1957 are thought to have immunity from exposure to naturally occurring mumps virus. Although most authorities assume that natural infection is associated with lifelong immunity, rare cases of recurrent mumps have been well documented in patients with a confirmed history of prior natural infection.

The annual incidence of mumps decreased by 98% and reached an all-time low in 1985. In 1986 a resurgence developed. In the past, most cases occurred in children aged 5 to 9 years; during the resurgence, the disease was more prevalent in 10- to 19-year-old patients. Outbreaks have been reported in high schools, on college campuses, and in the workplace. This increased incidence has been attributed to lack of vaccination, not vaccine failure. Subsequently, in the early 1990s, isolated outbreaks were reported in highly vaccinated populations and thought to be the result of large-scale vaccination failure. Not long after these reports, a second immunization as part of the MMR vaccine was recommended at 4 to 6 years of age. When compared with the prevaccine era, the two-dose MMR vaccination schedule has reduced the prevalence of mumps by 99%. In addition, in an attempt to decrease the prevalence in the older age groups, it is recommended that individuals lacking a history of mumps or MMR vaccination be immunized. This primarily affects those born between 1967 and 1977 and, to a lesser extent, those born between 1957 and 1967. For health care workers born before 1957, a single dose of MMR is recommended unless there is a physician's diagnosis of mumps or laboratory evidence of mumps immunity.

In 2006 an outbreak of mumps virus occurred in the United States, with an epicenter in Iowa and surrounding states. During this outbreak, only 7% of infected individuals were proven to be unvaccinated, and 49% had received at least the recommended two doses of the MMR. After two doses of MMR, the vaccine appears to be 98% effective against measles but only 90% effective against mumps. In spite of the vaccine failures in the recent outbreak, the high vaccination coverage most likely prevented thousands of additional cases of mumps. Some investigators wonder if such outbreaks may lead to a recommendation for a third dose of the MMR vaccine in the future.

The mumps virus can be transmitted through urine, saliva, or respiratory droplets. The incubation period usually is 16 to 18 days, with a range of about 2 to 4 weeks. Patients are contagious from 1 day before the clinical appearance of infection to 14 days after its clinical resolution.

CLINICAL FEATURES

Approximately 30% of mumps infections are subclinical. In symptomatic cases, prodromal symptoms of low-grade fever, headache, malaise, anorexia, and myalgia arrive first. Most frequently, these nonspecific findings are followed within 1 day by significant salivary gland changes. The parotid gland is involved most frequently, but the sublingual and submandibular glands also can be affected. Discomfort and swelling develop in the tissues surrounding the lower half of the external ear and extending down along the posterior inferior border of the adjacent mandible (Fig. 7-31). The enlargement typically peaks within 2 to 3 days, and the pain is most intense during this period of maximal enlargement. Chewing movements of the jaw or eating saliva-stimulating foods tends to increase the pain. Enlargement of the glands usually begins on one side and is followed by contralateral glandular changes within a few days. Unilateral involvement is seen in about 25% of patients.

The second most common finding is epididymo-orchitis, which occurs in about 25% of postpubertal males. In those affected the testicle exhibits rapid swelling, with significant pain and tenderness. The enlargement can range from a minimal swelling to a

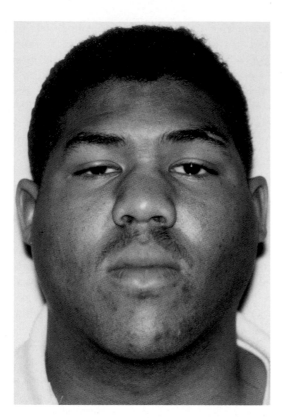

Fig. 7-31   Mumps. Bilateral parotid enlargement. *(From Neville BW, Damm DD, White DK: Color atlas of clinical oral pathology, ed 2, Hamilton, 1999, BC Decker.)*

fourfold increase in size. Unilateral involvement is most common. On resolution of the swelling, atrophy occurs in the affected testicle. Permanent sterility from testicular changes is rare. Less commonly, oophoritis and mastitis can be seen in postpubertal females. In addition, spontaneous abortion occurs in approximately 25% of women who contract mumps during the first trimester of pregnancy.

Less commonly, meningoencephalitis (from involvement of the choroid plexus), cerebellar ataxia, hearing loss, pancreatitis, arthritis, carditis, and decreased renal function may occur. The most common symptom associated with CNS involvement is headache, whereas involvement of the pancreas can lead to nausea and vomiting. Isolated changes, such as orchitis or meningitis, may occur in the absence of salivary gland involvement, thereby making diagnosis difficult in nonepidemic settings. Mumps-related mortality is exceedingly rare and most frequently associated with mumps encephalitis.

The most frequently reported oral manifestation is redness and enlargement of Wharton's and Stensen's salivary gland duct openings. In addition, involvement of the sublingual gland may produce bilateral enlargements of the floor of the mouth.

DIAGNOSIS

The diagnosis of mumps can be made easily from the clinical presentation when the infection is occurring in an epidemic fashion; however, isolated cases must be differentiated from other causes. The most frequently used confirmatory measures are demonstration of mumps-specific IgM or a fourfold rise of mumps-specific IgG titers when measured during the acute phase and about 2 weeks later. In addition, a swab of secretions obtained from parotid or other affected salivary gland ducts can be used for viral isolation or reverse-transcriptase–polymerase chain reaction testing.

TREATMENT AND PROGNOSIS

The treatment of mumps is palliative in nature. Frequently, nonaspirin analgesics and antipyretics are administered. In an attempt to minimize orchitis, bed rest is recommended for males until the fever breaks. Avoidance of sour foods and drinks helps to decrease the salivary gland discomfort. As with measles and rubella, the best results come from prior vaccination, thereby preventing the infection.

HUMAN IMMUNODEFICIENCY VIRUS AND ACQUIRED IMMUNODEFICIENCY SYNDROME

During the last 2 decades, more articles have been written on **human immunodeficiency virus** (HIV) and its related disease states than any other infectious process. A complete bibliography alone easily would be thicker than this chapter. Entire texts dedicated to HIV infection and **acquired immunodeficiency syndrome** (AIDS) are available and should be consulted for more detailed information.

The first cases of AIDS reported in the United States were documented by the Centers for Disease Central and Prevention (CDC) in the *Morbidity and Mortality Weekly Report* on June 5, 1981. This publication detailed *Pneumocystis carinii* pneumoniae in five previously healthy men from Los Angeles, California. More than 25 years have passed. During this time, 65 million individuals worldwide have become infected with HIV and more than 25 million individuals have died of AIDS. Through 2004, a total of 529,113 deaths as a result of AIDS in the United States have been reported to the CDC, and more than 1 million individuals are living with HIV. Worldwide in 2005 alone, 4.1 million new infections occurred, 38.6 million were living with HIV, and an estimated 2.8 million individuals died of AIDS.

At the time of publication of the first edition of this text, the infection was thought to be nearly 100% fatal. Through treatment advances, the annual incidence of

Table **7-1** Race/Ethnicity, Sex, and Transmission Category of AIDS Cases, 1981-1995 and 2001-2004

	1981-1995 (%)	2001-2004 (%)
RACE		
White, non-Hispanic	46.5	28.3
Black, non-Hispanic	34.6	49.5
Hispanic	17.9	20.3
Asian/Pacific Islander	0.7	1.1
Native American/Alaska Native	0.3	0.5
SEX		
Male	84.7	73.4
Female	15.3	26.6
TRANSMISSION CATEGORY		
Male-to-male sexual contact	51.2	40.8
Injection-drug use	26.8	22.8
Male-to-male sexual contact/Injection-drug use	7.8	4.9
Heterosexual contact	10.1	30.1
Perinatal	1.3	0.2
Other	2.9	1.3

AIDS and related deaths have been altered dramatically in the United States. Cases of AIDS in the United States expanded rapidly during the 1980s, peaked in 1992 (estimated 78,000), and decreased each year from that time until 1998 when the annual incidence stabilized at about 40,000. Highly active anti-retroviral therapy (HAART) (see Treatment and Prognosis section) is changing the face of HIV infection, with affected individuals demonstrating extended survival (resulting in an increased percentage of the population living with the virus). The percentage of individuals surviving 2 years after the diagnosis of AIDS has increased from 44% in 1981 to 1992, to 64% in 1993 to 1995, to 85% in 1996 to 2000.

In infected individuals, the virus can be found in most bodily fluids. HIV has been recovered from serum, blood, saliva, semen, tears, urine, breast milk, ear secretions, and vaginal secretions. The most frequent routes of transmission are sexual contact, parenteral exposure to blood, or transmission from mother to fetus during the perinatal period. Infection also has been documented to be caused by artificial insemination, breast-feeding from infected mothers, and organ transplantation. Although heterosexual transmission is increasing, most of the adults infected in the United States have been homosexual or bisexual men, intravenous (IV) drug abusers, hemophiliac patients receiving factor VIII before 1985, recipients of blood products, or heterosexual contacts with one of the other high-risk groups.

Researchers have debated the infectiousness of oral fluids. HIV has been found to be present in oral fluids,

but saliva appears to reduce the ability of HIV to infect its target cells, lymphocytes. Reports of transmission by oral fluids are rare, and it appears this is not a significant source for the transmission of AIDS. In spite of this, anecdotal reports have documented the transmission of AIDS during breast-feeding from the oral fluids of postpartum infected infants to their previously noninfected mothers. In addition, rare examples have been documented reporting the transmission of HIV infection by contamination of the oral fluids during cunnilingus or repeated passionate kissing. These rare anecdotal reports point out that oral fluids can be infectious and are not completely protective against oral introduction of HIV. Although saliva is known to contain a number of anti-HIV inhibitory factors, the presence of aphthae, erosions, ulcerations, and hemorrhagic inflammatory pathoses (e.g., gingivitis, periodontitis) may predispose an individual to oral transmission. In summary, the best precaution against infection is avoidance of all body fluids of infected patients.

Initially in the United States, AIDS was thought to be a disease that primarily affected whites and male homosexuals. Although men who have sex with men (MSM) remains the largest single risk factor, the nature of the epidemic is shifting because of numerous public health interventions directed against particularly vulnerable populations. These changing patterns are demonstrated well by comparing the data related to the early years of the infection with those noted in the initial portion of the twenty-first century (Table 7-1).

Since the initial years of the epidemic, blood-screening methods have improved dramatically and reduced the risk for HIV infection to as low as 1 in 2 million blood donations. The risk of transmission from infected mothers to newborns has been reduced from 25%-30% to 2% (95% reduction) because of widespread prenatal HIV testing, prophylactic use of antivirals, elective cesarean section performed before onset of labor, and avoidance of breast-feeding.

In the early years, non-Hispanic whites were the predominant ethnic group diagnosed with AIDS; however, with evolution of the epidemic, non-Hispanic blacks have become the predominant racial group. In addition, an increasing prevalence of HIV infection is being seen in females and heterosexuals. Of 35 areas reported to the CDC in 2004, 51% of all HIV infections and cases of AIDS were documented in blacks, even though this group accounted for only 13% of the population in the United States. Of these, 11% of the black men and 54% of the black women were infected through heterosexual contact. During this time, HIV infection was the leading cause of death for black women aged 25 to 34 years; the rates of infection per 100,000 in blacks, Hispanics, and whites were 76.3, 29.5, and 9.0, respectively. In comparing the racial rates of infection in the sexes in 2004, black males were affected seven times more frequently than whites, whereas black females demonstrated prevalence 21 times higher than white females.

The primary target cell of HIV is the CD4+ helper T lymphocyte. The DNA of HIV is incorporated into the DNA of the lymphocyte and is present for the life of the cell. In most viral infections, host antibodies that are protective against the organism usually are formed. In people with HIV infection, antibodies are developed but are not protective. The virus may remain silent, cause cell death, or produce syncytial fusion of the cells, which disrupts their normal function. A subsequent decrease in T-helper cell numbers occurs, with a resultant loss in immune function. The normal response to viruses, fungi, and encapsulated bacteria is diminished.

On introduction of HIV, an indefinite percentage of those infected will have an acute self-limited viral syndrome. This is followed by an asymptomatic stage, which averages 8 to 10 years. The length of the asymptomatic period is variable and may be affected by the nature of the virus, the host immune reaction, or external factors that may delay or accelerate the process. Almost inevitably, the final symptomatic stage develops.

CLINICAL FEATURES

HIV infection initially may be asymptomatic, or an acute response may be seen. The acute viral syndrome that occurs typically develops within 1 to 6 weeks after

exposure in 50% to 70% of infected patients. The symptoms bear some resemblance to those of infectious mononucleosis (e.g., generalized lymphadenopathy, sore throat, fever, maculopapular rash, headache, myalgia, arthralgia, diarrhea, photophobia, peripheral neuropathies). Oral changes may include mucosal erythema and focal ulcerations.

The acute viral syndrome clears within a few weeks; during this period, HIV infection usually is not considered or investigated. A variable asymptomatic period follows. Some patients have persistent generalized lymphadenopathy (PGL), which may later resolve. In some patients (before development of overt AIDS), there is a period of chronic fever, weight loss, diarrhea, oral candidiasis, herpes zoster, and/or oral hairy leukoplakia (OHL). This has been termed **AIDS-related complex** (ARC).

The presentation of symptomatic, overt AIDS is highly variable and often is affected by a person's prior exposure to a number of chronic infections. The signs and symptoms described under ARC are often present, along with an increasing number of opportunistic infections or neoplastic processes. In 50% of the cases, pneumonia caused by the protozoan *Pneumocystis carinii* is the presenting feature leading to the diagnosis. Other infections of diagnostic significance include disseminated cytomegalovirus (CMV) infection, severe herpes simplex virus (HSV) infection, atypical mycobacterial infection, cryptococcal meningitis, and central nervous system (CNS) toxoplasmosis. Persistent diarrhea is commonplace and may be bacterial or protozoal in origin. Clinically significant neurologic dysfunction is present in 30% to 50% of patients, and the most common manifestation is a progressive encephalopathy known as **AIDS-dementia complex.**

The most widely accepted classification of the oral manifestations of AIDS was compiled by the EC-Clearinghouse on Problems Related to HIV Infection and the WHO Collaborating Centre on Oral Manifestations of the Immunodeficiency Virus. This classification divided the manifestations into three groups: (1) strongly associated, (2) less commonly associated, and (3) seen in patients HIV infection (Box 7-1). The discussion here concentrates primarily on the clinical presentations. (For detailed information on the histopathology, diagnosis, and treatment of each condition, see the text covering the individual disease.) When the infections are treated differently in HIV-infected patients, these variations are presented here. The most common manifestations are presented first, followed by a selection of the less frequently encountered disorders.

The prevalence and mixture of oral manifestations noted in HIV-infected patients has been altered dramatically by the current antiretroviral therapies.

EC-Clearinghouse Classification of the Oral Manifestations of HIV Disease in Adults

GROUP 1: STRONGLY ASSOCIATED WITH HIV INFECTION

- Candidiasis: erythematous, pseudomembranous, angular cheilitis
- Hairy leukoplakia
- Kaposi's sarcoma (KS)
- Non-Hodgkin's lymphoma
- Periodontal diseases: linear gingival erythema, necrotizing gingivitis, necrotizing periodontitis

GROUP 2: LESS COMMONLY ASSOCIATED WITH HIV INFECTION

- Bacterial infections: *Mycobacterium avium-intracellulare, Mycobacterium tuberculosis*
- Melanotic hyperpigmentation
- Necrotizing ulcerative stomatitis
- Salivary gland disease: dry mouth, unilateral or bilateral swelling of major salivary glands
- Thrombocytopenia purpura
- Oral ulcerations NOS (not otherwise specified)
- Viral infections: herpes simplex, human papillomavirus, varicella-zoster

GROUP 3: SEEN IN HIV INFECTION

- Bacterial infections: *Actinomyces israelii, Escherichia coli, Klebsiella pneumonia*
- Cat-scratch disease (*Bartonella henselae*)
- Epithelioid (bacillary) angiomatosis (*Bartonella henselae*)
- Drug reactions: ulcerative, erythema multiforme, lichenoid, toxic epidermolysis
- Fungal infections other than candidiasis: *Cryptococcus neoformans, Geotrichum candidum, Histoplasma capsulatum, Mucoraceae* (mucormycosis/zygomycosis), *Aspergillus flavus*
- Neurologic disturbances: facial palsy, trigeminal neuralgia
- Recurrent aphthous stomatitis
- Viral infections: cytomegalovirus, molluscum contagiosum

HIV, Human immunodeficiency virus.

Numerous investigations of patients receiving HAART (see Treatment and Prognosis section) have demonstrated an increase in CD4+ count and a reduction in viral load that appear to be correlated with a reduced prevalence of many oral manifestations. Other factors that appear to affect the frequency of oral manifestations include xerostomia, poor oral hygiene, and smoking. Subsequent to HAART, the overall prevalence of oral manifestations decreased, including sig-

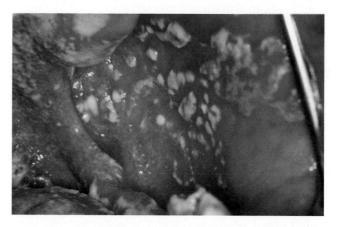

Fig. 7-32 **HIV-associated candidiasis.** Extensive removable white plaques of the left buccal mucosa.

nificant reductions in the frequency of oral candidiasis, OHL, HIV-associated periodontal disease, and Kaposi's sarcoma. Although the prevalence of certain lymphomas has decreased because of HAART, the frequency of all HIV-related lymphomas has not demonstrated significant change. In contrast, many researchers have reported an increased prevalence of benign human papillomavirus (HPV)-induced pathoses. A similar increased frequency of HIV-related salivary gland disease has been noted by some, but disputed by others.

The detection of oral manifestations can be critical, because it may suggest possible HIV infection in an unaware individual. The discovery in a patient with known HIV infection who is not yet on active therapy may signal progression of HIV disease. Finally, if new oral manifestations surface in a patient receiving antiretroviral therapy, it may lead to reevaluation and possible adjustment of the therapeutic regimen

ORAL AND MAXILLOFACIAL LESIONS STRONGLY ASSOCIATED WITH HIV INFECTION

CANDIDIASIS

Oral **candidiasis** is the most common intraoral manifestation of HIV infection and often is the presenting sign that leads to the initial diagnosis (Fig. 7-32). Although a number of *Candida* species have been encountered intraorally, the most common organism identified in association with oral candidiasis is *Candida albicans*. The presence of oral candidiasis in a patient infected with HIV is not diagnostic of AIDS but appears to be predictive for the subsequent development of full-blown AIDS in untreated patients within 2 years. Prevalence studies vary widely, but approximately one third of HIV-infected individuals and more than 90% of patients with AIDS develop oral candidiasis at some time during their disease course. The following four clinical patterns are seen:

1. Pseudomembranous candidiasis
2. Erythematous candidiasis
3. Hyperplastic candidiasis
4. Angular cheilitis

The first two variants constitute most of the cases (see page 213). Although infrequently seen in immunocompetent patients, chronic multifocal oral involvement is common in patients who are infected with HIV. Erythematous candidiasis typically begins to appear when the CD4 lymphocyte count drops below 400 cells/mm^3, with the pseudomembranous pattern being noted when the counts drop below 200 cells/mm^3. When comparing immunocompromised patients of different causations, those secondary to HIV infection have a greater prevalence of oral candidiasis, suggesting that HIV may play a role in initiation of the infection. Some studies have shown that development of candidiasis may be associated more closely with viral load than CD4 cell count. Oral candidiasis can be painful and associated with a reduction in taste and smell, which may lead to decreased intake of food and further wasting.

The diagnosis of candidiasis often is obvious from the clinical presentation but can be confirmed by cytologic smear or biopsy. Biopsy specimens of involved mucosa demonstrate the candidal organisms embedded in the superficial keratin, but the typical inflammatory reaction often is deficient (Fig. 7-33). Because *C. albicans* is a portion of the normal flora in 60% of healthy adults, positive microbiological cultures do not necessarily imply an active infection.

Treatment is much more difficult in patients with AIDS. Nystatin often is ineffective. Topical clotrimazole is associated with an improved response and typically produces a clinical cure rate that equals that of the systemic azoles. In spite of this success, topical therapy is associated with a high recurrence rate. The systemic azoles (i.e., fluconazole, ketoconazole, itraconazole) produce longer disease-free intervals but are associated with another set of problems. Itraconazole and ketoconazole require gastric acidity for adequate absorption, and all three agents are associated with a number of drug interactions. In addition, widespread use of systemic azoles has led to an increased prevalence of drug-resistant candidiasis in this patient population. In an attempt to reduce recurrences, patients have been encouraged to improve oral hygiene and assist mechanical cleansing of the mouth by rinsing with normal saline or home-made salt water several times daily.

In patients who are receiving effective antiretroviral therapy, have a CD4+ count exceeding 50 cells/mm^3, and have no signs of esophageal involvement, topical clotrimazole is the treatment of choice. Systemic therapy is recommended for patients not receiving effective antiretroviral therapy or for those with either esophageal involvement, a CD4+ count below 50 cells/mm^3, or a high viral load. Fluconazole is considered by many to be the drug of choice and has been shown to be the most effective prophylactic medication. In spite of this, non-*albicans* species such as *Candida glabrata* and *Candida krusei* have been isolated in HIV-infected patients, and these organisms are less susceptible to fluconazole. In many patients, itraconazole in an oral solution has been shown to be particularly effective in a swish-and-swallow method. Although gentian violet is not widely used, its effectiveness is better than nystatin and approaches the azoles, making this therapy a low-cost alternative in areas with inadequate funding or insufficient access to many of the newer medications. In several studies, antiretroviral protease inhibitors have been shown to exhibit a synergistic effect with the antifungal azoles and are thought possibly to interfere directly with candidal secretory aspartyl protease, an important virulence factor. Patients failing systemic azole therapy are candidates for intravenous amphotericin B if the patient's health supports its use. Amphotericin B oral suspension is available but reserved by many for azole-resistant candidiasis. Prophylactic antifungal therapy is not recommended unless frequent and severe recurrences are present.

ORAL HAIRY LEUKOPLAKIA

Although EBV is thought to be associated with several forms of lymphoma in HIV-infected patients, the most common EBV-related lesion in patients with AIDS is **oral hairy leukoplakia** (OHL). This lesion clinically presents as a white mucosal plaque that does not rub off and is characterized histopathologically by a some-

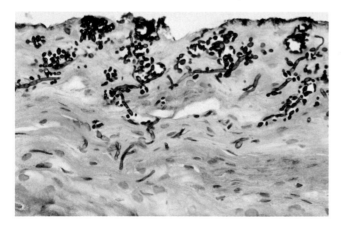

Fig. 7-33 HIV-associated candidiasis. Periodic acid-Schiff (PAS) stain of histopathologic section exhibiting numerous fungal organisms embedded in superficial keratin.

what distinctive (but not diagnostic) pattern of hyperkeratosis and epithelial hyperplasia.

Most cases of OHL occur on the lateral border of the tongue and range in appearance from faint white vertical streaks to thickened and furrowed areas of leukoplakia, exhibiting a shaggy keratotic surface (Fig. 7-34). The lesions infrequently may become extensive and cover the entire dorsal and lateral surfaces of the tongue. Rarely, the buccal mucosa, soft palate, pharynx, or esophagus may be involved.

Histopathologically, OHL exhibits thickened parakeratin that demonstrates surface corrugations or thin projections (Fig. 7-35). The epithelium is acanthotic and exhibits a bandlike zone of lightly stained cells with abundant cytoplasm ("balloon cells") in the upper spinous layer (Fig. 7-36). Close examination of the superficial epithelium reveals scattered cells with

nuclear clearing and a characteristic pattern of peripheral margination of chromatin termed *nuclear beading* (see Fig. 7-36, *inset*), caused by extensive EBV replication that displaces the chromatin to the nuclear margin. Dysplasia is not noted. Heavy candidal infestation of the parakeratin layer is typical, although the normal inflammatory reaction to the fungus usually is absent.

In the routine management of patients with HIV infection, the clinical features of OHL typically are sufficient for a presumptive diagnosis. When definitive diagnosis is necessary, demonstration of EBV within the lesion is required and can be achieved by *in situ* hybridization, PCR, immunohistochemistry, Southern blotting, or electron microscopy (Fig. 7-37).

Treatment of OHL usually is not needed, although slight discomfort or aesthetic concerns may necessitate therapy. Systemic antiherpesviral drugs produce rapid

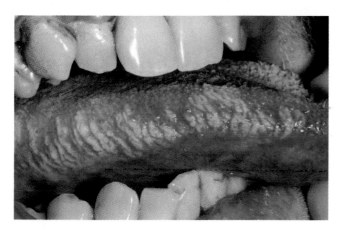

Fig. 7-34   HIV-associated oral hairy leukoplakia (OHL). Vertical streaks of keratin along the lateral border of the tongue.

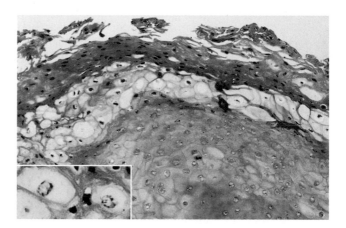

Fig. 7-36   HIV-associated oral hairy leukoplakia (OHL). Oral epithelium exhibiting hyperparakeratosis and layer of "balloon cells" in the upper spinous layer. *Inset* reveals high-power magnification of epithelial cells that demonstrate nuclear beading.

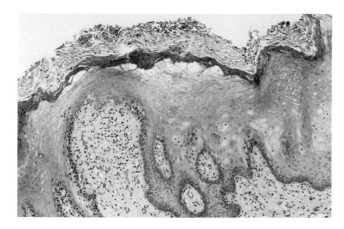

Fig. 7-35   HIV-associated oral hairy leukoplakia (OHL). Oral mucosa exhibiting hyperparakeratosis with surface corrugations.

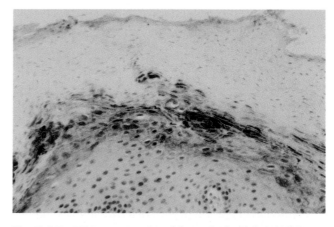

Fig. 7-37   HIV-associated oral hairy leukoplakia (OHL). Immunoperoxidase evaluation for Epstein-Barr virus (EBV) revealing positive reaction within numerous epithelial cells.

resolution, but recurrence is expected with discontinuation of therapy. Topical treatment with retinoids or podophyllum resin has resulted in temporary remissions. Surgical excision or cryotherapy has been used by some. A significantly reduced prevalence of OHL has been noted in patients on HAART who have demonstrated decreased viral load and an improved CD4 count. In underdeveloped countries with patients located great distances from urban health centers, the presence or absence of OHL can be used along with oral candidiasis as a clinical guide to assist in judging the effectiveness of antiviral therapy.

Although rare instances of OHL have been reported in immunocompetent individuals, most cases arise in immunocompromised persons. OHL also has been reported in heart, kidney, liver, and bone marrow transplant recipients, but its presence in the absence of a known cause of immunosuppression strongly suggests HIV infection. Discovery of OHL in "normal" patients mandates a thorough physical evaluation to rule out immunocompromised status. The presence of OHL in HIV-infected patients is a signal of severe immune suppression and more advanced disease.

KAPOSI'S SARCOMA

Kaposi's sarcoma (KS) is a multifocal neoplasm of vascular endothelial cell origin that was described initially in patients over the age of 60 (see page 557). However, since the beginning of the AIDS epidemic, most cases in the United States have been seen in association with HIV infection, with about 15% to 20% of patients with AIDS demonstrating KS. Human herpesvirus type 8 (HHV-8, Kaposi's sarcoma–associated herpesvirus [KSHV]) is noted within the tumor and believed to be responsible for the neoplasm's development. In Western countries, AIDS-associated KS has been reported primarily in homosexuals and is thought to be related to sexual transmission of HHV-8. Further evidence from Africa has demonstrated acquisition of HHV-8 infection before sexual activity and suggests alternate transmission pathways. HHV-8 has been found in saliva, serum, plasma, throat swabs, and bronchoalveolar lavage fluids. In Africa, HIV-related KS does not demonstrate a strong association with homosexual activity, exhibits an equal prevalence in men and women, and is not rare in children. In a recent North American study of healthy adults, HHV-8 was detected in oral epithelial cells and in the oropharynx, suggesting that the oral cavity may represent the predominant reservoir of infectious virus. These studies suggest that saliva represents an important route for transmission of HHV-8 in both heterosexual and homosexual populations.

KS typically manifests as multiple lesions of the skin or oral mucosa, although occasionally a solitary lesion

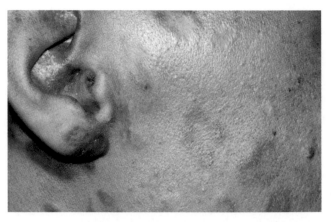

Fig. 7-38 **HIV-associated Kaposi's sarcoma (KS).** Multiple purple macules on the right side of the face.

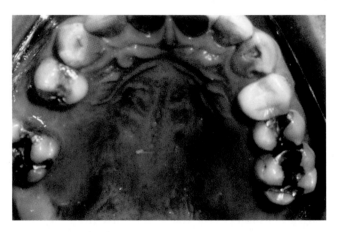

Fig. 7-39 **HIV-associated Kaposi's sarcoma (KS).** Large zones of KS exhibiting as a flat, brownish, and M-shaped discoloration of the hard palate.

is identified first. The trunk, arms, head, and neck are the most commonly involved anatomic sites (Fig. 7-38). Approximately 70% of individuals with HIV-related KS of skin or viscera demonstrate oral lesions; in 22% the oral cavity is the initial site of involvement. Although any mucosal site may be involved, the hard palate, gingiva, and tongue are affected most frequently (Figs. 7-39 and 7-40). When present on the palate or gingiva, the neoplasm can invade bone and create tooth mobility. The lesions begin as brown or reddish purple macular lesions that do not blanch with pressure. With time, the macules typically develop into plaques or nodules (Fig. 7-41). Pain, bleeding, and necrosis may become a problem and necessitate therapy (Fig. 7-42).

A biopsy is required to make the definitive diagnosis, although a presumptive diagnosis is sometimes made from the clinical presentation and history. Lesions that have a similar clinical appearance can

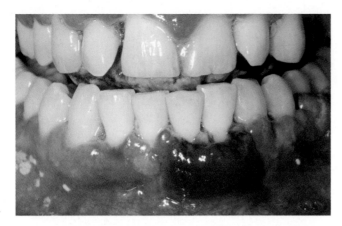

Fig. 7-40   HIV-associated Kaposi's sarcoma (KS). Raised, dark-red enlargement of the mandibular anterior facial gingiva on the left side.

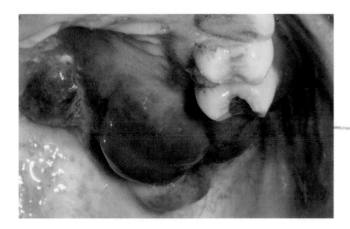

Fig. 7-41   HIV-associated Kaposi's sarcoma (KS). Diffuse, red-blue nodular enlargement of the left hard palate.

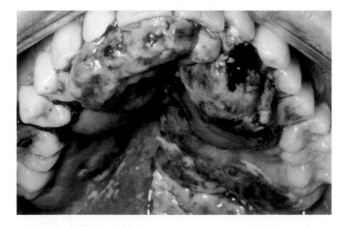

Fig. 7-42   HIV-associated Kaposi's sarcoma (KS). Diffuse, red-blue gingival enlargement that demonstrates widespread necrosis.

occur in HIV-infected patients who exhibit bacillary angiomatosis, the multifocal vascular proliferation associated with the cat-scratch bacillus (see page 206). HIV-related lymphomas also may resemble KS at times.

Before HAART, KS was considered a progressive malignancy that often disseminated widely to lymph nodes and various organ systems. HAART with protease inhibitors has been associated with a 30% to 50% reduction in the prevalence of KS and has produced significant regression of lesions in patients already affected. Because KS typically arises in immunocompromised patients and frequently demonstrates regression on return of immunocompetence, many researchers question whether KS is a true sarcoma. In cases not responding to HAART, single-agent chemotherapy such as alkaloids, bleomycin, doxorubicin, epirubicin, etoposide, and paclitaxel have shown effectiveness. Multiagent combinations have an increased effect but are associated with more severe adverse reactions and poor results in patients with widespread disease.

Oral lesions are frequently a cause of major morbidity, as a result of pain, bleeding, and functional interferences. Problematic lesions may be removed surgically or with cryotherapy. Intralesional injection of oral lesions with vinblastine (a chemotherapeutic agent) is effective. Intralesional injection of sodium tetradecyl sulfate, a sclerosing agent, has been effective for problematic intraoral lesions less than 2.5 cm in diameter. Laser ablation or electrosurgery have been used to treat KS, although theoretical concerns have been raised with respect to aerosolization of viral particles, which may place the surgical team at risk.

PERSISTENT GENERALIZED LYMPHADENOPATHY

After seroconversion, HIV disease often remains silent except for **persistent generalized lymphadenopathy** (PGL). The prevalence of this early clinical sign varies; however, in several studies it approaches 70%. PGL consists of lymphadenopathy that has been present for longer than 3 months and involves two or more extrainguinal sites. The most frequently involved sites are the posterior and anterior cervical, submandibular, occipital, and axillary nodes. Nodal enlargement fluctuates, usually is larger than 1 cm, and varies from 0.5 to 5.0 cm (Fig. 7-43).

Because lymphoma is known to occur in this population, a lymph node biopsy may be indicated for localized or bulky adenopathy, when cytopenia or an elevated erythrocyte sedimentation rate is present, or when requested for patient reassurance. Histopathologic examination reveals florid follicular hyperplasia. Although not as predictive as oral candidiasis or hairy

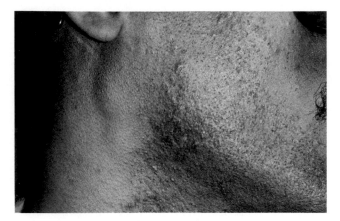

Fig. 7-43   HIV-associated lymphadenopathy. Enlarged cervical lymph nodes in a patient with persistent generalized lymphadenopathy (PGL).

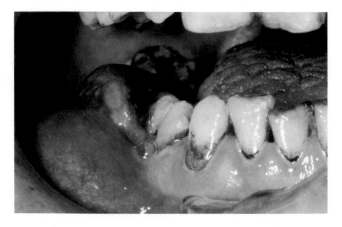

Fig. 7-44   HIV-associated lymphoma. Erythematous and ulcerated soft tissue enlargement of the posterior mandibular gingiva and mucobuccal fold on the right side.

leukoplakia, PGL does warn of progression to AIDS; almost one third of affected and untreated patients will have diagnostic features of AIDS within 5 years.

NON-HODGKIN'S LYMPHOMA

Non-Hodgkin's lymphoma (NHL) is the second most common malignancy in HIV-infected individuals. This neoplasm occurs in approximately 3% to 5% of those with the virus, a prevalence 60 times greater than the normal population. Typically, NHL in patients with AIDS presents as a high-grade and aggressive disease that frequently is associated with widespread involvement and short survival times. In AIDS the relative risk for developing a low-grade NHL is 15 times greater, compared with a 400 times greater risk for a high-grade NHL. The majority of the NHLs are B-cell lymphomas and include AIDS Burkitt's lymphoma, anaplastic large cell lymphoma, diffuse large cell lymphoma, immunoplasmacytoid lymphoma, primary effusion lymphoma, and plasmablastic lymphoma. Although a large number of these neoplasms demonstrate a relationship with EBV, studies have suggested that plasmablastic lymphoma and primary effusion lymphoma may be associated with both EBV and HHV-8.

Lymphoma in patients with AIDS usually occurs in extranodal locations, with the CNS being the most common site. Oral lesions are seen in approximately 4% of patients with AIDS-related NHL and most frequently involve the gingiva, palate, tongue, tonsil, or maxillary sinus (Fig. 7-44). Intraosseous involvement also has been documented and may resemble diffuse progressive periodontitis with loss of periodontal attachment and loosening of teeth. In these cases, widening of the periodontal ligament and loss of lamina dura frequently are noted and represent clues to the diagnosis.

The treatment usually is combination chemotherapy, and radiation is reserved for local control of the disease. These malignancies are aggressive, and survival usually is measured in months from the date of discovery. Although HAART has dramatically reduced the prevalence of many opportunistic infections and KS in HIV-infected patients, the effect on NHL appears to vary with the type of lymphoma and has been inconsistent. Although many forms of NHL continue to contribute to the morbidity and mortality of HIV-infected patients, others categories of NHL, such as plasmablastic lymphoma, have declined significantly because of HAART.

HIV-ASSOCIATED PERIODONTAL DISEASE

Three atypical patterns of periodontal disease are associated strongly with HIV infection:
1. Linear gingival erythema
2. Necrotizing ulcerative gingivitis
3. Necrotizing ulcerative periodontitis

Linear gingival erythema initially was termed *HIV-related gingivitis*, but ultimately was noted in association with other disease processes. This unusual pattern of gingivitis appears with a distinctive linear band of erythema that involves the free gingival margin and extends 2 to 3 mm apically (Fig. 7-45). In addition, the alveolar mucosa and gingiva may demonstrate punctate or diffuse erythema in a significant percentage of the cases. This diagnosis should be reserved for gingivitis that does not respond to improved plaque control and exhibits a greater degree of erythema than would be expected for the amount of plaque in the area. The literature related to linear gingival erythema is difficult to evaluate, because it appears that conventional marginal gingivitis often is misinterpreted as linear gingival erythema. Although some investigators

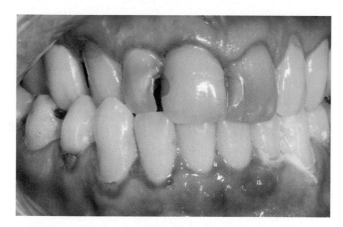

Fig. 7-45   HIV-associated gingivitis. Band of erythema involving the free gingival margin.

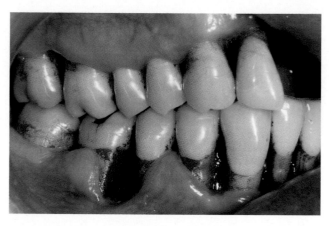

Fig. 7-47   HIV-associated periodontitis. Extensive loss of periodontal support without deep pocketing.

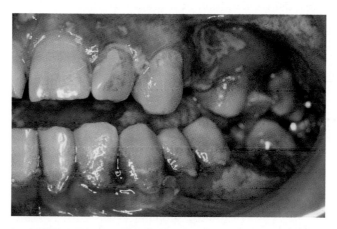

Fig. 7-46   HIV-associated necrotizing ulcerative gingivitis (NUG). Multiple punched-out interdental papillae of the mandibular gingiva. Note diffuse pseudomembranous candidiasis of the surrounding mucosa.

believe linear gingival erythema results from an abnormal host immune response to subgingival bacteria, data suggest that this pattern of gingivitis may represent an unusual pattern of candidiasis. Most instances respond to systemic antifungal medications such as fluconazole or ketoconazole.

Necrotizing ulcerative gingivitis (NUG) (see page 157) refers to ulceration and necrosis of one or more interdental papillae with no loss of periodontal attachment. Patients with NUG have interproximal gingival necrosis, bleeding, pain, and halitosis (Fig. 7-46).

Necrotizing ulcerative periodontitis (NUP) previously was termed *HIV-associated periodontitis*; however, it has not been deemed to be specific for HIV infection. NUP is characterized by gingival ulceration and necrosis associated with rapidly progressing loss of periodontal attachment. Although severe cases can affect all teeth, multiple isolated defects often are seen and con-

trast with the diffuse pattern associated with typical chronic periodontitis. Edema, severe pain, and spontaneous hemorrhage are common and often lead affected patients to seek care. Deep pocketing usually is not seen because extensive gingival necrosis typically coincides with loss of the adjacent alveolar bone (Fig. 7-47). Loss of more than 6 mm of attachment within a 6-month period is not unusual. HIV-associated periodontitis does not respond to conventional periodontal therapy.

The treatment of NUG and NUP revolves around débridement, antimicrobial therapy, immediate follow-up care, and long-term maintenance. The initial removal of necrotic tissue is necessary, combined with povidone-iodine irrigation. The use of systemic antibiotics usually is not necessary, but metronidazole (narrow spectrum to suppress periodontal pathogens without strongly promoting candidal overgrowth) has been administered to patients with extensive involvement that is associated with severe acute pain. All patients should use chlorhexidine mouth rinses initially and for long-term maintenance. After initial débridement, follow-up removal of additional diseased tissue should be performed within 24 hours and again every 7 to 10 days for two to three appointments, depending on the patient's response. At this point, monthly recalls are necessary until the process stabilizes; evaluations then are performed every 3 months.

In patients with gingival necrosis, the process occasionally extends away from the alveolar ridges and creates massive areas of tissue destruction termed **necrotizing stomatitis** (Fig. 7-48). The process clinically resembles noma (see page 201) and may involve predominantly soft tissue or extend into the underlying bone, resulting in extensive sequestration (Fig. 7-49). Although this process initially was thought to be an extension of NUP, necrotizing stomatitis has arisen on

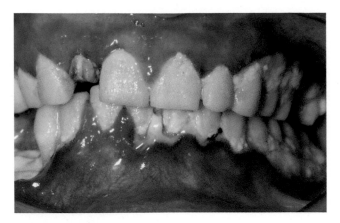

Fig. 7-48   HIV-associated periodontitis with necrotizing stomatitis. Diffuse gingival necrosis with extension onto alveolar mucosa.

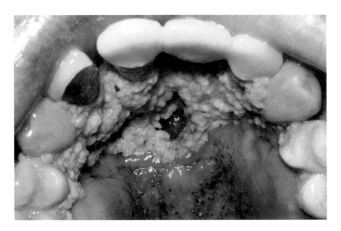

Fig. 7-49   HIV-associated necrotizing stomatitis. Massive necrosis of soft tissue and bone of the anterior maxilla.

the oral mucosa separate from the gingiva (not overlying bone).

In the absence of gingival involvement, the clinical features of necrotizing stomatitis are nonspecific and mandate biopsy. In many instances, the areas of soft tissue ulceration and necrosis demonstrate infection with one of more agents, such as HSV, CMV, and EBV.

In addition to these three atypical forms of HIV-related periodontal disease, patients also may demonstrate conventional gingivitis, chronic periodontitis, and progressive nonnecrotizing periodontitis. Studies have shown that periodontal attachment loss can be combated successfully with regular professional removal of supra- and subgingival plaque in patients who optimize their personal oral hygiene techniques. Because smoking has been associated strongly with all forms of periodontal disease, patients should be encouraged to discontinue their tobacco habit.

LESS COMMON ORAL AND MAXILLOFACIAL MANIFESTATIONS OF HIV INFECTION

MYCOBACTERIAL INFECTION

The best known mycobacterial infection is **tuberculosis** (TB), which typically is caused by *Mycobacterium tuberculosis* (see page 195). Infections with other mycobacteria include *M. avium* and *M. intracellulare* (*M. avium-intracellulare* complex), *M. bovis*, *M. scrofulaceum*, *M. africanum*, and *M. haemophilum*, although these usually are found only in the immunocompromised patient. Worldwide, one in three individuals contracts TB sometime during their life, with more than 2 million associated deaths each year. Those coinfected with HIV are at greater risk of death and account for 15% of AIDS-related deaths worldwide. It is estimated that more than 4.4 million individuals are coinfected with TB and HIV, with more than half a million individuals exhibiting active TB.

Oral lesions are uncommon and occur in less than 5% of individuals with active TB. When present, the tongue is affected most frequently, but lesions also can develop on the buccal mucosa, gingiva, floor of mouth, lips, and palate. The affected areas present as chronic ulcerations, granular leukoplakias, or exophytic proliferative masses. Jaw involvement also has been reported. Confirming the diagnosis of TB often can be difficult in AIDS patients, because up to 80% do not react to tuberculin skin tests. In such cases, identifying the organism by examining AFB-stained sections of biopsy material and confirming its presence on culture of infected tissue are important.

Management is difficult because of increasing drug resistance and difficulty in ensuring patient compliance with the extended treatment protocols. Agents frequently used in the triple-drug regimens include rifampicin, isoniazid, and pyrazinamide, with ethambutol added when isoniazid resistance is likely.

HYPERPIGMENTATION

Hyperpigmentation of the skin, nails, and mucosa has been reported in HIV-infected patients. The changes are similar microscopically to focal melanosis, with increased melanin pigmentation observed in the basal cell layer of the affected epithelium. Several medications taken by AIDS patients (e.g., ketoconazole, clofazimine, pyrimethamine, zidovudine) may cause the increased melanin pigmentation. Adrenocortical destruction has been reported from several of the infections associated with AIDS, resulting in an addisonian pattern of pigmentation. Finally, pigmentation with no apparent cause has arisen in HIV-infected patients, and some investigators have theorized that this may be a direct result of the HIV infection.

HIV-ASSOCIATED SALIVARY GLAND DISEASE

HIV-associated salivary gland disease also can arise anytime during infection. Clinically obvious salivary gland disease is noted in approximately 5% to 10% of HIV-infected patients, with a greater prevalence noted in children. The main clinical sign is salivary gland enlargement, particularly affecting the parotid. Bilateral involvement is seen in about 60% of patients with glandular changes and often is associated with cervical lymphadenopathy.

As a result of a genetically influenced alteration of the immune response to HIV infection, some patients develop **diffuse infiltrative lymphocytosis syndrome** (DILS), which is associated with a more favorable prognosis for their HIV infection but also associated with a forty-fourfold greater chance of lymphoma. Affected individuals reveal CD8 lymphocytosis and lymphadenopathy, along with salivary gland enlargement. Although the pathosis may involve any of the major or minor salivary glands, the parotid is affected most commonly. Other sites of involvement include the lacrimal glands, kidneys, muscles, nerves, and lungs. The glandular involvement arises from CD8-lymphocytic infiltration and often is followed by lymphoepithelial cyst formation in the parotid.

The most widely accepted therapy for DILS is oral prednisone or antiretroviral therapy, although some patients have been treated with parotidectomy or radiation therapy. The effect of HAART is unclear. Some investigators have reported an increased prevalence (possibly because of partial immune reconstitution), whereas others have noted regression after initiation of antiviral therapy. Because of the increased risk for B-cell lymphoma, observation with histopathologic monitoring by fine-needle aspiration is recommended by some. In patients with large lymphoepithelial cysts, aspiration or sclerotherapy with tetracycline or doxycycline has been associated with temporary improvement. Associated xerostomia is variable and treated in a manner similar to that of cases associated with non-HIV disease (i.e., maintenance of good oral health and the use of sialogogues and saliva substitutes).

THROMBOCYTOPENIA

Thrombocytopenia (see page 584) has been reported in up to 40% of patients with HIV infection, may occur at any time during the course of the disease, and frequently is the first clinical manifestation of HIV infection. The causes are diverse and include direct infection by HIV, immune dysfunction, alteration of platelet production, loss because of associated infectious diseases, and drug reactions. Cutaneous lesions are present in most cases, but oral lesions do occur

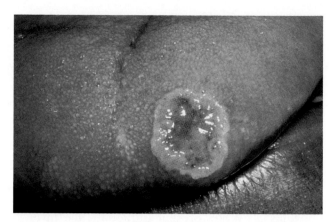

Fig. 7-50 HIV-associated recurrent herpetic infection. Mucosal erosion of the anterior dorsal surface of the tongue on the left side. Note the yellowish circinate border.

with petechiae, ecchymosis, or spontaneous gingival hemorrhage.

Platelets have been shown to engulf HIV and play an important role in the immune response to the virus. HIV-infected patients with extended thrombocytopenia have demonstrated decreased survival. HAART has reduced the prevalence of thrombocytopenia and is the first line of defense. Additional therapies used in nonresponsive patients include splenectomy, intravenous immunoglobulin (IVIG), IV anti-Rho immunoglobulin (anti-D), and transfusion of platelets. Corticosteroids, danazol, and vinca alkaloids are additional approaches proven to be effective in the general population but associated with increased risks in HIV-infected patients.

HERPES SIMPLEX VIRUS

Recurrent HSV infections occur in about the same percentage of HIV-infected patients as they do in the immunocompetent population (10% to 15%); however, the lesions are more widespread, occur in an atypical pattern, and may persist for months (Fig. 7-50). The prevalence of HSV lesions increases significantly once the CD4+ count drops below 50 cells/mm³. Herpes labialis may extend to the facial skin and exhibit extensive lateral spread. Persistence of active sites of HSV infection for more than 1 month in a patient infected with HIV is one accepted definition of AIDS. The clinical presentations of recurrences in immunocompromised patients and appropriate therapy and maintenance have been discussed in the text on herpesvirus (see page 244).

As mentioned in the discussion of necrotizing stomatitis, evaluation for HSV should be performed in all persistent oral ulcerations in HIV-infected individuals. In these ulcerations, investigators have discovered HSV in 10% to 19% (with an additional 10% to 28% exhibiting coinfection by HSV and CMV).

VARICELLA-ZOSTER VIRUS

Recurrent varicella-zoster virus (VZV) infection **(herpes zoster)** is fairly common in HIV-infected patients, but the course is more severe, with increased morbidity and mortality rates. Many of these patients are younger than age 40, in contrast to cases in immunocompetent patients that usually arise later in life. In the early stages of HIV-related immunosuppression, herpes zoster usually is confined to a dermatome but persists longer than usual. In full-blown AIDS, herpes zoster usually begins in a classic dermatomal distribution; however, subsequent cutaneous dissemination is not unusual. When present intraorally, the involvement often is severe and occasionally leads to bone sequestration and loss of teeth. In many instances, the associated osteonecrosis and tooth exfoliation may be delayed a month or more after the initial onset of the herpes zoster. Associated pain typically is intense. Although peroral antiviral medications are beneficial in immunocompetent patients, intravenous acyclovir is recommended for severe herpes zoster in the absence of an intact immune system.

HUMAN PAPILLOMAVIRUS

Human papillomavirus (HPV) is responsible for several facial and oral lesions in immunocompetent patients, the most frequent of which are the **verruca vulgaris (common wart)** (see page 364) and **oral squamous papilloma** (see page 362). An increased prevalence of HPV-related lesions is noted in HIV-infected patients, and most are located in the anogenital areas. Oral involvement also may be seen. Although usual types of HPV may be present in intraoral lesions, HIV-infected patients often demonstrate more unusual variants such as HPV-7 (associated with butcher's warts) or HPV-32 (often noted in multifocal epithelial hyperplasia) (see page 367).

An increased prevalence of HPV-related lesions has been reported from several centers in patients responding to HAART. Although the exact cause is not clear, some wonder if the virus remains latent in many patients until partial immune reconstitution leads to a local inflammatory response, viral reactivation, and the initiation of clinically evident lesions. In several cohorts, the risk of oral HPV lesions increased with the effectiveness of the antiretroviral therapy.

The oral lesions usually are multiple and may be located on any mucosal surface. The labial mucosa, tongue, buccal mucosa, and gingiva are frequent sites. The lesions may exhibit a cluster of white, spikelike projections, pink cauliflower-like growths, or slightly elevated sessile papules (Fig. 7-51).

Histopathologically, the lesions may be sessile or papillary and covered by acanthotic or even hyperplastic stratified squamous epithelium (Fig. 7-52). The

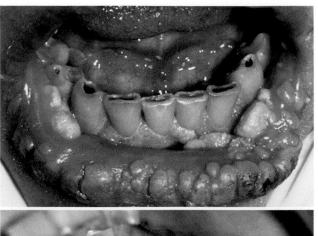
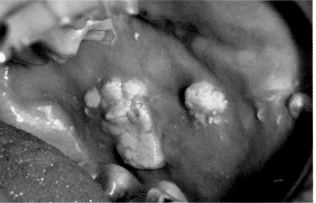

Fig. 7-51   HIV-associated human papillomavirus (HPV) infection. Multiple exophytic and somewhat papillary nodules of the lip, buccal mucosa, and gingiva.

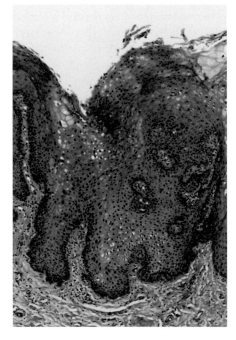

Fig. 7-52   HIV-associated human papillomavirus (HPV) infection. Oral mucosa exhibiting acanthosis and mild nuclear pleomorphism.

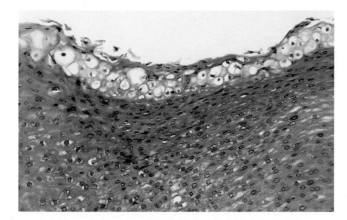

Fig. 7-53   **HIV-associated human papillomavirus (HPV) infection.** Oral mucosa exhibiting extensive koilocytosis in the superficial spinous cell layer.

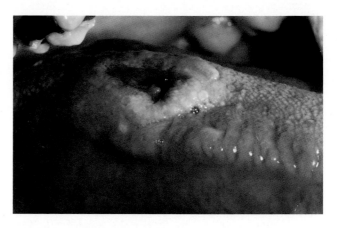

Fig. 7-55   **HIV-associated histoplasmosis.** Indurated ulceration with a rolled border on the dorsal surface of the tongue on the right side.

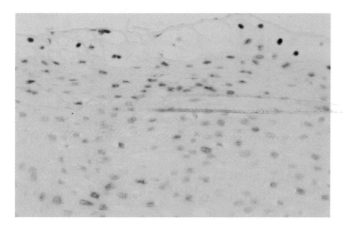

Fig. 7-54   **HIV-associated human papillomavirus (HPV) infection.** DNA *in situ* hybridization of oral mucosal biopsy that reveals diffuse cellular positivity for HPV.

affected epithelium often demonstrates vacuolization of numerous epithelial cells (i.e., koilocytosis) and occasionally may exhibit mild variation in nuclear size (Fig. 7-53). Immunohistochemistry or DNA *in situ* hybridization often is used to confirm the presence and type of HPV within histopathologic specimens (Fig. 7-54).

Dysplasia has been noted within HPV-related lesions in patients with AIDS and mandates close observation of affected patients for development of squamous cell carcinoma. The treatment of choice is surgical removal; however, recurrences are common, especially in patients with significant immune deficiency. Other therapeutic modalities that have been used include topical podophyllin, imiquimod, interferon, cryosurgery, laser ablation, and electrocoagulation. If one of the latter two choices is used, the surgical team must be wary of the resultant plume that may contain infectious HPV.

OTHER ORAL AND MAXILLOFACIAL LESIONS SEEN IN HIV INFECTION

HISTOPLASMOSIS

Histoplasmosis, the most common endemic respiratory fungal infection in the United States, is produced by *Histoplasma capsulatum* (see page 224). In healthy patients the infection typically is subclinical and self-limiting, but clinically evident infections do occur in immunocompromised individuals. Although a number of deep fungal infections are possible in patients with AIDS, histoplasmosis is the most common, with disseminated disease noted in approximately 5% of AIDS patients residing in areas where the fungus is endemic. In patients with AIDS, diagnosis of histoplasmosis also has been documented in nonendemic areas, possibly from reactivation of a previous subclinical infection.

The signs and symptoms associated with dissemination are nonspecific and include fever, weight loss, splenomegaly, and pulmonary infiltrates. Oral lesions are not uncommon and usually are caused by blood-borne organisms or spread from pulmonary involvement. On occasion, the initial diagnosis is made from the oral changes, with some patients demonstrating involvement isolated to the oral cavity. Although intrabony infection in the jaws has been reported, the most common oral presentation of histoplasmosis is a chronic, indurated mucosal ulceration with a raised border (Fig. 7-55). The oral lesions may be single or multiple, and any area of the oral mucosa may be involved.

Microscopically, the small fungal organisms are visible within the cytoplasm of histiocytes and

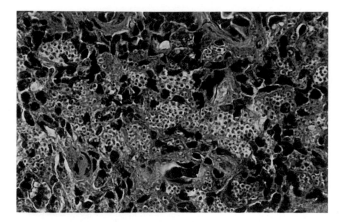

Fig. 7-56   HIV-associated histoplasmosis. Mucosal biopsy in which the connective tissue is filled with numerous clusters of small fungal organisms.

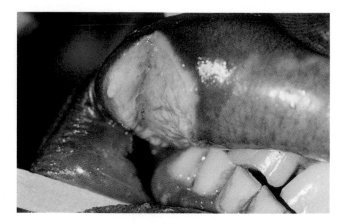

Fig. 7-58   HIV-associated ulceration. Atypical mucosal ulceration that mandates biopsy and may be attributable to a variety of causes.

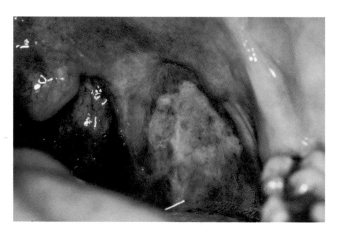

Fig. 7-57   HIV-associated aphthous ulceration. Large superficial ulceration of the posterior soft palate.

multinucleated giant cells. These phagocytic cells may be present in sheets or in organized granulomas (Fig. 7-56). The therapy of choice for disseminated histoplasmosis has been intravenous amphotericin B, but itraconazole has been shown to be effective with fewer adverse reactions and better patient compliance. Ketoconazole is another alternative, but its hepatotoxicity makes this approach a less desirable form of therapy.

APHTHOUS ULCERATIONS

Lesions that are clinically similar to **aphthous ulcerations** occur with increased frequency in patients infected with HIV. All three forms (minor, major, and herpetiform) are seen; surprisingly, however, almost two thirds of the patients have the usually uncommon herpetiform and major variants (Fig. 7-57). As immunosuppression becomes more profound, major aphthous ulcerations demonstrate an increased prevalence.

Treatment with potent topical or intralesional corticosteroids has been successful in a number of patients. Not all lesions respond, and recurrences are common. Secondary candidiasis may be a complication of therapy. Systemic corticosteroid drugs also may prove beneficial but typically are avoided in an attempt to prevent further immune depression. For lesions nonresponsive to topical corticosteroids, thalidomide has been found to be advantageous in many patients. Thalidomide must be used cautiously for only a short term because of its association with an irreversible peripheral neuropathy and its ability to enhance the production of HIV. In a limited number of patients, granulocyte colony-stimulating factor (G-CSF) has produced rapid and sustained resolution of aphthous ulcerations that were resistant to therapy with topical corticosteroids, cyclosporine, and thalidomide.

Biopsy of any chronic mucosal ulceration clinically diagnosed as an aphthous ulceration should be considered if the lesion is atypical clinically or does not respond to therapy (Fig. 7-58). In such cases, biopsy often reveals another cause, such as HSV, CMV, deep fungal infection, or neoplasia. (For further information on aphthous ulcerations and the pathogenesis of these lesions in patients infected with HIV, see page 331.)

MOLLUSCUM CONTAGIOSUM

Molluscum contagiosum is an infection of the skin caused by a poxvirus (see page 371). The lesions are small, waxy, dome-shaped papules that often demonstrate a central depressed crater. In immunocompetent individuals, the lesions are self-limiting and typically involve the genital region or trunk. In patients with AIDS, hundreds of lesions may be present, with many exhibiting little tendency to undergo spontaneous resolution, and some occasionally obtaining large size. Approximately 5% to 10% of HIV-infected patients

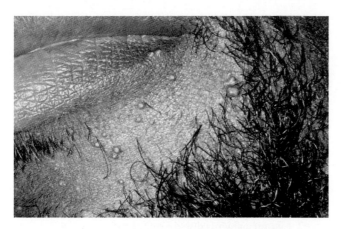

Fig. 7-59 HIV-associated molluscum contagiosum. Numerous perioral papules.

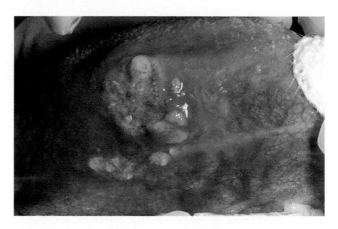

Fig. 7-61 HIV-associated squamous cell carcinoma. Ulceration with raised, indurated borders on the lateral tongue.

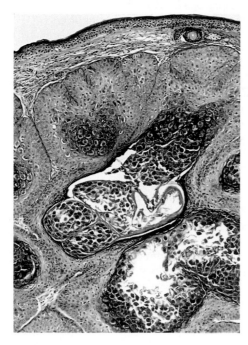

Fig. 7-60 HIV-associated molluscum contagiosum. Downgrowth of surface epithelium exhibiting numerous "molluscum bodies."

are affected, and the facial skin commonly is involved (Fig. 7-59). Rare intraoral examples of molluscum contagiosum have been reported, appearing as erythematous papules. These lesions may involve either the keratinized or nonkeratinized mucosa.

Histopathologically, the surface epithelium forms several hyperplastic downgrowths. This involuting epithelium contains numerous large, intracytoplasmic inclusions known as **molluscum bodies** (Fig. 7-60). In the center of the lesion, the keratin layer often disintegrates and releases the adjacent molluscum bodies, hence the central crater.

Numerous reports have documented resolution of widespread and recalcitrant lesions after successful initiation of HAART. It is not known if these responses are secondary to immune reconstitution or the antiviral effects of the therapy. Because viral particles have been identified in perilesional skin of HIV-infected patients, local therapy (e.g., curettage, cryosurgery, cautery, photodynamic therapy, podophyllotoxin) often is associated with recurrences. Anecdotal reports of positive responses to immunomodulatory (imiquimod) or antiviral therapy (cidofovir) have been documented in severely immunocompromised patients with previously recalcitrant disease.

ORAL SQUAMOUS CELL CARCINOMA

Squamous cell carcinoma of the oral cavity, pharynx, and larynx has been reported in HIV-infected patients. These neoplasms are associated with the same cancer risk factors as the general population but tend to occur at a younger age. Similar clinical presentations and anatomic distribution of these carcinomas are noted (Fig. 7-61). It appears that HIV infection may accelerate the development of squamous cell carcinoma, possibly because of impaired immune surveillance.

Treatment of squamous cell carcinoma is not significantly different for HIV-infected patients and consists of surgical resection, radiation therapy, or combined radiation and chemotherapy. Clinical staging can be problematic because of HIV-related cervical lymphadenopathy. In these cases, cross-sectional computed tomography (CT) or magnetic resonance imaging (MRI) could be performed in an attempt to distinguish lymph nodes enlarged by lymphoproliferative disease from those containing metastatic carcinoma. The majority of HIV-infected patients with a diagnosis of squamous cell carcinoma have advanced disease and exhibit a less favorable prognosis.

DIAGNOSIS

Confirmation of HIV infection can be made by viral culture or by detection of HIV antibodies or antigens. The standard screening tool is the enzyme immunoassay (EIA) for antibodies to HIV. This test can have false-positive results or cross-reactions; therefore, it should be repeated and followed by the more accurate Western blot antibody assay. Other alternatives include radioimmunoprecipitation (RIPA), rapid latex agglutination assay, and dot-blot immunobinding assay. All of these evaluations are used to detect antibodies to HIV.

In an attempt to improve the safety of the blood supply, a few assays have been approved by the FDA to detect viral antigens before development of anti-HIV antibodies. These tests are not used widely and include the p24 antigen capture assay and polymerase chain reaction (PCR) for detection of HIV DNA that may be integrated into the host DNA. This latter method may be used to identify someone who was infected recently or HIV carriers who otherwise have negative antigen or antibody findings.

The diagnosis of AIDS is indicated if the patient has laboratory evidence of HIV infection combined with documentation of less than 200 CD4+ T lymphocytes per microliter or a CD4+ T-lymphocyte percentage of total lymphocytes that is less than 14. In addition, the diagnosis of AIDS can be made in an HIV-infected person if one of the indicator diseases listed in Box 7-2 has been documented.

TREATMENT AND PROGNOSIS

As mentioned previously, HIV infection initially was considered fatal; however, the introduction of HAART has altered the course of the epidemic. A wide variety of antiretroviral agents is available and continues to expand (Box 7-3), increasing the effectiveness of medical therapy. Although numerous drug combinations are possible, HAART often consists of two nucleoside analogue reverse-transcriptase inhibitors, at least one protease inhibitor, and/or one nonnucleoside analogue reverse-transcriptase inhibitor. Alternatively, one nucleoside analogue reverse-transcriptase inhibitor can be combined with one nonnucleoside analogue reverse-transcriptase inhibitor and one protease inhibitor.

The current therapeutic approaches have driven HIV to undetectable levels in many patients, with a resultant clinically significant reconstitution of the immune system. With the current antiretroviral medications, total HIV eradication would take at least a decade and presently is not a realistic goal. Although no cure exists, survival times are increasing as a result of earlier diagnosis and improved therapy.

Box 7-2

Indicator Diseases Used in the Diagnosis of Acquired Immunodeficiency Syndrome

1. Candidiasis of bronchi, trachea, or lungs
2. Candidiasis, esophageal
3. Cervical cancer, invasive
4. Coccidioidomycosis, disseminated or extrapulmonary
5. Cryptococcosis, extrapulmonary
6. Cryptosporidiosis, chronic intestinal (>1 month's duration)
7. Cytomegalovirus disease (other than liver, spleen, or nodes)
8. Cytomegalovirus-induced retinitis (with loss of vision)
9. Encephalopathy, HIV-related
10. Herpes simplex: chronic ulcer or ulcers (>1 month's duration) or bronchitis, pneumonitis, or esophagitis
11. Histoplasmosis, disseminated or extrapulmonary
12. Isosporiasis, chronic intestinal (>1 month's duration)
13. Kaposi's sarcoma (KS)
14. Lymphoma, Burkitt's (or equivalent term)
15. Lymphoma, immunoblastic (or equivalent term)
16. Lymphoma, primary, of brain
17. *Mycobacterium avium* complex or *M. kansasii*, disseminated or extrapulmonary
18. *Mycobacterium tuberculosis*, any site (pulmonary or extrapulmonary)
19. *Mycobacterium*, other species or unidentified species, disseminated, or extrapulmonary
20. *Pneumocystis carinii* pneumonia
21. Pneumonia, recurrent
22. Progressive multifocal leukoencephalopathy
23. *Salmonella* septicemia, recurrent
24. Toxoplasmosis of brain
25. Wasting syndrome as a result of AIDS

HIV, Human immunodeficiency virus.

Although antiretroviral therapy is effective for many patients, it is expensive. In addition, this treatment often is associated with significant adverse reactions, may not be effective in all patients, or may fail after a period of initial success. Work is proceeding toward the development of a safe and effective vaccine against HIV infection, but complex issues slow the progress. Advances in therapy and prevention of HIV infection occur daily; however, the best defense against the disease is prevention of the initial infection.

Despite the continuing advances in medical therapy and the ongoing work toward a successful vaccine, many of the positive gains against the epidemic have been achieved through epidemiologically directed public health interventions. The ever-changing data

Box 7-3

Antiretroviral Therapy

1. Nucleoside reverse-transcriptase inhibitors
   - Abacavir, didanosine, emtricitabine, lamivudine, stavudine, tenofovir, zalcitabine, or zidovudine
2. Nucleotide reverse-transcriptase inhibitors
   - Adefovir or tenofovir
3. Nonnucleoside reverse-transcriptase inhibitors
   - Capravirine, delavirdine, efavirenz, emivirine, or nevirapine
4. Protease inhibitors
   - Amprenavir, atazanavir, darunavir, fosamprenavir, indinavir, lopinavir/ritonavir, nelfinavir, ritonavir, saquinavir, saquinavir-SGC, or tipranavir
5. Fusion inhibitors
   - Enfuvirtide
6. Integrase inhibitors
   - MK-0518 (experimental)
7. CCR5 inhibitors
   - Maraviroc (experimental), vicriviroc (experimental)

continue to be important and highlight increasingly important areas (e.g., increasing prevalence in heterosexuals and blacks) for present and future interventions. Routine HIV testing is critical, because it represents the best avenue toward life-saving early therapy and prevention of HIV transmission to others. It is estimated that more than 300,000 individuals in the United States are unaware that they are infected with HIV. To appropriately emphasize early diagnosis and prevention, the CDC recommends HIV testing as a part of routine clinical care in all health care settings.

Some health professionals have been concerned about the risk of occupational transmission of HIV. The average risk of seroconversion after a percutaneous exposure to HIV-infected blood is estimated to be approximately 0.3%. Mucous membrane exposure to HIV-infected blood results in seroconversion in only 0.09% of cases, and the rate is even lower after a nonintact skin exposure. The risk of transmission after exposure to fluids or tissues other than blood has not been quantified but most likely is considerably lower. On exposure to HIV-contaminated material, the risk of seroconversion can be reduced by greater than 75% through postexposure prophylaxis (PEP) with antiretroviral medications if initiated within hours of the event. Four weeks of therapy is recommended; however, this often is difficult to complete because of adverse reactions; therefore, the regimen probably should not be used for exposures that pose a negligible risk for transmission. The basic PEP consists of a two-drug regimen that may be expanded to a three-drug

combination for more severe exposures. Because of the complexity of choosing and administering the regimen, involvement of an infectious disease specialist or a physician experienced in antiretroviral therapy is strongly recommended. Regardless, promptness in the initiation of the therapy is paramount.

BIBLIOGRAPHY

Herpes Simplex Virus

Amir J: Clinical aspects and antiviral therapy in primary herpetic gingivostomatitis, *Paediatr Drugs* 3:593-597, 2001.

Arduino PG, Porter SR: Oral and perioral herpes simplex virus type I (HSV-I) infection: review of its management, *Oral Dis* 12:254-270, 2006.

Chilukuri S, Rosen T: Management of acyclovir-resistant herpes simplex virus, *Dermatol Clin* 21:311-320, 2003.

Cohen PR, Kazi S, Grossman ME: Herpetic geometric glossitis: a distinctive pattern of lingual herpes simplex virus infection, *South Med J* 88:1231-1235, 1995.

Cohen SG, Greenberg MS: Chronic oral herpes simplex virus infection in immunocompromised patients, *Oral Surg Oral Med Oral Pathol* 59:465-471, 1985.

Flaitz CM, Nichols CM, Hicks MJ: Herpesviridae-associated persistent mucocutaneous ulcers in acquired immunodeficiency syndrome: a clinicopathologic study, *Oral Surg Oral Med Oral Pathol Oral Radiol Endod* 81:433-441, 1996.

Hess GP, Walson PD: Seizures secondary to oral viscous lidocaine, *Ann Emerg Med* 17:725-727, 1988.

Huber MA: Herpes simplex type-1 virus infection, *Quintessence Int* 34:453-457, 2003.

Juretić M: Natural history of herpetic infection, *Helv Paediatr Acta* 21(4):356-368, 1966.

Kameyama T, Futami M, Nakayoshi N et al: Shedding of herpes simplex virus type I into saliva in patients with orofacial fracture, *J Med Virol* 28:78-80, 1989.

Kameyama T, Sujaku C, Yamamoto S et al: Shedding of herpes simplex virus type 1 into saliva, *J Oral Pathol* 17:478-481, 1988.

Kolokotronis A, Doumas S: Herpes simplex virus infection, with particular reference to the progression and complications of primary herpetic gingivostomatitis, *Clin Microbiol Infect* 12:202-211, 2006.

Krause PR, Straus SE: Herpesvirus vaccines. Development, controversies, and applications, *Infec Dis Clin North Am* 13:61-81, 1999.

Jensen LA, Hoehns JD, Squires CL: Oral antivirals for the acute treatment of recurrent herpes labialis, *Ann Pharmacother* 38:705-709, 2004.

Nahmias AJ: Sero-epidemiological and -sociological patterns of herpes simplex virus infection in the world, *Scand J Infect Dis Suppl* 69:19-36, 1990.

Nesbit SP, Gobetti JP: Multiple recurrence of oral erythema multiforme after secondary herpes simplex: report of case and review of literature, *J Am Dent Assoc* 112:348-352, 1986.

Overall JC: Oral herpes simplex: pathogenesis, clinical and virologic course, approach to treatment. In Hooks JJ, Jordan G: *Viral infections in oral medicine*, pp 53-78, New York, 1982, Elsevier.

Park JB, Park N: Effect of chlorhexidine on the in vitro and in vivo herpes simplex virus infection, *Oral Surg Oral Med Oral Pathol* 67:149-153, 1989.

Parlette EC, Polo JM: Inoculation herpes barbae, *Skinmed* 4:186-187, 2005.

Raborn GW, Grace MGA: Recurrent herpes simplex labialis: selected therapeutic options, *J Can Dent Assoc* 69:498-503, 2003.

Raborn GW, Martel AY, Lassonde M et al: Effective treatment of herpes simplex labialis with penciclovir cream. Combined results of two trials, *J Am Dent Assoc* 133:303-309, 2002.

Scott DA, Coulter WA, Lamey P-J: Oral shedding of herpes simplex virus type 1: a review, *J Oral Pathol Med* 26:441-447, 1997.

Spruance SL, Freeman DJ, Stewart JC et al: The natural history of ultraviolet radiation–induced herpes simplex labialis and response to therapy with perioral and topical formulations of acyclovir, *J Infect Dis* 163:728-734, 1991.

Spruance SL, Nett R, Marbury T et al: Acyclovir cream for treatment of herpes simplex labialis: results of two randomized, double-blind, vehicle-controlled, multicenter clinical trials, *Antimicrob Agents Chemother* 46:2238-2243, 2002.

Starr JR, Daling JR, Fitzgibbons ED et al: Serologic evidence of herpes simplex virus 1 infection and oropharyngeal cancer risk, *Cancer Res* 61:8459-8464, 2001.

Stanberry LR: Herpes: vaccines for HSV, *Dermatol Clin* 16:811-816, 1998.

Stoopler ET, Greenberg MS: Update on herpesvirus infections, *Dent Clin North Am* 47:517-532, 2003.

Weathers DR, Griffin JW: Intraoral ulcerations of recurrent herpes simplex and recurrent aphthae: two distinct clinical entities, *J Am Dent Assoc* 81:81-88, 1970.

Woo, S-K, Challacombe SJ: Management of recurrent oral herpes simplex infections, *Oral Surg Oral Med Oral Pathol Oral Radiol Endod* 103(suppl 1):S12.e1-S12.e18, 2007.

Wormser GP, Mack L, Lenox T et al: Lack of effect of oral acyclovir on prevention of aphthous stomatitis, *Otolaryngol Head Neck Surg* 98:14-17, 1988.

Varicella-Zoster Virus

Alper BS, Lewis PR: Does treatment of acute herpes zoster prevent or shorten postherpetic neuralgia? *J Fam Pract* 49:255-264, 2000.

Badger GR: Oral signs of chickenpox (varicella): report of two cases, *J Dent Child* 47:349-351, 1980.

Balfour HH Jr, Bean B, Laskin OL et al: Acyclovir halts progression of herpes zoster in immunocompromised patients, *N Engl J Med* 308:1448-1453, 1983.

Barrett AP, Katelaris CH, Morris JGL et al: Zoster sine herpete of the trigeminal nerve, *Oral Surg Oral Med Oral Pathol* 75:173-175, 1993.

Centers for Disease Control and Prevention: Decline in annual incidence of varicella-selected states, *MMWR Morb Mortal Wkly Rep* 52:884-885, 2003.

Centers for Disease Control and Prevention: A new product (VariZIG) for postexposure prophylaxis of varicella available under an investigational new drug application expanded access protocol, *MMWR Morb Mortal Wkly Rep* 55:209-210, 2006.

Centers for Disease Control and Prevention: *CDC's advisory committee recommends "shingles" vaccination.* Available at http://www.cdc.gov/od/media/pressrel/r061026.htm. Accessed December 21, 2007.

Dunkle LM, Arvin AM, Whitley RJ et al: A controlled trial of acyclovir for chickenpox in normal children, *N Engl J Med* 325:1539-1544, 1991.

Furuta Y, Ohtani F, Aizawa H et al: Varicella-zoster virus reactivation is an important cause of acute peripheral facial paralysis in children, *Pedatric Infect Dis* 24:97-101, 2005.

Gilden DH, Cohrs RJ, Hayward AR et al: Chronic varicella-zoster virus ganglionitis–possible cause of postherpetic neuralgia, *J Neurovirol* 9:404-407, 2003.

Kolokotronis A, Louloudiadis K, Fotiou G et al: Oral manifestations of infections due to varicella zoster virus in otherwise healthy children, *J Clin Pediatr Dent* 25:107-112, 2001.

Lieberman JM, Williams WR, Miller JM et al: The safety and immunogenicity of a quadrivalent measles, mumps, rubella and varicella vaccine in healthy children. A study of manufacturing consistency and persistence of antibody, *Pediatr Infect Dis J* 25:615-622, 2006.

Meer S, Coleman H, Altini M et al: Mandibular osteomyelitis and tooth exfoliation following zoster-CMV co-infection, *Oral Surg Oral Med Oral Pathol Oral Radiol Endod* 101:70-75, 2006.

Mendieta C, Miranda J, Brunet LI et al: Alveolar bone necrosis and tooth exfoliation following herpes zoster infection: a review of the literature and case report, *J Periodontol* 76:148-153, 2005.

Ogita S, Terada K, Niizuma T et al: Characteristics of facial nerve palsy during childhood in Japan: frequency of varicella-zoster virus association, *Pediatr Int* 48:245-249, 2006.

Oxman MN, Levin MJ, Johnson GR et al: A vaccine to prevent herpes zoster and postherpetic neuralgia in older adults, *N Engl J Med* 352:2271-2284, 2005.

Stankus SJ, Dlugopolski M, Packer D: Management of herpes zoster (shingles) and postherpetic neuralgia, *Am Fam Physician* 61:2437-2448, 2000.

Straus SE, Ostrove JM, Inchauspe G et al: NIH conference. Varicella-zoster virus infections. Biology, natural history, treatment and prevention, *Ann Intern Med* 108:221-237, 1988.

Wutzler P: Antiviral therapy of herpes simplex and varicella-zoster virus infections, *Intervirology* 40:343-356, 1997.

Infectious Mononucleosis

Courant P, Sobkov T: Oral manifestations of infectious mononucleosis, *J Periodontol* 40:279-283, 1979.

Fraser-Moodie W: Oral lesions in infectious mononucleosis, *Oral Surg Oral Med Oral Pathol* 12:685-691, 1959.

Har-EI G, Josephsen JS: Infectious mononucleosis complicated by lingual tonsillitis, *J Laryngol Otol* 104:651-653, 1990.

Niedobitek G, Meru N, Delecluse H-J: Epstein-Barr virus infection and human malignancies, *Int J Exp Pathol* 82:149-170, 2001.

Roberge RJ, Simon M, Russell M et al: Lingual tonsillitis: an unusual presentation of mononucleosis, *Am J Emerg Med* 19:173-175, 2001.

Ryan C, Dutta C, Simo R: Role of screening for infectious mononucleosis in patients admitted with isolated, unilateral peritonsillar abscess, *J Laryngol Otol* 118:362-365, 2004.

Slote J, Saygun I, Sabeti M et al: Epstein-Barr virus in oral diseases, *J Periodontol Res* 41:235-244, 2006.

Torre D, Tambini R: Acyclovir for treatment of infectious mononucleosis: a meta-analysis, *Scand J Infect Dis* 31:543-547, 1999.

van der Horst C, Joncas J, Ahronheim G et al: Lack of effect of peroral acyclovir for the treatment of acute infectious mononucleosis, *J Infect Dis* 164:788-791, 1991.

Cytomegalovirus

Bonnet F, Neau D, Viallard J-F et al: Clinical and laboratory findings of cytomegalovirus infection in 115 hospitalized non-immunocompromised adults, *Ann Med Interne (Paris)* 152:227-235, 2001.

Epstein JB, Scully C: Cytomegalovirus: a virus of increasing relevance to oral medicine and pathology, *J Oral Pathol Med* 22:348-353, 1993.

Epstein JB, Sherlock CH, Wolber RA: Oral manifestations of cytomegalovirus infection, *Oral Surg Oral Med Oral Pathol* 75:443-451, 1993.

Flaitz CM, Nichols CM, Hicks MJ: Herpesviridae-associated persistent mucocutaneous ulcers in acquired immunodeficiency syndrome: a clinicopathologic study, *Oral Surg Oral Med Oral Pathol Oral Radiol Endod* 81:433-441, 1996.

Guntinas-Lichius O, Wagner M, Krueger GRF et al: Severe acute cytomegalovirus sialadenitis in an immunocompetent adult: case report, *Clin Infect Dis* 22:1117-1118, 1996.

Jones AC, Freedman PD, Phelan JA et al: Cytomegalovirus infections of the oral cavity: a report of six cases and review of the literature, *Oral Surg Oral Med Oral Pathol* 75:76-85, 1993.

Regezi JA, Eversole LR, Barker BF et al: Herpes simplex and cytomegalovirus coninfected oral ulcers in HIV-infected patients, *Oral Surg Oral Med Oral Pathol Oral Radiol Endod* 81:55-62, 1996.

Schubert MM, Epstein JB, Lloid ME: Oral infections due to cytomegalovirus in immunocompromised patients, *J Oral Pathol Med* 22:268-273, 1993.

Slots J: Update on human cytomegalovirus in destructive periodontal disease, *Oral Microbiol Immunol* 19:217-223, 2004.

Stagno S, Pass RF, Thomas JP et al: Defects of tooth structure in congenital cytomegalovirus infection, *Pediatrics* 69:646-648, 1982.

Torres R, Cottrell D, Reebye UN: Ulcerative tongue lesion secondary to cytomegalovirus, *J Mass Dent Soc* 53:36-37, 2004.

Enteroviruses

Buchner A: Hand, foot, and mouth disease, *Oral Surg Oral Med Oral Pathol* 41:333-337, 1976.

Khetsuriani N, Lamonte-Fowlkes A, Oberst S et al: Enterovirus surveillance—United States, 1970-2005, *MMWR Surveill Summ* 55:1-20, 2006.

Chang L-Y, Lin T-Y, Huang Y-C et al: Comparison of enterovirus 71 and coxsackievirus A16 clinical illnesses during the Taiwan enterovirus epidemic, 1998, *Pediatr Infect Dis J* 18:1092-1096, 1999.

Ho M, Hsu K-H, Twu S-J et al: An epidemic of enterovirus 71 infection in Taiwan, *N Engl J Med* 341:929-935, 1999.

Ornoy A, Tenenbaum A: Pregnancy outcome following infections by coxsackie, echo, measles, mumps, hepatitis, polio and encephalitis viruses, *Reprod Toxicol* 21:446-457, 2006.

Steigman AJ, Lipton MM, Braspennickx H: Acute lymphonodular pharyngitis: a newly described condition due to coxsackie virus, *J Pediatr* 61:331-336, 1962.

Rubeola

Kaplan LJ, Daum RS, Smaron M et al: Severe measles in immunocompromised patients, *JAMA* 267:1237-1241, 1992.

Koplik H: The diagnosis of the invasion of measles from a study of the exanthema as it appears on the buccal mucosa membrane, *Arch Pediatr* 13:918-922, 1896.

Nozawa Y, Ono N, Abe M et al: An immunohistochemical study of Warthin-Finkeldey cells in measles, *Pathol Int* 44:442-447, 1994.

Pomerance HH: The usual childhood diseases: forgotten but not gone, *Fetal Pediatr Pathol* 24:169-189, 2005.

Roberts GBS, Bain AD: The pathology of measles, *J Pathol Bacteriol* 76:111-118, 1958.

Suringa DWR, Bank LJ, Ackerman AB: Role of measles virus in skin lesions and Koplik's spots, *N Engl J Med* 283:1139-1142, 1970.

Warthin AS: Occurrence of numerous large giant cells in the tonsils and pharyngeal mucosa in the prodromal stage of measles, *Arch Pathol* 11:864-874, 1931.

Rubella

Centers for Disease Control and Prevention: Elimination of rubella and congenital rubella syndrome—United States, 1969-2004, *MMWR Morb Mortal Wkly Rep* 54:279-282, 2005.

Forchheimer F: German measles (Rubella). In Stedman TL: *Twentieth century practice, an international encyclopedia of modern medical science by leading authorities of Europe and America*, pp 175-188, New York, 1898, W Wood.

Pomerance HH: The usual childhood diseases: forgotten but not gone, *Fetal Pediatr Pathol* 24:169-189, 2005.

Watson JC, Hadler SC, Dykewicz CA et al: Measles, mumps, and rubella—vaccine use and strategies for elimination of measles, rubella, and congenital rubella syndrome and control of mumps: recommendations of the Advisory Committee on Immunization Practices (ACIP), *Morb Mortal Wkly Rep* 47(RR-8):1-57, 1998.

Mumps

Anonymous: Global status of mumps immunization and surveillance, *Wkly Epidemiol Rec* 80:418-424, 2005.

Campos-Outcalt D: Mumps epidemic in 2006: are you prepared to detect and prevent it? *J Fam Pract* 55:500-502, 2006.

Centers for Disease Control and Prevention: Update: mumps activity—United States, January 1-October 7, 2006, *MMWR Morb Mortal Wkly Rep* 55:1152-1153, 2006.

Centers for Disease Control and Prevention: Updated recommendations of the Advisory Committee on Immunization Practices (ACIP) for the control and elimination of mumps, *MMWR Morb Mortal Wkly Rep* 55:629-630, 2006.

Linder TE, Brestel R, Schlegel C: Mumps virus infection: case report of an unusual head and neck manifestation, *Am J Otolaryngol* 17:420-423, 1996.

van Loon FP, Holmes SJ, Sirotkin BI et al: Mumps surveillance—United States 1988-1993, *MMWR CDC Surveill Summ* 44:1-14, 1995.

Human Immunodeficiency Virus and Acquired Immunodeficiency Syndrome

Baccaglini L, Atkinson JC, Patton LL et al: Management of oral lesions in HIV-positive patients, *Oral Surg Oral Med Oral Pathol Oral Radiol* 103(suppl 1):S50.e1-S50.e23, 2007.

Blignaut E, Patton LL, Nittayananta W et al: HIV phenotypes, oral lesions, and management of HIV-related disease, *Adv Dent Res* 19:122-129, 2006.

Campo J, Perea MA, del Romero J et al: Oral transmission of HIV, reality or fiction? An update, *Oral Dis* 12:219-228, 2006.

Centers for Disease Control and Prevention: Twenty-five years of HIV/AIDS—United States, 1981-2006, *MMWR Morb Mortal Wkly Rep* 55:585-589, 2006.

Centers for Disease Control and Prevention: Revised recommendations for HIV testing of adults, adolescents, and pregnant women, *MMWR Recomm Rep* 55:1-7, 2006.

Centers for Disease Control and Prevention: Updated U.S. public health service guidelines for the management of occupational exposures to HIV and recommendations for postexposure prophylaxis, *MMWR Recomm Rep* 54:1-17, 2005.

Cherry-Peppers G, Daniels CO, Meeks V et al: Oral manifestations in the era of HAART, *J Nat Med Assoc* 95:21S-32S, 2003.

Cioc AM, Allen C, Kalmar JR et al: Oral plasmablastic lymphoma in AIDS patients are associated with human herpesvirus 8, *Am J Surg Pathol* 28:41046, 2004.

Cohen PT, Sande MA, Volberding PA: *The AIDS knowledge base: a textbook on HIV disease from the University of California, San Francisco, and the San Francisco General Hospital*, ed 3, Waltham, Mass, 1999, Medical Publishing Group.

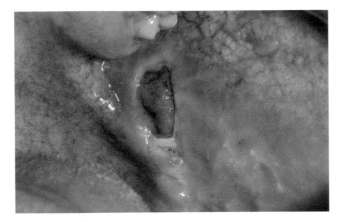

Fig. 8-5   Traumatic ulceration. Well-circumscribed ulceration of the posterior buccal mucosa on the left side.

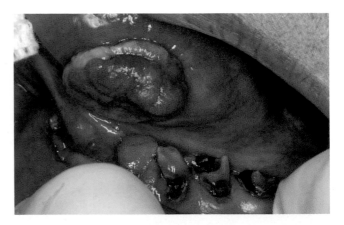

Fig. 8-7   Traumatic granuloma. Exophytic ulcerated mass on the ventrolateral tongue associated with multiple jagged teeth.

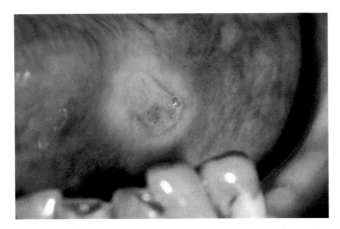

Fig. 8-6   Traumatic ulceration. Mucosal ulceration with a hyperkeratotic collar located on the ventral surface of the tongue.

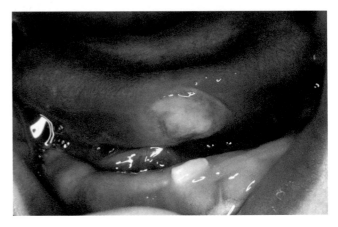

Fig. 8-8   Riga-Fede disease. Newborn with traumatic ulceration of anterior ventral surface of the tongue. Mucosal damage occurred from contact of tongue with adjacent tooth during breastfeeding.

CLINICAL FEATURES

Most injuries are unintentional and arise from a variety of causes. As would be expected, simple chronic traumatic ulcerations occur most often on the tongue, lips, and buccal mucosa—sites that may be injured by the dentition (Fig. 8-5). Lesions of the gingiva, palate, and mucobuccal fold may occur from other sources of irritation. Overzealous toothbrushing can create linear erosions along the free gingival margins. Although these areas may superficially resemble a number of the chronic vesiculoerosive processes, thorough questioning of the patient often leads to the appropriate diagnosis. The individual lesions appear as areas of erythema surrounding a central removable, yellow fibrinopurulent membrane. In many instances, the lesion develops a rolled white border of hyperkeratosis immediately adjacent to the area of ulceration (Fig. 8-6).

Eosinophilic ulcerations are not uncommon but frequently are not reported. The lesions occur in people of all ages, with a significant male predominance. Most have been reported on the tongue, although cases have been seen on the gingiva, buccal mucosa, floor of mouth, palate, and lip. The lesion may last from 1 week to 8 months. The ulcerations appear very similar to the simple traumatic ulcerations; however, on occasion, underlying proliferative granulation tissue can result in a raised lesion similar to a pyogenic granuloma (see page 517) (Fig. 8-7).

Riga-Fede disease typically appears between 1 week and 1 year of age. The condition often develops in association with natal or neonatal teeth (see page 81). The anterior ventral surface of the tongue is the most common site of involvement, although the dorsal surface also may be affected (Fig. 8-8). Ventral lesions contact the adjacent mandibular anterior incisors; lesions on the dorsal surface are associated with the maxillary incisors. A presentation similar to Riga-Fede disease can be the initial finding in a variety of neuro-

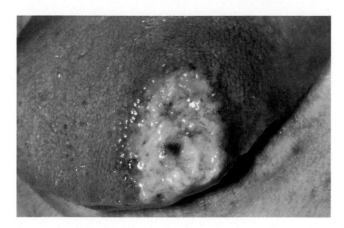

Fig. 8-9 Atypical histiocytic granuloma. Large ulceration of the anterior dorsal surface of the tongue.

logic conditions related to self-mutilation, such as familial dysautonomia (Riley-Day syndrome), congenital indifference to pain, Lesch-Nyhan syndrome, Gaucher disease, cerebral palsy, or Tourette syndrome.

The atypical eosinophilic ulceration occurs in older adults, with most cases developing in patients older than age 40. Surface ulceration is present, and an underlying tumefaction also is seen. The tongue is the most common site, although the gingiva, alveolar mucosa, mucobuccal fold, buccal mucosa, and lip may be affected (Fig. 8-9).

HISTOPATHOLOGIC FEATURES

Simple traumatic ulcerations are covered by a fibrino-purulent membrane that consists of fibrin intermixed with neutrophils. The membrane is of variable thickness, and the adjacent surface epithelium may be normal or may demonstrate slight hyperplasia with or without hyperkeratosis. The ulcer bed consists of granulation tissue that supports a mixed inflammatory infiltrate of lymphocytes, histiocytes, neutrophils, and, occasionally, plasma cells. In patients with eosinophilic ulcerations, the pattern is very similar; however, the inflammatory infiltrate extends into the deeper tissues and exhibits sheets of lymphocytes and histiocytes intermixed with eosinophils. In addition, the vascular connective tissue deep to the ulceration may become hyperplastic and cause surface elevation.

Atypical eosinophilic ulcerations exhibit numerous features of the traumatic eosinophilic ulceration, but the deeper tissues are replaced by a highly cellular proliferation of large lymphoreticular cells. The infiltrate is pleomorphic, and mitotic features are somewhat common. Intermixed with the large atypical cells are mature lymphocytes and numerous eosinophils.

Although an associated immunohistochemical profile rarely has been reported, several investigators have shown the large cells to be T lymphocytes, the majority of which react with CD30 (Ki-1). In many instances, molecular studies for T-cell clonality by polymerase chain reaction (PCR) have been performed on the CD30+ cells and demonstrated monoclonal rearrangement. Whether this monoclonal infiltrate represents a true low-grade lymphoma or an unusual reactive lymphoproliferative process has not been determined.

TREATMENT AND PROGNOSIS

For traumatic ulcerations that have an obvious source of injury, the irritating cause should be removed. Dyclonine HCl or hydroxypropyl cellulose films can be applied for temporary pain relief. If the cause is not obvious, or if a patient does not respond to therapy, then biopsy is indicated. Rapid healing after a biopsy is typical even with large eosinophilic ulcerations (Fig. 8-10). Recurrence is not expected.

The use of corticosteroids in the management of traumatic ulcerations is controversial. Some clinicians have suggested that use of such medications may delay healing. In spite of this, other investigators have reported success using corticosteroids to treat chronic traumatic ulcerations.

Although extraction of the anterior primary teeth is not recommended, this procedure has resolved the ulcerations in Riga-Fede disease. The teeth should be retained if they are stable. Grinding the incisal mamelons, coverage of the teeth with a light-cured composite or cellulose film, construction of a protective shield, or discontinuation of nursing have been tried with variable success.

In patients demonstrating histopathologic similarities to the cutaneous CD30+ lymphoproliferative disorder, a thorough evaluation for systemic lymphoma is mandatory, along with lifelong follow-up. Although recurrence frequently is seen, the ulcerations typically heal spontaneously, and the vast majority of patients do not demonstrate dissemination of the process. Further documentation is critical to define more fully this poorly understood process.

ELECTRICAL AND THERMAL BURNS

Electrical burns to the oral cavity are fairly common, constituting approximately 5% of all burn admissions to hospitals. Two types of electrical burns can be seen: (1) **contact** and (2) **arc**.

Contact burns require a good ground and involve electrical current passing through the body from the point of contact to the ground site. The electric current can cause cardiopulmonary arrest and may be fatal.

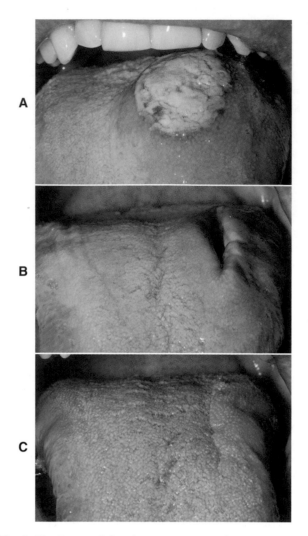

Fig. 8-10   Eosinophilic ulceration. A, Initial presentation of a large ulceration of the dorsal surface of the tongue. **B,** Significant resolution noted 2 weeks after incisional biopsy. **C,** Subsequent healing noted 4 weeks after biopsy.

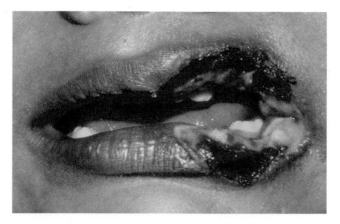

Fig. 8-11   Electrical burn. Yellow charred area of necrosis along the left oral commissure. *(Courtesy of Dr. Patricia Hagen.)*

CLINICAL FEATURES

Most electrical burns occur in children younger than 4 years of age. The lips are affected most frequently, and the commissure commonly is involved. Initially, the burn appears as a painless, charred, yellow area that exhibits little to no bleeding (Fig. 8-11). Significant edema often develops within a few hours and may persist up to 12 days. Beginning on the fourth day, the affected area becomes necrotic and begins to slough. Bleeding may develop during this period from exposure of the underlying vital vasculature, and the presence of this complication should be monitored closely. The adjacent mucobuccal fold, the tongue, or both also may be involved. On occasion, adjacent teeth may become nonvital, with or without necrosis of the surrounding alveolar bone. Malformation of developing teeth also has been documented. In patients receiving high-voltage electrical injury, resultant facial nerve paralysis is infrequently reported and typically resolves over several weeks to months.

The injuries related to thermal food burns usually appear on the palate or posterior buccal mucosa (Fig. 8-12). The lesions appear as zones of erythema and ulceration that often exhibit remnants of necrotic epithelium at the periphery. If hot beverages are swallowed, swelling of the upper airway can occur and lead to dyspnea, which may develop several hours after the injury.

TREATMENT AND PROGNOSIS

For patients with electrical burns of the oral cavity, tetanus immunization, if not current, is required. Most clinicians prescribe a prophylactic antibiotic, usually penicillin, to prevent secondary infection in severe cases. The primary problem with oral burns is contracture of the mouth opening during healing. Without

Most electrical burns affecting the oral cavity are the arc type, in which the saliva acts as a conducting medium and an electrical arc flows between the electrical source and the mouth. Extreme heat, up to 3000° C, is possible with resultant significant tissue destruction. Most cases result from chewing on the female end of an extension cord or from biting through a live wire.

Most **thermal burns** of the oral cavity arise from ingestion of hot foods or beverages. Microwave ovens have been associated with an increased frequency of thermal burns because of their ability to cook food that is cool on the exterior but extremely hot in the interior.

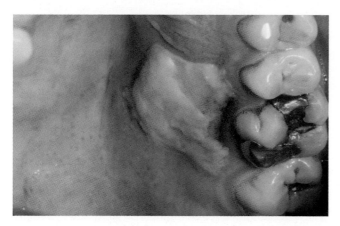

Fig. 8-12   Thermal food burn. Area of yellow-white epithelial necrosis of the left posterior hard palate. Damage was the result of attempted ingestion of a hot pizza roll.

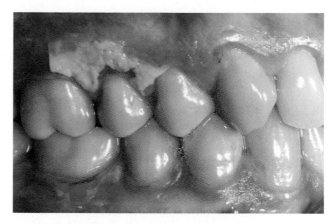

Fig. 8-13   Mucosal burn from tooth-whitening strips. Sharply demarcated zone of epithelial necrosis on the maxillary facial gingiva, which developed from the use of tooth-whitening strips. Less severe involvement also is present on the mandibular gingiva.

intervention, significant microstomia can develop and may produce such restricted access to the mouth that hygiene and eating become impossible in severe cases. Extensive scarring and disfigurement are typical in untreated patients.

To prevent the disfigurement, a variety of microstomia prevention appliances can be used to eliminate or reduce the need for subsequent surgical reconstruction. Compliance is the most important consideration when choosing the most appropriate device. Tissue-supported appliances appear most effective for infants and young children; older, more cooperative patients usually benefit from tooth-supported devices. In most cases, splinting is maintained for 6 to 8 months to ensure proper scar maturation. Evaluation for possible surgical reconstruction is usually performed after a 1-year follow-up.

Most thermal burns are of little clinical consequence and resolve without treatment. When the upper airway is involved and associated with breathing difficulties, antibiotics and corticosteroids often are administered. In rare cases, swelling of the airway mandates intubation or tracheotomy to resolve the associated dyspnea. In these severe cases, oral intake of food often is discontinued temporarily with nutrition provided by a nasogastric tube.

CHEMICAL INJURIES OF THE ORAL MUCOSA

A large number of chemicals and drugs come into contact with the oral tissues. A percentage of these agents are caustic and can cause clinically significant damage.

Patients often can be their own worst enemies. The array of chemicals that have been placed within the mouth in an attempt to resolve oral problems is amazing. Aspirin, sodium perborate, hydrogen peroxide, gasoline, turpentine, rubbing alcohol, and battery acid are just a few of the more interesting examples.

Certain patients, typically children or those under psychiatric care, may hold medications within their mouths rather than swallow them. A surprising number of medications are potentially caustic when held in the mouth long enough. Aspirin, bisphosphonates, and two psychoactive drugs, chlorpromazine and promazine, are well-documented examples.

Topical medications for mouth pain can compound the problem. Mucosal damage has been documented from many of the topical medicaments sold as treatments for toothache or mouth sores. Products containing isopropyl alcohol, phenol, hydrogen peroxide, or eugenol have produced adverse reactions in patients. Over-the-counter tooth-whitening products also contain hydrogen peroxide or one of its precursors, carbamide peroxidase, which has been shown to create mucosal necrosis (Fig. 8-13).

Health care practitioners are responsible for the use of many caustic materials. Silver nitrate, formocresol, sodium hypochlorite, paraformaldehyde, chromic acid, trichloroacetic acid, dental cavity varnishes, and acid-etch materials all can cause patient injury. Education and use of the rubber dam have reduced the frequency of such injuries.

The improper use of aspirin, hydrogen peroxide, silver nitrate, phenol, and certain endodontic materials deserves further discussion because of their frequency of misuse, the severity of related damage, and the lack of adequate documentation of these materials as harmful agents.

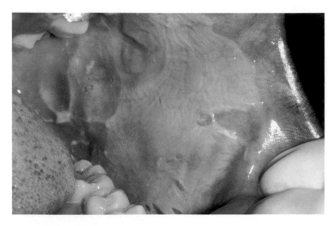

Fig. 8-14   Aspirin burn. Extensive area of white epithelial necrosis of the left buccal mucosa caused by aspirin placement in an attempt to alleviate dental pain.

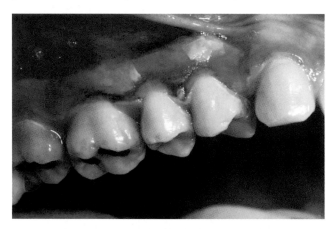

Fig. 8-15   Hydrogen peroxide burn. Extensive epithelial necrosis of the anterior maxillary gingiva secondary to interproximal placement of hydrogen peroxide with cotton swabs.

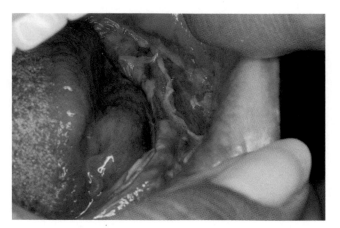

Fig. 8-16   Phenol burn. Extensive epithelial necrosis of the mandibular alveolar mucosa on the left side. Damage resulted from placement of an over-the-counter, phenol-containing, antiseptic and anesthetic gel under a denture. *(Courtesy of Dr. Dean K. White.)*

ASPIRIN

Mucosal necrosis from aspirin being held in the mouth is not rare (Fig. 8-14). Aspirin is available not only in the well-known tablets but also as powder.

HYDROGEN PEROXIDE

Hydrogen peroxide became a popular intraoral medication for prevention of periodontitis in the late 1970s. Since that time, mucosal damage has been seen more frequently as a result of this application. Concentrations at 3% or greater are associated most often with adverse reactions. Epithelial necrosis has been noted with dilutions as low as 1%, and many over-the-counter oral medications exceed this concentration (Fig. 8-15).

SILVER NITRATE

Silver nitrate remains a popular treatment for aphthous ulcerations, because the chemical cautery brings about rapid pain relief by destroying nerve endings. In spite

of this, its use should be strongly discouraged. In all cases the extent of mucosal damage is increased by its use. In some patients an abnormal reaction is seen, with resultant significant damage and enhanced pain. In one report, an application of a silver nitrate stick to a small aphthous ulceration led to a necrotic defect that exceeded 2×2 cm and had to be débrided surgically. In addition, rare reports have documented irreversible systemic argyria secondary to habitual intraoral use of topical silver nitrate after recommendation by a dentist (see page 315).

PHENOL

Phenol has occasionally been used in dentistry as a cavity-sterilizing agent and cauterizing material. It is extremely caustic, and judicious use is required. Over-the-counter agents advertised as "canker sore" treatments may contain low concentrations of phenol, often combined with high levels of alcohol. Extensive mucosal necrosis and (rarely) underlying bone loss have been seen in patients who placed this material (phenol concentration 0.5%) in attempts to resolve minor mucosal sore spots (Fig. 8-16).

A prescription therapy containing 50% sulfuric acid, 4% sulfonated phenol, and 24% sulfonated phenolic agents is being marketed heavily to dentists for treatment of aphthous ulcerations. Because extensive necrosis has been seen from use of medicaments containing 0.5% phenol, this product must be closely monitored and used with great care.

ENDODONTIC MATERIALS

Some endodontic materials are dangerous because of the possibility of soft tissue damage (Fig. 8-17) or their injection into hard tissue with resultant deep spread

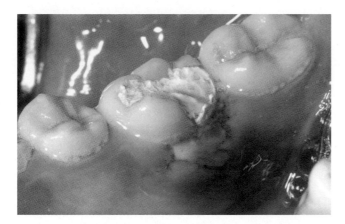

Fig. 8-17   Formocresol burn. Tissue necrosis secondary to leakage of endodontic material between a rubber dam clamp and the tooth.

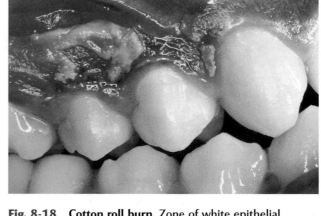

Fig. 8-18   Cotton roll burn. Zone of white epithelial necrosis and erythema of the maxillary alveolar mucosa.

and necrosis. Because of the past difficulty of obtaining profound anesthesia in some patients undergoing root canal therapy, some clinicians have used arsenical paste or paraformaldehyde formulations to devitalize the inflamed pulp. Gingival and bone necrosis have been documented as a consequence of leakage of this material from the pulp chamber into the surrounding tissues. In addition, extrusion of filling material containing paraformaldehyde into the periapical tissues has led to significant difficulties, and its use should be discouraged. Sodium hypochlorite produces similar results when it leaks into the surrounding supporting tissues or is injected past the apex, leading some to suggest chlorhexidine as a safer irrigant. The following can reduce the chances of tissue damage:

- Using a rubber dam
- Avoiding excessive pressure during application
- Keeping the syringe needle away from the apex

CLINICAL FEATURES

The previously discussed caustic agents produce similar damage. With short exposure, the affected mucosa exhibits a superficial white, wrinkled appearance. As the duration of exposure increases, the necrosis proceeds and the affected epithelium becomes separated from the underlying tissue and can be desquamated easily. Removal of the necrotic epithelium reveals red, bleeding connective tissue that subsequently will be covered by a yellowish, fibrinopurulent membrane. Mucosa bound to bone is keratinized and more resistant to damage, whereas the nonkeratinized movable mucosa is destroyed more quickly. In addition to mucosal necrosis, significant tooth erosion has been seen in patients who chronically chew aspirin or hold the medication in their teeth as it dissolves.

The use of the rubber dam can dramatically reduce iatrogenic mucosal burns. When cotton rolls are used for moisture control during dental procedures, two problems may occur. On occasion, caustic materials can leak into the cotton roll and be held in place against the mucosa for an extended period, with mucosal injury resulting from the chemical absorbed by the cotton. In addition, oral mucosa can adhere to dry cotton rolls, and rapid removal of the rolls from the mouth often can cause stripping of the epithelium in the area. The latter pattern of mucosal injury has been termed **cotton roll burn (cotton roll stomatitis)** (Fig. 8-18).

Caustic materials injected into bone during endodontic procedures can result in significant bone necrosis, pain, and perforation into soft tissue. Necrotic surface ulceration and edema with underlying areas of soft tissue necrosis may occur adjacent to the site of perforation.

HISTOPATHOLOGIC FEATURES

Microscopic examination of the white slough removed from areas of mucosal chemical burns reveals coagulative necrosis of the epithelium, with only the outline of the individual epithelial cells and nuclei remaining (Fig. 8-19). The necrosis begins on the surface and moves basally. The amount of epithelium affected depends on the duration of contact and the concentration of the offending agent. The underlying connective tissue contains a mixture of acute and chronic inflammatory cells.

TREATMENT AND PROGNOSIS

The best treatment of chemical injuries is prevention of exposure of the oral mucosa to caustic materials. When using potentially caustic drugs (e.g., aspirin,

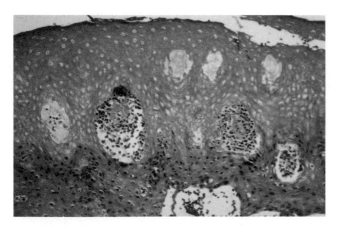

Fig. 8-19 Chemical-related epithelial necrosis. Oral mucosa exhibiting superficial coagulative necrosis of the epithelial cells.

chlorpromazine), the clinician must instruct the patient to swallow the medication and not allow it to remain in the oral cavity for any significant length of time. Children should not use chewable aspirin immediately before bedtime, and they should rinse after use.

Superficial areas of necrosis typically resolve completely without scarring within 10 to 14 days after discontinuation of the offending agent. For temporary protection, some clinicians have recommended coverage with a protective emollient paste or a hydroxypropyl cellulose film. Topical dyclonine HCl provides excellent but temporary pain relief. When large areas of necrosis are present, such as that related to the use of silver nitrate or accidental intrabony injection of offending materials, surgical débridement and antibiotic coverage often are required to promote healing and prevent spread of the necrosis.

NONINFECTIOUS ORAL COMPLICATIONS OF ANTINEOPLASTIC THERAPY

No systemic anticancer therapy currently available is able to destroy tumor cells without causing the death of at least some normal cells, and tissues with rapid turnover (e.g., oral epithelium) are especially susceptible. The mouth is a common site (and one of the most visible areas) for complications related to cancer therapy. Both radiation therapy and systemic chemotherapy may cause significant oral problems. The more potent the treatment, the greater the risk of complications. Each year almost 400,000 patients in the United States suffer acute or chronic oral side effects from anticancer treatments. With the advancement of medical practice, these complications are becoming more common as more patients have longer survival times and as intense therapies, such as bone marrow transplantation, become more commonplace. Oral complications are noted almost uniformly in patients receiving head and neck radiation, and close to 75% of bone marrow transplant patients are affected. The prevalence of chemotherapy-associated oral complications varies from 10% to 75%, depending on the type of associated cancer and the form of chemotherapy used.

CLINICAL FEATURES

A variety of noninfectious oral complications are seen regularly as a result of both radiation and chemotherapy. Two acute changes, **mucositis** and **hemorrhage,** are the predominant problems associated with chemotherapy, especially in cancers, such as leukemia, that involve high treatment doses.

Painful acute mucositis and dermatitis are the most frequently encountered side effects of radiation, but several chronic alterations continue to plague patients long after their courses of therapy are completed. Depending on the fields of radiation, the radiation dose, and the age of the patient, the following outcomes are possible:

- Xerostomia
- Loss of taste (hypogeusia)
- Osteoradionecrosis
- Trismus
- Chronic dermatitis
- Developmental abnormalities

HEMORRHAGE

Intraoral **hemorrhage** is typically secondary to thrombocytopenia, which develops from bone marrow suppression. Intestinal or hepatic damage, however, may cause lower vitamin K–dependent clotting factors, with resultant increased coagulation times. Conversely, tissue damage related to therapy may cause release of tissue thromboplastin at levels capable of producing potentially devastating disseminated intravascular coagulation (DIC). Oral petechiae and ecchymosis secondary to minor trauma are the most common presentations. Any mucosal site may be affected, but the labial mucosa, tongue, and gingiva are involved most frequently.

MUCOSITIS

Recent research suggests that mucosal damage secondary to cancer therapy is much more complex than previously thought and appears to arise from an extended series of molecular and cellular events that take place not only in the epithelium but also in the underlying stroma. Genetic differences in the rate of tissue apop-

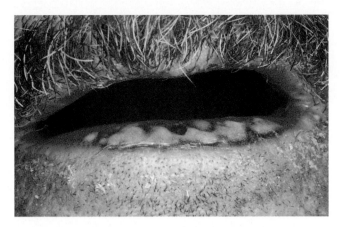

Fig. 8-20   Chemotherapy-related epithelial necrosis. Vermilion border of the lower lip exhibiting epithelial necrosis and ulceration in a patient receiving systemic chemotherapy.

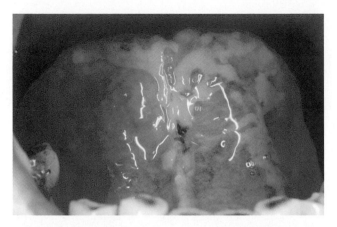

Fig. 8-21   Chemotherapy-related epithelial necrosis. Large, irregular area of epithelial necrosis and ulceration of the anterior ventral surface of the tongue in a patient receiving systemic chemotherapy.

tosis, microvascular injury from endothelial apoptosis, and increased peripheral blood levels of tumor necrosis factor α and interleukin-6 appear to be involved. Beyond the direct effects of the antineoplastic agent, additional risk factors include young age, female sex, poor oral hygiene, oral foci of infection, poor nutrition, impaired salivary function, tobacco use, and alcohol consumption.

Cases of oral **mucositis** related to radiation or chemotherapy are similar in their clinical presentations. The manifestations of chemotherapy develop after a few days of treatment; radiation mucositis may begin to appear during the second week of therapy. Both chemotherapy and radiation-induced mucositis will resolve slowly 2 to 3 weeks after cessation of treatment. Oral mucositis associated with chemotherapy typically involves the nonkeratinized surfaces (i.e., buccal mucosa, ventrolateral tongue, soft palate, floor of the mouth), whereas radiation therapy primarily affects the mucosal surfaces within the direct portals of radiation.

The earliest manifestation is development of a whitish discoloration from a lack of sufficient desquamation of keratin. This is soon followed by loss of this layer with replacement by atrophic mucosa, which is edematous, erythematous, and friable. Subsequently, areas of ulceration develop with formation of a removable yellowish, fibrinopurulent surface membrane (Figs. 8-20 to 8-22). Pain, burning, and discomfort are significant and can be worsened by eating and oral hygiene procedures.

DERMATITIS

Acute **dermatitis** of the skin in the fields of radiation is common and varies according to the intensity of the therapy. Patients with mild radiation dermatitis experi-

ence erythema, edema, burning, and pruritus. This condition resolves in 2 to 3 weeks after therapy and is replaced by hyperpigmentation and variable hair loss. Moderate radiation causes erythema and edema in combination with erosions and ulcerations. Within 3 months these alterations resolve, and permanent hair loss, hyperpigmentation, and scarring may ensue. Necrosis and deep ulcerations can occur in severe acute reactions. Radiation dermatitis also may become chronic and be characterized by dry, smooth, shiny, atrophic, necrotic, telangiectatic, depilated, or ulcerated areas.

XEROSTOMIA

Salivary glands are very sensitive to radiation, and **xerostomia** is a common complication. When a portion of the salivary glands is included in the fields of radiation, the remaining glands undergo compensatory hyperplasia in an attempt to maintain function. The changes begin within 1 week of initiation of radiation therapy, with a dramatic decrease in salivary flow noted during the first 6 weeks of treatment. Even further decreases may be noted for up to 3 years.

Serous glands exhibit an increased radiosensitivity when compared with the mucous glands. On significant exposure, the parotid glands are affected dramatically and irreversibly. In contrast, the mucous glands partially recover and, over several months, may achieve flow that approaches 50% of preradiation levels. Symptomatic dry mouth appears most strongly associated with a decrease in palatal mucous secretions, with the loss of parotid serous secretion exerting a less noticeable effect. In addition to the discomfort of a mouth that lacks proper lubrication, diminished flow of saliva leads to a significant decrease of the bactericidal action and self-cleansing properties of saliva.

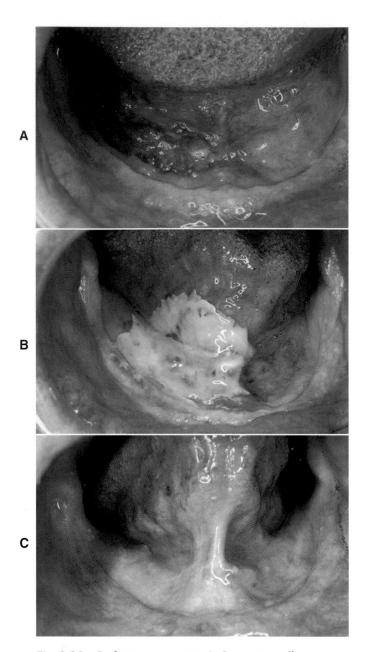

Fig. 8-22 Radiation mucositis. A, Squamous cell carcinoma before radiation therapy. Granular erythroplakia of the floor of the mouth on the patient's right side. **B,** Same lesion after initiation of radiation therapy. Note the large, irregular area of epithelial necrosis and ulceration of the anterior floor of the mouth on the patient's right side. **C,** Normal oral mucosa after radiation therapy. Note resolution of the tumor and the radiation mucositis.

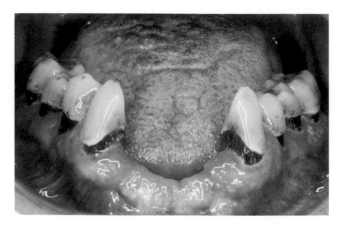

Fig. 8-23 Xerostomia-related caries. Extensive cervical caries of mandibular dentition secondary to radiation-related xerostomia.

Without intervention, patients often develop symptomatic dry mouth that affects their ability to eat comfortably, wear dentures, speak, and sleep. In addition, there often is an increase in the caries index **(xerostomia-related caries),** regardless of the patient's past caries history (Fig. 8-23). The decay is predominantly cervical in location and secondary to xerostomia (not a direct effect of the radiation).

LOSS OF TASTE

In patients who receive significant radiation to the oral cavity, a substantial loss of all four tastes **(hypogeusia)** often develops within several weeks. Although these tastes return within 4 months for most patients, some patients are left with permanent hypogeusia; others may have persistent **dysgeusia** (altered sense of taste) (see page 875).

OSTEORADIONECROSIS

Osteoradionecrosis is one of the most serious complications of radiation to the head and neck; however, it is seen less frequently today because of better treatment modalities and prevention. The current prevalence rate is approximately 5%, whereas the frequency approached 15% less than 20 years ago. Although the risk is low, it increases dramatically if a local surgical procedure is performed within 21 days of therapy initiation or within 12 months after therapy.

In the past, many researchers believed that radiation induced an osseous endarteritis that led to tissue hypoxia, hypocellularity, and hypovascularity and created a predisposition to necrosis if a minor injury occurred. This theory led to widespread use of hyperbaric oxygen in the prevention and treatment of this pathosis. However, many now believe the process is more complex and may involve radiation damage to osseous cells; when these cells lose normal function, bone turnover is suppressed in a manner similar to the effect on osteoclasts associated with use of bisphosphonates (see page 299). Researchers believe that damage to these cells not only disrupts their primary function but also affects bone vascularity

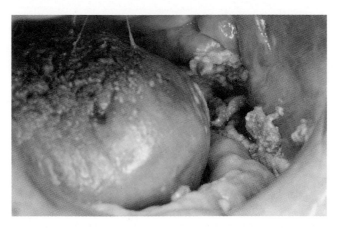

Fig. 8-24   Osteoradionecrosis. Ulceration overlying left body of the mandible with exposure and sequestration of superficial alveolar bone.

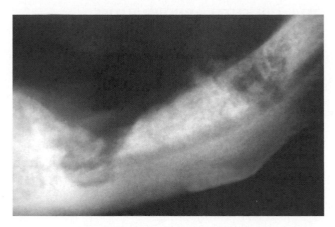

Fig. 8-25   Osteoradionecrosis. Multiple ill-defined areas of radiolucency and radiopacity of the mandibular body.

through a complex interaction of cytokines and growth factors.

Previously, investigators suggested that radiation-associated reduction in healing capacity might be permanent, with the risk for osteonecrosis remaining high for many years. Currently, others have proposed that repair of damaged osseous cells occurs as they are replaced by future cellular generations. Investigations have suggested that significant recovery does occur, and the prevalence of osteonecrosis is reduced significantly after a 1-year recovery period, with or without use of hyperbaric oxygen. More recent clinical trials of irradiated patients have shown a low prevalence of osteonecrosis if a period of postradiation healing (1 year or longer) is combined with atraumatic surgical technique.

Although most instances of osteoradionecrosis arise secondary to local trauma, a minority appear spontaneous. The mandible is involved most frequently, although a few cases have involved the maxilla (Fig. 8-24). Affected areas of bone reveal ill-defined areas of radiolucency that may develop zones of relative radiopacity as the dead bone separates from the residual vital areas (Fig. 8-25). Intractable pain, cortical perforation, fistula formation, surface ulceration, and pathologic fracture may be present (Fig. 8-26).

The radiation dose is the main factor associated with bone necrosis, although the proximity of the tumor to bone, the presence of remaining dentition, and the type of treatment also exert an effect. Additional factors associated with an increased prevalence include older age, male sex, poor health or nutritional status, and continued use of tobacco or alcohol.

Prevention of bone necrosis is the best course of action. Before therapy, all questionable teeth should be extracted or restored, and oral foci of infection should

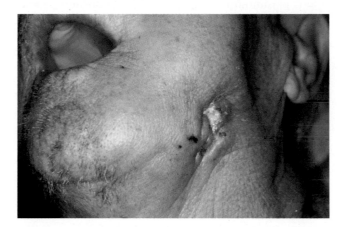

Fig. 8-26   Osteoradionecrosis. Same patient as depicted in Fig. 8-24. Note fistula formation of the left submandibular area resulting from osteoradionecrosis of the mandibular body.

be eliminated; excellent oral hygiene should be initiated and maintained. A healing time of at least 3 weeks between extensive dental procedures and the initiation of radiotherapy significantly decreases the chance of bone necrosis. Extraction of teeth or any bone trauma is strongly contraindicated during radiation therapy.

TRISMUS

Trismus may develop and can produce extensive difficulties concerning access for hygiene and dental treatment. Tonic muscle spasms with or without fibrosis of the muscles of mastication and the temporomandibular joint (TMJ) capsule can cause difficulties in jaw opening. When these structures are radiated heavily, jaw-opening exercises may help to decrease or prevent problems.

DEVELOPMENTAL ABNORMALITIES

Antineoplastic therapy during childhood can affect growth and development. The changes vary according to the age at treatment and the type and severity of therapy. Radiation can alter the facial bones and result in micrognathia, retrognathia, or malocclusion. Developing teeth are very sensitive and can exhibit a number of changes, such as root dwarfism, blunting of roots, dilaceration of roots, incomplete calcification, premature closure of pulp canals in deciduous teeth, enlarged canals in permanent teeth, microdontia, and hypodontia (see page 58).

TREATMENT AND PROGNOSIS

Optimal treatment planning involves the oral health practitioner before initiation of antineoplastic therapy. Elimination of all current or potential oral foci of infection is paramount, along with patient education about maintaining ultimate oral hygiene. Proper nutrition, cessation of tobacco use, and alcohol abstinence will minimize oral complications. Once cancer therapy is initiated, efforts must be directed toward relieving pain, preventing dehydration, maintaining adequate nutrition, eliminating foci of infection, and ensuring continued appropriate oral hygiene.

MUCOSITIS

In an attempt to decrease the severity, duration, and symptoms associated with oral mucositis, a large number of treatments such as anesthetic, analgesic, antimicrobial, and coating agents have been tried with mixed reviews. Few have been proven to be consistently beneficial in well-designed placebo-controlled trials. A low-cost salt and soda rinse often has demonstrated similar effectiveness and a lower adverse reaction profile when compared with many other interventions. When all treatments fail, the degree of mucositis and associated pain may mandate systemic morphine therapy.

Cryotherapy (placement of ice chips in the mouth 5 minutes before chemotherapy and continued for 30 minutes) has been shown to reduce significantly the prevalence and severity of oral mucositis secondary to bolus injection of chemotherapeutic drugs with a short half-life, such as 5-fluorouracil or edatrexate. Although limited by the hardware expense and necessity for specialized training, low-level helium-neon laser therapy also appears to reduce the frequency and severity of chemotherapy-associated mucositis.

A new avenue of research is concentrating on growth factors that may affect the prevalence of oral mucositis. Recently, intravenous (IV) recombinant human keratinocyte growth factor (palifermin) became the first compound approved by the U.S. Food and Drug Administration (FDA) for reduction of oral mucositis related to myelotoxic chemotherapy. In clinical studies, this expensive biologic response modifier provided a modest, but statistically significant, reduction in the severity of mucositis, severity of oral pain, use of narcotic analgesia, and need for total parenteral nutrition.

One of the more effective mechanisms to reduce radiation-associated mucositis has been placement of midline radiation blocks or use of three-dimensional radiation treatment to limit the volume of irradiated mucosa. Although not approved in the United States but available in Canada and Europe, topical benzydamine reduces the frequency, severity, and pain of radiation-associated oral mucositis. This unique nonsteroidal antiinflammatory drug (NSAID) also exhibits analgesic, anesthetic, and antimicrobial properties.

XEROSTOMIA

Xerostomic patients should be counseled to avoid all agents that may decrease salivation, especially the use of tobacco products and alcohol. To combat xerostomia-related caries, a regimen of daily topical fluoride application should be instituted.

The problem of chronic xerostomia has been approached through the use of salivary substitutes and sialagogues. Because the mucous glands often demonstrate significant recovery after radiation, the sialagogues show promise because they stimulate the residual functional glands. Moisturizing gels, sugarless candies, and chewing gum are used, but the most efficacious product in controlled clinical studies has been systemic use of one of the cholinergic drugs, pilocarpine or cevimeline. Although these drugs may be beneficial for many patients, they are contraindicated in patients with asthma, gastrointestinal ulcerations, labile hypertension, glaucoma, chronic obstructive pulmonary disease, and significant cardiovascular disease. Adverse reactions are uncommon but include excess sweating, rhinitis, headache, nausea, uropoiesis, flatulence, and circulatory disorders.

Other systemic salivary stimulants that are associated with a less dramatic influence on flow include bethanechol and anetholetrithione. Anetholetrithione appears to act by increasing the number of salivary gland receptors. Although somewhat effective when used alone, this medication has been combined with one of the cholinergic medications and achieved improvement in patients who failed to respond to the use of a single agent.

LOSS OF TASTE

Although the taste buds often regenerate within 4 months after radiation therapy, the degree of long-term impairment is highly variable. In those with continuing symptoms, zinc sulfate supplements greater than the usual recommended daily doses appear to be beneficial.

OSTEORADIONECROSIS

Although prevention must be stressed, cases of osteoradionecrosis do occur. Use of hyperbaric oxygen has numerous contraindications and possible adverse reactions. Because of the newer theories of pathogenesis for osteoradionecrosis, many clinicians are less inclined to use hyperbaric oxygen except in selected cases. Therapy consists of antibiotics, débridement, irrigation, and removal of diseased bone. The amount of bone removed is determined by clinical judgment, with the surgery extended until brightly bleeding edges are seen.

BISPHOSPHONATE-ASSOCIATED OSTEONECROSIS

The initial association between use of bisphosphonates and subsequent development of gnathic osteonecrosis was documented in 2003. Bisphosphonates comprise a unique class of medications that has been shown to inhibit osteoclasts and possibly interfere with angiogenesis through actions such as inhibition of vascular endothelial growth factor. These medications can be delivered by mouth (PO) or intravenously (IV) and are used primarily to slow osseous involvement of a number of cancers (multiple myeloma and metastatic breast or prostate carcinoma), to treat Paget's disease (see page 623), and to reverse osteoporosis.

The first-generation bisphosphonates have a relatively low potency and are readily metabolized by osteoclasts. Addition of a nitrogen side chain was added subsequently, creating a more potent second generation of these drugs, designated **aminobisphosphonates** (Box 8-1). In contrast to the first generation, these formulations are incorporated into the skeleton and demonstrate an extended half-life (e.g., estimated to be 12 years for alendronate). Currently, strong association with gnathic osteonecrosis has been limited to the aminobisphosphonates.

Although bone may seem to be a stable tissue, it constantly is undergoing a process of resorption and reapposition throughout life. The typical lifespan of an osteoblast/osteocyte is approximately 150 days. Osteoclasts also play a critical role in the maintenance of normal bone by repairing microfractures and resorbing areas of bone that contain foci of older nonvital osteocytes. On resorption of bone, cytokines and growth factors such as bone morphogenetic protein are released and induce formation of active bone-forming osteoblasts. If osteoclastic function declines, then microfractures accumulate and the lifespan of the

Box 8-1

Bisphosphonate Medications

FIRST-GENERATION DRUGS
- Bonefos (clodronate)
  Relative potency of 10
  PO and IV formulations
- Didronel (etidronate disodium)
  Relative potency of 1
  PO
- Skelid (tiludronic disodium)
  Relative potency of 10
  PO

AMINOBISPHOSPHONATE DRUGS
- Actonel (risedronate sodium)
  Relative potency of 5000
  PO
- Aredia (pamidronate disodium)
  Relative potency 100
  IV
- Boniva (ibandronate sodium)
  Relative potency 10,000
  PO and IV formulations
- Fosamax (alendronate sodium)
  Relative potency 1000
  PO
- Reclast (zoledronic acid)
  Relative potency 100,000
  IV formulation
  Infused annually for osteoporosis
  FDA approval pending
- Zometa (zoledronic acid)
  Relative potency 100,000
  IV

PO, By mouth; *IV*, Intravenous; *FDA*, U.S. Food and Drug Administration.

entrapped osteocytes is exceeded, creating areas of vulnerable bone. When osteoclasts ingest bisphosphonate-treated bone, the medication is cytotoxic and induces osteoclastic apoptosis, a reduction in recruitment of additional osteoclasts, and a stimulation of osteoblasts to release an osteoclast-inhibiting factor. The incorporation of the medication is highest in areas of active remodeling, such as the jaws. Although the vast majority of osteonecrosis cases have occurred in the jaws, extragnathic involvement has been documented (e.g., osteonecrosis of ear after removal of exostosis of the external ear canal).

CLINICAL AND RADIOGRAPHIC FEATURES

In an excellent systematic review of 368 reported cases of **bisphosphonate-associated osteonecrosis** (BON), 94% were discovered in patients who were treated with

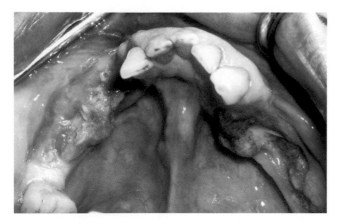

Fig. 8-27 Bisphosphonate-associated osteonecrosis.
Bilateral necrotic exposed bone of the mandible in a patient
receiving zoledronic acid for metastatic breast cancer. (*Courtesy
of Dr. Brent Mortenson.*)

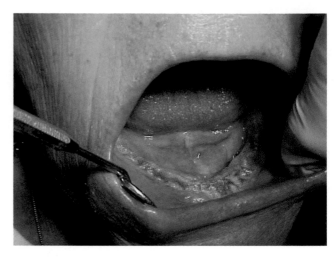

Fig. 8-28 Bisphosphonate-associated osteonecrosis.
Extensive necrosis of the mandible, which followed extraction
of multiple teeth. The patient was receiving zoledronic acid
for metastatic breast cancer. (*Courtesy of Dr. Benny Bell.*)

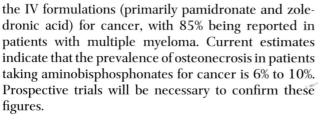

the IV formulations (primarily pamidronate and zoledronic acid) for cancer, with 85% being reported in
patients with multiple myeloma. Current estimates
indicate that the prevalence of osteonecrosis in patients
taking aminobisphosphonates for cancer is 6% to 10%.
Prospective trials will be necessary to confirm these
figures.

Osteonecrosis related to use of oral aminobisphosphonates is most uncommon (conservative estimate by
drug industry: annual incidence is 0.7 per 100,000);
however, prospective trials for the true incidence of
this complication have yet to be performed. Risk factors
for BON associated with the PO formulations include
advanced patient age (older than 65 years), corticosteroid use, use of chemotherapy drugs, diabetes, smoking
or alcohol use, poor oral hygiene, and duration of drug
use exceeding 3 years. A predictive test for those at risk
for bisphosphonate osteonecrosis has not been confirmed. Some investigators recently have suggested
use of a serum marker for bone turnover, serum C-
telopeptide (CTX), but additional prospective studies
are needed to confirm the utility of this test.

Although a mandibular predominance has been
noted, involvement of the maxilla or both jaws is not
uncommon (Fig. 8-27). In 60% of these patients, the
necrosis has followed an invasive dental procedure,
with the remainder occurring spontaneously (Fig.
8-28). On occasion, the necrosis can occur after minor
trauma to bony prominences, such as tori or other
exostoses (Fig. 8-29). Affected patients have areas of
exposed, necrotic bone that is asymptomatic in approximately one third.

Investigators have suggested that bone at imminent
risk for osteonecrosis often will demonstrate increased

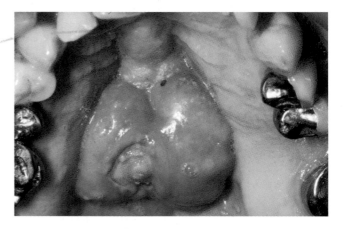

Fig. 8-29 Bisphosphonate-associated osteonecrosis.
Lobulated palatal torus with an area of exposed necrotic
bone in a patient taking alendronate for osteoporosis.

radiopacity before clinical evidence of frank necrosis.
These changes typically occur predominantly in areas
of high bone remodeling, such as the alveolar ridges.
Panoramic radiographs often will reveal a marked
radiodensity of the crestal portions of each jaw, with a
more normal appearance of the bone away from tooth-
bearing portions. Periosteal hyperplasia also is not rare.
In more severe cases, the osteonecrosis creates a moth-
eaten and ill-defined radiolucency with or without
central radiopaque sequestra (Fig. 8-30). In some cases
the necrosis can lead to development of a cutaneous
sinus or pathologic fracture (Fig. 8-31).

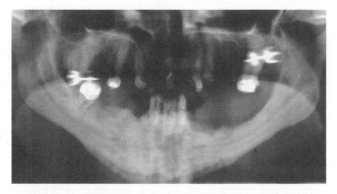

Fig. 8-30   Bisphosphonate-associated osteonecrosis.
Panoramic radiograph of patient depicted in Fig. 8-27. Note sclerosis of tooth-bearing areas along with multiple radiolucencies and periosteal hyperplasia of the lower border of the mandible. *(Courtesy of Dr. Brent Mortenson.)*

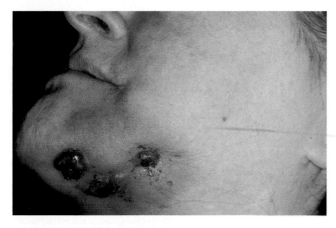

Fig. 8-31   Bisphosphonate-associated osteonecrosis.
Patient with multiple cutaneous sinuses associated with extensive necrosis of the left side of the mandible. The patient was taking zoledronic acid for multiple myeloma.
(Courtesy of Dr. Molly Rosebush.)

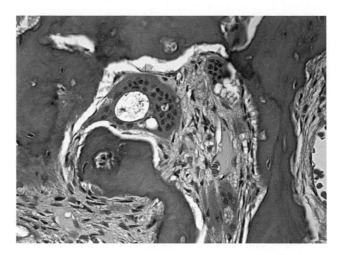

Fig. 8-32   Bisphosphonate-associated osseous changes.
Pagetoid bone exhibiting enlarged, irregular osteoclasts that contain numerous intracytoplasmic vacuoles. *(Courtesy of Dr. Don Cohen.)*

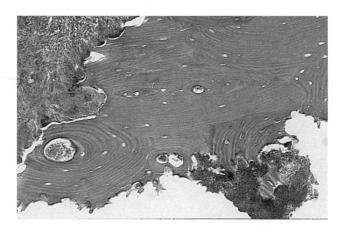

Fig. 8-33   Bisphosphonate-associated osteonecrosis.
Sclerotic lamellar bone exhibiting loss of the osteocytes from their lacunae and peripheral resorption with bacterial colonization.

HISTOPATHOLOGIC FEATURES

Biopsy of vital bone altered by aminobisphosphonates is not common. In such cases the specimen often reveals irregular trabeculae of pagetoid bone, with adjacent enlarged and irregular osteoclasts that often demonstrate numerous intracytoplasmic vacuoles (Fig. 8-32). Specimens of active areas of BON reveal trabeculae of sclerotic lamellar bone, which demonstrate loss of the osteocytes from their lacunae and frequent peripheral resorption with bacterial colonization (Fig. 8-33). Although the peripheral bacterial colonies often resemble actinomycetes, the infestation is not consistent with cervicofacial actinomycosis.

TREATMENT AND PROGNOSIS

The clinical approach to patients treated with aminobisphosphonates varies according to the formulation of the drug, the disease being treated, and the duration of drug use. All patients who take these medications should be warned of the risks and instructed to obtain and maintain ultimate oral hygiene. The oral medications are extremely caustic; patients should be warned to minimize oral mucosal contact and ensure the medication is swallowed completely.

Routine dental therapy, in most cases, should not be modified solely on the basis of oral aminobisphosphonate use. All restorative, prosthodontic, conventional endodontic, and routine periodontic procedures can be implemented as needed. Although orthodontic treatment is not contraindicated, progress should be evaluated after 2 to 3 months of active therapy. At that point, therapy can proceed if the tooth movement is occurring predictably with normal forces. Invasive orthodontic techniques such as orthognathic surgery, four-tooth extraction cases, and miniscrew anchorage should be avoided, if possible. Because the medication is drawn to sites of active bone remodeling, a drug holiday (or switching to a nonaminobisphosphonate agent) during active orthodontics may be advantageous.

When manipulation of bone is considered (e.g., surgical endodontics, periodontal bone recontouring, oral surgery, implant placement), the patient should be advised of the potential complications of aminobisphosphonate use and the risk of BON. Written informed consent and documentation of a discussion of the benefits, risks, and alternative therapies are highly advised. For elective surgical procedures in patients with a duration of drug use exceeding 3 years, discontinuation of the medication 3 months before and 3 months after surgery has been suggested. Because of the reduced angiogenesis, osseous grafts should be used judiciously. If multiple sites require surgery, then one sextant should be treated with a 2-month disease-free follow-up before completion of the remaining sextants. During this interval, use of chlorhexidine twice daily is recommended. The sextant-by-sextant approach is not necessary for periapical inflammatory disease or abscesses, both of which can lead directly to osteonecrosis and demand immediate resolution.

Dental therapy in patients taking an IV formulation for cancer is much more problematic. Prevention is paramount. In patients evaluated before initiation of an IV aminobisphosphonate, the goal is to eliminate all dental infections and improve dental health to prevent future invasive therapy; this includes removal of large tori or partially impacted teeth. If only noninvasive therapy is necessary, then the initiation of the medication need not be delayed. If surgical procedures are performed, then a month-long delay in initiation of the medication is recommended, along with prophylactic antibiotic therapy (i.e., penicillin; quinolone and metronidazole, or erythromycin and metronidazole for those allergic to penicillin).

For patients presenting in the midst of active IV therapy, a number of clinicians have suggested that manipulation of bone should be avoided. Conventional endodontics is a better option than extraction. If a nonvital tooth is not restorable, then endodontics should be performed and followed by crown amputation. Teeth with 1+ or 2+ mobility should be splinted; those with 3+ mobility can be extracted.

For patients with BON, the goal of therapy is to stop pain. A number of clinicians believe that removal of bone typically results in further bone necrosis, and hyperbaric oxygen has not been beneficial. Asymptomatic patients should rinse daily with chlorhexidine and

be monitored closely. Any rough edges of exposed bone should be smoothed. If the exposed bone irritates adjacent tissues, then coverage with a soft splint may prove beneficial. In symptomatic patients, systemic antibiotic therapy (i.e., penicillin with or without metronidazole, ciprofloxacin or erythromycin and metronidazole for those allergic to penicillin) and chlorhexidine usually lead to pain relief. If the antibiotics fail to stop the pain, then hospitalization with IV therapy is indicated. In recalcitrant cases the bulk of the dead bone is reduced surgically, followed by administration of systemic antibiotics. Because of the long half-life of bisphosphonates, discontinuation of the drug offers no short-term benefit. In isolated anecdotal reports of recalcitrant cases, discontinuation of the medication for 6 to 12 months occasionally has been associated with spontaneous sequestration and resolution.

As mentioned in the discussion of the radiographic features, the alveolar ridges of patients affected with osteonecrosis exhibit significant sclerosis because of increased drug deposition in areas of high remodeling. Some investigators have successfully treated patients with BON by resection of all of the osteosclerotic areas with extension to the underlying more lucent and normally bleeding bone. As adjunctive therapy to enhance healing, the osseous defect can be covered with a resorbable collagen membrane impregnated with platelet-rich plasma.

Overall, the benefits of aminobisphosphonate therapy for osteoporosis and metastatic cancer appear to greatly outweigh the risk of developing BON. However, the oral medications should be prescribed only for those individuals with inadequate bone density and should be discontinued or switched to a nonaminobisphosphonate once the bone density returns to an acceptable level.

Increased bone density does not correlate necessarily to good bone quality. The negative effects of oversuppression of bone metabolism must be considered in all patients prescribed oral aminobisphosphonates. Several reports have documented spontaneous nontraumatic stress fractures with associated delayed healing in patients on long-term aminobisphosphonate therapy. Many physicians now believe that aminobisphosphonate therapy should be stopped after 5 years and not reinitiated until bone density studies confirm redevelopment of significant osteoporosis.

Dentists should be proactive and strongly encourage patients to speak to their attending physicians for consideration of these factors during planning and execution of long-term care. For individuals scheduled to receive IV aminobisphosphonate therapy as part of their cancer management, the involved oncologist should recommend pretreatment dental evaluation and preventive care, with long-term, close follow-up.

OROFACIAL COMPLICATIONS OF METHAMPHETAMINE ABUSE

Methamphetamine ("meth") is a drug with stimulant effects on the central nervous system (CNS). In 1937 the drug was approved in the United States for the treatment of narcolepsy and attention deficit hyperactivity disorder. Within a few years, many began to use the drug to increase alertness, control weight, and combat depression. Because methamphetamine users perceive increased physical ability, greater energy, and euphoria, illegal use and manufacture of the drug began to develop. Because of greater control over the main ingredient, pseudoephedrine, production of homemade methamphetamine is decreasing but often being replaced by illegal importation of the finished product. The drug is a powdered crystal that dissolves easily in liquid and can be smoked, snorted, injected, or taken orally. The drug is known by nicknames that include *chalk, crank, crystal, fire, glass, ice, meth,* and *speed.*

CLINICAL FEATURES

Although methamphetamine abuse may occur throughout society, most users are men between the ages of 19 and 40 years. The effects of the medication last up to 12 hours, and the typical abuser reports use that exceeds 20 days per month, creating an almost continuous effect of the drug. The short-term effects of methamphetamine include insomnia, aggressiveness, agitation, hyperactivity, decreased appetite, tachycardia, tachypnea, hypertension, hyperthermia, vomiting, tremors, and xerostomia. Long-term effects additionally include strong psychologic addiction, violent behavior, anxiety, confusion, depression, paranoia, auditory hallucinations, delusions, mood changes, skin lesions, and a number of cardiovascular, CNS, hepatic, gastrointestinal, renal, and pulmonary disorders.

Many addicts develop delusions of **parasitosis (formication, from the** Latin word *formica,* which translates to *ant*), a neurosis that produces the sensation of snakes or insects crawling on or under the skin. This sensation causes the patient to attempt to remove the perceived parasites, usually by picking at the skin with fingernails, resulting in widespread traumatic injury. The factitial damage can alter dramatically the facial appearance in a short period of time, and these lesions have been nicknamed *speed bumps, meth sores,* or *crank bugs.*

Rampant dental caries is another common manifestation and exhibits numerous similarities with milk-bottle caries. The carious destruction initially affects

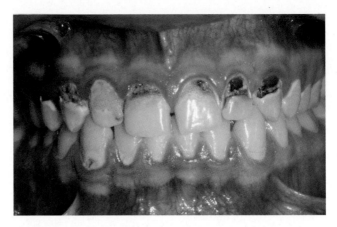

Fig. 8-34   Methamphetamine-related dental caries. Extensive smooth-surface decay of the anterior dentition.

the facial smooth and interproximal surfaces, but without intervention, the coronal structure of the entire dentition can be destroyed (Fig. 8-34). The carious destruction appears to be caused by poor oral hygiene combined with extreme drug-related xerostomia, which leads to heavy consumption of acidic and sugar-filled soft drinks or other refined carbohydrates.

TREATMENT AND PROGNOSIS

The oral health practitioner should be alerted when an emaciated, agitated, and nervous young adult presents with tachycardia, tachypnea, hypertension, hyperthermia, and rampant smooth surface and interproximal caries. Failure to recognize these signs can be serious. For up to 6 hours after ingestion, methamphetamine potentiates the effects of sympathomimetic amines. Use of local anesthetics with epinephrine or levonordefrin can lead to a hypertensive crisis, cerebral vascular accident, or myocardial infarction. Caution also should be exercised when administering sedatives, general anesthesia, nitrous oxide, or prescriptions for narcotics. Although cessation of the illicit drug use is paramount, patients should be encouraged during periods of xerostomia to discontinue use of highly acidic and sugar-filled soft drinks and to avoid diuretics such as caffeine, tobacco, and alcohol. In addition, the importance of personal and oral hygiene should be stressed. Preventive measures such as topical fluorides may assist in protecting the remaining dentition. A medical consultation with referral to a substance abuse center should be encouraged.

ANESTHETIC NECROSIS

Administration of a local anesthetic agent can, on rare occasions, be followed by ulceration and necrosis at the site of injection. Researchers believe that this

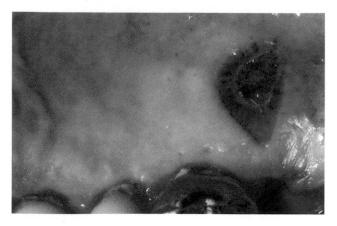

Fig. 8-35   Anesthetic necrosis. Mucosal necrosis of the hard palate secondary to palatal injection with a local anesthetic agent containing epinephrine.

necrosis results from localized ischemia, although the exact cause is unknown and may vary from case to case. Faulty technique, such as subperiosteal injection or administration of excess solution in tissue firmly bound to bone, has been blamed. The epinephrine contained in many local anesthetics also has received attention as a possible cause of ischemia and secondary necrosis.

CLINICAL FEATURES

Anesthetic necrosis usually develops several days after the procedure and most commonly appears on the hard palate (Fig. 8-35). A well-circumscribed area of ulceration develops at the site of injection. The ulceration often is deep, and, on occasion, healing may be delayed. One report has documented sequestration of bone at the site of tissue necrosis.

TREATMENT AND PROGNOSIS

Treatment of anesthetic necrosis usually is not required unless the ulceration fails to heal. Minor trauma, such as that caused by performing a cytologic smear, has been reported to induce resolution in these chronic cases. Recurrence is unusual but has been reported in some patients in association with use of epinephrine-containing anesthetics. In these cases the use of a local anesthetic without epinephrine is recommended.

EXFOLIATIVE CHEILITIS

Exfoliative cheilitis is a persistent scaling and flaking of the vermilion border, usually involving both lips. The process arises from excessive production and subsequent desquamation of superficial keratin. A significant percentage of cases appears related to chronic injury secondary to habits such as lip licking, biting, picking, or sucking. Those cases proven to arise from chronic injury are termed **factitious cheilitis.**

Many patients deny chronic self-irritation of the area. The patient may be experiencing associated personality disturbances, psychologic difficulties, or stress. In a review of 48 patients with exfoliative cheilitis, 87% exhibited psychiatric conditions and 47% also demonstrated abnormal thyroid function. Evidence suggests that there may be a link between thyroid dysfunction and some psychiatric disturbances.

In other cases, no evidence of chronic injury is evident. In these patients other causes should be ruled out (e.g., atopy, chronic candidal infection, actinic cheilitis, cheilitis glandularis, hypervitaminosis A, photosensitivity). In a review of 165 patients with acquired immunodeficiency syndrome (AIDS), more than one quarter had alterations that resembled exfoliative cheilitis. In this group the lip alterations appeared secondary to chronic candidal infestation. The most common presentation of bacterial or fungal infections of the lips is **angular cheilitis** (see page 216). Diffuse primary infection of the entire lip is very unusual; most diffuse cases represent a secondary candidal infection in areas of low-grade trauma of the vermilion border of the lip **(cheilocandidiasis).**

In one review of 75 patients with chronic cheilitis, a thorough evaluation revealed that more than one third represented irritant contact dermatitis (often secondary to chronic lip licking). In 25% of the patients, the cheilitis was discovered to be an allergic contact mucositis (see page 350). Atopic eczema was thought to be the cause in 19% of cases; the remaining portion was related to a wide variety of pathoses.

In spite of a thorough investigation, there often remain a number of patients with classic exfoliative cheilitis for which no underlying cause can be found. These idiopathic cases are most troublesome and often resistant to a wide variety of interventions.

CLINICAL FEATURES

A marked female predominance is seen in cases of factitious origin, with most cases affecting those younger than 30 years of age. Mild cases feature chronic dryness, scaling, or cracking of the vermilion border of the lip (Fig. 8-36). With progression, the vermilion can become covered with a thickened, yellowish hyperkeratotic crust that can be hemorrhagic or that may exhibit extensive fissuring. The perioral skin may become involved and exhibit areas of crusted erythema (Fig. 8-37). Although this pattern may be confused with perioral dermatitis (see page 352), the most appropri-

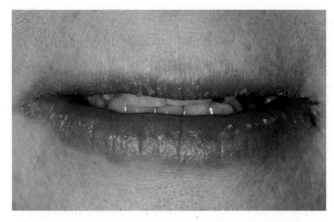

Fig. 8-36   Exfoliative cheilitis. Scaling and erythema of the vermilion border of the lower lip.

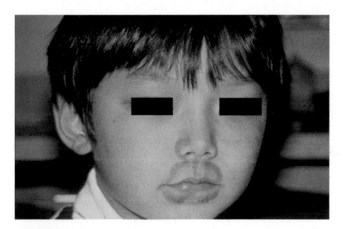

Fig. 8-37   Circumoral dermatitis. Crusting and erythema of the skin surface adjacent to the vermilion border in a child who chronically sucked on both lips.

ate name for this process is *circumoral dermatitis.* Both lips or just the lower lip may be involved.

In patients with chronic cheilitis, development of fissures on the vermilion border is not rare. In a prevalence study of more than 20,000 patients, these fissures involved either lip and were slightly more common in the upper lip. In contrast to typical exfoliative cheilitis, these fissures demonstrate a significant male predilection and a prevalence rate of approximately 0.6%. The majority arise in young adults, with rare occurrence noted in children and older adults.

Although the cause is unknown, proposed contributing factors include overexposure to sun, wind, and cold weather; mouth breathing; bacterial or fungal infections; and smoking. An increased prevalence of lip fissures has been noted in patients with Down syndrome and may be the result of the high frequency of mouth breathing or the tendency to develop orofacial candidiasis. Application of lipstick or lip balm appears to be

protective. Fissure occurrence also may be related to a physiologic weakness of the tissues. Those affecting the lower lip typically occur in the midline, whereas fissures on the upper vermilion most frequently involve a lateral position. These are the sites of prenatal merging of the mandibular and maxillary processes.

TREATMENT AND PROGNOSIS

In those cases associated with an obvious cause, elimination of the trigger typically results in resolution of the changes. In those cases with no underlying physical, infectious, or allergic cause, psychotherapy (often combined with mild tranquilization or stress reduction) may achieve resolution. In cases for which no cause can be found, therapeutic interventions often are not successful.

Cases that result from candidal infections often do not resolve until the chronic trauma also is eliminated. Initial topical antifungal agents, antibiotics, or both can be administered to patients in whom chronic trauma is not obvious or is denied. If the condition does not resolve, then further investigation is warranted in an attempt to discover the true source of the lip alterations.

Hydrocortisone and iodoquinol (antibacterial and antimycotic) cream has been used to resolve chronic lip fissures in some patients (Fig. 8-38). Other reported therapies include various corticosteroid preparations, topical tacrolimus, sunscreens, and moisturizing preparations. In many cases, resistance to topical therapy or frequent recurrence is noted. In these cases, cryotherapy or excision with or without Z-plasty has been used successfully.

SUBMUCOSAL HEMORRHAGE

Everyone has experienced a bruise from minor trauma. This occurs when a traumatic event results in hemorrhage and entrapment of blood within tissues. Different terms are used, depending on the size of the hemorrhage:
- Minute hemorrhages into skin, mucosa, or serosa are termed **petechiae.**
- If a slightly larger area is affected, the hemorrhage is termed a **purpura.**
- Any accumulation greater than 2 cm is termed an **ecchymosis.**
- If the accumulation of blood within tissue produces a mass, this is termed a **hematoma.**

Blunt trauma to the oral mucosa often results in hematoma formation. Less well known are petechiae and purpura, which can arise from repeated or prolonged increased intrathoracic pressure (Valsalva maneuver) associated with such activities as repeated

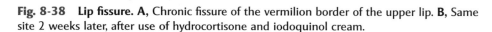

Fig. 8-38   Lip fissure. A, Chronic fissure of the vermilion border of the upper lip. **B,** Same site 2 weeks later, after use of hydrocortisone and iodoquinol cream.

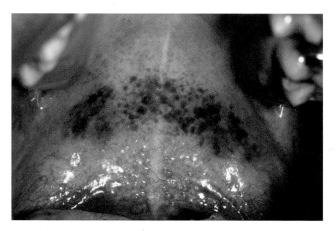

Fig. 8-39   Petechiae. Submucosal hemorrhage of the soft palate caused by violent coughing.

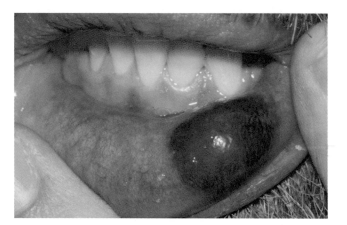

Fig. 8-40   Purpura. Submucosal hemorrhage of the lower labial mucosa on the left side secondary to blunt trauma.

coughing, vomiting, convulsions, or giving birth (Fig. 8-39). When considering a diagnosis of traumatic hemorrhage, the clinician should keep in mind that hemorrhages can result from nontraumatic causes, such as anticoagulant therapy, thrombocytopenia, disseminated intravascular coagulation (DIC), and a number of viral infections, especially infectious mononucleosis and measles.

With the increased frequency of dental implant placement, a number of reports have surfaced related to potentially life-threatening floor of mouth hemorrhage secondary to a tear in the lingual periosteum or perforation of the cortical plate during implant site preparation. Similar spontaneous sublingual hemorrhage has been documented in patients with severe hypertension or a systemic coagulopathy. Another unusual hemorrhagic event involves the development of an organized hematoma within the maxillary sinus. The blood originates from a variety sources, the most

common of which is intranasal hemorrhage that drains through the ostia and collects in the antrum.

CLINICAL FEATURES

Submucosal hemorrhage appears as a nonblanching flat or elevated zone with a color that varies from red or purple to blue or blue-black (Fig. 8-40). As would be expected, traumatic lesions are located most frequently on the labial or buccal mucosa. Blunt facial trauma often is responsible, but injuries such as minor as cheek biting may produce a hematoma or areas of purpura (Fig. 8-41). Mild pain may be present.

The hemorrhage associated with increased intrathoracic pressure usually is located on the skin of the face and neck and appears as widespread petechiae that clear within 24 to 72 hours. Although it has not been as well documented as the cutaneous lesions, mucosal hemorrhage can be seen in the same setting

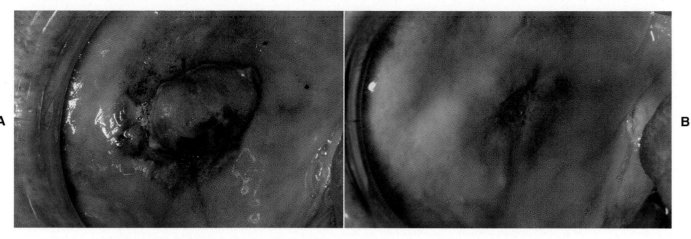

Fig. 8-41   Hematoma. A, Dark-purple nodular mass of the buccal mucosa in a patient on coumadin therapy. **B,** Near resolution of the lesion 8 days later after discontinuation of the medication. *(Courtesy of Dr. Charles Ferguson.)*

and most often appears as soft palatal petechiae or purpura.

Hematoma formation associated with surgical implant preparation usually is associated with damage of the soft tissues adjacent to the lingual surface of the mandible and produces swelling and elevation of the floor of the mouth. Although the hemorrhage is noticeable immediately in most patients, the problem may not become evident clinically for 4 to 6 hours. Distension, elevation, and protrusion of the tongue may occur and be associated with inability to swallow or significant dyspnea.

Patients with antral hematomas typically complain of frequent nasal bleeding but also may experience unilateral nasal obstruction, hyposmia, headache, and malar swelling. Facial paresthesia and vision problems occur less frequently. Computed tomography (CT) typically demonstrates a soft tissue mass filling and expanding the antrum, often associated with proptosis and partial destruction or displacement of the sinus walls. In many instances, the radiographic appearance is worrisome for a malignant neoplasm.

TREATMENT AND PROGNOSIS

Often, no treatment is required if the hemorrhage is not associated with significant morbidity or related to systemic disease. The areas should resolve spontaneously. Large hematomas may require several weeks to resolve. If the hemorrhage occurs secondary to an underlying disorder, then treatment is directed toward control of the associated disease.

In cases of emergent hemorrhage associated with surgical implant placement, the first priority is to secure the airway. Although the hemorrhage can be controlled with conservative measures in some cases, the majority require surgical exploration with isolation and repair of the damaged vessel. Antral hematomas usually are removed via a Caldwell-Luc procedure for both therapeutic and diagnostic purposes. After successful removal, a search for the bleeding source or any underlying coagulopathy is recommended to prevent recurrence.

ORAL TRAUMA FROM SEXUAL PRACTICES

Although orogenital sexual practices are illegal in many jurisdictions, they are extremely common. Among homosexual men and women, orogenital sexual activity almost is universal. For married heterosexual couples younger than age 25, the frequency has been reported to be as high as 90%. Considering the prevalence of these practices, the frequency of associated traumatic oral lesions is surprisingly low.

CLINICAL FEATURES

The most commonly reported lesion related to orogenital sex is submucosal palatal hemorrhage secondary to fellatio. The lesions appear as erythema, petechiae, purpura, or ecchymosis of the soft palate. The areas often are asymptomatic and resolve without treatment in 7 to 10 days (Fig. 8-42). Recurrences are possible with repetition of the inciting (exciting?) event. The erythrocytic extravasation is thought to result from the musculature of the soft palate elevating and tensing against an environment of negative pressure. Similar lesions have been induced from coughing, vomiting, or forceful sucking on drinking straws and glasses.

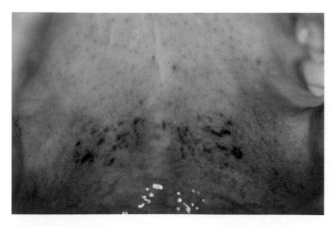

Fig. 8-42   Palatal petechiae from fellatio. Submucosal hemorrhage of the soft palate resulting from the effects of negative pressure.

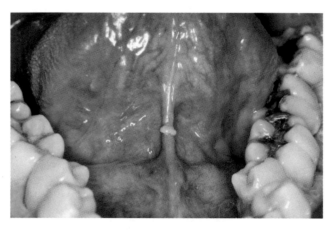

Fig. 8-43   Fibrous hyperplasia from repeated cunnilingus. Linear fibrous hyperplasia of the lingual frenum caused by repeated irritation from lower incisors.

Forceful thrusting against the vascular soft palate has been suggested as another possible cause.

Oral lesions also can occur from performing cunnilingus, resulting in horizontal ulcerations of the lingual frenum. As the tongue is thrust forward, the taut frenum rubs or rakes across the incisal edges of the mandibular central incisors. The ulceration created coincides with sharp tooth edges when the tongue is in its most forward position. The lesions resolve in 7 to 10 days but may recur with repeated performances. Linear fibrous hyperplasia has been discovered in the same pattern in individuals who chronically perform the act (Fig. 8-43).

HISTOPATHOLOGIC FEATURES

With an appropriate index of suspicion, biopsy usually is not required; however, a biopsy has been performed in some cases of palatal lesions secondary to fellatio.

These suction-related lesions reveal subepithelial accumulations of red blood cells that may be extensive enough to separate the surface epithelium from underlying connective tissue. Patchy degeneration of the epithelial basal cell layer can occur. The epithelium classically demonstrates migration of erythrocytes and leukocytes from the underlying lamina propria.

TREATMENT AND PROGNOSIS

No treatment is required, and the prognosis is good. In patients who request assistance, palatal petechiae can be prevented through the use of less negative pressure and avoidance of forceful thrusting. Smoothing and polishing the rough incisal edges of the adjacent mandibular teeth can minimize the chance of lingual frenum ulceration.

AMALGAM TATTOO AND OTHER LOCALIZED EXOGENOUS PIGMENTATIONS

A number of pigmented materials can be implanted within the oral mucosa, resulting in clinically evident pigmentations. Implantation of dental amalgam (**amalgam tattoo**) occurs most often, with a frequency that far outdistances that for all other materials. *Localized argyrosis* has been used as another name for amalgam tattoo, but this nomenclature is inappropriate because amalgam contains not only silver but also mercury, tin, copper, zinc, and other metals.

Amalgam can be incorporated into the oral mucosa in several ways. Previous areas of mucosal abrasion can be contaminated by amalgam dust within the oral fluids. Broken amalgam pieces can fall into extraction sites. If dental floss becomes contaminated with amalgam particles of a recently placed restoration, then linear areas of pigmentation can be created in the gingival tissues as a result of hygiene procedures (Fig. 8-44). Amalgam from endodontic retrofill procedures can be left within the soft tissue at the surgical site (Fig. 8-45). Finally, fine metallic particles can be driven through the oral mucosa from the pressure of high-speed air turbine drills.

Theoretically, the use of the rubber dam should decrease the risk; however, immediately after removal of the dam, the occlusion often is adjusted with the potential for amalgam contamination of any areas of mucosal damage. Submucosal implantation of pencil graphite, coal and metal dust, fragments of broken carborundum disks, dental burs, and, in the past, charcoal dentifrices, have resulted in similar-appearing areas of discoloration.

Intentional tattooing, which can be found in approximately 25% of the world's population, also may be

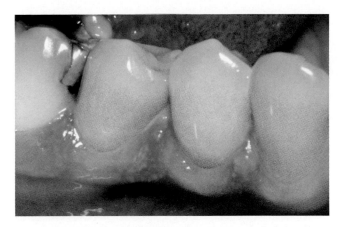

Fig. 8-44 Floss-related amalgam implantation. Linear strips of mucosal pigmentation that align with the interdental papillae. The patient used dental floss on the mandibular first molar immediately after the placement of the amalgam restoration. Because the area was still anesthetized, the patient impaled the floss on the gingiva, then continued forward using the amalgam-impregnated floss in the bicuspid area to create additional amalgam tattoos.

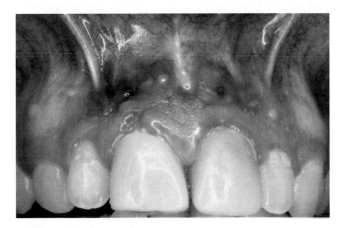

Fig. 8-45 Endodontic-related amalgam implantation. Multifocal areas of mucosal discoloration overlying the maxillary anterior incisors, which have been treated with apical retrofill procedures.

performed in the oral cavity. Although some cases are culturally related, health professionals also are responsible for a number of intentional oral and facial tattoos for the purpose of demonstrating landmarks, judging tumor response to antineoplastic therapies, repigmenting areas of vitiligo, cosmetically disguising disfigured areas, and applying permanent cosmetic makeup. Injudicious intraoral use of these marking agents can cause diffusion of the pigment with discoloration of the adjacent skin surface.

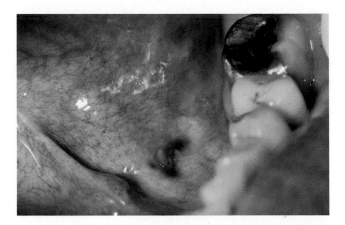

Fig. 8-46 Amalgam tattoo. Area of mucosal discoloration of the floor of the mouth on the patient's left side.

CLINICAL AND RADIOGRAPHIC FEATURES

Amalgam tattoos appear as macules or, rarely, as slightly raised lesions. They may be black, blue, or gray. The borders can be well defined, irregular, or diffuse (Fig. 8-46). Lateral spread may occur for several months after the implantation. In most cases, only one site is affected, although multiple tattoos in a single patient may be present. Any mucosal surface can be involved, but the most common sites are the gingiva, alveolar mucosa, and buccal mucosa (Fig. 8-47).

Periapical radiographs, when taken, are negative in many cases. When metallic fragments are visible radiographically, the clinical area of discoloration typically extends beyond the size of the fragment. The fragments are densely radiopaque, varying from several millimeters to pinpoint in size (see Fig. 8-47). On occasion, the pattern of the amalgam dispersal has been sufficiently unique to be used as a distinctive characteristic in the identification of unknown deceased individuals.

The pattern of accidental localized foreign body tattoo other than amalgam is diverse and depends on the associated trauma that impacted the material. Mucosal graphite implantation is rarely documented, but it most likely occurs with a higher frequency than indicated by the number of cases reported. Examples in the literature have been presented as grayish areas of mucosal discoloration of the hard palate, the most likely site for pencil-related trauma.

Cosmetic tattooing is gaining in popularity and may include injection of permanent cosmetic inks into the eyelids and vermilion border of the upper and lower lips. On occasion, patients may react to the material and experience swelling, burning, and itching at the site, followed by enlargement and induration. In such cases, biopsy often reveals a granulomatous reaction to the foreign material.

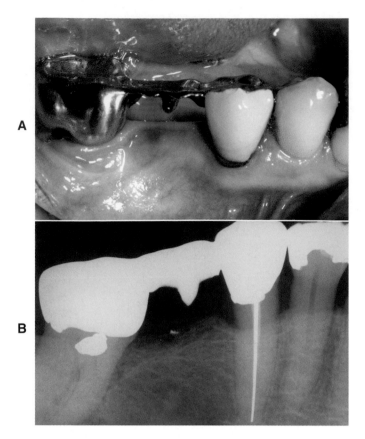

Fig. 8-47   Amalgam tattoo. A, Area of mucosal discoloration of the mandibular alveolar ridge immediately below the bridge pontic. **B,** Radiograph of the same patient showing radiopaque metallic fragment present at the site of mucosal discoloration.

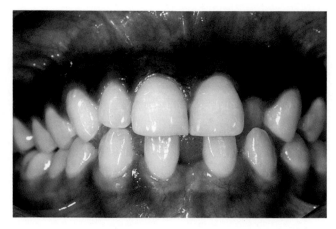

Fig. 8-48   Intentional intraoral tattoo. Cultural tattoo of the maxillary facial gingiva in a patient from Senegal. *(Courtesy of Dr. Kristin McNamara.)*

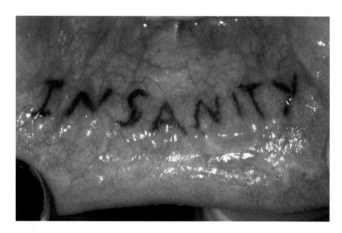

Fig. 8-49   Intentional intraoral tattoo. Amateur tattoo of the lower labial mucosa. *(Courtesy of Dr. Edward Herschaft.)*

The intentional intraoral tattoos that are not placed by health professionals occur most frequently on the anterior maxillary facial gingiva of individuals from a number of African countries and have been documented at institutions in the United States (Fig. 8-48). In these cases the anterior maxillary facial gingiva is given a heavy blue-black discoloration. Occasionally, tattoos (usually blue or black) are placed on the labial mucosa of adults in the United States to convey a personal, often vulgar, message (Fig. 8-49).

HISTOPATHOLOGIC FEATURES

Microscopic examination of amalgam tattoos reveals pigmented fragments of the metal within the connective tissue. Scattered, large, dark, solid fragments or numerous fine, black, or dark-brown granules may be seen (Fig. 8-50). The silver salts of the dental amalgam preferentially stain the reticulin fibers, especially those encircling nerves and vascular channels (Fig. 8-51).

The biologic response to amalgam appears related to particle size and the elemental composition of the amalgam. Large fragments often become surrounded by dense fibrous connective tissue with mild inflammation. Smaller particles typically are associated with a more significant inflammatory response that may be granulomatous or a mixture of lymphocytes and plasma cells. Graphite implantation appears similar microscopically to amalgam but can be differentiated by its pattern of birefringence after treatment with ammonium sulfide and by the lack of staining of the reticulin fibers. In addition, energy dispersive x-ray microanalysis can be used to identify the type of material present within areas of foreign body tattoos.

TREATMENT AND PROGNOSIS

To confirm the diagnosis of amalgam tattoo, the clinician can obtain radiographs of the areas of mucosal discoloration in an attempt to demonstrate the metallic

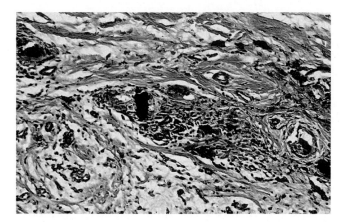

Fig. 8-50 Amalgam tattoo. Numerous dark, solid fragments of amalgam are surrounded by a lymphohistiocytic inflammatory infiltrate.

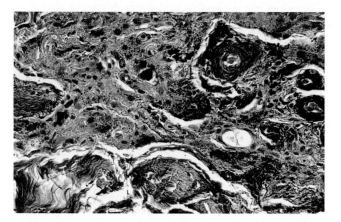

Fig. 8-51 Amalgam tattoo. Dark amalgam stain encircling numerous vascular channels.

fragments. The films should be capable of high detail, because many of the fragments are no larger than the point of a pin.

No treatment is required if the fragments can be detected radiographically. If no metallic fragments are found and the lesion cannot be diagnosed clinically, then biopsy may be needed to rule out the possibility of melanocytic neoplasia. On occasion, the amalgam implantation may create pigmentation in a cosmetically objectionable location such as the anterior maxillary facial gingiva. In such cases, conservative surgical excision can be performed; alternatively amalgam tattoos have been removed successfully with Q-switched ruby or alexandrite lasers. With respect to cosmetic tattoos, a variety of treatments such as corticosteroids and lasers have been used with variable results.

ORAL PIERCINGS AND OTHER BODY MODIFICATIONS

Historical evidence from almost every continent shows that body piercing is an ancient practice with a strong association with religious, cultural, or superstitious beliefs. In the Western world, body piercing beyond the earlobes has become increasingly popular as a method of self-expression during the past decade. In a 2001 survey of 481 college students in the United States, 51% admitted body piercing, and the prevalence still appears to be rising. Usually, the piercing is performed to place jewelry in sites such as the eyebrows, helix of the ears, nose, navel, nipples, genitals, and a number of intraoral sites.

Forked tongue (split tongue, bifid tongue) is a rather recent addition to the art of body modification, with few associated publications. In this practice the anterior one third of the tongue is split down the middle. This has been performed slowly by pulling fishing line through a pierced hole and tightening the loop over a period of 3 weeks or using a surgical instrument or laser to quickly separate the two halves. Some form of cautery is necessary to prevent the halves from reuniting. Forked tongue also has been reported as a complication of tongue piercing.

Another practice with unique orofacial manifestations is implantation of a form of **talisman** (magical charm) called **susuk (charm needles, charm pins).** This practice is common in southeast Asia, especially Malaysia, Thailand, Singapore, Indonesia, and Brunei. The susuk is placed by a native magician or medicine man termed *bomoh* and is thought to enhance or preserve beauty, relieve pain, bring success in business, or provide protection against harm. The majority of the individuals with susuk are Muslims, although Islam strictly prohibits black magic. Therefore, many affected individuals will deny placement of susuk, even when confronted directly with hard evidence.

CLINICAL AND RADIOGRAPHIC FEATURES

Intraoral piercings are noted most frequently in adolescents and young adults, with a female predominance. The most commonly affected sites are the tongue, lips, buccal mucosa, and, rarely, the uvula. The selected site typically is pierced with a 14- to 16-gauge sheeted needle, then the jewelry of choice is threaded through the wound. The jewelry most often is gold, silver, or stainless steel; in the tongue, the most frequent adornment is a **barbell** (dumbbell might be a better name!) consisting of a metal rod with a ball that screws onto each end (Fig. 8-52). The lip jewelry is termed a **labret** and most often consists of a ring or a rod with a flat end attached to the

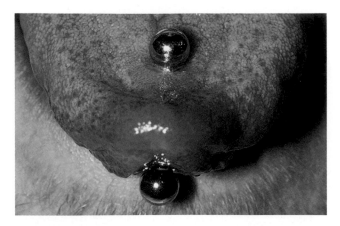

Fig. 8-52 Lingual piercing. Tongue pierced with a jewelry item known as a *barbell*.

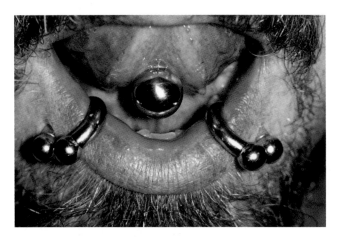

Fig. 8-53 Labial piercing. Lower lip pierced bilaterally with labrets consisting of a circular rod with terminating balls. The patient also has a lingual barbell.

mucosal side and a round ball for the cutaneous surface (Fig. 8-53).

If no complications occur, healing of the piercing site takes place within 4 to 6 weeks. Potential acute complications include pain, prolonged or profuse bleeding, swelling (to the point of airway obstruction in rare cases), infection including Ludwig's angina and cerebellar brain abscess, lingual nerve damage, speech impediment, and allergy to the jewelry. Chronic complications include mucosal or gingival trauma, chipped or fractured teeth, hypersalivation, aspiration or swallowing of jewelry, tissue hyperplasia around the posts, and embedded jewelry. Gingival recession (labrets, barbells) and tooth fracture (barbells) are extremely common, with the prevalence closely related to the duration of use. Molars and premolars are fractured most frequently, with the damage associated more often with a short-stem barbell, whereas greater severity of gingival recession is associated with long-stem barbells and labrets.

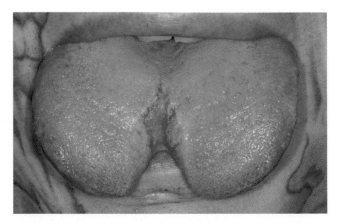

Fig. 8-54 Forked tongue. Anterior portion of the tongue divided into two separate lobes, each of which can be controlled independently. *(Courtesy Dr. Fleming Chisholm.)*

In individuals with forked tongues, the anterior half of the tongue is split down the middle (Fig. 8-54). Risks of the procedure include inflammation, infection, profuse or prolonged hemorrhage, and permanent neurovascular damage. After healing, some individuals have developed the ability to control each half independently.

Susuk usually is shaped like a needle that is pointed on one end and blunt on the other. Most are made from silver or gold, measure 0.5 mm in diameter, and vary from 0.5 to 1.0 cm in length. Rarely, they are made from diamonds. The pins vary in number from one to many and are inserted subcutaneously, often in a symmetrical fashion. The orofacial region is the most common location, but some choose the chest, arms, breasts, and pubic region. In most instances, the individuals are middle-aged adults. Normally, no clinical evidence exists, either visually or by palpation, and the pins are discovered during routine radiography for unrelated medical or dental problems (Fig. 8-55).

TREATMENT AND PROGNOSIS

As mentioned, intraoral barbells and labrets are associated with an increasing prevalence of oral complications that relate closely with duration of use. The patient should be strongly encouraged to remove the jewelry. On removal, if the site demonstrates significant inflammation, local débridement, antibiotic therapy, and chlorhexidine mouthwash may be appropriate.

Except for slight sibilant distortions and shortening of the protrusive length of the tongue, few long-term adverse events have been noted in patients with forked tongues.

Susuk have not been associated with harmful effects, and no treatment is required. If the needles have a

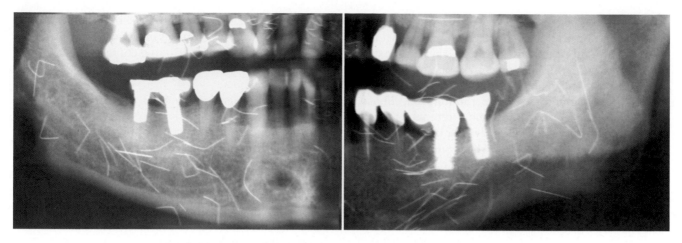

Fig. 8-55   Susuk (charm needles). Panoramic radiograph showing multiple radiopaque needles superimposed on the jaws. *(Courtesy of Dr. Jeff Bayme.)*

ferrous content, then magnetic resonance imaging (MRI) would be contraindicated. On occasion, affected individuals request removal of the susuk before they die because they believe their death will be excruciatingly painful.

SYSTEMIC METALLIC INTOXICATION

Ingestion or exposure to any one of several heavy metals can cause significant systemic and oral abnormalities. Exposure to heavy metals may be massive, resulting in acute reactions, or it may be minimal over a longer period, producing chronic changes. Oral alterations from ingestion of lead, mercury, silver, bismuth, arsenic, and gold are rare but may occur and warrant discussion. Oral complications from excessive zinc, iron, tin, and manganese are extremely rare.

LEAD

Little is known about the prevalence of lead poisoning (plumbism), but lead is one of the most widespread environmental toxins affecting children in the United States. Lead solder for plumbing was not banned until 1986. Homes built before then have the potential for significant water contamination, and one of the primary causes of lead intoxication in infants is formula preparation using tap water tainted by the metal.

Another significant source of lead poisoning in children is lead-based paint; children may ingest chips of the paint in older homes or be exposed to the fumes or dust during sanding and renovation. Paint with a high lead content was not restricted until 1977 and still remains in many homes. Removal of lead from gasoline began in 1972 but was not completed until 1995. These sources of lead combined with previous indus-

trial emissions have resulted in sites with highly contaminated soil, especially in urban areas. Despite the widespread publicity and significant efforts to restrict exposure to lead during childhood, significant risk remains.

Adult exposure also occurs and often is related to industry. The potential for exposure exists during handling of lead oxide batteries, in lead-processing industries, and from the welding of lead-covered surfaces. Some food and drink containers or vegetables grown in lead-contaminated soil also may contain inappropriate levels of the metal. Lead contamination in illicit alcohol has made the distinction between symptoms of lead intoxification and chronic alcohol abuse very difficult in certain sections of the American Deep South. Lead also can be found in brass fixtures, ceramics, crystal, electrical cable, radiation shielding, folk remedies, and cosmetics. Rarely, plumbism arises from retained lead bullet fragments in gunshot victims.

MERCURY

The danger of mercury exposure is well known. Elemental mercury is poorly absorbed, and its ingestion is relatively harmless. In contrast, inhalation of mercury vapor is very hazardous, with a high rate of absorption and systemic retention. Ingestion of mercury salts (e.g., mercurous chloride) also is associated with significant adverse reactions. Exposure has occurred in association with the use of mercury in teething powders, cathartic agents, and anthelmintic preparations.

A great deal of attention has been directed toward the mercury released from dental amalgams, but no well-documented adverse health effects have been identified (except for relatively rare contact hypersensitivity to mercury, see page 354). The level of mercury that is released from amalgams does not appear sufficiently high to cause disease and has been shown not to exceed the range expected from background exposure to environmental mercury. In an attempt to shed light on this controversy, the National Institutes of Health (NIH) funded two large randomized clinical trials that compared the neurologic and renal effects of dental amalgam in a 7-year study of a large cohort of children. In these pivotal investigations, no adverse effects from dental amalgam were seen. Interestingly, the control group that received only composite restorations demonstrated a 50% higher need for additional restorative treatment because of the failure of their restorations during the long-term study.

SILVER

Silver has known antibacterial properties and has been associated with a number of additional health benefits. In the past, silver compounds were used topically in nose drops and systemically for a variety of disorders including mental illness, epilepsy, nicotine addition, common colds, sinusitis, gastrointestinal ulcerations, syphilis, and gonorrhea. Because of the numerous complications, including silver intoxification, the FDA concluded that the risk of systemic silver products exceeded their benefits. In 1999 the use of colloidal silver or silver salts was banned in over-the-counter products. Several silver nitrate and silver sulfadiazine formulations remain available by prescription. These products should be used only under strict supervision. Well-documented examples of generalized argyria have been seen secondary to long-term treatment of aphthous ulcerations, denture sores, and minor gingival hemorrhage with topical silver nitrate.

Devices for production of homemade colloidal silver suspension and a number of colloidal silver proteins continue to be marketed over the Internet and in health food stores as essential mineral supplements for diseases such as arthritis, cancer, diabetes, AIDS, and herpes. These unregulated silver products have no known physiologic function, and their continued use cannot be supported.

BISMUTH AND ARSENIC

In the United States, exposure to bismuth and arsenic currently is rare. The medical use of these metals has diminished dramatically; most current cases arise from occupational exposure. Bismuth was used in the past for treatment of venereal diseases and various dermatoses, whereas arsenic compounds were prescribed for asthma and skin disorders such as psoriasis. Bismuth iodoform paraffin paste continues to be used by otolaryngologists and oral surgeons as a surgical pack, with rare reports of associated toxicity. In addition, bismuth subsalicylate tablets (Pepto-Bismol) have been reported to produce localized mucosal discoloration. Chronic exposure to arsenic continues in some lesser developed areas of the world from drinking contaminated water.

GOLD

Gold has been used in medical treatment in the past and continues to be used today in selected cases of active rheumatoid arthritis and other immunologically mediated diseases. In these cases the side effects are well known, and physicians observe the patients closely. In reviews of large-scale skin testing, gold has been found to be among the top 10 most frequent allergens, with positive reactions seen in about 10% of the population, including increased prevalence in patients who have gold dental restorations.

CLINICAL FEATURES

LEAD

Lead poisoning results in nonspecific systemic signs and symptoms, thereby making the ultimate diagnosis very difficult. The presentation is extremely variable and determined by the type of lead (organic or inorganic) and the age of the patient. Patients with acute cases most often have abdominal colic, which may occur along with anemia, fatigue, irritability, and weakness. Encephalopathy and renal dysfunction also may occur. Chronic exposure causes dysfunction of the nervous system, kidneys, marrow, bone, and joints. Symptoms generally include fatigue, musculoskeletal pain, and headache. Bones and teeth represent a major reservoir in patients with chronic plumbism, with 90% of the body's deposition being within bone. In radiographs of the long bones in infants, a radiopaque lead line often is noted along the epiphyseal plates. In addition, abdominal radiographs often will reveal small radiopaque paint chips in the gastrointestinal tract.

Oral manifestations include ulcerative stomatitis and a gingival lead line (**Burton's line**). The lead line appears as a bluish line along the marginal gingiva resulting from the action of bacterial hydrogen sulfide on lead in the gingival sulcus to produce a precipitate of lead sulfide. Gray areas also may be noted on the buccal mucosa and tongue. Additional manifestations include the following:

- Tremor of the tongue on thrusting
- Advanced periodontal disease
- Excessive salivation
- Metallic taste

MERCURY

Mercury poisoning also may be acute or chronic. With acute cases, abdominal pain, vomiting, diarrhea, thirst, pharyngitis, and gingivitis typically are present. With chronic cases, gastrointestinal upset and numerous neurologic symptoms occur. Oral changes include a metallic taste and ulcerative stomatitis combined with inflammation and enlargement of the salivary glands, gingiva, and tongue. The gingiva may become blue-gray to black. Mercuric sulfide can be generated by the bacterial action on the metal and can cause significant destruction of the alveolar bone with resultant exfoliation of teeth.

Chronic mercury exposure in infants and children is termed **acrodynia (pink disease, Swift disease).** The children have cold, clammy skin, especially on the hands, feet, nose, ears, and cheeks. An erythematous and pruritic rash is present. Severe sweating, increased lacrimation, irritability, insomnia, photophobia, hypertension, weakness, tachycardia, and gastrointestinal upset also may be present. On occasion, these highly irritable children have torn out patches of their hair. Oral signs include excessive salivation, ulcerative gingivitis, bruxism, and premature loss of teeth. Because mercury salts were formerly used in the processing of felt, hat makers in past centuries were exposed to the metal and experienced similar symptoms, giving rise to the phrase "mad as a hatter."

SILVER

Acute silver intoxication can produce coma, pleural edema, hemolysis, and bone marrow failure. Chronic systemic silver intoxication is known as **argyria.** Silver is disseminated throughout the body with substantial amounts accumulating as subepithelial deposits in the skin. These deposits result in a diffuse grayish discoloration that develops primarily in the sun-exposed areas (Fig. 8-56). The sclerae and nails also may be pigmented. One of the first signs of argyria occurs in the oral cavity and appears as a slate-blue silver line along the gingival margins. This discoloration is secondary to deposition of metallic silver and silver sulfide pigments. In addition, the oral mucosa often exhibits a diffuse blue-black discoloration.

BISMUTH

Chronic bismuth exposure can result in a diffuse blue-gray discoloration of the skin. The conjunctiva and oral cavity also may be involved. A blue-gray line along the gingival margin similar to that seen from lead intoxication is the most common intraoral presentation. Bismuth combines with bacterial hydrogen sulfide to form bismuth sulfide, which is irritating locally but not as destructive as mercuric sulfide. Associated ptyalism, burning, stomatitis, and ulceration may be seen. Intoxication from bismuth-containing surgical packs has been associated with CNS symptoms such as delirium. Chronic use of bismuth subsalicylate tablets can create a removable black discoloration of the otherwise normal filiform papillae. Although the lingual alteration may resemble black hairy tongue, the papillae are not elongated.

ARSENIC

In addition to widespread effects on numerous organ systems, significant dermatologic alterations frequently occur. Prolonged ingestion of arsenic often results in a diffuse macular hyperpigmentation. The discoloration is due to both the presence of the metal and an increased melanin production. In addition, palmar and plantar hyperkeratosis often is noted, as well as numerous premalignant skin lesions called **arsenical keratoses.** Development of basal cell carcinoma and cutaneous squamous cell carcinoma has been seen after years of exposure. Oral manifestations are rare and typically appear as excessive salivation and painful areas of necrotizing ulcerative stomatitis. In the past, extensive dorsal hyperkeratosis of the tongue was seen in patients with syphilis and may be related to arsenic therapy used before the advent of antibiotic therapy.

GOLD

The most common complication of gold therapy is dermatitis, which often is preceded by a warning signal: pruritus. Although a generalized exfoliative dermatitis with resultant alopecia and loss of nails can be seen, dermatitis about the face, eyelids, and at direct sites of skin contact is the most common presentation. Because of the high frequency of allergy to gold, skin testing often is performed before administration of gold drug therapy.

The second most common adverse reaction to gold is severe oral mucositis, which most frequently involves

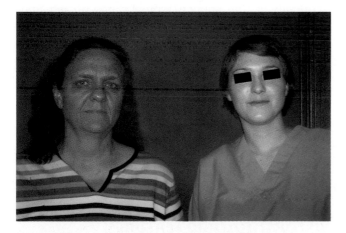

Fig. 8-56 Argyria. Grayish discoloration of the face compared with a more normal facial complexion in an individual who used a silver-containing nutritional supplement. Before development of silver intoxication, this blue-eyed, red-haired individual had a very light complexion. *(Courtesy of Bradford R. Williams.)*

the buccal mucosa, lateral border of the tongue, palate, and pharynx. These mucosal changes represent a systemic allergic reaction and are different from intraoral contact gold hypersensitivity (see page 347). A metallic taste often precedes development of the oral lesions and should be considered another warning signal. Therapy with gold rarely can bring about a slate-blue discoloration of sun-exposed skin (**chrysiasis**).

TREATMENT AND PROGNOSIS

The management of heavy metal intoxication involves removal from further exposure to the agent, supportive care, decontamination, and use of chelating agents. In some cases a medication may be responsible and can be discontinued; however, sometimes the source of the metal may be difficult to determine. In infants with radiographic evidence of gastrointestinal lead-containing paint chips, bowel irrigation with a polyethylene glycol electrolyte lavage solution may be warranted. In the past, two chelators, ethylenediaminetetraacetic acid (EDTA) (calcium disodium ethylenediaminetetraacetate) and BAL (2,3-dimercaptopropanol), were first-line therapy in the treatment of lead poisoning, whereas arsenic and mercury intoxication were treated with BAL. These medications may have significant side effects, and less toxic alternatives such as DMSA (2,3-dimercaptosuccinic acid) and DMPS (2,3-dimercaptopropane-1-sulfonate) now are available. No antidote exists for silver intoxication, and treatment is limited to supportive measures. Attempts to remove the bluish discoloration of facial argyria with dermabrasion have been unsuccessful. Encephalopathy associated with use of bismuth-containing surgical packs clears on removal of the material.

SMOKER'S MELANOSIS

Oral pigmentations are increased significantly in heavy smokers. In one investigation of more than 31,000 whites, 21.5% of tobacco smokers exhibited areas of melanin pigmentation compared with 3% among those not using tobacco. In another study of an ethnically pigmented population, smokers had more oral surfaces exhibiting melanin pigmentation.

Melanin pigmentation in the skin exerts a well-known protective effect against ultraviolet (UV) damage. Investigations of melanocytes located away from sun-exposed areas have shown the ability of melanin to bind to noxious substances. Exposure to polycyclic amines (e.g., nicotine and benzpyrene) has been shown to stimulate melanin production by melanocytes that also are known to bind strongly to nicotine. Research has suggested that melanin production in the oral mucosa of smokers serves as a protective

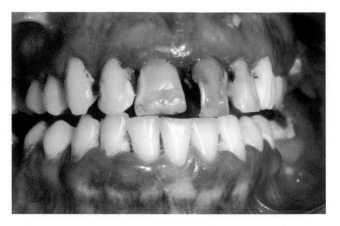

Fig. 8-57 Smoker's melanosis. Light, diffuse melanin pigmentation in a white female who is a heavy smoker. Pigmentary changes are limited to the anterior facial gingiva.

response against some of the harmful substances in tobacco smoke. This concept is supported by the findings in "reverse" smokers, who smoke with the lit end of the cigarette inside the mouth and demonstrate heavy melanin pigmentation of the palate. In some reverse smokers, areas of melanocytes are lost and zones of depigmented red mucosa can develop. Cancer is found in 12% of patients with these red zones, further delineating the probable protective effects of melanocytes against toxic substances.

CLINICAL FEATURES

Although any mucosal surface may be affected, smoker's melanosis most commonly affects the anterior facial gingiva (Fig. 8-57). Most people affected by this condition are cigarette users. In contrast, pipe smokers frequently exhibit pigmentations located on the commissural and buccal mucosae. Reverse smokers show alterations of the hard palate.

The areas of pigmentation significantly increase during the first year of smoking and appear correlated to the number of cigarettes smoked each day. A higher frequency is seen in females, and researchers have suggested that female sex hormones exert a synergistic effect when combined with smoking. Reports from Sweden, Germany, and Japan have shown tobacco smoking to be the most common cause for mucosal pigmentation in light-skinned adult populations.

HISTOPATHOLOGIC FEATURES

Biopsy specimens of affected areas in people with smoker's melanosis reveal increased melanin pigmentation of the basal cell layer of the surface epithelium, similar to a melanotic macule (see page 379). In addition, collections of incontinent melanin pigmentation are seen free within the superficial connective tissue and in scattered melanophages.

DIAGNOSIS

The clinician can make the diagnosis by correlating the smoking history with the clinical presentation and medical history. Other causes of melanin pigmentation, such as trauma, neurofibromatosis, Peutz-Jeghers syndrome, drug-related pigmentation, endocrine disturbances, hemochromatosis, chronic pulmonary disease, and racial pigmentation should be excluded.

TREATMENT AND PROGNOSIS

Cessation of smoking results in gradual disappearance of the areas of related pigmentation over a 3-year period. Biopsy should be considered when the pigmentation is in unexpected locations, such as the hard palate, or when there are unusual clinical changes, such as increased melanin density or surface elevation.

DRUG-RELATED DISCOLORATIONS OF THE ORAL MUCOSA

An expanding number of medications have been implicated as a cause of oral mucosal discolorations. Although many medications stimulate melanin production by melanocytes, deposition of drug metabolites is responsible for the color change in others. These pigmentary alterations have been associated with use of phenolphthalein, minocycline, tranquilizers, antimalarial medications, estrogen, chemotherapeutic agents, and some medications used in the treatment of patients with AIDS.

The antimalarial agents that are most frequently implicated are chloroquine, hydrochloroquine, quinidine, and quinacrine; chlorpromazine represents the most frequently implicated tranquilizer. Besides treating malaria, antimalarial agents are used for many other disorders, including lupus erythematosus and rheumatoid arthritis.

Oral mucosal pigmentation associated with chemotherapeutic medications is most commonly reported with use of doxorubicin, busulfan, cyclophosphamide, or 5-fluorouracil. Although idiopathic hyperpigmentation also may occur, AIDS patients receiving zidovudine (AZT), clofazimine, or ketoconazole have demonstrated increased melanin pigmentation.

CLINICAL FEATURES

The clinical presentations of pigmentations related to drug use vary. Most agents produce a diffuse melanosis of the skin and mucosal surfaces, but others may cause

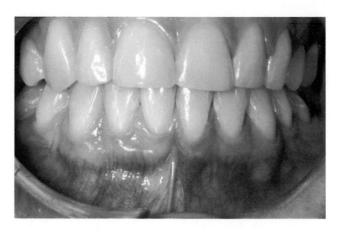

Fig. 8-58 Minocycline-related discoloration. Blue-gray discoloration of the facial surface of the anterior mandibular alveolus because stained alveolar bone is visible through the thin mucosa.

a unique pattern. As in many cases of increased melanin pigmentation, females are more sensitive, most likely as a result of an interaction with sex hormones.

Use of phenolphthalein as a laxative has been associated with numerous small, well-circumscribed areas of hyperpigmentation on the skin. Similar areas of oral mucosal melanosis also can occur.

Long-term use of minocycline, a semisynthetic derivative of tetracycline, results in discoloration of the bone and developing teeth. The affected bone is dark green but creates a blue-gray discoloration as seen through the translucent oral mucosa. The most common presentations include a linear band above the facial attached gingiva near the mucogingival junction and a broad zone of discoloration on the hard palate (Fig. 8-58).

Rare soft tissue pigmentation of the lips, tongue, eyes, and skin also has been reported with use of minocycline. The cutaneous pigmentation appears to be dose-dependent and is seen in up to 15% of patients being treated for acne and as many as 70% of those treated for rheumatoid arthritis. The pigmentation presents in three patterns, two of which are thought to be caused by deposition of drug metabolites that become chelated with iron. In the third pattern, the medication triggers a diffuse muddy-brown or gray cutaneous pigmentation resulting from increased melanosis of the epithelial basal cell layer and superficial connective tissue. This latter pattern is accentuated in sun-exposed areas, and the diagnosis can be made only when there is a direct association between initiation and cessation of the medication and the appearance and fading of the pigmentation. Minocycline-related pigmentation of the oral mucosa unrelated to discoloration of the underlying bone also has been reported,

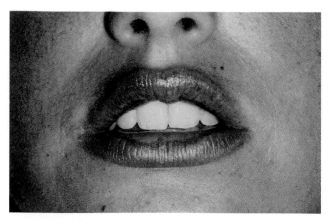

Fig. 8-59   Minocycline-associated pigmentation. Sharply demarcated brown pigmentation on the vermilion border of the lips, which arose in association with long-term minocycline use and is the result of increased melanin deposition.

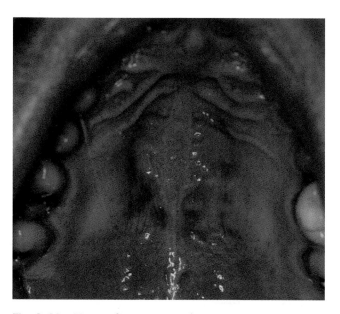

Fig. 8-60   Minocycline-associated pigmentation. Multifocal areas of palatal pigmentation secondary to deposition of drug metabolites chelated to iron in association with long-term minocycline use. *(From Treister NS, Magalnick D, Woo S-B: Oral mucosal pigmentation secondary to minocycline therapy: report of two cases and a review of the literature, Oral Surg Oral Med Oral Pathol Oral Radiol Endod 97:718-725, 2004.)*

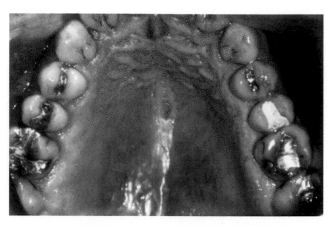

Fig. 8-61   Chlorpromazine pigmentation. Diffuse grayish pigmentation of the hard palate.

cations may occasionally lead to a more diffuse brown melanosis of the oral mucosa and skin.

Estrogen, chemotherapeutic agents, and medications used in the treatment of AIDS patients may result in a diffuse brown melanosis of the skin and mucosal surfaces. Any mucosal surface may be involved, but the attached gingiva and buccal mucosa are most frequently affected. The pattern and appearance of the oral mucosal involvement are similar to those seen in racial pigmentation.

TREATMENT AND PROGNOSIS

Although the discolorations of the oral mucosa may be aesthetically displeasing, they cause no long-term problems. In most instances, discontinuing the medication results in gradual fading of the areas of hyperpigmentation.

REACTIVE OSSEOUS AND CHONDROMATOUS METAPLASIA (CUTRIGHT LESION)

On occasion, cartilage or bone may be discovered within soft tissue specimens removed from the oral cavity. Cartilaginous rests are known to exist in the area of the nasopalatine duct. In the past, several investigators have reported the presence of cartilage within flabby soft tissue removed from maxillary edentulous alveolar ridges of long-term denture wearers. This finding was thought to represent cartilaginous metaplasia secondary to chronic denture trauma. In retrospect, the islands of cartilage within these cases most likely represent embryologic remnants, not traumatic metaplasia. These rests are also occasionally discovered during histopathologic examination of nasopalatine duct cysts and maxillary gingivectomy specimens.

with patients exhibiting either widespread increased melanosis or focal accumulations of iron-containing particles (Figs. 8-59 and 8-60). Although the cutaneous and oral mucosal staining fade after discontinuation of the medication, the dental discoloration remains.

The classic presentation of intraoral pigmentation from use of antimalarial medications or tranquilizers is a blue-black discoloration limited to the hard palate (Fig. 8-61). In addition, the intake of antimalarial medi-

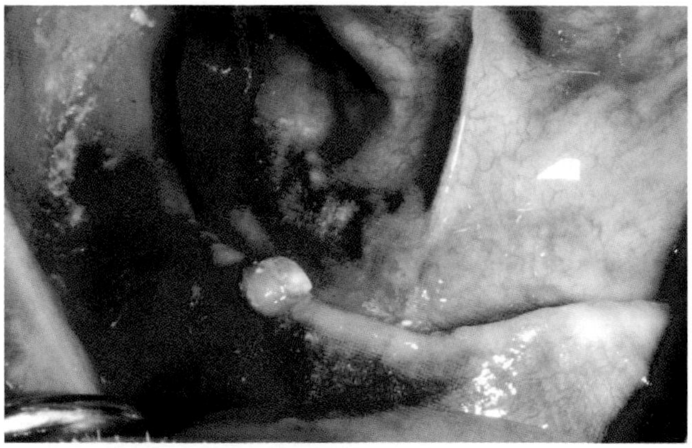

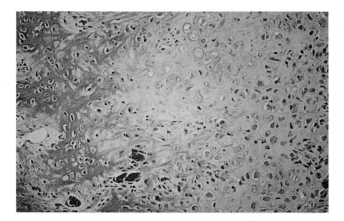

Fig. 8-62   Periosteal hyperplasia with osseous and chondromatous metaplasia. Tender, elevated nodule along the thin crest of the mandibular alveolar ridge. *(Courtesy of Dr. Steven Tucker.)*

Fig. 8-63   Osseous and chondromatous metaplasia. High-power photomicrograph demonstrating cellular woven bone and metaplastic cartilage.

Despite the suggestion that the anterior maxillary lesions are embryologic and not traumatic, development of **osseous** and **chondromatous metaplasia** from mechanical denture irritation does occur. Although such metaplasia is probably uncommon in the anterior maxilla, its development is not rare along the crest of the posterior mandibular alveolar ridge in long-term denture wearers with atrophic ridges.

CLINICAL AND RADIOGRAPHIC FEATURES

In patients with reactive osseous and chondromatous metaplasia, an extremely tender and localized area of the alveolar ridge is typically noted that may be associated with local enlargement (Fig. 8-62). These changes almost always arise in patients with extensive atrophy of the mandibular alveolar ridge leading to a knife edge-like crest. Although most examples involve the posterior mandible, similar areas may rarely be seen overlying the maxillary alveolar ridge or associated with anterior portions of the mandible. Because of significant associated symptoms and occasional enlargement, biopsy is frequently performed.

HISTOPATHOLOGIC FEATURES

Histopathologic examination of reactive osseous and chondromatous metaplasia typically demonstrates a mass of hypercellular periosteum that blends into areas of osseous and chondromatous tissue. The bone and cartilage frequently exhibit atypical features, such as hypercellularity, pleomorphism, nuclear hyperchromatism, and occasional binucleated or multinucleated cells (Fig. 8-63). These alterations are worrisome for sarcoma, but the appropriate diagnosis can be made

when an appropriate clinicopathologic correlation is made. In contrast, the cartilaginous rest discovered incidentally in maxillary specimens is usually very bland without any atypical features that would suggest malignancy.

TREATMENT AND PROGNOSIS

The thin mandibular ridges may be recontoured or supplemented with graft material to improve shape and to alleviate the symptoms associated with the localized periosteal hyperplasia. Implants also may reduce the traumatic injury to the ridge and lessen the chance of recurrence. If the ridge modification is not made, then the continued injury to the site occasionally results in recurrence of the lesion.

ORAL ULCERATION WITH BONE SEQUESTRATION (SPONTANEOUS SEQUESTRATION; TRAUMATIC SEQUESTRATION)

Focal superficial sequestration of a fragment of cortical bone not related to systemic disease, infection, or a major traumatic event is uncommon. In such instances the cause of the focal osteonecrosis is not known, although many believe the primary event is a traumatic or aphthous ulceration that leads to osteitis and necrosis of a small focus of adjacent cortical bone. Others have suggested the blood supply of the peripheral cortical plate may be delivered by the periosteal microvasculature, and loss of this supply leads to focal bone necrosis and sequestration. Such lesions tend to occur in anatomically unique sites in which a bony prominence is covered by a thin mucosal surface.

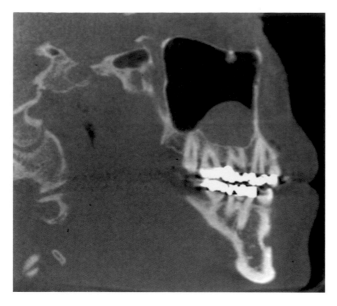

Fig. 8-67   Antral pseudocyst. Three-dimensional cone-beam sagittal section of same patient depicted in Fig. 8-66. Note that the floor of the sinus remains intact below the lesion. *(Courtesy of Dr. Scott Jenkins and Dr. Nick Morrow.)*

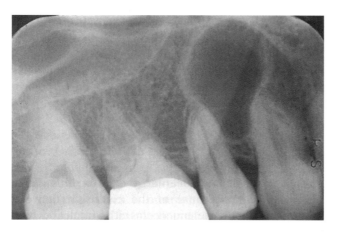

Fig. 8-68   Surgical ciliated cyst. Well-defined radiolucency between vital maxillary bicuspids. *(Courtesy of Dr. Patrick Coleman.)*

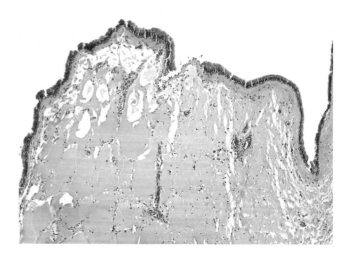

Fig. 8-69   Antral pseudocyst. Medium-power photomicrograph demonstrating sinus lining overlying edematous connective tissue.

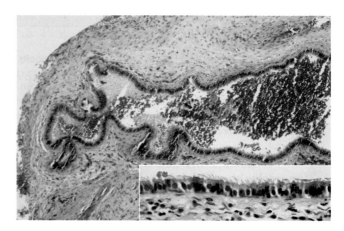

Fig. 8-70   Surgical ciliated cyst. True cyst lined by respiratory epithelium. Inset provides high-power view of the ciliated pseudostratified columnar epithelium that lines the cyst.

thinned and eventually eroded. Surgical ciliated cysts are spherical lesions that are separate from the sinus and lack the dome-shaped appearance of pseudocysts (Fig. 8-68). As these postoperative cysts enlarge, they too can lead to perforation of the sinus walls. Retention cysts rarely reach a size that would produce detectable radiographic changes.

HISTOPATHOLOGIC FEATURES

Antral pseudocysts are covered by sinus epithelium and demonstrate a subepithelial inflammatory exudate that consists of serum occasionally intermixed with inflammatory cells (Fig. 8-69). Collections of cholesterol clefts and scattered small dystrophic calcifications may be seen. True sinus mucoceles and surgical ciliated cysts are true cystic structures lined by ciliated pseudostratified columnar epithelium, squamous epithelium with mucous cells, or metaplastic squamous epithelium (Fig. 8-70). A sinus retention cyst shows focal dilatation of a duct associated with the seromucous glands of the sinus lining. The lumen of the dilated duct is filled with thick mucus, often intermixed with chronic inflammatory cells.

TREATMENT AND PROGNOSIS

Typically, pseudocysts of the maxillary sinus are harmless, and no treatment is necessary. The adjacent teeth should be evaluated thoroughly, and any foci of infection should be eliminated. A few clinicians prefer to confirm their radiographic impression and rule out a tumor through drainage of the inflammatory exudate. Removal by means of a Caldwell-Luc operation should be performed on any radiographically diagnosed lesion that produces significant expansion or is associated definitively with symptoms such as headache.

Because sinus mucoceles and surgical ciliated cysts are expansile and destructive lesions, the traditional therapy for these pathoses is assured surgical removal. Numerous investigators also have shown that sinus mucoceles arising from ostial obstruction often do not require surgical excision and respond well to endoscopic middle meatal antrostomy and marsupialization of the mucocele.

CERVICOFACIAL EMPHYSEMA

Cervicofacial emphysema arises from the introduction of air into subcutaneous or fascial spaces of the face and neck. The forced air may spread through the spaces to the retropharyngeal and mediastinal areas. The first case was reported almost 100 years ago and occurred as a result of blowing into a bugle a short time after tooth extraction.

Cervicofacial emphysema of dental origin may arise in several ways:

- After the use of compressed air by the clinician
- After difficult or prolonged extractions
- As a result of increased intraoral pressure (e.g., sneezing, blowing) after an oral surgical procedure
- From no obvious cause

Introduction of air within tissue has been seen after a large number of dental procedures, but most instances involve either surgical extraction of teeth, osteotomies, significant trauma, or the use of air or water syringes. In addition, the prevalence has increased as a result of the use of air-driven handpieces during oral surgery. On occasion, cervicofacial emphysema has resulted from compressed air being accidentally forced into small intraoral lacerations located away from the field of operation. Conservative surgical flap design without extension into fascial planes and limited use of air-driven handpieces during surgical procedures may minimize the chance of occurrence. Rare reports of cervicofacial emphysema after self-induced oral injury have been reported in prisoners attempting to escape by simulation of a medical emergency and a drug abuser with Munchausen syndrome who was trying to access unnecessary medical intervention.

An analogous problem termed **pneumoparotid** can arise when air enters the parotid duct, leading to enlargement of the parotid gland caused by air insufflation. This can be accidental, self-induced, or occupa-

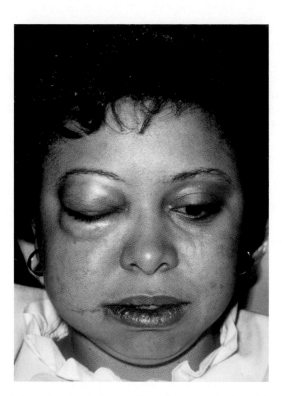

Fig. 8-71 Cervicofacial emphysema. Periorbital and facial enlargement caused by use of an air-driven handpiece during third molar removal.

tional (e.g., glassblowers, wind instrument players). Stensen's duct has numerous redundant mucosal folds that seal as intraoral pressure is increased; in addition, contraction of the buccinator muscle further prevents entrance of air by compressing the duct. In spite of this protection, dramatic increases in intraoral pressures can result in air filling the parotid ductal system.

CLINICAL AND RADIOGRAPHIC FEATURES

More than 90% of cases of cervicofacial emphysema develop during surgery or within the first postoperative hour. Cases with delayed onset are associated with increased postoperative pressure created by the patient. The initial change is one of soft tissue enlargement from the presence of the air in deeper tissues (Fig. 8-71). Pain is usually minimal, and crepitus is detected easily with gentle palpation. Subsequently, the enlargement increases and spreads because of secondary inflammation and edema. Variable pain, facial erythema, dysphagia, dysphonia, vision difficulties, and mild fever may occur. The facial enlargement often is confused with an angioedema, but the diagnosis can be made by identifying crepitus within the swelling.

Significant spread into the mediastinum can result in dysphonia, dysphagia, or dyspnea. Cardiac auscultation often reveals crepitus synchronous with the heart beat (**Hamman's crunch**) in cases with mediastinal involvement. Pneumomediastinum can be confirmed on chest radiographs by observing displacement of the mediastinal pleura.

Pneumoparotid typically appears as a unilateral enlargement of the parotid that demonstrates crepitus on gentle palpation. Milking the parotid duct produces a frothy, air-filled saliva, rather than the typical clear, waterlike secretion.

TREATMENT AND PROGNOSIS

Broad-spectrum antibiotic coverage is recommended in all dental-related cases of cervicofacial emphysema. The body gradually removes the entrapped air during a 2- to 5-day period. Most cases spontaneously resolve without significant difficulty. Rare cases of respiratory distress have been noted, and assisted ventilation was required.

The first goal of therapy for pneumoparotid is discovery of the inciting event. In occupation-related cases, such as those seen in trumpet players, the individual should be coached to compress the cheeks during playing. This procedure contracts the buccinator muscle and compresses the parotid duct. Acute symptoms are treated with antibiotics, massage, hydration, sialogogues, and warm compresses.

MYOSPHERULOSIS

Placement of topical antibiotic in a petrolatum base into a surgical site may occasionally result in a unique foreign body reaction, known as **myospherulosis.** The resultant histopathologic pattern is most unusual and was thought initially to represent a previously undescribed endosporulating fungus.

CLINICAL AND RADIOGRAPHIC FEATURES

Myospherulosis may occur at any site within soft tissue or bone where the antibiotic has been placed. The initial report described involvement of the arms, legs, and gluteal and scapular regions. Most cases in the dental literature have occurred within bone at previous extraction sites where an antibiotic had been placed in an attempt to prevent alveolar osteitis. Although maxillary and oral soft tissue examples have been documented, most cases have occurred within mandibular surgical sites. In addition, myospherulosis is reported occasionally in a paranasal sinus after a surgical proce-

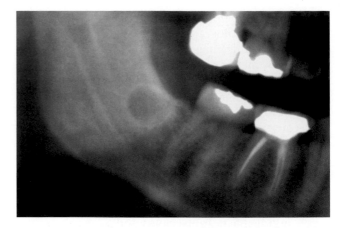

Fig. 8-72   Myospherulosis. Radiolucency has persisted after extraction of the mandibular third molar. An antibiotic ointment was placed at the time of initial surgery.

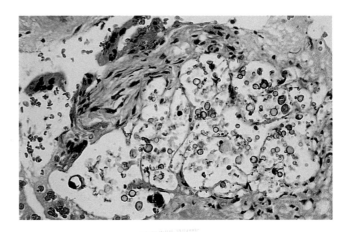

Fig. 8-73   Myospherulosis. High-power photomicrograph exhibiting multiple cystlike spaces containing numerous brown-stained spherules.

dure in which a gauze packing coated with an antibiotic ointment was used.

The involved area may exhibit swelling or be discovered as an asymptomatic and circumscribed radiolucency in a previous extraction site (Fig. 8-72). In some cases pain and purulent drainage have resulted. On exploration of the lesion, a black, greasy, tarlike material is found.

HISTOPATHOLOGIC FEATURES

The histopathologic pattern is unique; it is the result of a tissue interaction with both the petroleum base and the antibiotic, typically tetracycline. Dense collagenous tissue is intermixed with a granulomatous inflammatory response showing macrophages and multinucleated giant cells. Within the connective tissue are multiple cystlike spaces that contain numerous brown- to black-staining spherules (Fig. 8-73). The collections of spherules sometimes are surrounded by an outer membrane known as a *parent body,* forming structures that resemble a "bag of marbles." The spherules represent red blood cells that have been altered by the medication. The unusual dark coloration is due to the degradation of hemoglobin. To complicate matters, myospherulosis arising in a paranasal sinus occasionally is contaminated with respiratory fungal organisms, such as the zygomycetes or aspergillus.

TREATMENT AND PROGNOSIS

Myospherulosis is treated by surgical removal of the foreign material and associated tissue. Histopathologic examination of the altered tissue provides the definitive diagnosis. Recurrence is not expected. Those arising in a paranasal sinus and exhibiting fungal infestation respond well to local measures and do not require systemic antimicrobial therapy. Some investigators have recommended discontinuation of nasal packing with antibiotic ointment, because patients with antral myospherulosis have been found to be almost three times more likely than controls to develop adhesions and require revision of their sinus surgery.

A similar clinical and radiographic pattern has been seen in association with the use of powdered tetracycline in a polymer dressing. Although somewhat different histopathologically, this formulation also leads to a granulomatous foreign body reaction. Because of complications associated with both formulations, the practice of applying topical antibiotics to oral wounds should be approached with caution, and other methods of delivery should be considered. If topical antibiotics are used, then they should be accompanied by close follow-up to ensure appropriate clinical and radiographic evidence of healing of the surgical site.

BIBLIOGRAPHY

Linea Alba
Kashani HG, Mackenzie IC, Kerber PE: Cytology of linea alba using a filter imprint technique, *Clin Prev Dent* 2:21-24, 1980.
Parlak AH, Koybasi S, Yavuz et al: Prevalence of oral lesions in 13- to 16-year old students in Duzce, Turkey, *Oral Dis* 12:553-558, 2006.
Wood NK, Goaz PW: *Differential diagnosis of oral and maxillofacial lesions,* ed 5, pp 98-99, St Louis, 1997, Mosby.

Morsicatio Buccarum
Bouquot JE: Common oral lesions found during a mass screening examination, *J Am Dent Assoc* 112:50-57, 1986.
Hjørting-Hansen E, Holst E: Morsicatio mucosae oris and suctio mucosae oris: an analysis of oral mucosal changes due to

biting and sucking habits, *Scand J Dent Res* 78:492-499, 1970.
Kocsard E, Schwarz L, Stephen BS et al: Morsicatio buccarum, *Br J Dermatol* 74:454-457, 1962.
Reichart PA, Philipsen HP: Betel chewer's mucosa—a review, *J Oral Pathol Med* 27:239-242, 1998.
Romero M, Vicente A, Bravo LA: Prevention of habitual cheek biting: a case report, *Spec Care Dentist* 25:214-216, 2005.
Schiödt M, Larsen V, Bessermann M: Oral findings in glassblowers, *Community Dent Oral Epidemiol* 8:195-200, 1980.
Sewerin I: A clinical and epidemiologic study of morsicatio buccarum/labiorum, *Scand J Dent Res* 79:73-80, 1971.
Van Wyk CW, Staz J, Farman AG: The chewing lesion of the cheeks and lips: its features and the prevalence among a selected group of adolescents, *J Dent* 5:193-199, 1977.

Eosinophilic Ulcerations
Aloebeid B, Pan L-X, Milligan L et al: Eosinophil-rich CD30+ lymphoproliferative disorder of the oral mucosa, *Am J Clin Pathol* 121:43-50, 2004.
Baghdadi ZD: Riga-Fede disease: report of a case and review, *J Clin Pediatr Dent* 25:209-213, 2001.
Bhaskar SN, Lilly GE: Traumatic granuloma of the tongue (human and experimental), *Oral Surg Oral Med Oral Pathol* 18:206-218, 1964.
El-Mofty SK, Swanson PE, Wick MR et al: Eosinophilic ulcer of the oral mucosa: report of 38 new cases with immunohistochemical observations, *Oral Surg Oral Med Oral Pathol* 75:716-722, 1993.
Eversole LR, Leider AS, Jacobsen PL et al: Atypical histiocytic granuloma: light microscopic, ultrastructural, and histochemical findings in an unusual pseudomalignant reactive lesion of the oral cavity, *Cancer* 55:1722-1729, 1985.
Ficarra G, Prignano F, Romagnoli P: Traumatic eosinophilic granuloma of the oral mucosa: a CD30+ (Ki-1) lymphoproliferative disorder, *Oral Oncol* 33:375-379, 1997.
Hirshberg A, Amariglio N, Akrish S et al: Traumatic ulcerative granuloma with stromal eosinophilia, *Am J Clin Pathol* 126:522-529, 2006.
Kabani S, Cataldo E, Folkerth R et al: Atypical lymphohistiocytic infiltrate (pseudolymphoma) of the oral cavity, *Oral Surg Oral Med Oral Pathol* 66:587-592, 1988.
Regezi JA, Zarbo RJ, Daniels TE et al: Oral traumatic granuloma: characterization of the cellular infiltrate, *Oral Surg Oral Med Oral Pathol* 75:723-727 1993.
Throndson RR, Wright JM, Watkins D: Atypical histiocytic granuloma of the oral mucosa: an unusual clinicopathologic entity simulating malignancy, *J Oral Maxillofac Surg* 59:822-826, 2001.
Zaenglein AL, Chang MU, Meehan SA et al: Extensive Riga-Fede disease of the lip and tongue, *J Am Acad Dermatol* 47:445-447, 2002.

Electrical Burns
Czerepak CS: Oral splint therapy to manage electrical burns of the mouths in children, *Clin Plast Surg* 11:685-692, 1984.
Goto R, Miyabe K, Mori N: Thermal burn of the pharynx and larynx after swallowing hot milk, *Auris Nasus Larynx* 29:301-303, 2002.
Gormley MB, Marshall J, Jarrett W et al: Thermal trauma: a review of 22 electrical burns of the lip, *J Oral Surg* 30:531-533, 1972.
Leake JE, Curtin JW: Electrical burns of the mouth in children, *Clin Plast Surg* 11:669-683, 1986.
Taylor LB, Walker J: A review of selected microstomia prevention appliances, *Pediatr Dent* 19:413-418, 1997.

Oral Adverse Reactions to Chemicals

Baruchin AM, Lustig JP, Nahlieli O et al: Burns of the oral mucosa: report of 6 cases, *J Craniomaxillofac Surg* 19:94-96, 1991.

Buck IF, Zeff S, Kalnins L et al: The treatment of intraoral chemical burns, *J Oral Ther* 2:101-106, 1965.

Frost DE, Barkmeier WW, Abrams H: Aphthous ulcer—a treatment complication, *Oral Surg Oral Med Oral Pathol* 45:863-869, 1978.

Gernhardt CR, Eppendorf K, Kozlowski A et al: Toxicity of concentrated sodium hypochlorite used as an endodontic irrigant, *Int Endod J* 37:272-280, 2004.

Grace EG, Sarlani E, Kaplan S: Tooth erosion caused by chewing aspirin, *J Am Dent Assoc* 135:911-914, 2004.

Kawakami J, Muto T, Shigeo K et al: Tooth exfoliation and necrosis of the crestal bone caused by use of formocresol, *Oral Surg Oral Med Oral Pathol Oral Radiol Endod* 95:736-738, 2003.

Özgöz, M, Yağiz H, Çiçek Y et al: Gingival necrosis following the use of a paraformaldehyde-containing paste: a case report, *Int Endod J* 37:157-161, 2004.

Rawal SY, Claman LJ, Kalmar JR et al: Traumatic lesions of the gingiva: a case series, *J Periodontol* 75:762-769, 2004.

Rees TD, Orth CF: Oral ulcerations with use of hydrogen peroxide, *J Periodontol* 57:689-692, 1986.

Noninfectious Complications of Antineoplastic Therapy

Annane D, Depondt J, Aubert P et al: Hyperbaric oxygen therapy for radionecrosis of the jaw: a randomized, placebo-controlled, double-blind trial from the ORN96 study group, *J Clin Oncol* 22:4893-4900, 2004.

Dreizen S: Description and incidence of oral complications. Consensus Development Conference on Oral Complications of Cancer Therapies: Diagnosis, Prevention, and Treatment, *NCI Monogr* 9:11-15, 1990.

Epstein JB, Klasser GD: Emerging approaches for prophylaxis and management of oropharyngeal mucositis in cancer therapy, *Expert Opin Emerging Drugs* 11:353-373, 2006.

Keller EE: Placement of dental implants in the irradiated mandible: a protocol without adjunctive hyperbaric oxygen, *J Oral Maxillofac Surg* 55:972-980, 1997.

Marx RE, Johnson RP, Kline SN: Prevention of osteoradionecrosis: a randomized prospective clinical trial of hyperbaric oxygen versus penicillin, *J Am Dent Assoc* 111:49-54. 1985.

Rubenstein EB, Peterson DE, Schubert M et al: Clinical practice guidelines for the prevention and treatment of cancer therapy-induced oral and gastrointestinal mucositis, *Cancer* 100(suppl 9):2026-2046, 2004.

Scully C, Sonis S, Diz PD: Oral mucositis, *Oral Dis* 12:229-241, 2006.

Sulaiman F, Huryn JM, Zlotolow IM: Dental extraction in the irradiated head and neck patient: a retrospective analysis of Memorial Sloan-Kettering Cancer Center protocols, criteria, and end results, *J Oral Maxillofac Surg* 61:1123-1131, 2003.

Teng MS, Futran ND: Osteonecrosis of the mandible, *Curr Opin Otolaryngol Head Neck Surg* 13:217-221, 2005.

Bisphosphonate-Related Osteonecrosis

Adornato MC, Morcos I, Rozanski J: The treatment of bisphosphonate-associated osteonecrosis of the jaws with bone resection and autologous platelet-derived growth factors, *J Am Dent Assoc* 138:971-977, 2007.

American Dental Association Council on Scientific Affairs: Dental management of patients receiving oral bisphosphonate therapy. Expert panel recommendations, *J Am Dent Assoc* 137:1144-1150, 2006.

Cohen D, Bhattacharyya N, Islam J et al: *Case based evidence for expanding the criteria for the diagnosis of bisphosphonate induced*

osteochemonecrosis, Abstract 31, American Academy of Oral and Maxillofacial Pathology, Kansas City, Mo, May 8, 2007.

Odvina CV, Zerwekh JE, Rao DS et al: Severely suppressed bone turnover: a potential complication of alendronate therapy, *J Clin Endocrinol Metab* 90:1294-1301, 2005.

Ott SM: Long-term safety of bisphosphonates, *J Clin Endocrinol Metab* 90:1897-1899, 2005.

Marx RE: Pamidronate (Aredia) and zoledronate (Zometa) induced avascular necrosis of the jaws: a growing epidemic (letter to the editor), *J Oral Maxillofac Surg* 61:1115-1117, 2003.

Marx RE, Cillo JE Jr, Ulloa JJ: Oral bisphosphonate-induced osteonecrosis: risk factors, prediction of risk using serum CTX testing, prevention, and treatment, *J Oral Maxillofac Surg* 65:2397-2410, 2007.

Marx RE, Sawatari Y, Fortin M et al: Bisphosphonate-induced exposed bone (osteonecrosis/osteopetrosis) of the jaws: risk factors, recognition, prevention, and treatment, *J Oral Maxillofac Surg* 63:1567-1575, 2005.

Ruggiero SL, Fantasia J, Carlson E: Bisphosphonate-related osteonecrosis of the jaw: background and guidelines for diagnosis, staging and management, *Oral Surg Oral Med Oral Pathol Oral Radiol Endod* 102:433-441, 2006.

Ruggiero SL, Mehrotra B, Rosenberg TJ et al: Osteonecrosis of the jaws associated with the use of bisphosphonates: a review of 63 cases, *J Oral Maxillofac Surg* 62:527-534, 2004.

Schneider JP: Should bisphosphonates be continued indefinitely? An unusual fracture in a healthy woman on long-term alendronate, *Geriatrics* 61:31-33, 2006.

Woo S-B, Hellstein JW, Kalmar JR: Systematic review: bisphosphonates and osteonecrosis of the jaws, *Ann Intern Med* 144:753-761, 2006.

Orofacial Complications of Methamphetamine Abuse

Curtis EK: Meth mouth: a review of methamphetamine abuse and its oral manifestations, *Gen Dent* 54:125-129, 2006.

Goodchild JH, Donaldson M, Mangini DJ: Methamphetamine abuse and the impact on dental health, *Dent Today* 26:124-131, 2007.

Rhodus NL, Little JW: Methamphetamine abuse and "meth mouth," *Northwest Dent* 84:29, 31, 33-37, 2005.

Richards JR, Brofeldt BT: Patterns of tooth wear associated with methamphetamine use, *J Periodontol* 71:1371-1374, 2000.

Shaner JW, Kimmes N, Saini T et al: "Meth mouth": rampant caries in methamphetamine abusers, *AIDS Patient Care STDs* 20:146-150, 2006.

Anesthetic Necrosis

Carroll MJ: Tissue necrosis following a buccal infiltration, *Br Dent J* 149:209-210, 1980.

Giunta J, Tsamsouris A, Cataldo E et al: Postanesthetic necrotic defect, *Oral Surg Oral Med Oral Pathol* 40:590-593, 1975.

Schaffer J, Calman HI, Levy B: Changes in the palate color and form (case 9), *Dent Radiogr Photogr* 39:3-6, 19-22, 1966.

Exfoliative Cheilitis

Axéll T, Skoglund A: Chronic lip fissures. Prevalence, pathology and treatment, *Int J Oral Surg* 10:354-358, 1981.

Connolly M, Kennedy C: Exfoliative cheilitis successfully treated with topical tacrolimus, *Br J Dermatol* 151:241-242, 2004.

Daley TD, Gupta AK: Exfoliative cheilitis, *J Oral Pathol Med* 24:177-179, 1995.

Freeman S, Stephens R: Cheilitis: analysis of 75 cases referred to a contact dermatitis clinic, *Am J Contact Dermat* 7:146-151, 1996.

Leyland L, Field EA: Case report: exfoliative cheilitis managed with antidepressant medication, *Dent Update* 31:524-526, 2004.

Reade PC, Sim R: Exfoliative cheilitis–a factitious disorder? *Int J Oral Maxillofac Surg* 15:313-317, 1986.

Rosenquist B: Median lip fissure: etiology and suggested treatment, *Oral Surg Oral Med Oral Pathol* 72:10-14, 1991.

Scully C, van-Bruggen W, Diz-Dios P et al: Down syndrome: lip lesions (angular stomatitis and fissures) and *Candida albicans*, *Br J Dermatol* 147:37-40, 2002.

Taniguchi S, Kono T: Exfoliative cheilitis: a case report and review of the literature, *Dermatology* 196:253-255, 1998.

Submucosal Hemorrhage

Kalpidis CDR, Setayesh RM: Hemorrhaging associated with endosseous implant placement in the anterior mandible: a review of the literature, *J Periodontol* 75:631-645, 2004.

Kravitz P: The clinical picture of "cough purpura," benign and nonthrombocytopenic eruption, *Va Med* 106:373-374, 1979.

Lee B-J, Park H-J, Heo S-C: Organized hematoma of the maxillary sinus, *Acta Otolaryngol* 123:869-872, 2003.

Tabaee A, Kacker A: Hematoma of the maxillary sinus presenting as a mass–a case report and review of the literature, *Int J Pediatr Otorhinolaryngol* 65:153-157, 2002.

Woo BM, Al-Bustani S, Ueeck BA: Floor of mouth haemorrhage and life-threatening airway obstruction during immediate implant placement in the anterior mandible, *Int J Oral Maxillofac Surg* 35:961-964, 2006.

Oral Trauma from Sexual Practices

Damm DD, White DK, Brinker CM: Variations of palatal erythema secondary to fellatio, *Oral Surg Oral Med Oral Pathol* 52:417-421, 1981.

Elam AL: Sexually related trauma: a review, *Ann Emerg Med* 15:576-584, 1986.

Farman AG, Van Wyk CW: The features of non-infectious oral lesions caused by fellatio, *J Dent Assoc S Afr* 32:53-55, 1977.

Leider AS: Intraoral ulcers of questionable origin, *J Am Dent Assoc* 92:1177-1178, 1976.

Mader CL: Lingual frenum ulcer resulting from orogenital sex, *J Am Dent Assoc* 103:888-890, 1981.

Terezhalmy GT: Oral manifestations of sexually related diseases, *Ear Nose Throat J* 62:287-296, 1983.

Van Wyk CW: Oral lesions caused by habits, *Forensic Sci* 7:41-49, 1976.

Localized Exogenous Pigmentations

Buchner A, Hansen LS: Amalgam pigmentation (amalgam tattoo) of the oral mucosa: a clinicopathologic study of 268 cases, *Oral Surg Oral Med Oral Pathol* 49:139-147, 1980.

Daley TD, Gibson D: Practical applications of energy dispersive x-ray microanalysis in diagnostic oral pathology, *Oral Surg Oral Med Oral Pathol* 69:339-344, 1990.

Kaufman T, Bloch C, Schmidt W et al: Chronic inflammation and pain inside the mandibular jaw and a 10-year forgotten amalgam filling in an alveolar cavity of an extracted molar tooth, *Ultrastruct Pathol* 29:405-413, 2005.

Klontz KC, Lambert LA, Jewell RE et al: Adverse effects of cosmetic tattooing: an illustrative case of granulomatous dermatitis following the application of permanent makeup, *Arch Dermatol* 141:918-919, 2005.

Mani NJ: Gingival tattoo: a hitherto undescribed mucosal pigmentation, *Quintessence Int* 16:157-159, 1985.

Muller H, van der Velden, Samderubun EM: Tattooing in maxillofacial surgery, *J Craniomaxillofac Surg* 16:382-384, 1988.

Peters E, Gardner DG: A method of distinguishing between amalgam and graphite in tissue, *Oral Surg Oral Med Oral Pathol* 62:73-76, 1986.

Shah G, Alster TS: Treatment of an amalgam tattoo with a Q-switched alexandrite (755 nm) laser, *Dermatol Surg* 28:1180-1181, 2002.

Slabbert H, Ackermann GL, Altini M: Amalgam tattoo as a means for person identification, *J Forensic Odontostomatol* 9:17-23, 1991.

Weaver T, Auclair PL, Taybos GM: An amalgam tattoo causing local and systemic disease? *Oral Surg Oral Med Oral Pathol* 63:137-140, 1987.

Oral Piercings and Forked Tongue

Benecke M: First report of nonpsychotic self-cannibalism (autophagy), tongue splitting, and scar patterns (scarification) as an extreme form of cultural body modification in a western civilization, *Am J Forensic Med* 20:281-285, 1999.

Brennan M, O'Connell B, O'Sullivan M: Multiple dental fractures following tongue barbell placement: a case report, *Dent Traumatol* 22:41-43, 2006.

Bressmann T: Self-inflicted cosmetic tongue split: a case report, *J Can Dent Assoc* 70:156-157, 2004.

Campbell A, Moore A, Williams E et al: Tongue piercing: impact of time and barbell stem length on lingual gingival recession and tooth chipping, *J Periodontol* 73:289-297, 2002.

Fleming PS, Flood TR: Bifid tongue–a complication of tongue piercing, *Br Dent J* 198:265-266, 2005.

Kapferer I, Benesch T, Gregoric N et al: Lip piercing: prevalence of associated gingival recession and contributing factors. A cross-sectional study, *J Periodontol Res* 42:177-183, 2007.

Loh FC, Yeo JF: Talisman in the orofacial region, *Oral Surg Oral Med Oral Pathol* 68:252-255, 1989.

Nor MM, Yushar A, Razali M et al: Incidental radiologic findings of susuk in the orofacial region, *Dentomaxillofac Radiol* 35:473-474, 2006.

Systemic Metal Intoxication

Ahnlide I, Ahlgren C, Björkner B et al: Gold concentration in blood in relation to the number of gold restorations and contact allergy to gold, *Acta Odontol Scand* 60:301-305, 2002.

Bellinger DC, Trachtenberg F, Barregard L et al: Neuropsychological and renal effects of dental amalgam in children. A randomized trial, *J Am Med Assoc* 295:1775-1783, 2006.

DeRouen TA, Martin MD, Leroux BG et al: Neurobehavioral effects of dental amalgam in children. A randomized trial, *J Am Med Assoc* 295:1784-1792, 2006.

Dodes JE: The amalgam controversy. An evidence-based analysis, *J Am Dent Assoc* 132:348-356, 2001.

Drake PL, Hazelwood KJ: Exposure-repeated health effects of silver and silver compounds: a review, *Ann Occup Hyg* 49:575-585, 2005.

Dummet CO: Systemic significance of oral pigmentation and discoloration, *Postgrad Med J* 49(1):78-82, 1971.

Eisler R: Mammalian sensitivity to elemental gold (Au degrees), *Biol Trace Elem Res* 100:1-18, 2004.

Fowler J Jr, Taylor J, Storrs F et al: Gold allergy in North America, *Am J Contact Dermat* 12:3-5, 2001.

Gordon NC, Brown S, Khosla VM et al: Lead poisoning: a comprehensive review and report of a case, *Oral Surg Oral Med Oral Pathol* 47:500-512, 1979.

Harris RA, Poole A: Beware of bismuth: post maxillectomy delirium, *ANZ J Surg* 72:846-847, 2002.

Ioffreda MD, Gordon CA, Adams DR et al: Black tongue, *Arch Dermatol* 137:968-969, 2001.

Jacobs R: Argyria: my life story, *Clin Dermatol* 24:66-69, 2006.

Langworth S, Björkman L, Elinder C-G et al: Multidisciplinary examination of patients with illness attributed to dental fillings, *J Oral Rehabil* 29:705-713, 2002.

Lee SM, Lee SH: Generalized argyria after habitual use of AgNO₃, *J Dermatol* 21:50-53, 1994.

Marshall JP, Schneider RP: Systemic argyria secondary to topical silver nitrate, *Arch Dermatol* 113:1077-1179, 1977.

Martin MD, Williams BJ, Charleston JD et al: Spontaneous exfoliation of teeth following severe elemental mercury poisoning: case report and histological investigation for mechanism, *Oral Surg Oral Med Oral Pathol Oral Radiol Endod* 84:495-501, 1997.

Mirsattari SM, Hammond RR, Sharpe MD et al: Myoclonic status epilepticus following repeated oral ingestion of colloidal silver, *Neurology* 62:1408-1410, 2004.

Su M, Barrueto F Jr, Hoffman RS: Childhood lead poisoning from paint chips: a continuing problem, *J Urban Health* 79:491-501, 2002.

Wadhera A, Fung M: Systemic argyria associated with ingestion of colloidal silver, *Dermatol Online J* 11(1):12, 2005.

Smoker's Melanosis

Axéll T, Hedin CA: Epidemiologic study of excessive oral melanin pigmentation with special reference to the influence of tobacco habits, *Scand J Dent Res* 90:434-442, 1982.

Hedin CA: Smokers' melanosis, *Arch Dermatol* 113:1533-1538, 1977.

Hedin CA, Axéll T: Oral melanin pigmentation in 467 Thai and Malaysian people with special emphasis on smoker's melanosis, *J Oral Pathol Med* 20:8-12, 1991.

Hedin CA, Larsson Å: The ultrastructure of the gingival epithelium in smokers' melanosis, *J Periodontal Res* 19:177-190, 1984.

Hedin CA, Pindborg JJ, Daftary DK et al: Melanin depigmentation of the palatal mucosa in reverse smokers: a preliminary study, *J Oral Pathol Med* 21:440-444, 1992.

Ramer M, Burakoff RP: Smoker's melanosis, *N Y State Dent J* 63:20-21, 1997.

Drug-Related Discolorations of the Oral Mucosa

Birek C, Main JHP: Two cases of oral pigmentation associated with quinidine therapy, *Oral Surg Oral Med Oral Pathol* 66:59-61, 1988.

Cale AE, Freedman PD, Lumerman H: Pigmentation of the jawbones and teeth secondary to minocycline hydrochloride therapy, *J Periodontol* 59:112-114, 1988.

Cockings JM, Savage NW: Minocycline and oral pigmentation, *Aust Dent J* 43:14-16, 1998.

Dummet CO: Oral mucosal discolorations related to pharmacotherapeutics, *J Oral Ther Pharmacol* 1:106-110, 1964.

Granstein RD, Sober AJ: Drug- and heavy metal-induced hyperpigmentation, *J Am Acad Dermatol* 5:1-18, 1981.

Hood AF: Cutaneous side effects of cancer chemotherapy, *Med Clin North Am* 70:187-209, 1986.

Langford A, Pohle H-D, Gelderblom H et al: Oral hyperpigmentation in HIV-infected patients, *Oral Surg Oral Med Oral Pathol* 67:301-307, 1989.

LaPorta VN, Nikitakis NG, Sindler AJ et al: Minocycline-associated intra-oral soft-tissue pigmentation: clinicopathologic correlations and review, *J Clin Periodontol* 32:119-122, 2005.

Pérusse R, Morency R: Oral pigmentation induced by Premarin, *Cutis* 48:61-64, 1991.

Treister NS, Magalnick D, Woo S-B: Oral mucosal pigmentation secondary to minocycline therapy: report of two cases and a review of the literature, *Oral Surg Oral Med Oral Pathol Oral Radiol Endod* 97:718-725, 2004.

Traumatic Osseous and Chondromatous Metaplasia

Cutright DE: Osseous and chondromatous metaplasia caused by dentures, *Oral Surg Oral Med Oral Pathol* 34:625-633, 1972.

Daley TD, Damm DD, Wysocki GP et al: Atypical cartilage in reactive osteocartilagenous metaplasia of the traumatized edentulous mandibular ridge, *Oral Surg Oral Med Oral Pathol Oral Radiol Endod* 83:26-29, 1997.

Lello GE, Makek M: Submucosal nodular chondrometaplasia in denture wearers, *J Prosthet Dent* 54:237-240, 1985.

Magnusson BC, Engström H, Kahnberg K-E: Metaplastic formation of bone and chondroid in flabby ridges, *Br J Oral Maxillofac Surg* 24:300-305, 1986.

Oral Ulceration with Bone Sequestration

Farah CS, Savage NW: Oral ulceration with bone sequestration, *Aust Dent J* 48:61-64, 2003.

Kessler HP: Lingual mandibular sequestration with ulceration, *Tex Dent J* 122:198-199, 206-207, 2005.

Peters E, Lovas GL, Wysocki GP: Lingual mandibular sequestration and ulceration, *Oral Surg Oral Med Oral Pathol Oral Radiol Endod* 75:739-743, 1993.

Scully C: Oral ulceration: a new and unusual complication, *Br Dent J* 192:139-140, 2002.

Sonnier KE, Horning GM: Spontaneous bony exposure: a report of 4 cases of idiopathic exposure and sequestration of alveolar bone, *J Periodontol* 68:758-762, 1997.

Pseudocysts and Cysts of the Maxillary Sinus

Allard RHB, van der Kwast WAM, van der Waal I: Mucosal antral cysts: review of the literature and report of a radiographic survey, *Oral Surg Oral Med Oral Pathol* 51:2-9, 1981.

Bockmühl U, Kratzsch B, Benda K et al: Surgery for paranasal sinus mucoceles: efficacy of endonasal micro-endoscopic management and long-term results of 185 patients, *Rhinology* 44:62-67, 2006.

Bourgeois SL, Nelson BL: Surgical ciliated cyst of the mandible secondary to simultaneous LeFort I osteotomy and genioplasty: report of case and review of the literature, *Oral Surg Oral Med Oral Pathol Oral Radiol Endod* 100:36-39, 2005.

Carter LC, Calamel A, Haller A et al: Seasonal variation in maxillary antral pseudocyst in a general clinical population, *Dentomaxillofac Radiol* 27:22-24, 1998.

Gardner DG: Pseudocysts and retention cysts of the maxillary sinus, *Oral Surg Oral Med Oral Pathol* 58:561-567, 1984.

Gardner DG, Gullane PJ: Mucoceles of the maxillary sinus, *Oral Surg Oral Med Oral Pathol* 62:538-543, 1986.

Kaneshiro S, Nakajima T, Yoshikawa Y et al: The postoperative maxillary cyst: report of 71 cases, *J Oral Surg* 39:191-198, 1981.

Cervicofacial Emphysema

Horowitz I, Hirshberg A, Freedman A: Pneumomediastinum and subcutaneous emphysema following surgical extraction of mandibular third molars: three case reports, *Oral Surg Oral Med Oral Pathol* 63:25-28, 1987.

Karras SC, Sexton JJ: Cervicofacial and mediastinal emphysema as the result of a dental procedure, *J Emerg Med* 14:9-13, 1996.

López-Peláez MF, Roldán J, Mateo S: Cervical emphysema, pneumomediastinum, and pneumothorax following self-induced oral injury: report of four cases and review of the literature, *Chest* 120:306-309, 2001.

Martín-Granizo R, Herrera M, Garcìa-Gonzàlez D et al: Pneumoparotid in childhood: report of two cases, *J Oral Maxillofac Surg* 57:1468-1471, 1999.

Stanton DC, Balasanian E, Yepes JF: Subcutaneous cervicofacial emphysema and pneumo-mediastinum: a rare complication after a crown preparation, *Gen Dent* 53:122-124, 2005.

Tosun F, Ozer C, Akcam T et al: A patient with severe cervicofacial subcutaneous emphysema associated with Munchausen's syndrome, *J Craniofac Surg* 16:661-664, 2005.

Myospherulosis

Dunlap CL, Barker BF: Myospherulosis of the jaws, *Oral Surg Oral Med Oral Pathol* 50:238-243, 1980.

Lynch DP, Newland JR, McClendon JL: Myospherulosis of the oral hard and soft tissues, *J Oral Maxillofac Surg* 42:349-355, 1984.

Moore JW, Brekke JH: Foreign body giant cell reaction related to placement of tetracycline-treated polylactic acid: report of 18 cases, *J Oral Maxillofac Surg* 48:808-812, 1990.

Sarkar S, Gangane N, Sharma S: Myospherulosis of maxillary sinus—a case report with review of literature, *Indian J Pathol Microbiol* 41:491-493, 1998.

Sindwani R, Cohen JT, Pilch BZ et al: Myospherulosis following sinus surgery: pathological curiosity or important clinical entity, *Laryngoscope* 113:1123-1127, 2003.

Wallace ML, Neville BW: Myospherulosis: report of a case, *J Periodontol* 61:55-57, 1990.

9

Allergies and Immunologic Diseases

CHAPTER OUTLINE

TRANSIENT LINGUAL PAPILLITIS

Transient lingual papillitis (lie bumps, tongue torches) represents a common oral pathosis that, for some reason, rarely has been documented. Affected patients experience clinical alterations that involve a variable number of fungiform papillae of the tongue. The pathogenesis currently is unknown, but the lesions most likely arise from a variety of influences. Suggested causes include local irritation, stress, gastrointestinal disease, hormonal fluctuation, upper respiratory tract infection, viral infection, and topical hypersensitivity to foods, drinks, or oral hygiene products.

CLINICAL FEATURES

Three patterns of transient lingual papillitis have been documented. The first pattern is localized and involves one to several fungiform papillae that become enlarged and present as elevated papules that are red but may demonstrate a yellow, ulcerated cap (Fig. 9-1). The lesions appear most frequently on the anterior portion of the dorsal surface, are associated with mild to moderate pain, and resolve spontaneously within hours to several days. In a survey of 163 dental school staff members, 56% reported previous episodes of transient lingual papillitis. There was a female predominance, and the vast majority reported a single affected papilla.

In one report the occurrence of the lesions appeared to be associated with a food allergy.

In the second pattern the involvement is more generalized and affects a large percentage of the fungiform papillae on the tip and lateral portions of the dorsal surface (Fig. 9-2). Individual papillae are very sensitive, enlarged, erythematous, and occasionally display focal surface erosion. Fever and cervical lymphadenopathy are not rare. In these cases, spread of the process among family members has been reported, suggesting a possible correlation to an unknown virus. Spontaneous resolution occurs in about 7 days, with occasional recurrences reported.

The third pattern of transient lingual papillitis also demonstrates more diffuse involvement. The altered papillae are asymptomatic, appear as elevated white to yellow papules, and have been termed the *papulokeratotic variant* because of a thickened parakeratotic cap (Fig. 9-3). Although these lesions could be the result of a topical allergy, the histopathology demonstrates features similar to chronic nibbling and suggests the possibility of an unusual pattern of frictional hyperkeratosis.

HISTOPATHOLOGIC FEATURES

On histopathologic examination of the first two variants, affected papillae demonstrate normal surface epithelium that may reveal focal areas of exocytosis or

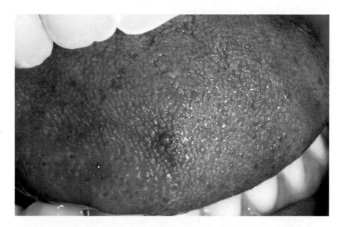

Fig. 9-1 Transient lingual papillitis. Tender, yellow-pink papule on the dorsum of the tongue.

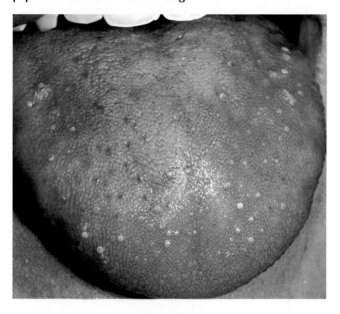

Fig. 9-2 Transient lingual papillitis. Multiple painful white papules on the lateral dorsum and tip of tongue.

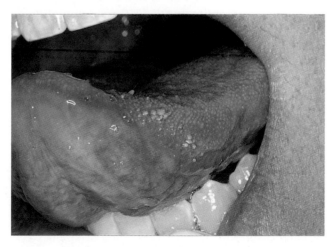

Fig. 9-3 Transient lingual papillitis. Clusters of asymptomatic, elevated, yellow papules on the dorsolateral surface of the tongue. *(Courtesy of Dr. Craig Fowler.)*

ulceration. The underlying lamina propria exhibits a proliferation of numerous small vascular channels and a mixed inflammatory cellular infiltrate. Investigation for evidence of human papillomavirus (HPV), herpes simplex, and fungal infestation has been negative. The papulokeratotic variant demonstrates marked hyperparakeratosis in which the surface is ragged and reveals bacterial colonization. A chronic lymphocytic infiltrate is noted in the superficial lamina propria with extension into the basilar portion of the adjacent epithelium.

TREATMENT AND PROGNOSIS

Although transient lingual papillitis resolves without therapy, topical corticosteroids, anesthetics, and coating agents have been used to reduce the pain or duration. In an attempt to eliminate the pain, occasional patients have reported removing the affected papillae with devices such as fingernail clippers. The papulokeratotic variant is asymptomatic and requires no therapy. Although frequently unsuccessful, search for a local or systemic triggering event seems prudent.

RECURRENT APHTHOUS STOMATITIS (RECURRENT APHTHOUS ULCERATIONS; CANKER SORES)

Recurrent aphthous stomatitis is one of the most common oral mucosal pathoses. The reported prevalence in the general population varies from 5% to 66%, with a mean of 20%. The hypotheses of its pathogenesis are numerous. As soon as one investigator claims to have discovered the definitive cause, a subsequent report discredits the discovery. Different subgroups of patients appear to have different causes for the occurrence of aphthae. These factors suggest a disease process that is triggered by a variety of causative agents, each of which is capable of producing the disease in certain subgroups of patients. To state it simply, the cause appears to be "different things in different people."

Although no single triggering agent is responsible, the mucosal destruction appears to represent a T cell–mediated immunologic reaction. Analysis of the peripheral blood in patients with aphthae shows a decreased ratio of CD4+ to CD8+ T lymphocytes, increased T cell–receptor $\gamma\delta^+$ cells, and increased tumor necrosis factor-α (TNF-α). Many investigators agree that the epithelial destruction appears to be a local T cell–mediated response and involves T cells with TNF-α generated by these cells, macrophages, and mast cells. Evidence of the destruction of the oral mucosa mediated by these lymphocytes is strong, but the initiating causes are elusive and most likely highly variable.

The following all have been reported to be responsible in certain subgroups of patients (and each discounted in other subgroups!):

- Allergies
- Genetic predisposition
- Hematologic abnormalities
- Hormonal influences
- Immunologic factors
- Infectious agents
- Nutritional deficiencies
- Smoking cessation
- Stress
- Trauma

When all the various subgroups are combined, the various causes cluster into three categories:

1. Primary immunodysregulation
2. Decrease of the mucosal barrier
3. Increase in antigenic exposure

One or more of these three factors may be involved in subgroups of patients.

Recurrent aphthous stomatitis demonstrates a definite tendency to occur along family lines. When both parents have a history of aphthous ulcers, there is a 90% chance that their children will develop the lesions. In addition, several investigators have shown an association with certain histocompatibility antigen (HLA) types in subgroups of patients. Stress, with its presumed effects on the immune system, directly correlates with the presence of aphthous stomatitis in some groups. In studies of professional students, recurrences clustered around stressful periods of the academic year; conversely, periods of vacation were associated with a low frequency of lesions.

Aphthouslike ulcerations have occurred in patients with systemic immunodysregulations. Patients with cyclic neutropenia (see page 583) occasionally have cycles of aphthouslike ulcerations that correspond to the periods of severe immunodysregulation. In addition, patients with acquired immunodeficiency syndrome (AIDS) have an increased frequency of severe aphthous stomatitis (see page 278), a fact that is not surprising considering the elevated CD8+/CD4+ ratio as the result of the reduction of CD4+ T lymphocytes.

The mucosal barrier appears to be important in the prevention of aphthous stomatitis and might explain the almost exclusive presence of aphthous stomatitis on nonkeratinized mucosa. Numerous factors that decrease the mucosal barrier increase the frequency of occurrence (e.g., trauma, nutritional deficiencies, smoking cessation); conversely, those associated with an increased mucosal barrier have been correlated with decreased ulcerations (e.g., smoking, hormonal changes, marked absence of aphthae on mucosa bound

---

Box 9-1

Systemic Disorders Associated With Recurrent Aphthous Stomatitis

- Behçet's syndrome
- Celiac disease
- Cyclic neutropenia
- Nutritional deficiencies (iron, folate, zinc, B_1, B_2, B_6, B_{12})
- IgA deficiency
- Immunocompromised conditions, including human immunodeficiency virus (HIV) disease
- Inflammatory bowel disease
- MAGIC syndrome (mouth and genital ulcers with inflamed cartilage)
- PFAPA syndrome (periodic fever, aphthous stomatitis, pharyngitis, cervical adenitis)
- Reactive arthritis
- Sweet's syndrome
- Ulcus vulvae acutum

---

to bone). In a small subset of female patients, a negative association was reported between the occurrence of aphthae and the luteal phase of the menstrual cycle—a period of mucosal proliferation and keratinization. In addition, these same patients often experience ulcer-free periods during pregnancy.

An antigenic stimulus appears to be the primary initiating factor in the immune-mediated cytotoxic destruction of the mucosa in many patients. The list seems endless, and every item on the list may be important in small subsets of patients. Commonly mentioned potential antigens include sodium lauryl sulfate in toothpaste, many systemic medications (e.g., nonsteroidal antiinflammatory drugs [NSAIDs], various beta blockers, nicorandil), microbiologic agents (e.g., L forms of streptococci, *Helicobacter pylori*, herpes simplex virus [HSV], varicella-zoster virus [VZV], adenovirus, and cytomegalovirus [CMV]), and many foods (e.g., cheese, chocolate, coffee, cow's milk, gluten, nuts, strawberries, tomatoes, dyes, flavoring agents, preservatives).

An increased prevalence of aphthouslike ulcerations has been noted in a variety of systemic disorders (Box 9-1). These ulcerations typically are identical clinically and histopathologically to those noted in otherwise healthy individuals. In many cases, resolution of the systemic disorder produces a decreased frequency and severity of the mucosal ulcerations.

Three clinical variations of aphthous stomatitis are recognized:

1. Minor
2. Major
3. Herpetiform

Minor aphthous ulcerations (Mikulicz's aphthae) are the most common and represent the pattern present in more than 80% of those affected. **Major aphthous ulcerations (Sutton's disease** or **periadenitis mucosa necrotica recurrens** [PMNR]) occur in approximately 10% of the patients referred for treatment. The remaining patients have **herpetiform aphthous ulcerations.** The minor and major forms most likely represent variations of the same process, although herpetiform aphthae demonstrate a unique pattern. Some investigators differentiate the herpetiform variant because of supposed evidence of a viral cause, but the proof is weak and does not justify its distinction from the other aphthous ulcerations. Some authors include Behçet's syndrome as an additional variation of aphthous stomatitis, but this multisystem disorder is more complex and is considered later in this chapter.

CLINICAL FEATURES

Aphthous ulcerations are noted more frequently in children and young adults, with approximately 80% of affected individuals reporting their first ulceration before the age of 30. In one large series of 17,235 adults older than 17 years of age, the point prevalence of aphthous ulcerations was 0.89%, with the annual incidence in adults younger than 40 years old being almost twice that of older adults (22.5% versus 13.4%).

MINOR APHTHOUS ULCERATIONS

Patients with minor aphthous ulcerations experience the fewest recurrences, and the individual lesions exhibit the shortest duration of the three variants. The ulcers arise almost exclusively on nonkeratinized mucosa and may be preceded by an erythematous macule in association with prodromal symptoms of burning, itching, or stinging. The ulceration demonstrates a yellow-white, removable fibrinopurulent membrane that is encircled by an erythematous halo (Fig. 9-4). Classically, the ulcerations measure between 3 and 10 mm in diameter and heal without scarring in 7 to 14 days (Fig. 9-5). From one to five lesions typically are present during each episode, and the pain often is out of proportion for the size of the ulceration. The buccal and labial mucosae are affected most frequently, followed by the ventral surface of the tongue, mucobuccal fold, floor of the mouth, and soft palate (Fig. 9-6). Involvement of keratinized mucosa (e.g., hard palate, gingiva, dorsal surface of the tongue, and vermilion border) is rare and usually represents extension from adjacent nonkeratinized epithelium. The recur-

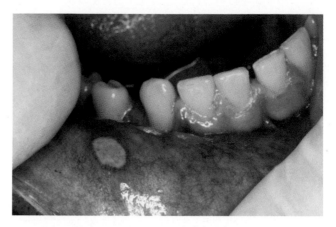

Fig. 9-4   Minor aphthous ulceration. Erythematous halo encircling a yellowish ulceration of the lower labial mucosa. *(Courtesy of Dr. Dean K. White.)*

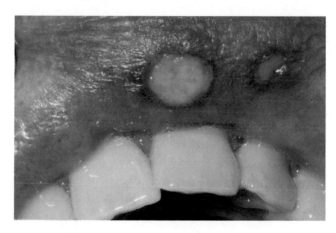

Fig. 9-5   Minor aphthous ulcerations. Two ulcerations of different sizes located on the maxillary labial mucosa.

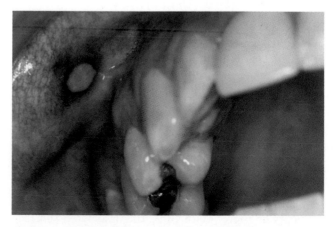

Fig. 9-6   Minor aphthous ulceration. Single ulceration of the anterior buccal mucosa.

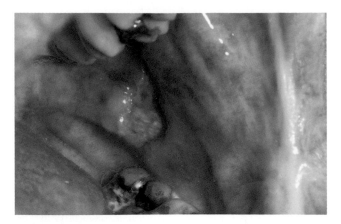

Fig. 9-7   Major aphthous ulceration. Large, deep, and irregular ulceration of the posterior buccal mucosa. Note extensive scarring of the anterior buccal mucosa from previous ulcerations.

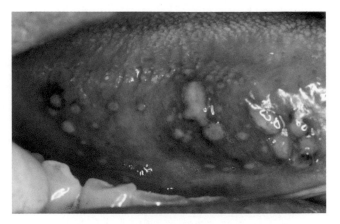

Fig. 9-9   Herpetiform aphthous ulcerations. Numerous pinhead ulcerations of the ventral surface of the tongue, several of which have coalesced into larger, more irregular areas of ulceration.

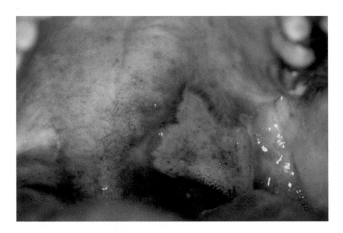

Fig. 9-8   Major aphthous ulceration. Large, irregular ulceration of the soft palate.

HERPETIFORM APHTHOUS ULCERATIONS

Herpetiform aphthous ulcerations demonstrate the greatest number of lesions and the most frequent recurrences. The individual lesions are small, averaging 1 to 3 mm in diameter, with as many as 100 ulcers present in a single recurrence. Because of their small size and large number, the lesions bear a superficial resemblance to a primary HSV infection, leading to the confusing designation, **herpetiform.** It is common for individual lesions to coalesce into larger irregular ulcerations (Fig. 9-9). The ulcerations heal within 7 to 10 days, but the recurrences tend to be closely spaced. Many patients are affected almost constantly for periods as long as 3 years. Although the nonkeratinized, movable mucosa is affected most frequently, any oral mucosal surface may be involved. There is a female predominance, and typically the onset is in adulthood.

Further classification of all three types is valuable when planning the most appropriate diagnostic evaluation and therapy. The lesions are diagnosed as **simple aphthosis** when they appear in patients with few lesions that heal within 1 to 2 weeks and recur infrequently. In contrast, patients with **complex aphthosis** have multiple (≥3) and almost constant oral ulcerations that often develop as older lesions resolve. Severe pain and large size are common. Although associated genital or perianal lesions also may be present, there is no other evidence of an associated systemic disease.

HISTOPATHOLOGIC FEATURES

The histopathologic picture of aphthous stomatitis is characteristic but not pathognomonic. The early ulcerative lesions demonstrate a central zone of ulceration,

rence rate is highly variable, ranging from one ulceration every few years to two episodes per month.

MAJOR APHTHOUS ULCERATIONS

Major aphthous ulcerations are larger than minor aphthae and demonstrate the longest duration per episode. The number of lesions usually is intermediate between that seen in the minor and herpetiform variants. The ulcerations are deeper than the minor variant, measure from 1 to 3 cm in diameter, take from 2 to 6 weeks to heal, and may cause scarring (Fig. 9-7). The number of lesions varies from 1 to 10. Any oral surface area may be affected, but the labial mucosa, soft palate, and tonsillar fauces are involved most commonly (Fig. 9-8). The onset of major aphthae is after puberty, and recurrent episodes may continue to develop for up to 20 years or more. With time, the associated scarring can become significant, and in rare instances may lead to a restricted mouth opening.

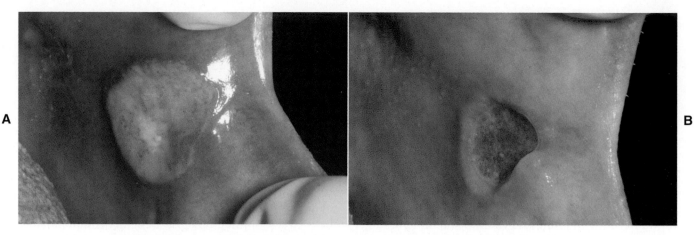

Fig. 9-10   Major aphthous ulceration. A, Large ulceration of the left anterior buccal mucosa. **B,** Same lesion after 5 days of therapy with betamethasone syrup used in a swish-and-swallow method. The patient was free of pain by the second day of therapy. The ulceration healed completely during the next week.

which is covered by a fibrinopurulent membrane. Deep to the area of ulceration, the connective tissue exhibits an increased vascularity and a mixed inflammatory cellular infiltrate that consists of lymphocytes, histiocytes, and polymorphonuclear leukocytes. The epithelium at the margin of the lesion demonstrates spongiosis and numerous mononuclear cells in the basilar one third. A band of lymphocytes intermixed with histiocytes is present in the superficial connective tissue and surrounding deeper blood vessels.

DIAGNOSIS

No laboratory procedure provides definitive diagnosis. The diagnosis is made from the clinical presentation and from exclusion of other diseases that produce ulcerations that closely resemble aphthae (see Box 9-1). In patients with complex aphthous ulcerations, a systematic evaluation for an underlying trigger or associated systemic condition is prudent. In a review of 244 patients with complex aphthous ulcerations, an associated triggering condition (e.g., hematologic deficiency, gastrointestinal disease, immunodeficiency, drug reaction) was discovered in almost 60%. Because the histopathologic features are nonspecific, a biopsy is useful only in eliminating differential possibilities and is not beneficial in arriving at the definitive diagnosis.

TREATMENT AND PROGNOSIS

The patient's medical history should be reviewed for signs and symptoms of any systemic disorder that may be associated with aphthouslike ulcerations. Most patients with mild aphthosis receive either no treatment, therapy with a number of over-the-counter anes-

thetics or protective bioadhesive products, or periodic topical medicaments that minimize the frequency and severity of the attacks.

In patients with mild disease, the mainstay of therapy is the use of topical corticosteroids, and the list of possible choices is long. Most patients with diffuse minor or herpetiform aphthae respond well to 0.01% dexamethasone elixir used in a rinse-and-expectorate method. Patients with localized ulcerations can be treated successfully with 0.05% augmented betamethasone dipropionate gel or 0.05% fluocinonide gel. Adrenal suppression does not occur with appropriate use of these medications. Major aphthous ulcerations are more resistant to therapy and often warrant more potent corticosteroids (Fig. 9-10). The individual lesions may be injected with triamcinolone acetonide or covered with 0.05% clobetasol propionate gel or 0.05% halobetasol propionate ointment. Triamcinolone tablets also can be dissolved directly over the lesions. In hard-to-reach areas, such as the tonsillar pillars, beclomethasone dipropionate aerosol spray can be used. In resistant cases, systemic corticosteroids may be required to supplement the topical medications and gain control. In such instances, prednisolone or betamethasone syrup in a swish-and-swallow method is preferable to prednisone tablets. In this way the ulcerations will receive both topical and systemic therapy.

Numerous alternatives to corticosteroid agents have been used to treat patients suffering from aphthous ulcerations (the most widely accepted are highlighted in bold). Caution should be exercised, however, because many of these agents have not been examined in a double-blind, placebo-controlled fashion to assess the degree of effectiveness compared with placebo. Furthermore, some of these treatments may have significant side effects or may be quite expensive. Included within the list of therapies are acyclovir, **amlexanox,** topical 5-aminosalicylic acid, azelastine hydrochloride, benzydamine hydrochloride, carbenoxolone sodium, chemical cauterizing agents, **chlorhexidine, colchicine,** cyclosporine, **dapsone,** deglycyrrhizinated liquorice, gamma globulin, hydrogen peroxide, hydroxypropyl cellulose films, interferon-α, irsogladine maleate, levamisole, LongoVital, monoamine oxidase (MAO) inhibitors, pentoxifylline, prostaglandin E-2 gel, sucralfate, sodium cromoglycate (cromolyn), tacrolimus, **tetracyclines, thalidomide,** transfer factor (extract of immunocytes), triclosan, and vitamin and mineral supplements (especially zinc sulfate). The success of these therapies is highly variable. These treatments do not resolve the underlying problem and are merely an attempt to "beat back brush fires." Recurrences often continue, although breaking up the cycle may induce longer disease-free intervals between attacks. Surgical removal of aphthous ulcerations has been used but is an inappropriate therapy. Although laser ablation shortens the duration and decreases associated symptoms, its use is of very limited practical benefit because patients cannot return on each recurrence.

Chemical cautery with silver nitrate continues to be suggested as an effective therapy, but it can no longer be recommended because of the numerous safer alternatives and its rare association with massive necrosis (see page 292) and systemic argyria (see page 315). An over-the-counter cautery that uses sulfuric acid and phenolic agents is indicated in certain situations, but patients must be warned of the potential for significant local tissue necrosis related to its misuse.

Patients with complex aphthosis require a more extensive evaluation for occult systemic disease and a search for possible triggers of the immune-mediated mucosal destruction. To go beyond the management of individual recurrences is difficult, expensive, and often frustrating. In spite of this, patients with severe disease should be offered the opportunity to investigate the underlying causes.

As previously mentioned, the immune attacks are usually a result of immunodysregulation, a decreased mucosal barrier, or an elevated antigenic stimulus. The evaluation for systemic disorders usually eliminates the first two causes. Typically, this is followed by patch tests for antigen stimuli or an elimination diet for possible offending foods. Therapeutic trials might be instituted against the viruses and bacteria that have been implicated in subsets of patients with aphthous stomatitis. The investigator should explain to the patient that the underlying causation is diverse; even with the most exhaustive search, the answer may be elusive. In many cases, stress appears involved, and all evaluations in these patients will be within normal limits. In spite of the high likelihood of an expensive and negative evaluation, discovery of an underlying abnormality that can be treated often leads to permanent resolution or dramatic improvement in the course of the recurrences.

BEHÇET'S SYNDROME (BEHÇET'S DISEASE; ADAMANTIADES SYNDROME)

The combination of chronic ocular inflammation and orogenital ulcerations was reported as early as the era of the ancient Greeks and later described in 1931 by a Greek ophthalmologist, Benedict Adamantiades. The classic triad was not delineated until 1937, when a Turkish dermatologist, Hulusi Behçet, defined the disease that bears his name. Although the disease has been traditionally thought primarily to affect the oral, genital, and ocular regions, it now is recognized to be a multisystem disorder.

Although no clear causation has been established, **Behçet's syndrome** has an immunogenetic basis because of strong associations with certain HLA types. As in aphthous stomatitis, the disorder appears to be an immunodysregulation that may be primary or secondary to one or more triggers. Investigators have correlated attacks to a number of environmental antigens, including bacteria (especially streptococci), viruses, pesticides, and heavy metals.

Histocompatibility antigen B-51 (HLA-B51) has been linked closely to Behçet's syndrome, and the frequency of both the disease (approximately 1 in 1000) and the haplotype is high in Turkey, Japan, and the Eastern Mediterranean countries. This distribution appears correlated to the ancient "Silk Route" that extended from China to Rome and was traveled by the Turks. Sexual reproduction between immigrants and locals along the route appears to have spread the genetic vulnerability. Interestingly, when predisposed populations migrate to nonendemic locations, the prevalence decreases, suggesting environmental factors also are involved.

CLINICAL FEATURES

As mentioned previously, the highest prevalence occurs in the Middle East and Japan, with a much lower frequency noted in northern Europe, the United States, and the United Kingdom. At the time of discovery, most patients are young adults, with the disease diagnosed uncommonly in blacks, children, and older adults.

Oral involvement is an important component of Behçet's syndrome, and it is the first manifestation in 25% to 75% of the cases. Oral lesions occur at some

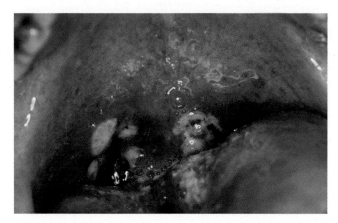

Fig. 9-11   Behçet's syndrome. Diffuse erythema surrounding numerous irregular ulcerations of the soft palate.

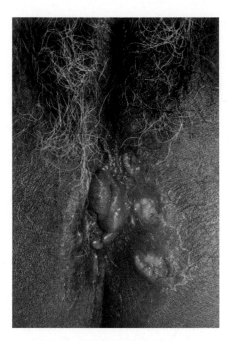

Fig. 9-12   Behçet's syndrome. Numerous irregular ulcerations of the labia majora and perineum. *(From Helm TN, Camisa C, Allen C et al: Clinical features of Behçet's disease, Oral Surg Oral Med Oral Pathol 72:30, 1991.)*

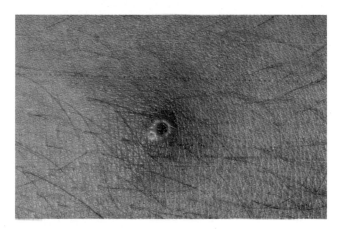

Fig. 9-13   Behçet's syndrome. Sterile pustule of the skin that developed 1 day after injection of saline. This reaction is termed *cutaneous pathergy*.

point during the disease in 99% of the patients and typically precede other sites of involvement.

The lesions are similar to aphthous ulcerations occurring in otherwise healthy individuals and demonstrate the same duration and frequency. In spite of this, investigators have shown several statistically significant clinical variations that are different from typical aphthous ulcerations and may be used to increase the index of suspicion for Behçet's syndrome. When compared with patients with aphthae, a larger percentage of those with Behçet's syndrome demonstrate six or more ulcerations. The lesions commonly involve the soft palate and oropharynx, which are usually infrequent sites for the occurrence of routine aphthae. The individual lesions vary in size, have ragged borders, and are surrounded by a larger zone of diffuse erythema (Fig. 9-11).

All three forms of oral aphthous stomatitis may be seen. Although the majority of affected patients have lesions that resemble minor aphthous ulcerations, some reports have documented a prevalence of major aphthae that approaches 40% in patients affected with Behçet's syndrome. The herpetiform variant remains uncommon and is noted in approximately 3%. Patients with major aphthae often demonstrate more frequent recurrences and more ulcerations per relapse. In spite of more severe oral disease, the presence of major aphthae in Behçet's syndrome does not correlate with an increased risk for more severe systemic expression.

The genital lesions are similar in appearance to the oral ulcerations. They occur in 75% of the patients and appear on the vulva, vagina, glans penis, scrotum, and perianal area (Fig. 9-12). These lesions recur less frequently than do the oral ulcerations, are deeper, and tend to heal with scarring. The genital ulcerations cause more symptoms in men than in women and

may be discovered only by a routine examination in women.

Common cutaneous lesions include erythematous papules, vesicles, pustules, pyoderma, folliculitis, acneiform eruptions, and erythema nodosum–like lesions. From a diagnostic standpoint, one of the most important skin manifestations is the presence of positive "pathergy." One or 2 days after the oblique insertion of a 20-gauge or smaller needle under sterile conditions, a tuberculin-like skin reaction or sterile pustule develops (Fig. 9-13). This skin hyperreactivity (pathergy)

Table **9-1**   **International Study Group Criteria for the Diagnosis of Behçet's Disease**

Recurrent oral ulceration	Minor, major, or herpetiform aphthae
Plus two of the following:	
Recurrent genital ulcerations	Aphthaelike ulcerations
Eye lesions	Anterior or posterior uveitis, cells in vitreous on slit-lamp examination, or retinal vasculitis
Skin lesions	Erythema nodosum, pseudofolliculitis or papulopustular lesions, or acneiform nodules noted in postadolescent patients not receiving corticosteroids
Positive pathergy test	Read by physician at 24-48 hours

appears to be unique to Behçet's syndrome and is present in 40% to 88% of patients with this disorder.

Ocular involvement is present in 70% to 85% of the cases and is more frequent and severe in males. The most common findings are posterior uveitis, conjunctivitis, corneal ulceration, papilledema, and arteritis. Although Behçet originally described hypopyon (pus in the anterior chamber) as a cause of blindness, this finding currently is rare. The most common secondary ocular complications are cataracts, glaucoma, and neovascularization of the iris and retina.

Arthritis is one of the more common minor manifestations of the disease and is usually self-limiting and nondeforming. The knees, wrists, elbows, and ankles are affected most frequently.

Central nervous system (CNS) involvement is not common but, when present, is associated with a poor prognosis. From 10% to 25% of the patients demonstrate CNS involvement, and the alterations produced result in a number of changes that include paralysis and severe dementia.

Other alterations may be seen that involve the cardiovascular, gastrointestinal, hematologic, pulmonary, muscular, and renal systems. These most likely occur secondary to vasculitis and create a variety of clinical presentations.

DIAGNOSIS

No laboratory finding is diagnostic of Behçet's syndrome. In an attempt to standardize diagnoses, definitive criteria have been developed. Table 9-1 delineates the requirements proposed by the Behçet's International Study Group. Although this system is used widely, many authorities exclude acneiform skin lesions in young adults from the criteria because of the high prevalence of this finding in an otherwise normal population.

HISTOPATHOLOGIC FEATURES

The histopathologic features are not specific for Behçet's syndrome and can be seen in many disorders, including aphthous stomatitis. The pattern most frequently seen is called *leukocytoclastic vasculitis*. The ulceration is similar in appearance to that seen in aphthous stomatitis, but the small blood vessels classically demonstrate intramural invasion by neutrophils, karyorrhexis of neutrophils, extravasation of red blood cells, and fibrinoid necrosis of the vessel wall.

TREATMENT AND PROGNOSIS

The oral and genital ulcerations typically respond well to potent topical or intralesional corticosteroids or topical tacrolimus. In more severe cases, this therapy can be combined with oral colchicine or dapsone. Patients who fail this initial conservative approach often respond to thalidomide, low-dose methotrexate, systemic corticosteroids, or infliximab (anti-TNF-α antibody). Severe ocular or systemic disease often necessitates combined use of systemic immunosuppressive and immunomodulatory agents (e.g., corticosteroids, cyclosporine, azathioprine, interferon-α2a, cyclophosphamide).

Behçet's syndrome has a highly variable course. A relapsing and remitting pattern is typical, with attacks becoming more intermittent after 5 to 7 years. The major morbidity and mortality of the disease appear confined to the years immediately after the initial diagnosis; therefore, early aggressive therapy is recommended for patients with severe clinical manifestations. Mortality is typically low; when noted, it most frequently is secondary to pulmonary hemorrhage, CNS hemorrhage, or bowel perforation. In the absence of CNS disease or significant vascular complications, the prognosis is generally good.

SARCOIDOSIS

Sarcoidosis is a multisystem granulomatous disorder of unknown cause. Jonathan Hutchinson initially described the disease in 1875, but Boeck coined the term *sarcoidosis* (Greek meaning "fleshlike condition") 14 years later. The evidence implicates improper degradation of antigenic material with the formation of noncaseating granulomatous inflammation. The nature of the antigen is unknown, and probably several different antigens may be responsible. Possible involved antigens include infectious agents (e.g., mycobacterium, propionibacteria, Epstein-Barr virus, human herpesvirus 8 [HHV-8]) and a number of environmental factors (e.g., wood dust, pollen, clay, mold, silica). The inappropriate defense response may result from prolonged or heavy antigenic exposure, an immunodysregulation (genetic or secondary to other factors) that prevents an adequate cell-mediated response, a defective regulation of the initial immune reaction, or a combination of all three of these factors. Several investigators have confirmed a genetic predisposition and positive associations with certain HLA types.

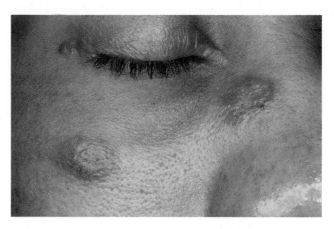

Fig. 9-14 Sarcoidosis. Violaceous indurated plaques of the right malar area and bridge of nose. *(Courtesy of Dr. George Blozis.)*

CLINICAL FEATURES

Sarcoidosis has a worldwide distribution but is recognized more commonly in the developed world. In North America, blacks are affected 10 to 17 times more frequently than whites. There is a slight female predominance, and the disease exhibits a bimodal age distribution, with the first peak between 25 and 35 years of age and the second peak between 45 and 65 years of age.

Sarcoidosis most commonly appears acutely over a period of days to weeks, and the symptoms are variable. Common clinical symptoms include dyspnea, dry cough, chest pain, fever, malaise, fatigue, arthralgia, and weight loss. Less frequently, sarcoidosis arises insidiously over months to years, without significant symptoms; when clinically evident, pulmonary symptoms are most common. Approximately 20% of patients have no symptoms, and the disease is discovered on routine chest radiographs.

Although any organ may be affected, the lungs, lymph nodes, skin, eyes, and salivary glands are the predominant sites. Lymphoid tissue is involved in almost all cases. The mediastinal and paratracheal lymph nodes are involved commonly, and chest radiographs frequently reveal bilateral hilar lymphadenopathy. Approximately 90% of affected patients will reveal an abnormal chest radiograph sometime during the course of the disease. Cutaneous manifestations occur about 25% of the time. These often appear as chronic, violaceous, indurated lesions that are termed **lupus pernio** and frequent the nose, ears, lips, and face (Fig. 9-14). Symmetrical, elevated, indurated, purplish plaques also are seen commonly on the limbs, back, and buttocks. Scattered, nonspecific, tender erythematous nodules, known as **erythema nodosum**, frequently occur on the lower legs.

Ocular involvement is noted in 25% of the cases and most often appears as anterior uveitis. Lesions of the conjunctiva and retina may occur. Involvement of the lacrimal glands often produces keratoconjunctivitis sicca; the salivary glands can be altered similarly, with resultant clinical enlargement and xerostomia. Significant enlargement can occur in any major or minor salivary gland. Removal of intraoral mucoceles that occur in the salivary glands affected by the granulomatous process has led to the initial diagnosis in some cases. The salivary gland enlargement, xerostomia, and keratoconjunctivitis sicca can combine to mimic Sjögren syndrome (see page 466).

Although lymphoid, pulmonary, cutaneous, and ocular lesions are most common, virtually any organ system may be affected. Other potential sites include the endocrine system, gastrointestinal tract, heart, kidneys, liver, nervous system, and spleen. Intraosseous lesions may occur and most commonly involve the phalanges, metacarpals, and metatarsals. Less frequently, the skull, nasal bones, ribs, and vertebrae are affected.

Two distinctive clinical syndromes are associated with acute sarcoidosis. **Löfgren's syndrome** consists of erythema nodosum, bilateral hilar lymphadenopathy, and arthralgia. Patients with **Heerfordt's syndrome (uveoparotid fever)** have parotid enlargement, anterior uveitis of the eye, facial paralysis, and fever.

If salivary gland and lymph node involvement are excluded, clinically evident oral manifestations in sarcoidosis are uncommon. Any oral mucosal site can be affected, most often appearing as a submucosal mass, an isolated papule, an area of granularity, or an ulceration. The mucosal lesions may be normal in color, brown-red, violaceous, or hyperkeratotic (Figs. 9-15 and 9-16). The most frequently affected intraoral soft tissue site is the buccal mucosa, followed by the gingiva, lips, floor of mouth, tongue, and palate. Most cases appearing in the floor of the mouth involve salivary

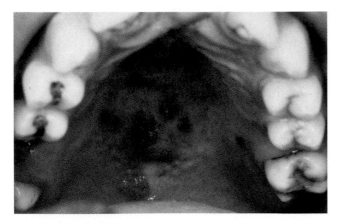

Fig. 9-15   Sarcoidosis. Multiple erythematous macules of the hard palate. *(Courtesy of Dr. George Blozis.)*

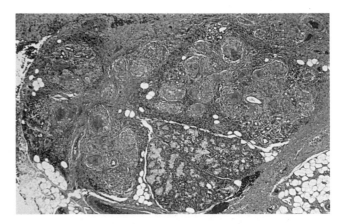

Fig. 9-17   Sarcoidosis. Photomicrograph of a labial minor salivary gland demonstrating granulomatous inflammation characterized by circumscribed collections of histiocytes, lymphocytes, and multinucleated giant cells.

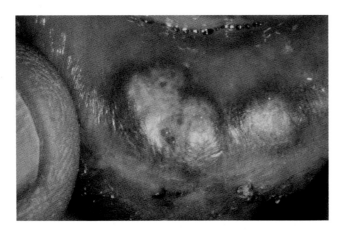

Fig. 9-16   Sarcoidosis. Erythematous macules with central hyperkeratosis of the lower labial mucosa.

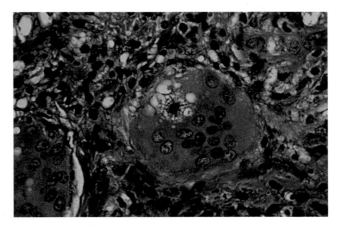

Fig. 9-18   Sarcoidosis. Photomicrograph illustrating multinucleated giant cell with intracytoplasmic asteroid body.

glands and create mucus extravasation. Intraosseous lesions affect either jaw and represent approximately one fourth of all reported intraoral cases. Of these cases, most appeared as ill-defined radiolucencies that occasionally eroded the cortex but never created expansion. In a literature review of 45 reported cases of intraoral sarcoidosis, the oral lesion was the first documented clinical manifestation of the disease in the majority of patients.

HISTOPATHOLOGIC FEATURES

Microscopic examination of sarcoidosis exhibits a classic picture of granulomatous inflammation. Tightly clustered aggregates of epithelioid histiocytes are present, with a surrounding rim of lymphocytes. Intermixed with the histiocytes are scattered Langhans' or foreign body type giant cells (Fig. 9-17). The granulomas often contain laminated basophilic calcifications, known as **Schaumann bodies** (degenerated lyso-

somes), or stellate inclusions, known as **asteroid bodies** (entrapped fragments of collagen) (Fig. 9-18). In lymph nodes, small yellow-brown structures called **Hamazaki-Wesenberg bodies** (large lysosomes) may be noted in the subcapsular sinus. None of these structures are specific for sarcoidosis. Special stains for fungal and bacterial organisms are negative. No polarizable, dissolvable, or pigmented foreign material can be detected.

DIAGNOSIS

The diagnosis is established by the clinical and radiographic presentations, the histopathologic appearance, and the presence of negative findings with both special stains and cultures for organisms. Elevated serum angiotensin-converting enzyme (ACE) levels and appropriate documentation of pulmonary involvement strongly support the diagnosis. Other laboratory abnormalities that may be seen include eosinophilia;

Table **9-2**   **Systemic Evaluation of Patients with Orofacial Granulomatosis**

Systemic Cause	Preliminary Screening Procedure
Chronic granulomatous disease	Neutrophil nitroblue tetrazolium reduction test (perform if medical history of chronic infections is noted)
Crohn's disease	Hematologic evaluation for evidence of gastrointestinal malabsorption (e.g., low albumin, calcium, folate, iron, and red blood cell count; elevated erythrocyte sedimentation rate) or leukocyte scintigraphy using ^{99m}Tc-HMPAO (hexamethylpropylene amine oxime); if initial screen is positive, then recommend esophagogastroduodenoscopy, ileocolonoscopy, and small-bowel radiographs
Sarcoidosis	Serum angiotensin-converting enzyme and chest radiograph (hilar lymphadenopathy)
Tuberculosis	Skin test and chest radiograph (negative acid-fast bacteria [AFB] stain on biopsy specimen does not rule out mycobacterial infection)

leukopenia; anemia; thrombocytopenia; and elevation of the serum alkaline phosphatase level, erythrocyte sedimentation rate, serum calcium concentration, and urinary calcium level.

A skin test for sarcoidosis, the **Kveim test,** can be performed by intradermal injection of a sterilized suspension of human sarcoid tissue. The procedure is no longer widely used because of difficulty in obtaining material for the test, concern related to its accuracy, and the inability to guarantee the absence of contamination (e.g., prions) in this human tissue.

Minor salivary gland biopsy has been promoted as a diagnostic aid in suspected cases of sarcoidosis (see Fig. 9-17). Investigators have documented success rates between 38% and 58%. The misdiagnosis of Sjögren syndrome from minor salivary gland biopsy specimens has been reported in patients with sarcoidosis. Previously, biopsy of the parotid was avoided because of the fear of salivary fistula formation and damage to the facial nerve. These concerns have been reduced through biopsy of the posterior superficial lobe of the parotid gland, and confirmation of sarcoidosis has been reported in 93% of patients from this procedure.

TREATMENT AND PROGNOSIS

In approximately 60% of patients with sarcoidosis, the symptoms resolve spontaneously within 2 years without treatment. Most initial diagnoses are followed by a 3- to 12-month period of observation to define the general course of the disease. Active intervention is recommended for progressive disease and patients with cardiac or neurologic involvement, hypercalcemia, disfiguring skin disease, or serious ocular lesions that do not respond to local therapy. In patients requiring treatment, corticosteroids remain first-line therapy, but resistance and relapses are common. Medications used in patients with refractory disease include methotrexate, azathioprine, chlorambucil, and cyclophospha-

mide. Several studies have shown promising results with TNF-α antagonists such as etanercept, infliximab, pentoxyphylline, and thalidomide. Antimalarial medications, such as chloroquine, have demonstrated effectiveness in resolving mucocutaneous sarcoidosis that was resistant to steroids. In 10% to 20% of those affected by sarcoidosis, resolution does not occur even with treatment. CNS and chronic extrathoracic involvement are associated with a poor response to therapy. Approximately 4% to 10% of patients die of pulmonary, cardiac, or CNS complications.

OROFACIAL GRANULOMATOSIS

Since Wiesenfeld introduced it 1985, **orofacial granulomatosis** has become a well-accepted and unifying term encompassing a variety of clinical presentations that, on biopsy, reveal the presence of nonspecific granulomatous inflammation. The conditions previously designated as Melkersson-Rosenthal syndrome and cheilitis granulomatosa of Miescher are subsets of orofacial granulomatosis, and neither represents a specific disease.

The disorder is somewhat analogous to aphthous stomatitis, in that the cause is idiopathic but appears to represent an abnormal immune reaction. Sometimes oral lesions are seen that are identical to idiopathic orofacial granulomatosis but represent a secondary reaction to one or more of a variety of factors. Table 9-2 delineates systemic diseases that may mimic orofacial granulomatosis, and Table 9-3 lists possible local causes. Although many researchers have presented evidence that the immune response appears secondary to a chronic antigenic stimulus, the pathosis most likely has numerous triggers, resulting in various theories that are correct only in subsets of patients.

The majority of patients are adults; however, the process may occur at any age. When noted in children and adults younger than 30 years old, some investiga-

Table **9-3**   **Interventions to Rule Out Local Causes for Orofacial Granulomatosis**

Local Cause	Intervention
Chronic oral infection	Eliminate all oral foci of infection.
Foreign material	The foreign debris noted in iatrogenic gingivitis is often subtle and difficult to associate definitively with the diffuse inflammatory process. If lesions are nonmigrating and isolated to gingiva, then response to local excision of a single focus should be evaluated.
Allergy	Cosmetics, foods, food additives, flavorings, oral hygiene products (e.g., toothpaste, mouth rinses), and dental restorative metals have been implicated. Patch testing (i.e., contact dermatitis standard series with oral battery) or elimination diet may discover the offending antigen.

tors have found an increased association with an asymptomatic gastrointestinal inflammatory process that is not consistent with Crohn's disease and possibly may be associated with a dietary trigger. A positive response has been seen in patients maintaining a diet free of two common food allergens, cinnamon and benzoate. In another cohort, allergy testing and dietary restriction also proved beneficial.

Because clinical and histopathologic features of orofacial granulomatosis can be produced by a variety of underlying causes, this diagnosis is the beginning, not the end, of the patient's evaluation. After initial diagnosis, the patient should be evaluated for several systemic diseases and local processes (see Tables 9-2 and 9-3) that may be responsible for similar oral lesions. If features diagnostic of one of these more specific disorders are discovered, then the final diagnosis is altered appropriately.

CLINICAL FEATURES

The clinical presentation of orofacial granulomatosis is highly variable. By far, the most frequent site of involvement is the lips. The labial tissues demonstrate a nontender, persistent swelling that may involve one or both lips (Fig. 9-19). On rare occasions, superficial amber vesicles, resembling lymphangiomas, are found. When these signs are combined with facial paralysis and a fissured tongue, the clinical presentation is called **Melkersson-Rosenthal syndrome** (Figs. 9-20 and 9-21). Involvement of the lips alone is called **cheilitis granulomatosa (of Miescher).** Some consider cheilitis granulomatosa an oligosymptomatic form of Melkersson-Rosenthal syndrome, but it appears best to include all of these under the term *orofacial granulomatosis.* In addition to labial edema, swelling of other parts of the face may be seen, and cervical lymphadenopathy rarely has been noted.

Intraoral sites also can be affected, and the predominant lesions are edema, ulcers, and papules. The tongue may develop fissures, edema, paresthesia, erosions, or

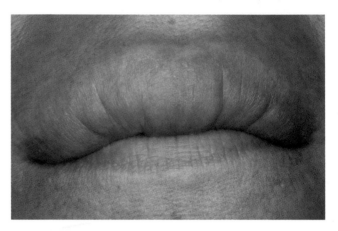

Fig. 9-19   Orofacial granulomatosis (cheilitis granulomatosa). Nontender, persistent enlargement of the upper lip. *(From: Allen CM, Camisa C: Diseases of the mouth and lips. In Sams WM, Lynch P, editors: Principles of dermatology, New York, 1990, Churchill Livingstone.)*

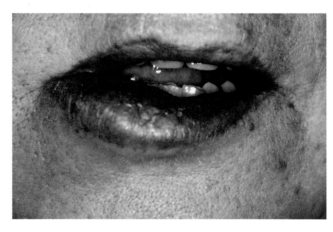

Fig. 9-20   Melkersson-Rosenthal syndrome. Persistent enlargement of the lower lip. *(Courtesy of Dr. Richard Ziegler.)*

taste alteration. The gingiva can develop swelling, erythema, pain, or erosions. The buccal mucosa often exhibits a cobblestone appearance of edematous mucosa or focal areas of submucosal enlargement. Linear hyperplastic folds may occur in the mucobuccal

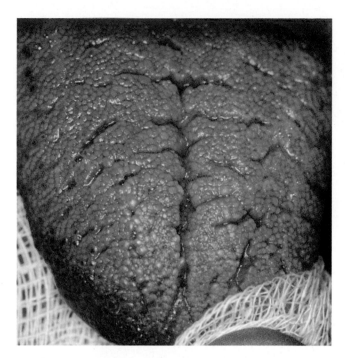

Fig. 9-21   Melkersson-Rosenthal syndrome. Same patient as depicted in Fig. 9-20. Note numerous furrows on the dorsal surface of the tongue. *(Courtesy of Dr. Richard Ziegler.)*

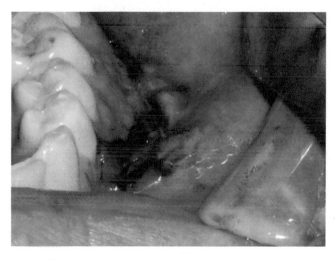

Fig. 9-22   Orofacial granulomatosis. Hemorrhagic and hyperplastic mucosa of the posterior mandibular mucobuccal fold. *(Courtesy of Dr. Russell Spinazze.)*

fold, with linear ulcerations appear in the base of these folds (Fig. 9-22). The palate may have papules or large areas of hyperplastic tissue. Hyposalivation rarely is reported.

HISTOPATHOLOGIC FEATURES

In classic cases of cheilitis granulomatosa, edema is present in the superficial lamina propria with dilation of lymphatic vessels and scattered lymphocytes seen

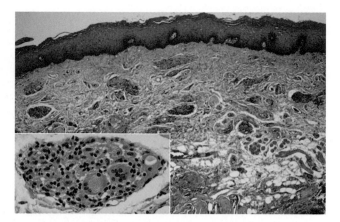

Fig. 9-23   Orofacial granulomatosis. Clusters of granulomatous inflammation around scattered vessels. The inset illustrates the histiocytes and multinucleated giant cells within the granulomas.

diffusely and in clusters. Fibrosis may be present in long-term lesions. Scattered aggregates of noncaseating granulomatous inflammation, consisting of lymphocytes and epithelioid histiocytes, are present, with or without multinucleated giant cells. Typically, the granulomas appear to cluster around scattered vessels and are not as well formed or discrete as those seen in sarcoidosis (Fig. 9-23).

Special stains for fungal organisms and acid-fast bacteria are negative. No dissolvable, pigmented, or polarizable foreign material should be present. When the lesions are confined to the gingiva, a thorough search should be made, because many cases of granulomatous gingivitis are due to subtle collections of foreign material (see page 160).

DIAGNOSIS

The initial diagnosis of orofacial granulomatosis is made on histopathologic demonstration of granulomatous inflammation that is associated with negative special stains for organisms and no foreign material. Based on the clinical and historical findings, one or more conditions may have to be considered in the differential diagnosis. It should be stressed that no one cause for the granulomas will be found when large groups of patients with orofacial granulomatosis are studied. (See Tables 9-2 and 9-3 for a list of conditions and suggested procedures that may be appropriate to arrive at a more definitive diagnosis.)

TREATMENT AND PROGNOSIS

The first goal of management should be discovery of the initiating cause, although this may be difficult because the trigger often is elusive. In children and

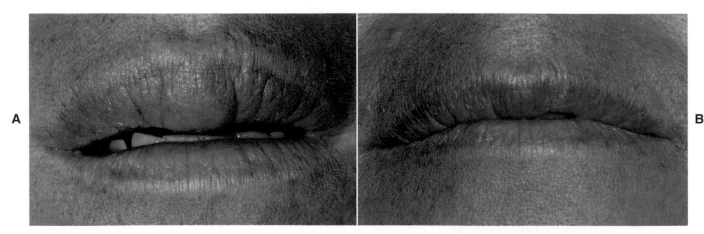

Fig. 9-24   Orofacial granulomatosis. A, Diffuse enlargement of the upper lip. **B,** Same patient after intralesional triamcinolone injections.

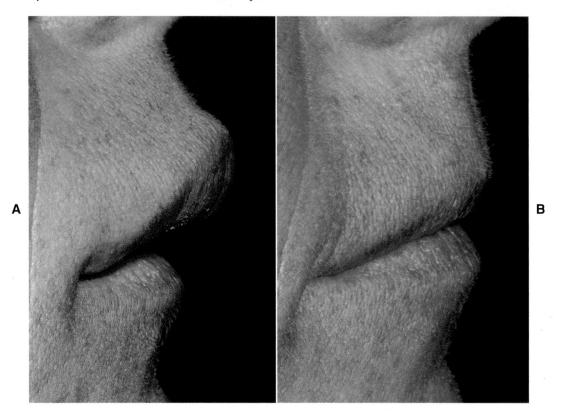

Fig. 9-25   Orofacial granulomatosis. Same patient depicted in Fig. 9-24. **A,** Clinical appearance before local therapy. **B,** Significant resolution after intralesional corticosteroid therapy.

young adults, the search for a dietary allergen or an association with underlying gastrointestinal disease should be considered. Local measures to resolve the clinical manifestations can be attempted but, as would be expected, recurrences are common. The individual lesions have been treated with a variety of interventions, with variable results. Topical or intralesional corticosteroids, radiotherapy, salazosulfapyridine (sulfasalazine), hydroxychloroquine sulfate, azathioprine, cyclosporine A, methotrexate, danazol, dapsone, TNF-

α antagonists (infliximab, thalidomide), clofazimine, metronidazole, and numerous other antibiotics have been tried. Currently, most investigators administer intralesional delayed-release high-concentrate triamcinolone to control the progression of this disease (Figs. 9-24 and 9-25). Of the alternatives, clofazimine (antileprosy agent with antigranulomatous properties) is mentioned most frequently as the second choice after corticosteroids. Because of the natural variability of the disease's progression and the occurrence of spontaneous remissions, therapies are difficult to assess. In the absence of a response to other treatments, surgical recontouring has been used by some but carries a considerable risk of recurrence and rarely appears to be warranted. After excision, some clinicians recommend intralesional steroids to slow recurrences.

The prognosis is highly variable. No therapy has proved to be the "silver bullet" in resolving the individual lesions. In some cases, lesions resolve spontaneously, with or without therapy; in others, they continue to progress in spite of a myriad of therapeutic attempts to stop the progression. The "lucky" subset of patients includes those who have found an initiating causation and have resolved their problems by the exclusion of the offending agent.

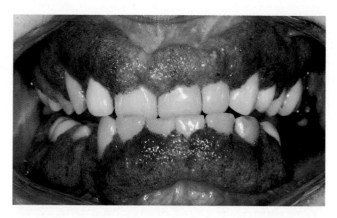

Fig. 9-26   Wegener's granulomatosis. Hemorrhagic and friable gingiva (strawberry gingivitis). *(Courtesy of Dr. Sam McKenna.)*

WEGENER'S GRANULOMATOSIS

Wegener's granulomatosis is a well-recognized, although uncommon, disease process of unknown cause. The initial description of the syndrome by Wegener included necrotizing granulomatous lesions of the respiratory tract, necrotizing glomerulonephritis, and systemic vasculitis of small arteries and veins. Hypotheses about the cause of the disease include an abnormal immune reaction secondary to a nonspecific infection or an aberrant hypersensitivity response to an inhaled antigen. A possible hereditary predisposition has been mentioned in some cases.

Before the current treatment modalities were initiated, the disorder was uniformly fatal. The disease begins as a localized process, which may become more widely disseminated if left untreated. Most patients respond favorably to treatment; consequently, early diagnosis and appropriate therapy are critical.

CLINICAL FEATURES

Wegener's granulomatosis demonstrates a wide age range from childhood to old age, with a mean of approximately 40 years and no sex predilection. The disease can involve almost every organ system in the body. With classic Wegener's granulomatosis, patients initially show involvement of the upper and lower respiratory tract; if the condition remains untreated, then renal involvement often rapidly develops (**generalized Wegener's granulomatosis**).

Limited Wegener's granulomatosis is diagnosed when there is involvement of the respiratory system without rapid development of renal lesions. One subset of patients exhibits lesions primarily of the skin and mucosa, a condition termed **superficial Wegener's granulomatosis**. In this form of the disease, systemic involvement develops slowly. These three different clinical patterns highlight the variability of the clinical aggressiveness that can occur in patients with Wegener's granulomatosis.

Purulent nasal drainage, chronic sinus pain, nasal ulceration, congestion, and fever are frequent findings from upper respiratory tract involvement. Persistent otitis media, sore throat, and epistaxis also are reported. With progression, destruction of the nasal septum can result in a saddle-nose deformity. Patients with lower respiratory tract involvement may be asymptomatic, or they may have dry cough, hemoptysis, dyspnea, or chest pain. Renal involvement usually occurs late in the disease process and is the most frequent cause of death. The glomerulonephritis results in proteinuria and red blood cell casts. Occasionally, the eyes, ears, and skin also are involved.

Oral lesions are seen in the minority of those affected; occasionally, the oral changes may be the only clinically evident finding. The most characteristic oral manifestation is **strawberry gingivitis**. This distinctive but uncommon pattern of gingival alteration appears to be an early manifestation of Wegener's granulomatosis and has been documented before renal involvement in most cases. The affected gingiva demonstrates a florid and granular hyperplasia. The surface forms numerous short bulbous projections, which are hemorrhagic and friable; this red, bumpy surface is responsible for the strawberry-like appearance (Fig. 9-26). The buccal surfaces are affected more frequently, and the alterations are classically confined to the attached gingiva. The process appears to begin in the interdental region and demonstrates lateral spread to adjacent areas. At the time of diagnosis, the involvement may be localized or generalized to multiple quadrants. Destruction of underlying bone with the development of tooth mobility has been reported.

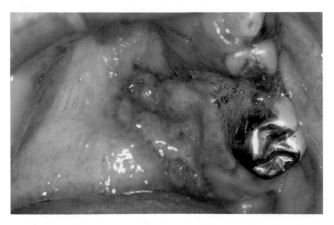

Fig. 9-27   Wegener's granulomatosis. Deep, irregular ulceration of the hard palate on the left side. *(From Allen CM, Camisa C, Salewski C et al: Wegener's granulomatosis: report of three cases with oral lesions, J Oral Maxillofac Surg 49:294-298, 1991.)*

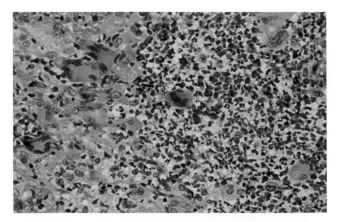

Fig. 9-28   Wegener's granulomatosis. Connective tissue containing proliferation of numerous vascular channels and a heavy inflammatory infiltrate consisting of lymphocytes, neutrophils, eosinophils, and multinucleated giant cells.

Oral ulceration also may be a manifestation of Wegener's granulomatosis. Unlike the strawberry gingiva, the ulcerations do not form a pattern that is unique. These lesions are clinically nonspecific and may occur on any mucosal surface (Fig. 9-27). In contrast to the gingival changes, the oral ulcerations are diagnosed at a later stage of the disease, with more than 60% of the affected patients demonstrating renal involvement. Other less common orofacial manifestations include facial paralysis, labial mucosal nodules, sinusitis-related toothache, arthralgia of the temporomandibular joint (TMJ), jaw claudication, palatal ulceration from nasal extension, oral-antral fistulae, and poorly healing extraction sites.

Enlargement of one or more major salivary glands from primary involvement of the granulomatous process also has been reported. The glandular involvement also appears early in the course of the disease and may lead to early diagnosis and treatment.

HISTOPATHOLOGIC FEATURES

Wegener's granulomatosis appears as a pattern of mixed inflammation centered around blood vessels. Involved vessels demonstrate transmural inflammation, often with areas of heavy neutrophilic infiltration, necrosis, and nuclear dust (leukocytoclastic vasculitis). The connective tissue adjacent to the vessel has an inflammatory cellular infiltrate, which contains a variable mixture of histiocytes, lymphocytes, eosinophils, and multinucleated giant cells (Fig. 9-28). Special stains for organisms are negative, and no foreign material can be found. In oral biopsy specimens, the oral epithelium may demonstrate pseudoepitheliomatous hyperplasia and subepithelial abscesses. Because of the paucity of large vessels in many oral mucosal biopsies,

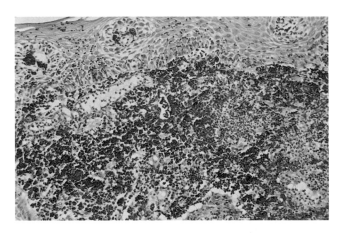

Fig. 9-29   Wegener's granulomatosis. Gingival biopsy specimen showing a mixed inflammatory cellular infiltrate obscured by extensive extravasation of red blood cells.

vasculitis may be difficult to demonstrate, and the histopathologic presentation may be one of ill-defined collections of epithelioid histiocytes intermixed with eosinophils, lymphocytes, and multinucleated giant cells. In addition, the lesions of strawberry gingivitis typically demonstrate prominent vascularity with extensive red blood cell extravasation (Fig. 9-29).

DIAGNOSIS

The diagnosis of Wegener's granulomatosis is made from the combination of the clinical presentation and the microscopic finding of necrotizing and granulomatous vasculitis. Radiographic evaluation of the chest and sinuses is recommended to document possible involvement of these areas. The serum creatinine and urinalysis results are used to rule out significant renal alterations.

A laboratory marker for Wegener's granulomatosis has been identified. Indirect immunofluorescence for serum antibodies directed against cytoplasmic components of neutrophils has been used to support a diagnosis of Wegener's granulomatosis. There are two reaction patterns of these antineutrophil cytoplasm antibodies (ANCA):

1. Perinuclear (p-ANCA)
2. Cytoplasmic (c-ANCA)

Cytoplasmic localization (c-ANCA) is the most useful in the diagnosis of Wegener's granulomatosis. Positive immunofluorescence for c-ANCA should be confirmed with a specific enzyme-linked immunosorbent assay (ELISA) test for antibodies against proteinase 3 (PR3), the major antigen for c-ANCA that resides in the azurophilic granules of neutrophils. These combined tests are associated with a sensitivity of 73% and a diagnostic specificity of 99% for Wegener's granulomatosis. False positives are uncommon and may be associated with a variety of other diseases. In contrast, p-ANCAs are detected in several vasculitides that typically do not present in the oral cavity. With ELISA testing, antibodies directed against myeloperoxidase, a lysosomal enzyme in neutrophils, will be identified.

TREATMENT AND PROGNOSIS

The mean survival of untreated patients with disseminated classic Wegener's granulomatosis is 5 months; 80% of the patients are dead at 1 year and 90% within 2 years. The prognosis is better for the limited and superficial forms of the disease, although a proportion of patients with localized disease eventually will develop classic Wegener's granulomatosis.

The first line of therapy is oral prednisone and cyclophosphamide. On remission, the prednisone is gradually discontinued, with continuation of the cyclophosphamide for at least 1 year. Relapse is not uncommon, especially during tapering of the therapy. Although high response rates are noted, serious side effects related to the therapy are not rare. Trimethoprim-sulfamethoxazole has been used successfully in localized cases and when the immunosuppressive regimen has failed. Low-dose methotrexate and corticosteroids also have been used in patients whose disease is not immediately life threatening or has not responded appropriately to cyclophosphamide. Additional treatment options under study for generalized Wegener's granulomatosis include cyclosporine, tacrolimus, mycophenolate mofetil, plasmapheresis, antilymphocytic monoclonal antibodies, and intravenous pooled immunoglobulin.

Treatment has a profound effect on the progression of the disease. With appropriate therapy, prolonged remission is noted in up to 75% of affected patients; a cure often is attainable when the disease is diagnosed and appropriately treated while the involvement is localized. Because of a relapse rate up to 30%, maintenance therapy is necessary in many patients. The c-ANCA levels can be used to monitor the disease activity. Patients appear less likely to have relapses if their antineutrophilic antibodies disappear during treatment; in contrast, patients whose levels of antibodies persist are at greater risk for relapse.

ALLERGIC MUCOSAL REACTIONS TO SYSTEMIC DRUG ADMINISTRATION

The future of dentistry and medicine will involve a high volume of patients suffering from adverse drug reactions. By 2030, 20% of the population will be more than 65 years old. As the population ages and those affected with chronic diseases increase, patients taking multiple medications most likely will escalate. In the United States during the year 2000, more than 2.8 billion prescriptions were filled, enough to supply each inhabitant with 10 prescriptions annually. Although use of two medications is associated with a 6% risk of an adverse reaction, the frequency rises to 50% with five drugs and almost a 100% when eight or more medications are used simultaneously.

The list of offending medications and their resultant side effects appears almost endless. In a short and highly beneficial article, Matthews listed more than 150 frequently prescribed medications and related them to 46 oral and perioral side effects associated with their use. Despite such excellent articles, it may be helpful for health care practitioners to use one of the excellent drug reference programs available on compact disk or online to create an adverse reaction and drug interaction document for patients in their practice and to update these on a regular basis.

In addition to common drug-related problems such as xerostomia (see page 464), dysgeusia (see page 875), and gingival hyperplasia (see page 163), medications can induce a wide variety of mucosal ulcerations and erosions. An allergic reaction of the oral mucosa to the systemic administration of a medication is called **stomatitis medicamentosa**. Besides **erythema multiforme** (see page 776), several different patterns of oral mucosal disease can be seen:

- Anaphylactic stomatitis
- Intraoral fixed drug eruptions
- Lichenoid drug reactions
- Lupus erythematosus–like eruptions
- Pemphigus-like drug reactions
- Nonspecific vesiculoerosive or aphthouslike lesions

Anaphylactic stomatitis arises after the allergen enters the circulation and binds to IgE–mast cell

Box 9-2

Medications Implicated in Fixed Drug Eruptions

- Analgin
- Barbiturates
- Co-trimoxazole
- Dapsone
- Phenazone derivatives
- Phenolphthalein
- Salicylates
- Sulfonamides
- Tetracycline

Box 9-3

Medications Implicated in Lichenoid Eruptions

- Allopurinol
- Amiphenazole
- Amphotericin
- Arsenicals
- Bismuth
- Captopril
- Carbamazepine
- Chloroquine
- Chlorothiazide
- Chlorpropamide
- Cimetidine
- Cyanamide
- Dapsone
- Fenclofenac
- Furosemide
- Gold salts
- Hydroxychloroquine
- Ketoconazole
- Levamisole
- Lithium
- Lorazepam
- Mercury
- Methyldopa
- Metopromazine
- Oxyprenolol
- Palladium
- Paraaminosalicylic acid
- Penicillamine
- Phenothiazines
- Phenylbutazone
- Practolol
- Propranolol
- Pyrimethamine
- Pyritinol
- Quinacrine
- Quinidine
- Spironolactone
- Streptomycin
- Sulfonylureas
- Tetracycline
- Tolbutamide
- Triprolidine

Box 9-4

Medications Implicated in Lupus Erythematosus-Like Eruptions

- Carbamazepine
- Chlorpromazine
- Etanercept
- Ethosuximide
- Gold
- Griseofulvin
- Hydantoins
- Hydralazine
- Infliximab
- Isoniazid
- Lithium
- Methyldopa
- Penicillamine
- Primidone
- Procainamide
- Quinidine
- Reserpine
- Streptomycin
- Thiouracil
- Trimethadione

Box 9-5

Medications Implicated in Pemphigus-Like Eruptions

- α-Mercaptopropionyl glycine
- Ampicillin
- Captopril
- Cephalexin
- Ethambutol
- Glibenclamide
- Gold
- Heroin
- Ibuprofen
- Penicillamine
- Phenobarbital
- Phenylbutazone
- Piroxicam
- Practolol
- Propranolol
- Pyritinol chlorhydrate
- Rifampin
- Thiopromine

Box 9-6

Drugs Associated with Nonspecific Vesiculoerosive or Aphthouslike Lesions

- Captopril
- Gold salts
- Hydroxyurea
- Indomethacin
- Losartan
- Meprobamate
- Methyldopa
- Naproxen
- Nicorandil
- Penicillamine
- Phenylbutazone
- Propranolol
- Spironolactone
- Thiazide diuretics
- Tolbutamide

complexes. Although systemic anaphylactic shock can result, localized alterations also occur. Fixed drug eruptions are inflammatory alterations of the mucosa or skin that recur at the same site after the administration of any allergen, often a medication.

The vast number of medications capable of producing anaphylactic stomatitis precludes their listing, but common culprits are antibiotics (especially penicillin) and sulfa drugs. Medications reported to be associated with fixed drug eruptions are listed in Box 9-2, lichenoid drug eruptions in Box 9-3, lupus erythematosus-like drug eruptions in Box 9-4, pemphigus-like drug reactions in Box 9-5, and nonspecific vesiculoerosive or aphthouslike eruptions in Box 9-6.

CLINICAL FEATURES

The patterns of mucosal alterations associated with the systemic administration of medications are varied, almost as much as the number of drugs that result in these changes. Anaphylactic stomatitis may occur alone or in conjunction with urticarial skin lesions or other signs and symptoms of anaphylaxis (e.g., hoarseness, respiratory distress, vomiting). The affected mucosa

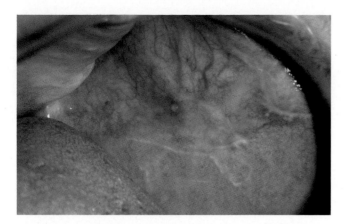

Fig. 9-30 Allergic mucosal reaction to systemic drug administration. Mucosal lesions associated with use of oxybutynin chloride (anticholinergic therapy for urinary incontinence). Note lichen planus-like striae. In addition, multiple superficial mucoceles occurred on the soft palate, floor of the mouth, and bilaterally on the buccal mucosa.

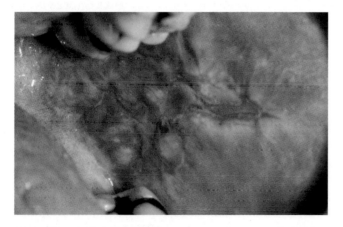

Fig. 9-31 Lichenoid drug reaction to allopurinol. Irregular area of superficial erosion of the left buccal mucosa. Lesions were also present on the contralateral buccal mucosa and bilaterally on the lateral borders of the tongue.

may exhibit multiple zones of erythema or numerous aphthouslike ulcerations. Mucosal fixed drug eruptions appear as localized areas of erythema and edema, which can develop into vesiculoerosive lesions and are located most frequently on the labial mucosa. Lichenoid, lupuslike, and pemphigus-like drug reactions resemble their namesakes clinically, histopathologically, and immunologically (Fig. 9-30). These latter chronic drug reactions may involve any mucosal surface, but the most common sites are the posterior buccal mucosa and the lateral borders of the tongue (Figs. 9-31 and 9-32). Bilateral and symmetrical lesions are fairly common.

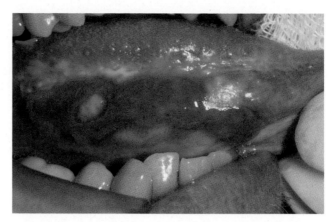

Fig. 9-32 Allergic mucosal reaction to systemic drug administration. Large irregular erosion of the right ventral surface of the tongue. The lesion arose secondary to use of oxaprozin, a nonsteroidal antiinflammatory drug (NSAID).

HISTOPATHOLOGIC FEATURES

Anaphylactic stomatitis typically reveals a nonspecific pattern of subacute mucositis that contains lymphocytes intermixed with eosinophils and neutrophils. Fixed drug eruptions also reveal a mixed inflammatory cellular infiltrate that consists of lymphocytes, eosinophils, and neutrophils, often combined with spongiosis and exocytosis of the epithelium. Vacuolar change of the basal cell layer and individual necrotic epithelial cells are occasionally noted. The drug reactions that simulate lichen planus, lupus erythematosus, and pemphigus resemble their namesakes. The histopathologic and immunologic features of these chronic drug reactions cannot be used reliably to separate them from their associated primary immunologic disease.

Immunofluorescence has been used in an attempt to separate drug reactions from primary vesiculoerosive disease. In most instances, this technique has proven to be unsatisfactory. In spite of these findings, a unique pattern of reaction has been seen when indirect immunofluorescence for IgG has been performed in patients with lichenoid drug reactions. In many of these patients, a distinctive annular fluorescent pattern, termed **string of pearls,** has been noted along the cell membrane of the basal cell layer of stratified squamous epithelium. The detected circulating antibody has been termed **basal cell cytoplasmic antibody.** Although further study is desirable, this technique may prove to be a useful adjunct during evaluation of oral lichenoid lesions.

DIAGNOSIS

A detailed medical history must be obtained, and the patient should be questioned closely concerning the use of both prescription and over-the-counter medications. Once a potentially offending medication is discovered, a temporal relationship between the drug's use and the mucosal alteration must be established. The association may be acute and obvious, or the onset of the oral lesions may be delayed. If more than one medication is suspected, then serial elimination of the medications can be performed in collaboration with the patient's physician until the offending agent is discovered.

In chronic drug reactions, definitive diagnosis can be made if the mucosal alterations resolve after resolution of the medication and recur on reintroduction of the agent. Presumptive diagnosis is usually sufficient and justified when the mucosal alterations clear after cessation of the offending medication.

In possible lupuslike drug reactions, serum evaluation for generic antinuclear antibodies (ANAs) and antibodies against double-stranded DNA and histones often can be beneficial. Lupuslike drug reactions typically are associated with circulating generic ANAs and antibodies against histones, whereas lupus erythematosus also reveals antibodies to double-stranded DNA (a finding not typically noted in drug reactions). This pattern does not hold true in reactions associated with the TNF-α antagonists, infliximab and etanercept, which simulate systemic lupus erythematosus (SLE) very closely and are associated with antibodies to double-stranded DNA.

TREATMENT AND PROGNOSIS

The responsible medication should be discontinued and, if necessary, replaced with another drug that provides a similar therapeutic result. Localized acute reactions can be resolved with topical corticosteroids. When systemic manifestations are present, anaphylactic stomatitis often warrants systemic administration of adrenaline (epinephrine), corticosteroids, or antihistamines. Chronic oral lesions often resolve on cessation of the offending drug, but topical corticosteroids may sometimes be required for complete resolution.

If discontinuation of the medication is contraindicated, palliative care can be provided; however, corticosteroids often are ineffective as long as the offending medication is continued.

ALLERGIC CONTACT STOMATITIS (STOMATITIS VENENATA)

The list of agents reported to cause **allergic contact stomatitis** reactions in the oral cavity is extremely diverse. Numerous foods, food additives, chewing gums, candies, dentifrices, mouthwashes, glove and rubber dam materials, topical anesthetics, restorative

metals, acrylic denture materials, dental impression materials, and denture adhesive preparations have been mentioned. Two types of allergens, cinnamon and dental restorative materials, demonstrate clinical and histopathologic patterns that are sufficiently unique to justify separate descriptions.

Although the oral cavity is exposed to a wide variety of antigens, the frequency of a true allergic reaction to any one antigen from this contact appears to be rare. This was verified in a prospective study of 13,325 dental patients, in which only seven acute and 15 chronic cases of adverse effects were attributed to dental materials. The oral mucosa is much less sensitive than the surface of the skin; this is most likely because of the following:

- The period of contact is often brief.
- The saliva dilutes, digests, and removes many antigens.
- The limited keratinization of oral mucosa makes hapten binding more difficult, and the high vascularity tends to remove any antigen quickly.
- The allergen may not be recognized (because of the lower density of Langerhans cells and T lymphocytes).

If the skin has been sensitized originally, the mucosa may or may not demonstrate future clinical sensitization. In contrast, if the mucosa is sensitized initially, then the skin usually demonstrates similar changes with future exposure. Long-term oral exposure may induce tolerance and reduce the prevalence of cutaneous sensitivity in some instances. For example, exposure to nickel-containing orthodontic hardware has been associated with a reduced prevalence of future cutaneous sensitivity to nickel jewelry.

In addition to oral lesions, allergic contact reactions may produce exfoliative cheilitis (see page 304) or perioral dermatitis (see next section). As mentioned in Chapter 8, most cases of chronic cheilitis represent local irritation, usually from chronic lip licking. In spite of this, investigation has revealed that approximately 25% of affected cases are allergic contact cheilitis from a variety of antigens that include medications, lipsticks, sunscreens, toothpaste, dental floss, nail polishes, and cosmetics.

CLINICAL FEATURES

Allergic contact stomatitis can be acute or chronic. Of those cases diagnosed, there is a distinct female predominance in both forms. After eliminating focal trauma, localized signs and symptoms suggest mucositis from an isolated allergen (e.g., dental metal); in contrast, widespread mouth pain suggests an association with a more diffuse trigger such as food, drink, flavorings, or oral hygiene materials.

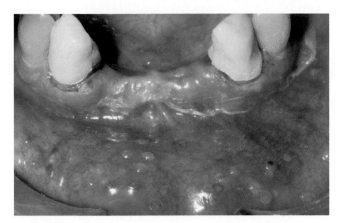

Fig. 9-33   Allergic contact stomatitis to aluminum chloride. Mucosal erythema and vesicles of the lower labial mucosa caused by use of aluminum chloride on gingival retraction cord.

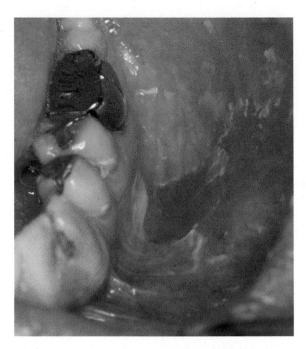

Fig. 9-34   Allergic contact stomatitis to toothpaste. Erythematous mucosa with superficial epithelial desquamation.

In patients with acute contact stomatitis, burning is the most frequent symptom. The appearance of the affected mucosa is variable, from a mild and barely visible redness to a brilliantly erythematous lesion with or without edema. Vesicles are rarely seen and, when present, rapidly rupture to form areas of erosion (Fig. 9-33). Superficial ulcerations that resemble aphthae occasionally arise. Itching, stinging, tingling, and edema may be noted.

In chronic cases the affected mucosa is typically in contact with the causative agent and may be erythematous or white and hyperkeratotic. Periodically, erosions may develop within the affected zones. Some allergens, especially toothpastes, can cause widespread erythema, with desquamation of the superficial layers of the epithelium (Fig. 9-34). Allergic contact cheilitis demonstrates clinical features identical to those cases created through chronic irritation, and it most frequently appears as chronic dryness, scaling, fissuring, or cracking of the vermilion border of the lip. Rarely, symptoms identical to orolingual paresthesia can be present without any clinically evident signs. One distinctive pattern, plasma cell gingivitis, is discussed elsewhere (see page 159).

DIAGNOSIS

Usually, the diagnosis of acute contact stomatitis is straightforward because of the temporal relationship between the use of the agent and the resultant eruption. If an acute oral or circumoral reaction is noted within 30 minutes of a dental visit, then allergy to all used dental materials, local anesthetics, and gloves should be investigated.

The diagnosis of chronic contact stomatitis is much more difficult. Most investigators require good oral health, elimination of all other possible causes, and visible oral signs, together with a positive history of allergy and a positive skin test result to the suspected allergen. If allergic contact stomatitis is strongly suspected but skin test results are negative, then direct testing of the oral mucosa can be attempted. The antigen can be placed on the mucosa in a mixture with Orabase or in a rubber cup that is fixed to the mucosa.

TREATMENT AND PROGNOSIS

In mild cases of acute contact stomatitis, removal of the suspected allergen is all that is required. In more severe cases, antihistamine therapy, which is combined with topical anesthetics (e.g., dyclonine HCl), is usually beneficial. Chronic reactions respond to removal of the antigenic source and application of a topical corticosteroid, such as fluocinonide gel or dexamethasone elixir.

When attempting to discover the source of a diffuse allergic mucositis, use of plain baking soda or toothpaste that is free of flavoring or preservatives is recommended. The patient also should be instructed to avoid mouthwash, gum, mints, chocolate, cinnamon-containing products, carbonated drinks, and excessively salty, spicy, or acidic foods. If an association cannot be found, then cutaneous patch testing may provide helpful information.

PERIORAL DERMATITIS

Perioral dermatitis refers to a unique inflammatory skin disease that involves the circumoral area. Although the exact mechanism is uncertain, many investigators believe the process arises from an idiosyncratic response to a variety of exogenous substances; once this process is initiated, potent topical corticosteroid use worsens the condition. Although the vast majority of affected patients report topical corticosteroid use, only a minority initiate this therapy before initial development of the dermatitis. Exogenous substances reported to initiate the rash include tartar-control toothpaste, bubble gum, moisturizers, night creams, and other cosmetic products (e.g., foundation). Some of these substances may initially induce an irritant or allergic contact dermatitis, whereas others are thought to produce inappropriate occlusion of the skin surface with subsequent proliferation of skin flora.

CLINICAL FEATURES

Perioral dermatitis appears with persistent erythematous papules and papulopustules that involve the skin surrounding the vermilion border of the upper and lower lips (Fig. 9-35). Classically, there is a zone of spared skin immediately adjacent to the vermilion border. Pruritus is variable. In adults, more than 90% of affected patients are women, lending further support to the association with cosmetic use. The prevalence of perioral dermatitis appears to be increasing and may be related to the greater percentage of cosmetic-wearing women in the workforce. In children, the female predominance is dramatically reduced or is nonexistent in some studies. In addition, an identical pattern of periorbital and perinasal dermatitis often

is present in younger patients with classic perioral lesions.

Some investigators have reported perioral dermatitis that has arisen solely from use of tartar-control toothpaste (irritant contact dermatitis from pyrophosphate compounds), but close inspection reveals a different clinical presentation. In these reports the dermatitis appears as a zone of erythema without papules or pustules; it involves only the skin immediately adjacent to the vermilion border, without the classic sparing of this area. This pathosis is classified most appropriately as circumoral dermatitis and does not fulfill the classic criteria for perioral dermatitis.

HISTOPATHOLOGIC FEATURES

Biopsy of perioral dermatitis demonstrates a variable pattern. In many cases there is a chronic lymphohistiocytic dermatitis that often exhibits spongiosis of the hair follicles. In other patients a rosacea-like pattern is noted in which there is perifollicular granulomatous inflammation. On occasion, this histopathologic pattern has been misdiagnosed as sarcoidosis.

TREATMENT AND PROGNOSIS

The first step in management is discontinuation of potent topical corticosteroid use, if present. Often, this is followed by a period of exacerbation, which can be minimized by substitution of a less potent corticosteroid before total cessation. Oral tetracycline has been shown to be effective by many investigators, with erythromycin substituted during childhood and pregnancy. Topical metronidazole or erythromycin also has been used successfully in several studies. The pathosis typically demonstrates significant improvement within several weeks and total resolution in a few months. Recurrence is uncommon.

CONTACT STOMATITIS FROM ARTIFICIAL CINNAMON FLAVORING

Mucosal abnormalities secondary to the use of artificially flavored cinnamon products are fairly common, but the range of changes was not widely recognized until the late 1980s. Cinnamon oil is used as a flavoring agent in confectionery, ice cream, soft drinks, alcoholic beverages, processed meats, gum, candy, toothpaste, breath fresheners, mouthwashes, and even dental floss. Concentrations of the flavoring are up to 100 times that in the natural spice. The reactions are documented most commonly in those products associated with prolonged or frequent contact, such as candy, chewing gum, and toothpaste. The anticalculus components of tartar-control toothpastes have a strong bitter flavor

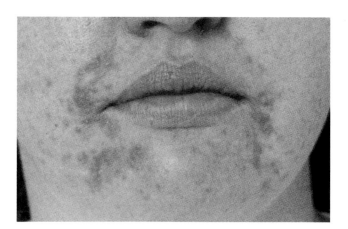

Fig. 9-35   Perioral dermatitis. Multiple erythematous papules of the skin surrounding the vermilion border of the lips. *(Courtesy of Dr. Charles Camisa.)*

and require a significant concentration of flavoring agents including cinnamon to hide the taste, resulting in a greater chance these formulations will cause oral mucosal lesions. Although much less common, reactions to cinnamon in its natural spice form have been documented.

CLINICAL FEATURES

The clinical presentations of contact stomatitis vary somewhat, according to the medium of delivery. Toothpaste results in a more diffuse pattern; the signs associated with chewing gum and candy are more localized. Pain and burning are common symptoms in all cases.

The gingiva is the most frequent site affected by toothpaste, often resembling **plasma cell gingivitis** (see page 159); enlargement, edema, and erythema are common. Sloughing of the superficial oral epithelium without creation of an erosion is seen commonly. Erythematous mucositis, occasionally combined with erosion, has been reported on the buccal mucosa and tongue. Exfoliative cheilitis and circumoral dermatitis also may occur.

Reactions from chewing gum and candy are more localized and typically do not affect the lip vermilion or perioral skin. Most of the lesions appear on the buccal mucosa and lateral borders of the tongue. Buccal mucosal lesions often are oblong patches that are aligned along the occlusal plane (Fig. 9-36). Individual lesions have an erythematous base but often are predominantly white as a result of hyperkeratosis of the surface epithelium. Ulceration within the lesions may occur. Hyperkeratotic examples often exhibit a ragged surface and occasionally may resemble the pattern seen in morsicatio (see page 286). Lingual involvement may become extensive and spread to the dorsal surface

(Fig. 9-37). Significant thickening of the surface epithelium can occur and may raise clinical concern for oral hairy leukoplakia (OHL) (see page 268) or carcinoma (Fig. 9-38).

HISTOPATHOLOGIC FEATURES

Usually, the epithelium in contact stomatitis from artificial cinnamon flavoring is acanthotic, often with elongated rete ridges and thinning of the suprapapillary plates. Hyperkeratosis and extensive neutrophilic exocytosis may be present. The superficial lamina propria demonstrates a heavy inflammatory cell infiltrate that consists predominantly of lymphocytes that may be intermixed with plasma cells, histiocytes, or eosinophils. This infiltrate often obscures the epithelium and connective tissue interface (Fig. 9-39). A characteristic

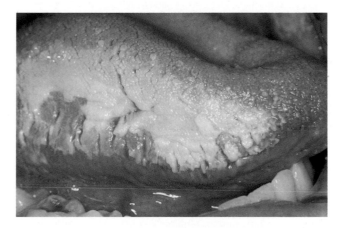

Fig. 9-37 Contact stomatitis from cinnamon flavoring. Sensitive and thickened hyperkeratosis of the lateral and dorsal surface of the tongue on the right side.

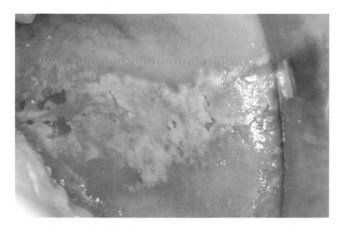

Fig. 9-36 Contact stomatitis from cinnamon flavoring. Oblong area of sensitive erythema with overlying shaggy hyperkeratosis.

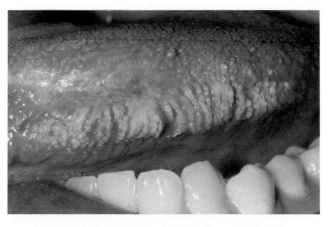

Fig. 9-38 Contact stomatitis from cinnamon flavoring. Left lateral border of the tongue demonstrating linear rows of hyperkeratosis that resemble oral hairy leukoplakia (OHL).

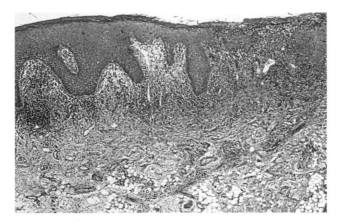

Fig. 9-39 Contact stomatitis from cinnamon flavoring.
Oral mucosa demonstrating significant interface mucositis and deeper perivascular inflammation.

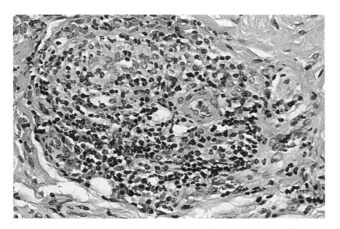

Fig. 9-40 Contact stomatitis from cinnamon flavoring.
Perivascular inflammatory infiltrate consisting predominantly of lymphocytes and plasma cells.

feature in localized cases caused by gum, mints, or candies is the frequent presence of an obvious perivascular inflammatory infiltrate that extends well below the interface zone (Fig. 9-40).

DIAGNOSIS

With a high index of suspicion and knowledge of the variations of the clinical pattern, the diagnosis of localized contact stomatitis often can be made from the clinical appearance and the history of cinnamon use. Often biopsies are performed for atypical or extensive cases because of the differential diagnosis, which includes several significant vesiculoerosive and neoplastic conditions. The histopathologic features are not specific, but they are sufficient to raise a high index of suspicion in an oral and maxillofacial pathologist who is familiar with the pattern. Use of cinnamon-containing toothpaste should be investigated in every

patient with an atypical pattern of gingivitis. Diet-related examples often are the most difficult to diagnose and may necessitate cutaneous allergy patch testing or a diet diary to isolate the cause.

TREATMENT AND PROGNOSIS

Typically, the signs and symptoms disappear within 1 week after the discontinuation of the cinnamon product. If the patient resumes intake of the product, then the lesions reappear, usually within 24 hours. On occasion, resolution is more gradual and the patient may benefit from short-term use of a topical corticosteroid.

LICHENOID CONTACT STOMATITIS FROM DENTAL RESTORATIVE MATERIALS

Since the nineteenth century when dental amalgam began to have widespread use, the material has been associated in the lay press with almost every medical ailment known to man. Such accusations tend to occur in cycles. Mercury within amalgam has been accused of producing Alzheimer's disease, neurotoxicity, kidney dysfunction, reduced immunocompetence, alterations of oral and intestinal bacteria, birth defects, and adverse effects on general health. In spite of intense scrutiny, there appears to be no relationship between any of these physical disorders and the use of amalgam restorations (see the discussion of systemic intoxification from mercury, page 313). An investigation of patients with concerns associated with their amalgam restorations reveals that most of their complaints can be associated with oral, dental, or medical problems unrelated to the restorations.

A review of the ill effects of mercury in dental amalgam demonstrates that the occurrence of toxicity is negligible, but a small percentage (1% to 2%) of those who are allergic to mercury can react to the mercury released from dental amalgams. The frequency of adverse effects to dental amalgam is estimated to be one case per million. Acute hypersensitivity reactions typically appear 2 to 24 hours after the removal and replacement of dental amalgam, and the symptoms disappear after 10 to 14 days.

In contrast, chronic reactions are not rare and may arise from hypersensitivity or a chronic toxic reaction from almost any dental metal. When the reaction is related to hypersensitivity, the most frequent antigen is mercury or a mercury compound; gold is a distant second. Even less commonly, copper, palladium, silver, tin, zinc, beryllium, chromium, cobalt, or platinum is responsible. Some investigators have called these alterations "galvanic lesions," but neither clinical nor experi-

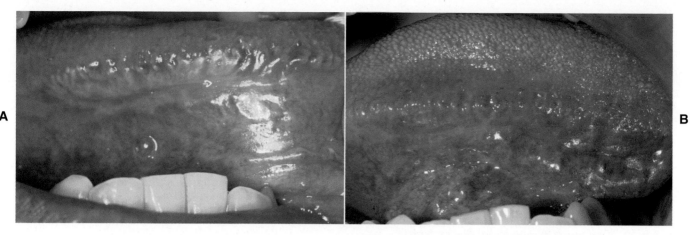

Fig. 9-41   Oral mucosal contact reaction to dental amalgam. A, Hyperkeratotic lesion with a peripheral radiating pattern on the lateral border of the tongue on the right side; the altered mucosa contacted the amalgams of the adjacent mandibular molar teeth. The lesion remained in the same location for 5 years and periodically became erosive and symptomatic. Smoothing and polishing of the adjacent restorations had no effect. **B,** Appearance of previously altered area of the tongue 14 days after removal of adjacent amalgams. Note total resolution of the mucosal alterations.

mental studies support the electrogalvanic hypothesis of origin.

Hypersensitivity to dental resins is quite rare, and many cases have been proven to be secondary to excess monomer in cold-cure denture resin, not a true allergy. Reports have documented resin-induced contact stomatitis that resolved after boiling of the denture (which removed the residual free monomer). Free monomer is unusual in heat-cured denture resin and composite restorations, making true contact hypersensitivity very rare.

Contact stomatitis appears clinically and histopathologically similar to lichen planus (see page 782) but demonstrates a difference in evolution. When patients with true oral lichen planus are examined, the lesions migrate and exhibit no direct correlation to contact with dental materials. In addition, these patients do not demonstrate a significantly increased positive patch testing to dental restorative materials and exhibit minimal-to-no clinical improvement on removal of their amalgams.

However, there is a subgroup of patients whose lichenoid lesions do not migrate and usually involve only the mucosa adjacent to a dental metal. On patch testing, the vast majority of these patients react to the offending metal, and the lesions resolve rapidly after removal of adjacent amalgams. This pathosis should be diagnosed as **lichenoid contact stomatitis** to a dental restorative material, not as true lichen planus.

The results of cutaneous patch testing cannot be applied uniformly to the oral cavity. For a metal to become allergenic, it must undergo corrosion and release of metallic ions. Amalgams that have been in place for many years typically are responsible for the vast majority of lichenoid contact stomatitis lesions. Positive cutaneous patch testing to gold and nickel is common and greatly outnumbers reactivity to mercury compounds. In spite of this, intraoral reactions to gold and nickel are very uncommon, most likely the result of the low level of corrosion in these metals. Patients with lichenoid contact stomatitis to a single amalgam support this concept, although their mucosa contacts numerous other similar restorations. When such a patient also demonstrates positive patch testing, the anomaly most likely is due to variable corrosion of the restorations. On occasion, patients can demonstrate a contact reaction but reveal negative patch testing. In these cases, the mucosal alterations most likely are due to local irritation of the old restoration (Koebner phenomenon), and studies of these patients have shown a lower long-term response to replacement of the metallic restorations.

CLINICAL FEATURES

The most commonly affected sites for lichenoid contact stomatitis are the posterior buccal mucosa and the ventral surface of the lateral borders of the tongue. Gingival cuffs adjacent to subgingival metallic restorations and porcelain-fused-to-metal (PFM) crowns with metal collars also may be affected. The lesions usually are confined to the area of contact but may extend up to 1 cm beyond the point of mucosal association. The affected mucosa may be white or erythematous, with or without peripheral striae (Fig. 9-41). Most patients have no symptoms, but periodic erosion may be noted.

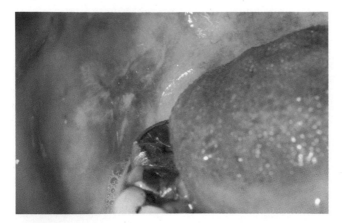

Fig. 9-42   Oral mucosal contact reaction to dental amalgam. Radiating pattern of hyperkeratotic striae on the posterior buccal mucosa that contacts a large distobuccal amalgam of the permanent mandibular second molar.

In all likelihood, many of the lesions previously reported as the so-called plaque type of lichen planus were, in reality, lichenoid contact stomatitis.

DIAGNOSIS

The diagnosis is made from the clinical appearance of the lesions, the lack of migration, and the correlation to adjacent dental metal (Fig. 9-42). Although the histopathologic features may be indistinguishable from lichen planus, biopsy occasionally is performed to confirm the clinical impression and to rule out other pathoses such as epithelial dysplasia. Although patch testing is not necessary for a strong presumptive diagnosis, the procedure does help identify patients who are predisposed to react to the metal (possibly advantageous in a patient with a single site of lichenoid stomatitis who also has numerous similar, but less corroded, restorations demonstrating mucosal contact). In addition, the patch testing will include a battery of additional dental metals that will assist in the choice of material for future restorations.

HISTOPATHOLOGIC FEATURES

Biopsy of allergic contact stomatitis from dental materials exhibits numerous features of lichen planus. The surface epithelium may be hyperkeratotic, atrophic, or ulcerated. Areas of hydropic degeneration of the basal cell layer often are present. The superficial lamina propria contains a dense bandlike chronic inflammatory cellular infiltrate consisting predominantly of lymphocytes, but there may be scattered plasma cells. On occasion, deeper lymphoid aggregates may be noted, often in a perivascular orientation.

TREATMENT AND PROGNOSIS

Local measures, such as improved oral hygiene, smoothing, polishing, and recontouring, should be attempted before more aggressive measures, because clinically similar lesions have been noted as a result of surface plaque accumulation. If this is unsuccessful, then the amalgam in question should be replaced with a nonmetallic restoration, if possible. Other material choices include yellow gold, white gold, and PFM crowns. As mentioned, cutaneous patch testing not only confirms the diagnosis but also can be used as a guide during the selection of future restorative materials.

ANGIOEDEMA (ANGIONEUROTIC EDEMA; QUINCKE'S DISEASE)

Angioedema is a diffuse edematous swelling of the soft tissues that most commonly involves the subcutaneous and submucosal connective tissues but may affect the gastrointestinal or respiratory tract, occasionally with fatal results. The disorder has been referred to as **Quincke's disease,** after the clinician who initially related the changes to an alteration in vascular permeability. The outdated term **angioneurotic edema** also has been used, because affected patients often complained of a choking sensation and were labeled neurotic.

The most common cause is mast cell degranulation, which leads to histamine release and the typical clinical alterations. IgE-mediated hypersensitivity reactions caused by drugs, foods, plants, dust, and inhalants produce mast cell degranulation and are fairly common. Contact allergic reactions to foods, cosmetics, topical medications, and even dental rubber dams also have been responsible. Mast cell degranulation can even result from physical stimuli, such as heat, cold, exercise, emotional stress, solar exposure, and significant vibration.

An unusual pattern of drug reaction that can produce severe forms of angioedema that are not mediated by IgE is the type associated with use of drugs called *angiotensin-converting enzyme (ACE) inhibitors.* These medications are a popular treatment of essential hypertension and chronic heart failure; commonly prescribed ACE inhibitors include captopril, enalapril, and lisinopril. The swelling associated with these drugs does not respond well to antihistamines and was thought to be the result of excess bradykinin (ACE degrades bradykinin). In an attempt to avoid this angioedema, a second generation of medications called *angiotensin II receptor blockers* (e.g., losartan, valsartan) was developed specifically to avoid any inhibition of bradykinin degradation. These newer medications lower the frequency of angioedema, but do not eliminate the adverse reaction.

The prevalence of this pattern of angioedema is estimated to be 0.1% to 0.2% of those who use ACE inhibitors. In the majority of affected patients, the angioedema arises within hours of initial use of the drug. In up to 30% of the cases, the angioedema is delayed, with the longest reported interval between drug use initiation and the initial attack being 7 years. Attacks precipitated by dental procedures have been reported in long-term users of ACE inhibitors. Many clinicians overlook the association between angioedema and ACE inhibitors, with studies demonstrating continued administration of the medication in more than 50% of affected patients.

Angioedema also can result from activation of the complement pathway. This may be hereditary or acquired. Two rare autosomal dominant hereditary forms are seen. Type I, comprising 85% of the hereditary cases, is caused by a quantitative reduction in the inhibitor that prevents the transformation of C1 to C1 esterase. Without adequate levels of C1 esterase inhibitor (C1-INH), C1 esterase cleaves C4 and C2 and results in angioedema. Type II exhibits normal levels of C1-INH, but the inhibitor is dysfunctional.

The acquired type of C1-INH deficiency is seen in association with certain types of lymphoproliferative diseases or in patients who develop specific autoantibodies. In lymphoproliferative diseases, monoclonal antibodies directed against the tumor cells activate C1 and lead to consumption of C1-INH. In the autoimmune variant, the antibody attaches to the C1 receptor on the C1-INH molecule, leading to decreased functional C1-INH and consumption of C1. In both the acquired and the hereditary forms of abnormal C1-INH activity, minor trauma, such as a dental procedure, can precipitate an attack.

Finally, angioedema has been seen in the presence of high levels of antigen-antibody complexes (e.g., lupus erythematosus, viral or bacterial infections) and in patients with grossly elevated peripheral blood eosinophil counts.

CLINICAL FEATURES

Angioedema is characterized by the relatively rapid onset of soft, nontender tissue swelling, which may be solitary or multiple (Fig. 9-43). In the hereditary forms, the initial onset typically is noted in childhood or adolescence. The episodes are unpredictable and intermixed with edema-free intervals. Recurrent skin swelling and abdominal pain are the most frequent presentations. The extremities are the most common cutaneous sites of involvement, although the face, genitals, trunk, and neck also can be affected. Although not individually frequent, edema of the larynx, pharynx, uvula, or soft palate may be noted when patients are

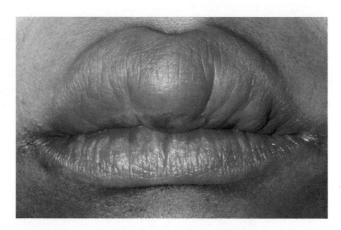

Fig. 9-43   Angioedema. Diffuse upper lip swelling that arose rapidly.

monitored for extended periods (and may be associated with respiratory distress). A deeper voice, hoarseness, aphonia, and dyspnea are important warning signs. Recurrent snoring-induced edema of the soft palate has been reported and associated with severe dyspnea. Isolated tongue involvement is uncommon. Involvement of the skin and mucous membranes can cause enlargements that may measure up to several centimeters in diameter (Fig. 9-44). Although pain is unusual, itching is common and erythema may be present. The enlargement typically resolves over 24 to 72 hours. In contrast to the hereditary variants, allergic, acquired, and ACE inhibitor–associated angioedema demonstrate significant involvement of the head and neck, such as the face, lips, tongue, floor of mouth, pharynx, and larynx. The risk of angioedema associated with ACE inhibitors is significantly greater in blacks (three to four times that of other races), and this pattern is the type most frequently encountered by oral health practitioners.

DIAGNOSIS

In cases of allergic causation, the diagnosis of angioedema often is made from the clinical presentation in conjunction with the known antigenic stimulus. When multiple antigenic exposures occur, the diagnosis of the offending agent can be difficult and involves dietary diaries and antigenic testing.

Those patients whose conditions cannot be related to antigenic exposure or medications should be evaluated for the presence of adequate functional C1-INH. In the hereditary types, both forms exhibit normal levels of C1 and decreased levels of *functional* C1-INH. Type I demonstrates a decreased quantity of C1-INH; type II exhibits normal levels of the inhibitor (but it is not functional). Both acquired forms demonstrate low levels of both C1-INH and C1.

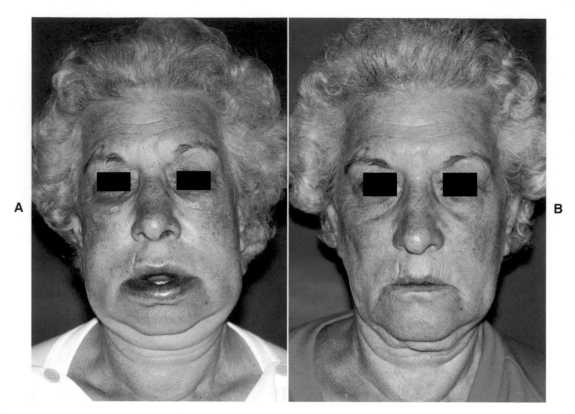

Fig. 9-44   Angioedema. A, Soft, nontender tissue swelling of the face arose relatively rapidly after dental treatment. **B,** Facial appearance after resolution of edematous facial enlargement.

TREATMENT AND PROGNOSIS

The treatment of allergic angioedema usually consists of oral antihistamine therapy. If the attack is not controlled or if laryngeal involvement is present, then intramuscular epinephrine should be administered. If the epinephrine does not stop the attack, then intravenous corticosteroids and antihistamines should be given.

Cases of angioedema related to ACE inhibitors are not IgE-mediated and often do not respond to antihistamines and corticosteroids. Because the airway may have to be opened, affected patients are kept under close observation until the swelling begins to subside. Although the mechanism is unclear, some patients with ACE inhibitor–associated angioedema have responded to C1-INH concentrate. Patients experiencing ACE inhibitor–associated angioedema should avoid all medications in this class of drugs, and their physicians should consider alternative hypertension management strategies. Angiotensin II receptor blockers do not appear to be safe alternatives.

Those cases related to C1-INH deficiency also do not respond to antihistamine, corticosteroid, or adrenergic therapy. Intubation and tracheostomy may be required for laryngeal involvement. Fresh freeze-dried plasma has been used; however, some investigators do not recommend its use because there is a risk of transmitting infection, and it replaces not only C1-INH but also potentially harmful C1 esterase, C1, C2, and C4. C1-INH concentrate and esterase-inhibiting drugs (aprotinin or tranexamic acid) are the treatments of choice for acute attacks. Because acute attacks of hereditary angioedema are not only unpleasant but also potentially life threatening, prevention is paramount. Patients should avoid violent physical activity and trauma. Medical prophylaxis is recommended before any dental or surgical procedure. All patients should carry medical warning cards that state the diagnosis and list elementary precautions. Prophylaxis for C1-INH deficiency is recommended in patients who have more than three attacks per year. Androgens induce hepatic synthesis of C1-INH, and either of the attenuated androgens (danazol or stanozolol) is used for both the hereditary forms and the acquired type that is related to lymphoproliferative disorders. The autoimmune acquired type is best prevented through the use of corticosteroids.

BIBLIOGRAPHY

Transient Lingual Papillitis

Brannon RB, Flaitz CM: Transient lingual papillitis: a papulo-keratotic variant, *Oral Surg Oral Med Oral Pathol Oral Radiol Endod* 96:187-191, 2003.

Flaitz CM, Chavarria C: Painful tongue lesions associated with a food allergy, *Pediatr Dent* 23:506-507, 2001.

Lacour J-P, Perrin C: Eruptive familial lingual papillitis: a new entity, *Pediatr Dermatol* 14:13-16, 1997.

Roux O, Lacour JP: Eruptive lingual papillitis with household transmission: a prospective clinical study, *Br J Dermatol* 150:299-303, 2004.

Whitaker SB, Krupa JJ, Singh BB: Transient lingual papillitis, *Oral Surg Oral Med Oral Pathol Oral Radiol Endod* 82:441-445, 1996.

Recurrent Aphthous Stomatitis

Brooke RI, Sapp JP: Herpetiform ulceration, *Oral Surg Oral Med Oral Pathol* 12:182-188, 1976.

Eisen D, Lynch DP: Selecting topical and systemic agents for recurrent aphthous stomatitis, *Cutis* 68:201-206, 2001.

Hay KD, Reade PC: The use of an elimination diet in the treatment of recurrent aphthous ulceration of the oral cavity, *Oral Surg Oral Med Oral Pathol* 57:504-507, 1984.

Jurge S, Kuffer R, Scully C et al: Mucosal disease series. Number IV. Recurrent aphthous stomatitis, *Oral Dis* 12:1-21, 2006.

Natah SS, Konttinen YT, Enattah NS et al: Recurrent aphthous ulcers today: a review of the growing knowledge, *Int J Oral Maxillofac Surg* 33:221-234, 2004.

Nolan A, Lamey P-J, Milligan KA et al: Recurrent aphthous ulceration and food sensitivity, *J Oral Pathol Med* 20:473-475, 1991.

Pedersen A, Hougen HP, Kenrad B: T-lymphocyte subsets in oral mucosa of patients with recurrent aphthous ulceration, *J Oral Pathol Med* 21:176-180, 1992.

Rivera-Hidalgo F, Shulman JD, Beach MM: The association of tobacco and other factors with recurrent aphthous in a U.S. adult population, *Oral Dis* 10:335-345, 2004.

Rogers RS: Complex aphthosis, *Adv Exp Med Biol* 528:311-316, 2003.

Scully C, Gorsky M, Lozada-Nur F: The diagnosis and management of recurrent aphthous stomatitis, *J Am Dent Assoc* 134:200-207, 2003.

Ship JA: Recurrent aphthous stomatitis: an update, *Oral Surg Oral Med Oral Pathol Oral Radiol Endod* 81:141-147, 1996.

Vincent SD, Lilly GE: Clinical, historic, and therapeutic features of aphthous stomatitis: literature review and open clinical trial employing steroids, *Oral Surg Oral Med Oral Pathol* 74:79-86, 1992.

Wray D, Graykowski EA, Notkins AL: Role of mucosal injury in initiating recurrent aphthous stomatitis, *Br Med J* 283:1569-1570, 1981.

Behçet's Syndrome

Escudier M, Bagan J, Scully C: Mucosal disease series. Number VII. Behçet's disease (Adamantiades syndrome), *Oral Dis* 12:78-84, 2006.

Evereklioglu C: Managing the symptoms of Behçet's disease, *Expert Opin Pharmacother* 5:317-328, 2004.

Helm TN, Camisa C, Allen C et al: Clinical features of Behçet's disease: report of four cases, *Oral Surg Oral Med Oral Pathol* 72:30-34, 1991.

International Study Group for Behçet's Disease: Criteria for diagnosis for Behçet's disease, *Lancet* 335:1078-1080, 1990.

Krause I, Rosen Y, Kaplan I et al: Recurrent aphthous stomatitis in Behçet's disease: clinical features and correlation with systemic disease expression and severity, *J Oral Pathol Med* 28:193-196, 1999.

McCarty MA, Garton RA, Jorizzo JL: Complex aphthosis and Behçet's disease, *Dermatol Clin* 21:41-48, 2003.

Sarcoidosis

Batal H, Chou LL, Cottrell DA: Sarcoidosis: medical and dental implications, *Oral Surg Oral Med Oral Pathol Oral Radiol Endod* 88:386-390, 1999.

Marx RE, Hartman KS, Rethman KV: A prospective study comparing incisional labial to incisional parotid biopsies in the detection and confirmation of sarcoidosis, Sjögren's disease, sialosis and lymphoma, *J Rheumatol* 15:621-629, 1988.

Saboor SA, Johnson NM: Sarcoidosis, *Br J Hosp Med* 48:293-302, 1992.

Suresh L, Aguirre A, Buhite RJ et al: Intraosseous sarcoidosis of the jaws mimicking aggressive periodontitis: a case report and literature review, *J Periodontol* 75:478-182, 2004.

Suresh L, Radfar L: Oral sarcoidosis: a review of the literature, *Oral Dis* 11:138-145, 2005.

Tozman ECS: Sarcoidosis: clinical manifestations, epidemiology, therapy, and pathophysiology, *Curr Opin Rheumatol* 3:155-159, 1991.

Orofacial Granulomatosis

Allen CM, Camisa C, Hamzeh S et al: Cheilitis granulomatosa: report of six cases and review of the literature, *J Am Acad Dermatol* 23:444-450, 1990.

Gibson J, Neilly JB, Wray APM et al: ^{99}Tc^m-HMPAO leucocyte labelling in orofacial granulomatosis and gastrointestinal Crohn's disease in childhood and early adulthood, *Nucl Med Commun* 21:155-158, 2000.

Kauzman A, Quesnel-Mercier A, Lalonde B: Orofacial granulomatosis: 2 case reports and literature review, *J Can Dent Assoc* 72:325-329, 2006.

Leão JC, Hodgson T, Scully C et al: Review article: orofacial granulomatosis, *Aliment Pharmacol Ther* 20:1019-1027, 2004.

Mignogna MD, Fedele S, LoRusso L et al: Effectiveness of small-volume, intralesional, delayed-release triamcinolone injections in orofacial granulomatosis: a pilot study, *J Am Acad Dermatol* 51:265-268, 2004.

Patton DW, Ferguson MM, Forsyth A et al: Oro-facial granulomatosis: a possible allergic basis, *Br J Oral Maxillofac Surg* 23:235-242, 1985.

Rees TD: Orofacial granulomatosis and related conditions, *Periodontol 2000* 21:145-157, 1999.

Sanderson J, Numes C, Escudier M et al: Oro-facial granulomatosis: Crohn's disease or a new inflammatory bowel disease, *Inflamm Bowel Dis* 11:840-846, 2005.

van der Waal RIF, Schulten EAJM, van der Meij EH et al: Cheilitis granulomatosa: overview of 13 patients with long-term follow-up—results of management, *Int J Dermatol* 41:225-229, 2002.

White A, Nunes C, Escudier M et al: Improvement of orofacial granulomatosis on a cinnamon- and benzoate-free diet, *Inflamm Bowel Dis* 12:508-514, 2006.

Wiesenfeld D, Ferguson MM, Mitchell DN et al: Oro-facial granulomatosis—a clinical and pathological analysis, *Q J Med* 54:101-113, 1985.

Worsaae N, Christensen KC, Schiødt M et al: Melkersson-Rosenthal and cheilitis granulomatosa: a clinicopathologic study of thirty-three patients with special reference to their oral lesions, *Oral Surg Oral Med Oral Pathol* 54:404-413, 1982.

Wray D, Rees SR, Gibson J et al: The role of allergy in oral mucosal diseases, Q J Med 93:507-511, 2000.

Wysocki GP, Brooke RI: Oral manifestations of chronic granulomatous disease, Oral Surg Oral Med Oral Pathol 46:815-819, 1978.

Zimmer WM, Rogers RS, Reeve CM et al: Orofacial manifestations of Melkersson-Rosenthal syndrome: a study of 42 patients and review of 220 cases from the literature, Oral Surg Oral Med Oral Pathol 74:610-619, 1992.

Wegener's Granulomatosis

Ah-See KW, McLaren K, Maran AGD et al: Wegener's granulomatosis presenting as major salivary gland enlargement, J Laryngol Otol 110:691-693, 1996.

Allen CM, Camisa C, Salewski C et al: Wegener's granulomatosis: report of three cases with oral lesions, J Oral Maxillofac Surg 49:294-298, 1991.

Chegar BE, Kelley RT: Wegener's granulomatosis presenting as unilateral parotid enlargement, Laryngoscope 114:1730-1733, 2004.

Eufinger H, Machtens E, Akuamoa-Boateng E: Oral manifestations of Wegener's granulomatosis: review of the literature and report of a case, Int J Oral Maxillofac Surg 21:50-53, 1992.

Fauci AS, Haynes BF, Katz P et al: Wegener's granulomatosis: prospective clinical and therapeutic experience with 85 patients for 21 years, Ann Intern Med 98:76-85, 1983.

Handlers JP, Waterman J, Abrams AM et al: Oral features of Wegener's granulomatosis, Arch Otolaryngol 111:267-270, 1985.

Knight JM, Hayduk MJ, Summerlin D-J et al: "Strawberry" gingival hyperplasia. A pathognomonic mucocutaneous finding in Wegener's granulomatosis, Arch Dermatol 136:171-173, 2000.

Magliulo G, Varacalli S, Sepe C: Wegener's granulomatosis presenting as facial palsy, Am J Otolaryngol 20:43-45, 1999.

Patten SF, Tomecki JT: Wegener's granulomatosis: cutaneous and oral mucosal disease, J Am Acad Dermatol 28:710-718, 1993.

Ponniah I, Shaheen A, Shankar KA et al: Wegener's granulomatosis: the current understanding, Oral Surg Oral Med Oral Pathol Oral Radiol Endod 100:265-270, 2005.

Allergic Mucosal Reactions to Systemic Drug Administration

Eversole LR: Allergic stomatitides, J Oral Med 34:93-102, 1979.

Felder RS, Millar SB, Henry RH: Oral manifestations of drug therapy, Spec Care Dent 8:119-124, 1988.

Jacobsen PL, Chávez EM: Clinical management of the dental patient taking multiple drugs, J Contemp Dent Pract 6:144-151, 2005.

Jain VK, Dixit VB, Archana: Fixed drug eruption of the oral mucous membrane, Ann Dent 50:9-11, 1991.

Kane M, Zacharczenko N: Oral side effects of drugs, N Y State Dent J 59:37-40, 1993.

Lamey P-J, McCartan BE, MacDonald DG et al: Basal cell cytoplasmic autoantibodies in oral lichenoid reactions, Oral Surg Oral Med Oral Pathol Oral Radiol Endod 79:44-49, 1995.

Matthews TG: Medication side effects of dental interest, J Prosthet Dent 64:219-226, 1990.

McCartan BE, McCreary CE: Oral lichenoid drug eruptions, Oral Dis 3:58-63, 1997.

Parks ET: Disorders affecting the oral cavity. Lesions associated with drug reactions, Dermatol Clin 14:327-337, 1996.

Scully C, Azul AM, Crighton A et al: Nicorandil can induce severe oral ulceration, Oral Surg Oral Med Oral Pathol Oral Radiol Endod 91:189-193, 2001.

Wright JM: Oral manifestations of drug reactions, Dent Clin North Am 28:529-543, 1984.

Allergic Contact Stomatitis

De Rossi SS, Greenberg MS: Intraoral contact allergy: a literature review and case reports, J Am Dent Assoc 129:1435-1441, 1998.

Eversole LR: Allergic stomatitides, J Oral Med 34:93-102, 1979.

Fisher AA: Contact stomatitis, glossitis, and cheilitis, Otolaryngol Clin North Am 7:827-843, 1974.

Fisher AA: Reactions of the mucous membrane to contactants, Clin Dermatol 5:123-136, 1987.

Kallus T, Mjör IA: Incidence of adverse effects of dental materials, Scand J Dent Res 99:236-240, 1991.

LeSueur BW, Yiannias JA: Contact stomatitis, Dermatol Clin 21:105-114, 2003.

Ophaswongse S, Maibach HI: Allergic contact cheilitis, Contact Dermatitis 33:365-370, 1995.

Shah M, Lewis FM, Gawkrodger DJ: Contact allergy in patients with oral symptoms: a study of 47 patients, Am J Contact Dermat 7:146-151, 1996.

Stenman E, Bergman M: Hypersensitivity reactions to dental materials in a referred group of patients, Scand J Dent Res 97:76-83, 1989.

Tosti A, Piraccini BM, Peluso AM: Contact and irritant stomatitis, Semin Cutan Med Surg 16:314-319, 1997.

van Loon LAJ, Bos JD, Davidson CL: Clinical evaluation of fifty-six patients referred with symptoms tentatively related to allergic contact stomatitis, Oral Surg Oral Med Oral Pathol 74:572-575, 1992.

Perioral Dermatitis

Beacham BE, Kurgansky D, Gould WM: Circumoral dermatitis and cheilitis caused by tartar control dentifrices, J Am Acad Dermatol 22:1029-1032, 1990.

Boeck K, Abeck D, Werfel S et al: Perioral dermatitis in children—clinical presentation, pathogenesis-related factors and response to topical metronidazole, Dermatology 195:235-238, 1997.

Hafeez ZH: Perioral dermatitis: an update, Int J Dermatol 42:514-517, 2003.

Hogan DJ: Perioral dermatitis, Curr Probl Dermatol 22:98-104, 1995.

Malik R, Quirk CJ: Topical applications and perioral dermatitis, Aust J Dermatol 41:34-38, 2000.

Nguyen V, Eichenfield LF: Periorificial dermatitis in children and adolescents, J Am Acad Dermatol 55:781-785, 2006.

Weber K, Thurmayr R: Critical appraisal of reports on the treatment of perioral dermatitis, Dermatology 210:300-307, 2005.

Cinnamon-Induced Contact Stomatitis

Allen CM, Blozis GG: Oral mucosal reactions to cinnamon-flavored chewing gum, J Am Dent Assoc 116:664-667, 1988.

Drake TE, Maibach HI: Allergic contact dermatitis and stomatitis caused by a cinnamic aldehyde-flavored toothpaste, Arch Dermatol 112:202-203, 1976.

Endo H, Rees TD: Clinical features of cinnamon-induced contact stomatitis, Compend Contin Educ Dent 27:403-409, 2006.

Lamey P-J, Ress TD, Forsyth A: Sensitivity reaction to the cinnamaldehyde component of toothpaste, Br Dent J 168:115-118, 1990.

Mihail RC: Oral leukoplakia caused by cinnamon food allergy, J Otolaryngol 21:366-367, 1992.

Miller RL, Gould AR, Bernstein ML: Cinnamon-induced stomatitis venenata. Clinical and characteristic histopathologic features, Oral Surg Oral Med Oral Pathol 73:708-716, 1992.

Lichenoid Contact Stomatitis from Dental Restorative Materials

Bergman M: Side-effects of amalgam and its alternatives: local, systemic and environmental, *Int Dent J* 40:4-10, 1990.

Bolewska J, Hansen HJ, Holmstrup P et al: Oral mucosal lesions related to silver amalgam restorations, *Oral Surg Oral Med Oral Pathol* 70:55-58, 1990.

Eley BM: The future of dental amalgam: a review of the literature. Part 6: possible harmful effects of mercury from dental amalgam, *Br Dent J* 182:455-459, 1997.

Holmstrup P: Oral mucosa and skin reactions related to amalgam, *Adv Dent Res* 6:120-124, 1992.

Holmstrup P: Reaction of the oral mucosa related to silver amalgam: a review, *J Oral Pathol Med* 20:1-7, 1991.

Jameson MW, Kardos TB, Kirk EE et al: Mucosal reactions to amalgam restorations, *J Oral Rehabil* 17:293-301, 1990.

Laeijendecker R, Dekker SK, Burger PM et al: Oral lichen planus and allergy to dental amalgam restorations, *Arch Dermatol* 140:1434-1438, 2004.

Mallo-Pérez L, Diaz-Donado C: Intraoral contact allergy to materials used in dental practice. A critical review, *Med Oral* 8:334-347, 2003.

Meurman JH, Porko C, Murtomaa H: Patients complaining about amalgam-related symptoms suffer more often from illnesses and chronic craniofacial pain than their controls, *Scand J Dent Res* 98:167-172, 1990.

Rogers RS, Bruce AJ: Lichenoid contact stomatitis. Is organic mercury the culprit? *Arch Dermatol* 140:1524-1525, 2004.

Angioedema

Abdi R, Dong VM, Lee CJ et al: Angiotensin II receptor blocker-associated angioedema: on the heels of ACE inhibitor angioedema, *Pharmacotherapy* 22:1173-1175, 2002.

Angostoni A, Cicardi M: Hereditary and acquired C1-inhibitor deficiency: biological and clinical characteristics in 235 patients, *Medicine* 71:206-215, 1992.

Bork K, Meng G, Staubach P et al: Hereditary angioedema: new findings concerning symptoms, affected organs, and course, *Am J Med* 119:267-274, 2006.

Dobson G, Edgar D, Trinder J: Angioedema of the tongue due to acquired C1 esterase inhibitor deficiency, *Anaesth Intensive Care* 31:99-102, 2003.

Greaves M, Lawlor F: Angioedema: manifestations and management, *J Am Acad Dermatol* 25:155-165, 1991.

Megerian CA, Arnold JE, Berer M: Angioedema: 5 years' experience, with a review of the disorder's presentation and treatment, *Laryngoscope* 102:256-260, 1992.

Nielsen EW, Gramstad S: Angioedema from angiotensin-converting enzyme (ACE) inhibitor treated with complement 1 (C1) inhibitor concentrate, *Acta Anaesthesiol Scand* 50: 120-122, 2006.

Rees SR, Gibson J: Angioedema and swellings of the orofacial region, *Oral Dis* 3:39-42, 1997.

10

Epithelial Pathology

Revised by ANGELA C. CHI

CHAPTER OUTLINE

SQUAMOUS PAPILLOMA

The **squamous papilloma** is a benign proliferation of stratified squamous epithelium, resulting in a papillary or verruciform mass. Presumably, this lesion is induced by the human papillomavirus (HPV). HPV comprises a large family (more than 100 types) of double-stranded DNA viruses of the papovavirus subgroup A. Research has shown that 81% of normal adults have buccal epithelial cells that contain at least one type of HPV, although case control studies using more rigorous criteria usually have shown distinct differences, with high levels of HPV in oral lesions and low levels in normal controls. The virus is capable of becoming totally integrated with the DNA of the host cell, and at least 24 types are associated with lesions of the head and neck. HPV can be identified by *in situ* hybridization, immu-

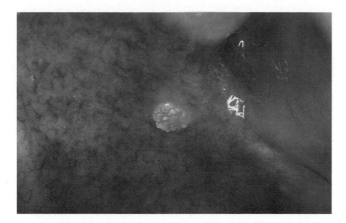

Fig. 10-1 **Squamous papilloma.** An exophytic lesion of the soft palate with multiple short, white surface projections.

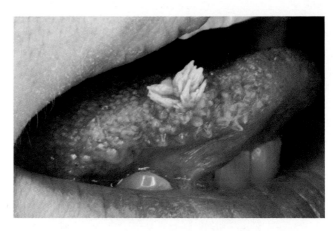

Fig. 10-2 **Squamous papilloma.** A pedunculated lingual mass with numerous long, pointed, and white surface projections. Note the smaller projections around the base of the lesion.

nohistochemical analysis, and polymerase chain reaction (PCR) techniques, but it is not visible with routine histopathologic staining. Viral subtypes 6 and 11 have been identified in up to 50% of oral papillomas, as compared with less than 5% in normal mucosal cells.

The exact mode of transmission is unknown. Transmission by sexual and nonsexual person-to-person contact, contaminated objects, saliva, or breast milk has been proposed. In contrast to other HPV-induced lesions, the viruses in oral squamous papillomas appear to have an extremely low virulence and infectivity rate. A latency or incubation period of 3 to 12 months has been suggested.

The squamous papilloma occurs in one of every 250 adults and makes up approximately 3% of all oral lesions submitted for biopsy. In addition, researchers have estimated that oral squamous papillomas comprise 7% to 8% of all oral masses or growths in children.

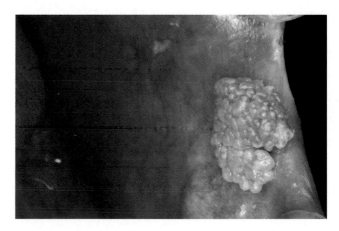

Fig. 10-3 **Squamous papilloma.** A pedunculated mass of the buccal commissure, exhibiting short or blunted surface projections and minimal white coloration.

CLINICAL FEATURES

The squamous papilloma occurs with equal frequency in both men and women. Some authors have asserted that it develops predominantly in children, but epidemiologic studies indicate that it can arise at any age and, in fact, is diagnosed most often in persons 30 to 50 years of age. Sites of predilection include the tongue, lips, and soft palate, but any oral surface may be affected. This lesion is the most common of the soft tissue masses arising from the soft palate.

The squamous papilloma is a soft, painless, usually pedunculated, exophytic nodule with numerous fingerlike surface projections that impart a "cauliflower" or wartlike appearance (Fig. 10-1). Projections may be pointed or blunted (Figs. 10-2 and 10-3), and the lesion may be white, slightly red, or normal in color, depend-

ing on the amount of surface keratinization. The papilloma is usually solitary and enlarges rapidly to a maximum size of about 0.5 cm, with little or no change thereafter. However, lesions as large as 3.0 cm in greatest diameter have been reported.

It is sometimes difficult to distinguish this lesion clinically from verruca vulgaris (see page 364), condyloma acuminatum (see page 366), verruciform xanthoma (see page 372), or multifocal epithelial hyperplasia (see page 367). In addition, extensive coalescing papillary lesions **(papillomatosis)** of the oral mucosa may be seen in several skin disorders, including nevus unius lateris, acanthosis nigricans, and focal dermal hypoplasia (Goltz-Gorlin) syndrome. **Laryngeal papillomatosis,** a rare and potentially devastating disease of the larynx and hypopharynx, has two distinct types: (1) **juvenile-onset** and (2) **adult-**

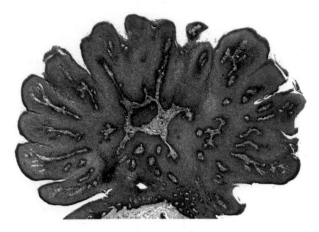

Fig. 10-4 **Squamous papilloma.** Low-power view showing a pedunculated squamous epithelial proliferation. There are multiple papillary projections with fibrovascular connective tissue cores.

onset. Hoarseness is the usual presenting feature, and rapidly proliferating papillomas in the juvenile-onset type may obstruct the airway. The strongest risk factor for juvenile-onset laryngeal papillomatosis is a maternal history of genital warts; transmission of HPV infection via the birth canal, the placenta, or amniotic fluid has been hypothesized.

HISTOPATHOLOGIC FEATURES

The papilloma is characterized by a proliferation of keratinized stratified squamous epithelium arrayed in fingerlike projections with fibrovascular connective tissue cores (Fig. 10-4). The connective tissue cores may show inflammatory changes, depending on the amount of trauma sustained by the lesion. The keratin layer is thickened in lesions with a whiter clinical appearance, and the epithelium typically shows a normal maturation pattern. Occasional papillomas demonstrate basilar hyperplasia and mitotic activity, which can be mistaken for mild epithelial dysplasia. **Koilocytes,** virus-altered epithelial clear cells with small dark (pyknotic) nuclei, are sometimes seen high in the prickle cell layer.

TREATMENT AND PROGNOSIS

Conservative surgical excision, including the base of the lesion, is adequate treatment for the oral squamous papilloma, and recurrence is unlikely. Frequently, lesions have been left untreated for years with no reported transformation into malignancy, continuous enlargement, or dissemination to other parts of the oral cavity.

Although spontaneous remission is possible, juvenile-onset laryngeal papillomatosis tends to be continu-

ously proliferative, sometimes leading to death by asphyxiation. Some investigators have noted especially aggressive behavior among cases associated with HPV type 11 infection. The papillomatosis is treated by repeated surgical debulking procedures to relieve airway obstruction. Adjuvant therapy with agents such as α-interferon may be used for cases exhibiting rapid regrowth or distant spread. Adult-onset lesions are typically less aggressive and tend to be single. Conservative surgical removal may be necessary to eliminate hoarseness from vocal cord involvement. In rare instances, squamous cell carcinoma will develop in long-standing laryngeal papillomatosis, sometimes in a smoker or a patient with a history of irradiation to the larynx.

A vaccine targeted against HPV types 6, 11, 16, and 18 has been introduced recently for the prevention of cervical cancer and genital warts. It is possible that this vaccine may prevent HPV-related lesions of the head and neck as well, such as oral squamous papilloma, laryngeal papillomatosis, and perhaps some cases of oral and oropharyngeal squamous cell carcinoma.

VERRUCA VULGARIS (COMMON WART)

Verruca vulgaris is a benign, virus-induced, focal hyperplasia of stratified squamous epithelium. One or more of the associated human papillomavirus (HPV) types 2, 4, 6, and 40 are found in virtually all examples. Verruca vulgaris is contagious and can spread to other parts of a person's skin or mucous membranes by way of autoinoculation. It infrequently develops on oral mucosa but is extremely common on the skin.

CLINICAL FEATURES

Verruca vulgaris is frequently discovered in children, but occasional lesions may arise even into middle age. The skin of the hands is usually the site of infection (Fig. 10-5). When the oral mucosa is involved, the lesions are usually found on the vermilion border, labial mucosa, or anterior tongue.

Typically, the verruca appears as a painless papule or nodule with papillary projections or a rough pebbly surface (Figs. 10-6 and 10-7). It may be pedunculated or sessile. Cutaneous lesions may be pink, yellow, or white; oral lesions are almost always white. Verruca vulgaris enlarges rapidly to its maximum size (usually <5 mm), and the size remains constant for months or years thereafter unless the lesion is irritated. Multiple or clustered lesions are common. On occasion, extreme accumulation of compact keratin may result in a hard surface projection several millimeters in height, termed a **cutaneous horn** or **keratin horn.** Other cutaneous

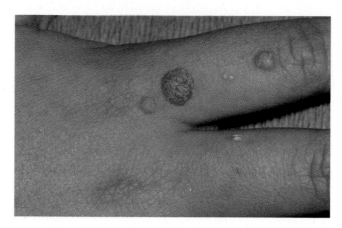

Fig. 10-5 Verruca vulgaris. Several warts on the finger, exhibiting a rough, papillary surface.

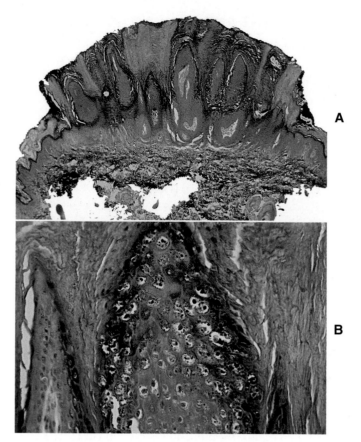

A

B

Fig. 10-8 Verruca vulgaris. A, Numerous papillary projections are covered by hyperkeratotic stratified squamous epithelium. Elongated rete ridges at the edge of the lesion converge toward the center. **B,** High-power view showing clear koilocytes in the upper epithelial layers.

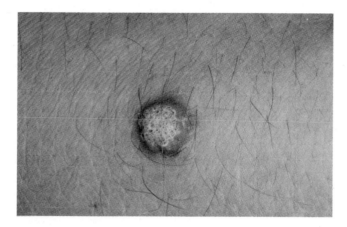

Fig. 10-6 Verruca vulgaris. Nodular lesion of the skin exhibiting numerous short papillary projections.

lesions, including seborrheic keratosis (see page 374), actinic keratosis (see page 404), and squamous cell carcinoma, may also create a cutaneous horn.

HISTOPATHOLOGIC FEATURES

The verruca vulgaris is characterized by a proliferation of hyperkeratotic stratified squamous epithelium arranged into fingerlike or pointed projections with connective tissue cores (Fig. 10-8). Chronic inflammatory cells often infiltrate the supporting connective tissue. Elongated rete ridges tend to converge toward the center of the lesion, producing a "cupping" effect. A prominent granular cell layer (hypergranulosis) exhibits coarse, clumped keratohyaline granules. Abundant koilocytes are often seen in the superficial spinous layer. Koilocytes are HPV-altered epithelial cells with perinuclear clear spaces and small, dark nuclei (pyknosis). Eosinophilic intranuclear viral inclusions are often noted within the cells of the granular layer.

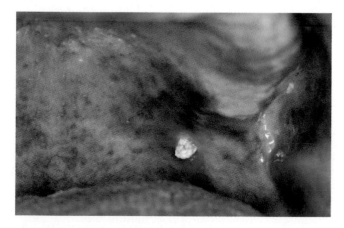

Fig. 10-7 Verruca vulgaris. Exophytic, white, papillary lesion of the lateral soft palate.

TREATMENT AND PROGNOSIS

Skin verrucae are treated effectively by topical salicylic acid, topical lactic acid, or liquid nitrogen cryotherapy. Surgical excision is indicated only for cases with an atypical clinical presentation in which the diagnosis is uncertain. Skin lesions that recur or are resistant to standard therapy may be treated by alternative methods, such as intralesional bleomycin, topical or intralesional 5-fluorouracil, or photodynamic therapy.

Oral lesions are usually surgically excised, or they may be destroyed by a laser, cryotherapy, or electrosurgery. Cryotherapy induces a subepithelial blister that lifts the infected epithelium from the underlying connective tissue, allowing it to slough away. All destructive or surgical treatments should extend to include the base of the lesion.

Recurrence is seen in a small proportion of treated cases. Without treatment, verrucae do not transform into malignancy, and two thirds will disappear spontaneously within 2 years, especially in children.

CONDYLOMA ACUMINATUM (VENEREAL WART)

Condyloma acuminatum is a virus-induced proliferation of stratified squamous epithelium of the genitalia, perianal region, mouth, and larynx. One or more of the human papillomavirus (HPV) types 2, 6, 11, 53, and 54 are usually detected in the lesion. However, the high-risk types 16, 18, and 31 also may be present, especially in anogenital lesions. Condyloma is considered to be a sexually transmitted disease (STD), with lesions developing at a site of sexual contact or trauma. This lesion represents 20% of all STDs diagnosed in STD clinics and may be an indicator of sexual abuse when diagnosed in young children. In addition, studies of oral and pharyngeal HPV infection in infants have suggested that vertical transmission from mothers with genital HPV infection may occur perinatally or perhaps *in utero*; however, reported transmission rates have varied widely (ranging from 4% to >80%). It is not unusual for oral and anogenital condylomata to be present concurrently. The incubation period for a condyloma is 1 to 3 months from the time of sexual contact. Once present, autoinoculation to other mucosal sites is possible.

CLINICAL FEATURES

Condylomata are usually diagnosed in teenagers and young adults, but people of all ages are susceptible. Oral lesions most frequently occur on the labial mucosa, soft palate, and lingual frenum. The typical condyloma appears as a sessile, pink, well-demarcated, nontender exophytic mass with short, blunted surface projections (Fig. 10-9). The condyloma tends to be larger than the papilloma and is characteristically clustered with other

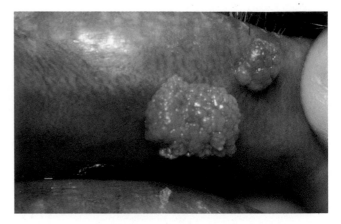

Fig. 10-9   Condyloma acuminatum. Two lesions of the upper lip mucosa exhibit short, blunted projections. *(Courtesy of Dr. Brian Blocher.)*

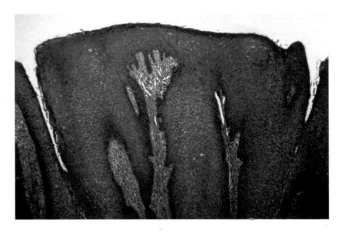

Fig. 10-10   Condyloma acuminatum. Medium-power photomicrograph showing acanthotic stratified squamous epithelium forming a blunted projection.

condylomata. The average lesional size is 1.0 to 1.5 cm, but oral lesions as large as 3 cm have been reported.

HISTOPATHOLOGIC FEATURES

Condyloma acuminatum appears as a benign proliferation of acanthotic stratified squamous epithelium with mildly keratotic papillary surface projections (Fig. 10-10). Thin connective tissue cores support the papillary epithelial projections, which are more blunted and broader than those of squamous papilloma and verruca vulgaris, imparting an appearance of keratin-filled crypts between prominences. In some cases, lesions extending from the surface mucosa to involve underlying salivary ductal epithelium have been reported; such lesions should be distinguished from salivary ductal papillomas (see page 485).

The covering epithelium is mature and differentiated, but the prickle cells often demonstrate pyknotic, crinkled (or "raisinlike") nuclei surrounded by clear zones **(koilocytes)**, a microscopic feature of HPV infec-

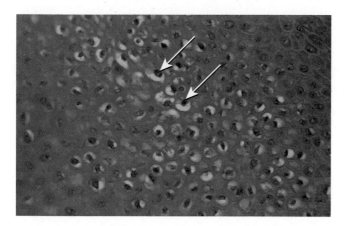

Fig. 10-11   Condyloma acuminatum. High-power photomicrograph demonstrating koilocytes (*arrows*) in the spinous layer.

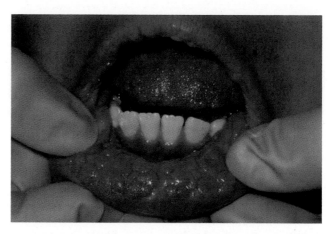

Fig. 10-12   Multifocal epithelial hyperplasia. Multiple, flat-topped papules and nodules of normal coloration are seen on the lower lip of a child. (*Courtesy of Dr. Mark Casafrancisco.*)

tion (Fig. 10-11). Koilocytes may be less prominent in oral lesions compared with genital lesions, in which case distinction from squamous papilloma may be difficult. Ultrastructural examination reveals virions within the cytoplasm or nuclei of koilocytes, and the virus also can be demonstrated by immunohistochemical analysis, *in situ* hybridization, and PCR techniques.

TREATMENT AND PROGNOSIS

The oral condyloma is usually treated by conservative surgical excision. Laser ablation also has been used, but this treatment has raised some question as to the airborne spread of HPV through the aerosolized microdroplets created by the vaporization of lesional tissue. Nonsurgical, patient-applied topical agents such as imiquimod or podophyllotoxin are becoming the mainstay of treatment for anogenital condylomata, although such treatments are not typically used for oral lesions. Regardless of the method used, a condyloma should be removed because it is contagious and can spread to other oral surfaces and to other persons through direct (usually sexual) contact. In the anogenital area, condylomata infected with HPV-16 or HPV-18 are associated with an increased risk of malignant transformation to squamous cell carcinoma, but this has not been demonstrated in oral lesions.

MULTIFOCAL EPITHELIAL HYPERPLASIA (HECK'S DISEASE; MULTIFOCAL PAPILLOMA VIRUS EPITHELIAL HYPERPLASIA; FOCAL EPITHELIAL HYPERPLASIA)

Multifocal epithelial hyperplasia is a virus-induced, localized proliferation of oral squamous epithelium that was first described in Native Americans and Inuit.

Currently, it is known to exist in many populations and ethnic groups and is apparently produced by human papillomavirus (HPV) types 13 and 32. In some populations, as many as 39% of children are affected. The condition often affects multiple members of a given family; this familial tendency may be related to either genetic susceptibility or HPV transmission between family members. An association with the HLA-DR4 (DRB1*0404) allele was found in a recent study of Mexican patients with this condition. Lower socio-economic status, crowded living conditions, and poor hygiene appear to be additional risk factors. Multiple papillary lesions similar to multifocal epithelial hyperplasia arise with increased frequency in patients with acquired immunodeficiency syndrome (AIDS) (see page 276).

CLINICAL FEATURES

Although multifocal epithelial hyperplasia is usually a childhood condition, it occasionally affects young and middle-aged adults. Previous studies have reported either a slight female predilection or no significant gender bias. The most common sites of involvement include the labial, buccal, and lingual mucosa, but gingival, palatal, and tonsillar lesions also have been reported. In addition, involvement of the conjunctiva has been described very rarely.

This disease typically appears as multiple soft, nontender, flattened or rounded papules, which are usually clustered and the color of normal mucosa, although they may be scattered, pale, or rarely white (Fig. 10-12). Occasional lesions show a slight papillary surface change (Fig. 10-13). Individual lesions are small (0.3 to 1.0 cm), discrete, and well demarcated, but they frequently cluster so closely together that the entire area takes on a cobblestone or fissured appearance.

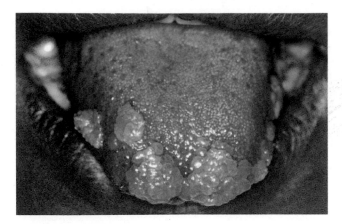

Fig. 10-13   Multifocal epithelial hyperplasia. The lesions may demonstrate a papillary surface change and paleness, as demonstrated on this child's tongue. *(Courtesy of Dr. Román Carlos.)*

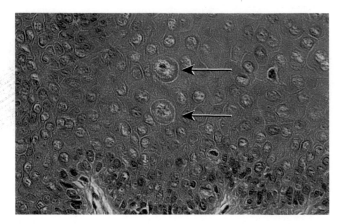

Fig. 10-15   Multifocal epithelial hyperplasia. Mitosoid cells *(arrows)* contain altered nuclei in this otherwise mature and well-differentiated stratified squamous epithelium.

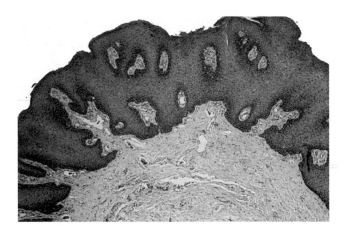

Fig. 10-14   Multifocal epithelial hyperplasia. Prominent acanthosis of the epithelium with broad and elongated rete ridges. The slightly papillary surface alteration noted here may or may not be present.

HISTOPATHOLOGIC FEATURES

The hallmark of multifocal epithelial hyperplasia is an abrupt and sometimes considerable acanthosis of the oral epithelium (Fig. 10-14). Because the thickened mucosa extends upward, not down into underlying connective tissues, the lesional rete ridges are at the same depth as the adjacent normal rete ridges. The ridges themselves are widened, often confluent, and sometimes club shaped. Some superficial keratinocytes show a koilocytic change similar to that seen in other HPV infections. Others occasionally demonstrate an altered nucleus that resembles a mitotic figure **(mitosoid cell)** (Fig. 10-15). Viruslike particles have been noted ultrastructurally within both the cytoplasm and the nuclei of cells within the prickle cell layer, and the presence of HPV has been demonstrated with both DNA *in situ* hybridization and immunohistochemical analysis.

TREATMENT AND PROGNOSIS

Spontaneous regression of multifocal epithelial hyperplasia has been reported after months or years and is inferred from the rarity of the disease in adults. Conservative surgical excision may be performed for diagnostic or aesthetic purposes or for lesions subject to recurrent trauma. Lesions also can be removed by cryotherapy or carbon dioxide (CO_2) laser ablation. Use of topical interferon-β and systemic interferon-α has been reported in a few cases, although with variable results. The risk of recurrence after therapy is minimal, and there seems to be no malignant transformation potential.

SINONASAL PAPILLOMAS

Papillomas of the sinonasal tract are benign, localized proliferations of the respiratory mucosa of this region. This mucosa gives rise to three histomorphologically distinct papillomas:

1. Fungiform
2. Inverted
3. Cylindrical cell

Lesions exhibiting features of both the inverted and the cylindrical cell types may be termed *mixed* or *hybrid* papillomas. In addition, a keratinizing **squamous papilloma,** similar to the oral squamous papilloma (see page 362), rarely may occur in the nasal vestibule.

Collectively, **sinonasal papillomas** represent 10% to 25% of all tumors of the nasal and paranasal region. Half of the sinonasal papillomas arise from the mucosa of the lateral nasal wall; the remainder predominantly involve the maxillary and ethmoid sinuses and the nasal septum. Multiple lesions may be present.

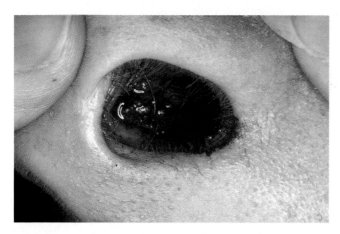

Fig. 10-16   Fungiform papilloma. Erythematous, papillary growth on the nasal septum.

The cause of sinonasal papillomas remains controversial and unclear. Some authorities say that these lesions represent neoplasms; others consider them to be a reactive hyperplasia secondary to a variety of environmental stimulants, such as allergy, chronic bacterial or viral (HPV type 11) infection, and tobacco smoking. Recent molecular genetic investigations have shown that inverted papillomas arise from a single progenitor cell (i.e., monoclonal), suggesting that these lesions are neoplastic and recurrence may result from growth of residual transformed cells.

FUNGIFORM (SEPTAL; SQUAMOUS; EXOPHYTIC) PAPILLOMA

The **fungiform papilloma** bears some similarity to the oral squamous papilloma, although it has a somewhat more aggressive biologic behavior and more varied epithelial types. It represents 18% to 50% of all sinonasal papillomas in various investigations. Almost all examples are positive for HPV type 6 or 11.

CLINICAL FEATURES

The fungiform papilloma arises almost exclusively on the nasal septum and is twice as common in men as in women. It occurs primarily in people 20 to 50 years of age. Typically, it exhibits unilateral nasal obstruction or epistaxis and appears as a pink or tan, broad-based nodule with papillary or warty surface projections (Fig. 10-16).

HISTOPATHOLOGIC FEATURES

The fungiform papilloma has a microscopic appearance similar to that of the oral squamous papilloma, although the stratified squamous epithelium covering

the fingerlike projections seldom is keratinized. Respiratory epithelium or "transitional" epithelium (intermediate between squamous and respiratory) may be seen in some lesions. Mucous (goblet) cells and intraepithelial microcysts containing mucus often are present. Mitoses are infrequent, and dysplasia is rare. The underlying connective tissue consists of delicate fibrous tissue with a minimal inflammatory component, unless it is irritated.

TREATMENT AND PROGNOSIS

Complete surgical excision is the treatment of choice for the fungiform papilloma. Recurrence is common, developing in approximately one third of all cases; however, this may be caused by incomplete excision. Most authorities consider this lesion to have minimal or no potential for malignant transformation.

INVERTED PAPILLOMA (INVERTED SCHNEIDERIAN PAPILLOMA)

The most common (50% to 78%) sinonasal papilloma, the **inverted papilloma,** is also the variant with the greatest potential for local destruction and malignant transformation. HPV types 6, 11, 16, and 18 have been identified, with considerable variability in the reported proportion of cases positive for HPV. This variability is likely due to differences in detection methods used; however, more recent studies using quantitative real-time polymerase chain reaction (PCR) suggest that HPV is present in approximately 18 to 30% of lesions.

CLINICAL AND RADIOGRAPHIC FEATURES

The inverted papilloma seldom occurs in patients younger than 20 years of age; the median age is 55 years. A strong male predilection is noted (3:1 male-to-female ratio). This lesion arises predominantly from the lateral nasal cavity wall or a paranasal sinus, usually the antrum. Typically, the inverted papilloma results in unilateral nasal obstruction; additional symptoms may include pain, epistaxis, purulent discharge, or local deformity. The papilloma appears as a soft, pink or tan, polypoid or nodular growth. Multiple lesions may be present.

Pressure erosion of the underlying bone is usually present and may be visible radiographically as an irregular radiolucency. Primary sinus lesions may be distinguishable only as a soft tissue radiodensity or mucosal thickening on radiographs; sinus involvement generally represents extension from the nasal cavity. Magnetic resonance imaging (MRI) can help to identify the extent of the lesion (Fig. 10-17).

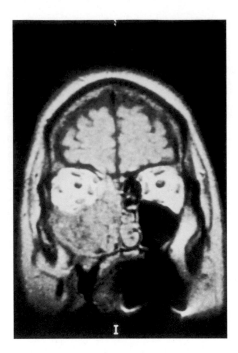

Fig. 10-17   Inverted papilloma. T1-weighted coronal magnetic resonance image (MRI) showing a tumor of the right lateral nasal fossa. The tumor fills the right maxilla and ethmoid sinuses and involves the floor of the orbit. *(Courtesy of Dr. Pamela Van Tassel.)*

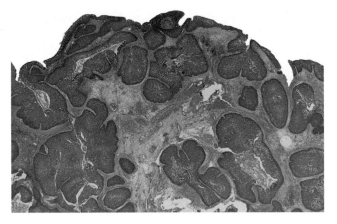

Fig. 10-18   Inverted papilloma. Low-power photomicrograph showing a squamous epithelial proliferation, with multiple "inverting" islands of epithelium extending into the underlying connective tissue.

HISTOPATHOLOGIC FEATURES

Microscopically, the inverted papilloma is characterized by squamous epithelial proliferation into the submucosal stroma (Fig. 10-18). The basement membrane remains intact, and the epithelium appears to be "pushing" into underlying connective tissue. Goblet (mucous) cells and mucin-filled microcysts frequently are noted within the epithelium. Keratin production is uncommon, but thin surface keratinization may be

seen. Mitoses often are noted within the basilar or parabasilar cells, and varying degrees of dysplasia may be seen. Papillary surface projections are present, and deep clefts may be seen between projections. The stroma consists of dense fibrous or loose myxomatous connective tissue with or without inflammatory cells.

Destruction of underlying bone frequently is noted. Immunohistochemical expression of CD44, a cell adhesion molecule, is increased in this papilloma, which may help to distinguish it from invasive papillary squamous cell carcinoma, which lacks this feature. Although some authors have suggested that hyperkeratosis, prominent epithelial hyperplasia, and high mitotic index are negative prognostic indicators, no histopathologic parameters have been found to be reliably predictive of recurrence or malignant transformation among inverted papillomas.

TREATMENT AND PROGNOSIS

The inverted papilloma has a significant growth potential and, if neglected, may extend into the nasopharynx, middle ear, orbit, or cranial base. In some studies, recurrence after conservative surgical excision has occurred in nearly 75% of all cases. However, with more aggressive surgical therapy, consisting of medial maxillectomy via a lateral rhinotomy or midfacial degloving approach, recurrence rates of less than 14% have been reported. Although an open surgical approach historically has been regarded as the standard of care, advances in transnasal endoscopic surgery have led to wider acceptance of this method as an alternative, particularly for patients with limited and easily accessible disease. Several investigators, using modern endoscopic techniques and careful patient selection, have reported recurrence rates comparable to those for conventional lateral rhinotomy with medial maxillectomy. Recurrences are usually noted within 2 years of surgery but can happen much later. Hence, long-term follow-up is essential. Continued tobacco smoking is associated with an increased risk of multiple recurrences.

The inverted papilloma also is associated with malignancy, usually squamous cell carcinoma, in 3% to 24% of cases. In such an eventuality, of course, the lesion is treated as a malignancy, typically by performing more radical surgery, with or without adjunctive radiotherapy.

CYLINDRICAL CELL PAPILLOMA (ONCOCYTIC SCHNEIDERIAN PAPILLOMA)

The **cylindrical cell papilloma** accounts for less than 7% of sinonasal papillomas. This lesion is considered by some authorities to be a variant of the **inverted**

papilloma because of the similarity in clinical and histopathologic features and a similarly low frequency of HPV.

CLINICAL FEATURES

Cylindrical cell papilloma typically occurs in adults 20 to 50 years of age. There is a strong male predominance, with a predilection for the maxillary antrum, lateral nasal cavity wall, and ethmoid sinus. The presenting symptom is usually unilateral nasal obstruction, and it appears as a beefy-red or brown mass with a multinodular surface.

HISTOPATHOLOGIC FEATURES

Microscopically, the cylindrical cell papilloma demonstrates both endophytic and exophytic growth. Surface papillary projections have a fibrovascular connective tissue core and are covered by a multilayered epithelium of tall columnar cells with small, dark nuclei and eosinophilic, occasionally granular, cytoplasm. The lesional epithelial cell is similar to an oncocyte. Cilia may be seen on the surface, and there are numerous intraepithelial microcysts filled with mucin, neutrophils, or both.

TREATMENT AND PROGNOSIS

Cylindrical cell papilloma is treated in the same manner as inverted papilloma (see previous topic). The potential for recurrence and malignant transformation seems to be lower than that of the inverted papilloma.

MOLLUSCUM CONTAGIOSUM

Molluscum contagiosum is a virus-induced epithelial hyperplasia produced by the molluscum contagiosum virus, a member of the DNA poxvirus group. At least 6% of the population (more in older age groups) has antibodies to this virus, although few ever develop lesions. After an incubation period of 14 to 50 days, infection produces multiple papules of the skin or, rarely, mucous membranes. These remain small for months or years and then spontaneously involute.

During its active phase, the molluscum contagiosum virus is sloughed from a central core in each papule. Routes of transmission include sexual contact (in adults) and such nonsexual contacts (in children and teenagers) as sharing clothing, wrestling, communal bathing, and swimming. Lesions have a predilection for warm portions of the skin and sites of recent injury. Florid cases have been reported in immunocompromised patients, and the prevalence among the human

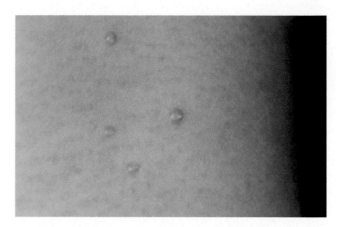

Fig. 10-19   Molluscum contagiosum. Multiple, smooth-surfaced papules, with several demonstrating small keratin-like plugs, are seen on the neck of a child.

immunodeficiency virus (HIV)-positive patient population is estimated to be 5% to 18% (see page 278). Patients with atopic dermatitis and Darier's disease also are at risk for developing severe and extensive disease.

CLINICAL FEATURES

Molluscum contagiosum is usually seen in children and young adults. The papules almost always are multiple and occur predominantly on the skin of the neck, face (particularly eyelids), trunk, and genitalia. Infrequently, oral involvement occurs, usually on the lips, buccal mucosa, palate, or gingiva.

Lesions are pink, smooth-surfaced, sessile, nontender, and nonhemorrhagic papules that are 2 to 4 mm in diameter (Fig. 10-19). Many show a small central indentation or keratin-like plug from which a curdlike substance can be expressed. Some are surrounded by a mild inflammatory erythema and may be slightly tender or pruritic. Eczematous eruptions occasionally may develop in the vicinity of molluscum contagiosum lesions, particularly in patients with atopic dermatitis.

In immunocompromised patients, atypical lesions that are unusually large, verrucous, or markedly hyperkeratotic have been described.

HISTOPATHOLOGIC FEATURES

Molluscum contagiosum appears as a localized lobular proliferation of surface stratified squamous epithelium (Fig. 10-20). The central portion of each lobule is filled with bloated keratinocytes that contain large, intranuclear, basophilic viral inclusions called **molluscum bodies** (or **Henderson-Paterson bodies**) (Fig. 10-21). These bodies begin as small eosinophilic structures in cells just above the basal layer. As they

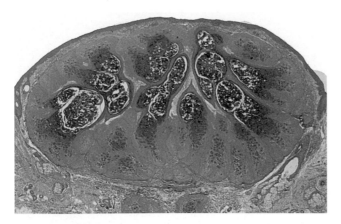

Fig. 10-20 Molluscum contagiosum. Well-defined epidermal proliferation demonstrating a central craterlike depression filled with virally altered keratinocytes.

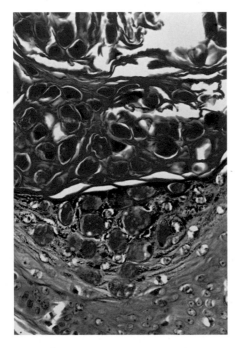

Fig. 10-21 Molluscum contagiosum. Higher-power photomicrograph showing keratinocytes with large, basophilic viral inclusions (molluscum bodies) being sloughed into the central crater (*top*).

approach the surface, these bodies increase so much in size that they frequently become larger than the original size of the invaded cells. A central crater is formed at the surface as stratum corneum cells disintegrate to release their molluscum bodies. These unique features make the diagnosis readily apparent.

TREATMENT AND PROGNOSIS

In most cases of molluscum contagiosum, spontaneous remission occurs within 6 to 9 months. For immuno-competent patients, there is ongoing debate as to whether the disease should be treated or allowed to resolve on its own. Treatment may be performed to decrease the risk of disease transmission, prevent auto-inoculation, or provide symptomatic relief.

Few controlled studies of treatment efficacy have been performed, but lesions most commonly are removed by curettage or cryotherapy. Alternative treatment methods include CO_2 or pulsed dye laser therapy, electrodessication, trichloroacetic acid, silver nitrate, potassium hydroxide, or the topical blistering agent cantharidin. Topical agents such as tretinoin, podophyllotoxin, and imiquimod are additional alternatives, although generally not as effective or rapid as in-office cryotherapy or curettage

In immunosuppressed patients with recalcitrant lesions, the antiviral agent cidofivir may be effective. Moreover, in patients with AIDS, highly active antiretroviral therapy indirectly counteracts molluscum contagiosum infection by increasing CD4+ T cell counts and improving the immune response.

There is no apparent potential to transform into carcinoma, and the lesions tend not to recur after treatment.

VERRUCIFORM XANTHOMA

Verruciform xanthoma is a hyperplastic condition of the epithelium of the mouth, skin, and genitalia, with a characteristic accumulation of lipid-laden histiocytes beneath the epithelium. First reported in 1971, it remains largely an oral disease; its cause is still unknown. Although verruciform xanthoma is a papillary lesion, human papillomavirus (HPV) has been identified in only a small number of cases, and no definitive role for this virus in the pathogenesis of these lesions has been established. The lesion probably represents an unusual reaction or immune response to localized epithelial trauma or damage. This hypothesis is supported by cases of verruciform xanthoma that have developed in association with disturbed epithelium (e.g., lichen planus, lupus erythematosus, epidermolysis bullosa, epithelial dysplasia, squamous cell carcinoma, pemphigus vulgaris, warty dyskeratoma, graft-versus-host disease [GVHD]). The lesion is histopathologically similar to other dermal xanthomas, but it is not associated with diabetes, hyperlipidemia, or any other metabolic disorder.

CLINICAL FEATURES

Verruciform xanthoma is typically seen in whites, 40 to 70 years of age, with a slight male predilection. Approximately half of the intraoral lesions occur on the gingiva and alveolar mucosa, but any oral site may be involved.

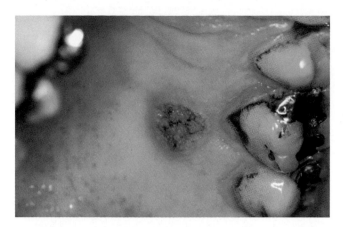

Fig. 10-22   Verruciform xanthoma. A well-demarcated, slightly elevated lesion of the hard palate that demonstrates a roughened or papillary surface.

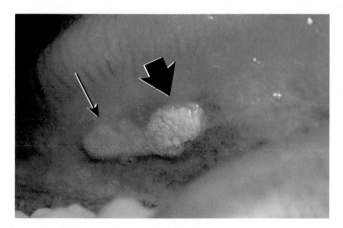

Fig. 10-23   Verruciform xanthoma. A lesion of the ventral tongue exhibits a biphasic appearance. The anterior aspect demonstrates elongated white (well-keratinized) projections *(large arrow)*. The posterior aspect demonstrates a surface of yellow, blunted projections *(small arrow)*.

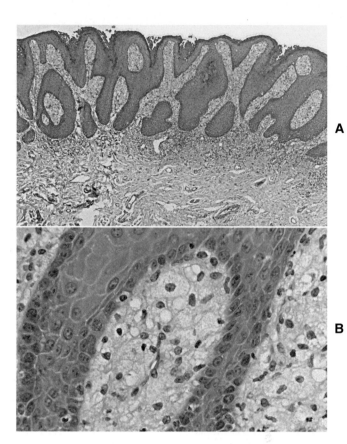

Fig. 10-24   Verruciform xanthoma. A, A slight papillary appearance is produced by hyperparakeratosis, and the rete ridges are elongated to a uniform depth. Note the parakeratin plugging between the papillary projections. **B,** The connective tissue papillae are composed almost exclusively of xanthoma cells—large macrophages with foamy cytoplasm.

The lesion appears as a well-demarcated, soft, painless, sessile, slightly elevated mass with a white, yellow-white, or red color and a papillary or roughened (verruciform) surface (Figs. 10-22 and 10-23). Rarely, flat-topped nodules are seen without surface projections. Most lesions are smaller than 2 cm in greatest diameter; no oral lesion larger than 4 cm has been reported. Multiple lesions occasionally have been described. Clinically, verruciform xanthoma may be similar to squamous papilloma, condyloma acuminatum, or early carcinoma.

HISTOPATHOLOGIC FEATURES

Verruciform xanthoma demonstrates papillary, acanthotic surface epithelium covered by a thickened layer of parakeratin. On routine hematoxylin and eosin (H&E) staining, the keratin layer often exhibits a distinctive orange coloration (Fig. 10-24). Clefts or crypts between the epithelial projections are filled with parakeratin, and rete ridges are elongated to a uniform depth. The most important diagnostic feature is the accumulation of numerous large macrophages with foamy cytoplasm, which typically are confined to the connective tissue papillae. These foam cells, also known as **xanthoma cells,** contain lipid and periodic acid-Schiff (PAS)-positive, diastase-resistant granules. With immunohistochemical stains, the xanthoma cells are positive for markers consistent with monocyte-macrophage lineage, including CD68 (KP1) and cathepsin B.

TREATMENT AND PROGNOSIS

The verruciform xanthoma is treated with conservative surgical excision. Recurrence after removal of the lesion is rare, and no malignant transformation has

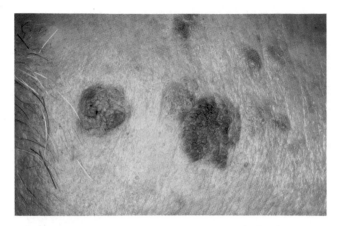

Fig. 10-25   Seborrheic keratosis. Multiple brown plaques on the face of an older man exhibit a fissured surface. They had been slowly enlarging for several years.

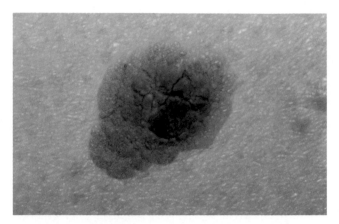

Fig. 10-26   Seborrheic keratosis. Crusted and pigmented epidermal plaque.

been reported. However, two cases have been reported in which a verruciform xanthoma occurred in association with carcinoma *in situ* or squamous cell carcinoma. This does not necessarily imply that verruciform xanthoma is a potentially malignant lesion; however, it may indicate that hyperkeratotic or dysplastic oral lesions can undergo degenerative changes to form a verruciform xanthoma.

SEBORRHEIC KERATOSIS

Seborrheic keratosis is an extremely common skin lesion of older people and represents an acquired, benign proliferation of epidermal basal cells. The cause is unknown, although there is a positive correlation with chronic sun exposure, sometimes with a hereditary (autosomal dominant) tendency. In addition, recent genetic studies have suggested that somatic mutations in the FGFR3 (fibroblast growth factor receptor 3) gene are important in the development of these lesions. Seborrheic keratosis does not occur in the mouth.

CLINICAL FEATURES

Seborrheic keratoses begin to develop on the skin of the face, trunk, and extremities during the fourth decade of life, and they become more prevalent with each passing decade. Lesions are usually multiple, beginning as small tan to brown macules that are indistinguishable clinically from **actinic lentigines** (see page 377), and which gradually enlarge and elevate (Figs. 10-25 and 10-26). Individual lesions are sharply demarcated plaques and have surfaces that are finely fissured, pitted, or verrucous, but may be smooth. They tend to appear "stuck onto" the skin and are usually less than 2 cm in diameter.

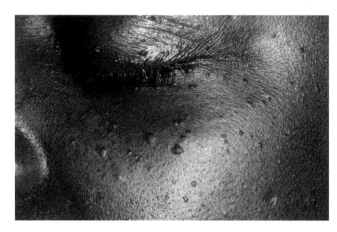

Fig. 10-27   Dermatosis papulosa nigra. Multiple small pigmented papules of the malar area.

Dermatosis papulosa nigra is a form of seborrheic keratosis that occurs in approximately 30% of blacks and frequently has an autosomal dominant inheritance pattern. This condition typically appears as multiple, small (1 to 2 mm), dark-brown to black papules scattered about the zygomatic and periorbital region (Fig. 10-27).

HISTOPATHOLOGIC FEATURES

Seborrheic keratosis consists of an exophytic proliferation of basilar epithelial cells that exhibit varying degrees of surface keratinization, acanthosis, and papillomatosis (Fig. 10-28). Characteristically, the entire epithelial hyperplasia extends upward, above the normal epidermal surface. The lesion usually exhibits deep, keratin-filled invaginations that appear cystic on cross-section; hence, they are called **horn cysts** or **pseudo-horn cysts** (Fig. 10-29). Melanin pigmentation often is seen within the basal layer.

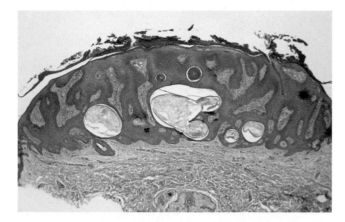

Fig. 10-28   Seborrheic keratosis. The acanthotic form demonstrates considerable acanthosis, surface hyperkeratosis, and numerous pseudocysts. The epidermal proliferation extends upward, above the normal epidermal surface.

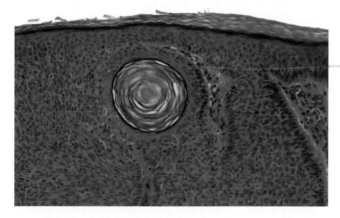

Fig. 10-29   Seborrheic keratosis. Pseudocysts are actually keratin-filled invaginations, as seen toward the left in this high-power photomicrograph. The surrounding epithelial cells are basaloid in appearance.

Several histopathologic patterns may be seen in seborrheic keratoses. The most common is the **acanthotic** form, which exhibits little papillomatosis and marked acanthosis with minimal surface keratinization. The **hyperkeratotic** form is characterized by prominent papillomatosis and hyperkeratosis with minimal acanthosis. The **adenoid** form consists of anastomosing trabeculae of lesional cells with little hyperkeratosis or papillomatosis. The lesions of dermatosis papulosa nigra are predominantly of the adenoid and acanthotic types.

Chronic trauma may alter these histopathologic features, and the lesion known as **inverted follicular keratosis of Helwig** is thought to represent an irritated seborrheic keratosis. This lesion shows a mild degree of proliferation into the connective tissue and a chronic inflammatory cell infiltrate adjacent to the lesion. Squamous metaplasia of the lesional cells results in whorled epithelial patterns called **squamous eddies**. Inflamed seborrheic keratosis may show enough nuclear atypia and mitotic activity to cause confusion with squamous cell carcinoma, but enough of the basic attributes of seborrheic keratosis typically remain to allow a proper diagnosis.

TREATMENT AND PROGNOSIS

Except for aesthetic purposes, a seborrheic keratosis seldom is removed. Cryotherapy with liquid nitrogen or simple curettage is the treatment of choice for lesions that are removed. Although the keratosis has no malignant potential, other more significant skin lesions may develop in areas contiguous to it. In rare cases, melanomas may resemble seborrheic keratoses clinically; thus it is important for a dermatologist or other qualified clinician to determine whether it is most appropriate to treat a lesion by cryotherapy or to excise and submit it for histopathologic confirmation. Moreover, the sudden appearance of numerous seborrheic keratoses with pruritus has been associated with internal malignancy, a rare event called the **Leser-Trélat sign.**

SEBACEOUS HYPERPLASIA

Sebaceous hyperplasia is characterized by a localized proliferation of sebaceous glands of the skin. It has no known cause and is common on the facial skin. In some cases an association with cyclosporine, systemic corticosteroids, hemodialysis, and Muir-Torre syndrome (a rare autosomal dominant disorder characterized by visceral malignancies, sebaceous adenomas and carcinomas, and keratoacanthomas) has been described. The major significance of this entity is its clinical similarity to more serious facial tumors, such as basal cell carcinoma.

CLINICAL FEATURES

Cutaneous sebaceous hyperplasia usually affects adults older than 40 years of age. It occurs most commonly on the skin of the face, especially the nose, cheeks, and forehead. Less commonly, lesions may involve the genital area, chest, and areola. The condition is characterized by one or more soft, nontender papules with white, yellow, or normal coloration (Fig. 10-30). Lesions are usually umbilicated, with a small central depression, representing the area where the ducts of the involved sebaceous lobules terminate. Most lesions are smaller than 5 mm in greatest diameter and take considerable time to reach even this small size.

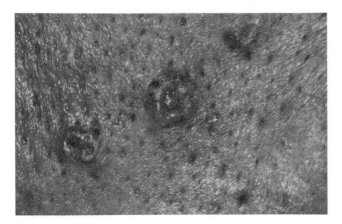

Fig. 10-30   Sebaceous hyperplasia. Multiple soft papules of the midface are umbilicated and small. Sebum can often be expressed from the central depressed area.

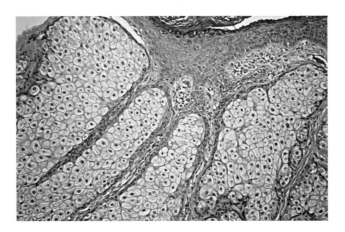

Fig. 10-31   Sebaceous hyperplasia. Sebaceous glands are enlarged and more numerous than normal, but they demonstrate no other pathologic changes.

Compression of the lesion usually causes sebum, the thick yellow-white product of the sebaceous gland, to be expressed in the central depressed area. This feature helps clinically to distinguish sebaceous hyperplasia from basal cell carcinoma. An oral counterpart, which probably has no relation to the skin lesion, appears as a white to yellow papule or nodular mass with a "cauliflower" appearance, usually of the buccal mucosa.

HISTOPATHOLOGIC FEATURES

Histopathologically, sebaceous hyperplasia is characterized by a collection of enlarged but otherwise normal sebaceous gland lobules grouped around one or more centrally located sebaceous ducts (Fig. 10-31).

TREATMENT AND PROGNOSIS

No treatment is necessary for sebaceous hyperplasia except for aesthetic reasons or unless basal cell carcinoma cannot be eliminated from the clinical dif-

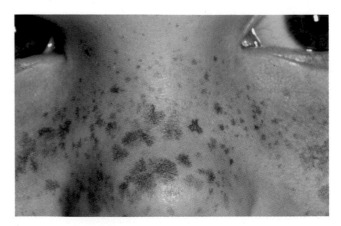

Fig. 10-32   Ephelides. Multiple brown macules over the bridge of the nose.

ferential diagnosis of cutaneous lesions. Excisional biopsy is curative. Cryosurgery, electrodessication, laser therapy, and photodynamic therapy are alternative methods for removal.

EPHELIS (FRECKLE)

An **ephelis** is a common small hyperpigmented macule of the skin that represents a region of increased melanin production. Ephelides are seen most often on the face, arms, and back of fair-skinned, blue-eyed, red- or light-blond haired persons; they may be associated with a strong genetic predilection (autosomal dominant). Recent studies have demonstrated a strong relationship between certain variants of the *MC1R* (melanocortin-1-receptor) gene and the development of ephelides. The skin discoloration is produced by a relative excess of melanin deposition in the epidermis, not by a local increase in the number of melanocytes.

CLINICAL FEATURES

Ephelides become noticeable during the first decade of life, and new macules seldom arise after the teenage years. During adult life the macules typically become less prominent. There is no sex predilection; however, persons with blond or red hair are more likely to have ephelides. The lesions become more pronounced after sun exposure and are associated closely with a history of painful sunburns in childhood.

Each individual macule is round or oval, and typically remains less than 3 mm in diameter (Fig. 10-32). It has a uniform light-brown coloration and is sharply demarcated from the surrounding skin. There is great variability in the numbers of ephelides present. Many individuals have less than 10, whereas some have hundreds of macules. The brown color is not as dark as the lentigo simplex (see page 378), and there is never elevation above the surface of the skin, as may occur in a melanocytic nevus (see page 382).

HISTOPATHOLOGIC FEATURES

The ephelis is composed of stratified squamous epithelium with abundant melanin deposition in the basal cell layer. Despite the increased melanin, the number of melanocytes is normal or may be somewhat reduced. In contrast to lentigo simplex, there is no elongation of rete ridges.

TREATMENT AND PROGNOSIS

No treatment is necessary for ephelides. The use of sunscreens can prevent the appearance of new freckles and help prevent the darkening of existing lesions.

ACTINIC LENTIGO (LENTIGO SOLARIS; SOLAR LENTIGO; AGE SPOT; LIVER SPOT; SENILE LENTIGO)

Actinic lentigo is a benign brown macule that results from chronic ultraviolet (UV) light damage to the skin. It is found in more than 90% of whites older than 70 years of age and rarely is seen before age 40. It does not occur within the mouth but is seen frequently on the facial skin. Persons who have facial ephelides (freckles) in childhood are more likely to develop actinic lentigines later in life. In a recent study of actinic lentigines in older whites, patients with multiple facial lesions typically were dark-skinned individuals who repeatedly received intermittent, intense sun exposure during their lifetime and whose facial lesions were preceded by the development of multiple actinic lentigines on the upper back.

CLINICAL FEATURES

Actinic lentigo is common on the dorsa of the hands, on the face, and on the arms of older whites (Figs. 10-33 and 10-34). It is typically multiple, but individual lesions appear as uniformly pigmented brown to tan macules with well-demarcated but irregular borders. Although the lesion may reach more than 1 cm in diameter, most examples are smaller than 5 mm. Adjacent lesions may coalesce, and new ones continuously arise with age. Unlike ephelides, no change in color intensity is seen after exposure to UV light.

HISTOPATHOLOGIC FEATURES

Rete ridges are elongated and club shaped in actinic lentigines, with thinning of the epithelium above the connective tissue papillae (Fig. 10-35). The ridges

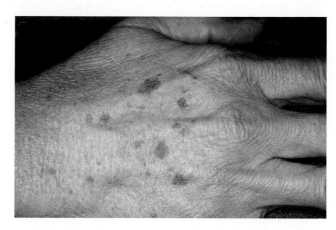

Fig. 10-33 **Actinic lentigines.** Multiple lesions on the sun-exposed skin of the hand of an older adult. Lesions are brown macules with irregular borders.

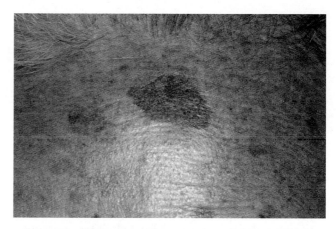

Fig. 10-34 **Actinic lentigo.** Large, flat, evenly pigmented lesion on the forehead of an older adult man.

sometimes seem to coalesce with one another. Within each rete ridge, melanin-laden basilar cells are intermingled with excessive numbers of heavily pigmented melanocytes.

TREATMENT AND PROGNOSIS

No treatment is required for actinic lentigo, except for aesthetic reasons. Lesions may be treated by cryotherapy, although hypopigmentation is a potential side effect. Laser therapy or intense pulsed light also can be effective. In addition, there is a wide range of topical therapies currently available, including hydroquinone, tretinoin, tazarotene, adapalene, and, more recently, a stable fixed combination of mequinol and tretinoin. Generally, sunscreens are recommended as preventive treatment and for maintenance of treatment success. Actinic lentigo does not undergo malignant transfor-

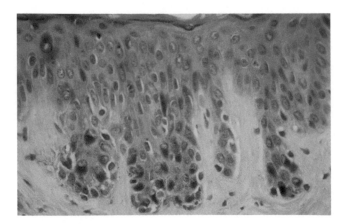

Fig. 10-35   Actinic lentigo. Rete ridges are elongated and occasionally intertwining. Pigmented melanocytes (with clear cytoplasm) are excessive and commingled with melanin-laden basilar cells.

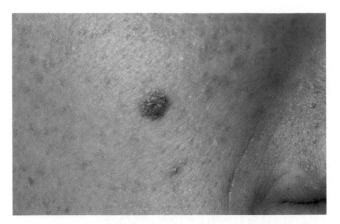

Fig. 10-36   Lentigo simplex. A sharply demarcated lesion of uniform brown coloration is seen on the midface.

mation; if removed, then it rarely recurs. New lesions, however, can arise in adjacent or distant skin at any time.

LENTIGO SIMPLEX

Lentigo simplex is one of several forms of benign cutaneous melanocytic hyperplasia of unknown cause. It usually occurs on skin that is not exposed to sunlight, but it may occur on any skin surface and at any age. Its color intensity does not change with variations in sun exposure. Lentigo simplex is darker in color than the common ephelis (see page 376). Ephelides, moreover, are found predominantly on sun-exposed skin, become more pronounced with increased sun exposure, and represent merely an increase in local melanin production rather than an increase in the number of productive melanocytes.

Some investigators believe that lentigo simplex represents the earliest stage of another common skin lesion, the melanocytic nevus (see page 382). Oral lesions have been reported, but they are rare and may be examples of the oral melanotic macule (see page 379).

CLINICAL FEATURES

Lentigo simplex usually occurs in children but may occur at any age. The typical lesion is a sharply demarcated macule smaller than 5 mm in diameter, with a uniformly tan to dark-brown color (Fig. 10-36). It is usually solitary, although some patients may have several lesions scattered on the skin of the trunk and extremities. Lentigo simplex reaches its maximum size in a matter of months and may remain unchanged indefinitely thereafter.

Clinically, individual lesions of lentigo simplex are indistinguishable from the nonelevated melanocytic nevus. With multiple lesions, conditions such as lentiginosis profusa, Peutz-Jeghers syndrome (see page 753), and the multiple lentigines or LEOPARD* syndrome must be considered as diagnostic possibilities.

HISTOPATHOLOGIC FEATURES

Lentigo simplex shows an increased number of benign melanocytes within the basal layer of the epidermis, and these often are clustered at the tips of the rete ridges. Abundant melanin is distributed among the melanocytes and basal keratinocytes, as well as within the papillary dermis in association with melanophages **(melanin incontinence).**

TREATMENT AND PROGNOSIS

Lentigo simplex may fade spontaneously after many years, but most lesions remain constant over time. Treatment is not required, except for aesthetic reasons. Conservative surgical excision is curative, and no malignant transformation potential has been documented for lesions not removed.

MELASMA (MASK OF PREGNANCY)

Melasma is an acquired, symmetrical hyperpigmentation of the sun-exposed skin of the face and neck. The cause is unknown, but it is classically associated with pregnancy. Exposure to exogenous estrogen and progesterone in the form of either oral contraceptives

---

*Lentigines (multiple), electrocardiographic abnormalities, ocular hypertelorism, pulmonary stenosis, abnormalities of genitalia, retardation of growth, and deafness (sensorineural).

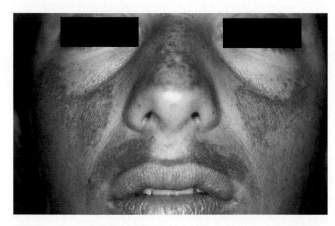

Fig. 10-37   Melasma. Diffuse hyperpigmentation of the facial skin in a pregnant woman.

or hormone replacement therapy also may cause melasma. Dark-complexioned persons—particularly Asian and Hispanic women—are more likely to develop this condition.

CLINICAL FEATURES

Melasma appears in adult women as bilateral light- to dark-brown cutaneous macules that vary in size from a few millimeters to more than 2 cm in diameter (Fig. 10-37). Lesions develop slowly with sun exposure and occur primarily on the midface, forehead, upper lip, chin, and (rarely) the arms. It is not unusual for the entire face to be involved. The pigmentation may remain faint or darken over time. Rarely, melasma is seen in men.

HISTOPATHOLOGIC FEATURES

Melasma is characterized by increased melanin deposition within an otherwise unremarkable epidermis. Pigment also may be seen within numerous melanophages in the dermis.

TREATMENT AND PROGNOSIS

Melasma is difficult to treat. First-line therapy typically consists of triple-combination topical therapy, such as Tri-Luma cream (a combination of 4% hydroquinone, 0.05% tretinoin, and 0.01% fluocinolone acetonide). Dual-ingredient topical agents (e.g., hydroquinone combined with glycolic acid or kojic acid) or single topical agents (e.g., 4% hydroquinone, 0.1% retinoic acid, or 20% azelaic acid) are alternatives for patients who are sensitive to triple-combination therapy. Options for second-line therapy include glycolic acid chemical peel, laser therapy, and dermabrasion,

although variable results have been reported with these alternative therapies. Because sun exposure is an important etiologic factor, sun avoidance and the use of sunscreens containing zinc oxide or titanium dioxide are crucial for effective clinical management. The lesions may resolve after parturition or after discontinuing oral contraceptives. There is no potential for malignant transformation.

ORAL MELANOTIC MACULE (FOCAL MELANOSIS)

The **oral melanotic macule** is a flat, brown, mucosal discoloration produced by a focal increase in melanin deposition and possibly a concomitant increase in the number of melanocytes. The cause remains unclear. Unlike the cutaneous ephelis (freckle), the melanotic macule is not dependent on sun exposure. Some authorities have questioned the purported lack of an association with actinic irradiation for the melanotic macule located on the vermilion border and prefer to consider it a distinct entity (**labial melanotic macule**). In one recent study of more than 773 solitary oral melanocytic lesions submitted to an oral pathology laboratory for histopathologic examination, oral and labial melanotic macules were the most common and comprised 86% of cases; oral and labial melanotic macules were encountered much more frequently than oral melanocytic nevi, melanoacanthomas, and melanomas.

CLINICAL FEATURES

The oral melanotic macule occurs at any age in both men and women; however, biopsy samples demonstrate a 2:1 female predilection. The average age of patients is 43 years at the time of diagnosis. The vermilion zone of the lower lip is the most common site of occurrence (33%), followed by the buccal mucosa, gingiva, and palate. Rare examples have been reported on the tongue in newborns.

The typical lesion appears as a solitary (17% are multiple), well-demarcated, uniformly tan to dark-brown, asymptomatic, round or oval macule with a diameter of 7 mm or smaller (Figs. 10-38 and 10-39). Occasional lesions may be blue or black. Lesions are not reported to enlarge after diagnosis, which suggests that the maximum dimension is achieved rather rapidly and remains constant thereafter.

HISTOPATHOLOGIC FEATURES

The oral melanotic macule is characterized by an increase in melanin (and perhaps melanocytes) in the basal and parabasal layers of an otherwise normal

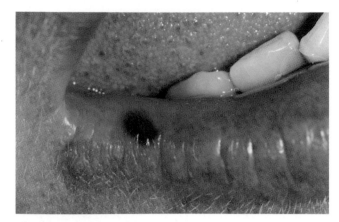

Fig. 10-38 Oral melanotic macule. A single small, uniformly pigmented brown macule on the lower lip vermilion.

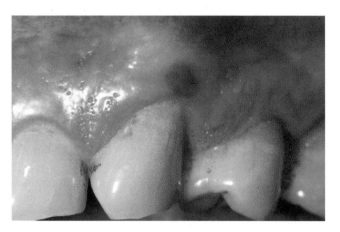

Fig. 10-39 Oral melanotic macule. A well-demarcated brown macule of the gingival mucosa.

stratified squamous epithelium (Fig. 10-40). Melanin also may be seen free or within melanophages in the subepithelial connective tissue **(melanin incontinence).** The lesion typically does not show elongated rete ridges like actinic lentigo (see page 377).

TREATMENT AND PROGNOSIS

Treatment is usually not required for the melanotic macule, except for aesthetic considerations. When necessary, excisional biopsy is the preferred treatment. Electrocautery, laser ablation, or cryosurgery is effective, but no tissue remains for histopathologic examination after these procedures. The intraoral melanotic macule has no malignant transformation potential, but an early melanoma can have a similar clinical appearance. For this reason, all oral pigmented macules of recent onset, large size, irregular pigmentation, unknown duration, or recent enlargement should be submitted for microscopic examination.

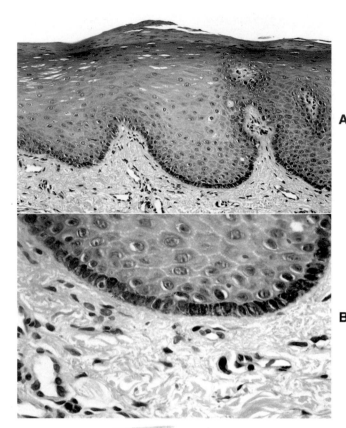

Fig. 10-40 Oral melanotic macule. A, Low-power view showing increased melanin pigmentation distributed along basal epithelial layer. **B,** High-power view showing granular brown melanin pigment in the basilar cells.

On occasion, flat pigmented lesions are encountered that are clinically and microscopically similar to the melanotic macule; however, these lesions represent a sign of systemic or genetic disease or may be a consequence of the use of certain medications. A list of these conditions is shown in Box 10-1.

ORAL MELANOACANTHOMA (MELANOACANTHOSIS)

Oral melanoacanthoma is a benign, relatively uncommon acquired pigmentation of the oral mucosa characterized by dendritic melanocytes dispersed throughout the epithelium. The lesion appears to be a reactive process; in some cases an association with trauma has been reported. Oral melanoacanthoma appears to be unrelated to the melanoacanthoma of skin, which most authorities believe represents a variant of seborrheic keratosis.

CLINICAL FEATURES

Oral melanoacanthoma is seen almost exclusively in blacks, shows a female predilection, and is most common during the third and fourth decades of life.

Associations with Melanin Pigmentation of Oral Mucosa

PHYSIOLOGIC OR SYNDROMIC ASSOCIATIONS

- Racial or physiologic pigmentation
- Peutz-Jeghers syndrome
- McCune-Albright syndrome
- LEOPARD syndrome (lentiginosis profusa, no intra-oral melanosis)
- Laugier-Hunziker syndrome
- Cronkhite-Canada syndrome
- Bloom syndrome
- Dunnigan syndrome
- Dyskeratosis congenita
- Endocrine candidiasis syndrome
- Incontinentia pigmenti
- Oculo-cerebro-cutaneous syndrome
- Rothmund-Thomson syndrome
- Trisomy 14 mosaicism
- Unusual facies, vitiligo, spastic paraplegia syndrome
- Xeroderma pigmentosum
- Addison's disease
- Neurofibromatosis type I

CHRONIC TRAUMA OR IRRITATION OR ENVIRONMENTAL POLLUTANT

- Chronic mucosal trauma or irritation (chronic cheek bite)
- Chronic autoimmune disease (erosive lichen planus, pemphigoid)
- Smoker's melanosis
- Yusho (chronic exposure to high levels of polychlorinated biphenyls [PCBs])

SYSTEMIC MEDICATIONS

- Chloroquine and other quinine derivatives
- Phenolphthalein
- Estrogen
- AIDS-related medications

From Bouquot JE, Nikai H: Lesions of the oral cavity. In Gnepp DR: *Diagnostic surgical pathology of the head and neck*, pp 141-238, Philadelphia, 2001, WB Saunders.

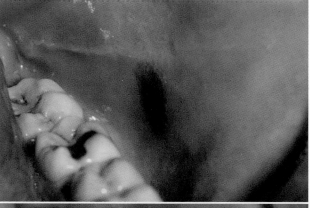
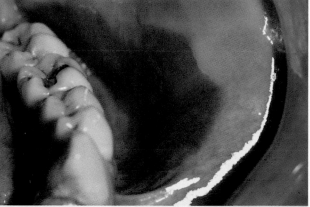
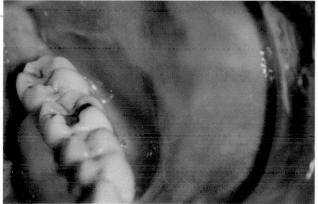

Fig. 10-41   Oral melanoacanthoma. A, Smooth, darkly pigmented macule of the buccal mucosa in a young adult. **B,** Appearance of the lesion 2 months later showing dramatic enlargement. **C,** Resolution of the lesion 3 months after incisional biopsy. *(From Park SK, Neville BW: AAOMP case challenge: rapidly enlarging pigmented lesion of the buccal mucosa, J Contemp Dent Pract 3:69-73, 2002.)*

The buccal mucosa is the most common site of occurrence. The lips, palate, gingiva, and alveolar mucosa also may be involved. Most patients exhibit solitary lesions, although bilateral or multifocal involvement is possible as well. Oral melanoacanthomas typically are asymptomatic; however, pain, burning, and pruritus have been reported in a few unusual cases. The lesion is smooth, flat or slightly raised, and dark-brown to black in color (Fig. 10-41). Lesions often demonstrate a rapid increase in size, and they occasionally reach a diameter of several centimeters within a period of a few weeks.

HISTOPATHOLOGIC FEATURES

The oral melanoacanthoma is characterized by numerous benign dendritic melanocytes (cells that are normally confined to the basal cell layer) scattered

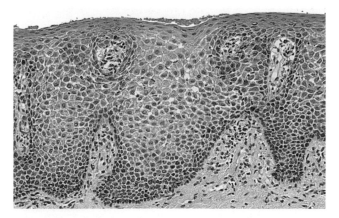

Fig. 10-42   Oral melanoacanthoma. Medium-power photomicrograph showing acanthosis of the epithelium. Spongiosis is demonstrated by intercellular spaces between the keratinocytes.

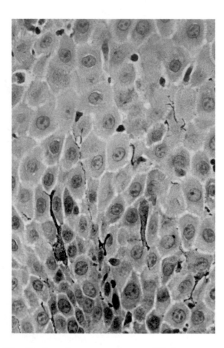

Fig. 10-43   Oral melanoacanthoma. High-power view showing numerous dendritic melanocytes extending between the spinous epithelial cells.

throughout the lesional epithelium (Figs. 10-42 and 10-43). Basal layer melanocytes are also present in increased numbers. Spongiosis and mild acanthosis are typically noted. In addition, eosinophils and a mild to moderate chronic inflammatory cell infiltrate are usually seen within the underlying connective tissue.

TREATMENT AND PROGNOSIS

Because of the alarming growth rate of oral melanoacanthoma, incisional biopsy is usually indicated to rule out the possibility of melanoma. Once the diagnosis has

> ### Box 10-2
>
> ## Types of Developmental Nevi
>
> - Epidermal nevus
> - Nevus sebaceus
> - Nevus flammeus (see page 543)
> - Basal cell nevus (nevoid basal cell carcinoma) (see page 688)
> - White sponge nevus (see page 743)

been established, no further treatment is necessary. In several instances, lesions have undergone spontaneous resolution after incisional biopsy. Recurrence or development of additional lesions has been reported only rarely. There is no potential for malignant transformation.

ACQUIRED MELANOCYTIC NEVUS (NEVOCELLULAR NEVUS; MOLE)

The generic term *nevus* refers to malformations of the skin (and mucosa) that are congenital or developmental in nature. Nevi may arise from the surface epithelium or any of a variety of underlying connective tissues. The most commonly recognized nevus is the **acquired melanocytic nevus,** or common **mole**—so much so that the simple term *nevus* is often used synonymously for these pigmented lesions. However, many other developmental nevi also are recognized (Box 10-2).

The acquired melanocytic nevus represents a benign, localized proliferation of cells from the neural crest, often called *nevus cells.* Although there is little debate as to their neural crest origin and their ability to produce melanin, various authorities are divided on the issue of whether these cells represent melanocytes or are merely "first cousins" of melanocytes. These melanocytic cells migrate to the epidermis during development, and lesions may first appear shortly after birth. The acquired melanocytic nevus is probably the most common of all human "tumors," and white adults have an average of 10 to 40 cutaneous nevi per person. Intraoral lesions occur but are not common.

CLINICAL FEATURES

Acquired melanocytic nevi begin to develop on the skin during childhood, and most cutaneous lesions are present before 35 years of age. They occur in both men and women, although women usually have a few more than men. Racial differences are seen. Whites have more nevi than Asians or blacks. Most lesions are distributed above the waist, and the head and neck region is a common site of involvement.

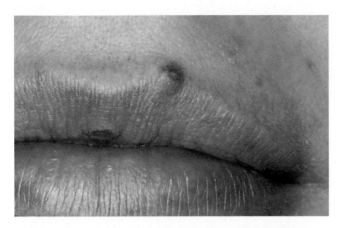

Fig. 10-44   Melanocytic (intradermal) nevus. A well-demarcated, dome-shaped papule is seen at the edge of the vermilion border of the upper lip.

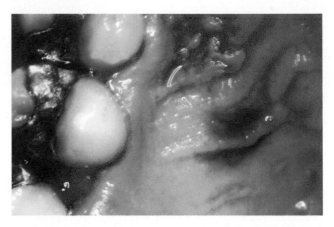

Fig. 10-46   Intramucosal melanocytic nevus. Pigmented lesion of the anterior hard palate. *(Courtesy of Dr. Lewis Claman.)*

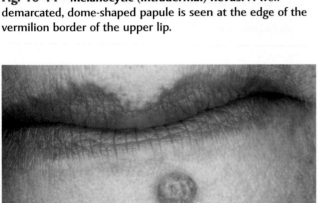

Fig. 10-45   Melanocytic (intradermal) nevus. Small nodule on the skin of the lower lip.

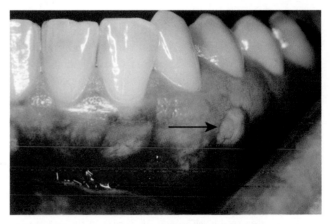

Fig. 10-47   Intramucosal melanocytic nevus. This intramucosal nevus *(arrow)* of the mandibular gingiva is nonpigmented. *(Courtesy of Dr. John Lenox.)*

Acquired melanocytic nevi evolve through several clinical stages, which tend to correlate with specific histopathologic features. The earliest presentation (known microscopically as a **junctional nevus**) is that of a sharply demarcated, brown or black macule, typically less than 6 mm in diameter. Although this lesional appearance may persist into adulthood, more often the nevus cells proliferate over a period of years to produce a slightly elevated, soft papule with a relatively smooth surface (**compound nevus**). The degree of pigmentation becomes less; most lesions appear brown or tan.

As time passes, the nevus gradually loses its pigmentation, the surface may become somewhat papillomatous, and hairs may be seen growing from the center (**intradermal nevus**) (Figs. 10-44 and 10-45). However, the nevus usually remains less than 6 mm in diameter. Ulceration is not a feature unless, for example, the nevus is situated in an area where a belt or bra strap traumatizes it easily. Throughout the

adult years, many acquired melanocytic nevi will involute and disappear; therefore, fewer of these lesions can be detected in older persons.

Intraoral melanocytic nevi are distinctly uncommon. Most arise on the palate, mucobuccal fold, or gingiva, although any oral mucosal site may be affected (Fig. 10-46). Intraoral melanocytic nevi have an evolution and appearance similar to skin nevi, although mature lesions typically do not demonstrate a papillary surface change. More than one in five intraoral nevi lack clinical pigmentation (Fig. 10-47). Approximately two thirds of intraoral examples are found in females; the average age at diagnosis is 35 years.

HISTOPATHOLOGIC FEATURES

The acquired melanocytic nevus is characterized by a benign, unencapsulated proliferation of small, ovoid cells (nevus cells). The lesional cells have small, uniform

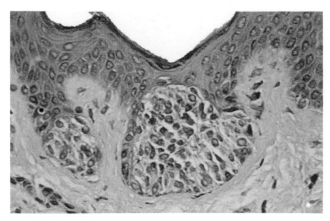

Fig. 10-48 Junctional nevus. Nests of melanocytic nevus cells along the basal layer of the epithelium.

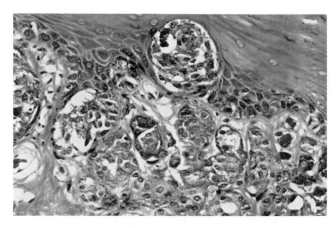

Fig. 10-49 Compound nevus. High-power view showing nests of pigmented nevus cells within the epithelium and the superficial lamina propria.

nuclei and a moderate amount of eosinophilic cytoplasm, with indistinct cell boundaries. These cells demonstrate a variable capacity to produce melanin, with the pigment primarily evident in the superficial aspects of the lesion. Nevus cells typically lack the dendritic processes that melanocytes possess. A characteristic microscopic feature is that the superficial nevus cells tend to be organized into small, round aggregates (*thèques*).

Melanocytic nevi are classified histopathologically according to their stage of development, which is reflected by the relationship of the nevus cells to the surface epithelium and underlying connective tissue. In the early stages, thèques of nevus cells are found only along the basal cell layer of the epithelium, especially at the tips of the rete ridges. Because the lesional cells are found at the junction between the epithelium and the connective tissue, this stage is known as a **junctional nevus** (Fig. 10-48). As the nevus cells proliferate, groups of cells begin to drop off into the underlying dermis or lamina propria. Because cells are now present along the junctional area and within the underlying connective tissue, the lesion then is called a **compound nevus** (Fig. 10-49).

In the later stages, nests of nevus cells are no longer found within the epithelium but are found only within the underlying connective tissue. Because of the connective tissue location of the lesional cells, on the skin this stage is called an **intradermal nevus.** The intraoral counterpart is called an **intramucosal nevus** (Fig. 10-50). Zones of differentiation often are seen throughout the lesion. The superficial cells typically appear larger and epithelioid, with abundant cytoplasm, frequent intracellular melanin, and a tendency to cluster into thèques. Nevus cells of the middle portion of the lesion have less cytoplasm, are seldom pigmented, and appear much like lymphocytes. Deeper nevus cells

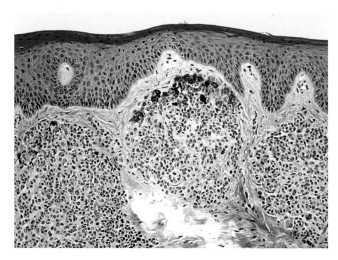

Fig. 10-50 Intramucosal nevus. Collections of melanocytic nevus cells within the lamina propria.

appear elongated and spindle shaped, much like Schwann cells or fibroblasts. Some authorities classify these variations as *type A* (epithelioid), *type B* (lymphocyte-like), and *type C* (spindle shaped) nevus cells.

Most intraoral melanocytic nevi are classified microscopically as *intramucosal nevi*. However, this probably reflects the age (average, 35 years) at which most oral nevi undergo biopsy and diagnosis, because these lesions would have earlier evolved through junctional and compound stages.

TREATMENT AND PROGNOSIS

No treatment is indicated for a cutaneous melanocytic nevus unless it is cosmetically unacceptable, is chronically irritated by clothing, or shows clinical evidence of a change in size or color. By midlife, cutaneous

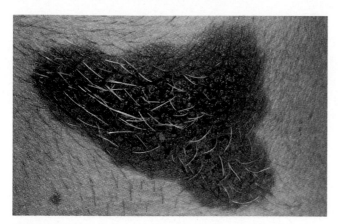

Fig. 10-51   Congenital melanocytic nevus. Pigmented lesion of the skin showing hypertrichosis.

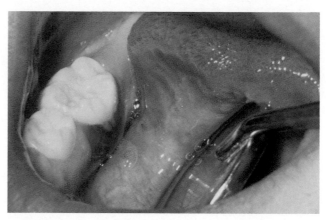

Fig. 10-52   Congenital melanocytic nevus. Deeply pigmented lesion of the lingual mandibular gingiva in a 3-year-old child.

melanocytic nevi tend to regress; by age 90, very few remain. If removal is elected, then conservative surgical excision is the treatment of choice; recurrence is unlikely.

At least some skin **melanomas** arise from long-standing or irritated nevi of the skin. Overall, the risk of transformation of a particular acquired melanocytic nevus to melanoma is approximately 1 in 1 million. However, because oral melanocytic nevi clinically can mimic an early melanoma, it is generally advised that biopsy be performed for all unexplained pigmented oral lesions, especially because of the extremely poor prognosis for oral melanoma discovered in its later stages.

VARIANTS OF MELANOCYTIC NEVUS

CONGENITAL MELANOCYTIC NEVUS

Congenital melanocytic nevus affects approximately 1% of newborns in the United States. This entity is usually divided into two types: (1) small (<20 cm in diameter) and (2) large (>20 cm in diameter). Approximately 15% of congenital nevi are found in the head and neck area, although intraoral involvement is quite rare.

CLINICAL FEATURES

The small congenital melanocytic nevus may be similar in appearance to an acquired melanocytic nevus, but it is frequently larger in diameter (Figs. 10-51 and 10-52). The large congenital lesion classically appears as a brown to black plaque, usually with a rough surface or multiple nodular areas. However, the clinical appearance often changes with time. Early lesions are flat and light tan, becoming elevated, rougher, and darker with age. A common feature is the presence of **hypertricho-**

sis (excess hair) within the lesion, which may become more prominent with age **(giant hairy nevus).** A very large congenital nevus sometimes may be referred to as **bathing trunk nevus** or **garment nevus,** because it gives the appearance of the patient wearing an article of clothing.

HISTOPATHOLOGIC FEATURES

The histopathologic appearance of the congenital melanocytic nevus is similar to that of the acquired melanocytic nevus, and some small congenital nevi cannot be distinguished microscopically from the acquired nevus. Both congenital and acquired types are composed of nevus cells, which may have a junctional, compound, or intradermal pattern. The congenital nevus is usually of the compound or intradermal type. In contrast to the acquired melanocytic nevus, the congenital nevus often shows extension of nevus cells into the deeper levels of the dermis, with "infiltration" of cells between collagen bundles. In addition, congenital nevus cells often are seen intermingled with neurovascular bundles in the reticular dermis and surrounding normal adnexal skin structures (e.g., hair follicles, sebaceous glands). Large congenital melanocytic nevi may show extension of nevus cells into the subcutaneous fat.

TREATMENT AND PROGNOSIS

Many congenital melanocytic nevi are excised for aesthetic purposes. In addition, 3% to 15% of large congenital nevi may undergo malignant transformation into melanoma. Therefore, whenever feasible, these lesions should be removed completely by conservative surgical excision. Close follow-up is required for lesions not removed. Patients with multiple large congenital nevi also are at risk for developing neurocutaneous

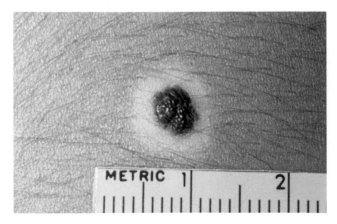

Fig. 10-53   Halo nevus. Elevated brown lesion of the skin showing surrounding depigmentation.

melanosis, a rare congenital syndrome in which patients may develop melanotic neoplasms of the central nervous system (CNS), including meningeal melanosis or melanoma. Unfortunately, no effective therapy is currently available for patients with symptomatic neurocutaneous melanosis.

HALO NEVUS

Halo nevus is a melanocytic nevus with a pale hypopigmented border or "halo" of the surrounding epithelium, apparently as a result of nevus cell destruction by the immune system. The halo develops because the immune cells also attack the melanocytes adjacent to the nevus. The cause of the immune attack is unknown, but regression of the nevus usually results. Interestingly, the development of multiple halo nevi has been seen in patients who have had a recent excision of a melanoma.

CLINICAL FEATURES

The halo nevus is typically an isolated phenomenon associated with a preexisting acquired melanocytic nevus. It is most common on the skin of the trunk during the second decade of life. The lesion typically appears as a central pigmented papule or macule, surrounded by a uniform, 2- to 3-mm zone of hypopigmentation (Fig. 10-53). Sometimes this peripheral zone is much wider.

HISTOPATHOLOGIC FEATURES

Histopathologically, the halo nevus differs from the routine acquired melanocytic nevus only in the presence of an intense chronic inflammatory cell infiltrate, which surrounds and infiltrates the nevus cell population.

TREATMENT AND PROGNOSIS

Usually, treatment is not required for halo nevus because it eventually will regress entirely. If treatment is elected, then conservative surgical removal is curative and recurrence is unlikely.

SPITZ NEVUS (BENIGN JUVENILE MELANOMA; SPINDLE AND EPITHELIOID CELL NEVUS)

Spitz nevus is an uncommon type of melanocytic nevus that shares many histopathologic features with melanoma. It was, in fact, first described as a *juvenile melanoma*. The distinctly benign biologic behavior of the lesion was first emphasized by Spitz in 1948. The first oral example was not reported until 1990.

CLINICAL FEATURES

The Spitz nevus typically develops on the skin of the extremities or the face during childhood. It appears as a solitary, dome-shaped, pink to reddish-brown papule, usually smaller than 6 mm in greatest diameter. The young age at presentation and the relatively small size of the Spitz nevus are useful features to help distinguish it from melanoma.

HISTOPATHOLOGIC FEATURES

The Spitz nevus has the overall microscopic architecture of a compound nevus, showing a zonal differentiation from the superficial to deep aspects of the lesion and good symmetry. Lesional cells are either spindle shaped or plump (epithelioid), and the two types often are intermixed. The epithelioid cells may be multinucleated and appear somewhat bizarre, often lacking cell cohesiveness. Mitotic figures, all normal in appearance, may be seen in the superficial aspects of the lesion. Ectatic superficial blood vessels, which probably impart much of the reddish color of some lesions, are seen frequently. The nevocellular nature of the lesional cells is demonstrated by immunohistochemical reactivity for S-100 protein and neuron-specific enolase.

TREATMENT AND PROGNOSIS

Conservative surgical excision is the treatment of choice for a Spitz nevus. There is little chance of recurrence after the nevus is removed.

BLUE NEVUS (DERMAL MELANOCYTOMA; JADASSOHN-TIÈCHE NEVUS)

Blue nevus is an uncommon, benign proliferation of dermal melanocytes, usually deep within subepithelial connective tissue. Two major types of blue nevus

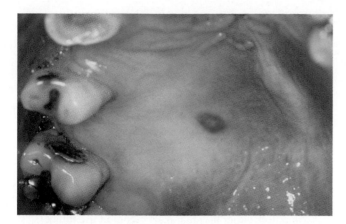

Fig. 10-54 Blue nevus. A well-circumscribed, deep-blue macular lesion is seen on palatal mucosa.

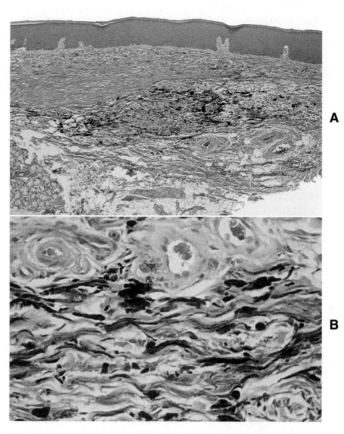

Fig. 10-55 Blue nevus. A, Abundant melanin is seen within spindle-shaped melanocytes located relatively deep within the lamina propria and parallel to the surface epithelium. **B,** High-power view showing heavily pigmented spindle-shaped cells.

are recognized: (1) the **common** blue nevus and (2) the **cellular** blue nevus. The common blue nevus is the second most frequent melanocytic nevus encountered in the mouth. The blue color of this melanin-producing lesion can be explained by the **Tyndall effect,** which relates to the interaction of light with particles in a colloidal suspension. In the case of a blue nevus, the melanin particles are deep to the surface, so that the light reflected back has to pass through the overlying tissue. Colors with long wavelengths (reds and yellows) tend to be more readily absorbed by the tissues; the shorter-wavelength blue light is more likely to be reflected back to the observer's eyes.

CLINICAL FEATURES

The common blue nevus may affect any cutaneous or mucosal site, but it has a predilection for the dorsa of the hands and feet, the scalp, and the face. Mucosal lesions may involve the oral mucosa, conjunctiva, and, rarely, sinonasal mucosa. Oral lesions are found almost always on the palate. The lesion usually occurs in children and young adults, and a female predilection is seen. It appears as a macular or dome-shaped, blue or blue-black lesion smaller than 1 cm in diameter (Fig. 10-54).

The cellular blue nevus is much less common and usually develops during the second to fourth decades of life, but it may be congenital. More than 50% of cellular blue nevi arise in the sacrococcygeal or buttock region, although they may be seen on other cutaneous or mucosal surfaces. Clinically, this nevus appears as a slow-growing, blue-black papule or nodule that sometimes attains a size of 2 cm or more. Occasional lesions remain macular.

HISTOPATHOLOGIC FEATURES

Histopathologically, the common blue nevus consists of a collection of elongated, slender melanocytes with branching dendritic extensions and numerous melanin globules. These cells are located deep within the dermis or lamina propria (Fig. 10-55) and usually align themselves parallel to the surface epithelium. The cellular blue nevus appears as a well-circumscribed, highly cellular aggregation of plump, melanin-producing spindle cells within the dermis or submucosa. More typical pigmented dendritic spindle cells are seen at the periphery of the lesional tissue. Occasionally, a blue nevus is found in conjunction with an overlying melanocytic nevus, in which case the term **combined nevus** is used.

TREATMENT AND PROGNOSIS

If clinically indicated, conservative surgical excision is the treatment of choice for the blue nevus of the skin. Recurrence is minimal with this treatment. Malignant transformation to melanoma is rare but has been reported. However, because an oral blue nevus clinically can mimic an early melanoma, it is usually advisable to perform a biopsy of intraoral pigmented lesions, especially because of the extremely poor prognosis for oral melanoma (see page 433).

LEUKOPLAKIA (LEUKOKERATOSIS; ERYTHROLEUKOPLAKIA)

Oral **leukoplakia** (*leuko* = white; *plakia* = patch) is defined by the World Health Organization (WHO) as "a white patch or plaque that cannot be characterized clinically or pathologically as any other disease." The term is strictly a clinical one and does not imply a specific histopathologic tissue alteration.

The definition of leukoplakia is unusual in that it makes the diagnosis dependent not so much on definable appearances as on the *exclusion* of other entities that appear as oral white plaques. Such lesions as lichen planus, morsicatio (chronic cheek nibbling), frictional keratosis, tobacco pouch keratosis, nicotine stomatitis, leukoedema, and white sponge nevus must be ruled out before a clinical diagnosis of leukoplakia can be made. As with most oral white lesions, the clinical color results from a thickened surface *keratin* layer, which appears white when wet, or a thickened *spinous* layer, which masks the normal vascularity (redness) of the underlying connective tissue.

Although leukoplakia is not associated with a specific histopathologic diagnosis, it is typically considered to be a precancerous or premalignant lesion. When the outcome of a large number of leukoplakic lesions is reviewed, the frequency of transformation into malignancy is greater than the risk associated with normal or unaltered mucosa. Because there is considerable misunderstanding of this concept, Box 10-3 provides definitions that are used throughout the chapter.

INCIDENCE AND PREVALENCE

Although leukoplakia is considered a premalignant lesion, the use of the clinical term in no way suggests that histopathologic features of epithelial dysplasia are present in all lesions. Dysplastic epithelium or frankly invasive carcinoma is, in fact, found in only 5% to 25% of biopsy samples of leukoplakia. The precancerous nature of leukoplakia has been established, not so much on the basis of this association or on the fact that more than one third of oral carcinomas have leukoplakia in close proximity, as on the results derived from clinical investigations that monitored numerous leukoplakic lesions for long periods. The latter studies suggest a malignant transformation potential of 4% (estimated lifetime risk). Specific clinical subtypes or phases, men-

---

Box 10-3

Precancer Terminology Used in This Text

- **Precancerous lesion (precancer, premalignancy).** A benign, morphologically altered tissue that has a greater than normal risk of malignant transformation.
- **Precancerous condition.** A disease or patient habit that does not necessarily alter the clinical appearance of local tissue but is associated with a greater than normal risk of precancerous lesion or cancer development in that tissue.
- **Malignant transformation potential.** The risk of cancer being present in a precancerous lesion or condition, either at initial diagnosis or in the future (usually expressed in percentages). The potential for mucosa without precancerous lesions or conditions is called *normal*.
- **Relative risk.** A specific epidemiologic measure of the association between exposure to a particular factor and the risk of acquiring a disease, expressed as a ratio of the incidence or prevalence of a disease among those exposed and those not exposed to the factor.

---

tioned later, are associated with potential rates as high as 47%. These figures may be artificially low because many lesions are surgically removed at the beginning of follow-up.

Leukoplakia is by far the most common oral precancer, representing 85% of such lesions. Based on pooled, weighted data from previously reported studies, the worldwide prevalence of leukoplakia has been estimated to fall within a range of 1.5% to 4.3%. There is a strong male predilection (70%), except in regional populations in which women use tobacco products more than men. A slight decrease in the proportion of affected males, however, has been noted over the past half century. The disease is diagnosed more frequently now than in the past, probably because of an enhanced awareness on the part of health professionals (rather than because of a real increase in frequency).

CAUSE

The cause of leukoplakia remains unknown, although hypotheses abound.

TOBACCO

The habit of tobacco smoking appears most closely associated with leukoplakia development. More than 80% of patients with leukoplakia are smokers. When large groups of adults are examined, smokers are much more likely to have leukoplakia than nonsmokers. Heavier smokers have greater numbers of lesions and

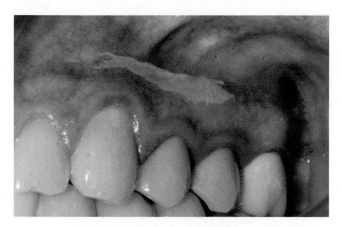

Fig. 10-56   Sanguinaria-associated keratosis. Thin white plaque on the maxillary alveolar mucosa.

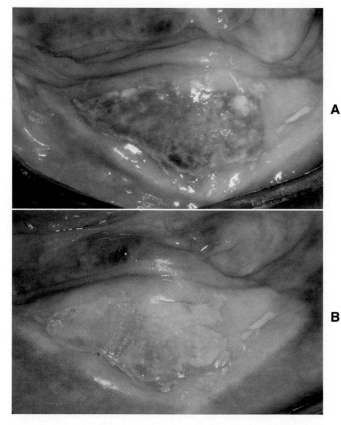

Fig. 10-57   Candidal leukoplakia. A, Well-circumscribed red and white plaque on the anterior floor of mouth, which showed candidal infestation on cytology smears. **B,** After antifungal therapy, the erythematous component resolved, resulting in a homogeneous white plaque.

larger lesions than do light smokers, especially after many years of tobacco use. In addition, a large proportion of leukoplakias in persons who stop smoking either disappear or become smaller within the first year of habit cessation.

The smokeless tobacco habit produces a somewhat different result. It often leads to a clinically distinctive white oral plaque called **tobacco pouch keratosis** (see page 398). This lesion probably is not a true leukoplakia.

ALCOHOL

Alcohol, which seems to have a strong synergistic effect with tobacco relative to oral cancer production, has not been associated with leukoplakia. People who excessively use mouth rinses with an alcohol content greater than 25% may have grayish buccal mucosal plaques, but these are not considered true leukoplakia.

SANGUINARIA

Persons who use toothpaste or mouth rinses containing the herbal extract, sanguinaria, may develop a true leukoplakia. This type of leukoplakia (**sanguinaria-associated keratosis**) is usually located in the maxillary vestibule or on the alveolar mucosa of the maxilla (Fig. 10-56). More than 80% of individuals with vestibular or maxillary alveolar leukoplakia have a history of using products that contain sanguinaria, compared with 3% of the normal population.

The affected epithelium may demonstrate dysplasia identical to that seen in other leukoplakias, although the potential for the development of cancer is uncertain. The leukoplakic plaque may not disappear even after the patient stops using the product; some lesions have persisted for years afterwards.

ULTRAVIOLET RADIATION

Ultraviolet radiation is accepted as a causative factor for leukoplakia of the lower lip vermilion. This is usually associated with actinic cheilosis (see page 405). Immunocompromised persons, especially transplant patients, are especially prone to the development of leukoplakia and squamous cell carcinoma of the lower lip vermilion.

MICROORGANISMS

Several microorganisms have been implicated in the cause of leukoplakia. *Treponema pallidum*, for example, produces glossitis in the late stage of syphilis, with or without the arsenic therapy in popular use before the advent of modern antibiotics. The tongue is stiff and frequently has extensive dorsal leukoplakia.

Tertiary syphilis is rare today, but oral infections by another microorganism, *Candida albicans*, are not. *Candida* organisms can colonize the superficial epithelial layers of the oral mucosa, often producing a thick, granular plaque with a mixed white and red coloration (Fig. 10-57). The terms **candidal leukoplakia** and

candidal hyperplasia have been used to describe such a lesion, and biopsy may show dysplastic or hyperplastic histopathologic changes. It is not known whether this yeast produces dysplasia or secondarily infects previously altered epithelium, but some of these lesions disappear or become less extensive, even less severely dysplastic, after antifungal therapy. Tobacco smoking may cause the leukoplakia and also predispose the patient to develop candidiasis.

Human papillomavirus (HPV), in particular subtypes 16 and 18, has been identified in some oral leukoplakias. These are the same HPV subtypes associated with uterine cervical carcinoma and a subset of oral squamous cell carcinomas. Such viruses, unfortunately, also can be found in normal oral epithelial cells, and so their presence is perhaps no more than coincidental. It may be significant, however, that HPV-16 has been shown to induce dysplasia-like changes in normally differentiating squamous epithelium in an otherwise sterile *in vitro* environment.

TRAUMA

Several keratotic lesions, which until recently had been viewed as variants of leukoplakia, are now considered not to be precancers. Nicotine stomatitis is a generalized white palatal alteration that seems to be a hyperkeratotic response to the heat generated by tobacco smoking (usually a pipe), rather than a response to the carcinogens within the smoke (see page 403). Its malignant transformation potential is so low as to be about the same as that of normal palatal mucosa.

In addition, chronic mechanical irritation can produce a white lesion with a roughened keratotic surface, termed **frictional keratosis.** Although the resulting lesion is clinically similar to true leukoplakia, such a lesion is now thought to be no more than a normal hyperplastic response (similar to a callus on the skin). Keratoses of this type are readily reversible after elimination of the trauma, and obviously traumatic lesions such as linea alba (see page 285), morsicatio (see page 286), and toothbrush gingival "abrasion" have not been documented to have transformed into malignancy. In addition, the presence of dentures or broken and missing teeth has not been shown to increase the cancer risk. Alveolar ridge keratoses (Fig. 10-58)—involving the retromolar pad or crest of an edentulous alveolar ridge—represent another form of frictional keratosis caused by masticatory function or denture trauma. Frictional keratosis should be differentiated from the group of oral precancers.

CLINICAL FEATURES

Leukoplakia usually affects persons older than 40 years of age. Prevalence increases rapidly with age, especially for males, and as many as 8% of men older than

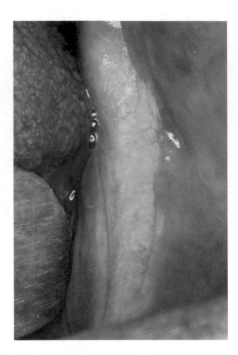

Fig. 10-58 Frictional keratosis. There is a rough, hyperkeratotic change to the posterior mandibular alveolar ridge ("alveolar ridge keratosis"), because this area is now edentulous and becomes traumatized from mastication. Such frictional keratoses should resolve when the source of irritation is eliminated and should not be mistaken for true leukoplakia.

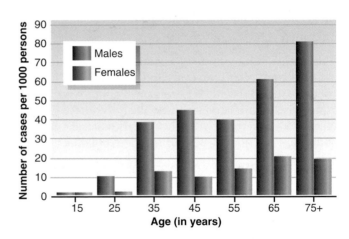

Fig. 10-59 Leukoplakia. Age-specific prevalence (number of new cases per 1000 adults examined at various ages) for oral leukoplakia demonstrates increasing prevalence with increasing age, especially for men.

70 years of age reportedly are affected (Fig. 10-59). The average age of affected persons (60 years) is similar to the average age for patients with oral cancer; however, in some studies, leukoplakia has been found to occur about 5 years earlier (on average) than oral squamous cell carcinoma.

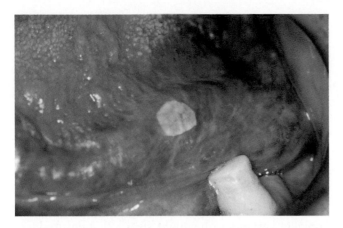

Fig. 10-60   Early or thin leukoplakia. This early lesion of the ventral tongue is smooth, white, and well demarcated from the surrounding normal mucosa.

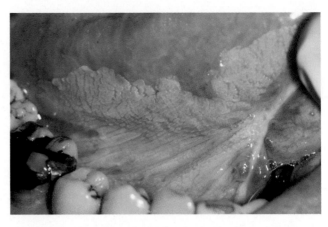

Fig. 10-61   Homogeneous or thick leukoplakia. A diffuse, corrugated white patch on the right ventral surface of the tongue and floor of mouth.

Approximately 70% of oral leukoplakias are found on the lip vermilion, buccal mucosa, and gingiva. Lesions on the tongue, lip vermilion, and oral floor, however, account for more than 90% of those that show dysplasia or carcinoma. Individual lesions may have a varied clinical appearance and tend to change over time. Early and mild lesions appear as slightly elevated gray or gray-white plaques, which may appear somewhat translucent, fissured, or wrinkled and are typically soft and flat (Fig. 10-60). They usually have sharply demarcated borders but occasionally blend gradually into normal mucosa.

Mild or **thin leukoplakia,** which seldom shows dysplasia on biopsy, may disappear or continue unchanged. For tobacco smokers who do not reduce their habit, as many as two thirds of such lesions slowly extend laterally, become thicker, and acquire a distinctly white appearance. The affected mucosa may become leathery to palpation, and fissures may deepen and become more numerous. At this stage or phase, the lesion is often called a **homogeneous** or **thick leukoplakia** (Figs. 10-61 and 10-62). Most thick, smooth lesions remain indefinitely at this stage. Some, perhaps as many as one third, regress or disappear; a few become even more severe, develop increased surface irregularities, and are then called **granular** or **nodular leukoplakia** (Figs. 10-63 and 10-64). Some lesions demonstrate sharp or blunt projections and have been called **verrucous** or **verruciform leukoplakia** (Fig. 10-65).

A special high-risk form of leukoplakia, **proliferative verrucous leukoplakia** (PVL), is characterized by the development of multiple keratotic plaques with roughened surface projections (Fig. 10-66). The relationship of PVL to cases described as *verrucous leukoplakia* is uncertain. The multiple PVL plaques tend to

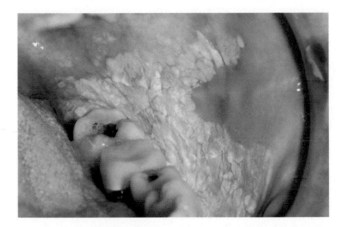

Fig. 10-62   Homogeneous or thick leukoplakia. Extensive buccal mucosa lesion with an uneven whiteness and fissures. Moderate epithelial dysplasia was noted on histopathologic evaluation, and squamous cell carcinoma later developed in this area.

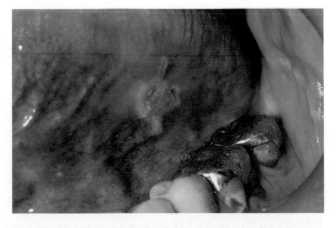

Fig. 10-63   Granular leukoplakia. Focal leukoplakic lesion with a rough, granular surface on the posterior lateral border of the tongue. Biopsy of the lesion revealed an early invasive squamous cell carcinoma.

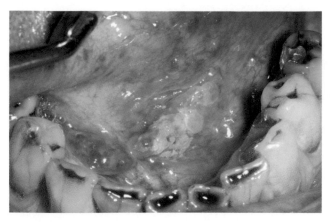

Fig. 10-64   Granular leukoplakia. Irregular white patch in the floor of the mouth of a heavy smoker. Early invasive squamous cell carcinoma was found on biopsy.

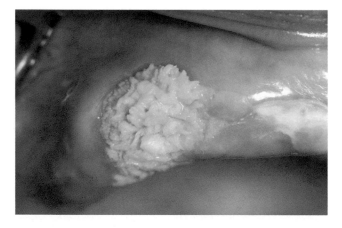

Fig. 10-65   Verruciform leukoplakia. Exophytic papillary lesion of the anterior maxillary alveolar ridge. Biopsy revealed a well-differentiated squamous cell carcinoma.

slowly spread and involve additional oral mucosal sites. The gingiva frequently is involved, although other sites may be affected as well. Although the lesions typically begin as simple, flat hyperkeratoses that are indistinguishable from ordinary leukoplakic lesions, PVL exhibits persistent growth, eventually becoming exophytic and verrucous in nature. As the lesions progress, they may go through a stage indistinguishable from **verrucous carcinoma** (see page 422), but they later usually develop dysplastic changes and transform into full-fledged **squamous cell carcinoma** (usually within 8 years of initial PVL diagnosis). These lesions rarely regress despite therapy. PVL is unusual among the leukoplakia variants in having a strong female predilection (1:4 male-to-female ratio) and minimal association with tobacco use.

Leukoplakia may become dysplastic, even invasive, with no change in its clinical appearance. However, some lesions eventually demonstrate scattered patches of redness, called **erythroplakia** (see page 397). Such areas usually represent sites in which epithelial cells are so immature or atrophic that they can no longer produce keratin. This intermixed red-and-white lesion, called **erythroleukoplakia** or **speckled leukoplakia**, represents a pattern of leukoplakia that frequently reveals advanced dysplasia on biopsy (Fig. 10-67).

Of course, many leukoplakic lesions are a mixture of the previously mentioned phases or subtypes. Because it is important to perform a biopsy of the lesional site with the greatest potential to contain dysplastic cells, Figs. 10-68 and 10-69 provide a clinical and graphic representation of such a lesion. Biopsy sites should be taken from areas with clinical lesional appearances that are most similar to those toward the right in Fig. 10-69.

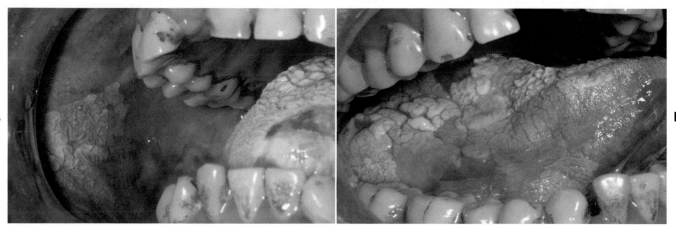

A   B

Fig. 10-66   Proliferative verrucous leukoplakia (PVL). A, Large, diffuse, and corrugated white lesions of the buccal mucosa and tongue. **B,** Same patient showing the extensive thickened and fissured alteration of the tongue.

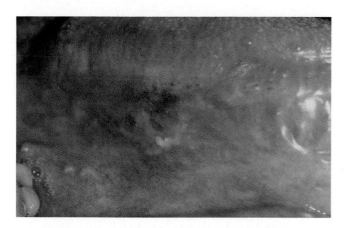

Fig. 10-67   Erythroleukoplakia. Mixed red-and-white lesion of the lateral border of the tongue. Biopsy revealed carcinoma *in situ.*

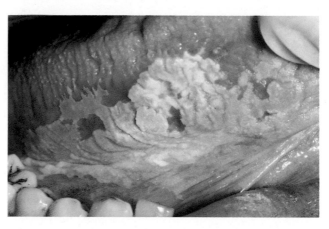

Fig. 10-68   Leukoplakia. Extensive ventral and lateral tongue lesion containing multiple areas representing various possible phases or clinical appearances (compare with Fig. 10-69).

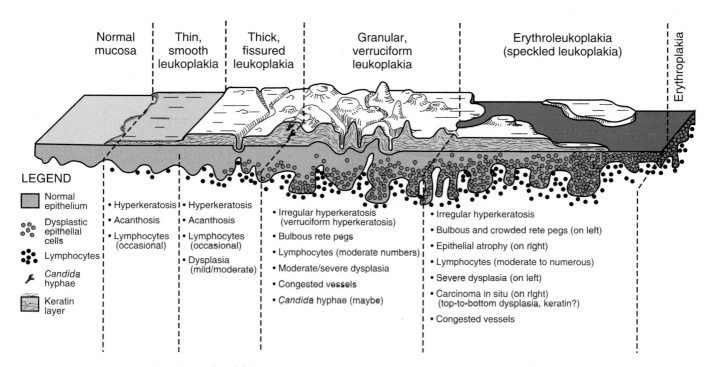

Fig. 10-69   Leukoplakia. Composite representation of the various phases or clinical appearances of oral leukoplakia, with anticipated underlying histopathologic changes. Lesions have increasing malignant transformation potentials as their appearances approach those toward the right. *(From Bouquot JE, Gnepp DR: Laryngeal precancer—a review of the literature, commentary and comparison with oral leukoplakia,* Head Neck *13:488-497, 1991.)*

In recent years, attempts have been made to develop new techniques to aid in the identification and diagnosis of premalignant and malignant oral lesions. However, at the present time, careful clinical evaluation with directed conventional biopsy remains the best and most accurate means of assessing oral leukoplakic lesions (see Fig. 10-101). In their excellent article, Alexander, Wright, and Thiebaud support this approach when they state, "Noninvasive screening techniques such as cytologic testing (including brush biopsy) and lesion staining with supravital dyes have many pitfalls and should not be considered as substitutes for biopsy when there is concern about malignancy."

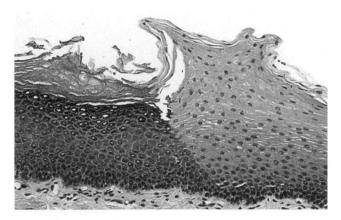

Fig. 10-70   Hyperorthokeratosis. This medium-power photomicrograph demonstrates hyperorthokeratosis with a well-defined granular cell layer on the left side. The right side shows normal parakeratinized epithelium without a granular cell layer.

HISTOPATHOLOGIC FEATURES

Microscopically, leukoplakia is characterized by a thickened keratin layer of the surface epithelium **(hyperkeratosis),** with or without a thickened spinous layer **(acanthosis).** Some leukoplakias demonstrate surface hyperkeratosis but show atrophy or thinning of the underlying epithelium. Frequently, variable numbers of chronic inflammatory cells are noted within the subjacent connective tissue.

The keratin layer may consist of parakeratin **(hyperparakeratosis),** orthokeratin **(hyperorthokeratosis),** or a combination of both (Fig. 10-70). With parakeratin, there is no granular cell layer and the epithelial nuclei are retained in the keratin layer. With orthokeratin, the epithelium demonstrates a granular cell layer and the nuclei are lost in the keratin layer.

Verrucous leukoplakia has papillary or pointed surface projections, varying keratin thickness, and broad, blunted rete ridges. It may be difficult to differentiate it from early verrucous carcinoma.

PVL shows a variable microscopic appearance, depending on the stage of the lesions. Early PVL appears as a benign hyperkeratosis that is indistinguishable from other simple leukoplakic lesions. With time, the condition progresses to a papillary, exophytic proliferation that is similar to localized lesions of verrucous leukoplakia (or what is sometimes termed **verrucous hyperplasia**). In later stages this papillary proliferation exhibits downgrowth of well-differentiated squamous epithelium with broad, blunt rete ridges. This epithelium demonstrates invasion into the underlying lamina propria; at this stage it is indistinguishable from verrucous carcinoma. In the final stages the invading epithelium becomes less differentiated,

transforming into a full-fledged squamous cell carcinoma. Because of the variable clinical and histopathologic appearance of PVL, careful correlation of the clinical and microscopic findings is required for diagnosis.

Most leukoplakic lesions demonstrate no dysplasia on biopsy. Evidence of epithelial dysplasia is found in only 5% to 25% of cases if all oral sites are considered. When present, these dysplastic changes typically begin in the basilar and parabasilar portions of the epithelium. The more dysplastic the epithelium becomes, the more the atypical epithelial changes extend to involve the entire thickness of the epithelium. The histopathologic alterations of dysplastic epithelial cells are similar to those of squamous cell carcinoma and may include the following:

- Enlarged nuclei and cells
- Large and prominent nucleoli
- Increased nuclear-to-cytoplasmic ratio
- Hyperchromatic (excessively dark-staining) nuclei
- Pleomorphic (abnormally shaped) nuclei and cells
- Dyskeratosis (premature keratinization of individual cells)
- Increased mitotic activity (excessive numbers of mitoses)
- Abnormal mitotic figures (tripolar or star-shaped mitoses or mitotic figures above the basal layer)

In addition, histomorphologic alterations of dysplastic epithelium are evident at low-power magnification, including the following:

- Bulbous or teardrop-shaped rete ridges
- Loss of polarity (lack of progressive maturation toward the surface)
- Keratin or epithelial pearls (focal, round collections of concentrically layered keratinized cells)
- Loss of typical epithelial cell cohesiveness

When epithelial dysplasia is present, the pathologist provides a descriptive adjective relating to its "severity" or intensity. **Mild epithelial dysplasia** refers to alterations limited principally to the basal and parabasal layers (Fig. 10-71). **Moderate epithelial dysplasia** demonstrates involvement from the basal layer to the midportion of the spinous layer (Fig. 10-72). **Severe epithelial dysplasia** demonstrates alterations from the basal layer to a level above the midpoint of the epithelium (Fig. 10-73). Sometimes dysplasia will be seen to extend down the duct of a minor salivary gland, especially in lesions of the floor of the mouth (Fig. 10-74).

When the entire thickness of the epithelium is involved, the term **carcinoma *in situ*** is used. Carcinoma *in situ* is defined as dysplastic epithelial cells that extend from the basal layer to the surface of the mucosa

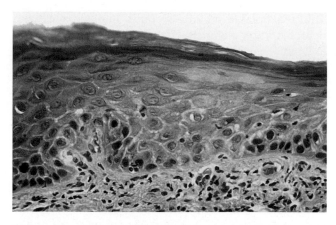

Fig. 10-71   Mild epithelial dysplasia. Hyperchromatic and slightly pleomorphic nuclei are noted in the basal and parabasal cell layers of this stratified squamous epithelium.

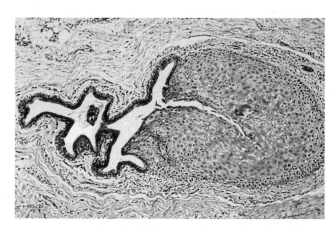

Fig. 10-74   Ductal dysplasia. Salivary gland duct exhibiting squamous metaplasia and dysplasia that originated from an overlying surface epithelial dysplasia.

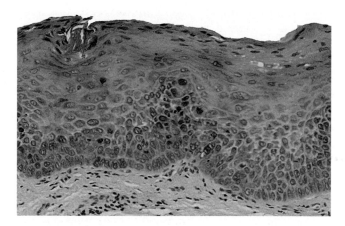

Fig. 10-72   Moderate epithelial dysplasia. Dysplastic changes extend to the midpoint of the epithelium and are characterized by nuclear hyperchromatism, pleomorphism, and cellular crowding.

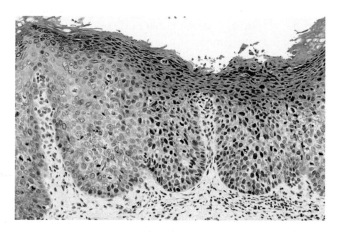

Fig. 10-75   Carcinoma *in situ*. Dysplastic changes extend throughout the entire thickness of the epithelium.

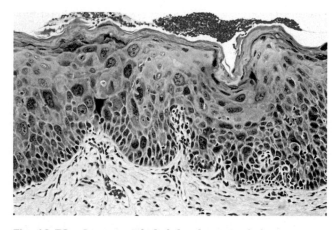

Fig. 10-73   Severe epithelial dysplasia. Epithelium exhibiting marked pleomorphism, hyperchromatism, and scattered mitotic figures. Atypical cells involve most of the epithelial thickness.

("top-to-bottom" change) (Fig. 10-75). There may or may not be a thin layer of keratin on the surface. The epithelium may be hyperplastic or atrophic. Some authorities consider this entity to be a precancerous lesion; others believe that it represents a genuine malignancy discovered before invasion. Regardless of the concept preferred, the important feature of carcinoma *in situ* is that no invasion has occurred, despite the fact that the atypical epithelial cells look exactly like those of squamous cell carcinoma (see page 419). Without invasion, the most serious aspect of malignant transformation, metastasis, cannot occur. In this light, it should be mentioned that keratin pearl formation is rare in carcinoma *in situ* and may indicate the presence of a focus of invasive squamous cell carcinoma in the adjacent tissue.

Sometimes dysplasia will be seen extending down the ducts of the minor salivary glands, especially in lesions in the floor of the mouth. When ductal dysplasia occurs in a precancerous surface dysplasia, the recurrence rate is increased. The depth of ductal dysplasia does not appear to be a significant factor.

TREATMENT AND PROGNOSIS

Because leukoplakia represents a clinical term only, the first step in treatment is to arrive at a definitive histopathologic diagnosis. Therefore, a biopsy is mandatory and will guide the course of treatment. Tissue obtained for biopsy, moreover, should be taken from the clinically most "severe" areas of involvement (with features toward the right side of Fig. 10-69). Multiple biopsies of large or multiple lesions may be required.

Leukoplakia exhibiting moderate epithelial dysplasia or worse warrants complete destruction or removal, if feasible. The management of leukoplakia exhibiting less severe change is guided by the size of the lesion and the response to more conservative measures, such as smoking cessation.

Complete removal can be accomplished with equal effectiveness by surgical excision, electrocautery, cryosurgery, or laser ablation. Long-term follow-up after removal is extremely important because recurrences are frequent and because additional leukoplakias may develop. This is especially true for the verruciform or granular types, 83% of which recur and require additional removal or destruction. Leukoplakia not exhibiting dysplasia often is not excised, but clinical evaluation every 6 months is recommended because of the possibility of progression toward epithelial dysplasia. Additional biopsies are recommended if smoking continues or if the clinical changes increase in severity.

Overall, 4% of oral leukoplakias become squamous cell carcinoma after diagnosis, according to follow-up studies. As previously stated, this figure, and those mentioned later, may be artificially low because so many monitored cases are treated early in an investigation. Not to do so, of course, raises certain ethical questions; hence, more accurate data may never become available. Other confounding features of leukoplakia follow-up investigations include variations in diagnostic definitions and periods of observation. Typically, the latter extend for 5 to 10 years, but several studies have observed patients with lesions for more than 20 years—one study for more than half a century.

With these caveats in mind, follow-up investigations have demonstrated that carcinomatous transformation usually occurs 2 to 4 years after the onset of the white plaque, but it may occur within months or after decades. Transformation does not appear to depend on the age of the affected patient.

Although dysplasia may be present in any leukoplakia, each clinical appearance or phase of leukoplakia has a different malignant transformation potential.

Thin leukoplakia seldom becomes malignant without demonstrating a clinical change. Homogeneous, thick leukoplakia undergoes malignant transformation in 1% to 7% of cases. Once the surface becomes granular or verruciform, the malignant transformation potential becomes 4% to 15%. Erythroleukoplakia carries an average transformation potential of 28%, but the rates have varied from 18% to 47% in different investigations.

The increased frequency of transformation of the different phases of leukoplakia is related closely to the degree of dysplasia present. The greater the clinical severity, the greater the chance of significant dysplasia and malignant transformation. Estimates of the malignant potential for histopathologically proven dysplastic lesions are, unfortunately, open to question because so many are excised completely. Thus their true biologic behavior in an unaltered state may not be appreciated fully. With this understanding, however, lesions diagnosed as moderate and severe dysplasia reportedly have malignant transformation potentials of 4% to 11% and 20% to 35%, respectively. Cancers from dysplastic lesions usually develop within 3 years of the dysplasia diagnosis, but they can occur much later. Additionally, one in three dysplasias will recur after complete removal.

In addition to the clinical and histopathologic appearance at diagnosis, several factors may increase the risk for cancer in leukoplakic lesions. These include persistence over several years, occurrence in a female patient, occurrence in a nonsmoker, and occurrence on the oral floor or ventral tongue. Leukoplakia of the latter two locations has shown malignant transformation in 16% to 39% of all cases and 47% of those occurring in females.

There is much interest in the identification of chromosomal, genetic, and molecular alterations that may aid in predicting the risk of malignant transformation for oral leukoplakia. Cytogenetic studies have suggested that loss of heterozygosity (LOH) of chromosome arms 3p and 9p is associated with increased risk of malignant transformation, and additional LOH at 4q, 8p, 11q, 13q, and 17p further increases this risk. Additional alterations such as microsatellite instability (insertion or deletion of base pairs in repetitive stretches of short DNA sequences), increased telomerase activity (important for cellular longevity), and changes in expression of various molecular markers (e.g., p53 and other markers of apoptosis, p16 and other markers of cell cycle regulation, epidermal growth factor receptor [EGFR], matrix metalloproteinases, vascular endothelial growth factor) have been found to correlate with histopathologic progression in oral premalignant lesions. Despite these interesting observations, many of the previously discussed analyses require fresh tissue or labor-intensive techniques that are not widely available, which limits their use in routine clinical practice. Thus histopathologic grading of dysplasia remains the standard method for predicting the risk of progression to malignancy.

Some smoking-related leukoplakias with no or minimal dysplasia may disappear or diminish in size within 3 months after the patient stops smoking. Thus habit cessation is recommended. Chemoprevention also may be useful, but it remains primarily experimental. Isotretinoin (13-*cis*-retinoic acid, a form of vitamin A)—alone or in combination with betacarotene—has been reported to reduce or eliminate some leukoplakic lesions in short-term studies. Toxic reactions to systemic retinoid agents are frequent, however, as is lesion recurrence after the conclusion of therapy. Agents such as bleomycin, lycopene, and cyclooxgenase-2 (COX-2) inhibitors have been investigated as potential chemopreventive agents as well. However, to date there is insufficient evidence from well-designed clinical trials to support the effectiveness of such medical therapies in treating oral dysplasia or preventing the progression of oral dysplasia to squamous cell carcinoma.

ERYTHROPLAKIA (ERYTHROPLASIA; ERYTHROPLASIA OF QUEYRAT)

As with leukoplakia, **erythroplakia** is defined as a red patch that cannot be clinically or pathologically diagnosed as any other condition. Queyrat originally used the term *erythroplasia* to describe a precancerous red lesion that develops on the penis. Oral erythroplakia is clinically and histopathologically similar to the genital process. Almost all true erythroplakias demonstrate significant epithelial dysplasia, carcinoma *in situ*, or invasive squamous cell carcinoma. The causes of erythroplakia are unknown, but they are presumed to be the same as those associated with invasive squamous cell carcinoma of the mouth (see page 409).

The point prevalence rate (number of persons with active lesions at a given point in time) of oral erythroplakia has been estimated as 1 per 2500 adults. The reported prevalence among several large-scale epidemiologic surveys—most of which were conducted in South and Southeast Asia—ranges from 0.02% to 0.83%. The incidence is not known, but the average annual incidence for microscopically proven oral carcinoma *in situ*, which represents the great majority of erythroplakias, has been estimated to be 1.2 per 100,000 population (2.0 in males and 0.5 in females) in the United States.

Erythroplakia also may occur in conjunction with leukoplakia (see page 388) and has been found concurrently with a large proportion of early invasive oral carcinomas. Although erythroplakia is less common

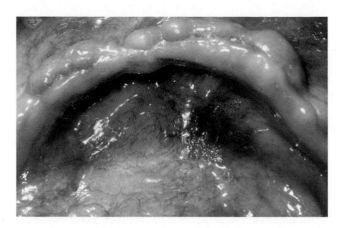

Fig. 10-76   Erythroplakia. An erythematous macular lesion is seen on the right floor of the mouth with no associated leukoplakia. Biopsy showed early invasive squamous cell carcinoma.

than leukoplakia, it has a much greater potential to be severely dysplastic at the time of biopsy or to develop invasive malignancy at a later time.

CLINICAL FEATURES

Erythroplakia is predominantly a disease of middle-aged to older adults with no significant gender predilection. In the United States, a peak prevalence of 65 to 74 years has been reported. In India, the peak prevalence is in a somewhat younger age range of 45 to 54 years. The floor of mouth, tongue, and soft palate are the most common sites of involvement, and multiple lesions may be present.

The altered mucosa appears as a well-demarcated erythematous macule or plaque with a soft, velvety texture (Figs. 10-76 and 10-77). It is usually asymptomatic and may be associated with an adjacent leukoplakia (**erythroleukoplakia**) (see Fig. 10-67). Nonspecific mucositis, candidiasis, psoriasis, or vascular lesions may clinically mimic erythroplakia, and biopsy often is required to distinguish between them.

HISTOPATHOLOGIC FEATURES

According to one large clinicopathologic investigation, 90% of erythroplakic lesions histopathologically represent severe epithelial dysplasia (see page 394), carcinoma *in situ* (see page 394), or superficially invasive squamous cell carcinoma (see page 419). The epithelium shows a lack of keratin production and often is atrophic, but it may be hyperplastic. This lack of keratinization, especially when combined with epithelial thinness, allows the underlying microvasculature to show through, thereby explaining the red color. The

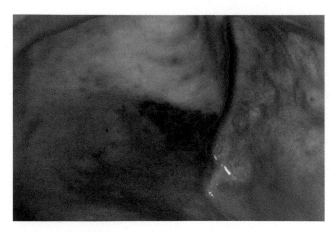

Fig. 10-77 Erythroplakia. Well-circumscribed red patch on the posterior lateral hard and soft palate. *(From Neville BW, Chi AC, Jeter M: Diagnostic challenge: a red lesion on the palate, J Am Dent Assoc 137:1537-1538, 2006.)*

underlying connective tissue often demonstrates chronic inflammation.

TREATMENT AND PROGNOSIS

Red lesions of the oral mucosa, especially those of the oral floor and ventral or lateral tongue, should be viewed with suspicion, and a biopsy should be performed. If a source of irritation can be identified and removed, then biopsy of such a lesion may be delayed for 2 weeks to allow a clinically similar inflammatory lesion time to regress.

As with leukoplakia, the treatment of erythroplakia is guided by the definitive diagnosis obtained by biopsy. Lesions exhibiting moderate dysplasia or worse must be removed completely or destroyed by the methods used for leukoplakia (see page 396). It is best, however, to preserve most of the specimen for microscopic examination because of the possibility that a focal invasive carcinoma might be missed in the initial biopsy material. Recurrence and multifocal oral mucosal involvement are common with erythroplakia; hence, long-term follow-up is suggested for treated patients.

SMOKELESS TOBACCO USE AND SMOKELESS TOBACCO KERATOSIS (SNUFF POUCH; SNUFF DIPPER'S LESION; TOBACCO POUCH KERATOSIS; SPIT TOBACCO KERATOSIS)

The three main types of smokeless tobacco used in the United States include chewing tobacco, moist snuff, and dry snuff. Moist snuff is the most popular, with a 77% increase in sales over the past 15 years, whereas dry snuff and chewing tobacco have been declining in popularity. The increase in popularity of moist snuff may be related in part to the convenience of small, prepackaged pouches that can be used discreetly. Chewing tobacco often is used by men in conjunction with outdoor activities, and dry snuff is used primarily by women in the southern United States. Smokeless tobacco use also has been referred to as **spit tobacco use**—a term preferred by the U.S. federal government in its attempt to diminish the appeal of the habit.

As part of its *Healthy People 2010* objectives, the U.S. Department of Health and Human Services has set a goal to reduce the prevalence of smokeless tobacco use among U.S. adults from 2.3% to 0.4%. At present, the proportion of adult men in the United States who regularly use smokeless tobacco approximates 4.5%. Among male high school students, the proportion is as high as 20% to 27% in some Southeastern and Midwestern states. However, over the past few decades, smokeless tobacco use has declined, particularly among young men 18 to 24 years of age. The habit is started early in life, usually at 8 to 14 years of age, and rarely is initiated after 20 years of age. A national survey detected smokeless tobacco lesions of all types in 1.5% (2.9% in males, 0.1% in females) of U.S. adolescents and teenagers.

In India, smokeless tobacco may be combined in a quid with other products, such as betel leaves, areca nuts, and slaked lime. Oral lesions associated with betel quid use are described separately (see the discussion of oral submucous fibrosis on page 401).

CLINICAL FEATURES

Several health and addiction hazards may be associated with the use of smokeless tobacco because of the ready absorption of nicotine and other molecules through the oral mucosa. A variety of local oral alterations also are found in chronic users. One of the most common local changes is a characteristic painless loss of gingival tissues in the area of tobacco contact (Fig. 10-78). This gingival recession may be accompanied by destruction of the facial surface of the alveolar bone and correlates well with the quantity of daily use and the duration of the smokeless tobacco habit. Although the association between smokeless tobacco and gingival recession is well known, there is some variability across studies regarding the association between smokeless tobacco and periodontal bone loss. Researchers have suggested that this variability may be related to the specific type of smokeless tobacco used or possible confounding by concurrent cigarette smoking.

Dental caries also has been reported to be more prevalent in smokeless tobacco users, perhaps because of the high sugar content of some brands; other reports

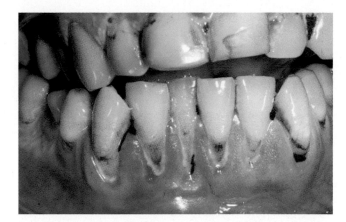

Fig. 10-78 Smokeless tobacco-related gingival recession. Extensive recession of the anterior mandibular facial gingiva.

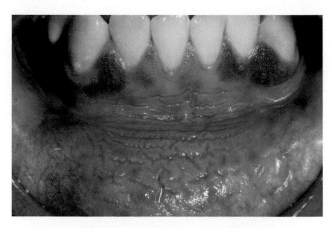

Fig. 10-79 Tobacco pouch keratosis, mild. A soft, fissured, gray-white lesion of the lower labial mucosa located in the area of chronic snuff placement. The gingival melanosis is racial pigmentation and not associated with the keratosis.

dispute caries susceptibility. Long-term use may lead to localized or generalized wear of occlusal and incisal surfaces, especially in those using the product in dusty environments. A brown-black extrinsic tobacco stain is typically found on the enamel and cementum surfaces of the teeth adjacent to the tobacco. In addition, halitosis is a frequent finding in chronic users.

A characteristic white plaque, the **smokeless tobacco keratosis,** also is produced on the mucosa in direct contact with snuff or chewing tobacco. In Western cultures, it affects 15% of chewing tobacco users and 60% of snuff users, if mild examples are included. The development of this lesion is most strongly influenced by habit duration and also by the brand of tobacco used, early onset of smokeless tobacco use, total hours of daily use, amount of tobacco consumed daily, and number of sites routinely used for tobacco placement. Smokeless tobacco keratosis in many Western cultures is usually noted in young adult men and in men older than 65 years of age, because the habit has not been popular among the generation that is now middle-aged. In some populations, the prevalence of smokeless tobacco keratosis (and the smokeless tobacco habit) is most frequent among older women. Individual lesions begin to develop shortly after heavy tobacco use begins, and new lesions seldom arise in persons with a long history of use. The lesion is confined to areas in direct contact with spit tobacco. It is typically a thin, gray or gray-white, almost "translucent," plaque with a border that blends gradually into the surrounding mucosa (Fig. 10-79). Sometimes mild peripheral erythema is present.

The altered mucosa typically has a soft velvety feel to palpation, and stretching of the mucosa often reveals a distinct "pouch" **(snuff pouch, tobacco pouch)** caused by flaccidity in the chronically stretched tissues in the area of tobacco placement. Because the tobacco is not in the mouth during a clinical examination, the usually stretched mucosa appears fissured or rippled, in a fashion resembling the sand on a beach after an ebbing tide. Similar alterations can occur when other bulky materials are held chronically in the vestibule (e.g., hard candy, sunflower seeds, beef jerky). Induration, ulceration, and pain are not associated with this lesion.

Smokeless tobacco keratosis usually takes 1 to 5 years to develop. Once it occurs, however, the keratosis typically remains unchanged indefinitely unless the daily tobacco contact time is altered. In some cases the white lesion gradually becomes thickened to the point of appearing leathery or nodular (Fig. 10-80).

HISTOPATHOLOGIC FEATURES

The histopathologic appearance of smokeless tobacco keratosis is not specific. The squamous epithelium is hyperkeratinized and acanthotic, with or without intracellular vacuolization or "edema" of glycogen-rich superficial cells. Parakeratin **chevrons** may be seen as pointed projections above or within superficial epithelial layers (Fig. 10-81). Increased subepithelial vascularity and vessel engorgement often are seen. In some cases an unusual deposition of amorphous eosinophilic material is noted within the subjacent connective tissue and salivary glands (Fig. 10-82). Epithelial dysplasia is uncommon in smokeless tobacco keratosis and, when present, is typically mild. Occasionally, however, significant dysplasia or squamous cell carcinoma may be present.

TREATMENT AND PROGNOSIS

Chronic use of smokeless tobacco in the United States is considered to be carcinogenic, although the risk is less than that associated with cigarette smoking and

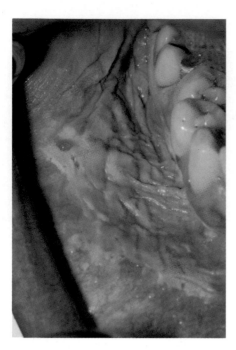

Fig. 10-80   Tobacco pouch keratosis, severe. A somewhat leathery, white, fissured plaque of the posterior mandibular vestibule, which is located in the area of chronic chewing tobacco placement.

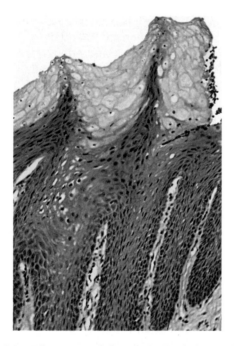

Fig. 10-81   Tobacco pouch keratosis. Epithelium exhibiting acanthosis, hyperparakeratosis, and "chevron" formation.

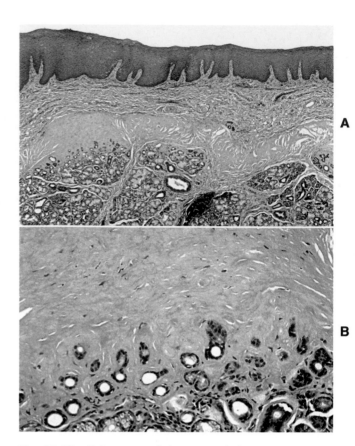

Fig. 10-82   Tobacco pouch keratosis. A, Low-power view showing mild hyperkeratosis and acanthosis. Note linear deposition of amorphous, eosinophilic material in the lamina propria above the minor salivary glands. **B,** Higher-power view of the amorphous material.

alcohol abuse. Fortunately, the clinical appearance of smokeless tobacco keratosis is distinct enough and the malignant transformation potential is low enough so that biopsy is needed for only the more severe lesions (i.e., those demonstrating an intense whiteness, a gran-ular or verruciform clinical appearance, ulceration, mass formation, induration, or hemorrhage). Obviously, treatment would then depend on the histopathologic diagnosis. Without microscopic evidence of dysplasia or malignancy, keratoses are not treated. Alternating the tobacco-chewing sites between the left and right sides will eliminate or reduce the keratotic lesion but may result in epithelial alteration or gingival and periodontal difficulties in two sites rather than one.

Squamous cell carcinoma (see page 410) related to smokeless tobacco use typically develops after a long latency period of several decades. In a recent review of case control studies performed in the United States and Western Europe, the reported relative risk of developing oral cancer from chronic smokeless tobacco use ranged from less than 2 to 26, with lower risk associated with chewing tobacco and moist snuff and higher risk associated with dry snuff. Recent studies from Sweden, however, have failed to show an increased risk for users of Swedish moist snuff (also known as *snus*). Many of the early reports of malignant

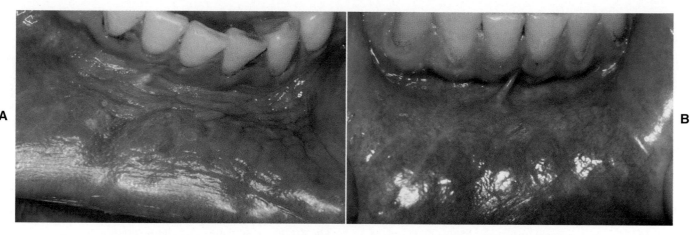

A

B

Fig. 10-83   **Tobacco pouch keratosis. A,** Moderately severe lesion of the lower anterior vestibule and lip in a 15-year-old male subject, which demonstrates a gray-white surface change and fissuring. The patient had been placing snuff in the area for several years. **B,** Two weeks after cessation of the tobacco habit, the mucosa has returned to an almost normal appearance.

transformation of snuff-related lesions described lesions among female dry snuff users in the southern United States. Only recently have epidemiologic studies tried to separate the various types of smokeless tobacco with respect to their carcinogenic potential. Squamous cell carcinoma is the most common malignancy resulting from this habit, but an uncommon low-grade oral malignancy, **verrucous carcinoma ("snuff dipper's" cancer),** also may be associated with smokeless tobacco use (see page 422).

Significantly, habit cessation leads to a normal mucosal appearance (usually within 2 weeks) in 98% of smokeless tobacco keratosis lesions that are not intensely white (Fig. 10-83). A lesion that remains after 6 weeks without smokeless tobacco contact should be considered to be a true leukoplakia and should be sampled for biopsy and managed accordingly.

ORAL SUBMUCOUS FIBROSIS

Oral submucous fibrosis is a chronic, progressive, scarring, high-risk precancerous condition of the oral mucosa seen primarily in the Indian subcontinent, Southeast Asia, Taiwan, southern China, and Papua New Guinea. It has been linked to the chronic placement in the mouth of a betel quid or *paan* and is found in 0.4% of India's villagers. The quid consists typically of a nut from the areca palm tree and slaked lime, usually with tobacco and sometimes with sweeteners and condiments, wrapped in a betel leaf. The slaked lime acts to release alkaloids (arecoline, arecaidine, guvacine, and guvacoline) from the areca nut, producing a feeling of euphoria and well-being in the user. Villagers habitu-

ally chew betel quids from an early age, frequently for 16 to 24 hours daily. Commercial freeze-dried betel quid substitutes (such as *pan masala, gutkha,* and *mawa*), conveniently packaged in portable sachets, have become increasingly popular because they have a long shelf life and do not require preparation before use. These products contain a higher concentration of areca nut and appear to cause oral submucous fibrosis more rapidly than conventionally prepared betel quid.

The condition is characterized by a mucosal rigidity of varied intensity caused by a fibroelastic hyperplasia and modification of the superficial connective tissue. The submucosal changes may be a response to the areca nut, whereas the epithelial alterations and carcinogenesis may be the result of tobacco contact. However, several studies suggest that even betel quid without tobacco may be carcinogenic, albeit probably less so than when combined with tobacco. Nutritional deficiency increases the risk and severity of fibrosis, and some persons seem to have a genetic predisposition to it. A few individuals have developed the disease after only a few contacts with areca nut.

The underlying pathogenetic mechanism for oral submucous fibrosis is hypothesized to involve the role of the areca nut in disrupting the homeostatic equilibrium between synthesis and degradation of the extracellular matrix. Cytokines and growth factors produced by activated inflammatory cells may promote fibrosis by inducing proliferation of fibroblasts, upregulating collagen synthesis, and downregulating collagenase production. In addition, considerable amounts of copper have been found in areca nut products; copper may upregulate collagen production by increasing the

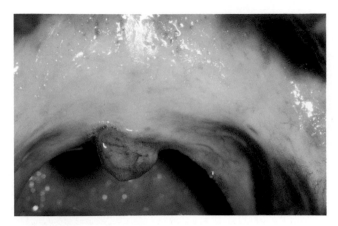

Fig. 10-84   Oral submucous fibrosis. Pallor and fibrosis of the soft palate in a betel quid chewer. The uvula has retained its normal color.

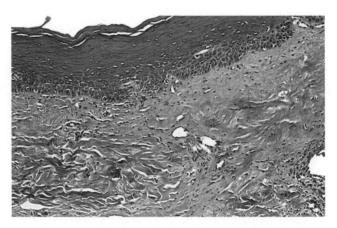

Fig. 10-85   Oral submucous fibrosis. Mucosal biopsy exhibiting hyperparakeratosis, basilar hyperplasia, and fibrosis in the lamina propria.

activity of the enzyme lysyl oxidase involved in collagen synthesis and cross-linking.

CLINICAL FEATURES

Oral submucous fibrosis often is first noted in young adult betel quid users, whose chief complaint is an inability to open the mouth **(trismus),** often accompanied by mucosal pain while eating spicy foods. An interincisal distance of less than 20 mm is considered severe; in advanced cases, the jaws may actually be inseparable. Females are more susceptible to these changes than males.

Vesicles, petechiae, melanosis, xerostomia, and a generalized oral burning sensation **(stomatopyrosis)** are usually the first signs and symptoms. The buccal mucosa, retromolar area, and soft palate are the most commonly affected sites. The mucosa in these regions develops a blotchy, marblelike pallor and a progressive stiffness of subepithelial tissues (Fig. 10-84). When the tongue is involved, it becomes rather immobile, is frequently diminished in size, and may be devoid of papillae. Submucosal fibrous bands are palpable on the buccal mucosa, soft palate, and labial mucosa of fully developed cases. Involvement may extend beyond the oral cavity to involve the oropharynx and upper esophagus. **Leukoplakia** of the surface mucosa often is noted.

Betel quid chewers also may exhibit a brown-red discoloration of the mucosa with an irregular surface that tends to desquamate. This particular change, known as **betel chewer's mucosa,** is not believed to be precancerous. In addition, some authors have reported **betel quid lichenoid lesions,** characterized by white, parallel, wavy striae resembling oral lichen planus (see page 782).

HISTOPATHOLOGIC FEATURES

Oral submucous fibrosis is characterized by the submucosal deposition of dense and hypovascular collagenous connective tissue with variable numbers of chronic inflammatory cells (Fig. 10-85). Epithelial changes include subepithelial vesicles in early lesions and hyperkeratosis with marked epithelial atrophy in older lesions. Epithelial dysplasia is found in 10% to 15% of cases submitted for biopsy, and carcinoma is found in at least 6% of sampled cases.

The lesions of so-called betel chewer's mucosa are histopathologically similar to morsicatio buccarum (see page 286), except that the ragged keratinaceous surface is covered by encrustations of betel quid ingredients.

TREATMENT AND PROGNOSIS

Unlike tobacco pouch keratosis, oral submucous fibrosis does not regress with habit cessation. Patients with mild cases may be treated with intralesional corticosteroids to reduce the symptoms; surgical splitting or excision of the fibrous bands may improve mouth opening and mobility in the later stages of the disease. One study showed that intralesional injections of interferon-γ improved maximum mouth opening, reduced mucosal burning, and increased suppleness of the buccal tissues. Additional agents that have been investigated for the treatment of oral submucous fibrosis include lycopene (alone or in combination with intralesional steroid injections) and pentoxifylline.

Frequent evaluation for development of oral squamous cell carcinoma is essential because a 17-year malignant transformation rate of 8% has been determined for betel quid users in India. Overall, persons

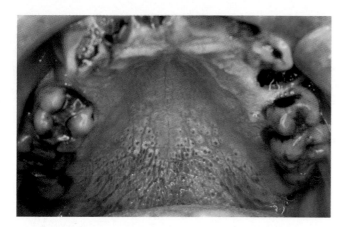

Fig. 10-86   Nicotine stomatitis. This extensive leathery, white change of the hard palate in a pipe smoker is sprinkled throughout with numerous red papules, which represent inflamed salivary duct openings. The gingival mucosa also is keratotic.

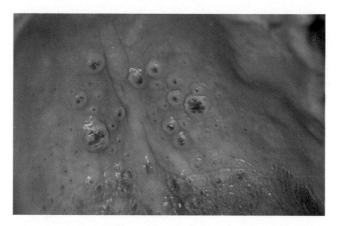

Fig. 10-87   Nicotine stomatitis. Close-up of the inflamed ductal openings of involved salivary glands of the hard palate. Note the white keratotic ring at the lip of many of the inflamed ducts.

with oral submucous fibrosis are at least 19 times more likely to develop oral cancer than persons without the disease.

NICOTINE STOMATITIS (NICOTINE PALATINUS; SMOKER'S PALATE)

Once a common mucosal change of the hard palate, **nicotine stomatitis** has become less common as cigar and pipe smoking have lost popularity. Although this lesion is a white keratotic change obviously associated with tobacco smoking, it does not appear to have a premalignant nature, perhaps because it develops in response to heat rather than the chemicals in tobacco smoke. Because pipe smoking generates more heat on the palate than other forms of smoking, nicotine stomatitis has been associated most often with this habit. Similar changes can also be produced by the long-term use of extremely hot beverages.

In some South American and Southeast Asian cultures, hand-rolled cigarettes and cigars are smoked with the lit end held within the mouth. This "reverse smoking" habit produces a pronounced palatal keratosis, or **reverse smoker's palate,** which has a significant potential to develop dysplasia or carcinoma.

CLINICAL FEATURES

Nicotine stomatitis most commonly is found in men older than 45 years of age. With long-term exposure to heat, the palatal mucosa becomes diffusely gray or white; numerous slightly elevated papules are noted, usually with punctate red centers (Figs. 10-86 and 10-87). Such papules represent inflamed minor salivary glands and their ductal orifices. The mucosa that

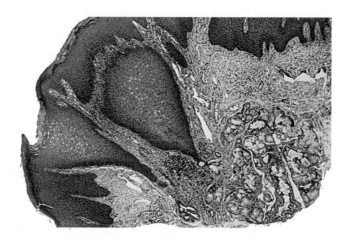

Fig. 10-88   Nicotine stomatitis. There is hyperkeratosis and acanthosis of the palatal epithelium. Note the squamous metaplasia of the minor salivary gland ducts.

covers the papules frequently appears whiter than the surrounding epithelium.

The palatal keratin may become so thickened that a fissured or "dried mud" appearance is imparted. The whiteness usually involves marginal gingiva and interdental papillae, and leukoplakia of the buccal mucosa is occasionally seen. A heavy brown or black tobacco stain may be present on the teeth.

HISTOPATHOLOGIC FEATURES

Nicotine stomatitis is characterized by hyperkeratosis and acanthosis of the palatal epithelium and mild, patchy, chronic inflammation of subepithelial connective tissue and mucous glands (Fig. 10-88). Squamous metaplasia of the excretory ducts is usually seen, and an inflammatory exudate may be noted within the duct lumina. In cases with papular elevation, hyperplastic ductal epithelium may be seen near the orifice. The degree of epithelial hyperplasia and hyperkeratosis appears to correlate positively with the duration and the level of heat exposure. Epithelial dysplasia rarely is seen.

TREATMENT AND PROGNOSIS

Nicotine stomatitis is completely reversible, even when it has been present for many decades. The palate returns to normal, usually within 1 to 2 weeks of smoking cessation. Although this is not a precancerous lesion and no treatment is needed, the patient nevertheless should be encouraged to stop smoking (and other high-risk areas should be examined closely). Any white lesion of the palatal mucosa that persists after 1 month of habit cessation should be considered a true leukoplakia and managed accordingly (see page 396).

ACTINIC KERATOSIS (SOLAR KERATOSIS)

Actinic keratosis is a common cutaneous premalignant lesion that is caused by cumulative ultraviolet (UV) radiation to sun-exposed skin, especially in fair-skinned people. A similar phenomenon, **actinic cheilosis,** is associated with sun damage to the lower lip vermilion (see page 405). UV light exposure can produce mutations in the p53 tumor suppressor gene, an alteration found frequently in this and other precancers and cancers of the head and neck region. Mutations in the telomerase gene represent another early event in lesion development, resulting in delayed apoptosis and immortalization of cells. Although UV light exposure is the major etiologic factor, additional potential risk factors include immunosuppression, arsenic exposure, and certain genetic abnormalities, such as albinism, Rothmund-Thompson syndrome, Cockayne syndrome, xeroderma pigmentosum (see page 747), and Bloom syndrome.

The lesion will develop on the skin of more than 50% of all white adults with significant lifetime sun exposure, and in the U.S. white population the prevalence rate is 15% for older men and 6% for older women. The prevalence increases with advancing age. According to the National Ambulatory Medical Care Survey, more than 47 million physician office visits were conducted in the United States over a 10-year period for the diagnosis of actinic keratosis.

CLINICAL FEATURES

Actinic keratosis seldom is found in persons younger than 40 years of age. The face and neck, the dorsum of the hands, the forearms, and the scalp of bald-headed men are the most common sites of occurrence. Indi-

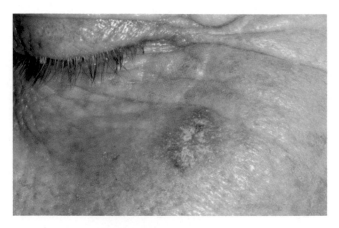

Fig. 10-89 Actinic keratosis. A plaque of the skin of the face with a rough, sandpaper-like surface.

vidual lesions are irregular scaly plaques, which vary in color from normal to white, gray, or brown, and may be superimposed on an erythematous background (Fig. 10-89). The keratotic scale peels off with varying degrees of difficulty. Palpation reveals a "sandpaper," roughened texture, and some lesions can be felt more easily than they can be seen. Typically, a lesion is smaller than 7 mm in diameter but may reach a size of 2 cm, usually with minimal elevation above the surface of the skin. Occasional lesions, however, produce so much keratin that a "horn" may be seen arising from the central area. Other skin lesions, such as verruca vulgaris or seborrheic keratosis, also may produce **keratin** or **cutaneous horns.**

HISTOPATHOLOGIC FEATURES

Histopathologically, actinic keratosis is characterized by hyperparakeratosis and acanthosis (Fig. 10-90). Teardrop-shaped rete ridges typically extend down from the epithelium; by definition, some degree of epithelial dysplasia is present. When full-thickness dysplasia is noted, this is termed **bowenoid actinic keratosis.** Suprabasilar acantholysis may be seen, as may melanosis and a lichenoid inflammatory infiltrate. The dermis exhibits a band of pale basophilic change, which represents sun-damaged collagen and elastic fibers **(solar elastosis).** In this band of sun-damaged connective tissue, there is a fourfold increase in the amount of elastic fibers, and band thickness is increased with increased exposure to actinic rays. Variable numbers of chronic inflammatory cells are typically present.

TREATMENT AND PROGNOSIS

Because of its precancerous nature, it is usually recommended that actinic keratosis be destroyed by liquid nitrogen cryotherapy, curettage, electrodesiccation, or

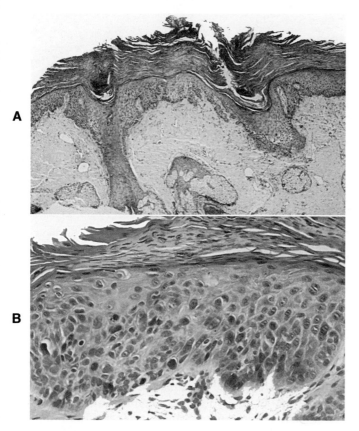

A

B

Fig. 10-90   Actinic keratosis. A, An extremely excessive amount of parakeratin is noted on the epidermal surface. **B,** High-power view showing hyperchromatism and pleomorphism of the epidermal cells.

surgical excision. Alternative treatment methods include topical agents (including 5-fluorouracil, imiquimod, and diclofenac) and photodynamic therapy. Recurrence is rare, but additional lesions frequently arise in adjacent sun-damaged skin. Long-term follow-up, therefore, is recommended.

Although the exact frequency of malignant transformation is unknown, it has been estimated that 10% of actinic keratoses will progress to squamous cell carcinoma, typically over a period of approximately 2 years.

ACTINIC CHEILOSIS (ACTINIC CHEILITIS)

Actinic cheilosis is a common premalignant alteration of the lower lip vermilion that results from long-term or excessive exposure to the ultraviolet component of sunlight. It is a problem confined predominantly to light-complexioned people with a tendency to sunburn easily. Outdoor occupation obviously is associated with this problem, leading to the popular use of terms such as *farmer's lip* and *sailor's lip.* A person with chronic

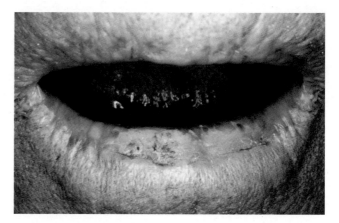

Fig. 10-91   Actinic cheilosis. A blurring of the interface between the vermilion mucosa and the skin of the lip is especially noted in this case.

sunlight exposure and compromised immunity, especially a transplant recipient, has an elevated risk of developing a cancer of the lower lip vermilion.

Actinic cheilosis is similar to **actinic keratosis** of the skin (see previous topic) in its pathophysiologic and biologic behavior.

CLINICAL FEATURES

Actinic cheilosis seldom occurs in persons younger than 45 years of age. It has a strong male predilection, with a male-to-female ratio as high as 10:1 in some studies.

The lesion develops so slowly that patients often are not aware of a change. The earliest clinical changes include atrophy of the lower lip vermilion border, characterized by a smooth surface and blotchy pale areas. Blurring of the margin between the vermilion zone and the cutaneous portion of the lip is typically seen (Fig. 10-91). As the lesion progresses, rough, scaly areas develop on the drier portions of the vermilion. These areas thicken and may appear as leukoplakic lesions, especially when they extend near the wet line of the lip. The patient may report that the scaly material can be peeled off with some difficulty, only to reform again within a few days.

With further progression, chronic focal ulceration may develop in one or more sites (Fig. 10-92). Such ulcerations may last for months and often suggest progression to early squamous cell carcinoma (Fig. 10-93).

HISTOPATHOLOGIC FEATURES

Actinic cheilosis is usually characterized by an atrophic stratified squamous epithelium, often demonstrating marked keratin production. Varying degrees of epithe-

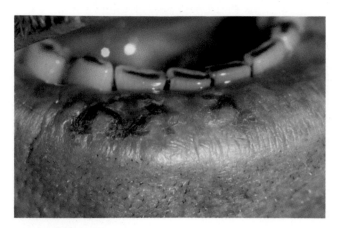

Fig. 10-92   Actinic cheilosis. Crusted and ulcerated lesions of the lower lip vermilion.

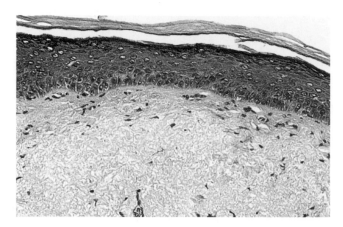

Fig. 10-94   Actinic cheilosis. Hyperorthokeratosis and epithelial atrophy. Note the striking underlying solar elastosis.

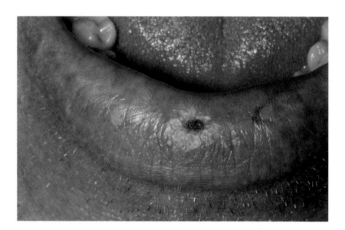

Fig. 10-93   Squamous cell carcinoma arising in actinic cheilosis. Patient with actinic cheilosis of the lower lip, who developed a small, chronic ulceration. Biopsy revealed early invasive squamous cell carcinoma.

lial dysplasia may be encountered. A mild chronic inflammatory cell infiltrate commonly is present subjacent to the dysplastic epithelium. The underlying connective tissue invariably demonstrates a band of amorphous, acellular, basophilic change known as **solar (actinic) elastosis**, an ultraviolet light–induced alteration of collagen and elastic fibers (Fig. 10-94).

TREATMENT AND PROGNOSIS

Many of the changes associated with actinic cheilosis are probably irreversible, but patients should be encouraged to use lip balms with sunscreens to prevent further damage. Areas of induration, thickening, ulceration, or leukoplakia should be submitted for biopsy to rule out carcinoma. In clinically severe cases without obvious malignant transformation, a lip shave procedure (**vermilionectomy**) may be performed. The ver-

milion mucosa is removed, and either a portion of the intraoral labial mucosa is pulled forward or the wound is allowed to heal by secondary intention. The advantage of this technique is that it provides tissue for histopathologic examination should areas of superficially invasive squamous cell carcinoma be present. Alternative treatments include CO_2 or erbium:YAG (Er:YAG) laser ablation, electrodesiccation, topical 5-fluorouracil, topical imiquimod, photodynamic therapy, and chemoexfoliation (or "chemical peel") with trichloroacetic acid. Long-term follow-up is recommended. Of course, if a squamous cell carcinoma is identified, then the involved lip is treated accordingly.

Squamous cell carcinoma, usually well-differentiated, develops over time in 6% to 10% of actinic cheilosis cases reported from medical centers. Such malignant transformation seldom occurs before 60 years of age, with the resulting carcinoma typically enlarging slowly and metastasizing only at a late stage.

KERATOACANTHOMA ("SELF-HEALING" CARCINOMA; PSEUDOCARCINOMA; KERATOCARCINOMA; SQUAMOUS CELL CARCINOMA, KERATOACANTHOMA TYPE)

Keratoacanthoma is a self-limiting, epithelial proliferation with a strong clinical and histopathologic similarity to well-differentiated **squamous cell carcinoma.** In fact, some authorities consider it to represent an extremely well-differentiated form of squamous cell carcinoma. Cutaneous lesions presumably arise from the infundibulum of hair follicles. Intraoral lesions have been reported, but they are rare; in fact, some authorities do not accept keratoacanthoma as an intraoral disease.

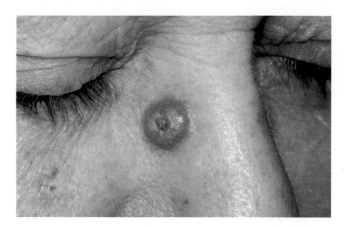

Fig. 10-95   Keratoacanthoma. A nontender, well-demarcated nodule of the skin of the nose in an older woman. The nodule demonstrates a central keratin plug.

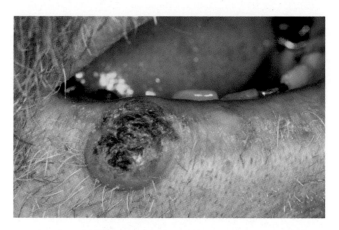

Fig. 10-96   Keratoacanthoma. This lesion, which is located at the outer edge of the vermilion border of the lip, demonstrates a prominent core or plug of keratin.

The cause of this lesion is unknown, but sun damage and human papillomavirus (HPV), possibly subtypes 26 or 37, have been proposed. The association with sun damage is suggested by the fact that most solitary lesions are found on sun-exposed skin, predominantly in older adults. Additional potential contributing factors include tar exposure, immunosuppression, and burns or other trauma. Keratoacanthoma-like lesions have been produced in animals by the cutaneous application of carcinogens.

There appears to be a hereditary predisposition for multiple lesions, and the lesions occur with increased frequency in patients with **Muir-Torre syndrome** (sebaceous neoplasms, keratoacanthomas, and gastrointestinal carcinomas).

A number of studies have examined potential genetic alterations or immunohistochemical markers for distinguishing between keratoacanthoma and squamous cell carcinoma. In general, these studies have shown that squamous cell carcinoma tends to have different chromosomal abnormalities and a greater number of genetic aberrations compared with keratoacanthoma, suggesting different pathogenetic mechanisms between these two lesions.

CLINICAL FEATURES

Keratoacanthoma rarely occurs in patients before 45 years of age and shows a male predilection. Almost 95% of solitary lesions are found on sun-exposed skin, and 8% of all cases are found on the outer edge of the vermilion border of the lips, with equal frequency on both the upper and the lower lips.

Keratoacanthoma appears as a firm, nontender, well-demarcated, sessile, dome-shaped nodule with a central plug of keratin (Figs. 10-95 and 10-96), although lesions reported as intraoral keratoacanthoma usually have lacked the central plug. The outer portion of the nodule has a normal texture and color but may be erythematous. The central keratin plug is yellowish, brown, or black and has an irregular, crusted, often verruciform surface.

The evolution of keratoacanthoma can be divided into three phases: (1) growth phase, (2) stationary phase, and (3) involution phase. During the growth phase, rapid enlargement is typical, with the lesion usually attaining a diameter of 1 to 2 cm within 6 weeks. This critical feature helps to distinguish it from the more slowly enlarging squamous cell carcinoma. The lesion stabilizes during the stationary phase, which usually is of a duration similar to that of the growth phase. Most lesions regress spontaneously within 6 to 12 months of onset, frequently leaving a depressed scar in the area (Fig. 10-97). The regression of these lesions is a curious phenomenon, which some investigators have theorized is related to a cytotoxic immune response to the tumor.

Occasional patients demonstrate large numbers of keratoacanthomas. One multiple-lesion variant, the **Ferguson Smith** type, manifests in early life and appears to be hereditary; the lesions are not likely to involute spontaneously. Another variant manifests as hundreds of small papules of the skin and upper digestive tract (**eruptive Grzybowski** type) and may be associated with internal malignancy.

HISTOPATHOLOGIC FEATURES

Keratoacanthoma of the skin and lip vermilion warrants excisional or large incisional biopsy with inclusion of adjacent, clinically normal epithelium for proper histopathologic interpretation; this is because the overall pattern of the tumor is diagnostically more important than the appearance of individual cells. The

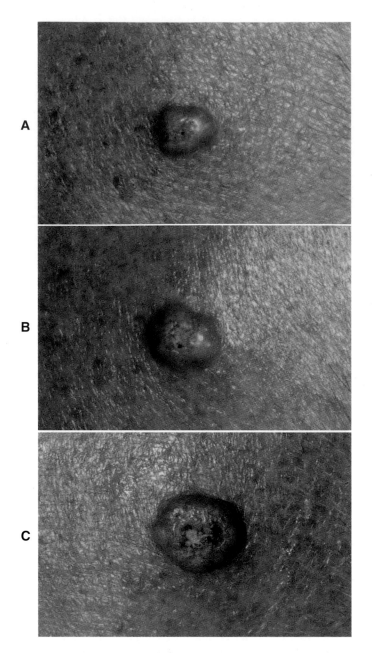

Fig. 10-97   Keratoacanthoma. A, Appearance on initial presentation. Note small, central keratin-filled invagination. **B,** Same lesion 1 week later showing slight enlargement. **C,** Same lesion showing further growth 3 weeks after initial presentation. All three photographs were taken at the same magnification. *(Courtesy of Dr. John Lovas.)*

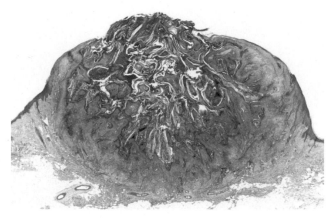

Fig. 10-98   Keratoacanthoma. Low-power microscopic view showing extensive epidermal proliferation with a central keratin plug.

cells appear mature, although considerable dyskeratosis (abnormal or premature keratin production) is typically seen in the form of deeply located individually keratinizing lesional cells and keratin pearls similar to those found in well-differentiated squamous cell carcinoma.

The surface epithelium at the lateral edge of the tumor appears normal; at the lip of the central crater, however, a characteristic acute angle (or "buttress") is formed between the overlying epithelium and the lesion. The crater is filled with keratin, and the epithelium at the base of the crater proliferates downward (Fig. 10-98). This action often elicits a pronounced chronic inflammatory cell response. Downward proliferation does not extend below the level of the sweat glands in skin lesions or into underlying muscle in vermilion lesions. Late-stage lesions show considerably more keratinization of the deeper aspects of the tumor than do early lesions.

TREATMENT AND PROGNOSIS

Despite the propensity of keratoacanthoma to involute of its own accord, surgical excision of large lesions is indicated for optimal aesthetic appearance because significant scarring may otherwise occur. After excision, 4% to 8% of treated patients experience recurrence. Although surgical excision is the preferred treatment, alternative therapies include cryosurgery (reserved for small early lesions), intralesional injection of chemotherapeutic agents (such as 5-fluorouracil, bleomycin, methotrexate, or interferon α-2a), and topical imiquimod. Systemic chemotherapy, often combined with cryotherapy, may be used to treat patients with multiple lesions of the Ferguson Smith or eruptive Grzybowski type.

Aggressive behavior and malignant transformation into carcinoma have been reported in a small proportion of keratoacanthomas—particularly those occurring in the setting of immunosuppression. However, the close histopathologic similarities between this lesion and squamous cell carcinoma sometimes make it difficult to rule out the possibility of misinterpretation of the microscopic section.

SQUAMOUS CELL CARCINOMA

In approximately one of every three Americans now living, a malignancy will develop at some point. It is estimated that in 2007, more than 1,444,000 cancer cases will be diagnosed in the United States, in addition to more than 1 million nonmelanoma skin cancers. Although 66% of affected persons now survive their disease, cancer still causes more than 559,000 deaths each year in the United States and accounts for more than 20% of all deaths. In addition, the current annual death rate from nondermal cancers (186 per 100,000 persons) has increased by 30% since 1930, partially because of a considerable increase in the incidence of lung cancer and partially because people are now less likely to die at an early age of other common disorders, such as cardiovascular disease and infection. From the 1990s through the present, however, this trend has reversed, and the average annual incidence and mortality rates for all cancers combined (excluding nonmelanoma skin cancers) have been declining.

Oral cancer accounts for less than 3% of all cancers in the United States, but it is the eighth most common cancer in males and the fifteenth most common in females. It is the eleventh most common cancer worldwide, with an especially high incidence reported in the Indian subcontinent, Australia, France, Brazil, and southern Africa. Approximately 94% of all oral malignancies are **squamous cell carcinoma.** In the United States, approximately 22,000 new cases of oral squamous cell carcinoma are diagnosed annually, and slightly more than 5300 individuals die of this disease each year. The average annual incidence and mortality rates, however, vary considerably between different races, genders, and age groups.

As with so many carcinomas, the risk of intraoral cancer increases with increasing age, especially for males. The annual incidence rate (the number of newly diagnosed cases per 100,000 persons each year) for this disease is 5 per 100,000 in the United States, although many texts report an 11 to 15 per 100,000 rate because of the inadvertent inclusion of pharyngeal and vermilion cancers with the intraoral cases. In the United States, white men have a higher risk of intraoral cancer after 65 years of age than does any other group. However, the highest annual incidence rate in middle age is seen in American men of African ancestry (Fig. 10-99). Although the annual incidence rate for intraoral cancer in black males has been decreasing slowly since the middle to late 1980s, marked disparities in survival and mortality rates between black and white males persist. Females, whether white or nonwhite, have a much lower annual incidence rate than males at all age levels. The overall male-to-female ratio is 3:1.

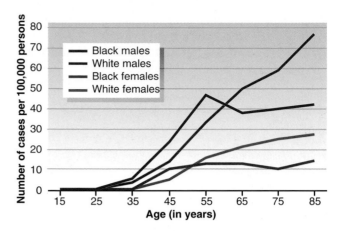

Fig. 10-99   Oral carcinoma. Age-specific incidence rates for intraoral squamous cell carcinoma (number of new cases diagnosed per 100,000 persons each year). Separate rates are provided for white and black men and women in the United States.

Carcinoma of the lip vermilion is somewhat different from intraoral carcinoma. It has a pathophysiology more akin to squamous cell carcinoma of the sun-exposed skin. The average annual incidence rate for white males in the United States is 4 per 100,000, but the rate increases dramatically with age, to almost 30 per 100,000 for men older than 75 years of age. Once the most common oral cancer, the cumulative lifetime risk for developing lip cancer today is only 0.15% for men and 0.07% for women. There was a considerable decrease in the annual incidence rate of this cancer in white males in the United States during the latter half of the twentieth century, because fewer and fewer of them held outdoor occupations. Few women or nonwhite men develop lip carcinoma; there has been little change in the incidence over time for these groups.

Outside the United States, exceptionally wide differences in annual incidence and mortality rates for oral carcinoma are found. These rates vary by as much as twentyfold among different countries. Many of these differences are undoubtedly caused by differing population habits, life expectancies, preventive education, and the quality of medical records in various countries. Despite the difficulties involved in interpreting such data, however, the data have been helpful in identifying potential causative factors.

ETIOLOGY OF ORAL CANCER

The cause of oral squamous cell carcinoma is multifactorial. No single causative agent or factor (carcinogen) has been clearly defined or accepted, but both extrinsic and intrinsic factors may be at work. It is likely that more than a single factor is needed to produce such a malignancy (cocarcinogenesis). *Extrinsic* factors include

Table **10-1**   **Precancerous Lesions of the Oral, Pharyngeal, and Laryngeal Mucosa (Clinical Terms Only)**

Disease Name	Malignant Transformation Potential
Proliferative verrucous leukoplakia (PVL)*	★★★★★★
Nicotine palatinus in reverse smokers†	★★★★★
Erythroplakia	★★★★★
Oral submucous fibrosis	★★★★★
Erythroleukoplakia	★★★★
Granular leukoplakia	★★★★
Laryngeal keratosis	★★★
Actinic cheilosis	★★★
Smooth, thick leukoplakia	★★
Smooth, red tongue of Plummer-Vinson syndrome	★★
Smokeless tobacco keratosis	★
Lichen planus (erosive forms)‡	★?
Smooth, thin leukoplakia	+/−

From Speight PM, Farthing PM, Bouquot JE: The pathology of oral cancer and precancer, *Curr Diag Pathol* 3:165-176, 1997.
*PVL: High-risk, high-recurrence form of oral leukoplakia affecting multiple sites.
†Reverse smoking: smoking with the lit end of the cigarette in one's mouth.
‡Precancer character is controversial.

such external agents as tobacco smoke, alcohol, syphilis, and (for vermilion cancers only) sunlight. *Intrinsic* factors include systemic or generalized states, such as general malnutrition or iron-deficiency anemia. Heredity does not appear to play a major causative role in oral carcinoma. Many oral squamous cell carcinomas have been documented to be associated with or preceded by a precancerous lesion, especially **leukoplakia** (Table 10-1).

TOBACCO SMOKING

Tobacco smoking reached its greatest popularity in the United States during the 1940s, when at least 65% of white men smoked and other population subgroups were beginning to smoke in large numbers. Today less than 21% of U.S. adults, men and women alike, smoke cigarettes. Unfortunately, the remaining smokers appear to be the heavier users; therefore, the effects on the mouth may be even greater than the typical effects noted in the past.

Much indirect clinical evidence implicates the habit of tobacco smoking in the development of oral squamous cell carcinoma. The proportion of smokers (80%) among patients with oral carcinoma is two to three times greater than the general population. The risk for a second primary carcinoma of the upper aerodigestive tract is two to six times greater for treated patients with oral cancer who continue to smoke than for those who quit after diagnosis.

In addition, case control studies have shown that pipe and cigar smoking carries a greater oral cancer risk than does cigarette smoking, and that the relative risk (smoker's risk for oral cancer compared with that of a nonsmoker) is dose dependent for cigarette smokers. It is at least five for persons who smoke 40 cigarettes daily, but increases to as much as 17 for persons who smoke 80 or more cigarettes daily. The risk, furthermore, increases the longer the person smokes.

The greatest risk of all probably is found in certain isolated Indian and South American cultures in which the practice of reverse smoking is popular, especially among women. In reverse smoking, the burning end of a handmade cigar or cigarette is held inside the mouth. This habit considerably elevates one's risk for oral cancer. Where reverse smoking is practiced, as many as 50% of all oral malignancies are found on the hard palate, a site usually spared by this disease.

It should be mentioned that there may be distinct differences between head and neck cancers that develop in smokers compared with those that develop in nonsmokers, although these differences do not appear to affect survival. Tumors in nonsmokers contain a lower frequency of common genetic alterations and have certain clinical differences. For example, affected nonsmokers are more likely to be female, to have oral (especially tongue) rather than pharyngeal or laryngeal disease, to be very young, and to demonstrate mutations of the p53 and other tumor suppressor genes.

SMOKELESS TOBACCO

Smokeless tobacco use in Western cultures may increase a chronic user's risk for oral carcinoma by a factor ranging from less than two to as high as 26. This variation in relative risk reported by different epidemiologic case control studies may be influenced by the type of smokeless tobacco used, with some studies suggesting a lower risk associated with wet snuff and chewing tobacco and a higher risk associated with dry snuff. This apparent increased risk is supported by clinicopathologic investigations that have found an abnormal male-to-female sex ratio for oral carcinoma (>1.0:1.5) in geographic areas where the habit is more popular among women than among men. These geographic areas are typically in the southern United States, where women use dry snuff. In addition, approximately 50% of all oral cancers in smokeless tobacco users occur at the site where the tobacco is habitually placed.

BETEL QUID (PAAN)

The betel quid or *paan* is a compound of natural substances (i.e., areca palm nuts, betel leaf, slaked lime, perhaps tobacco leaf) chewed for their psychostimulating effects. Among betel quid users in Asia, the lifetime risk of developing oral cancer is a remarkable 8%. This habit is also associated with significant development of precancers, such as leukoplakia. More than 600 million persons worldwide chew these quids on a regular basis.

ALCOHOL

Excessive alcohol consumption has been implicated in oral cancer development. It is uncertain whether alcohol alone can initiate carcinogenesis, although it is well established that alcohol in combination with tobacco is a significant risk factor for oral cancer development.

Case control studies have concluded that the risk is dose dependent and time dependent, and the combination of alcohol and tobacco abuse over long periods may increase a person's risk for oral cancer by a factor of 15 or more (relative risk is 15). In this light, it may be significant that the lowest annual oral cancer incidence rate in the United States is found in Utah, where 75% of the population follows Mormon doctrines that forbid the use of tobacco and alcohol.

Indirect evidence for alcohol's role in oral cancer production includes the fact that approximately one third of male patients with oral cancer are heavy alcohol users; less than 10% of the general population can be classified as such. Cirrhosis of the liver, likewise, is found in at least 20% of male patients with oral cancer. Nutritional deficiencies associated with heavy alcohol consumption also may contribute to an increased risk of oral cancer development.

PHENOLIC AGENTS

Recent evidence has pointed to an increased oral cancer risk for workers in the wood products industry chronically exposed to certain chemicals, such as phenoxyacetic acids. Moreover, it has long been known that these workers are at increased risk for nasal and nasopharyngeal carcinoma.

RADIATION

The effects of ultraviolet (UV) radiation on the lips are discussed elsewhere (actinic cheilosis, see page 405), but it is well known that another form of radiation, **x-irradiation,** decreases immune reactivity and produces abnormalities in chromosomal material. It should not seem surprising, then, that radiotherapy to the head and neck area increases the risk of the later development of a new primary oral malignancy, either a carcinoma or a sarcoma. This effect is dose dependent, but even low-dose radiotherapy for benign entities may increase the local risk to some extent. However, the small amount of radiation from routine diagnostic dental radiographs has not been associated with oral mucosal carcinomas.

IRON DEFICIENCY

Iron deficiency, especially the severe, chronic form known as the **Plummer-Vinson** or **Paterson-Kelly syndrome** (see page 828), is associated with an elevated risk for squamous cell carcinoma of the esophagus, oropharynx, and posterior mouth. Malignancies develop at an earlier age than in patients without iron deficiency anemia. People who are deficient in iron tend to have impaired cell-mediated immunity, and iron is essential to the normal functioning of epithelial cells of the upper digestive tract. In deficiency states, these epithelial cells turn over more rapidly and produce an atrophic or immature mucosa. Intertwining fibrous bands of scar tissue also may develop within the esophagus of severely affected patients **(esophageal webs).** Patients with such esophageal webbing seem to be especially susceptible to malignant transformation.

VITAMIN-A DEFICIENCY

Vitamin-A deficiency produces excessive keratinization of the skin and mucous membranes, and researchers have suggested that the vitamin may play a protective or preventive role in oral precancer and cancer. Some believe that blood levels of retinol and the amount of dietary betacarotene ingested are inversely proportional to the risk of oral squamous cell carcinoma and leukoplakia. Long-term therapy with retinoic acids and betacarotene also has been associated with a regression of at least some leukoplakic lesions and a concomitant reduction in the severity of dysplasia within such lesions.

SYPHILIS

Syphilis (tertiary stage) has long been accepted as having a strong association with the development of dorsal tongue carcinoma. The relative risk ratio approximates four. Conversely, a person with a lingual carcinoma is five times more likely to have a positive serology test for syphilis than someone without such a cancer. The arsenical agents and heavy metals that were used to treat syphilis before the advent of modern antibiotic therapy have carcinogenic properties themselves and may have been responsible for some of the earlier cancer development in this disease. Regardless of the pathophysiologic mechanism at work, however, syphilis-associated oral malignancies are rare today because the infection is typically diagnosed and treated before the onset of the tertiary stage.

CANDIDAL INFECTION

Hyperplastic candidiasis (see page 217) frequently is cited as an oral precancerous condition. Because this lesion appears as a white plaque that cannot be rubbed off, it also has been called *candidal leukoplakia*. Unfortunately, it is difficult both clinically and histopathologically to distinguish between a true hyperplastic candidiasis and a preexisting leukoplakia with superimposed candidiasis. Experimentally, some strains of *Candida albicans* have produced hyperkeratotic lesions of the dorsal rat tongue without any other contributing factor. In other studies, certain strains have been shown to produce **nitrosamines,** chemicals that have been implicated in carcinogenesis. Some candidal strains may have the potential to promote the development of oral cancer; to date, however, the evidence to suggest this role is largely circumstantial.

ONCOGENIC VIRUSES

Oncogenic (tumor producing) viruses may play a major role in a wide variety of cancers, although no virus has definitively been proven to cause oral cancer so far. Viral agents capable of integration into the host's genetic material may be particularly dangerous and potentially could commandeer the host's ability to regulate normal growth and proliferation of the infected cell. The oncogenic viruses may immortalize the host cell, thereby facilitating malignant transformation. In the past, retroviruses, adenoviruses, herpes simplex viruses (HSVs), and human papillomaviruses (HPVs) all have been suggested as playing a role in the development of oral carcinoma. It appears, however, that HPV is the only one still implicated, not only in oral cancer but also in carcinoma of the pharyngeal tonsil, larynx, esophagus, uterine cervix, vulva, and penis. HPV subtypes 16, 18, 31, and 33 are the strains most closely associated with dysplasia and squamous cell carcinoma. The underlying mechanisms by which HPV is believed to contribute to oral carcinogenesis primarily involve two virally encoded proteins: (1) E6 (which promotes degradation of the p53 tumor suppressor gene product) and (2) E7 (which promotes degradation of the pRb [retinoblastoma protein] tumor suppressor gene product).

HSV, especially type 2, once was thought to produce a large proportion of cancers of the uterine cervix, and it has been suggested as a causative factor in oral carcinoma. Evidence now suggests that it may be no more than a common companion infection in persons with HPV infections, and that the latter virus plays a much more important carcinogenic role than does HSV. Currently, the evidence gathered to prove a causal relationship between HSV and oral carcinoma is insufficient.

IMMUNOSUPPRESSION

Immunosuppression may play a role in the development of at least some malignancies of the upper aerodigestive tract. Without effective immunologic surveillance and attack, it is thought that newly created malignant cells cannot be recognized and destroyed at an early stage. Persons with AIDS and those who are undergoing immunosuppressive therapy for malignancy or organ transplantation are at increased risk for oral squamous cell carcinoma and other head and neck malignancies, especially when tobacco smoking and alcohol abuse are present.

ONCOGENES AND TUMOR SUPPRESSOR GENES

Oncogenes and tumor suppressor genes are chromosomal components capable of being acted on by a variety of causative agents. Normal genes, or **proto-oncogenes,** are transformed into activated oncogenes in certain malignancies through the actions of viruses, irradiation, or chemical carcinogens. Once oncogenes are activated, they may stimulate the production of an excessive amount of new genetic material through amplification or overexpression of the involved gene. Oncogenes probably are involved in the initiation and progression of a wide variety of neoplasms, including oral squamous cell carcinoma.

Tumor suppressor genes, on the other hand, allow tumor production indirectly when they become inactivated or mutated. Genetic aberrations commonly identified in oral squamous cell carcinomas include abnormalities of the *ras, myc,* and *EGFR* (epidermal growth factor receptor; also known as *c-erbB1*) oncogenes, and the *p53, pRb, p16,* and *E-cadherin* tumor suppressor genes. Most authorities feel that an accumulation of several of these various genetic aberrations is necessary before the affected cell expresses a malignant phenotype.

CLINICAL AND RADIOGRAPHIC FEATURES

Persons with oral squamous cell carcinoma are most often older men who have been aware of an alteration in an oral cancer site for 4 to 8 months

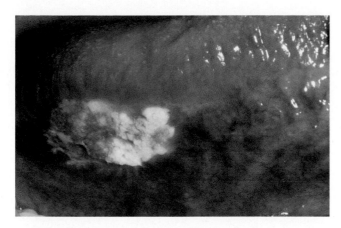

Fig. 10-100   Squamous cell carcinoma. Leukoplakic lesion on the right ventrolateral surface of the tongue.

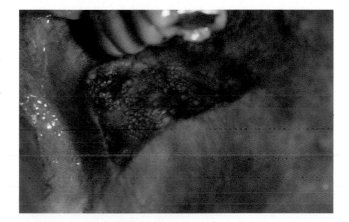

Fig. 10-101   Squamous cell carcinoma. Speckled erythroplakia of the left posterior buccal mucosa. Brush sampling had been reported to be negative for epithelial abnormality, but incisional biopsy revealed invasive squamous cell carcinoma. *(From Chi AC, Ravenel MC: AAOMP case challenge: a "speckled" lesion, J Contemp Dent Pract 6:168-172, 2005.)*

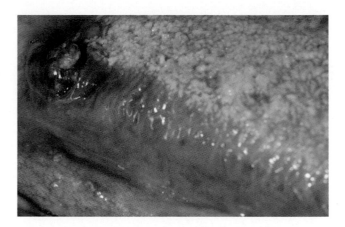

Fig. 10-102   Squamous cell carcinoma. An exophytic lesion of the posterior lateral tongue demonstrates surface nodularity and minimal surface keratin production. It is painless and indurated.

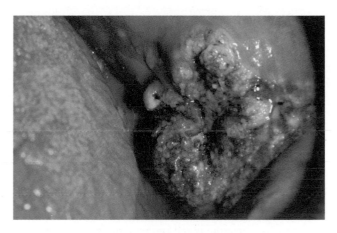

Fig. 10-103   Squamous cell carcinoma. An exophytic buccal lesion shows a roughened and irregular surface with areas of erythema admixed with small areas of white keratosis. Surface ulceration is evident.

before seeking professional help (8 to 24 months among lower socioeconomic groups). There is minimal pain during the early growth phase, and this may explain the delay in seeking professional care. If the health care professional does not have a high index of suspicion, then an additional several weeks or months may elapse before a biopsy is performed.

Oral squamous cell carcinoma has a varied clinical presentation, including the following:
- Exophytic (mass forming; fungating, papillary, verruciform)
- Endophytic (invasive, burrowing, ulcerated)
- Leukoplakic (white patch) (Fig. 10-100)
- Erythroplakic (red patch)
- Erythroleukoplakic (combined red-and-white patch) (Fig. 10-101)

The *leukoplakic* and *erythroplakic* examples are probably early cases that have not yet produced a mass or ulceration, and the clinical features are identical to those described for premalignant leukoplakia and erythroplakia (see pages 388 and 397). These mucosal surface changes typically are destroyed by the developing exophytic or endophytic carcinoma, but many cases are diagnosed before their complete destruction and show residual precancerous lesions involving adjacent mucosa.

An *exophytic* lesion typically has a surface that is irregular, fungating, papillary, or verruciform, and its color may vary from normal to red to white, depending on the amount of keratin and vascularity (Figs. 10-102 and 10-103). The surface is often ulcerated, and the tumor feels hard (**indurated**) on palpation (Fig. 10-104).

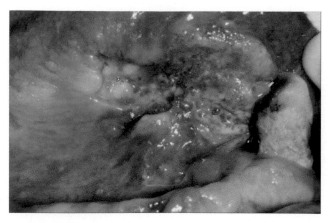

Fig. 10-104   Squamous cell carcinoma. Chronic ulcerated lesion on the right ventral surface of the tongue. The rolled anterior margin felt indurated on palpation.

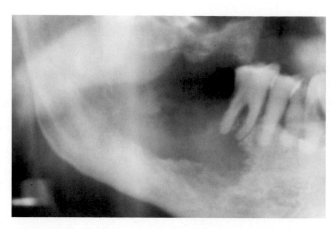

Fig. 10-106   Squamous cell carcinoma. Bone involvement is characterized by an irregular, "moth-eaten" radiolucency with ragged margins—an appearance similar to that of osteomyelitis.

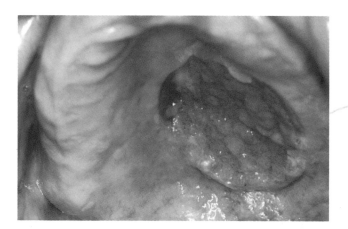

Fig. 10-105   Squamous cell carcinoma. An ulcerated or endophytic lesion of the hard palate demonstrates rolled borders and a necrotic ulcer bed. This cancer was painless, although it had partially destroyed underlying palatal bone.

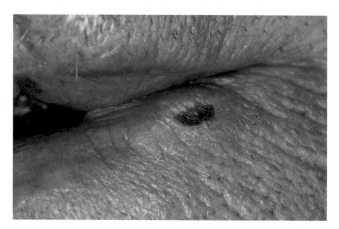

Fig. 10-107   Squamous cell carcinoma. Small, crusted ulcer of the lower lip vermilion.

The *endophytic* growth pattern has a depressed, irregularly shaped, ulcerated, central area with a surrounding "rolled" border of normal, red or white mucosa (Fig. 10-105). The rolled border results from invasion of the tumor downward and laterally under adjacent epithelium. This appearance is not unique to oral carcinoma because granulomatous lesions, such as deep fungal infections, tuberculosis, tertiary syphilis, oral lesions of Wegener's granulomatosis or Crohn's disease, and chronic traumatic ulcers, may look similar.

Destruction of underlying bone, when present, may be painful or completely painless, and it appears on radiographs as a "moth-eaten" radiolucency with ill-defined or ragged margins (an appearance similar to osteomyelitis) (Fig. 10-106). Carcinoma also can extend for many centimeters along a nerve (perineural invasion) without breaking away to form a true metastasis.

LIP VERMILION CARCINOMA

Carcinoma of the lip vermilion is typically found in light-skinned persons with either long-term exposure to UV radiation from sunlight or a history of acute sun damage (sunburn) early in life. Seventy percent of affected individuals have outdoor occupations. It is usually associated with **actinic cheilosis** (see page 405) and may arise at the site where the patient holds a cigarette, cigar, or pipe stem. Almost 90% of lesions are located on the lower lip.

The typical vermilion carcinoma is a crusted, oozing, nontender, indurated ulceration that is usually less than 1 cm in greatest diameter when discovered (Figs. 10-107 and 10-108). The tumor is characterized by a slow growth rate, and most patients have been aware

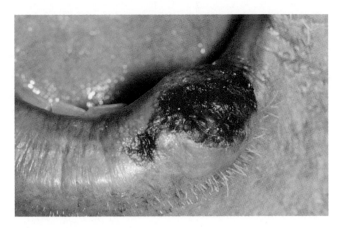

Fig. 10-108   Squamous cell carcinoma. Ulcerated mass of the lower lip vermilion.

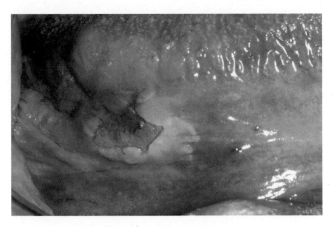

Fig. 10-110   Squamous cell carcinoma. Ulcerated lesion with surrounding leukoplakia on the posterior lateral and ventral tongue.

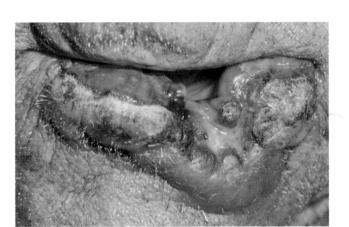

Fig. 10-109   Squamous cell carcinoma. Patient neglect can result in extensive involvement, even in a readily visible site such as the lip vermilion. This ulcerating lesion of the lower lip had been present for more than 1 year before diagnosis.

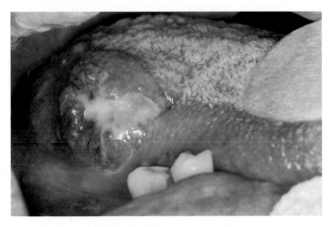

Fig. 10-111   Squamous cell carcinoma. Ulcerated, exophytic mass of the posterior lateral border of the tongue.

of a "problem" in the area for 12 to 16 months before a formal diagnosis is made. Metastasis is a late event; at diagnosis, fewer than 2% of patients have metastatically involved lymph nodes, usually in the submental region. Perineural invasion may result in extension of the tumor into the mandible through the mental foramen. Although this tumor is typically diagnosed and treated at an early stage, patient neglect can result in considerable destruction of normal tissue (Fig. 10-109).

INTRAORAL CARCINOMA

The most common site for intraoral carcinoma is the tongue, usually the posterior lateral and ventral surfaces. The oral floor is affected almost as frequently in men but is involved much less commonly in women.

Other sites of involvement (in descending order of frequency) are the soft palate, gingiva, buccal mucosa, labial mucosa, and hard palate.

Carcinoma of the tongue accounts for more than 50% of intraoral cancers in population studies in the United States (Figs. 10-110 and 10-111). Two thirds of lingual carcinomas appear as painless, indurated masses or ulcers of the posterior lateral border; 20% occur on anterior lateral or ventral surfaces, and only 4% occur on the dorsum. The tongue especially is the site of involvement in young patients and, in fact, is the site of the only congenital oral squamous cell carcinoma reported.

Carcinoma of the oral floor represents 35% of all intraoral cancers in epidemiologic surveys and appears to be increasing in frequency among females. It occurs a decade earlier in women than in men but is still usually a disease of older adults. Of all intraoral carcinomas, floor of mouth lesions are the most likely to

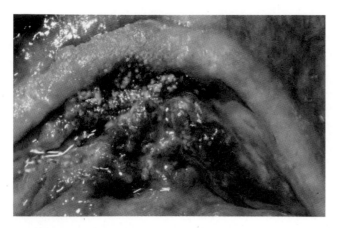

Fig. 10-112   Squamous cell carcinoma. Granular red and white lesion in the anterior floor of mouth.

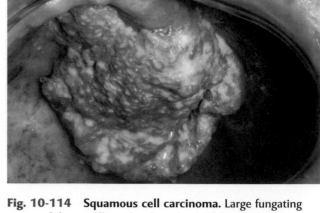

Fig. 10-114   Squamous cell carcinoma. Large fungating tumor of the maxillary alveolar ridge and hard palate.

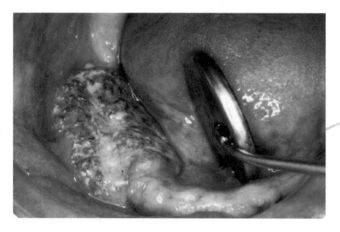

Fig. 10-113   Squamous cell carcinoma. An exophytic lesion with an irregular and pebbled surface has a linear indentation along its facial aspect resulting from pressure from the patient's lower denture. Underlying alveolar bone was extensively destroyed.

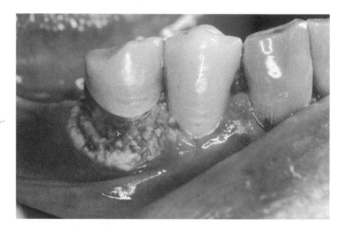

Fig. 10-115   Squamous cell carcinoma. An innocuous pebbled-surface change of the attached and marginal gingiva was interpreted as an inflammatory change until multifocal white keratoses occurred.

arise from a preexisting leukoplakia or erythroplakia (Fig. 10-112). It is also the oral cancer site most often associated with the development of a second primary malignancy of another aerodigestive tract location or of a distant organ. The most common site of involvement is the midline near the frenum.

Gingival and alveolar carcinomas are usually painless and most frequently arise from keratinized mucosa in a posterior mandibular site. This tumor has a special propensity to mimic the benign inflammatory and reactive lesions, such as pyogenic granuloma, that are so common to the gingiva. When the cancer develops in an edentulous area, it may give rise to a mass that "wraps around" a denture flange and superficially resembles inflammatory fibrous hyperplasia (epulis fissuratum) (Fig. 10-113). Tumors of the maxillary alveolar ridge may extend onto the hard palate (Fig. 10-114). If the tumor is adjacent to a tooth (Fig. 10-115), then

it may mimic periodontal disease or a pyogenic granuloma. Gingival carcinoma often destroys the underlying bone structure, causing tooth mobility. This lesion may not become clinically evident until after tooth extraction, when it proliferates out of the socket to mimic the hyperplastic granulation tissue of epulis granulomatosa. Of all the intraoral carcinomas, this one is least associated with tobacco smoking and has the greatest predilection for females.

OROPHARYNGEAL CARCINOMA

Carcinoma of the soft palate and oropharyngeal mucosa has the same basic clinical appearance as more anterior carcinomas, except that, in this posterior location, the patient often is unaware of its presence and the diagnosis may be delayed. Tumor size is typically greater than that of more anterior carcinomas, and the proportion of cases with cervical and distant metastasis

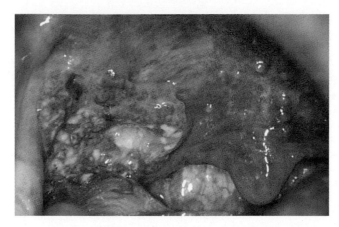

Fig. 10-116   Squamous cell carcinoma. Large, ulcerated lesion of the right lateral soft palate.

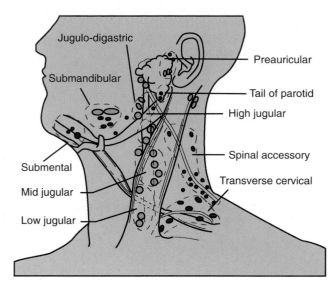

Fig. 10-117   Squamous cell carcinoma, metastatic spread. Diagram demonstrating potential sites for metastatic spread of oral carcinoma to regional lymph nodes.

at diagnosis is higher (Fig. 10-116). Three of every four oropharyngeal carcinomas arise from the tonsillar area or soft palate; most of the others originate on the base of the tongue. The initial symptoms are usually pain or difficulty in swallowing **(dysphagia).** The pain may be dull or sharp and frequently is referred to the ear.

As a general rule, the more posterior or inferior the oropharyngeal tumor location is, the larger is the lesion and the greater is the chance for lymphatic spread by the time of diagnosis. A soft palate lesion may present as a localized tumor, but 80% of posterior oropharyngeal wall lesions have metastasized or extensively involved surrounding structures by the time of diagnosis.

METASTASIS

The metastatic spread of oral squamous cell carcinoma is largely through the lymphatics to the ipsilateral cervical lymph nodes (Fig. 10-117). A cervical lymph node that contains a metastatic deposit of carcinoma is usually firm to stony hard, nontender, and enlarged (Fig. 10-118). If the malignant cells have perforated the capsule of the node and invaded into surrounding tissues, then the node will feel "fixed," or not easily movable. Extracapsular spread (extension of metastatic deposits outside of the lymph node capsule) is a microscopic feature associated with poor prognosis, including increased risk of locoregional recurrence, distant metastasis, and lower survival rates.

Occasionally, contralateral or bilateral metastatic deposits are seen, and at least 2% of patients have distant ("below the clavicles") metastasis at diagnosis; in some studies this figure is as high as 22%. The most common sites of distant metastasis are the lungs, liver, and bones, but any part of the body may be affected.

Carcinoma of the lower lip and oral floor tends to travel to the submental nodes; tumors from the poste-

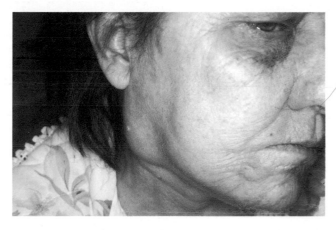

Fig. 10-118   Squamous cell carcinoma. Metastatic deposits within cervical lymph nodes present as firm, painless enlargements as seen in this patient with metastasis to a superior jugular node from a posterior lateral tongue carcinoma.

rior portions of the mouth travel to the superior jugular and digastric nodes. Lymphatic drainage from the oropharynx leads to the jugulodigastric chain of lymph nodes or to the retropharyngeal nodes, and metastatic deposits from oropharyngeal carcinoma are usually found there.

Metastasis is not an early event for carcinomas of the oral cavity proper. However, because of delay in the diagnosis, approximately 21% of patients have cervical metastases at diagnosis (60% in reports from tertiary care medical centers). In contrast, tumors that arise more posteriorly in the oropharynx are prone to early metastasis. More than 50% of all affected persons in

Table 10-2   Tumor-Node-Metastasis (TNM) Staging System for Oral Carcinoma

Primary Tumor Size (T)	
TX	No available information on primary tumor
T0	No evidence of primary tumor
Tis	Only carcinoma *in situ* at primary site
T1	Tumor 2 cm or less in greatest diameter
T2	Tumor more than 2 cm but not more than 4 cm in greatest diameter
T3	Tumor more than 4 cm in greatest diameter
T4a	(Lip) Tumor invades through cortical bone, inferior alveolar nerve, floor of mouth, or skin of face (i.e., chin, nose) Tumor is resectable
T4a	(Oral cavity) Tumor invades through cortical bone, into deep extrinsic tongue muscles (genioglossus, hyoglossus, palatoglossus, and styloglossus), maxillary sinus, or skin of face Tumor is resectable
T4b	Tumor involves masticator space, pterygoid plates, or skull base and/or encases internal carotid artery Tumor is unresectable

REGIONAL LYMPH NODE INVOLVEMENT (N)	
NX	Nodes could not be or were not assessed
N0	No regional lymph node metastasis
N1	Metastasis in a single ipsilateral node 3 cm or less in greatest diameter
N2	Metastasis in a single ipsilateral node more than 3 cm but not greater than 6 cm in greatest diameter; multiple ipsilateral nodes, none more than 6 cm in greatest diameter; or bilateral or contralateral nodes, none more than 6 cm in greatest diameter
N2a	Metastasis in a single ipsilateral node more than 3 cm but not greater than 6 cm in greatest diameter
N2b	Metastasis in multiple ipsilateral nodes, none more than 6 cm in greatest diameter
N2c	Metastasis in bilateral or contralateral nodes, none more than 6 cm in greatest diameter
N3	Metastasis in a node more than 6 cm in greatest diameter

Involvement by Distant Metastases (M)	
MX	Distant metastasis was not assessed
MO	No evidence of distant metastasis
M1	Distant metastasis is present

From Tumor-node-metastasis (TNM) staging system for oral carcinoma. In Greene FL, Page DL, Fleming ID et al, editors, *AJCC cancer staging manual*, ed 4, New York, 2002, Springer.

population studies have positive cervical nodes at diagnosis, and one in 10 already have distant metastasis by that time.

STAGING

Tumor size and the extent of metastatic spread of oral squamous cell carcinoma are the best indicators of the patient's prognosis. Quantifying these clinical parameters is called **staging** the disease. Table 10-2 summarizes the most popular staging protocol, the tumor-node-metastasis (TNM) system. Individualized TNM classifications are used for most human cancers, with each system pertaining exclusively to a specific anatomic site and a specific tumor type. This staging protocol depends on three basic clinical features:

1. T–Size of the primary tumor, in centimeters
2. N–Involvement of local lymph nodes
3. M–Distant metastasis

Once the three parameters are determined, they are tallied together to determine the appropriate stage. The higher the stage classification, the worse the prognosis (Table 10-3). In other words, a stage IV lesion is associated with a much worse prognosis than a stage I lesion. Most head and neck staging protocols do not use histopathologic or immunohistochemical findings beyond those needed for a determination of the diagnosis.

Table **10-3**   **TNM Clinical Staging Categories for Oral Squamous Cell Carcinoma**

		FIVE-YEAR RELATIVE SURVIVAL RATE	
Stage	**TNM Classification**	**Oral Cavity**	**Lip**
Stage I	T1 N0 M0	68%	83%
Stage II	T2 N0 M0	53%	73%
Stage III	T3 N0 M0, or T1, T2, or T3 N1 M0	41%	62%
Stage IV		27%	47%
IVA	T4a N0 or N1 M0, or T1, T2, T3, or T4a N2 M0		
IVB	Any T N3 M0, or T4b any N M0		
IVC	Any M1 lesion		

HISTOPATHOLOGIC FEATURES

Squamous cell carcinoma arises from dysplastic surface epithelium and is characterized histopathologically by invasive islands and cords of malignant squamous epithelial cells. When the tumor is sampled fortuitously at the earliest moment of invasion, the adjectives *superficially invasive* or *microinvasive* often are used. The features of epithelial dysplasia are discussed in more detail in the section pertaining to leukoplakia (see page 394).

Invasion is represented by irregular extension of lesional epithelium through the basement membrane and into subepithelial connective tissue. Individual squamous cells and sheets or islands of cells are seen to be thriving as independent entities within the connective tissues, without attachment to the surface epithelium. Invading cells and cell masses may extend deeply into underlying adipose tissue, muscle, or bone, destroying the original tissue as they progress. Lesional cells may surround and destroy blood vessels and may invade into the lumina of veins or lymphatics. There is often a strong inflammatory or immune cell response to invading epithelium, and focal areas of necrosis may be present. The lesional epithelium is capable of inducing the formation of new small blood vessels (**angiogenesis**) and, occasionally, dense fibrosis (**desmoplasia** or **scirrhous change**).

Whether the tumor is superficially or deeply invasive, lesional cells generally show abundant eosinophilic cytoplasm with large, often darkly staining (**hyperchromatic**) nuclei and an increased nuclear-to-cytoplasmic ratio. Varying degrees of cellular and nuclear pleomorphism are seen. The normal product of squamous epithelium is keratin, and **keratin pearls** (a round focus of concentrically layered keratinized cells) may be produced within lesional epithelium. Single cells also may undergo individual cell keratinization.

Histopathologic evaluation of the degree to which these tumors resemble their parent tissue (squamous epithelium) and produce their normal product (keratin) is called **grading**. Lesions are graded on a 3-point (grades I to III) or a 4-point (grades I to IV) scale. The less differentiated tumors receive the higher numerals. The histopathologic grade of a tumor is related somewhat to its biologic behavior. In other words, a tumor that is mature enough to closely resemble its tissue of origin seems to grow at a slightly slower pace and to metastasize later in its course. Such a tumor is called *low-grade, grade I,* or *well-differentiated* squamous cell carcinoma (Fig. 10-119). In contrast, a tumor with much cellular and nuclear pleomorphism and with little or no keratin production may be so immature that it becomes difficult to identify the tissue of origin. Such a tumor often enlarges rapidly, metastasizes early in its course, and is termed *high-grade, grade III/IV, poorly differentiated,* or *anaplastic* (Fig. 10-120). A tumor with a microscopic appearance somewhere between these two extremes is labeled a "moderately differentiated" carcinoma (Fig. 10-121).

To a certain extent, the grading of squamous cell carcinoma is a subjective process, depending on the area of the tumor sampled and the individual pathologist's criteria for evaluation. Moreover, clinical staging seems to correlate much better with the prognosis than microscopic grading. Over the past several decades, investigators have proposed various multiparameter histopathologic assessment systems in an attempt to provide more objective criteria that correlate with prognosis. Variables such as pattern of invasion, tumor thickness, degree of keratinization, nuclear pleomorphism, lymphocytic response, and mitotic rate have been included in such grading systems. However, widespread agreement regarding the use of such methods is lacking.

The diagnosis of squamous cell carcinoma almost always is made with routine light microscopy. Special studies that use monoclonal antibodies directed against cytokeratins may, however, be needed to distinguish

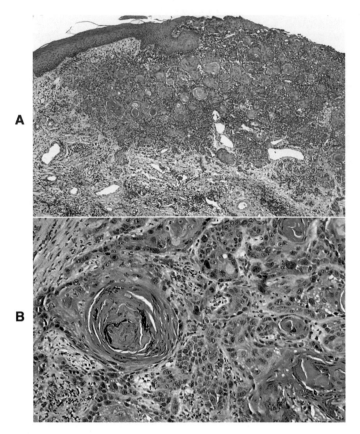

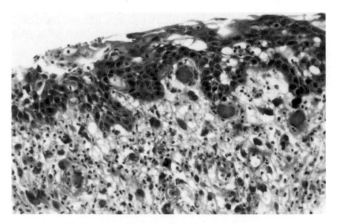

Fig. 10-120   Poorly differentiated squamous cell carcinoma. The numerous pleomorphic cells within the lamina propria represent anaplastic carcinoma.

Fig. 10-119   Well-differentiated squamous cell carcinoma. A, Low-power photomicrograph showing islands of malignant squamous epithelium invading into the lamina propria. **B,** High-power view showing dysplastic epithelial cells with keratin pearl formation.

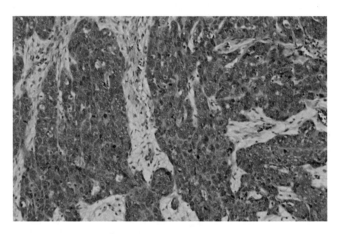

Fig. 10-121   Moderately differentiated squamous cell carcinoma. Although no keratinization is seen in this medium-power view, these malignant cells are still easily recognizable as being of squamous epithelial origin.

high-grade or poorly differentiated squamous cell carcinoma from other malignancies.

TREATMENT AND PROGNOSIS

Carcinoma of the vermilion zone of the lip is usually treated by surgical excision, typically a wedge resection, with excellent results. Only 8% recur, and 5-year survival rates are 95% to 100%. In one study that evaluated all vermilion cancers diagnosed in a population over six decades, not one patient died of his or her disease. Squamous cell carcinomas of the upper lip vermilion appear to have a different biologic behavior than do those of the lower lip. The 5-year survival rate is only 58%, and 25% of lesions recur after treatment. Fortunately, upper lip carcinoma is considerably less common than lower lip carcinoma.

The clinical stage of the disease guides the treatment of intraoral squamous cell carcinoma, which consists of wide (radical) surgical excision, radiation therapy, or a combination of surgery and radiation therapy. The tumor's location may influence the treatment plan.

Oropharyngeal lesions usually receive radiation therapy. Additional indications for radiation therapy include the presence of close or positive resection margins, regional metastasis, high-grade histopathologic features, and perineural or angiolymphatic invasion. A variety of chemotherapeutic agents are used as adjunctive therapy. Chemotherapy typically is administered concurrently with radiation, as induction chemotherapy followed by concurrent chemoradiation, or as palliative therapy. Commonly used agents include platinum-containing compounds (e.g., cisplatin, carboplatin), 5-fluorouracil, and taxanes (e.g., paclitaxel, docetaxel). In addition, clinical trials evaluating monoclonal antibodies or small molecule inhibitors directed against EGFR have shown promise, and molecular-based targeted therapies are anticipated to become important treatment strategies in the future. Although chemotherapeutic agents may reduce the size of a tumor mass temporarily, none has improved survival rates significantly.

For the small intraoral carcinoma, a single treatment modality is usually chosen. Patients with larger lesions or lesions with clinically palpable lymph nodes typically require combined therapy. In addition, patients with early-stage (clinically T1/T2 and N0) but deeply invasive (tumor thickness >3 or 4 mm) tongue carcinomas are at increased risk for subclinical nodal metastasis and thus may receive either postoperative neck irradiation or elective neck dissection. With suspected local lymph node metastasis, either a radical or modified radical neck dissection is performed. Radical neck dissection is essentially an *en bloc* removal of all fibrofatty tissues of the lateral triangle of the neck, including the superior, middle, and inferior jugular nodes, the supraclavicular group of nodes, and variable portions of the surrounding musculature. The use of sentinel-node biopsy (biopsy of the first lymph node in the lymphatic basin to receive drainage from the tumor) to identify patients with occult neck metastasis has shown promise but remains investigational for patients with oral cancer.

The prognosis for survival from oral cancer depends on tumor stage (see Table 10-3). The 5-year relative survival rate for intraoral carcinoma is 53% to 68% if the tumor is relatively small (<4 cm) and metastasis has not occurred by the time of diagnosis (stage I and II); 41% when the tumor is ≥4 cm and either without metastasis or with metastasis in a single ipsilateral regional lymph ≤3 cm (stage III); and only 27% when the tumor has invaded adjacent structures, has metastasized to a distant site, or is associated with regional metastasis of multiple nodes, a single ipsilateral node >3 cm and ≤6 cm, or a node >6 cm (stage IV). Although some patients die of their disease as many as 10 years after initial treatment, the great majority of deaths occur within the first 5 years.

The various molecular markers associated with carcinoma, such as mutation of the p53 tumor suppressor gene, have shown equivocal results as prognostic indicators. The relationship between HPV tumor status and prognosis is unclear. Some studies have suggested that HPV-positive tumors are associated with improved treatment response and prolonged survival; however, other studies have reported no significant difference in survival between patients with HPV-positive and HPV-negative tumors.

The overall 5-year survival rate for intraoral carcinoma in whites in the United States and Europe has increased from 40% in the 1950s to 59% today. During the same period, however, the rate for black Americans has increased only slightly from 36% to 39%. Researchers believe that this disparity in survival results from differences in access to health care services; in addition, some have hypothesized that lifestyle habits (e.g., tobacco and alcohol use, nutrition), cultural differences, and the presence of comorbid conditions may be contributing factors.

Despite advances in treatment and in the understanding of the underlying molecular pathogenesis of oral cancer, survival rates over the last several decades have not improved significantly and have remained in the range of 50% to 59%. Therefore, early diagnosis and prevention are essential for improving patient outcomes. In addition, there is much interest in the development of chemoprevention strategies for preventing the malignant transformation of oral dysplastic lesions or preventing the development of second primary or recurrent tumors in patients with a history of oral squamous cell carcinoma.

MULTIPLE CARCINOMAS

Patients with one carcinoma of the mouth or throat are at increased risk for additional concurrent (synchronous) or later (metachronous) primary surface epithelial malignancies of the upper aerodigestive tract, the esophagus, the stomach, the lungs, and other sites. This risk has been estimated to be as low as 6% and as high as 44% in affected individuals. The highest figures are associated with male patients who continue to smoke and abuse alcohol after therapy. Overall, in 9% to 25% of patients with oral carcinoma, additional mouth or throat malignancies develop.

In patients with more than one upper aerodigestive tract malignancy, approximately one third of the tumors arise simultaneously. Of the rest, the second lesion usually develops within 3 years after the initial cancer. This tendency toward the development of multiple mucosal cancers, sometimes called *field cancerization*, may reflect diffuse exposure to local carcinogens, a process that increases the malignant transformation potential of all exposed epithelial cells. Molecular analyses of various markers, including loss of heterozygosity (LOH), microsatellite alterations, p53 tumor suppressor gene mutations, and X-chromosome inactivation, have identified genetic alterations shared between tumor tissue and adjacent clinically normal-appearing tissue in one third to one half of cases examined. In addition, investigators have shown that a significant proportion of second primary tumors develop from the same preneoplastic precursor lesion or "field," with the remaining cases representing tumors that develop independently. Furthermore, researchers have proposed that patches of clonal cells can progress to develop additional mutations and give rise to subclones in a process known as *clonal divergence*, which would account for the genetic heterogeneity typically seen among these tumors.

VERRUCOUS CARCINOMA (SNUFF DIPPER'S CANCER; ACKERMAN'S TUMOR)

Verrucous carcinoma is a low-grade variant of oral **squamous cell carcinoma.** In 1948, Ackerman described this lesion in detail, although the term *verrucous carcinoma* had been used in 1944 in a series of cases reported by Burford, Ackerman, and Robinson. Ackerman postulated that some of these lesions might be associated with the use of smokeless tobacco, because 11 of his 31 patients were "tobacco chewers." However, there was no mention of the type of smokeless tobacco used and no mention of whether any of these patients also had smoked tobacco. In addition to the oral mucosa, verrucous carcinoma has been identified at several extraoral sites, including laryngeal, vulvovaginal, penile, anorectal, sinonasal, and esophageal mucosa, as well as the skin of the breast, axilla, ear canal, and soles of the feet. Tumors at anatomic sites other than the mouth are unrelated to tobacco use. Several investigators have identified human papillomavirus (HPV) subtypes 16 and 18 in a minority of oral verrucous carcinomas, but the significance of this is unclear because this virus often is associated with otherwise normal oral mucosa.

Verrucous carcinoma represents less than 1% to 10% of all oral squamous cell carcinomas, depending on the local popularity of smokeless tobacco use. The only epidemiologic assessment of this tumor in a Western culture reported an average annual incidence rate of one to three oral lesions per 1 million population each year. Among 411,534 cases of head and neck carcinoma recorded in the National Cancer Database from 1985 to 1996, only 0.6% of cases were diagnosed as verrucous carcinoma.

Some verrucous carcinomas arise from the oral mucosa in people who chronically use chewing tobacco or snuff, typically in the area where the tobacco is habitually placed. Cases also occur in nonusers, but the exact figure is difficult to assess because patients will often deny the tobacco habit. In smokeless tobacco users, conventional squamous cell carcinoma is much more likely to develop than this low-grade variant.

CLINICAL FEATURES

Verrucous carcinoma is found predominantly in men older than 55 years of age (average age, 65 to 70 years). In areas where women are frequent users of dry snuff, however, older females may predominate. The most common sites of oral mucosal involvement include the mandibular vestibule, gingiva, buccal mucosa, tongue, and hard palate. The site of occurrence often corresponds to the site of chronic tobacco placement. In

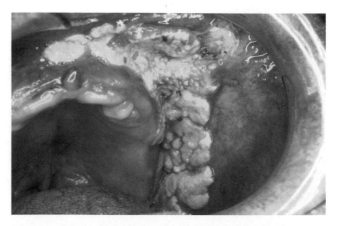

Fig. 10-122 Verrucous carcinoma. Extensive papillary, white lesion of the maxillary vestibule.

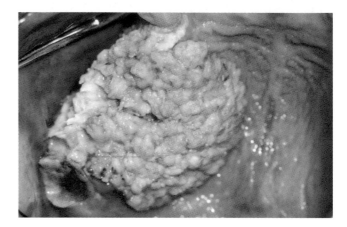

Fig. 10-123 Verrucous carcinoma. Large, exophytic, papillary mass of the maxillary alveolar ridge.

cultural groups who keep the tobacco in the maxillary vestibule or under the tongue, these locations are the most commonly involved sites.

Oral verrucous carcinoma is usually extensive by the time of diagnosis, and it is not unusual for a tumor to be present in the mouth for 2 to 3 years before definitive diagnosis. The lesion appears as a diffuse, well-demarcated, painless, thick plaque with papillary or verruciform surface projections (Figs. 10-122 and 10-123). Lesions are typically white but also may appear erythematous or pink. The color depends on the amount of keratin produced and the degree of host inflammatory response to the tumor. If left untreated, then lesions may destroy underlying structures, such as bone, cartilage, muscle, and salivary glands. Enlarged cervical lymph nodes in patients with verrucous carcinoma usually represent inflammatory reactive changes rather than nodal metastasis.

Leukoplakia or **tobacco pouch keratosis** may be seen on adjacent mucosal surfaces, and verrucous carcinoma is a lesion that may develop from the high-risk

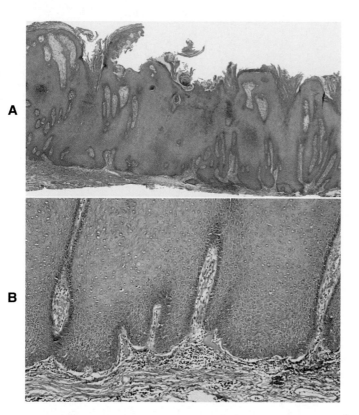

Fig. 10-124   Verrucous carcinoma. A, Low-power photomicrograph showing marked epithelial hyperplasia with a rough, papillary surface and keratin plugging. **B,** High-power view showing bulbous rete ridges without significant dysplasia.

precancer, proliferative verucous leukoplakia (PVL) (see page 391). PVL and verrucous carcinoma may have been reported in the past by the name **oral florid papillomatosis.**

HISTOPATHOLOGIC FEATURES

Verrucous carcinoma has a deceptively benign microscopic appearance; it is characterized by wide and elongated rete ridges that appear to "push" into the underlying connective tissue (Fig. 10-124). Lesions usually show abundant keratin (usually parakeratin) production and a papillary or verruciform surface. Parakeratin typically fills the numerous clefts or crypts **(parakeratin plugs)** between the surface projections. These projections may be long and pointed or short and blunted. The lesional epithelial cells generally show a normal maturation pattern with no significant degree of cellular atypia. There is frequently an intense infiltrate of chronic inflammatory cells in the subjacent connective tissue.

The histopathologic diagnosis of verrucous carcinoma requires an adequate incisional biopsy. Because the individual cells are not very dysplastic, the patholo-gist must evaluate the overall histomorphologic configuration of the lesion to arrive at an appropriate diagnosis. Adequate sampling also is important because as many as 20% of these lesions have a routine squamous cell carcinoma developing concurrently within the verrucous carcinoma.

TREATMENT AND PROGNOSIS

Because metastasis is an extremely rare event in verrucous carcinoma, the treatment of choice is surgical excision without radical neck dissection. The surgery generally need not be as extensive as that required for routine squamous cell carcinoma of a similar size. With this treatment, 90% of patients are disease free after 5 years, although some patients will require at least one additional surgical procedure during that time. The treatment failures usually occur in patients with the most extensive involvement or in those unable to tolerate extensive surgery because of unrelated systemic diseases. An additional cause of treatment failure is the initial inability to identify a focal squamous cell carcinoma arising concurrently within the less aggressive lesion. Verrucous carcinomas containing foci of conventional squamous cell carcinoma should be treated as conventional squamous cell carcinomas.

Radiotherapy is an alternative primary treatment modality but provides poorer local control and thus is considered less effective than surgery. In addition, radiotherapy has been unpopular because of published reports of poorly differentiated or anaplastic carcinoma developing within the lesion after treatment. However, more recent analysis suggests that this threat is seriously overexaggerated. Chemotherapy may temporarily reduce the size of verrucous carcinoma and may be an option for inoperable cases, but it is not considered a definitive, stand-alone treatment. In a limited number of cases, tumor regression after radiochemotherapy or photodynamic therapy has been reported, although these treatment alternatives require further study.

SPINDLE CELL CARCINOMA (SARCOMATOID SQUAMOUS CELL CARCINOMA; POLYPOID SQUAMOUS CELL CARCINOMA)

Spindle cell carcinoma is a rare variant of squamous cell carcinoma characterized by dysplastic surface squamous epithelium in conjunction with an invasive spindle cell element. It may be indistinguishable from connective tissue sarcomas or other spindle cell malignancies at the level of the light microscope.

In the past, this biphasic lesion was thought to be a "collision" tumor between a carcinoma and sarcoma, but most authorities now consider the spindle cells to

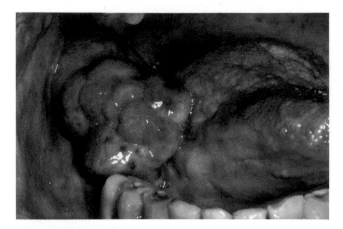

Fig. 10-125   Spindle cell carcinoma. Large polypoid mass arising from the right lateral tongue.

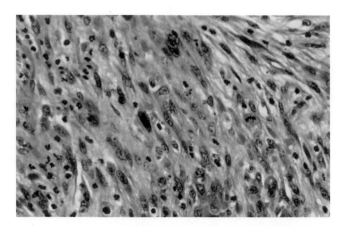

Fig. 10-126   Spindle cell carcinoma. Streaming fascicles of pleomorphic spindle cells that represent anaplastic epithelial cells.

be simply an anaplastic type of carcinoma cell. Electron microscopy and immunohistochemical analysis support the concept that these lesional cells are of epithelial origin, with the ability to produce mesenchymal intermediate filaments. Based on immunohistochemical studies, some investigators have hypothesized that a dysfunctional cadherin-catenin complex important for intercellular adhesion causes the tumor cells to shift from a squamous to a spindled type, with increased infiltrative behavior. More than one third of all mucosal cases develop as recurrences after radiotherapy for a more differentiated squamous cell carcinoma, a phenomenon known as **dedifferentiation.**

CLINICAL FEATURES

The mean age at diagnosis for spindle cell carcinoma is 57 years (range: 29 to 93 years). There is no sex predilection. The neoplasm occurs predominantly in the upper aerodigestive tract, especially the larynx, oral cavity, and esophagus. Within the mouth, the lower lip, lateral posterior tongue, and alveolar ridges are common sites, but other areas may be involved.

In contrast to other oral cancers, the spindle cell carcinoma typically appears as a pedunculated, polypoid mass, but it may occasionally appear as a sessile, nodular or fungating mass or as an ulcer (Fig. 10-125). Pain and paresthesia are prominent features. The tumor grows rapidly, tends to metastasize early, and is typically diagnosed in a late stage (stages III and IV). Lower lip lesions seem to have a special propensity to travel along nerves through the mental foramen and into the mandibular canal.

HISTOPATHOLOGIC FEATURES

The spindle cell carcinoma is composed predominantly of fascicles of anaplastic spindle-shaped cells (Fig. 10-126). Some spindle cells may appear as

obvious epithelial elements, but others strongly resemble atypical mesenchymal cells. On rare occasions, bone, cartilage, or muscle differentiation may be seen. Numerous mitotic figures often are present. The overall picture is similar to that of an anaplastic fibrosarcoma (see page 553), except for the often-inconspicuous squamous element.

The squamous component usually consists of carcinoma *in situ* of the overlying surface epithelium but may appear as islands of dysplastic squamous epithelium among the spindle cells. Direct transition between the two cell types may be seen. Metastatic lesions may show only spindle cells, only squamous cells, or a combination of spindle and squamous cells.

Serial sections may be needed to find areas of unequivocal squamous cell carcinoma, and immunohistochemical techniques can be particularly useful in distinguishing this tumor from mesenchymal spindle cell malignancies. The lesional cells of most mesenchymal tumors typically produce vimentin but not cytokeratin. Approximately two thirds of the cases of spindle cell carcinoma react with antibodies directed against cytokeratin, and an equivalent number show vimentin immunoreactivity. Some cases also will be positive for carcinoembryonic antigen (CEA).

TREATMENT AND PROGNOSIS

The treatment of choice for spindle cell carcinoma is radical surgery, with neck dissection when clinically positive nodes are present. Most authors agree that radiotherapy and chemotherapy are ineffective. However, adjuvant radiation therapy may be of benefit in cases where surgical margins are positive for tumor. The 5-year disease-free survival rate is approximately 30% for oral lesions, with most deaths occurring within

1 year of diagnosis. This is somewhat worse than the prognosis for the tumor when it occurs in other anatomic sites, but it is similar to the prognosis for high-grade oral squamous cell carcinoma. Surprisingly, tumor size seems to have little effect on the prognosis, although there is some evidence that the microscopic depth of invasion is a strong prognostic indicator in oral lesions, with superficial tumors demonstrating a better prognosis.

ADENOSQUAMOUS CARCINOMA

Adenosquamous carcinoma is a rare variant of **squamous cell carcinoma** that is characterized histopathologically by a combination of adenocarcinoma and squamous cell carcinoma. The adenoid (glandular) pattern, which includes mucus production, has been demonstrated clearly in metastatic deposits. Some authorities consider this carcinoma to be merely a high-grade **mucoepidermoid carcinoma** (see page 487). The cause is unknown.

CLINICAL FEATURES

Cases of adenosquamous carcinoma have been reported from the tongue, oral floor, and other mucosal surfaces, usually in older adults. There is a slight male predilection. The clinical appearance is that of a nodular, broad-based, variably painful mass with or without surface ulceration. Eighty percent of patients have metastatic deposits within the neck nodes at diagnosis.

HISTOPATHOLOGIC FEATURES

Adenosquamous carcinoma appears as an admixture of a surface squamous cell carcinoma and an underlying ductal adenocarcinoma. The glandular component tends to be most prominent in deeper portions of the tumor. Intracytoplasmic mucin is noted by mucicarmine staining in most cases, making differentiation from mucoepidermoid carcinoma difficult but helping to distinguish adenosquamous carcinoma from forms of squamous cell carcinoma that exhibit a pseudoglandular pattern of degeneration. Both squamous and glandular components immunoreact with antibodies directed against high molecular–weight cytokeratin (KL1).

TREATMENT AND PROGNOSIS

Radical surgical excision, with or without radiation therapy, is the treatment of choice for patients with adenosquamous carcinoma. The prognosis is poor; among previously reported cases involving the upper aerodigestive tract, the overall 5-year survival rate is 13%, with 42% of patients dying of disease after a mean period of 2 years after their diagnosis. Cervical lymph node metastasis develops in approximately 65% of patients, and distant metastasis develops in approximately 23% of patients, with the lung being the most common site of dissemination.

BASALOID SQUAMOUS CARCINOMA (BASALOID SQUAMOUS CELL CARCINOMA)

Basaloid squamous carcinoma is a lesion found primarily in the upper aerodigestive tract mucosa and represents the most recently described variant of squamous cell carcinoma. It has a tendency to develop in the hypopharynx, but dozens of oral lesions have been reported.

CLINICAL FEATURES

Basaloid squamous carcinoma of the head and neck occurs predominantly in men, although no significant gender predilection exists among previously reported oral cases. The neoplasm tends to occur in persons 40 to 85 years of age and in abusers of alcohol and smoked tobacco. It most commonly involves the larynx, pyriform sinus, and tongue base, but any region of the upper aerodigestive tract may be affected. The individual lesion clinically appears as a fungating mass or ulcer and may be painful or interfere with swallowing **(dysphagia)**. Almost 80% of patients have cervical metastases at the time of diagnosis of this high-grade, aggressive cancer.

HISTOPATHOLOGIC FEATURES

As its name connotes, basaloid squamous carcinoma has two microscopic components. The first is a superficial, well-differentiated or moderately differentiated squamous cell carcinoma, often with surface ulceration, multifocal origin, and areas of carcinoma *in situ*. The second, deeper component is an invasive basaloid epithelium arranged in islands, cords, and glandlike lobules. This deeper tumor often shows palisading of peripheral cells, necrosis of central regions, and occasional squamous differentiation (Fig. 10-127). This component appears similar to basal cell carcinoma, adenoid cystic carcinoma, basal cell adenocarcinoma, or neuroendocrine carcinoma. The interface between the two components is typically sharp and distinct, but transition from squamous to basaloid cells may occasionally be seen. Basaloid cells and islands of cells often are surrounded by mucoid stroma (basal lamina mate-

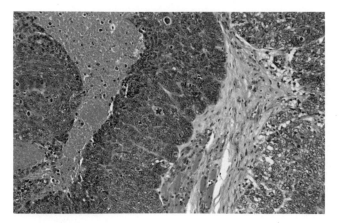

Fig. 10-127   Basaloid squamous carcinoma. Sheets of basaloid squamous epithelium exhibiting a high mitotic index and tumor necrosis.

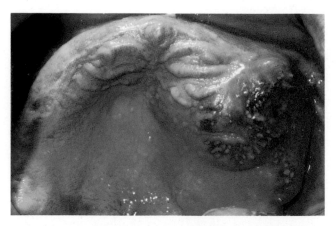

Fig. 10-128   Carcinoma of the maxillary sinus. The tumor has produced a bulge of the posterior maxillary alveolar ridge and is beginning to ulcerate through the surface mucosa.

rial). Microcystic spaces filled with PAS-positive basal lamina material may be interspersed among the tumor islands as well.

TREATMENT AND PROGNOSIS

Basaloid squamous carcinoma is an aggressive malignancy. Affected patients have a mean survival time of only 23 months. Although somewhat controversial, several recent studies have suggested that basaloid squamous cell carcinoma may have a similar outcome compared with conventional squamous cell carcinoma when cases are matched by clinical stage and anatomic location. Therefore, the poor prognosis for basaloid squamous cell carcinoma simply might be caused by a tendency for these patients to be diagnosed with late-stage disease. Surgery followed by radiotherapy is the recommended treatment, usually with adjuvant chemotherapy for the distant metastases.

CARCINOMA OF THE MAXILLARY SINUS

Carcinoma of the maxillary sinus or antrum is an uncommon malignancy of largely unknown cause. It does not appear to be related to sinusitis or nasal polyps. Unlike squamous cell carcinomas in other head and neck sites, squamous cell carcinomas of the paranasal sinuses have been associated only weakly with tobacco use. A strong causal relationship to occupational wood and leather dust exposure has been established for the rarely occurring sinonasal intestinal type of adenocarcinoma. Maxillary sinus carcinomas comprise only 3% of all head and neck carcinomas; however, among paranasal sinus carcinomas, the maxillary sinus is the most common site (accounting for 80% of lesions). Most lesions remain asymptomatic or mimic sinusitis for

long periods while the tumor grows to fill the sinus. Therefore, the diagnosis may not be made until the lesion has perforated through the surrounding bone.

The majority of maxillary sinus carcinomas are classified as *squamous cell carcinomas*. However, additional carcinomas that may arise in this location include sinonasal adenocarcinoma, **sinonasal undifferentiated carcinoma** (SNUC) (see next section), neuroendocrine (small cell undifferentiated) carcinoma, and salivary gland type of adenocarcinoma.

CLINICAL AND RADIOGRAPHIC FEATURES

Typically, carcinoma of the maxillary sinus is a disease of older adults. There is a slight predilection for males. More than 80% of cases are advanced (stage III or stage IV) at the time of diagnosis. Affected patients generally complain of a chronic unilateral nasal stuffiness or notice an ulceration or mass of the hard palate or alveolar bone (Fig. 10-128). When the second division of the trigeminal nerve is involved, intense pain or paresthesia of the midface or maxilla may occur, perhaps simulating a toothache. Teeth in the area of the tumor may become loosened, and dental radiographs often reveal a "moth-eaten" destruction of the lamina dura and surrounding bone. A panoramic radiograph shows a cloudy sinus with destruction of its bony wall; however, the extent of the tumor is best visualized by computed tomography (CT) or magnetic resonance imaging (MRI).

If the tumor perforates the lateral wall of the sinus, unilateral facial swelling and pain are usually present. If the extension is medial, then nasal obstruction or hemorrhage usually occurs. Extension superiorly results in displacement or protrusion of the eyeball. Approximately 4% of patients have cervical or submandibular lymph node metastasis at the time of diagnosis.

Distant metastasis is quite uncommon until late in the progression of disease.

HISTOPATHOLOGIC FEATURES

Although the antrum is lined by respiratory epithelium, the great majority of maxillary sinus carcinomas are **squamous cell carcinomas,** usually moderately or poorly differentiated.

TREATMENT AND PROGNOSIS

Carcinoma confined within the maxillary sinus usually is treated by hemimaxillectomy; those that have perforated through the surrounding bone are treated by radiotherapy or combined radical surgery and radiotherapy. However, even with radical treatment the prognosis is poor, with a 5-year survival rate of approximately 40%. The presence of metastatic deposits in local lymph nodes reduces the survival rate to less than 8%, as does involvement of the pterygopalatine fossa. With or without cervical node involvement, death usually occurs from local destruction and the inability to control the primary disease.

SINONASAL UNDIFFERENTIATED CARCINOMA

Sinonasal undifferentiated carcinoma (SNUC) is a rare, highly aggressive, and clinicopathologically distinctive neoplasm of the nasal cavity and paranasal sinuses. The tumor was first described in 1986, and since then fewer than 100 cases have been reported. In the earlier literature, tumors of this type were probably reported as anaplastic or undifferentiated carcinomas.

The histogenesis is uncertain; some investigators have theorized that the cell of origin may be related to the schneiderian membrane or olfactory epithelium. The pathogenesis of SNUC is poorly understood. A few cases have been associated with a history of smoking or the presence of Epstein-Barr virus (EBV), although a strong correlation with these factors has not been established. In some instances, patients have developed SNUC secondary to radiation therapy for nasopharyngeal carcinoma or retinoblastoma.

CLINICAL AND RADIOGRAPHIC FEATURES

Although a broad age range (third through ninth decades) has been reported, there is a tendency for older patients to be affected, with a median age at presentation in the sixth decade. Men are affected more commonly than women, with a male-to-female ratio of approximately 2:1 to 3:1.

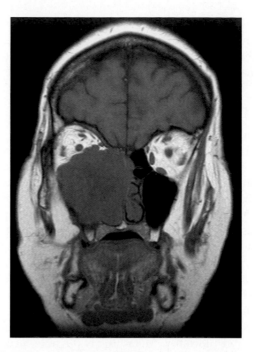

Fig. 10-129   Sinonasal undifferentiated carcinoma (SNUC). T1-weighted magnetic resonance image (MRI) showing a large destructive mass filling the right maxillary sinus with extension into the orbital region and nasal cavity. *(Courtesy of Dr. Zoran Rumboldt.)*

SNUC is well known for rapid development of locally extensive disease. The neoplasm typically appears as a large tumor mass that can involve multiple regions of the sinonasal tract, usually including the nasal cavity, maxillary sinus, and ethmoid sinuses. In addition, extension into contiguous sites—such as the nasopharynx, orbit, and cranial cavity—is common. Inferior penetration into the oral cavity is possible as well. There is usually relatively rapid development of multiple sinonasal symptoms, including nasal obstruction or discharge, epistaxis, swelling, and pain. Orbital involvement may lead to proptosis, periorbital swelling, diplopia, and vision loss. Cranial nerve palsies are a common finding as well.

Radiographic assessment is best performed by CT or MRI, which typically reveals a large, expansile sinonasal mass with bony destruction and invasion of adjacent structures (Fig. 10-129).

HISTOPATHOLOGIC FEATURES

Sinonasal undifferentiated carcinoma is characterized by trabeculae, ribbons, sheets, and nests of polygonal cells with minimal cytoplasm and pleomorphic, hyperchromatic to vesicular nuclei. No squamous or glandular differentiation should be observed. Mitotic figures are numerous. Tumor necrosis, apoptosis, and lymphovascular invasion usually are prominent. The surface epithelium overlying the tumor may exhibit dysplasia or carcinoma *in situ*. Immunohistochemical staining for cytokeratin or epithelial membrane antigen typically is positive.

TREATMENT AND PROGNOSIS

The standard approach has been aggressive multi-modal therapy, including complete surgical resection when feasible followed by adjuvant radiation and/or chemotherapy. The prognosis for this lesion is extremely poor, with an overall 5-year survival rate of less than 20%. However, a few centers recently have reported promising results with induction chemotherapy followed by radiation and surgical resection of any remaining disease. This newer treatment approach has been associated with 2-year survival rates of 64% to 75%. High-dose chemotherapy and bone marrow transplantation may extend the life of the patient. Local recurrence is common and is the major cause of morbidity and mortality. Metastasis is possible, usually to cervical lymph nodes, bone, liver, or brain.

NASOPHARYNGEAL CARCINOMA

Nasopharyngeal carcinoma refers to a group of malignancies that arise from the lining epithelium of the lymphoid tissue–rich nasopharynx; similar tumors are found in the palatine tonsil and base of tongue. These three anatomic sites are collectively called **Waldeyer's tonsillar tissue** or **Waldeyer's ring.**

Nasopharyngeal carcinoma is rare in most areas of the world. The average annual incidence rate in the United States is less than 1 case per 100,000 persons. In southern Chinese men, however, the rate is a startling 20 to 55 cases per 100,000. Among southern Chinese men who migrate to the United States, the rate is intermediate, which suggests an environmental causative agent. Intermediate rates also are observed among many indigenous people of Southeast Asia (including Thais, Vietnamese, Malays, and Filipinos), Inuits of Alaska and Greenland, and Arabs of North Africa. Infection with Epstein-Barr virus, diets deficient in vitamin C, and consumption of salt fish that contains potentially carcinogenic N-nitrosamines have been implicated as contributory factors. Tobacco also has been implicated as a risk factor; however, the magnitude of risk for carcinoma development for a given level of tobacco exposure is lower in the nasopharynx than in other parts of the upper aerodigestive tract.

CLINICAL FEATURES

Nasopharyngeal carcinoma occurs in all age groups, but most commonly affects those who are 40 to 60 years old. It also occurs three times more commonly in

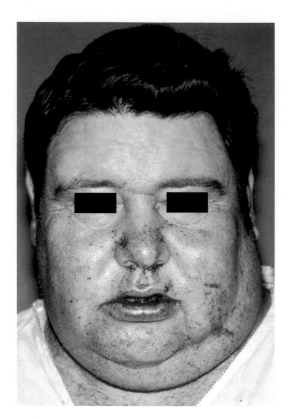

Fig. 10-130   Nasopharyngeal carcinoma. This patient initially appeared with metastatic carcinoma in the left lateral neck. Further evaluation revealed a primary tumor of the nasopharynx. *(Courtesy of Dr. D. E. Kenady.)*

men than in women. The primary lesion, which usually arises from the lateral nasopharyngeal wall, often is small and difficult to detect, even when the area is examined endoscopically. The first sign of disease for 50% to 60% of patients is an enlarged, firm to hard, cervical lymph node, which represents metastatic tumor (Fig. 10-130). Symptoms related to the ear are described by slightly less than half of these patients. If the tumor arises near the eustachian tube, then unilateral serous otitis media, otalgia, or hearing loss from obstruction may be the presenting complaint.

Epistaxis, nasal obstruction, and pharyngeal pain may be present. The tumor may invade through the foramen lacerum into the brain, producing CNS symptoms, or it may involve cranial nerves in the area, causing specific symptoms related to those nerves. Significantly, 5% to 10% of patients also have distant metastasis at the time of diagnosis.

HISTOPATHOLOGIC FEATURES

The surgeon often has difficulty finding the primary lesion of nasopharyngeal carcinoma clinically, and multiple, systematic biopsy samples of the nasopharyngeal mucosa may be necessary for tumor identification

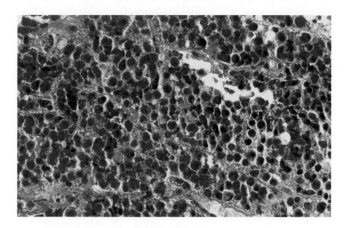

Fig. 10-131   Nasopharyngeal carcinoma. Poorly differentiated tumor exhibiting sheets of rounded tumor cells.

and diagnosis. Microscopic examination of a nasopharyngeal carcinoma typically shows one of three histopathologic patterns:

1. Squamous cell carcinoma (keratinizing squamous cell carcinoma)
2. Differentiated nonkeratinizing carcinoma (nonkeratinizing squamous cell carcinoma)
3. Undifferentiated nonkeratinizing carcinoma (poorly differentiated carcinoma, anaplastic carcinoma, lymphoepithelioma)

More than one histopathologic type may be present in the same biopsy sample, in which case the tumor is classified according to the predominant histologic type.

The histopathologic features of the **keratinizing squamous cell carcinoma** are identical to those of squamous cell carcinoma of other head and neck regions (see page 419). Evidence of keratinization must be seen at the light microscopic level.

The lesional cells of **differentiated nonkeratinizing carcinoma** are relatively mature and somewhat squamous in nature, but they produce no keratin. Broad interconnecting bands of oval or round cells are organized in plexiform and papillary patterns.

Undifferentiated nonkeratinizing carcinoma consists of sheets of lesional cells with less distinct margins that show virtually no differentiation in most instances (Fig. 10-131). They have very little cytoplasm and large vesicular nuclei. These tumor cells are often intermixed with the lymphoid cells normally found at this anatomic site. The term **lymphoepithelioma** has been used to describe this lesion because it was once thought to be a malignancy that originated from both epithelial and lymphoid tissues. This terminology should be discouraged, however, because the lymphoid tissue is not part of the neoplastic process. Such undifferentiated tumors may be difficult to distinguish from lymphoma by light microscopy alone, and immunohistochemical studies often are used to demonstrate

cytokeratins within the carcinoma cells. Some of these undifferentiated tumors currently are classified as sinonasal undifferentiated carcinomas (SNUC). Occasional neoplasms show neuroendocrine differentiation.

The less-differentiated lesions tend to occur in younger individuals. In fact, virtually all nasopharyngeal carcinomas in people younger than 40 years of age are poorly differentiated. Among southern Chinese patients, the vast majority (95%) of cases are classified as undifferentiated nonkeratinizing carcinomas, whereas in nonendemic areas, 30% to 50% of cases are keratinizing squamous cell carcinomas.

TREATMENT AND PROGNOSIS

Because of the inaccessibility of the nasopharynx and the high frequency of metastasis at diagnosis, nasopharyngeal carcinoma is treated most frequently with radiotherapy to the nasopharynx and neck. Although there has been some controversy regarding the benefit of adding chemotherapy to radiation therapy, emerging evidence favors concurrent chemoradiation over radiation alone for improved survival among patients with locally advanced disease.

The prognosis ranges from good to poor, depending on the stage of the disease. The overall 5-year disease-free survival rate reported in one large series of cases in the United States was 45.5%. For stage I patients, a 100% 5-year survival rate has been demonstrated. Stage II is associated with a 67% 5-year survival rate; stage III, 44%; and stage IV, 34%. Patients with two or more clinical symptoms tend to have a worse prognosis. When treated with radiation therapy, the differentiated and undifferentiated nonkeratinizing types exhibit a higher local control rate but a greater risk of distant metastasis compared with the keratinizing type. In the United States, higher survival rates have been observed among Chinese-American patients compared with other ethnic groups. This trend traditionally has been attributed to the prevalence of the more radiosensitive undifferentiated nonkeratinizing type among Chinese-American patients; however, for reasons unclear, Chinese ethnicity has been shown to be a favorable prognostic factor even independent of histopathologic type. Persons treated for nasopharyngeal carcinoma are also at increased risk of developing a second primary malignancy of the head and neck mucosa.

BASAL CELL CARCINOMA (BASAL CELL EPITHELIOMA; RODENT ULCER)

Basal cell carcinoma, the most common skin cancer (and the most common of all cancers), is a locally invasive, slowly spreading, primary epithelial malignancy that arises from the basal cell layer of the skin and its appendages. About 80% are found on the skin of the head and neck. More than 800,000 new cases of basal cell carcinoma are diagnosed annually in the United States, representing 80% of all skin cancers. The worldwide incidence is increasing by about 10% per year. Incidence generally increases with age, although a recent study suggests a disproportionate increase among young adults (particularly women) as well.

This cancer mainly results from chronic exposure to ultraviolet radiation. Frequent sunburns and tendency for freckling in childhood are associated with an increased risk, whereas occupational sun exposure and sunburns as an adult do not seem to be risk factors. Lesser risk factors include exposure to significant ionizing radiation, ingestion of arsenic, immunosuppressive therapy, and psoralen and ultraviolet A (PUVA) treatment (often used for psoriasis). In addition, several genodermatoses are associated with basal cell carcinoma development, including the nevoid basal cell carcinoma syndrome (see page 688), xeroderma pigmentosum (see page 747), albinism, Rasmussen syndrome, Rombo syndrome, and Bazex-Christol-Dupré syndrome.

Recent molecular genetic studies have shown that dysregulation of the hedgehog signaling pathway is a critical early event in the development of basal cell carcinoma. Inactivating mutations in the *patched (PTCH)* gene on chromosome 9q22 have been identified in both sporadic cases and patients with the nevoid basal cell carcinoma syndrome. Mutations in other genes participating in this pathway (e.g., *smoothened [SMO]*) occasionally may be found in sporadic cases as well. These mutations lead to constitutive activation of hedgehog signaling and enhanced cellular proliferation. In addition, mutations in p53 are found in more than 50% of sporadic basal cell carcinomas and may represent a later event in tumor development.

Oral lesions have been reported but are usually considered to be cases of misdiagnosed salivary or odontogenic neoplasms.

CLINICAL FEATURES

Basal cell carcinoma is a disease of adult whites, especially those with fair complexions. Although most patients are older than 40 years of age at the time of diagnosis, some lesions are detected as early as the second decade of life, particularly in patients with red or blonde hair and blue or green eyes. Approximately 80% of lesions occur on the head and neck, with the remainder involving the trunk and limbs.

The most common form of this lesion, the **nodular (noduloulcerative) basal cell carcinoma,** begins as a firm, painless papule that slowly enlarges and gradually develops a central depression and an umbilicated

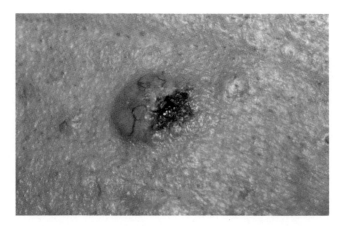

Fig. 10-132 **Basal cell carcinoma.** Early noduloulcerative basal cell carcinoma of the forehead showing raised, rolled borders and focal ulceration. Fine, telangiectatic blood vessels can be seen on the surface.

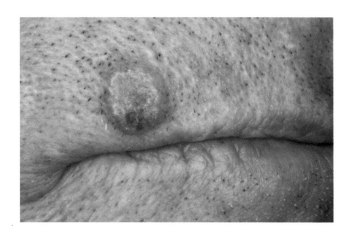

Fig. 10-133 **Basal cell carcinoma.** Noduloulcerative lesion of the upper lip demonstrating telangiectasia and small ulceration.

appearance. One or more telangiectatic blood vessels are usually seen coursing over the rolled border surrounding the central depression (Figs. 10-132 and 10-133). When the lesion is pressed, a characteristic pearly opalescent quality is discerned. Expanding ulceration often develops in the central depressed area, and the patient may give a history of intermittent bleeding followed by healing. Untreated lesions continue to enlarge slowly over months and years, with ulceration and destruction of underlying structures, hence their historical name, **rodent ulcer.** Destruction of underlying bone or cartilage may occur, but metastasis is extremely rare.

Several other clinicopathologic varieties of this tumor have also been described. **Pigmented basal cell carcinoma** is seen occasionally and represents a noduloulcerative tumor colonized by benign melano-

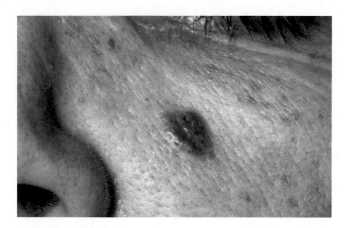

Fig. 10-134   Basal cell carcinoma. Pigmented basal cell carcinoma of the cheek.

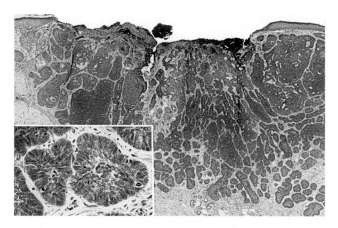

Fig. 10-135   Basal cell carcinoma. Low-power photomicrograph showing ulceration of the epidermal surface associated with an invading tumor of hyperchromatic epithelial cells. *Inset* demonstrates islands of basophilic epithelium with peripheral palisading.

cytes (Fig. 10-134). The melanin production imparts a tan, brown, black, or even bluish color to the lesion, and usually the pigment is not distributed uniformly, as it would be in a melanocytic nevus (see page 382).

Sclerosing (morpheaform) basal cell carcinoma is an insidious lesion that often mimics scar tissue. The overlying skin appears pale and atrophic, and the lesion is firm to palpation with poorly demarcated borders. A slight elevation may be noted at the edges of the tumor. Often a great deal of invasion has occurred before the patient becomes aware of a problem.

The **superficial basal cell carcinoma** occurs primarily on the skin of the trunk. Often, lesions are multiple and appear as well-demarcated, erythematous, scaly patches that may be mistaken clinically for psoriasis. A fine, elevated, "threadlike" border is seen at the margins.

Some investigators believe that the basal cell carcinoma associated with the **nevoid basal cell carcinoma syndrome** (see page 688) should be placed in a separate category. These lesions develop in both sun-exposed and protected areas of the skin and may number in the hundreds on a single patient. The tumors associated with this syndrome usually do not produce a significant degree of tissue destruction.

HISTOPATHOLOGIC FEATURES

The basal cell carcinoma displays a considerable diversity of appearances under the microscope: nodulocystic (noduloulcerative), superficial, adenoid, pigmented, infiltrative, morpheaform, and keratotic. The noduloulcerative, pigmented, and syndrome-related basal cell carcinomas are comprised of uniform ovoid, dark-staining basaloid cells with moderate-sized nuclei and relatively little cytoplasm (Fig. 10-135). The cells are arranged into well-demarcated islands and strands,

which appear to arise from the basal cell layer of the overlying epidermis and invade into the underlying dermal connective tissue. Epithelial islands typically demonstrate palisading of the peripheral cells; frequently, a clear zone of artifactual retraction is seen between the epithelial islands and the connective tissue. Although most of these neoplasms show no differentiation, some exhibit areas of keratin production, sebaceous differentiation, or interlacing strands of lesional cells that resemble duct formation ("adenoid"). Necrosis of epithelial islands may produce a cystic appearance. Actinic damage in the form of **solar elastosis** almost always is seen in adjacent stroma.

Pigmented basal cell carcinoma demonstrates dendritic melanocytes within tumor islands, and melanophages may be seen in the surrounding stroma. Sclerosing basal cell carcinoma is characterized by infiltrating thin strands of basaloid tumor cells set in a densely collagenous background. Superficial basal cell carcinoma includes lobules of tumor cells that drop from the epidermis in a multifocal pattern. Occasionally, basal cell carcinoma is seen admixed with an independent primary squamous cell carcinoma of the skin. The resulting "collision" tumor is called **basosquamous carcinoma.** Some authorities consider the basosquamous carcinoma to be a simple basal cell carcinoma with abundant squamous metaplasia.

TREATMENT AND PROGNOSIS

The treatment of basal cell carcinoma often depends on the size and site of the lesion. Small lesions (<1 cm) are treated by routine surgical excision, laser ablation, or electrodesiccation and curettage, with 3- to 5-mm margins of clinically normal-appearing skin beyond the visible lesion. These methods result in a cure rate of 95% to 98%. Radical surgical excision and radiation therapy are recommended for large or aggressive lesions. For sclerosing type of lesions, recurrent lesions, or lesions situated near embryonic planes of fusion (along which these tumor cells tend to invade), a procedure called **Mohs micrographic surgery** should be used. This technique essentially uses frozen-section evaluation of specially mapped and marked surgical specimens to determine whether tumor tissue has been left behind. If it has, then the surgeon can return immediately to that particular area and remove more tissue, repeating the process until the patient is free of disease.

Topical treatments have shown promise as an alternative for certain variants of basal cell carcinoma, although long-term follow-up data for these alternative therapies are lacking. Photodynamic therapy is effective for superficial basal cell carcinomas, with good cosmetic outcomes reported. Additional topical treatments include 5% fluorouracil cream for the management of multiple superficial basal cell carcinomas on the trunk and limbs and 5% imiquimod cream for superficial basal cell carcinomas on the trunk, neck, or limbs.

Recurrence of a properly treated basal cell carcinoma is uncommon, and metastasis is exceptionally rare. In patients with uncontrollable disease, death is usually the result of local invasion into vital structures. However, with early detection and the advent of Mohs surgery, such an outcome is unusual today.

Patients with a history of basal cell carcinoma must be evaluated periodically. There is a 30% chance of a second basal cell carcinoma and a 6% chance of a cutaneous squamous cell carcinoma developing within 3 years of treatment of the initial tumor.

MERKEL CELL CARCINOMA (MERKEL CELL TUMOR; NEUROENDOCRINE CARCINOMA OF SKIN; SMALL CELL CARCINOMA OF SKIN; TRABECULAR CARCINOMA OF SKIN)

The **Merkel cell carcinoma,** first described in 1972, is a rare, aggressive primary malignancy with neuroendocrine features. It occurs primarily on the skin of the head and neck region. As with other skin malignancies, ultraviolet (UV) light exposure is a major risk factor. In addition, an increased frequency has been reported among immunosuppressed individuals, including transplant recipients, patients with chronic lymphocytic leukemia, and patients with HIV infection. Lesional cells contain cytoplasmic granules that resemble the neurosecretory granules found within the epidermal Merkel cells of touch receptor regions. Intraoral and lip vermilion cases have been reported but are rare.

CLINICAL FEATURES

Merkel cell carcinoma typically appears in older people, with more than 76% of cases reported in individuals 65 years or older. The tumor exhibits a predilection for whites and a slight male predominance. It occurs primarily on the sun-exposed areas of fair-skinned individuals, most commonly (75%) on the skin of the face. The vermilion border of the lower lip is also a susceptible site. Merkel cell carcinoma only rarely (4.5%) arises from mucosal sites, including the oral, nasal, pharyngeal, laryngeal, and vaginal mucosa. The tumor usually appears as a slowly enlarging, dome-shaped nodule with a smooth surface and prominent surface vessels **(telangiectasias).** It is red or violaceous and ranges in size from 0.5 to 5.0 cm. Ulceration rarely is seen. Occasional lesions grow rapidly, and 25% demonstrate local metastasis at diagnosis, belying its innocuous clinical appearance.

HISTOPATHOLOGIC FEATURES

Merkel cell carcinoma consists of infiltrating sheets and anastomosing strands of moderately sized, uniform, undifferentiated basophilic cells in the dermis and subcutaneous fat (Fig. 10-136). Pseudoglandular, trabecular, cribriform ("Swiss cheese"), and sheetlike patterns may be seen. The surface epithelium is usually intact and otherwise unremarkable unless secondarily ulcerated by the tumor. Mitotic figures are abundant, and tumor cells have prominent nuclei, scant cytoplasm, and indistinct cell borders. Intracytoplasmic argyrophilic granules may be demonstrated by the Grimelius stain, and lesional cells typically exhibit a "perinuclear

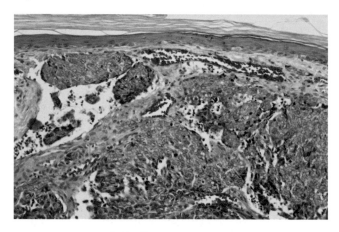

Fig. 10-136   Merkel cell carcinoma. A sheet of undifferentiated basophilic cells is seen beneath the epidermal surface.

dot" immunoreactivity pattern with antibodies directed against cytokeratin 20 (CK20). Immunopositivity for markers of neuroendocrine differentiation, such as chromogranin A, synaptophysin, and neuron-specific enolase, also may be helpful in establishing the diagnosis. Lack of immunoreactivity for antithyroid transcription factor 1 (anti-TTF-1) may help to exclude the possibility of metastatic small cell carcinoma of the lung, which may have similar histomorphologic features. At times, this entity is difficult to differentiate histopathologically from amelanotic melanoma, metastatic esthesioneuroblastoma, metastatic small cell carcinoma of the lung, malignant lymphoma, and other undifferentiated malignancies. In this situation, a panel of immunohistochemical studies should be used to exclude these other diagnostic possibilities. Careful physical examination of the patient also may provide useful diagnostic information.

TREATMENT AND PROGNOSIS

Merkel cell carcinoma is typically treated by wide local excision. For small primary skin tumors, removal by Mohs micrographic surgery with or without adjuvant radiation has been proven effective and less disfiguring than standard surgery. Lymph node dissection is performed when clinically palpable nodes are found. Sentinel lymph node biopsy may be used to determine whether regional lymph node dissection and/or radiation therapy is indicated in those patients with clinically negative nodes. Some controversy exists regarding adjuvant therapy in the management of Merkel cell carcinoma. Although some authors have not found adjuvant radiation to improve survival, most studies have shown improved survival and a significant decrease in risk of local recurrence and regional metastasis with postoperative radiation therapy. The role of adjuvant chemotherapy remains investigational.

Recurrence develops in 55% of cases, most commonly within the draining lymph nodes. In a recent analysis of U.S. Surveillance, Epidemiology, and End Results (SEER) Program data for a cohort of more than 1000 patients with Merkel cell carcinoma, the 5-year survival rates for patients with localized, regional, and distant disease were 75%, 59%, and 25%, respectively. The overall 5-year disease-specific survival rate is approximately 64%. Female sex, localized disease, limb involvement, and younger age have been found to be positive predictors of survival. In a few rare cases, complete spontaneous regression of the primary tumor has been reported, which suggests that immunologic therapy may be an alternative approach to investigate in the future.

Approximately 25% of patients with Merkel cell carcinoma develop additional malignancies (e.g., squamous cell carcinomas of the skin, hematologic malignancies, or adenocarcinomas of the breast or ovary) before, concurrent with, or after their diagnosis. Thus these patients should be monitored closely.

MELANOMA (MALIGNANT MELANOMA; MELANOCARCINOMA)

Melanoma is a malignant neoplasm of melanocytic origin that arises from a benign melanocytic lesion or *de novo* from melanocytes within otherwise normal skin or mucosa. Although most melanomas occur on the skin, they may develop at any site where melanocytes are present. Damage from UV radiation is considered a major causative factor, as suggested by the fact that the incidence of melanoma increases for light-complexioned populations as they approach the equator. However, chronic sun exposure does not seem to be as significant as it is for other cutaneous cancers, such as basal and squamous cell carcinoma. Acute sun damage may be of greater causative importance than chronic exposure in melanoma. Lesions of the oral mucosa, of course, are not related to sun exposure.

The risk of melanoma development is two to eight times greater when a relative has a history of the cancer. Additional risk factors include a fair complexion and light hair, a tendency to sunburn easily, a history of painful or blistering sunburns in childhood, an indoor occupation with outdoor recreational habits, a personal history of melanoma, and a personal history of dysplastic or congenital nevus.

Melanoma is the third most common skin cancer, but it accounts for only 5% of the total. Most deaths that are due to skin cancer, however, are caused by melanoma. In the United States for the year 2008, it is estimated that 62,480 people will be diagnosed with cutaneous melanoma and 8420 people will die of the disease. The age-adjusted incidence rate for skin melanoma (23.6 per 100,000 men and 14.9 per 100,000 women) has been increasing dramatically over the past several decades. Based on U.S. incidence rates from 2002 to 2004, it is estimated that 1 in 58 persons will be diagnosed with cutaneous melanoma during their lifetime. Controversy exists regarding this perceived increase in melanoma incidence. Some investigators contend that the increase is due to increased numbers of skin biopsies and improved diagnosis of early-stage disease, whereas others feel that there is a true increase in disease rate. Despite increasing incidence, the mortality rate for cutaneous melanoma has remained relatively constant since the 1990s, apparently because a large proportion of cases are diagnosed at an early stage. According to the *National Cancer Database Report on Cutaneous and Noncutaneous Melanoma*, 91.2% of all melanomas arise on the skin, whereas ocular, mucosal, and unknown primaries account for 5.2%, 1.3%, and 2.2% of cases, respectively. Almost 25% of cutaneous melanomas arise in the head and neck area, 40% occur on the extremities, and the rest occur on the trunk. More than half of mucosal melanomas occur in the head and neck area (including the oral and sinonasal regions), with the remainder involving the urogenital and rectal mucosa.

Oral mucosal melanoma is rare in the United States, where it occurs in only 1 in every 2 million persons annually and comprises much less than 1% of all melanomas. Several reports suggest it is more frequent in other countries, such as Japan and Uganda; however, other investigators have suggested that the true incidence of mucosal melanomas is not greater in these countries but only appears so because of the comparatively low incidence of cutaneous melanomas in these racial groups. The mucosal melanoma tends to present at a more advanced stage and is much more aggressive than its cutaneous counterpart. At least one in three patients with oral melanoma has a history of a pigmented macule in the region of the tumor for some time before melanoma diagnosis. Melanoma occasionally affects the parotid gland, usually as a metastatic deposit from a scalp, conjunctival, or paranasal tumor.

In recent years, there have been many discoveries regarding recurrent genetic alterations in melanomas, including those involving the *Ras-Raf-ERK*, mitogen-activating protein (MAP) kinase, and phosphatidylinositol 3-kinase (*Pl3K*) pathways. In particular, a high proportion (approximately 50% to 70%) of melanomas possess mutations in the gene encoding BRAF, a protein kinase involved in the *Ras-Raf-ERK* signaling pathway.

CLINICAL FEATURES

Most melanomas are seen in white adults. The average age of affected persons is 50 to 55 years, but cases are rather evenly distributed over the 30- to 80-year age bracket. A few melanomas occur in the second and third decades of life. Four clinicopathologic types of melanoma have been described:

1. Superficial spreading melanoma
2. Nodular melanoma
3. Lentigo maligna melanoma
4. Acral lentiginous melanoma

Melanomas tend to exhibit two directional patterns of growth: (1) the **radial growth phase** and (2) the **vertical growth phase.** In the early stages of melanoma development, the radial growth phase tends to predominate in lentigo maligna melanoma, superficial spreading melanoma, and acral lentiginous melanoma. In these lesions, the malignant melanocytes have a propensity to spread horizontally through the basal layer

Box 10-4

The "ABCDE" Clinical Features of Melanoma

- **A**symmetry (because of its uncontrolled growth pattern)
- **B**order irregularity (often with notching)
- **C**olor variegation (which varies from shades of brown to black, white, red, and blue, depending on the amount and depth of melanin pigmentation)
- **D**iameter greater than 6 mm (which is the diameter of a pencil eraser)
- **E**volving (lesions that have changed with respect to size, shape, color, surface, or symptoms over time)

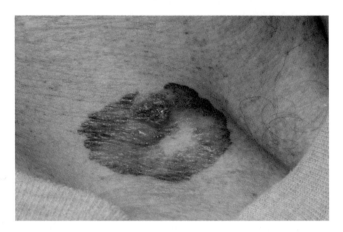

Fig. 10-137   Superficial spreading melanoma. This lesion on the neck demonstrates the ABCDE warning signs of melanoma: **A**symmetry, **B**order irregularity, **C**olor variegation, **D**iameter larger than a pencil eraser, and **E**volving larger size. *(Courtesy of Dr. Mark Bowden.)*

of the epidermis. Eventually, however, the malignant cells begin to invade the underlying connective tissue, thus initiating the vertical growth phase. With nodular melanoma, the radial growth phase is very short or nonexistent and the vertical growth phase predominates.

Because many clinical similarities exist between melanoma and its benign counterpart, the melanocytic nevus, an "ABCDE" system of evaluation has been developed to help distinguish a melanoma clinically from a melanocytic nevus (Box 10-4).

SUPERFICIAL SPREADING MELANOMA

Superficial spreading melanoma is the most common form of melanoma, representing 70% of cutaneous lesions (Fig. 10-137). The most common sites of origin are the interscapular area of males and the back of the legs of females. This form of melanoma appears as a macule with a variety of potential colors (i.e., tan, brown, gray, black, blue, white, pink). Typically, the lesion is smaller than 3 cm in greatest diameter at diagnosis, but it may be several times that size. Many lesions are slightly elevated. Clinically, invasion is indicated by the appearance of surface nodules or induration, and usually occurs within 1 year of discovery of the precursor macule. Satellite macules or nodules of malignant cells may develop around the primary lesion.

NODULAR MELANOMA

Nodular melanoma represents 15% of cutaneous melanomas, and one third of such lesions develop in the head and neck area. Nodular melanoma is thought to begin almost immediately in the vertical growth phase; therefore, it typically appears as a nodular elevation that rapidly invades into the connective tissue. Nodular melanoma is usually a deeply pigmented exophytic lesion, although sometimes the melanoma cells are so poorly differentiated that they no longer can produce melanin, resulting in a nonpigmented **amelanotic melanoma.**

LENTIGO MALIGNA MELANOMA

Lentigo maligna melanoma, which accounts for 5% to 10% of cutaneous melanomas, develops from a precursor lesion called **lentigo maligna (Hutchinson's freckle).** Lentigo maligna occurs almost exclusively on the sun-exposed skin of fair-complexioned older adults, particularly in the midfacial region, and represents a **melanoma *in situ*** in a purely radial growth phase.

The lesion appears as a large, slowly expanding macule with irregular borders and a variety of colors, including tan, brown, black, and even white (Fig. 10-138). Patients usually indicate that the lesion has been present and has slowly expanded laterally for years. The average duration of the radial growth phase

is 15 years. The appearance of nodularity within a lentigo maligna signals the onset of the invasive or vertical growth phase and the transition to lentigo maligna melanoma.

ACRAL LENTIGINOUS MELANOMA (MUCOSAL LENTIGINOUS MELANOMA)

Acral lentiginous melanoma is the most common form of melanoma in blacks, and it is also the most common form of **oral melanoma.** It typically develops on the palms of the hands, soles of the feet, subungual area, and mucous membranes. It begins as a darkly pigmented, irregularly marginated macule, which later develops a nodular invasive growth phase. Recently, some authorities have separated this lesion into two entities: (1) **acral lentiginous melanoma** and (2) **mucosal lentiginous melanoma.**

Oral melanoma is often nodular at the time of diagnosis, but early lesions may be flat. Affected persons are usually in their sixth or seventh decade of life. Two thirds of patients are men. Four of every five oral melanomas are found on the hard palate or maxillary alveolus.

An oral lesion typically begins as a brown to black macule with irregular borders (Figs. 10-139 and 10-140). The macule extends laterally, and a lobulated, exophytic mass develops once the vertical growth is initiated (Fig. 10-141). Ulceration may develop early, but many lesions are dark, lobulated, exophytic masses without ulceration at the time of diagnosis. More than 20% of oral melanomas contain so little pigment that they have an essentially normal mucosal tint. Pain is not a common feature except in ulcerated lesions, and most lesions remain relatively soft to palpation. Underlying or adjacent bone may show radiographic evidence of irregular or "moth-eaten" destruction.

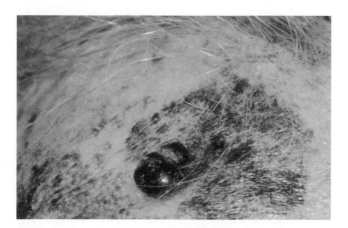

Fig. 10-138 Lentigo maligna melanoma. A slowly evolving pigmented lesion of the facial skin in an older adult man.

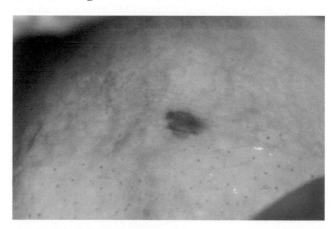

Fig. 10-139 Oral melanoma. This discrete area of pigmentation, measuring approximately 5 mm in diameter, was discovered on the posterior hard palate of a middle-aged woman during a routine oral examination. Biopsy revealed melanoma *in situ.*

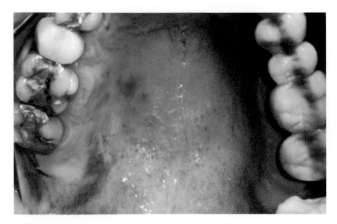

Fig. 10-140   Oral melanoma. Diffuse, splotchy area of pigmentation of the lateral hard palate. *(Courtesy of Dr. Len Morrow.)*

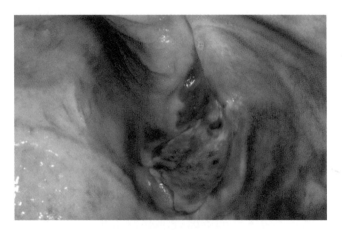

Fig. 10-141   Oral melanoma. Ulcerated pigmented mass of the posterior maxillary alveolar ridge.

HISTOPATHOLOGIC FEATURES

With cutaneous and oral melanomas, atypical melanocytes are initially seen at the epithelial and connective tissue junction. From here, they have the potential to proliferate throughout the epithelium, laterally along the basal cell layer, and downward into the connective tissue. In the early stages of the neoplasm, atypical melanocytes are seen either scattered singly among the basal epithelial cells or as nests within the basal cell layer. The atypical melanocytes are usually larger than normal melanocytes and have varying degrees of nuclear pleomorphism and hyperchromatism.

With superficial spreading melanoma, pagetoid spread often is seen. Large melanoma cells infiltrate the surface epithelium singly or in nests (Fig. 10-142). The resulting microscopic pattern is called *pagetoid* because it resembles an intraepithelial adenocarcinoma known as *Paget's disease of skin.*

The spreading of the lesional cells along the basal layer constitutes the radial growth phase of the neo-

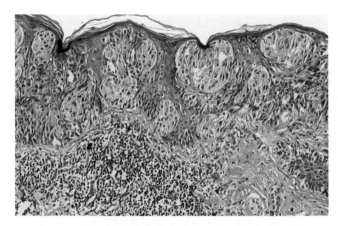

Fig. 10-142   Superficial spreading melanoma. The radial growth phase is characterized by the spread of atypical melanocytes along the basilar portion of the epidermis. Also note the presence of individual melanocytes invading the higher levels of the epithelium.

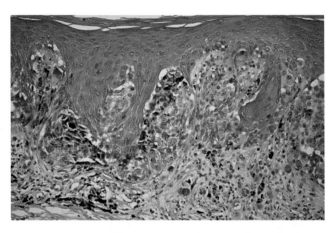

Fig. 10-143   Acral lentiginous melanoma. This palatal melanoma demonstrates numerous atypical melanocytes in the basilar portion of the epithelium with invasion into the superficial lamina propria. This represents the biopsy specimen from Fig. 10-140.

plasm. Such lateral spread of cells within the epithelium, which occurs before invasion into the underlying connective tissue, is characteristically seen in superficial spreading melanoma, lentigo maligna melanoma, and acral lentiginous melanoma. In acral lentiginous melanoma, many of the melanocytes have prominent dendritic processes (Fig. 10-143).

When malignant melanocytes are observed invading the connective tissue, the vertical growth phase has taken place. In nodular melanoma, this vertical growth phase occurs early in the course of the tumor. No radial growth of cells can be observed in the overlying epithelium beyond the edge of the invasive tumor (Fig. 10-144). The invasive melanoma cells usually appear either spindle-shaped or epithelioid and infiltrate the connective tissue as loosely aggregated cords or sheets of pleomorphic cells. Oral lesions tend to show invasion of lymphatic and blood vessels more readily than skin lesions. Several mucosal melanomas have been reported to contain unequivocal bone and cartilage, a feature that may cause diagnostic confusion with pleomorphic adenoma, sarcomatoid carcinoma, osteogenic sarcoma, and mesenchymal chondrosarcoma.

In most instances, the lesional cells of melanoma contain fine melanin granules, but they may demonstrate no melanin production (amelanotic melanoma). A lack of melanin production may cause diagnostic confusion at the light microscopic level because mela-

noma can mimic a variety of undifferentiated tumors. Immunohistochemical studies showing S-100 protein, HMB-45, Melan-A, and Mart-1 reactivity of the lesional cells are beneficial in distinguishing such melanomas from other malignancies.

TREATMENT AND PROGNOSIS

Microscopic measurement of the depth of invasion is an important component of the histopathologic evaluation of cutaneous melanoma because of its correlation with the prognosis. The Clark system of measurement assigns a "level" to the lesion that depends on the deepest anatomic cutaneous region that has been invaded by tumor cells (Table 10-4). The more recent Breslow classification, however, appears to show a more accurate correlation with the prognosis and is based on the actual measurement of the distance from the top of the granular cell layer to the deepest identifiable point of tumor invasion.

Clinical staging for cutaneous melanoma is performed using a TNM classification system that takes into account tumor thickness, ulceration, regional nodal metastasis, and distant metastasis (Table 10-5). In this system, tumor thickness as measured by the Breslow classification is an important determinant of tumor (T) classification, and the Clark system is used only to further subtype T1 lesions (thin melanomas ≤1 mm). Ulceration is an adverse prognostic factor; thus patients with stage I to III disease are upstaged (from A to B) when ulceration is present. Among patients with stage IV disease, elevated serum lactic dehydrogenase (LDH) is associated with an especially poor prognosis.

Although depth of invasion and presence of ulceration are correlated closely with patient outcome in cutaneous melanomas, such a close association has not been found in mucosal melanomas. In general, there is a marked deterioration in prognosis among patients with oral mucosal melanomas exceeding a depth of 0.5 mm.

Surgical excision is the mainstay of treatment, although the extent of the excision is somewhat controversial. Older literature suggests that surgical margins of 3 to 5 cm around the tumor are necessary to achieve

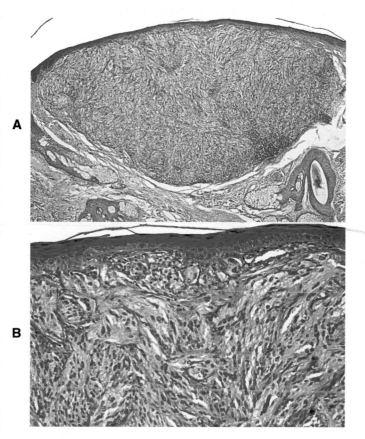

Fig. 10-144   Nodular melanoma. A, Low-power photomicrograph showing a nodular mass of malignant melanocytes invading into the dermis. Note the lack of radial growth in the adjacent overlying epidermis. **B,** Higher-power photomicrograph showing atypical spindle-shaped melanocytes.

Table **10-4**   **Clark's Classification in Cutaneous Melanoma**

Clark's Definition of Level of Tumor Invasion	Clark's Classification
Cells confined to epithelium	Level I
Cells penetrating papillary dermis	Level II
Cells filling papillary dermis	Level III
Cells extending into reticular dermis	Level IV
Cells invading subcutaneous fat	Level V

Table **10-5**   **TNM Classification System and Stage Groupings for Cutaneous Melanoma**[a]

T CLASSIFICATION	TUMOR THICKNESS (BRESLOW'S DEPTH OF INVASION)[b]	ULCERATION STATUS
T1	≤1.0 mm	a: Without ulceration or Clark's level II/III b: With ulceration or Clark's level IV/V
T2	1.01-2.0 mm	a: Without ulceration b: With ulceration
T3	2.01-4.0 mm	a: Without ulceration b: With ulceration
T4	>4.0 mm	a: Without ulceration b: With ulceration

N CLASSIFICATION	NUMBER OF METASTATIC REGIONAL LYMPH NODES	NODAL METASTATIC MASS
N0	0	
N1	One	a: Microscopic[c] b: Macroscopic[d]
N2	Two to three, or intralymphatic regional metastasis without nodal metastasis	a: Microscopic b: Macroscopic c: In-transit metastasis/satellite(s) without metastatic nodes
N3	Four or more, or matted nodes, or in-transit[e] metastasis/satellite(s)[f] with metastatic nodes	

M CLASSIFICATION	SITE OF DISTANT METASTASIS	SERUM LACTATE DEHYDROGENASE
M0	No distant metastasis	Normal
M1a	Distant skin, subcutaneous, or nodal metastasis	Normal
M1b	Lung metastasis	Normal
M1c	All other visceral metastases	Normal
	Any distant metastasis	Elevated

CLINICAL STAGE GROUPING	TNM CLASSIFICATION	FIVE-YEAR SURVIVAL RATE[g]
Stage IA	T1a N0 M0	95%
Stage IB	T1b N0 M0	91%
	T2a N0 M0	89%
Stage IIA	T2b N0 M0	77%
	T3a N0 M0	79%
Stage IIB	T3b N0 M0	63%
	T4a N0 M0	67%
Stage IIC	T4b N0 M0	45%
Stage III	Any T N1 M0	29%-70%
	Any T N2 M0	24%-63%
	Any T N3 M0	27%
Stage IV	Any M1	10%-19%

[a]Based on Greene FL, Page DL, Fleming ID et al, editors: *AJCC cancer staging manual*, ed 6, New York, 2002, Springer.
[b]Breslow's depth is measured from the top of the granular cell layer.
[c]Microscopic—clinically occult.
[d]Macroscopic—clinically apparent.
[e]In-transit—intralymphatic metastases occurring within 2 cm of the primary tumor.
[f]Satellite metastasis—intralymphatic metastases occurring >2 cm from the primary tumor but before the first echelon of regional lymph nodes.
[g]Survival data from Balch CM, Buzaid AC, Soong SJ et al: Final version of the American Joint Committee on Cancer staging system for cutaneous melanoma, *J Clin Oncol* 19:3635-3648, 2001.

control, regardless of the site of the lesion. More recent studies indicate that a 1-cm margin is adequate for small cutaneous tumors less than 2 mm in thickness. For larger, more deeply invasive tumors, wide surgical excision still is recommended.

Lymph node dissection is usually performed on patients with clinically evident regional metastasis in the absence of distant metastasis. Elective lymph node dissection for patients with intermediate thickness (1 to 4 mm) lesions in the absence of clinically palpable nodes is somewhat controversial. The rationale for this procedure is that these patients have a high probability of occult regional nodal disease and low probability of distant metastasis. However, the reported survival benefit of this treatment strategy is variable, and significant morbidity can be associated with lymph node dissection. To address this problem, sentinel-node biopsy (biopsy of the first lymph node in the lymphatic basin to receive drainage from the tumor) often is used as an alternative to elective lymph node dissection to identify patients with occult nodal metastases who would benefit from total lymphadenectomy.

Although melanomas traditionally are considered to be radioresistant, several clinical studies have demonstrated that radiation may be of some benefit as adjunctive—or less commonly primary—therapy for certain subsets of patients; newer radiotherapy techniques, such as hypofractionation and neutron beam therapy, may play a greater role in the future. In addition, adjunct chemotherapy and immunotherapy are showing promise. With advances in the understanding of the molecular pathogenesis of melanoma, rationally designed targeted therapies (e.g., tyrosine kinase inhibitors, farnesyltransferase inhibitors, *Pl3K* pathway inhibitors) are being developed as well.

The cutaneous melanoma that is detected early ($\leq$1.0-mm thick with or without ulceration, 1.01- to 2.0-mm thick without ulceration) and removed before metastasis has developed (stages IA and IB) is associated with an 89% to 95% 5-year survival rate. Cutaneous melanoma that is thicker (1.01 to 2.0 mm with ulceration, 2.01 to >4 mm with or without ulceration) but has not yet metastasized at the time of diagnosis (stages IIA to IIC) is associated with a 45% to 77% 5-year survival rate. If regional lymph node metastasis is present at the time of diagnosis (stages IIIA to IIIC), then 5-year survival rates in the range of 24% to 70% can be expected. The prognosis for patients with disseminated disease present at the time of diagnosis (stage IV) is dismal, with a 5-year survival rate of only 7% to 19%. Overall, the 5-year survival rate for cutaneous melanoma is 92%, and the 10-year survival rate is 79%. Current survival is much improved over past decades, primarily as a result of public education. Currently, the clinical features of cutaneous melanoma are

so widely known that many lesions are discovered and treated at an early stage.

Other factors may influence the outcome of the disease besides the depth of invasion. For reasons that are unclear, melanomas affecting certain cutaneous sites seem to carry a worse prognosis than those at other sites with a similar depth of invasion. The areas with a worse prognosis are designated **BANS** (interscapular area of the **B**ack, posterior upper **A**rm, posterior and lateral **N**eck, and **S**calp). In addition, the prognosis is better for patients younger than 50 years of age and for women. Follow-up of patients treated for melanoma is important not only to monitor for metastatic disease but also because, in 3% to 5% of these patients, a second primary melanoma will eventually develop.

The prognosis for **oral melanoma** is extremely poor. Although 5-year survival rates as high as 45% have been reported, in the majority of studies, 5-year survival rates are in the range of only 13% to 22%. The poor prognosis for oral melanoma appears to be related to difficulty in achieving wide resection and a tendency for early hematogenous metastasis. Younger patients have a better survival than older ones, and patients with nonpigmented or amelanotic lesions appear to have a particularly poor prognosis. Patients usually die from distant metastasis rather than from the lack of local control. Radical surgical removal is the treatment of choice; hemimaxillectomy is done for unilateral lesions that invade the overlying maxillary bone.

BIBLIOGRAPHY

Squamous Papilloma

Abbey LM, Page DG, Sawyer DR: The clinical and histopathologic features of a series of 464 oral squamous cell papillomas, *Oral Surg Oral Med Oral Pathol* 49:419-428, 1980.

Bouquot JE, Wrobleski GJ: Papillary (pebbled) masses of the oral mucosa, so much more than simple papillomas, *Pract Periodontics Aesth Dent* 8:533-543, 1996.

Carr J, Gyorfi T: Human papillomavirus. Epidemiology, transmission, and pathogenesis, *Clin Lab Med* 20:235-255, 2000.

Freed GL, Derkay CS: Prevention of recurrent respiratory papillomatosis: role of HPV vaccination, *Int J Pediatr Otorhinolaryngol* 70:1799-1803, 2006.

Kimberlin DW, Malis DJ: Juvenile onset recurrent respiratory papillomatosis: possibilities for successful antiviral therapy, *Antiviral Res* 45:83-93, 2000.

Lee HJ, Smith RJ: Recurrent respiratory papillomatosis: pathogenesis to treatment, *Curr Opin Otolaryngol Head Neck Surg* 13:354-359, 2005.

Stamataki S, Nikolopoulos TP, Korres S et al: Juvenile recurrent respiratory papillomatosis: still a mystery disease with difficult management, *Head Neck* 29:155-162, 2007.

Summersgill KF, Smith EM, Levy BT et al: Human papillomavirus in the oral cavities of children and adolescents, *Oral Surg Oral Med Oral Pathol Oral Radiol Endod* 91:62-69, 2001.

Graham-Brown RAC, McGibbon DH, Sarkany I: A papular plaque-like eruption on the face due to naevoid sebaceous gland hyperplasia, *Clin Exp Dermatol* 8:379-382, 1983.

Richey DF: Aminolevulinic acid photodynamic therapy for sebaceous gland hyperplasia, *Dermatol Clin* 25:59-65, 2007.

Ephelis

Bastiaens M, Hoefnagel J, Westendorp R et al: Solar lentigines are strongly related to sun exposure in contrast to ephelides, *Pigment Cell Res* 17:225-229, 2004.

Bastiaens M, ter Huurne J, Gruis N et al: The melanocortin-1-receptor gene is the major freckle gene, *Human Mol Genet* 10:1701-1708, 2001.

Bastiaens MT, Westendorp RG, Vermeer BJ et al: Ephelides are more related to pigmentary constitutional host factors than solar lentigines, *Pigment Cell Res* 12:316-322, 1999.

Bliss JM, Ford D, Swerdlow AJ et al: Risk of cutaneous melanoma associated with pigmentation characteristics and freckling: systematic overview of 10 case-control studies, *Int J Cancer* 62:367-372, 1995.

Actinic Lentigo

Andersen WK, Labadie RR, Bhawan J: Histopathology of solar lentigines of the face: a quantitative study, *J Am Acad Dermatol* 36:444-447, 1997.

Beacham BE: Solar-induced epidermal tumors in the elderly, *Am Fam Physician* 42:153-160, 1990.

Fleischer AB Jr, Schwartzel EH, Colby SI et al: The combination of 2% 4-hydroxyanisole (Mequinol) and 0.01% tretinoin is effective in improving the appearance of solar lentigines and related hyperpigmented lesions in two double-blind multicenter clinical studies, *J Am Acad Dermatol* 42:459-467, 2004.

Holzle E: Pigmented lesions as a sign of photodamage, *Br J Dermatol* 127:48-50, 1992.

Jarratt M: Mequinol 2%/tretinoin 0.01% solution: an effective and safe alternative to hydroquinone 3% in the treatment of solar lentigines, *Cutis* 74:319-322, 2004.

Kang S, Goldfarb MT, Weiss JS et al: Assessment of adapalene gel for the treatment of actinic keratoses and lentigines: a randomized trial, *J Am Acad Dermatol* 49:83-90, 2003.

Monestier S, Gaudy C, Gouvernet J et al: Multiple senile lentigos of the face, a skin ageing pattern resulting from a life excess of intermittent sun exposure in dark-skinned Caucasians: a case-control study, *Br J Dermatol* 154:438-444, 2006.

Ortonne JP, Pandya AG, Lui H et al: Treatment of solar lentigines, *J Am Acad Dermatol* 54:S262-S271, 2006.

Rafal ES, Griffiths CE, Ditre CM et al: Topical tretinoin (retinoic acid) treatment for liver spots associated with photodamage, *N Engl J Med* 326:368-374, 1992.

Shimbashi T, Kamide R, Hashimoto T: Long-term follow-up in treatment of solar lentigo and café-au-lait macules with Q-switch ruby laser, *Aesthetic Plast Surg* 21:445-448, 1997.

Lentigo Simplex

Buchner A, Merrell PW, Hansen LS et al: Melanocytic hyperplasia of the oral mucosa, *Oral Surg Oral Med Oral Pathol* 71:58-62, 1991.

Coleman WP 3rd, Gately LE 3rd, Krementz AB et al: Nevi, lentigines and melanomas in blacks, *Arch Dermatol* 116:548-551, 1980.

Gorlin RJ, Andersen RC, Blaw M: Multiple lentigines syndrome, *Am J Dis Child* 117:652-662, 1969.

Grichnik JM, Rhodes AR, Sober AJ: Lentigo simplex. In Freedberg IM, Eisen AZ, Wolff K et al, editors: *Fitzpatrick's dermatology in general medicine*, ed 6, pp 881-882, New York, 2003, McGraw-Hill.

Melasma

Aloi F, Solaroli C, Giovannini E: Actinic lichen planus simulating melasma, *Dermatology* 195:69-70, 1997.

Gupta AK, Gover MD, Nouri K et al: The treatment of melasma: a review of clinical trials, *J Am Acad Dermatol* 55:1048-1065, 2006.

Kauh YC, Zachian TF: Melasma, *Adv Exp Med Biol* 455:491-499, 1999.

Lim JT: Treatment of melasma using kojic acid in a gel containing hydroquinone and glycolic acid, *Dermatol Surg* 25:282-284, 1999.

Rendon M, Berneburg M, Arellano I et al: Treatment of melasma, *J Am Acad Dermatol* 54:S272-S281, 2006.

Sanchez NP, Pathuk MA, Sato S et al: Melasma: a clinical, light microscopic, ultrastructural and immunofluorescence study, *J Am Acad Dermatol* 4:698-703, 1981.

Victor FC, Gelber J, Rao B: Melasma: a review, *J Cutan Med Surg* 8:97-102, 2004.

Oral Melanotic Macule

Axéll T: A prevalence study of oral mucosal lesions in an adult Swedish population, *Odontol Revy* 27:1-103, 1976.

Bouquot JE: Common oral lesions found during a mass screening examination, *J Am Dent Assoc* 112:50-57, 1986.

Bouquot JE, Nikai H: Lesions of the oral cavity. In Gnepp DR, editor: *Diagnostic surgical pathology of the head and neck*, pp 141-238, Philadelphia, 2001, WB Saunders.

Buchner A, Hansen LS: Melanotic macule of the oral mucosa: a clinicopathologic study of 105 cases, *Oral Surg Oral Med Oral Pathol* 48:244-249, 1979.

Buchner A, Merrell PW, Carpenter WM: Relative frequency of solitary melanocytic lesions of the oral mucosa, *J Oral Pathol Med* 33:550-557, 2004.

Dohil MA, Billman G, Pransky S et al: The congenital lingual melanotic macule, *Arch Dermatol* 139:767-770, 2003.

Kaugars GE, Heise AP, Riley WT et al: Oral melanotic macules: a review of 353 cases, *Oral Surg Oral Med Oral Pathol* 76:59-61, 1993.

Weathers DR, Corio RL, Crawford BE et al: The labial melanotic macule, *Oral Surg Oral Med Oral Pathol* 42:196-205, 1976.

Yeh CJ: Simple cryosurgical treatment of the oral melanotic macule, *Oral Surg Oral Med Oral Pathol Oral Radiol Endod* 90:12-13, 2000.

Oral Melanoacanthoma

Andrews BT, Trask DK: Oral melanoacanthoma: a case report, a review of the literature, and a new treatment option, *Ann Otol Rhinol Laryngol* 114:677-680, 2005.

Chandler K, Chaudhry Z, Kumar N et al: Melanoacanthoma: a rare cause of oral hyperpigmentation, *Oral Surg Oral Med Oral Pathol Oral Radiol Endod* 84:492-494, 1997.

Contreras E, Carlos R: Oral melanoacanthosis (melanoachantoma): report of a case and review of the literature, *Med Oral Patol Oral Cir Bucal* 10:9-12, 2005.

Fatahzadeh M, Sirois DA: Multiple intraoral melanoacanthomas: a case report with unusual findings, *Oral Surg Oral Med Oral Pathol Oral Radiol Endod* 94:54-56, 2002.

Fornatora ML, Reich RF, Haber S et al: Oral melanoacanthoma: a report of 10 cases, review of literature, and immunohistochemical analysis of HMB-45 reactivity, *Am J Dermatopathol* 25:12-15, 2003.

Heine BT, Drummond JF, Damm DD et al: Bilateral oral melanoacanthoma, *Gen Dent* 44:451-452, 1996.

Landwehr DJ, Halkins LE, Allen CM: A rapidly growing pigmented plaque, *Oral Surg Oral Med Oral Pathol Oral Radiol Endod* 84:332-334, 1997.

Tomich CE, Zunt SL: Melanoacanthosis (melanoacanthoma) of the oral mucosa, *J Dermatol Surg Oncol* 16:231-236, 1990.

Melanocytic Nevus

Allen CM, Pellegrini A: Probable congenital melanocytic nevus of the oral mucosa: case report, *Pediatr Dermatol* 12:145-148, 1995.

Barnhill RL: The Spitzoid lesion: the importance of atypical variants and risk assessment, *Am J Dermatopathol* 28:75-83, 2006.

Bett BJ: Large or multiple congenital melanocytic nevi: occurrence of cutaneous melanoma in 1008 persons, *J Am Acad Dermatol* 52:793-797, 2005.

Brener MD, Harrison BD: Intraoral blue nevus: report of a case, *Oral Surg Oral Med Oral Pathol* 28:326-330, 1969.

Buchner A, Hansen LS: Pigmented nevi of the oral mucosa: a clinicopathologic study of 36 new cases and review of 155 cases from the literature. Part I: a clinicopathologic study of 36 new cases, *Oral Surg Oral Med Oral Pathol* 63:566-572, 1987.

Buchner A, Hansen LS: Pigmented nevi of the oral mucosa: a clinicopathologic study of 36 new cases and review of 155 cases from the literature. Part II: analysis of 191 cases, *Oral Surg Oral Med Oral Pathol* 63:676-682, 1987.

Buchner A, Leider AS, Merrell PW et al: Melanocytic nevi of oral mucosa: a clinicopathologic study of 130 cases from northern California, *J Oral Pathol Med* 19:197-201, 1990.

Casso EM, Grin-Jorgensen CM, Grant-Kels JM: Spitz nevi, *J Am Acad Dermatol* 27:901-913, 1992.

Chuang WY, Hao SP, Yeh CJ et al: Blue nevi of the sinonasal mucosa: a report of two cases and review of the literature, *Laryngoscope* 117:371-372, 2007.

Dorji T, Cavazza A, Nappi O et al: Spitz nevus of the tongue with pseudoepitheliomatous hyperplasia: report of three cases of a pseudomalignant condition, *Am J Surg Pathol* 26:774-777, 2002.

Fistarol SK, Itin PH: Plaque-type blue nevus of the oral cavity, *Dermatology* 211:224-233, 2005.

Flaitz CM, McCandless G: Palatal blue nevus in a child, *Pediatr Dent* 23:354-355, 2001.

Frank SB, Cohen HJ: The halo nevus, *Arch Dermatol* 89:367-373, 1964.

Hale EK, Stein J, Ben-Porat L et al: Association of melanoma and neurocutaneous melanocytosis with large congenital melanocytic naevi—results from the NYU-LCMN registry, *Br J Dermatol* 152:512-517, 2005.

Laskaris G, Kittas C, Triantafyllou A: Unpigmented intramucosal nevus of palate. An unusual clinical presentation, *Int J Oral Maxillofac Surg* 23:39-40, 1994.

LeBoit P: Spitz nevus: a look back and a look ahead, *Adv Dermatol* 16:81-109, 2000.

Mader CL, Konzelman JL: Intraoral blue nevus—a review, *Cutis* 24:165-166, 1979.

Marghoob, AA, Agero ALC, Benvenuto-Andrade C et al: Large congenital melanocytic nevi, risk of cutaneous melanoma, and prophylactic surgery, *J Am Acad Dermatol* 54:868-870, 2006.

Meleti M, Mooi WJ, Casparie MK et al: Melanocytic nevi of the oral mucosa—no evidence of an increased risk for oral malignant melanoma: an analysis of 119 cases, *Oral Oncol* 43: 976-981, 2007.

Mones JM, Ackerman AB: "Atypical" Spitz's nevus, "malignant" Spitz's nevus, and "metastasizing" Spitz's nevus: a critique in historical perspective of three concepts and flawed fatally, *Am J Dermatopathol* 26:310-333, 2004.

Mooi WJ: Spitz nevus and its histologic simulators, *Adv Anat Pathol* 9:209-221, 2002.

Nikia H, Miyauchi M, Ogawa I et al: Spitz nevus of the palate. Report of a case, *Oral Surg Oral Med Oral Pathol* 69:603-608, 1990.

Pinto A, Raghavendra S, Lee R et al: Epithelioid blue nevus of the oral mucosa: a rare histologic variant, *Oral Surg Oral Med Oral Pathol* 96:429-436, 2003.

Sulit DJ, Guardiano RA, Krivda S: Classic and atypical Spitz nevi: review of the literature, *Cutis* 79:141-146, 2007.

Takata M, Saida T: Genetic alterations in melanocytic tumors, *J Dermatol Sci* 43:1-10, 2006.

Weedon D, Little JH: Spindle and epithelioid cell nevi in children and adults: a review of 211 cases of the Spitz nevus, *Cancer* 40:217-225, 1977.

Zembowicz A, Mihm MC: Dermal dendritic melanocytic proliferations: an update, *Histopathology* 45:433-451, 2004.

Leukoplakia

Alexander RE, Wright JM, Thiebaud S: Evaluating, documenting and following up oral pathological conditions. A suggested protocol, *J Am Dent Assoc* 132:329-335, 2001.

Bagán JV, Jimenez Y, Sanchis JM: Proliferative verrucous leukoplakia: high incidence of gingival squamous cell carcinoma, *J Oral Pathol Med* 32:379-382, 2003.

Bagán JV, Murillo J, Poveda R et al: Proliferative verrucous leukoplakia: unusual locations of oral squamous cell carcinomas, and field cancerization as shown by the appearance of multiple OSCCs, *Oral Oncol* 40:440-443, 2004.

Bánóczy J: Follow-up studies in oral leukoplakia, *J Maxillofac Surg* 5:69-75, 1977.

Barrett AW, Kingsmill VJ, Speight PM: The frequency of fungal infection in biopsies of oral mucosal lesions, *Oral Dis* 4:26-31, 1998.

Bernstein ML: Oral mucosal white lesions associated with excessive use of Listerine mouthwash: report of two cases, *Oral Surg Oral Med Oral Pathol* 46:781-785, 1978.

Bouquot JE, Gorlin RJ: Leukoplakia, lichen planus and other oral keratoses in 23,616 white Americans over the age of 35 years, *Oral Surg Oral Med Oral Pathol* 61:373-381, 1986.

Bouquot J, Kurland L, Weiland L: Leukoplakia of the head and neck: characteristics of 568 lesions with 6,720 person-years of follow-up, *Oral Surg Oral Med Oral Pathol Oral Radiol Endod* 88:202, 1999.

Bouquot JE, Weiland LH, Kurland LT: Leukoplakia and carcinoma in situ synchronously associated with invasive oral/oropharyngeal carcinoma in Rochester, Minnesota, 1935-1984, *Oral Surg Oral Med Oral Pathol* 65:199-207, 1988.

Bouquot JE, Whitaker SB: Oral leukoplakia—rationale for diagnosis and prognosis of its clinical subtypes or "phases," *Quintessence Int* 25:133-140, 1994.

Brennan M, Migliorati CA, Lockhart PB et al: Management of oral epithelial dysplasia: a review, *Oral Surg Oral Med Oral Pathol Oral Radiol Endod* 103 (suppl 1):S19.e1-S19.e12, 2007.

Cabay RJ, Morton TH, Epstein JB: Proliferative verrucous leukoplakia and its progression to oral carcinoma: a review of the literature, *J Oral Pathol Med* 36:255-261, 2007.

Chi AC, Lambert PR 3rd, Pan Y et al: Is alveolar ridge keratosis a true leukoplakia? A clinicopathologic comparison of 2,153 lesions, *J Am Dent Assoc* 138:641-651, 2007.

Cowan CG, Gregg TA, Napier SS et al: Potentially malignant oral lesions in Northern Ireland: a 20-year population-based perspective of malignant transformation, *Oral Dis* 7:18-24, 2001.

Crissman JD, Zarbo RJ: Dysplasia, in situ carcinoma, and progression to invasive squamous cell carcinoma of the upper aerodigestive tract, *Am J Surg Pathol* 13(suppl 1):5-16, 1989.

Ranganathan K, Devi MU, Kirankumar K et al: Oral submucous fibrosis: a case-control study in Chennai, South India, *J Oral Pathol Med* 33:274-277, 2004.

Reichart PA, Philipsen HP: Betel chewer's mucosa—a review, *J Oral Pathol Med* 27:239-242, 1998.

Tilakaratne WM, Klinikowski MF, Saku T et al: Oral submucous fibrosis: review on aetiology and pathogenesis, *Oral Oncol* 42:561-568, 2006.

World Health Organization International Agency for Research on Cancer: *IARC monographs on the evaluation and carcinogenic risks to humans, betel-quid and areca-nut chewing and some areca-nut-derived nitrosamines*, vol 85, Lyon, France, 2004, IARC Press.

Zheng X, Reichart PA: A review of betel quid chewing, oral cancer and precancer in Mainland China, *Oral Oncol* 43:424-430, 2007.

Nicotine Stomatitis

Ortiz GM, Pierce AM, Wilson DF: Palatal changes associated with reverse smoking in Filipino women, *Oral Dis* 2:232-237, 1996.

Rossie KM, Guggenheimer J: Thermally induced "nicotine" stomatitis: a case report, *Oral Surg Oral Med Oral Pathol* 70:597-599, 1990.

Saunders WH: Nicotine stomatitis of the palate, *Ann Otol Rhinol Laryngol* 67:618-627, 1958.

Schwartz DL: Stomatitis nicotina of the palate: report of two cases, *Oral Surg Oral Med Oral Pathol* 20:306-315, 1965.

Actinic Keratosis

Alexiades-Armenakas M: Aminolevulinic acid photodynamic therapy for actinic keratoses/actinic cheilitis/acne: vascular lasers, *Dermatol Clin* 25:25-33, 2007.

Fu W, Cockerell CJ: The actinic (solar) keratosis: a 21st-century perspective, *Arch Dermatol* 139:66-70, 2003.

Fuchs A, Marmur E: The kinetics of skin cancer: progression of actinic keratosis to squamous carcinoma, *Dermatol Surg* 33:1099-1101, 2007.

Gupta AK, Cooper EA, Feldman SR et al: A survey of office visits for actinic keratosis as reported by NAMCS, 1990-1999. National Ambulatory Medical Care Survey, *Cutis* 70(suppl 2):8-13, 2002.

Gupta AK, Davey V, Mcphail H: Evaluation of the effectiveness of imiquimod and 5-fluorouracil for the treatment of actinic keratosis: critical review and meta-analysis of efficacy studies, *J Cutan Med Surg* 9:209-214, 2005.

Hadley G, Derry S, Moore RA: Imiquimod for actinic keratosis: systematic review and meta-analysis, *J Invest Dermatol* 126:1251-1255, 2006.

Jorizzo JL: Current and novel treatment options for actinic keratosis, *J Cutan Med Surg* 8:13-21, 2005.

Lober BA, Fenske NA: Optimum treatment strategies for actinic keratosis (intraepidermal squamous cell carcinoma), *Am J Clin Dermatol* 5:395-401, 2004.

Lober BA, Lober CW: Actinic keratosis is squamous cell carcinoma, *South Med J* 93:650-655, 2000.

Marks VJ: Actinic keratosis: a premalignant skin lesion, *Otolaryngol Clin North Am* 26:23-35, 1993.

Memon AA, Tomenson JA, Bothwell J et al: Prevalence of solar damage and actinic keratosis in a Merseyside population, *Br J Dermatol* 142:1154-1159, 2000.

Tran H, Chen K, Shumack S: Summary of actinic keratosis studies with imiquimod 5% cream, *Br J Dermatol* 149(suppl 66):37-39, 2003.

Wade TR, Ackerman AB: The many faces of solar keratoses, *J Dermatol Surg Oncol* 4:730-734, 1978.

Actinic Cheilosis

Alexiades-Armenakas M: Aminolevulinic acid photodynamic therapy for actinic keratoses/actinic cheilitis/acne: vascular lasers, *Dermatol Clin* 25:25-33, 2007.

Dufresne RG Jr, Curlin MU: Actinic cheilitis. A treatment review, *Dermatol Surg* 23:15-21, 1997.

Huber MA, Terezhalmy GT: The patient with actinic cheilitis, *Gen Dent* 54:274-282, 2006.

Kaugars GE, Pillion T, Svirsky JA et al: Actinic cheilitis: a review of 152 cases, *Oral Surg Oral Med Oral Pathol Oral Radiol Endod* 88:181-186, 1999.

Manganaro AM, Will MJ, Poulous E: Actinic cheilitis: a premalignant condition, *Gen Dent* 5:492-494, 1997.

Markopoulos A, Albanidou-Farmaki E, Kayavis I: Actinic cheilitis: clinical and pathologic characteristics in 65 cases, *Oral Dis* 10:212-216, 2004.

Menta Simonsen Nico M, Rivitti AE, Lourenço SV: Actinic cheilitis: histologic study of the entire vermilion and comparison with previous biopsy, *J Cutan Pathol* 34:309-314, 2007.

Orenstein A, Goldan O, Weissman O et al: A new modality in the treatment of actinic cheilitis using the Er:YAG laser, *J Cosmet Laser Ther* 9:23-25, 2007.

Smith KH, Germain M, Yeager J et al: Topical 5% imiquimod for the therapy of actinic cheilitis, *J Am Acad Dermatol* 47:497-501, 2002.

Keratoacanthoma

Cribier B, Asch P-H, Grosshans E: Differentiating squamous cell carcinoma from keratoacanthoma using histopathological criteria. Is it possible? A study of 296 cases, *Dermatology* 199:208-212, 1999.

Chen YK, Lin LM, Lin CC et al: Keratoacanthoma of the tongue: a diagnostic problem, *Otolaryngol Head Neck Surg* 128:581-582, 2003.

Clausen OPF, Aass HCD, Beigi M: Are keratoacanthomas variants of squamous cell carcinoma? A comparison of chromosomal aberrations by comparative genomic hybridization, *J Invest Dermatol* 126:2308-2315, 2006.

de Visscher JG, van der Wal JE, Starink TM et al: Giant keratoacanthoma of the lower lip. Report of a case of spontaneous regression, *Oral Surg Oral Med Oral Pathol Oral Radiol Endod* 81:193-196, 1996.

Eversole LR, Leider AS, Alexander G: Intraoral and labial keratoacanthoma, *Oral Surg Oral Med Oral Pathol* 54:663-667, 1982.

Griffiths RW: Keratoacanthoma observed, *Br J Plast Surg* 57:485-501, 2004.

Jaber PW, Cooper PH, Greer ICE: Generalized eruptive keratoacanthoma of Grzybowski, *J Am Acad Dermatol* 29:299-304, 1993.

Janette A, Pecaro B, Lonergan M et al: Solitary intraoral keratoacanthoma: report of a case, *J Oral Maxillofac Surg* 54:1026-1030, 1996.

Ponti G, Ponz de Leon M: Muir-Torre syndrome, *Lancet Oncol* 6:980-987, 2005.

Sanchez Yus E, Simon P, Requena L et al: Solitary keratoacanthoma: a self-healing proliferation that frequently becomes malignant, *Am J Dermatopathol* 22:305-310, 2000.

Schwartz RA: Keratoacanthoma, *J Am Acad Dermatol* 30:1-19, 1994.

Schwartz RA: Keratoacanthoma: a clinico-pathologic enigma, *Dermatol Surg* 30:326-333, 2004.

Weedon D: Keratoacanthoma: a personal perspective, *Curr Diagn Pathol* 9:259-265, 2003.

Squamous Cell Carcinoma

American Cancer Society: *Cancer facts & figures–2007*, pp 1-56, Atlanta, Ga, 2007, American Cancer Society.

Anneroth G, Hansen LS, Silverman S Jr: Malignancy grading in oral squamous cell carcinoma. 1. Squamous cell carcinoma of the tongue and floor of mouth: histologic grading in the clinical evaluation, *J Oral Pathol* 15:162-168, 1986.

Baker SR, Krause CJ: Carcinoma of the lip, *Laryngoscope* 90:19-27, 1980.

Ballantyne AJ, McCarten AB, Ibanez ML: The extension of cancer of the head and neck through peripheral nerves, *Am J Surg* 106:657-667, 1963.

Barasch A, Safford M, Eisenberg E: Oral cancer and oral effects of anticancer therapy, *Mt Sinai J Med* 65:370-377, 1998.

Black RJ, Gluckman JL, Shumrick DA: Multiple primary tumours of the upper aerodigestive tract, *Clin Otolaryngol* 8:277-281, 1983.

Blot WJ, McLaughlin JK, Winn DM et al: Smoking and drinking in relation to oral and pharyngeal cancer, *Cancer Res* 48:3282-3287, 1988.

Bouquot JE: Common oral lesions found during a mass screening examination, *J Am Dent Assoc* 112:50-57, 1986.

Bouquot JE: Epidemiology. In Gnepp DR: *Pathology of the head and neck*, pp 263-314, New York, 1988, Churchill Livingstone.

Bouquot JE, Meckstroth RL: Oral cancer in a tobacco-chewing U.S. population: incidence and mortality, *Oral Surg Oral Med Oral Pathol Oral Radiol Endod* 86:697-706, 1998.

Bouquot JE, Weiland LH, Kurland LT: Metastases to and from the upper aerodigestive tract in the population of Rochester, Minnesota, 1935-1984, *Head Neck* 11:212-218, 1989.

Braakhuis BJM, Leemans CR, Brakenhoff RH: Expanding fields of genetically altered cells in head and neck squamous carcinogenesis, *Semin Cancer Biol* 15:113-120, 2005.

Brandwein-Gensler M, Teixeira MS, Lewis CM et al: Oral squamous cell carcinoma: histologic risk assessment, but not margin status, is strongly predictive of local disease-free and overall survival, *Am J Surg Pathol* 29:167-178, 2005.

Brugere J, Guenel P, Leclerc A et al: Differential effects of tobacco and alcohol in cancer of the larynx, pharynx, and mouth, *Cancer* 57:391-395, 1986.

Bsoul SA, Huber MA, Terezhalmy GT: Squamous cell carcinoma of the oral tissues: a comprehensive review for oral healthcare providers, *J Contemp Dent Pract* 4:001-016, 2005.

Centers for Disease Control and Prevention: Tobacco use among adults–United States, 2005, *MMWR Morb Mortal Wkly Rep* 55:1145-1148, 2006.

Chang KW, Chang CS, Lai KS et al: High prevalence of human papillomavirus infection and possible association with betel quid chewing and smoking in oral epidermoid carcinomas in Taiwan, *J Med Virol* 28:57-61, 1989.

Choi SY, Kahyo H: Effect of cigarette smoking and alcohol consumption in the aetiology of cancer of the oral cavity, pharynx and larynx, *Int J Epidemiol* 20:878-885, 1991.

Choong NW, Cohen EEW: Epidermal growth factor receptor directed therapy in head and neck cancer, *Crit Rev Oncol Hematol* 57:25-42, 2006.

Cianfriglia F, Di Gregorio DA, Manieri A: Multiple primary tumours in patients with oral squamous cell carcinoma, *Oral Oncol* 35:157-163, 1999.

Cox MF, Scully C, Maitland N: Viruses in the aetiology of oral carcinoma? Examination of the evidence, *Br J Oral Maxillofac Surg* 29:381-387, 1991.

Davies L, Welch HG: Epidemiology of head and neck cancer in the United States, *Otolaryngol Head Neck Surg* 135:451-457, 2006.

de Visscher JG, Schaapveld M, Otter R et al: Epidemiology of cancer of the lip in the Netherlands, *Oral Oncol* 34:421-426, 1998.

Dickenson AJ, Currie WJ, Avery BS: Screening for syphilis in patients with carcinoma of the tongue, *Br J Oral Maxillofac Surg* 33:319-320, 1995.

Flaitz CM, Hicks MJ: Molecular piracy: the viral link to carcinogenesis, *Oral Oncol* 34:448-453, 1998.

Fukuzawa K, Noguchi Y, Yoshikawa T et al: High incidence of synchronous cancer of the oral cavity and the upper gastrointestinal tract, *Cancer Lett* 144:145-151, 1999.

Greene FL, Page DL, Fleming ID et al, editors: Lip and oral cavity. In *AJCC cancer staging manual*, ed 6, pp 23-32, New York, 2002, Springer-Verlag.

Ha PK, Califano JA: The molecular biology of mucosal field cancerization of the head and neck, *Crit Rev Oral Biol Med* 14:363-369, 2003.

Ha PK, Califano JA: The role of human papillomavirus in oral carcinogenesis, *Crit Rev Oral Biol Med* 15:188-196, 2004.

Hart AK, Karakla DW, Pitman KT et al: Oral and oropharyngeal squamous cell carcinoma in young adults: a report on 13 cases and review of the literature, *Otolaryngol Head Neck Surg* 120:828-833, 1999.

Hjortdal O, Naess A, Berner A: Squamous cell carcinomas of the lower lip, *J Craniomaxillofac Surg* 23:34-37, 1995.

Jemal A, Siegel R, Ward E et al: Cancer statistics, 2007, *CA Cancer J Clin* 57:43-66, 2007.

Kademani D: Oral cancer, *Mayo Clin Proc* 82:878-887, 2007.

Kalyankrishna S, Grandis JR: Epidermal growth factor receptor biology in head and neck cancer, *J Clin Oncol* 24:2666-2672, 2006.

Karja J, Syrjanen S, Usenius T et al: Oral cancer in children under 15 years of age: a clinicopathological and virological study, *Acta Otolaryngol Suppl* 449:145-149, 1988.

Kleinman DV, Crossett LS, Gloeckler Ries LA et al: *Cancer of the oral cavity and pharynx: a statistics review monograph, 1973-1987*, NIH Monograph, Bethesda, Md, 1992, National Institute of Dental Research.

Koch WM, Lango M, Sewell D et al: Head and neck cancer in nonsmokers: a distinct clinical and molecular entity, *Laryngoscope* 109:1544-1551, 1999.

Kowalski LP, Bagietto R, Lara JR et al: Prognostic significance of the distribution of neck node metastasis from oral carcinoma, *Head Neck* 22:207-214, 2000.

Kreimer AR, Clifford GM, Boyle P et al: Human papillomavirus types in head and neck squamous cell carcinomas worldwide: a systematic review, *Cancer Epidemiol Biomarkers Prev* 14:467-475, 2005.

Krogh P, Hald B, Holmstrup P: Possible mycological etiology of oral mucosal cancer: Catalytic potential of infecting *Candida albicans* and other yeasts in production of N-nitrosobenzylmethylamine, *Carcinogenesis* 8:1543-1548, 1987.

Kurumatani N, Kirita T, Zheng Y et al: Time trends in the mortality rates for tobacco- and alcohol-related cancers within the oral cavity and pharynx in Japan, 1950-94, *J Epidemiol* 9:46-52, 1999.

Lindqvist C, Teppo L: Epidemiological evaluation of sunlight as a risk factor of lip cancer, *Br J Cancer* 37:983-989, 1978.

Maserejian NN, Joshipura KJ, Rosner BA et al: Prospective study of alcohol consumption as risk of oral premalignant lesions in men, *Cancer Epidemiol Biomarkers Prev* 15:774-781, 2006.

Mashberg A, Samit AM: Early diagnosis of asymptomatic oral and oropharyngeal cancer, *CA Cancer J Clin* 45:328-351, 1995.

Massano J, Regateiro FS, Januário G et al: Oral squamous cell carcinoma: review of prognostic and predictive factors, *Oral*

Surg Oral Med Oral Pathol Oral Radiol Endod 102:67-76, 2006.

Mattson ME, Winn DM: *Smokeless tobacco: association with increased cancer risk*, NCI Monogr No 8, pp 13-16, Bethesda, Md, 1989, National Cancer Institute.

McDowell JD: An overview of epidemiology and common risk factors for oral squamous cell carcinoma, *Otolaryngol Clin North Am* 39:277-294, 2006.

Merchant A, Husain SS, Hosain M et al: Paan without tobacco: an independent risk factor for oral cancer, *Int J Cancer* 86:128-131, 2000.

Moreno-Lopez LA, Esparza-Gomez GC, Gonzalez-Navarro A et al: Risk of oral cancer associated with tobacco smoking, alcohol consumption and oral hygiene: a case-control study in Madrid, Spain, *Oral Oncol* 36:170-174, 2000.

Morse DE, Kerr AR: Disparities in oral and pharyngeal cancer incidence, mortality and survival among black and white Americans, *J Am Dent Assoc* 137:203-212, 2006.

Morse DE, Psoter WJ, Cleveland D et al: Smoking and drinking in relation to oral cancer and oral epithelial dysplasia, *Cancer Causes Control* 18:919-929, 2007.

Nair S, Pillai MR: Human papillomavirus and disease mechanisms: relevance to oral and cervical cancers, *Oral Dis* 11:350-359, 2005.

Neville BW, Day TA: Oral cancer and precancerous lesions, *CA Cancer J Clin* 52:195-215, 2002.

Niv A, Sion-Vardi N, Gatot A et al: Identification and typing of human papillomavirus (HPV) in squamous cell carcinoma of the oral cavity and oropharynx, *J Laryngol Otol* 114:41-46, 2000.

Notani PN, Jayant K: Role of diet in upper aerodigestive tract cancers, *Nutr Cancer* 10:103-113, 1987.

Paleri V, Rees G, Arullendran P et al: Sentinel node biopsy in squamous cell cancer of the oral cavity and oral pharynx: a diagnostic meta-analysis, *Head Neck* 27:739-747, 2005.

Partridge M, Kiguwa S, Emilion G et al: New insights into p53 protein stabilisation in oral squamous cell carcinoma, *Oral Oncol* 35:45-55, 1999.

Pentenero M, Gandolfo S, Carrozzo M: Importance of tumor thickness and depth of invasion in nodal involvement and prognosis of oral squamous cell carcinoma: a review of the literature, *Head Neck* 27:1080-1091, 2005.

Prince S, Bailey BM: Squamous cell carcinoma of the tongue: review, *Br J Oral Maxillofac Surg* 37:164-174, 1999.

Rodu B: Smokeless tobacco and oral cancer: a review of the risks and determinants, *Crit Rev Oral Biol Med* 15:252-263, 2004.

Rodu B, Cole P: Oral cavity and pharynx-throat cancer in the United States, 1973-2003, *Oral Surg Oral Med Oral Pathol Oral Radiol Endod* 104:653-658, 2007.

Rothman K, Keller A: The effect of joint exposure to alcohol and tobacco on risk of cancer of the mouth and pharynx, *J Chronic Dis* 25:711-716, 1972.

Sankaranarayanan R: Oral cancer in India: an epidemiologic and clinical review, *Oral Surg Oral Med Oral Pathol* 69:325-330, 1990.

Sciubba JJ: Oral cancer: the importance of early diagnosis and treatment, *Am J Clin Dermatol* 2:239-251, 2001.

Shaha AR, Patel S, Shasha D et al: Head and neck cancer. In Lenhard RE, Osteen RT, Gansler T: *Clinical oncology*, pp 297-331, Atlanta, Ga, 2000, American Cancer Society.

Shiboski CH, Schmidt BL, Jordan RC: Racial disparity in stage at diagnosis and survival among adults with oral cancer in the US, *Community Dent Oral Epidemiol* 35:233-240, 2007.

Silverman S Jr, Griffith M: Smoking characteristics of patients with oral carcinoma and the risk for second oral primary carcinoma, *J Am Dent Assoc* 85:637-640, 1972.

Specenier PM, Vermorken JB: Neoadjuvant chemotherapy in head and neck cancer: should it be revisited? *Cancer Lett* 256:166-177, 2007.

Speight PM, Farthing PM, Bouquot JE: The pathology of oral cancer and precancer, *Curr Diag Pathol* 3:165-176, 1997.

Spiro RH, Guillamondegui O Jr, Paulino AF et al: Pattern of invasion and margin assessment in patients with oral tongue cancer, *Head Neck* 21:408-413, 1999.

Stewart BW, Kleihues P, editors: Head and neck cancer. In *World Cancer Report*, pp 232-236, Lyon, France, 2003, IARC Press.

Syrjänen S: HPV infections and tonsillar carcinoma, *J Clin Pathol* 57:449-455, 2004.

Syrjänen S: Human papillomavirus (HPV) in head and neck cancer, *J Clin Virol* 32S:S59-S66, 2005.

Strome SE, To W, Strawderman M et al: Squamous cell carcinoma of the buccal mucosa, *Otolaryngol Head Neck Surg* 120:375-379, 1999.

Tabor MP, Brakenhoff RH, van Houten VMM et al: Persistence of genetically altered fields in head and neck cancer patients: biological and clinical implications, *Clin Cancer Res* 7:1523-1532, 2001.

Tralongo V, Rodolico V, Luciani A et al: Prognostic factors in oral squamous cell carcinoma. A review of the literature, *Anticancer Res* 19:3503-3510, 1999.

van Oijen MG, Leppers VD, Straat FG et al: The origins of multiple squamous cell carcinomas in the aerodigestive tract, *Cancer* 88:884-893, 2000.

Velly AM, Franco EL, Schlecht N et al: Relationship between dental factors and risk of upper aerodigestive tract cancer, *Oral Oncol* 34:284-291, 1998.

Watts JM: The importance of the Plummer-Vinson syndrome in the etiology of carcinoma of the upper gastrointestinal tract, *Postgrad Med J* 37:523-533, 1961.

Winn DM: Smokeless tobacco and cancer: the epidemiologic evidence, *CA Cancer J Clin* 38:236-243, 1988.

World Health Organization International Agency for Research on Cancer: *IARC monographs on the evaluation and carcinogenic risks to humans, Betel-quid and areca-nut chewing and some areca-nut-derived nitrosamines*, vol 85, Lyon, France, 2004, IARC Press.

Verrucous Carcinoma

Ackerman LV: Verrucous carcinoma of the oral cavity, *Surgery* 23:670-678, 1948.

Addante RR, McKenna SJ: Verrucous carcinoma, *Oral Maxillofac Surg Clin North Am* 18:513-519, 2006.

Bouquot JE: Oral verrucous carcinoma—incidence in two U.S. populations, *Oral Surg Oral Med Oral Pathol Oral Radiol Endod* 86:318-324, 1998.

Burford WN, Ackerman LV, Robinson HBG: Ellis Fischel State Cancer Hospital number: symposium on twenty cases of benign and malignant lesions of the oral cavity, from the Ellis Fischel State Cancer Hospital, Columbia, Missouri, *Am J Orthod Oral Surg* 30:353-372, 1944.

Jordan RC: Verrucous carcinoma of the mouth, *J Can Dent Assoc* 61:797-801, 1995.

Kamath VV, Varma RR, Gadewar DR et al: Oral verrucous carcinoma: an analysis of 37 cases, *J Craniomaxillofac Surg* 17:309-314, 1989.

Karthikeya P, Mahima VG, Bhavna G: Sinonasal verrucous carcinoma with oral invasion, *Indian J Dent Res* 17:82-86, 2006.

Koch BB, Trask DK, Hoffman HT et al: National survey of head and neck verrucous carcinoma: patterns of presentation, care, and outcome, *Cancer* 92:110-120, 2001.

McCoy JM, Waldron CA: Verrucous carcinoma of the oral cavity: a review of forty-nine cases, *Oral Surg Oral Med Oral Pathol* 52:623-629, 1981.

Medina JE, Dichtel W, Luna MA: Verrucous-squamous carcinomas of the oral cavity: a clinicopathologic study of 104 cases, *Arch Otolaryngol* 110:437-440, 1984.

Ogawa A, Fukua Y, Nakajima T et al: Treatment results of verrucous carcinoma and its biological behavior, *Oral Oncol* 40:793-797, 2004.

Oliveira DT, de Moraes RV, Filho JFF et al: Oral verrucous carcinoma: a retrospective study in Sao Paulo Region, Brazil, *Clin Oral Invest* 10:205-209, 2006.

Schwartz RA: Verrucous carcinoma of the skin and mucosa, *J Am Acad Dermatol* 32:1-24, 1995.

Strojan P, Soba E, Budihna M et al: Radiochemotherapy with vinblastine, methotrexate, and bleomycin in the treatment of verrucous carcinoma of the head and neck, *J Surg Oncol* 92:278-283, 2005.

Tharp II ME, Shidnia H: Radiotherapy in the treatment of verrucous carcinoma of the head and neck, *Laryngoscope* 105:391-396, 1995.

Spindle Cell Carcinoma

Batsakis JG, Suarez P: Sarcomatoid carcinomas of the upper aerodigestive tracts, *Adv Anat Pathol* 7:282-293, 2000.

Benninger MS, Kraus D, Sebek B et al: Head and neck spindle cell carcinoma: an evaluation of current management, *Cleve Clin J Med* 59:479-482, 1992.

Ellis GL, Langloss JM, Heffner DK et al: Spindle-cell carcinoma of the aerodigestive tract: an immunohistochemical analysis of 21 cases, *Am J Surg Pathol* 11:335-342, 1987.

Gupta R, Singh S, Hedau S et al: Spindle cell carcinoma of head and neck: an immunohistochemical and molecular approach to its pathogenesis, *J Clin Pathol* 60:472-475, 2007.

Lewis JE, Olsen KD, Sebo TJ: Spindle cell carcinoma of the larynx: review of 26 cases including DNA content and immunohistochemistry, *Hum Pathol* 28:664-673, 1997.

Rizzardi C, Frezzini C, Maglione M et al: A look at the biology of spindle cell squamous carcinoma of the oral cavity: report of a case, *J Oral Maxillofac Surg* 61:264-268, 2003.

Shibuya Y, Umeda M, Yokoo S et al: Spindle cell squamous carcinoma of the maxilla: report of a case with immunohistochemical analysis, *J Oral Maxillofac Surg* 58:1164-1169, 2000.

Slootweg PJ, Roholl PJ, Muller H et al: Spindle-cell carcinoma of the oral cavity and larynx. Immunohistochemical aspects, *J Craniomaxillofac Surg* 17:234-236, 1989.

Su HH, Chu ST, Hou YY et al: Spindle cell carcinoma of the oral cavity and oropharynx: factors affecting outcome, *J Chin Med Assoc* 69:478-483, 2006.

Adenosquamous Carcinoma

Abdelsayed RA, Sangueza OP, Newhouse RF et al: Adenosquamous carcinoma: a case report with immunohistochemical evaluation, *Oral Surg Oral Med Oral Pathol Oral Radiol Endod* 85:173-177, 1998.

Alos L, Castillo M, Nadal A et al: Adenosquamous carcinoma of the head and neck: criteria for diagnosis in a study of 12 cases, *Histopathology* 44:570-579, 2004.

Banks ER, Cooper PH: Adenosquamous carcinoma of the skin: a report of 10 cases, *J Cutan Pathol* 18:227-234, 1991.

Gerughty RM, Hennigar GB, Brown FM: Adenosquamous carcinoma of the nasal, oral and laryngeal cavities: a clinicopathologic survey of ten cases, *Cancer* 22:1140-1155, 1968.

Keelawat S, Liu CZ, Roehm PC et al: Adenosquamous carcinoma of the upper aerodigestive tract: a clinicopathologic study of 12 cases and review of the literature, *Am J Otolaryngol* 23:160-168, 2002.

Martinez-Madrigal F, Baden E, Casiraghi O et al: Oral and pharyngeal adenosquamous carcinoma: a report of four cases with immunohistochemical studies, *Eur Arch Otorhinolaryngol* 248:255-258, 1991.

Scully C, Porter SR, Speight PM et al: Adenosquamous carcinoma of the mouth: a rare variant of squamous cell carcinoma, *Int J Oral Maxillofac Surg* 28:125-128, 1999.

Sheahan P, Fitzgibbon J, Lee G et al: Adenosquamous carcinoma of the tongue in a 22-year-old female: report of a case with immunohistochemistry, *Eur Arch Otorhinolaryngol* 260:509-512, 2003.

Sheahan P, Toner M, Timon CV I: Clinicopathologic features of head and neck adenosquamous carcinoma, *ORL J Otorhinolaryngol Relat Spec* 67:10-15, 2005.

Yoshimura Y, Mishimma K, Ohara S et al: Clinical characteristics of oral adenosquamous carcinoma: report of a case and an analysis of the reported Japanese cases, *Oral Oncol* 39:309-315, 2003.

Basaloid Squamous Carcinoma

Altavilla G, Mannara GM, Rinaldo A et al: Basaloid squamous cell carcinoma of oral cavity and oropharynx, *ORL J Otorhinolaryngol Relat Spec* 61:169-173, 1999.

Banks ER, Frierson HF Jr, Mills SE et al: Basaloid squamous cell carcinoma of the head and neck: a clinicopathologic and immunohistochemical study of 40 cases, *Am J Surg Pathol* 16:939-946, 1992.

Barnes L, Ferlito A, Altavilla G et al: Basaloid squamous cell carcinoma of the head and neck: clinicopathological features and differential diagnosis, *Ann Otol Rhinol Laryngol* 105:75-82, 1996.

Coletta RD, Cotrim P, Vargas PA et al: Basaloid squamous carcinoma of the oral cavity: report of 2 cases and study of AgNOR, PCNA, p53, and MMP expression, *Oral Surg Oral Med Oral Pathol Oral Radiol Endod* 91:563-569, 2001.

Coletta RD, Cotrim P, Almeida OP et al: Basaloid squamous carcinoma of oral cavity: a histologic and immunohistochemical study, *Oral Oncol* 38:723-729, 2002.

De Sampaio Góes FC, Oliveira DT, Dorta RG et al: Prognoses of oral basaloid squamous cell carcinoma and squamous cell carcinoma: a comparison, *Arch Otolaryngol Head Neck Surg* 130:83-86, 2004.

Ide F, Shimoyama T, Horie N et al: Basaloid squamous cell carcinoma of the oral mucosa: a new case and review of 45 cases in the literature, *Oral Oncol* 38:120-124, 2002.

Ide F, Shimoyama T, Suzuki T et al: Polypoid carcinoma of the tongue, *J Oral Pathol Med* 25:90-92, 1996.

Oikawa k, Tabuchi K, Nomura M et al: Basaloid squamous cell carcinoma of the maxillary sinus: a report of two cases, *Auris Nasus Larynx* 34:119-123, 2007.

Paulino AF, Singh B, Shah JP et al: Basaloid squamous cell carcinoma of the head and neck, *Laryngoscope* 110:1479-1482, 2000.

Sampaio-Góes FCG, Oliveira DT, Dorta RG et al: Expression of PCNA, p53, Bax, and Bcl-X in oral poorly differentiated and basaloid squamous cell carcinoma: relationships with prognosis, *Head Neck* 27:982-989, 2005.

Zbären P, Nuyens M, Stauffer E: Basaloid squamous cell carcinoma of the head and neck, *Curr Opin Otolaryngol Head Neck Surg* 12:116-121, 2004.

Carcinoma of the Maxillary Sinus

Bhattacharyya N: Factors affecting survival in maxillary sinus cancer, *J Oral Maxillofac Surg* 61:1016-1021, 2003.

Carrillo JF, Guemes A, Ramierz-Ortega MC et al: Prognostic factors in maxillary sinus and nasal cavity carcinoma, *Eur J Surg Oncol* 31:1206-1212, 2005.

Doig TN, McDonald SW, McGregor IA: Possible routes of spread of carcinoma of the maxillary sinus to the oral cavity, *Clin Anat* 11:149-156, 1998.

Georgiou AF, Walker DM, Collins AP et al: Primary small cell undifferentiated (neuroendocrine) carcinoma of the maxillary sinus, *Oral Surg Oral Med Oral Pathol Oral Radiol Endod* 98:572-578, 2004.

Giri SP, Reddy EK, Gemer LS et al: Management of advanced squamous cell carcinomas of the maxillary sinus, *Cancer* 69:657-661, 1992.

Guntinas-Lichius O, Kreppel MP, Stuetzer H et al: Single modality and multimodality treatment of nasal and paranasal sinuses cancer: a single institution experience of 229 patients, *Eur J Surg Oncol* 33:222-228, 2007.

Hoppe BS, Stegman LD, Zelefsky MJ et al: Treatment of nasal cavity and paranasal sinus cancer with modern radiotherapy techniques in the postoperative setting—the MKSCC experience, *Int J Radiat Oncol Biol Phys* 67:691-702, 2007.

Indudharan R, Das PK, Thida T: Verrucous carcinoma of maxillary antrum, *Singapore Med J* 37:559-561, 1996.

Itami J, Uno T, Aruga M et al: Squamous cell carcinoma of the maxillary sinus treated with radiation therapy and conservative surgery, *Cancer* 82:104-107, 1998.

Paulino AC, Marks JE, Bricker P et al: Results of treatment of patients with maxillary sinus carcinoma, *Cancer* 83:457-465, 1998.

Smith SR, Som P, Fahmy A et al: A clinicopathological study of sinonasal neuroendocrine carcinoma and sinonasal undifferentiated carcinoma, *Laryngoscope* 110:1617-1622, 2000.

Tiwari R, Hardillo JA, Mehta D et al: Squamous cell carcinoma of maxillary sinus, *Head Neck* 22:164-169, 2000.

Waldron JN, O'Sullivan B, Gullane P et al: Carcinoma of the maxillary antrum: a retrospective analysis of 110 cases, *Radiother Oncol* 57:167-173, 2000.

Sinonasal Undifferentiated Carcinoma

Ejaz A, Wenig BM: Sinonasal undifferentiated carcinoma: clinical and pathologic features and a discussion on classification, cellular differentiation, and differential diagnosis, *Adv Anat Pathol* 12:134-143, 2005.

Frierson HF Jr, Mills SE, Fechner RE et al: Sinonasal undifferentiated carcinoma: an aggressive neoplasm derived from schneiderian epithelium and distinct from olfactory neuroblastoma, *Am J Surg Pathol* 10:771-779, 1986.

Gorelick J, Ross D, Marentette L et al: Sinonasal undifferentiated carcinoma: case series and review of literature, *Neurosurgery* 47:750-755, 2000.

Houston GD: Sinonasal undifferentiated carcinoma. Report of two cases and review of the literature, *Oral Surg Oral Med Oral Pathol Oral Radiol Endod* 85:185-188, 1998.

Houston GD, Gillies E: Sinonasal undifferentiated carcinoma: a distinctive clinicopathologic entity, *Adv Anat Pathol* 6:317-323, 1999.

Jeng YM, Sung MT, Fang CL et al: Sinonasal undifferentiated carcinoma and nasopharyngeal-type carcinoma: two clinically, biologically, and histopathologically distinct entities, *Am J Surg Pathol* 26:371-376, 2002.

Jones AV, Robinson I, Speight PM: Sinonasal undifferentiated carcinoma: report of a case and review of literature, *Oral Oncol* 41:299-302, 2005.

Kim BS, Vongtama R, Juillard G: Sinonasal undifferentiated carcinoma: case series and literature review, *Am J Otolaryngol* 25:162-166, 2004.

Levine PA, Frierson HF, Stewart FM et al: Sinonasal undifferentiated carcinoma: a distinctive and highly aggressive neoplasm, *Laryngoscope* 97:905-908, 1987.

Righi PD, Francis F, Aron BS et al: Sinonasal undifferentiated carcinoma: a 10-year experience, *Am J Otolaryngol* 17:167-171, 1996.

Rischin D, Porceddu S, Peters L et al: Promising results with chemoradiation in patients with sinonasal undifferentiated carcinoma, *Head Neck* 26:435-441, 2004.

Sharara N, Muller S, Olson J et al: Sinonasal undifferentiated carcinoma with orbital invasion: report of three cases, *Ophthal Plast Reconstr Surg* 17:288-292, 2001.

Smith SR, Som P, Fahmy A et al: A clinicopathological study of sinonasal neuroendocrine and sinonasal undifferentiated carcinoma, *Laryngoscope* 110:1617-1622, 2000.

Nasopharyngeal Carcinoma

Agulnik M, Siu LL: State-of-the-art management of nasopharyngeal carcinoma: current and future directions, *Br J Cancer* 92:799-806, 2005.

August M, Dodson TB, Nastri A et al: Nasopharyngeal carcinoma: clinical assessment and review of 176 cases, *Oral Surg Oral Med Oral Pathol Oral Radiol Endod* 91:205-214, 2001.

Chen CL, Hsu MM: Second primary epithelial malignancy of nasopharynx and nasal cavity after successful curative radiation therapy of nasopharyngeal carcinoma, *Hum Pathol* 31:227-232, 2000.

Epstein JB, Jones CK: Presenting signs and symptoms of nasopharyngeal carcinoma, *Oral Surg Oral Med Oral Pathol* 75:32-36, 1993.

Farrow DC, Vaughan TL, Berwick M et al: Diet and nasopharyngeal cancer in a low-risk population, *Int J Cancer* 78:675-679, 1998.

Ma BBY, Chan ATC: Recent perspectives in the role of chemotherapy in the management of advanced nasopharyngeal carcinoma, *Cancer* 103:22-31, 2005.

O'Meara WP, Lee N: Advances in nasopharyngeal carcinoma, *Curr Opin Oncol* 17:225-230, 2005.

Ou SHI, Zell JA, Ziogas A et al: Epidemiology of nasopharyngeal carcinoma in the United States: improved survival of Chinese patients within the keratinizing squamous cell carcinoma histology, *Ann Oncol* 18:29-35, 2007.

Wei WI, Sham JST: Nasopharyngeal carcinoma, *Lancet* 365:2041-2052, 2005.

Wenig BM: Nasopharyngeal carcinoma, *Ann Diagn Pathol* 3:374-385, 1999.

Yu MC, Yuan JM: Epidemiology of nasopharyngeal carcinoma, *Cancer Biol* 12:421-429, 2002.

Basal Cell Carcinoma

Bath-Hextall FJ, Perkins W, Bong J et al: Interventions for basal cell carcinoma of the skin, *Cochrane Database Syst Rev* 1: CD003412, 2007.

Ceilley RI, Del Rosso JQ: Current modalities and new advances in the treatment of basal cell carcinoma, *Int J Dermatol* 45:489-498, 2006.

Christenson LF, Borrowman TA, Vachon CM et al: Incidence of basal cell and squamous cell carcinomas in a population younger than 40 years, *JAMA* 294:681-690, 2005.

Crowson AN: Basal cell carcinoma: biology, morphology and clinical implications, *Mod Pathol* 19:S127-S147, 2006.

Daya-Grosjean L, Couvé-Privat S: Sonic hedgehog signaling in basal cell carcinomas, *Cancer Lett* 225:181-192, 2005.

Del Rosario RN, Barr RJ, Jensen JL et al: Basal cell carcinoma of the buccal mucosa, *Am J Dermatopathol* 23:203-205, 2001.

Gutierrez MM, Mora RG: Nevoid basal cell carcinoma syndrome: a review and case report of a patient with unilateral basal cell nevus syndrome, *J Am Acad Dermatol* 15:1023-1030, 1986.

Kato N, Endo Y, Tamura G et al: Ameloblastoma with basal cell carcinoma-like feature emerging as a nasal polyp, *Pathol Int* 49:747-751, 1999.

Kuijpers DIM, Thissen MRTM, Neumann MHA: Basal cell carcinoma. Treatment options and prognosis, a scientific approach to a common malignancy, *Am J Clin Dermatol* 3:247-259, 2002.

Martin RC 2nd, Edwards MJ, Cawte TG et al: Basosquamous carcinoma: analysis of prognostic factors influencing recurrence, *Cancer* 88:1365-1369, 2000.

Niederhagen B, Lindern J, Berge S et al: Staged operations for basal cell carcinoma of the face, *Br J Oral Maxillofac Surg* 38:477-479, 2000.

Rishiraj B, Epstein JB: Basal cell carcinoma: what dentists need to know, *J Am Dent Assoc* 130:375-380, 1999.

Rubin AI, Chen EH, Ratner D: Basal-cell carcinoma, *N Engl J Med* 353:2262-2269, 2005.

Telfer NR, Colver GB, Bowers PW: Guidelines for the management of basal cell carcinoma, *Br J Dermatol* 141:415-423, 1999.

Merkel Cell Carcinoma

Agelli M, Clegg LX: Epidemiology of primary Merkel cell carcinoma in the United States, *J Am Acad Dermatol* 49:832-841, 2003.

Bickle K, Glass LF, Messina JF et al: Merkel cell carcinoma: a clinical, histopathologic, and immunohistochemical review, *Semin Cutan Med Surg* 23:46-53, 2004.

Chan JK, Suster S, Wenig BM et al: Cytokeratin 20 immunoreactivity distinguishes Merkel cell (primary cutaneous neuroendocrine) carcinomas and salivary gland small cell carcinomas from small cell carcinomas of various sites, *Am J Surg Pathol* 21:226-234, 1997.

Dancey AL, Rayatt SS, Soon C et al: Merkel cell carcinoma: a report of 34 cases and literature review, *J Plast Reconstr Aesthet Surg* 59:1294-1299, 2006.

Garneski KM, Nghiem P: Merkel cell carcinoma adjuvant therapy: current data support radiation but not chemotherapy, *J Am Acad Dermatol* 57:166-169, 2007.

Gollard R, Weber R, Kosty MP et al: Merkel cell carcinoma. Review of 22 cases with surgical, pathologic, and therapeutic considerations, *Cancer* 8:1842-1851, 2000.

Hendrikx SMGA, de Wilde PCM, Kaanders JHAM et al: Merkel cell carcinoma in the oral cavity: a case presentation and review of the literature, *Oral Oncol* 41:202-206, 2005.

Jabbour J, Cumming R, Scolyer RA et al: Merkel cell carcinoma: assessing the effect of wide local excision, lymph node dissection, and radiotherapy on recurrence and survival in early-stage disease—results from a review of 82 consecutive cases diagnosed between 1992 and 2004, *Ann Surg Oncol* 14:1943-1952, 2007.

Lewis KG, Weinstock MA, Weaver AL et al: Adjuvant local irradiation for Merkel cell carcinoma, *Arch Dermatol* 142:693-700, 2006.

Longo F, Califano L, Mangone GM et al: Neuroendocrine (Merkel cell) carcinoma of the oral mucosa: report of a case with immunohistochemical study and review of the literature, *J Oral Pathol Med* 28:88-91, 1999.

Mendenhall WM, Mendenhall CM, Mendenhall NP: Merkel cell carcinoma, *Laryngoscope* 114:906-910, 2004.

Miller SJ, Alam M, Andersen J et al: Merkel cell carcinoma, *J Natl Compr Canc Netw* 4:704-712, 2006.

Pectasides D, Pectasides M, Economopoulos T: Merkel cell carcinoma of the skin, *Ann Oncol* 17:1489-1495, 2006.

Suárez C, Rodrigo JP, Ferlito et al: Merkel cell carcinoma of the head and neck, *Oral Oncol* 40:773-779, 2004.

Yom SS, Rosenthal DI, El-Naggar AK et al: Merkel cell carcinoma of the tongue and head and neck oral mucosal sites, *Oral Surg Oral Med Oral Pathol Oral Radiol Endod* 101:761-768, 2006.

Melanoma

Abassi NR, Shaw HM, Rigel DS et al: Early diagnosis of cutaneous melanoma. Revisiting the ABCD criteria, *JAMA* 292:2771-2776, 2004.

Balch CM, Buzaid AC, Soong SJ et al: Final version of the American Joint Committee on Cancer staging system for cutaneous melanoma, *J Clin Oncol* 19:3635-3648, 2001.

Barnhill RL, Mihm MC Jr: The histopathology of cutaneous malignant melanoma, *Semin Diagn Pathol* 10:47-75, 1993.

Barrett AW, Bennett JH, Speight PM: A clinicopathological and immunohistochemical analysis of primary oral mucosal melanoma, *Oral Oncol* 31:100-105, 1995.

Batsakis JG, Suarez P: Mucosal melanomas: a review, *Adv Anat Pathol* 7:167-180, 2000.

Chidzonga MM, Mahomva L, Marimo C et al: Primary malignant melanoma of the oral mucosa, *J Oral Maxillofac Surg* 65:1117-1120, 2007.

Curtin JA, Fridlyand J, Kageshita T et al: Distinct sets of genetic alterations in melanoma, *N Engl J Med* 353:2135-2147, 2005.

Garbe C, Eigentler TK: Diagnosis and treatment of cutaneous melanoma: state of the art 2006, *Melanoma Res* 17:117-127, 2007.

Garzino-Demo P, Fasolis M, Maggiore GM et al: Oral mucosal melanoma: a series of case reports, *J Craniomaxillofac Surg* 32:251-257, 2004.

Gorsky M, Epstein JB: Melanoma arising from the mucosal surfaces of the head and neck, *Oral Surg Oral Med Oral Pathol Oral Radiol Endod* 86:715-719, 1998.

Gray-Schopfer V, Wellbrock C, Marais R: Melanoma biology and new targeted therapy, *Nature* 445:851-857, 2007.

Greene FL, Page DL, Fleming ID et al, editors: Melanoma of the skin. In *AJCC cancer staging manual*, ed 6, pp 209-217, New York, 2002, Springer-Verlag.

Hall HI, Miller DR, Rogers JD et al: Update on the incidence and mortality from melanoma in the United States, *J Am Acad Dermatol* 40:35-42, 1999.

Hicks MJ, Flaitz CM: Oral mucosal melanoma: epidemiology and pathobiology, *Oral Oncol* 36:152-169, 2000.

Jemal A, Siegel R, Ward E et al: Cancer statistics, 2007, *CA Cancer J Clin* 57:43-66, 2007.

Kahn M, Weathers DR, Hoffman JG: Transformation of a benign oral pigmentation to primary oral mucosal melanoma, *Oral Surg Oral Med Oral Pathol Oral Radiol Endod* 100:454-459, 2005.

Kilpatrick SE, White WL, Browne JD: Desmoplastic malignant melanoma of the oral mucosa. An underrecognized diagnostic pitfall, *Cancer* 78:383-389, 1996.

Manganaro AM, Hammond HL, Dalton MJ et al: Oral melanoma: case reports and review of the literature, *Oral Surg Oral Med Oral Pathol Oral Radiol Endod* 80:670-677, 1995.

Markovic SN, Erickson LA, Rao RD et al: Malignant melanoma in the 21st century, part 1: epidemiology, risk factors, screening, prevention, and diagnosis, *Mayo Clin Proc* 82:364-380, 2007.

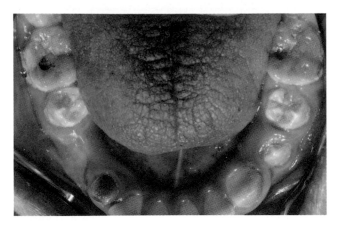

Fig. 11-1   Salivary gland aplasia. Dry, leathery tongue and diffuse enamel erosion in a child with aplasia of the major salivary glands.

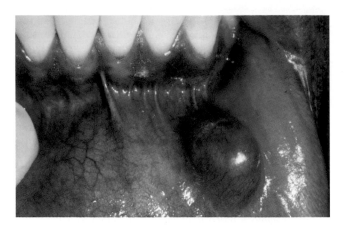

Fig. 11-2   Mucocele. Blue-pigmented nodule on the lower lip.

pertechnetate scintiscan, computed tomography (CT), or magnetic resonance imaging (MRI).

LADD syndrome is an autosomal dominant disorder that is caused by mutations in the fibroblast growth factor 10 (*FGF10*) gene. It is characterized by aplasia or hypoplasia of the lacrimal and salivary glands, cup-shaped ears, and dental and digital anomalies. Dental features may include hypodontia, microdontia, and mild enamel hypoplasia.

TREATMENT AND PROGNOSIS

Patient management is directed toward compensating for the saliva deficiency, and saliva substitutes are often necessary. If any residual functional salivary gland tissue is present, then sialagogue medications such as pilocarpine or cevimeline may be used to increase saliva production. Salivary flow also may be stimulated via the use of sugarless gum or sour candy. Regular preventive dental care is important to avoid xerostomia-related caries and enamel breakdown.

MUCOCELE (MUCUS EXTRAVASATION PHENOMENON; MUCUS ESCAPE REACTION)

The **mucocele** is a common lesion of the oral mucosa that results from rupture of a salivary gland duct and spillage of mucin into the surrounding soft tissues. This spillage is often the result of local trauma, although there is no known history of trauma in many cases. Unlike the salivary duct cyst (see page 457), the mucocele is not a true cyst because it lacks an epithelial lining. Some authors, however, have included true salivary duct cysts in their reported series of cases, sometimes under the classification of *retention mucocele*.

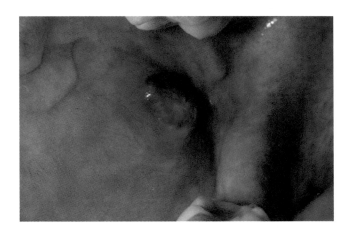

Fig. 11-3   Mucocele. Nodule on the posterior buccal mucosa.

Because these two entities exhibit distinctly different clinical and histopathologic features, they are discussed as separate topics in this chapter.

CLINICAL FEATURES

Mucoceles typically appear as dome-shaped mucosal swellings that can range from 1 or 2 mm to several centimeters in size (Figs. 11-2 to 11-4). They are most common in children and young adults, perhaps because younger people are more likely to experience trauma that induces mucin spillage. However, mucoceles have been reported in patients of all ages, including infants and older adults. The spilled mucin below the mucosal surface often imparts a bluish translucent hue to the swelling, although deeper mucoceles may be normal in color. The lesion characteristically is fluctuant, but some mucoceles feel firmer to palpation. The reported

Table **11-1**   **Location of Mucoceles**

Location	Number of Cases	Percentage of All Cases
Lower lip	1477	81.0
Floor of mouth	106	5.8
Ventral tongue	106	5.8
Buccal mucosa	87	4.8
Palate	26	1.4
Retromolar	10	0.5
Unknown	12	0.7
Upper lip	0	0.0
Total	**1824**	**100**

Data from Chi A, Lambert P, Richardson M et al: *Oral mucoceles: a clinicopathologic review of 1,824 cases including unusual variants,* Abstract No. 19. Paper presented at the annual meeting of the American Academy of Oral and Maxillofacial Pathology, Kansas City, Mo, 2007.

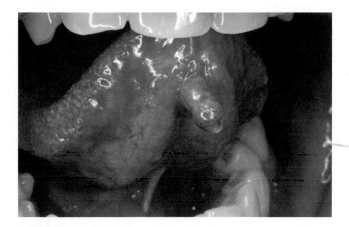

Fig. 11-4   Mucocele. Exophytic lesion on the anterior ventral tongue.

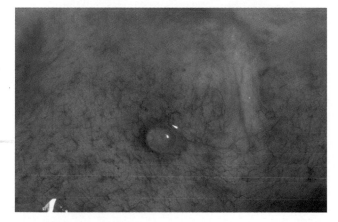

Fig. 11-5   Superficial mucocele. Vesicle-like lesion on the soft palate.

duration of the lesion can vary from a few days to several years; most patients report that the lesion has been present for several weeks. Many patients relate a history of a recurrent swelling that periodically may rupture and release its fluid contents.

The lower lip is by far the most common site for the mucocele; a recent large study of 1824 cases found that 81% occurred at this one site (Table 11-1). Lower lip mucoceles usually are found lateral to the midline. Less common sites include the floor of mouth (ranulas: 5.8%), anterior ventral tongue (from the glands of Blandin-Nuhn: 5.7%), buccal mucosa (4.7%), palate (1.4%), and retromolar pad (0.5%). Mucoceles rarely develop on the upper lip. In the large series summarized in Table 11-1, not a single example was identified from the upper lip. This is in contrast to salivary gland tumors, which are not unusual in the upper lip but are distinctly uncommon in the lower lip.

As noted, the soft palate and retromolar area are uncommon sites for mucoceles. However, one interesting variant, the **superficial mucocele,** does develop in these areas and along the posterior buccal mucosa.

Superficial mucoceles present as single or multiple tense vesicles that measure 1 to 4 mm in diameter (Fig. 11-5). The lesions often burst, leaving shallow, painful ulcers that heal within a few days. Repeated episodes at the same location are not unusual. Some patients relate the development of the lesions to mealtimes. Superficial mucoceles also have been reported to occur in association with lichenoid disorders, such as lichen planus, lichenoid drug eruptions, and chronic graft-versus-host disease (GVHD). The vesicular appearance is created by the superficial nature of the mucin spillage, which causes a separation of the epithelium from the connective tissue. The pathologist must be aware of this lesion and should not mistake it microscopically for a vesiculobullous disorder, especially mucous membrane (cicatricial) pemphigoid.

HISTOPATHOLOGIC FEATURES

On microscopic examination, the mucocele shows an area of spilled mucin surrounded by a granulation tissue response (Figs. 11-6 and 11-7). The inflamma-

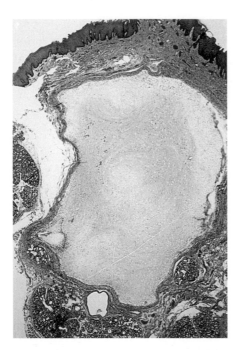

Fig. 11-6   Mucocele. Mucin-filled cystlike cavity beneath the mucosal surface. Minor salivary glands are present below and lateral to the spilled mucin.

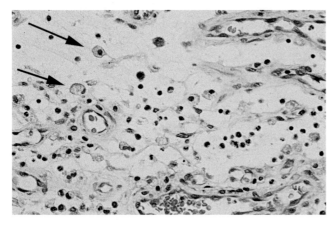

Fig. 11-7   Mucocele. High-power view showing spilled mucin that is associated with granulation tissue containing foamy histiocytes (*arrows*).

tion usually includes numerous foamy histiocytes (macrophages). In some cases a ruptured salivary duct may be identified feeding into the area. The adjacent minor salivary glands often contain a chronic inflammatory cell infiltrate and dilated ducts.

TREATMENT AND PROGNOSIS

Some mucoceles are short-lived lesions that rupture and heal by themselves. Many lesions, however, are chronic in nature, and local surgical excision is neces-

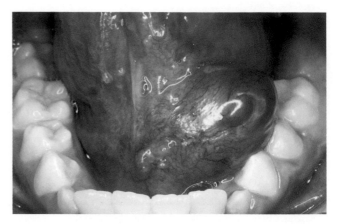

Fig. 11-8   Ranula. Blue-pigmented swelling in the left floor of the mouth.

sary. To minimize the risk of recurrence, the surgeon should remove any adjacent minor salivary glands that may be feeding into the lesion when the area is excised. The excised tissue should be submitted for microscopic examination to confirm the diagnosis and rule out the possibility of a salivary gland tumor. The prognosis is excellent, although occasional mucoceles will recur, necessitating reexcision, especially if the feeding glands are not removed.

RANULA

Ranula is a term used for mucoceles that occur in the floor of the mouth. The name is derived from the Latin word *rana*, which means "frog," because the swelling may resemble a frog's translucent underbelly. The term *ranula* also has been used to describe other similar swellings in the floor of the mouth, including true salivary duct cysts, dermoid cysts, and cystic hygromas. However, the term is best used for mucus escape reactions (mucoceles). The source of mucin spillage is usually from the sublingual gland, but ranulas also may arise from the submandibular duct or, possibly, from minor salivary glands in the floor of the mouth. Larger ranulas usually arise from the body of the sublingual gland, although smaller lesions can develop along the sublingual plica from the superficial ducts of Rivini of this gland.

CLINICAL FEATURES

The ranula usually appears as a blue, dome-shaped, fluctuant swelling in the floor of the mouth (Fig. 11-8), but deeper lesions may be normal in color. Ranulas are seen most frequently in children and young adults. They tend to be larger than mucoceles in other oral locations, often developing into large masses that fill the floor of the mouth and elevate the tongue. The

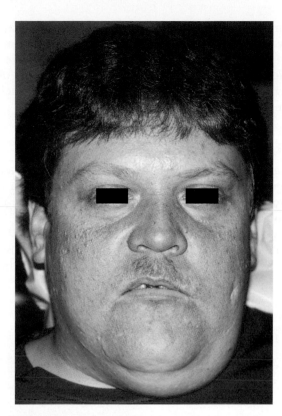

Fig. 11-9   Plunging ranula. Soft swelling in the neck.

ranula usually is located lateral to the midline, a feature that may help to distinguish it from a midline dermoid cyst (see page 33). Like other mucoceles, ranulas may rupture and release their mucin contents, only to re-form.

An unusual clinical variant, the **plunging** or **cervical ranula**, occurs when the spilled mucin dissects through the mylohyoid muscle and produces swelling within the neck (Fig. 11-9). A concomitant swelling in the floor of the mouth may or may not be present. If no lesion is produced in the mouth, then the clinical diagnosis of ranula may not be suspected. Imaging studies can be helpful in supporting a diagnosis of plunging ranula and in determining the origin of the lesion. CT and MRI images of plunging ranulas that arise from the sublingual gland often exhibit a slight extension of the lesion into the sublingual space ("tail sign")—an imaging feature not observed in lesions that develop from the submandibular gland.

HISTOPATHOLOGIC FEATURES

The microscopic appearance of a ranula is similar to that of a mucocele in other locations. The spilled mucin elicits a granulation tissue response that typically contains foamy histiocytes.

TREATMENT AND PROGNOSIS

Treatment of the ranula consists of removal of the feeding sublingual gland and/or marsupialization. Marsupialization (exteriorization) entails removal of the roof of the intraoral lesion, which often can be successful for small, superficial ranulas associated with the ducts of Rivini. However, marsupialization is often unsuccessful for larger ranulas developing from the body of the sublingual gland, and most authors emphasize that removal of the offending gland is the most important consideration in preventing a recurrence of the lesion. If the gland is removed, then meticulous dissection of the lining of the lesion may not be necessary for the lesion to resolve, even for the plunging ranula.

SALIVARY DUCT CYST (MUCUS RETENTION CYST; MUCUS DUCT CYST; SIALOCYST)

The **salivary duct cyst** is an epithelium-lined cavity that arises from salivary gland tissue. Unlike the more common mucocele (see page 454), it is a true developmental cyst that is lined by epithelium that is separate from the adjacent normal salivary ducts. The cause of such cysts is uncertain.

Cystlike dilatation of salivary ducts also may develop secondary to ductal obstruction (e.g., mucus plug), which creates increased intraluminal pressure. Although some authors refer to such lesions as mucus retention cysts, such lesions probably represent salivary ductal ectasia rather than a true cyst.

CLINICAL FEATURES

Salivary duct cysts usually occur in adults and can arise within either the major or minor glands. Cysts of the major glands are most common within the parotid gland, presenting as slowly growing, asymptomatic swellings. Intraoral cysts can occur at any minor gland site, but most frequently they develop in the floor of the mouth, buccal mucosa, and lips (Fig. 11-10). They often look like mucoceles and are characterized by a soft, fluctuant swelling that may appear bluish, depending on the depth of the cyst below the surface. Some cysts may feel relatively firm to palpation. Cysts in the floor of the mouth often arise adjacent to the submandibular duct and sometimes have an amber color.

On rare occasions, patients have been observed to develop prominent ectasia of the excretory ducts of many of the minor salivary glands throughout the mouth. Such lesions have been termed "mucus retention cysts," although they probably represent multifocal ductal dilatation. The individual lesions often present as painful nodules that demonstrate dilated ductal orifices on the mucosal surface. Mucus or pus may be expressed from these dilated ducts.

HISTOPATHOLOGIC FEATURES

The lining of the salivary duct cyst is variable and may consist of cuboidal, columnar, or atrophic squamous epithelium surrounding thin or mucoid secretions in the lumen (Fig. 11-11). In contrast, ductal ectasia secondary to salivary obstruction is characterized by oncocytic metaplasia of the epithelial lining. This epithelium often demonstrates papillary folds into the cystic lumen, somewhat reminiscent of a small Warthin tumor (see page 482) but without the prominent lymphoid stroma (Fig. 11-12). If this proliferation is extensive enough,

then these lesions sometimes are diagnosed as **papillary cystadenoma**, although it seems likely that most are not true neoplasms. The individual lesions of patients with multiple "mucus retention cysts" also show prominent oncocytic metaplasia of the epithelial lining.

TREATMENT AND PROGNOSIS

Isolated salivary duct cysts are treated by conservative surgical excision. For cysts in the major glands, partial or total removal of the gland may be necessary. The lesion should not recur.

For rare patients who develop multifocal salivary ductal ectasia ("mucus retention cysts"), local excision may be performed for the more problematic swellings;

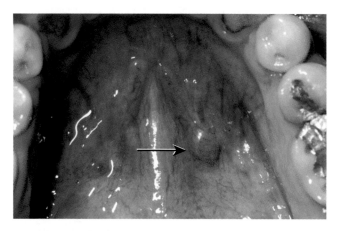

Fig. 11-10   Salivary duct cyst. Nodular swelling (arrow) overlying Wharton's duct.

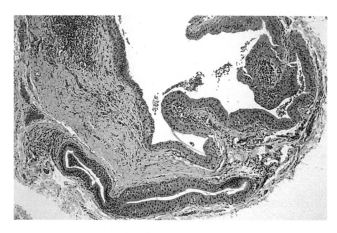

Fig. 11-12   Oncocytic salivary ductal ectasia. This dilated duct is lined by columnar eosinophilic oncocytes that exhibit papillary folds into the ductal lumen. Such lesions may develop secondary to ductal obstruction.

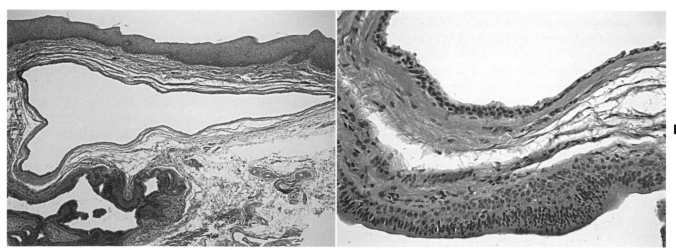

A   B

Fig. 11-11   Salivary duct cyst. A, Low-power photomicrograph showing a cyst below the mucosal surface. **B,** High-power view of cystic cavity (top) lined by thin cuboidal epithelium. Adjacent to the cyst is an excretory salivary gland duct lined by columnar epithelium (bottom).

however, surgical management does not appear feasible or advisable for all of the lesions, which may number as many as 100. In one reported case, systemic erythromycin and chlorhexidine mouth rinses were helpful in relieving pain and reducing drainage of pus. Sialagogue medications also may be helpful in stimulating salivary flow, thereby preventing the accumulation of inspissated mucus within the dilated excretory ducts.

SIALOLITHIASIS (SALIVARY CALCULI; SALIVARY STONES)

Sialoliths are calcified structures that develop within the salivary ductal system. Researchers believe that they arise from deposition of calcium salts around a nidus of debris within the duct lumen. This debris may include inspissated mucus, bacteria, ductal epithelial cells, or foreign bodies. The cause of sialoliths is unclear, but their formation can be promoted by chronic sialadenitis and partial obstruction. Their development is not related to any systemic derangement in calcium and phosphorus metabolism.

CLINICAL AND RADIOGRAPHIC FEATURES

Sialoliths most often develop within the ductal system of the submandibular gland; the formation of stones within the parotid gland system is distinctly less frequent. The long, tortuous, upward path of the submandibular (Wharton's) duct and the thicker, mucoid secretions of this gland may be responsible for its greater tendency to form salivary calculi. Sialoliths also can form within the minor salivary glands, most often within the glands of the upper lip or buccal mucosa. Salivary stones can occur at almost any age, but they are most common in young and middle-aged adults.

Major gland sialoliths most frequently cause episodic pain or swelling of the affected gland, especially at mealtime. The severity of the symptoms varies, depending on the degree of obstruction and the amount of resultant backpressure produced within the gland. If the stone is located toward the terminal portion of the duct, then a hard mass may be palpated beneath the mucosa (Fig. 11-13).

Sialoliths typically appear as radiopaque masses on radiographic examination. However, not all stones are visible on standard radiographs (perhaps because of the degree of calcification of some lesions). They may be discovered anywhere along the length of the duct or within the gland itself (Fig. 11-14). Stones in the terminal portion of the submandibular duct are best demonstrated with an occlusal radiograph. On panoramic or periapical radiographs, the calcification may appear superimposed on the mandible and care must

be exercised not to confuse it with an intrabony lesion (Fig. 11-15). Multiple parotid stones radiographically can mimic calcified parotid lymph nodes, such as might occur in tuberculosis. Sialography, ultrasound, and CT scanning may be helpful additional imaging studies for sialoliths.

Minor gland sialoliths often are asymptomatic but may produce local swelling or tenderness of the affected gland (Fig. 11-16). A small radiopacity often can be demonstrated with a soft tissue radiograph.

HISTOPATHOLOGIC FEATURES

On gross examination, sialoliths appear as hard masses that are round, oval, or cylindrical. They are typically yellow, although they may be a white or yellow-brown color. Submandibular stones tend to be larger than those of the parotid or minor glands. Sialoliths are usually solitary, although occasionally two or more stones may be discovered at surgery.

Microscopically, the calcified mass exhibits concentric laminations that may surround a nidus of

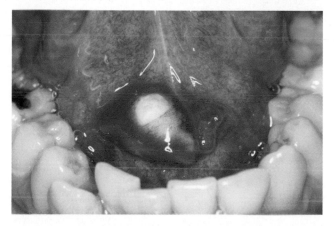

Fig. 11-13 **Sialolithiasis.** Hard mass at the orifice of Wharton's duct.

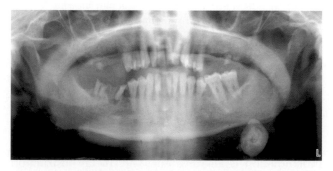

Fig. 11-14 **Sialolithiasis.** Radiopaque mass located at the left angle of the mandible. (*Courtesy of Dr. Roger Bryant.*)

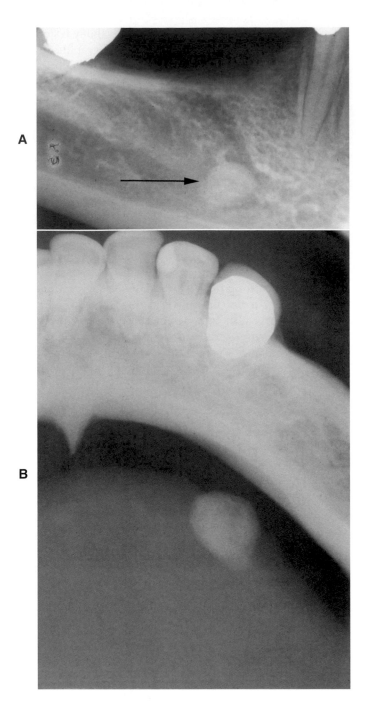

Fig. 11-15   Sialolithiasis. A, Periapical film showing discrete radiopacity (*arrow*) superimposed on the body of the mandible. Care must be taken not to confuse such lesions with intrabony pathosis. **B,** Occlusal radiograph of same patient demonstrating radiopaque stone in Wharton's duct.

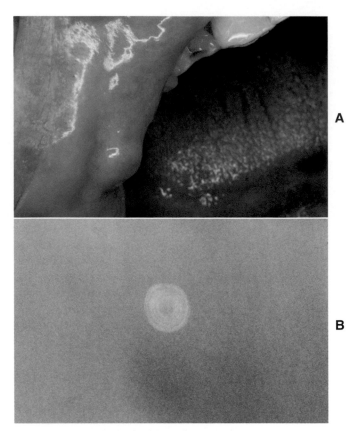

Fig. 11-16   Sialolithiasis. A, Minor salivary gland sialolith presenting as a hard nodule in the upper lip. **B,** A soft tissue radiograph of the same lesion revealed a laminated calcified mass.

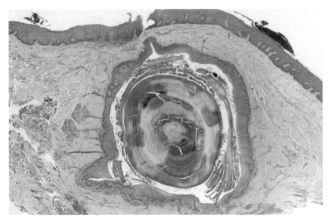

Fig. 11-17   Sialolithiasis. Intraductal calcified mass showing concentric laminations. The duct exhibits squamous metaplasia.

amorphous debris (Fig. 11-17). If the associated duct also is removed, then it often demonstrates squamous, oncocytic, or mucous cell metaplasia. Periductal inflammation is also evident. The ductal obstruction frequently is associated with an acute or chronic sial-adenitis of the feeding gland.

TREATMENT AND PROGNOSIS

Small sialoliths of the major glands sometimes can be treated conservatively by gentle massage of the gland in an effort to milk the stone toward the duct orifice. Sialagogues (drugs that stimulate salivary flow), moist heat, and increased fluid intake also may promote passage of the stone. Larger sialoliths usually need to be removed surgically. If significant inflammatory damage has occurred within the feeding gland, then the gland may need to be removed. Minor gland sialoliths are best treated by surgical removal, including the associated gland.

Shock wave lithotripsy (extracorporeal or intracorporeal), salivary gland endoscopy, and radiologically guided basket retrieval are newer techniques that have been shown to be effective in the removal of sialoliths from the major glands. These minimally invasive techniques have low morbidity and may preclude the necessity of gland removal.

SIALADENITIS

Inflammation of the salivary glands (**sialadenitis**) can arise from various infectious and noninfectious causes. The most common viral infection is mumps (see page 263), although a number of other viruses also can involve the salivary glands, including Coxsackie A, ECHO, choriomeningitis, parainfluenza, and cytomegalovirus (CMV) (in neonates). Most bacterial infections arise as a result of ductal obstruction or decreased salivary flow, allowing retrograde spread of bacteria throughout the ductal system. Blockage of the duct can be caused by sialolithiasis (see page 459), congenital strictures, or compression by an adjacent tumor. Decreased flow can result from dehydration, debilitation, or medications that inhibit secretions.

One of the more common causes of sialadenitis is recent surgery (especially abdominal surgery), after which an acute parotitis (*surgical mumps*) may arise because the patient has been kept without food or fluids (NPO) and has received atropine during the surgical procedure. Other medications that produce xerostomia as a side effect also can predispose patients to such an infection. Most cases of acute bacterial sialadenitis are caused by *Staphylococcus aureus*, but they also may arise from streptococci or other organisms. Noninfectious causes of salivary inflammation include Sjögren syndrome (see page 466), sarcoidosis (see page 338), radiation therapy (see page 295), and various allergens.

CLINICAL AND RADIOGRAPHIC FEATURES

Acute bacterial sialadenitis is most common in the parotid gland and is bilateral in 10% to 25% of cases. The affected gland is swollen and painful, and the overlying skin may be warm and erythematous (Fig. 11-18). An associated low-grade fever and trismus may be present. A purulent discharge often is observed from the duct orifice when the gland is massaged (Fig. 11-19).

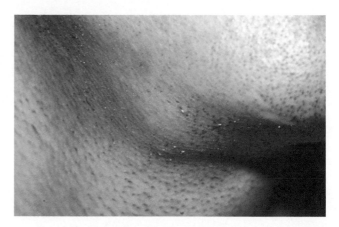

Fig. 11-18   Sialadenitis. Tender swelling of the submandibular gland.

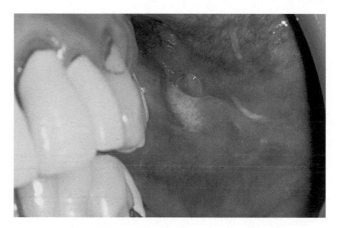

Fig. 11-19   Sialadenitis. A purulent exudate can be seen arising from Stensen's duct when the parotid gland is massaged.

Recurrent or persistent ductal obstruction (most commonly caused by sialoliths) can lead to a chronic sialadenitis. Periodic swelling and pain occur within the affected gland, usually developing at mealtime when salivary flow is stimulated. In the submandibular gland, persistent enlargement may develop (**Küttner tumor**), which is difficult to distinguish from a true neoplasm. Sialography often demonstrates sialectasia (ductal dilatation) proximal to the area of obstruction (Fig. 11-20). In chronic parotitis, Stensen's duct may show a characteristic sialographic pattern known as "sausaging," which reflects a combination of dilatation plus ductal strictures from scar formation. Chronic sialadenitis also can occur in the minor glands, possibly as a result of blockage of ductal flow or local trauma.

Subacute necrotizing sialadenitis is a form of salivary inflammation that occurs most commonly in teenagers and young adults. The lesion usually involves the minor salivary glands of the hard or soft palate,

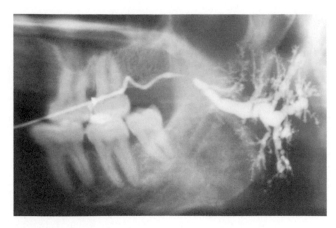

Fig. 11-20 Chronic sialadenitis. Parotid sialogram demonstrating ductal dilatation proximal to an area of obstruction. *(Courtesy of Dr. George Blozis.)*

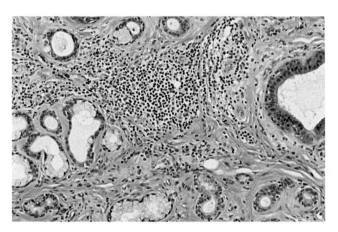

Fig. 11-21 Chronic sclerosing sialadenitis. Chronic inflammatory infiltrate with associated acinar atrophy, ductal dilatation, and fibrosis.

presenting as a painful nodule that is covered by intact, erythematous mucosa. Unlike necrotizing sialometaplasia (see page 471), the lesion does not ulcerate or slough necrotic tissue. An infectious or allergic cause has been hypothesized.

HISTOPATHOLOGIC FEATURES

In patients with acute sialadenitis, accumulation of neutrophils is observed within the ductal system and acini. Chronic sialadenitis is characterized by scattered or patchy infiltration of the salivary parenchyma by lymphocytes and plasma cells. Atrophy of the acini is common, as is ductal dilatation. If associated fibrosis is present, then the term **chronic sclerosing sialadenitis** is used (Fig. 11-21).

Subacute necrotizing sialadenitis is characterized by a heavy mixed inflammatory infiltrate consisting of neutrophils, lymphocytes, histiocytes, and eosinophils.

There is loss of most of the acinar cells, and many of the remaining ones exhibit necrosis. The ducts tend to be atrophic and do not show hyperplasia or squamous metaplasia.

TREATMENT AND PROGNOSIS

The treatment of acute sialadenitis includes appropriate antibiotic therapy and rehydration of the patient to stimulate salivary flow. Surgical drainage may be needed if there is abscess formation. Although this regimen is usually sufficient, a 20% to 50% mortality rate has been reported in debilitated patients because of the spread of the infection and sepsis.

The management of chronic sialadenitis depends on the severity of the condition and ranges from conservative therapy to surgical intervention. Initial management often includes antibiotics, analgesics, sialagogues, and glandular massage. Early cases that develop secondary to ductal blockage may respond to removal of the sialolith or other obstruction. However, if sialectasia is present, then the dilated ducts can lead to stasis of secretions and predispose the gland to further sialolith formation. Sialadenoscopy and ductal irrigation are newer techniques that can be used to dilate ductal strictures and to eliminate sialoliths and mucus plugs. Second-line treatment options for chronic parotitis have included ligation of Stensen's duct, but this method has a high failure rate. Tympanic neurectomy, which results in decreased secretion by the parotid gland via transection of the parasympathetic secretory fibers at the tympanic plexus, produces improvement in 75% of patients with chronic parotitis. If conservative methods cannot control chronic sialadenitis, then surgical removal of the affected gland may be necessary.

Subacute necrotizing sialadenitis is a self-limiting condition that usually resolves within 2 weeks of diagnosis without treatment.

CHEILITIS GLANDULARIS

Cheilitis glandularis is a rare inflammatory condition of the minor salivary glands. The cause is uncertain, although several etiologic factors have been suggested, including actinic damage, tobacco, syphilis, poor hygiene, and heredity.

CLINICAL FEATURES

Cheilitis glandularis characteristically occurs on the lower lip, although there are also purported cases involving the upper lip and palate. Affected individuals experience swelling and eversion of the lower lip as a result of hypertrophy and inflammation of the glands

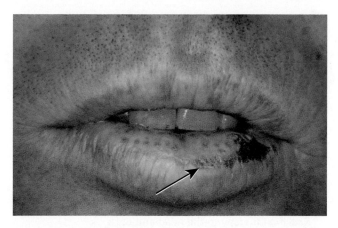

Fig. 11-22 **Cheilitis glandularis.** Prominent lower lip with inflamed openings of the minor salivary gland ducts. An early squamous cell carcinoma has developed on the patient's left side just lateral to the midline (***arrow***). *(Courtesy of Dr. George Blozis.)*

(Fig. 11-22). The openings of the minor salivary ducts are inflamed and dilated, and pressure on the glands may produce mucopurulent secretions from the ductal openings. The condition most often has been reported in middle-aged and older men, although cases also have been described in women and children. However, some of the childhood cases may represent other entities, such as exfoliative cheilitis (see page 304).

Historically, cheilitis glandularis has been classified into three types, based on the severity of the disease:
1. Simple
2. Superficial suppurative (Baelz's disease)
3. Deep suppurative (cheilitis glandularis apostematosa)

The latter two types represent progressive stages of the disease with bacterial involvement; they are characterized by increasing inflammation, suppuration, ulceration, and swelling of the lip.

HISTOPATHOLOGIC FEATURES

The microscopic findings of cheilitis glandularis are not specific and usually consist of chronic sialadenitis and ductal dilatation. Concomitant dysplastic changes may be observed in the overlying surface epithelium in some cases.

TREATMENT AND PROGNOSIS

The treatment of choice for most cases of persistent cheilitis glandularis associated with actinic damage is vermilionectomy (lip shave), which usually produces a satisfactory cosmetic result. A significant percentage of cases (18% to 35%) have been associated with the devel-

opment of squamous cell carcinoma of the overlying epithelium of the lip. Because actinic damage has been implicated in many cases of cheilitis glandularis, it is likely that this same solar radiation is responsible for the malignant degeneration.

SIALORRHEA

Sialorrhea, or excessive salivation, is an uncommon condition that has various causes. Minor sialorrhea may result from local irritations, such as aphthous ulcers or ill-fitting dentures. Patients with new dentures often experience excess saliva production until they become accustomed to the prosthesis. Episodic hypersecretion of saliva, or "water brash," may occur as a protective buffering system to neutralize stomach acid in individuals with gastroesophageal reflux disease. Sialorrhea is a well-known clinical feature of rabies and heavy-metal poisoning (see page 313). It also may occur as a consequence of certain medications, such as antipsychotic agents, especially clozapine, and cholinergic agonists used to treat dementia of the Alzheimer's type and myasthenia gravis.

Drooling can be a problem for patients who are mentally retarded, who have undergone surgical resection of the mandible, or who have various neurologic disorders such as cerebral palsy, Parkinson's disease, or amyotrophic lateral sclerosis (ALS). In these instances, the drooling is probably not caused by overproduction of saliva but by poor neuromuscular control.

In addition, there is a second group of patients who report complaints of drooling; however, no obvious clinical evidence of excessive saliva production is observed, and they do not have any of the recognized causes for sialorrhea. Personality analysis has suggested that the complaint of sialorrhea in such otherwise healthy patients does not have an organic basis but may be associated with high levels of neuroticism and a tendency to dissimulate.

CLINICAL FEATURES

The excess saliva production typically produces drooling and choking, which may cause social embarrassment. In children with mental retardation or cerebral palsy, the uncontrolled salivary flow may lead to macerated sores around the mouth, chin, and neck that can become secondarily infected. The constant soiling of clothes and bed linens can be a significant problem for the parents and caretakers of these patients.

An interesting type of supersalivation of unknown cause has been termed **idiopathic paroxysmal sialorrhea.** Individuals with this condition experience short episodes of excessive salivation lasting from 2 to 5 minutes. These episodes are associated with a prodrome of nausea or epigastric pain.

TREATMENT AND PROGNOSIS

Some causes of sialorrhea are transitory or mild, and no treatment is needed. For individuals with increased salivation associated with gastroesophageal reflux disease, medical management of their reflux problem may be beneficial.

For persistent severe drooling, therapeutic intervention may be indicated. Speech therapy can be used to improve neuromuscular control, but patient cooperation is necessary. Anticholinergic medications can decrease saliva production but may produce unacceptable side effects. Transdermal scopolamine has been tried with some success, but it should not be used in children younger than age 10. Intraglandular injection of botulinum toxin has been shown to be successful in reducing salivary secretions, with a duration of action that varies from 6 weeks to 6 months.

Several surgical techniques have been used successfully to control severe drooling in individuals with poor neuromuscular control:

- Relocation of the submandibular ducts (sometimes along with excision of the sublingual glands)
- Relocation of the parotid ducts
- Submandibular gland excision plus parotid duct ligation
- Ligation of the parotid and submandibular ducts
- Bilateral tympanic neurectomy with sectioning of the chorda tympani

In ductal relocation, the ducts are repositioned posteriorly to the tonsillar fossa, thereby redirecting salivary flow and minimizing drooling. The use of bilateral tympanic neurectomy and sectioning of the chorda tympani destroys parasympathetic innervation to the glands, reducing salivary secretions and possibly inducing xerostomia. However, this procedure also produces a loss of taste to the anterior two thirds of the tongue.

XEROSTOMIA

Xerostomia refers to a subjective sensation of a dry mouth; it is frequently, but not always, associated with salivary gland hypofunction. A number of factors may play a role in the cause of xerostomia, and these are listed in Box 11-1. Xerostomia is a common problem that has been reported in 25% of older adults. In the past, complaints of dry mouth in older patients often were ascribed to the predictable result of aging. However, it is now generally accepted that any reductions in salivary function associated with age are modest and probably are not associated with any significant

---

Box 11-1

Causes of Xerostomia

DEVELOPMENTAL ORIGIN
Salivary gland aplasia

WATER/METABOLITE LOSS
Impaired fluid intake
Hemorrhage
Vomiting/diarrhea

IATROGENIC ORIGIN
Medications
Radiation therapy to the head and neck
Chemotherapy

SYSTEMIC DISEASES
Sjögren syndrome
Diabetes mellitus
Diabetes insipidus
Sarcoidosis
Human immunodeficiency virus (HIV) infection
Hepatitis C infection
Graft-versus-host disease (GVHD)
Psychogenic disorders

LOCAL FACTORS
Decreased mastication
Smoking
Mouth breathing

---

reduction in salivary function. Instead, xerostomia in older adults is more likely to be the result of other factors, especially medications. More than 500 drugs have been reported to produce xerostomia as a side effect, including 63% of the 200 most frequently prescribed medicines in the United States. A list of the most common and significant drugs associated with xerostomia is provided in Table 11-2. Not only are specific drugs known to produce dry mouth, but the prevalence of xerostomia also increases in relation to the total number of drugs that a person takes, regardless of whether the individual medications are xerogenic or not.

CLINICAL FEATURES

Examination of the patient typically demonstrates a reduction in salivary secretions, and the residual saliva appears either foamy or thick and "ropey." The mucosa appears dry, and the clinician may notice that the examining gloves stick to the mucosal surfaces. The dorsal tongue often is fissured with atrophy of the filiform papillae (see Fig. 11-1). The patient may complain of difficulty with mastication and swallowing, and

Table **11-2**   **Medications That May Produce Xerostomia**

Class of Drug	Example
Antihistamine agents	Diphenhydramine
	Chlorpheniramine
Decongestant agents	Pseudoephedrine
Antidepressant agents	Amitriptyline
	Citalopram
	Fluoxetine
	Paroxetine
	Sertraline
	Bupropion
Antipsychotic agents	Phenothiazine derivatives
	Haloperidol
Sedatives and anxiolytic agents	Diazepam
	Lorazepam
	Alprazolam
Antihypertensive agents	Reserpine
	Methyldopa
	Chlorothiazide
	Furosemide
	Metoprolol
	Calcium channel blockers
Anticholinergic agents	Atropine
	Scopolamine

they may even indicate that food adheres to the oral membranes during eating. The clinical findings, however, do not always correspond to the patient's symptoms. Some patients who complain of dry mouth may appear to have adequate salivary flow and oral moistness. Conversely, some patients who clinically appear to have a dry mouth have no complaints. The degree of saliva production can be assessed by measuring both resting and stimulated salivary flow.

There is an increased prevalence of oral candidiasis in patients with xerostomia because of the reduction in the cleansing and antimicrobial activity normally provided by saliva. In addition, these patients are more prone to dental decay, especially cervical and root caries. This problem has been associated more often with radiation therapy, and it is sometimes called *radiation-induced caries* but more appropriately should be called *xerostomia-related caries* (see page 296).

TREATMENT AND PROGNOSIS

The treatment of xerostomia is difficult and often unsatisfactory. Artificial salivas are available and may help make the patient more comfortable, as may continuous sips of water throughout the day. In addition, sugarless candy can be used in an effort to stimulate salivary flow. One of the better patient-accepted man-

agement approaches includes the use of oral hygiene products that contain lactoperoxidase, lysozyme, and lactoferrin (e.g., Biotene toothpaste and mouth rinse, Oralbalance gel). If the dryness is secondary to the patient's medication, then discontinuation or dose modification in consultation with the patient's physician may be considered; a substitute drug can also be tried.

Systemic pilocarpine is a parasympathomimetic agonist that can be used as a sialagogue. At doses of 5 to 10 mg, three to four times daily, it can be an effective promoter of salivary secretion. Excess sweating is a common side effect, but more serious problems, such as increased heart rate and blood pressure, are uncommon. The U.S. Food and Drug Administration (FDA) has also approved cevimeline hydrochloride, an acetylcholine derivative, for use as a sialagogue. Both pilocarpine and cevimeline are contraindicated in patients with narrow-angle glaucoma.

Because of the increased potential for dental caries in patients with xerostomia, frequent dental visits are recommended. Office and daily home fluoride applications can be used to help prevent decay, and chlorhexidine mouth rinses minimize plaque buildup.

BENIGN LYMPHOEPITHELIAL LESION (MYOEPITHELIAL SIALADENITIS)

In the late 1800s, Johann von Mikulicz-Radecki described the case of a patient with an unusual bilateral painless swelling of the lacrimal glands and all of the salivary glands. Histopathologic examination of the involved glands showed an intense lymphocytic infiltrate, with features that today are recognized microscopically as the **benign lymphoepithelial lesion**. This clinical presentation became known as **Mikulicz disease**, and clinicians began using this term to describe a variety of cases of bilateral parotid and lacrimal enlargement. However, many of these cases were not examples of benign lymphoepithelial lesions microscopically; instead, they represented salivary and lacrimal involvement by other disease processes, such as tuberculosis, sarcoidosis, and lymphoma. These cases of parotid and lacrimal enlargement secondary to other diseases were later recognized as being different and termed **Mikulicz syndrome**, with the term **Mikulicz disease** reserved for cases associated with benign lymphoepithelial lesions. However, these two terms have become so confusing and ambiguous that they should no longer be used.

Many cases of so-called Mikulicz disease may be examples of what is now more commonly known as **Sjögren syndrome** (see page 466). Sjögren syndrome is an autoimmune disease that may produce bilateral salivary and lacrimal enlargement, with microscopic

Box 11-2

Revised International Classification Criteria for Sjögren Syndrome

I. Ocular symptoms: A positive response to at least one of the following questions:
  A. Have you had daily, persistent, troublesome dry eyes for more than 3 months?
  B. Do you have a recurrent sensation of sand or gravel in the eyes?
  C. Do you use tear substitutes more than three times a day?

II. Oral symptoms: A positive response to at least one of the following questions:
  A. Have you had a daily feeling of dry mouth for more than 3 months?
  B. Have you had recurrently or persistently swollen salivary glands as an adult?
  C. Do you frequently drink liquids to aid in swallowing dry food?

III. Ocular signs: Objective evidence of ocular involvement defined as a positive result for at least one of the following two tests:
  A. Schirmer I test, performed without anesthesia (≤5 mm in 5 minutes)
  B. Rose bengal score or other ocular dye score (≥4 according to van Bijsterveld's scoring system)

IV. Histopathology: In minor salivary glands (obtained through normal-appearing mucosa) focal lymphocytic sialadenitis, evaluated by an expert histopathologist, with a focus score ≥1, defined as a number of lymphocytic foci (which are adjacent to normal-appearing mucous acini and contain more than 50 lymphocytes) per 4 mm^2 of glandular tissue

V. Salivary gland involvement: Objective evidence of salivary gland involvement defined by a positive result for at least one of the following diagnostic tests:
  A. Unstimulated whole salivary flow (≤1.5 ml in 15 minutes)
  B. Parotid sialography showing the presence of diffuse sialectasias (punctate, cavitary, or destructive pattern), without evidence of obstruction in the major ducts
  C. Salivary scintigraphy showing delayed uptake, reduced concentration, and/or delayed excretion of tracer

VI. Autoantibodies: Presence in the serum of the following autoantibodies:
  A. Antibodies to Ro(SS-A) or La(SS-B) antigens, or both

RULES FOR CLASSIFICATION

Primary Sjögren Syndrome

In patients without any potentially associated disease, primary Sjögren syndrome is defined as follows:

I. Presence of any four of the six items is indicative of primary Sjögren syndrome, as long as either item IV (histopathology) or VI (serology) is positive

II. Presence of any three of the four objective criteria items (items III, IV, V, and VI)

Secondary Sjögren Syndrome

In patients with a potentially associated disease (e.g., another well-defined connective tissue disease), presence of item I or item II plus any two from among items III, IV, and V considered indicative of secondary Sjögren syndrome

Exclusion Criteria

Past head and neck radiation treatment
Hepatitis C infection
Acquired immunodeficiency syndrome (AIDS)
Preexisting lymphoma
Sarcoidosis
Graft-versus-host disease (GVHD)
Use of anticholinergic drugs

and may be intermittent or persistent in nature. The greater the severity of the disease, the greater the likelihood of this salivary enlargement. In addition, the reduced salivary flow places these individuals at increased risk for retrograde bacterial sialadenitis.

Although it is not diagnostic, sialographic examination often reveals punctate sialectasia and lack of normal arborization of the ductal system, typically demonstrating a "fruit-laden, branchless tree" pattern (Fig. 11-26). Scintigraphy with radioactive technetium-99m pertechnetate characteristically shows decreased uptake and delayed emptying of the isotope.

The term **keratoconjunctivitis sicca** describes not only the reduced tear production by the lacrimal glands but also the pathologic effect on the epithelial cells of the ocular surface. As in xerostomia, the severity of xerophthalmia can vary widely from one patient to the next. The lacrimal inflammation causes a decrease of the aqueous layer of the tear film; however, mucin production is normal and may result in a mucoid discharge. Patients often complain of a scratchy, gritty sensation or the perceived presence of a foreign body in the eye. Defects of the ocular surface epithelium develop and can be demonstrated with rose bengal dye. Vision may become blurred, and sometimes there is an aching pain. The ocular manifestations are least severe in the morning on wakening and become more pronounced as the day progresses.

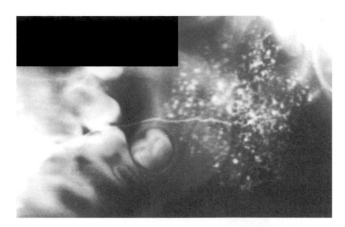

Fig. 11-26 **Sjögren syndrome.** Parotid sialogram demonstrating atrophy and punctate sialectasia ("fruit-laden, branchless tree"). *(Courtesy of Dr. George Blozis.)*

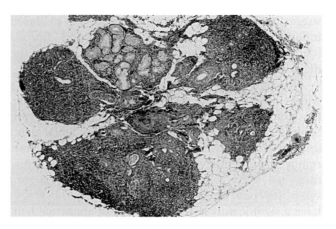

Fig. 11-27 **Sjögren syndrome.** Labial gland biopsy showing multiple lymphocytic foci.

A simple means to confirm the decreased tear secretion is the Schirmer test. A standardized strip of sterile filter paper is placed over the margin of the lower eyelid, between the medial and lateral third of the lid of the unanesthetized eye, so that the tabbed end rests just inside the lower lid. By measuring the length of wetting of the filter paper, tear production can be assessed. Values less than 5 mm (after a 5-minute period) are considered diagnostic of keratoconjunctivitis sicca.

Sjögren syndrome is a systemic disease, and the inflammatory process also can affect various other body tissues. The skin is often dry, as are the nasal and vaginal mucosae. Fatigue is fairly common, and depression sometimes can occur. Other possible associated problems include lymphadenopathy, primary biliary cirrhosis, Raynaud's phenomenon, interstitial nephritis, interstitial lung fibrosis, vasculitis, and peripheral neuropathies.

LABORATORY VALUES

In patients with Sjögren syndrome, the erythrocyte sedimentation rate is high and serum immunoglobulin (Ig) levels, especially IgG, typically are elevated. A variety of autoantibodies can be produced, and although none of these is specifically diagnostic, their presence can be another helpful clue to the diagnosis. A positive rheumatoid factor (RF) is found in approximately 60% of cases, regardless of whether the patient has rheumatoid arthritis. Antinuclear antibodies (ANAs) are also present in 75% to 85% of patients. Two particular nuclear autoantibodies—anti-SS-A (anti-Ro) and anti-SS-B (anti-La)—may be found, especially in patients with primary Sjögren syndrome. Anti-SS-A antibodies have been detected in approximately 40% of patients, whereas anti-SS-B antibodies have been discovered in

about 25% of these individuals. Occasionally, salivary duct autoantibodies also can be demonstrated, usually in secondary Sjögren syndrome. However, because these are infrequent in primary cases, they are believed to occur as a secondary phenomenon (rather than playing a primary role in pathogenesis).

HISTOPATHOLOGIC FEATURES

The basic microscopic finding in Sjögren syndrome is a lymphocytic infiltration of the salivary glands, with destruction of the acinar units. If the major glands are enlarged, then microscopic examination usually shows progression to a lymphoepithelial lesion (see page 466), with characteristic epimyoepithelial islands in a background lymphoid stroma. Lymphocytic infiltration of the minor glands also occurs, although epimyoepithelial islands are rarely seen in this location.

Biopsy of the minor salivary glands of the lower lip has become a useful test in the diagnosis of Sjögren syndrome. A 1.5- to 2.0-cm incision is made on clinically normal lower labial mucosa, parallel to the vermilion border and lateral to the midline, allowing the harvest of five or more accessory glands. These glands then are examined histopathologically for the presence of focal chronic inflammatory aggregates (50 or more lymphocytes and plasma cells). These aggregates should be adjacent to normal-appearing acini and should be found consistently in most of the glands in the specimen. The finding of more than one focus of 50 or more cells within a 4-mm^2 area of glandular tissue is considered supportive of the diagnosis of Sjögren syndrome (Fig. 11-27). The greater the number of foci (up to 10 or confluent foci) is, the greater is the correlation with this diagnosis. The focal nature of this chronic inflammation among otherwise normal acini is a highly

Table **11-3**   **Sites of Occurrence of Primary Epithelial Salivary Gland Tumors**

Author (Year)	Number of Cases	SITE OF OCCURRENCE			
		Parotid	Submandibular	Sublingual	Minor
Eveson and Cawson (1985)	2,410	73%	11%	0.3%	14%
Seifert et al. (1986)	2,579	80%	10%	1.0%	9%
Spiro (1986)	2,807	70%	8%	(Included with minor gland tumors)	22%
Ellis et al. (1991)	13,749	64%	10%	0.3%	23%

Table **11-4**   **Frequency of Malignancy for Salivary Tumors at Different Sites**

Author (Year)	Number of Cases	PERCENTAGE OF CASES THAT ARE MALIGNANT			
		Parotid	Submandibular	Sublingual	Minor
Eveson and Cawson (1985)	2,410	15%	37%	86%	46%
Seifert et al. (1986)	2,579	20%	45%	90%	45%
Spiro (1986)	2,807	25%	43%	(Included with minor gland tumors)	82%
Ellis et al. (1991)	13,749	32%	41%	70%	49%

Table **11-5**   **Parotid Tumors**

	Ellis et al. (United States, 1991)	Eveson & Cawson (Great Britain, 1985)	Thackray & Lucas (Great Britain, 1974)	Eneroth (Sweden, 1971)	Foote & Frazell (United States, 1953)
Total number of cases	8222	1756	651	2158	764
BENIGN TUMORS					
Pleomorphic adenoma	53.0%	63.3%	72.0%	76.8%	58.5%
Warthin tumor	7.7%	14.0%	9.0%	4.7%	6.5%
Oncocytoma	1.9%	0.9%	0.6%	1.0%	0.1%
Basal cell adenoma	1.4%	–	–	–	–
Other benign tumors	3.7%	7.1%*	1.8%	–	0.7%
TOTAL	**67.7%**	**85.3%**	**83.4%**	**82.5%**	**65.8%**
MALIGNANT TUMORS					
Mucoepidermoid carcinoma	9.6%	1.5%	2.3%	4.1%	11.8%
Acinic cell adenocarcinoma	8.6%	2.5%	1.2%	3.1%	2.7%
Adenoid cystic carcinoma	2.0%	2.0%	3.3%	2.3%	2.1%
Malignant mixed tumor	2.5%	3.2%	4.1%	1.5%	6.0%
Squamous cell carcinoma	2.1%	1.1%	1.0%	0.3%	3.4%
Other malignant tumors	7.5%	4.4%	4.7%	6.3%	8.1%
TOTAL	**32.3%**	**14.7%**	**16.6%**	**17.5%**	**34.2%**

*Includes all "other monomorphic adenomas."

Table **11-6**   **Submandibular Tumors**

	Ellis et al. (United States, 1991)	Eveson & Cawson (Great Britain, 1985)	Thackray & Lucas (Great Britain, 1974)	Eneroth (Sweden, 1971)	Foote & Frazell (United States, 1953)
Total number of cases	1235	257	60	170	107
BENIGN TUMORS					
Pleomorphic adenoma	53.3%	59.5%	68.0%	60.0%	43.9%
Warthin tumor	1.3%	0.8%	1.7%	2.4%	0.0%
Oncocytoma	1.5%	0.4%	0.0%	0.6%	0.0%
Basal cell adenoma	1.0%	–	–	–	–
Other benign tumors	1.7%	1.9%*	0.0%	–	0.0%
TOTAL	**58.8%**	**62.6%**	**69.7%**	**62.9%**	**43.9%**
MALIGNANT TUMORS					
Mucoepidermoid carcinoma	9.1%	1.6%	0.0%	3.5%	7.5%
Acinic cell adenocarcinoma	2.7%	0.4%	0.0%	0.6%	0.0%
Adenoid cystic carcinoma	11.7%	16.8%	17.0%	15.3%	15.9%
Malignant mixed tumor	3.5%	7.8%	1.7%	1.8%	10.3%
Squamous cell carcinoma	3.4%	1.9%	3.3%	7.1%	12.1%
Other malignant tumors	10.8%	8.9%	8.3%	8.8%	10.3%
TOTAL	**41.2%**	**37.4%**	**30.3%**	**37.1%**	**56.1%**

*Includes all "other monomorphic adenomas."

overwhelmingly the most common tumor (53% to 77% of all cases the parotid gland). Warthin tumors are also fairly common; they account for 6% to 14% of cases. A variety of malignant tumors occur, with the mucoepidermoid carcinoma appearing to be the most frequent overall. However, two studies from Great Britain show a significantly lower prevalence of this tumor, possibly indicative of a geographic difference, especially compared with reports of cases from the United States.

From 8% to 11% of all salivary tumors occur in the submandibular gland, but the frequency of malignancy in this gland is almost double that of the parotid gland, ranging from 37% to 45%. However, as shown in Table 11-6, the pleomorphic adenoma is still the most common tumor and makes up 44% to 68% of all neoplasms. Unlike its occurrence in the parotid gland, the Warthin tumor is unusual in the submandibular gland, making up no more than 1% to 2% of all tumors. Adenoid cystic carcinoma is the most common malignancy, ranging from 12% to 27% of all cases.

Tumors of the sublingual gland are rare, comprising no more than 1% of all salivary neoplasms. However, 70% to 90% of sublingual tumors are malignant.

Tumors of the various smaller minor salivary glands make up 9% to 23% of all tumors, which makes this group the second most common site for salivary neoplasia. Table 11-7 summarizes the findings of five large surveys of minor gland tumors. Unfortunately, a rela-

tively high proportion (almost 50%) of these have been malignant in most studies. Excluding rare sublingual tumors, it can be stated that the smaller the gland is, the greater is the likelihood of malignancy for a salivary gland tumor.

As observed in the major glands, the pleomorphic adenoma is the most common minor gland tumor and accounts for about 40% of all cases. Mucoepidermoid carcinoma and adenoid cystic carcinoma generally have been considered the two most common malignancies, although polymorphous low-grade adenocarcinoma also is becoming recognized as one of the more common minor gland tumors.

The palate is the most frequent site for minor salivary gland tumors, with 42% to 54% of all cases found there (Table 11-8). Most of these occur on the posterior lateral hard or soft palate, which have the greatest concentration of glands. Table 11-9 shows the relative prevalence of various tumors on the palate. The lips are the second most common location for minor gland tumors (21% to 25% of cases), followed by the buccal mucosa (11% to 15% of cases). Labial tumors are significantly more common in the upper lip, which accounts for 77% to 89% of all lip tumors (Table 11-10). Although mucoceles are commonly found on the lower lip, this is a surprisingly rare site for salivary gland tumors.

Significant differences in the percentage of malignancies and the relative frequency of various tumors

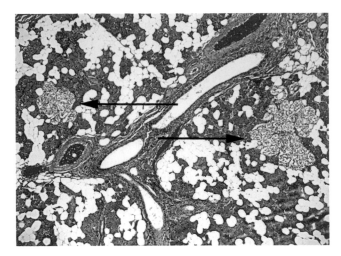

Fig. 11-44   Oncocytosis. Multifocal collections of clear oncocytes *(arrows)* in the parotid gland.

abundant granular, eosinophilic cytoplasm as a result of the proliferation of mitochondria. On occasion, these cells may have a clear cytoplasm from the accumulation of glycogen (Fig. 11-44). The multifocal nature of the proliferation may be confused with that of a metastatic tumor, especially when the oncocytes are clear in appearance.

TREATMENT AND PROGNOSIS

Oncocytosis is a benign condition and often is discovered only as an incidental finding. No further treatment is necessary, and the prognosis is excellent.

WARTHIN TUMOR (PAPILLARY CYSTADENOMA LYMPHOMATOSUM)

Warthin tumor is a benign neoplasm that occurs almost exclusively in the parotid gland. Although it is much less common than the pleomorphic adenoma, it represents the second most common benign parotid tumor, accounting for 5% to 14% of all parotid neoplasms. The name **adenolymphoma** also has been used for this tumor, but this term should be avoided because it overemphasizes the lymphoid component and may give the mistaken impression that the lesion is a type of lymphoma. Analyses of the epithelial and lymphoid components of the Warthin tumor have shown both to be polyclonal; this suggests that this lesion may not represent a true neoplasm but would be better classified as a tumorlike process.

The pathogenesis of these tumors is uncertain. The traditional hypothesis suggests that they arise from heterotopic salivary gland tissue found within parotid lymph nodes. However, researchers have also suggested that these tumors may develop from a prolifera-

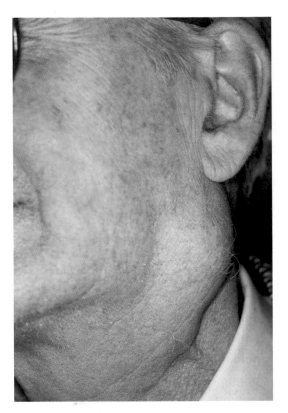

Fig. 11-45   Warthin tumor. Mass in the tail of the parotid **gland.** *(Courtesy of Dr. George Blozis.)*

tion of salivary gland ductal epithelium that is associated with secondary formation of lymphoid tissue. This latter theory is supported by studies that have found cytogenetic abnormalities in the epithelial component. A number of studies have demonstrated a strong association between the development of this tumor and smoking. Smokers have an eightfold greater risk for Warthin tumor than do nonsmokers.

CLINICAL FEATURES

The Warthin tumor usually appears as a slowly growing, painless, nodular mass of the parotid gland (Fig. 11-45). It may be firm or fluctuant to palpation. The tumor most frequently occurs in the tail of the parotid near the angle of the mandible, and it may be noted for many months before the patient seeks a diagnosis. One unique feature is the tendency of Warthin tumor to occur bilaterally, which has been noted in 5% to 17% of reported cases. Most of these bilateral tumors do not occur simultaneously but are metachronous (occurring at different times).

In rare instances, the Warthin tumor has been reported within the submandibular gland or minor salivary glands. However, because the lymphoid component is often less pronounced in these extraparotid sites, the pathologist should exercise caution to avoid

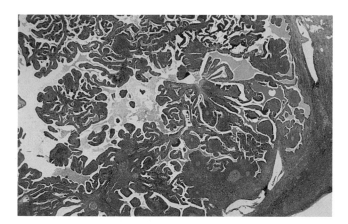

Fig. 11-46   Warthin tumor. Low-power view showing a papillary cystic tumor with a lymphoid stroma.

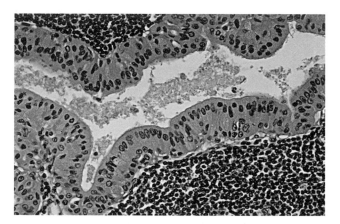

Fig. 11-47   Warthin tumor. High-power view of epithelial lining showing double row of oncocytes with adjacent lymphoid stroma.

overdiagnosis of a lesion better classified as a papillary cystadenoma or a salivary duct cyst with oncocytic ductal metaplasia.

Warthin tumor most often occurs in older adults, with a peak prevalence in the sixth and seventh decades of life. The observed frequency of this tumor is much lower in blacks than in whites. Most studies show a decided male predilection, with some early studies demonstrating a male-to-female ratio up to 10:1. However, more recent investigations show a more balanced sex ratio. Because Warthin tumors have been associated with cigarette smoking, this changing sex ratio may be a reflection of the increased prevalence of smoking in women over the past few decades. This association with smoking also may help explain the frequent bilaterality of the tumor, because any tumorigenic effects of smoking might be manifested in both parotids.

HISTOPATHOLOGIC FEATURES

The Warthin tumor has one of the most distinctive histopathologic patterns of any tumor in the body. Although the term **papillary cystadenoma lymphomatosum** is cumbersome, it accurately describes the salient microscopic features.

The tumor is composed of a mixture of ductal epithelium and a lymphoid stroma (Figs. 11-46 and 11-47). The epithelium is oncocytic in nature, forming uniform rows of cells surrounding cystic spaces. The cells have abundant, finely granular eosinophilic cytoplasm and are arranged in two layers. The inner luminal layer consists of tall columnar cells with centrally placed, palisaded, and slightly hyperchromatic nuclei. Beneath this is a second layer of cuboidal or polygonal cells with more vesicular nuclei. The lining epithelium demonstrates multiple papillary infoldings that pro-

trude into the cystic spaces. Focal areas of squamous metaplasia or mucous cell prosoplasia may be seen. The epithelium is supported by a lymphoid stroma that frequently shows germinal center formation.

TREATMENT AND PROGNOSIS

Surgical removal is the treatment of choice for patients with Warthin tumor. The procedure usually is easily accomplished because of the superficial location of the tumor. Some surgeons prefer local resection with minimal surrounding tissue; others opt for superficial parotidectomy to avoid violating the tumor capsule and because a tentative diagnosis may not be known preoperatively. A 6% to 12% recurrence rate has been reported. Many authors, however, believe that the tumor is frequently multicentric in nature; therefore, it is difficult to determine whether these are true recurrences or secondary tumor sites. Malignant Warthin tumors (**carcinoma ex papillary cystadenoma lymphomatosum**) have been reported but are exceedingly rare.

MONOMORPHIC ADENOMA

The term **monomorphic adenoma** originally was used to describe a group of benign salivary gland tumors demonstrating a more uniform histopathologic pattern than the common pleomorphic adenoma. In some classification schemes, a variety of tumors were included under the broad heading of monomorphic adenoma, including Warthin tumor, oncocytoma, basal cell adenoma, and canalicular adenoma. Other authors have used this term more specifically as a synonym just for the basal cell adenoma or canalicular adenoma. Because of its ambiguous nature, the term *monomorphic adenoma* probably should be avoided, and each of the

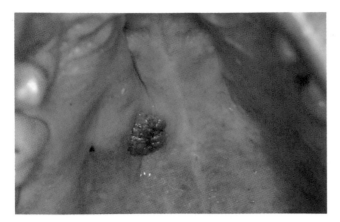

Fig. 11-51 Sialadenoma papilliferum. Exophytic papillary mass on the palate. *(Courtesy of Dr. Peter Lyu.)*

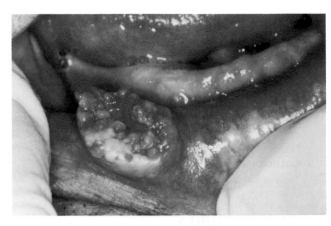

Fig. 11-52 Inverted ductal papilloma. Exophytic mass with central papillary projections on the lower labial mucosa. *(Courtesy of Dr. Amy Bogardus.)*

enoma lymphomatosum). The **sialadenoma papilliferum**, **intraductal papilloma**, and **inverted ductal papilloma** are three rare salivary tumors that also show unique papillomatous features.

It also should be mentioned that, on occasion, the common squamous papilloma (see page 362) of the oral mucosa will arise at the site where a minor salivary gland duct merges with the surface epithelium. Because of this location, such squamous papillomas also contain scattered mucous cells within the exophytic papillary growth, and these lesions have sometimes been called *ductal papillomas*. However, it should be emphasized that these lesions are viral (human papillomavirus [HPV]) surface papillomas and not primary salivary gland tumors.

CLINICAL FEATURES

The sialadenoma papilliferum most commonly arises from the minor salivary glands, especially on the palate, although it also has been reported in the parotid gland. It usually is seen in older adults and has a 1.5:1.0 male-to-female ratio. The tumor appears as an exophytic, papillary surface growth that is clinically similar to the common squamous papilloma (Fig. 11-51).

The intraductal papilloma is an ill-defined lesion that often has been confused with other salivary gland lesions, such as the papillary cystadenoma. It usually occurs in adults and is most common in the minor salivary glands, where it appears as a submucosal swelling.

The inverted ductal papilloma is a rare tumor that has been described only in the minor salivary glands of adults. The lower lip and mandibular vestibule are the most common locations. The lesion usually appears as an asymptomatic nodule, which sometimes

may show a pit or indentation in the overlying surface mucosa (Fig. 11-52).

HISTOPATHOLOGIC FEATURES

At low-power magnification, the sialadenoma papilliferum is somewhat similar to the squamous papilloma, exhibiting multiple exophytic papillary projections that are covered by stratified squamous epithelium. This epithelium is contiguous with a proliferation of papillomatous ductal epithelium found below the surface and extending downward into the deeper connective tissues (Fig. 11-53). Multiple ductal lumina are formed, which characteristically are lined by a double-rowed layer of cells consisting of a luminal layer of tall columnar cells and a basilar layer of smaller cuboidal cells. These ductal cells often have an oncocytic appearance. An inflammatory infiltrate of plasma cells, lymphocytes, and neutrophils is characteristically present. Because of their microscopic similarity, this tumor has been considered to be an analogue of the cutaneous syringocystadenoma papilliferum.

The intraductal papilloma exhibits a dilated, unicystic structure that is located below the mucosal surface. It is lined by a single or double row of cuboidal or columnar epithelium, which has multiple arborizing papillary projections into the cystic lumen. In contrast, the inverted ductal papilloma is composed primarily of a proliferation of squamoid epithelium with multiple thick, bulbous papillary projections that fill the ductal lumen (Fig. 11-54). This epithelium may be contiguous with the overlying mucosal epithelium, communicating with the surface through a small porelike opening. Although the tumor is primarily squamous in nature, the luminal lining cells of the papillary projections are often cuboidal or columnar in shape, with scattered mucus-producing cells.

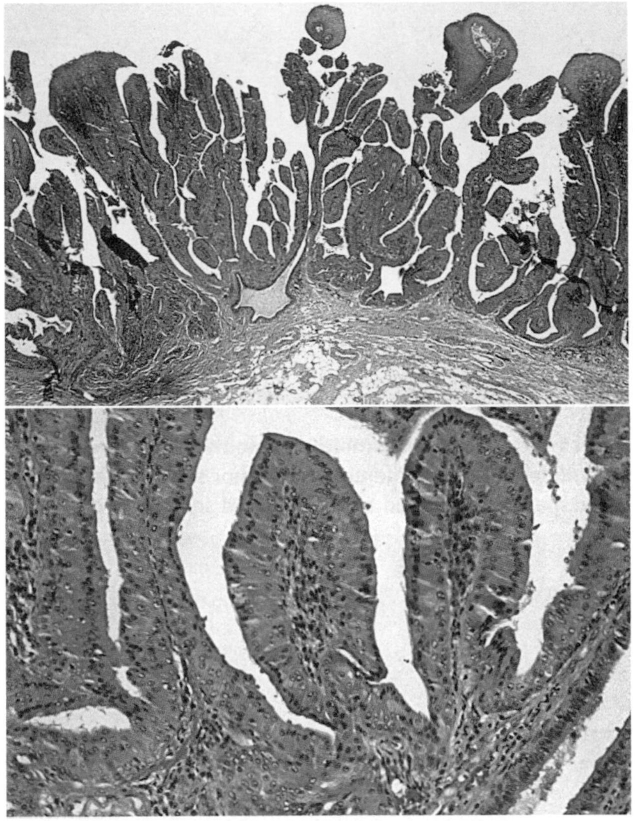

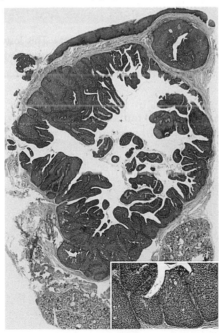

Fig. 11-53 Sialadenoma papilliferum. A, Low-power view showing a papillary surface tumor with associated ductal structures in the superficial lamina propria. **B,** High-power view of cystic areas lined by papillary, oncocytic epithelium.

Fig. 11-54 Inverted ductal papilla. Papillary intraductal proliferation located beneath the mucosal surface. Higher-power view shows both squamous cells and mucous cells *(inset). (Courtesy of Dr. Dean K. White.)*

TREATMENT AND PROGNOSIS

All three forms of ductal papilloma are best treated by conservative surgical excision. Recurrence is rare.

MUCOEPIDERMOID CARCINOMA

The **mucoepidermoid carcinoma** is one of the most common salivary gland malignancies. Because of its highly variable biologic potential, it was originally called **mucoepidermoid tumor.** The term recognized one subset that acted in a malignant fashion and a second group that appeared to behave in a benign fashion with favorable prognosis. However, researchers later recognized that even low-grade tumors occasionally could exhibit malignant behavior; therefore, the term *mucoepidermoid carcinoma* is the preferred designation.

CLINICAL FEATURES

Most studies show that the mucoepidermoid carcinoma is the most common malignant salivary gland neoplasm. In the United States, it makes up 10% of all major gland tumors and 15% to 23% of minor gland tumors. However, British studies have shown a much lower relative frequency, with mucoepidermoid carcinoma accounting for only 1% to 2% of major gland neoplasms and 9% of minor gland tumors. Perhaps a true geographic difference exists in the prevalence of this lesion.

The tumor occurs fairly evenly over a wide age range, extending from the second to seventh decades of life. Rarely is it seen in the first decade of life. However, mucoepidermoid carcinoma is the most common malignant salivary gland tumor in children. Some tumors have been associated with a previous history of radiation therapy to the head and neck region.

The mucoepidermoid carcinoma is most common in the parotid gland and usually appears as an asymptomatic swelling. Most patients are aware of the lesion for 1 year or less, although some report a mass of many years' duration. Pain or facial nerve palsy may develop, usually in association with high-grade tumors. The minor glands constitute the second most common site, especially the palate (Fig. 11-55). Minor gland tumors also typically appear as asymptomatic swellings, which are sometimes fluctuant and have a blue or red color that can be mistaken clinically for a mucocele. Although the lower lip, floor of mouth, tongue, and retromolar pad areas are uncommon locations for salivary gland neoplasia, the mucoepidermoid carcinoma is the most common salivary tumor in each of these sites (Fig. 11-56). Intraosseous tumors also may develop in the jaws (see page 490).

Fig. 11-65   Acinic cell adenocarcinoma. Parotid tumor demonstrating sheet of granular, basophilic serous acinar cells.

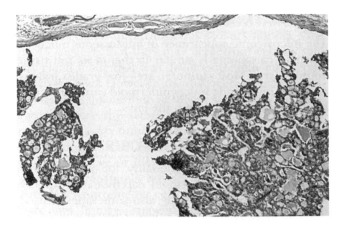

Fig. 11-67   Acinic cell adenocarcinoma. Papillary-cystic variant showing proliferation of tumor cells into a large cystic space.

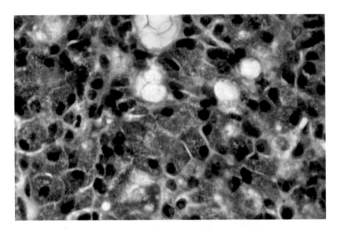

Fig. 11-66   Acinic cell adenocarcinoma. High-power view of serous cells with basophilic, granular cytoplasm.

similar to that of thyroid tissue. A lymphoid infiltrate, sometimes with germinal center formation, is not unusual.

TREATMENT AND PROGNOSIS

Acinic cell adenocarcinomas confined to the superficial lobe of the parotid gland are best treated by lobectomy; for those in the deep lobe, total parotidectomy is usually necessary. The facial nerve may need to be sacrificed if it is involved by tumor. Submandibular tumors are managed by total removal of the gland, and minor gland tumors are treated with assured surgical excision. Lymph node dissection is not indicated unless there is clinical evidence of metastatic disease. Adjunctive radiation therapy may be considered for uncontrolled local disease.

The acinic cell adenocarcinoma is associated with one of the better prognoses of any of the malignant salivary gland tumors. Approximately one third of patients have recurrences locally, and metastases develop in 10% to 15% of patients. From 6% to 26% of patients die of their disease. The prognosis for minor gland tumors is better than that for tumors arising in the major glands.

encapsulated; however, some tumors exhibit an infiltrative growth pattern. The most characteristic cell is one with features of the serous acinar cell, with abundant granular basophilic cytoplasm and a round, darkly stained eccentric nucleus. These cells are fairly uniform in appearance, and mitotic activity is uncommon. Other cells may resemble intercalated duct cells, and some tumors also have cells with a clear, vacuolated cytoplasm.

Several growth patterns may be seen. The **solid** variety consists of numerous well-differentiated acinar cells arranged in a pattern that resembles normal parotid gland tissue (Figs. 11-65 and 11-66). In the **microcystic** variety, multiple small cystic spaces are created that may contain some mucinous or eosinophilic material. In the **papillary-cystic** variety, larger cystic areas are formed that are lined by epithelium having papillary projections into the cystic spaces (Fig. 11-67). The **follicular** variety has an appearance

MALIGNANT MIXED TUMORS (CARCINOMA EX PLEOMORPHIC ADENOMA; CARCINOMA EX MIXED TUMOR; CARCINOSARCOMA; METASTASIZING MIXED TUMOR)

Malignant mixed tumors represent malignant counterparts to the benign mixed tumor or pleomorphic adenoma. These uncommon neoplasms constitute 2% to 6% of all salivary tumors and can be divided into three categories:

1. Carcinoma ex pleomorphic adenoma (carcinoma ex mixed tumor)
2. Carcinosarcoma
3. Metastasizing mixed tumor

The most common of these is the **carcinoma ex pleomorphic adenoma,** which is characterized by malignant transformation of the epithelial component of a previously benign pleomorphic adenoma. The **carcinosarcoma** is a rare "mixed" tumor in which both carcinomatous and sarcomatous elements are present. The **metastasizing mixed tumor** has histopathologic features that are identical to the common pleomorphic adenoma (mixed tumor). In spite of its benign appearance, however, the lesion metastasizes. The metastatic tumor also has a benign microscopic appearance, usually similar to that of the primary lesion.

CLINICAL FEATURES

CARCINOMA EX PLEOMORPHIC ADENOMA

There is fairly convincing evidence that the carcinoma ex pleomorphic adenoma represents a malignant transformation within what was previously a benign neoplasm. First of all, the mean age of patients with this tumor is about 15 years older than that for the benign pleomorphic adenoma. It is most common in middle-aged and older adults, with a peak prevalence in the sixth to eighth decades of life. In addition, patients may report that a mass has been present for many years, sometimes undergoing a recent rapid growth with associated pain or ulceration. However, some tumors may have a short duration. The histopathologic features, which are discussed later, also support malignant transformation of a benign pleomorphic adenoma. It has been noted that the risk for malignant change in a pleomorphic adenoma increases with the duration of the tumor.

More than 80% of cases of carcinoma ex pleomorphic adenoma are seen within the major glands, primarily the parotid gland (Fig. 11-68). Nearly two thirds of minor salivary gland cases occur on the palate (Fig. 11-69). Although pain or recent rapid growth is not unusual, many cases present as a painless mass that is indistinguishable from a benign tumor. Parotid tumors may produce facial nerve palsy.

CARCINOSARCOMA

The carcinosarcoma is an extremely rare tumor. Most cases have been reported in the parotid gland, but the lesion also has been seen in the submandibular gland and minor salivary glands. The clinical signs and symptoms are similar to those of the carcinoma ex pleomorphic adenoma. Some patients have a previous history of a benign pleomorphic adenoma, although other cases appear to arise *de novo.*

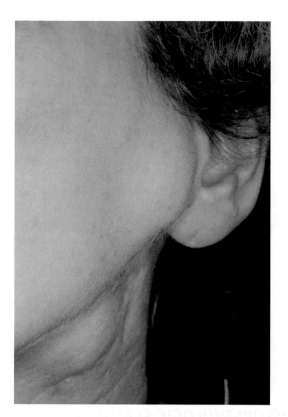

Fig. 11-68   Carcinoma ex pleomorphic adenoma. Mass of the parotid gland.

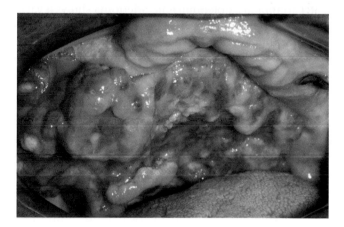

Fig. 11-69   Carcinoma ex pleomorphic adenoma. Granular exophytic and ulcerated mass filling the vault of the palate.

METASTASIZING MIXED TUMOR

The metastasizing mixed tumor is also quite rare. As with other malignant mixed tumors, most cases originate in the parotid gland, but the primary tumor also may occur in the submandibular gland or minor salivary glands. Metastases have been found most frequently in the bones or lung, but they also can occur in other sites, such as regional lymph nodes, skin, or the liver. Most patients have a history of a benign mixed

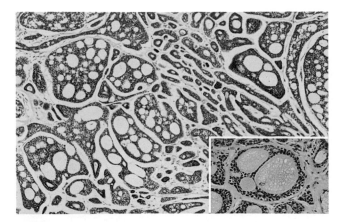

Fig. 11-73 Adenoid cystic carcinoma. Islands of hyperchromatic cells forming cribriform and tubular structures. *Inset* shows a high-power view of a small cribriform island.

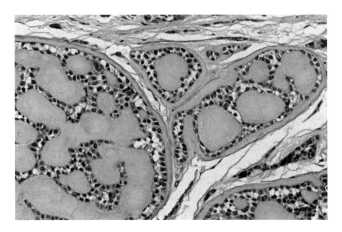

Fig. 11-74 Adenoid cystic carcinoma. The tumor cells are surrounded by hyalinized material.

are recognized: (1) cribriform, (2) tubular, and (3) solid. Usually a combination of these is seen, and the tumor is classified based on the predominant pattern.

The **cribriform pattern** is the most classic and best-recognized appearance, characterized by islands of basaloid epithelial cells that contain multiple cylindrical, cystlike spaces resembling Swiss cheese. These spaces often contain a mildly basophilic mucoid material, a hyalinized eosinophilic product, or a combined mucoid-hyalinized appearance. Sometimes the hyalinized material also surrounds these cribriform islands (Fig. 11-74), or small strands of tumor are found embedded within this hyalinized "stroma." The tumor cells are small and cuboidal, exhibiting deeply basophilic nuclei and little cytoplasm. These cells are fairly uniform in appearance, and mitotic activity is rarely seen. The pathologist should be mindful that other salivary tumors, especially polymorphous low-grade

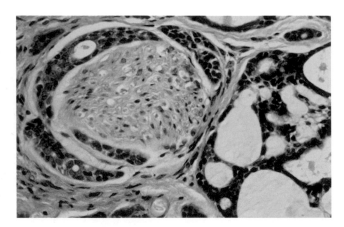

Fig. 11-75 Adenoid cystic carcinoma. Perineural invasion.

adenocarcinoma, also may exhibit areas with a cribriform pattern.

In the **tubular pattern,** the tumor cells are similar but occur as multiple small ducts or tubules within a hyalinized stroma. The tubular lumina can be lined by one to several layers of cells, and sometimes both a layer of ductal cells and myoepithelial cells can be discerned.

The **solid variant** consists of larger islands or sheets of tumor cells that demonstrate little tendency toward duct or cyst formation. Unlike the cribriform and tubular patterns, cellular pleomorphism and mitotic activity, as well as focal necrosis in the center of the tumor islands, may be observed.

A highly characteristic feature of adenoid cystic carcinoma is its tendency to show perineural invasion (Fig. 11-75), which probably corresponds to the common clinical finding of pain in these patients. Sometimes the cells appear to have a swirling arrangement around nerve bundles. However, perineural invasion is not pathognomonic for adenoid cystic carcinoma; it also may be seen in other salivary malignancies, especially polymorphous low-grade adenocarcinomas.

Positive immunostaining reactions for CD43 and c-kit (CD117) in adenoid cystic carcinoma have been reported to be useful diagnostic features that can help to distinguish this tumor from polymorphous low-grade adenocarcinoma, basal cell adenoma, and canalicular adenoma. In addition, the patterns of expression of a variety of other immunohistochemical markers have been suggested to be diagnostically relevant, including stains for vimentin, collagen IV, laminin, integrins, Ki-67, smooth muscle actin, and various cytokeratins.

TREATMENT AND PROGNOSIS

Adenoid cystic carcinoma is a relentless tumor that is prone to local recurrence and eventual distant metastasis. Surgical excision is usually the treatment of choice, and adjunct radiation therapy may slightly improve patient survival in some cases. Because metastasis to regional lymph nodes is uncommon, neck dissection typically is not indicated. Because of the poor overall prognosis, regardless of treatment, clinicians should be cautioned against needlessly aggressive and mutilating surgical procedures for large tumors or cases already showing metastases.

Because the tumor is prone to late recurrence and metastasis, the 5-year survival rate has little significance and does not equate to a cure. The 5-year survival rate may be as high as 70%, but this rate continues to decrease over time. The 10-year survival is approximately 50%, and by 20 years, only 25% of patients are still alive. Tumors with a solid histopathologic pattern are associated with a worse outlook than those with a cribriform or tubular arrangement. With respect to site, the prognosis is poorest for tumors arising in the maxillary sinus and submandibular gland. Most studies have shown that microscopic identification of perineural invasion has little effect on the prognosis. Tumor DNA ploidy analysis may help to predict the prognosis of adenoid cystic carcinoma; patients with diploid tumors have been shown to have a significantly better outcome than patients with aneuploid tumors.

Death usually results from local recurrence or distant metastases. Tumors of the palate or maxillary sinus eventually may invade upward to the base of the brain. Metastases occur in approximately 35% of patients, most frequently involving the lungs and bones.

POLYMORPHOUS LOW-GRADE ADENOCARCINOMA (LOBULAR CARCINOMA; TERMINAL DUCT CARCINOMA)

The **polymorphous low-grade adenocarcinoma** is a more recently recognized type of salivary malignancy that was first described in 1983. Before its identification as a distinct entity, examples of this tumor were categorized as pleomorphic adenoma, an unspecified form of adenocarcinoma, or sometimes as adenoid cystic carcinoma. Once recognized as a specific entity, however, it was realized that this tumor possesses distinct clinicopathologic features and is one of the more common minor salivary gland malignancies.

CLINICAL FEATURES

The polymorphous low-grade adenocarcinoma is almost exclusively a tumor of the minor salivary glands. However, rare examples also have been reported in the major glands, either arising *de novo* or as the malignant component of a carcinoma ex pleomorphic adenoma.

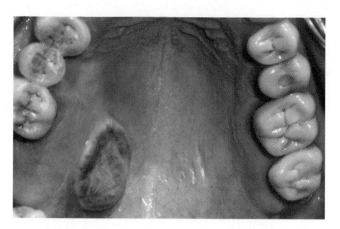

Fig. 11-76   Polymorphous low-grade adenocarcinoma. Ulcerated mass of the posterior lateral hard palate.

Sixty-five percent occur on the hard or soft palate (Fig. 11-76), with the upper lip and buccal mucosa being the next most common locations. It is most common in older adults, having a peak prevalence in the sixth to eighth decades of life. Two thirds of all cases occur in females.

The tumor most often appears as a painless mass that may have been present for a long time with slow growth. Occasionally, it is associated with bleeding or discomfort. Tumor can erode or infiltrate the underlying bone.

HISTOPATHOLOGIC FEATURES

The tumor cells of polymorphous low-grade adenocarcinomas have a deceptively uniform appearance. They are round to polygonal in shape, with indistinct cell borders and pale to eosinophilic cytoplasm. The nuclei may be round, ovoid, or spindled; these nuclei usually are pale staining, although they can be more basophilic in some areas. The cells can exhibit different growth patterns, hence, the *polymorphous* term. The cells may grow in a solid pattern or form cords, ducts, or larger cystic spaces. In some tumors, a cribriform pattern can be produced that mimics adenoid cystic carcinoma (Fig. 11-77). Mitotic figures are uncommon.

At low power, the tumor sometimes appears well circumscribed. However, the peripheral cells are usually infiltrative, invading the adjacent tissue in a single-file fashion (Fig. 11-78). Extension into underlying bone or skeletal muscle may be observed. The stroma is often mucoid in nature, or it may demonstrate hyalinization. Perineural invasion is common—another feature that may cause the tumor to be mistaken for adenoid cystic carcinoma (Fig. 11-79). However, a distinction between these two tumors is important because of their vastly different prognoses.

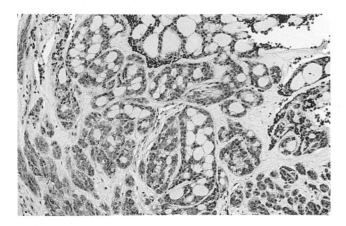

Fig. 11-77 Polymorphous low-grade adenocarcinoma.
This medium-power view shows a cribriform arrangement of
uniform tumor cells with pale-staining nuclei.

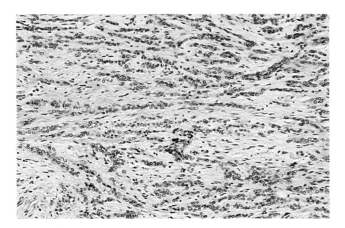

Fig. 11-78 Polymorphous low-grade adenocarcinoma.
Pale-staining cells that infiltrate as single-file cords.

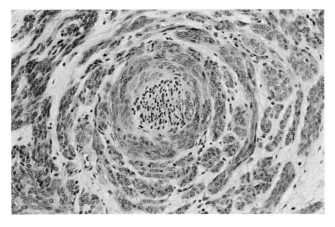

Fig. 11-79 Polymorphous low-grade adenocarcinoma.
Perineural invasion.

Immunohistochemical staining can be helpful in
distinguishing polymorphous low-grade adenocarcinoma from other salivary gland tumors that it may
mimic. When compared with adenoid cystic carcinoma, polymorphous low-grade adenocarcinoma
exhibits significantly weaker expression of CD43 and
c-kit (CD117). Likewise, lack of staining for glial fibrillary acidic protein (GFAP) can help to differentiate this
tumor from pleomorphic adenoma, which is almost
always strongly positive for GFAP.

TREATMENT AND PROGNOSIS

The polymorphous low-grade adenocarcinoma is best
treated by wide surgical excision, sometimes including
resection of the underlying bone. Metastasis to regional
lymph nodes is relatively uncommon, occurring in
just under 10% of patients. Therefore, neck dissection
seems unwarranted unless there is clinical evidence of
cervical metastases. Distant metastasis is rare.

The overall prognosis is relatively good. Recurrent
disease has been reported in 9% to 17% of all patients,
but this usually can be controlled with reexcision.
Death from tumor is rare but may occur secondary to
direct extension into vital structures. Microscopic identification of perineural invasion does not appear to
affect the prognosis.

SALIVARY ADENOCARCINOMA, NOT OTHERWISE SPECIFIED

In spite of the wide variety of salivary gland malignancies that have been specifically identified and categorized, some tumors still defy the existing classification
schemes. These tumors usually are designated as
salivary adenocarcinomas, not otherwise specified
(NOS).

CLINICAL AND HISTOPATHOLOGIC FEATURES

Because these adenocarcinomas represent such a
diverse group of neoplasms, it is difficult to generalize
about their clinical and microscopic features. Like most
salivary tumors, they appear to be most common in the
parotid gland, followed by the minor glands and the
submandibular gland (Figs. 11-80 and 11-81). They
may present as asymptomatic masses or cause pain or
facial nerve paralysis. The microscopic appearance is
highly variable but demonstrates features of a glandular malignancy with evidence of cellular pleomorphism, an infiltrative growth pattern, or both. These
tumors exhibit a wide spectrum of differentiation,
ranging from well-differentiated, low-grade neoplasms
to poorly differentiated, high-grade malignancies.

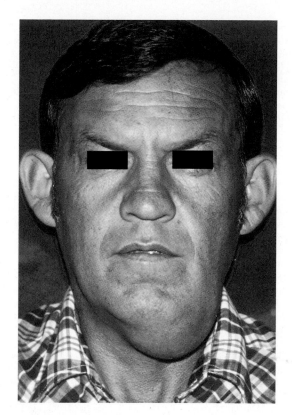

Fig. 11-80   Salivary adenocarcinoma. "Clear cell" adenocarcinoma of the submandibular gland.

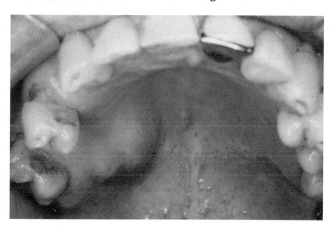

Fig. 11-81   Salivary adenocarcinoma. Mass of the posterior lateral hard palate.

As these tumors are studied more, it should be possible to classify some of them into separate, specific categories and allow more definitive analyses of their clinical and microscopic features.

TREATMENT AND PROGNOSIS

Because of their diversity, it is difficult to predict the prognosis for salivary adenocarcinoma (NOS), but patients with early-stage, well-differentiated tumors appear to have a better outcome. The survival rate is

better for tumors of the oral cavity than for those in the major salivary glands. The reported 10-year survival rate for parotid tumors ranges from 26% to 55%; in contrast, one study reported a 10-year survival rate of 76% for intraoral tumors.

BIBLIOGRAPHY

Salivary Gland Aplasia
Antoniades DZ, Markopoulos AK, Deligianni E et al: Bilateral aplasia of parotid glands correlated with accessory parotid tissue, *J Laryngol Otol* 120:327-329, 2006.

Mandel L: An unusual pattern of dental damage with salivary gland aplasia, *J Am Dent Assoc* 137:984-989, 2006.

Matsuda C, Matsui Y, Ohno K et al: Salivary gland aplasia with cleft lip and palate. A case report and review of the literature, *Oral Surg Oral Med Oral Pathol Oral Radiol Endod* 87:594-599, 1999.

Milunsky JM, Zhao G, Maher TA et al: LADD syndrome is caused by FGF10 mutations, *Clin Genet* 69:349-354, 2006.

Ramirez D, Lammer EJ: Lacrimoauriculodentodigital syndrome with cleft lip/palate and renal manifestations, *Cleft Palate Craniofac J* 41:501-506, 2004.

Mucocele
Baurmash HD: Mucoceles and ranulas, *J Oral Maxillofac Surg* 61:369-378, 2003.

Campana F, Sibaud V, Chauvel A et al: Recurrent superficial mucoceles associated with lichenoid disorders, *J Oral Maxillofac Surg* 64:1830-1833, 2006.

Cataldo E, Mosadomi A: Mucoceles of the oral mucous membrane, *Arch Otolaryngol* 91:360-365, 1970.

Chi A, Lambert P, Richardson M et al: *Oral mucoceles: a clinicopathologic review of 1,824 cases including unusual variants,* Abstract No. 19. Paper presented at the annual meeting of the American Academy of Oral and Maxillofacial Pathology, Kansas City, Mo, 2007.

Eveson JW: Superficial mucoceles: pitfall in clinical and microscopic diagnosis, *Oral Surg Oral Med Oral Pathol* 66:318-322, 1988.

Jensen JL: Superficial mucoceles of the oral mucosa, *Am J Dermatopathol* 12:88-92, 1990.

Jinbu Y, Kusama M, Itoh H et al: Mucocele of the glands of Blandin-Nuhn: clinical and histopathologic analysis of 26 cases, *Oral Surg Oral Med Oral Pathol Oral Radiol Endod* 95:467-470, 2003.

Jinbu Y, Tsukinoki K, Kusama M et al: Recurrent multiple superficial mucocele on the palate: histopathology and laser vaporization, *Oral Surg Oral Med Oral Pathol Oral Radiol Endod* 95:193-197, 2003.

Standish SM, Shafer WG: The mucous retention phenomenon, *J Oral Surg* 17:15-22, 1959.

Sugerman PB, Savage NW, Young WG: Mucocele of the anterior lingual salivary glands (glands of Blandin and Nuhn): report of 5 cases, *Oral Surg Oral Med Oral Pathol Oral Radiol Endod* 90:478-482, 2000.

Ranula
Anastassov GE, Haiavy J, Solodnik P et al: Submandibular gland mucocele: diagnosis and management, *Oral Surg Oral Med Oral Pathol Oral Radiol Endod* 89:159-163, 2000.

Baurmash HD: A case against sublingual gland removal as primary treatment of ranulas, *J Oral Maxillofac Surg* 65:117-121, 2007.

Baurmash HD: Mucoceles and ranulas, *J Oral Maxillofac Surg* 61:369-378, 2003.

Davison MJ, Morton RP, McIvor NP: Plunging ranula: clinical observations, *Head Neck* 20:63-68, 1998.

Galloway RH, Gross PD, Thompson SH et al: Pathogenesis and treatment of ranula: report of three cases, *J Oral Maxillofac Surg* 47:299-302, 1989.

Mahadevan M, Vasan N: Management of pediatric plunging ranula, *Int J Pediatr Otorhinolaryngol* 70:1049-1054, 2006.

Kurabayashi T, Ida M, Yasumoto M et al: MRI of ranulas, *Neuroradiology* 42:917-922, 2000.

Yoshimura Y, Obara S, Kondoh T et al: A comparison of three methods used for treatment of ranula, *J Oral Maxillofac Surg* 53:280-282, 1995.

Zhao Y-F, Jia Y, Chen X-M et al: Clinical review of 580 ranulas, *Oral Surg Oral Med Oral Pathol Oral Radiol Endod* 98:281-287, 2004.

Salivary Duct Cyst

Eversole LR: Oral sialocysts, *Arch Otolaryngol* 113:51-56, 1987.

Takeda Y, Yamamoto H: Salivary duct cyst: its frequency in a certain Japanese population group (Tohoku districts), with special reference to adenomatous proliferation of the epithelial lining, *J Oral Sci* 43:9-13, 2001.

Tal H, Altini M, Lemmer J: Multiple mucous retention cysts of the oral mucosa, *Oral Surg Oral Med Oral Pathol* 58:692-695, 1984.

Sialolithiasis

Arzoz E, Santiago A, Esnal F et al: Endoscopic intracorporeal lithotripsy for sialolithiasis, *J Oral Maxillofac Surg* 54:847-850, 1996.

Baurmash HD: Submandibular salivary stones: current management modalities, *J Oral Maxillofac Surg* 62:369-378, 2004.

Capaccio P, Ottaviani F, Manzo R et al: Extracorporeal lithotripsy for salivary calculi: a long-term clinical experience, *Laryngoscope* 114:1069-1073, 2004.

Jensen JL, Howell FV, Rick GM et al: Minor salivary gland calculi: a clinicopathologic study of forty-seven new cases, *Oral Surg Oral Med Oral Pathol* 47:44-50, 1979.

McGurk M, Escudier MP, Brown JE: Modern management of salivary calculi, *Br J Surg* 92:107-112, 2005.

Nahlieli O, Baruchin AM: Sialoendoscopy: three years' experience as a diagnostic and treatment modality, *J Oral Maxillofac Surg* 55:912-918, 1997.

Nahlieli O, Eliav E, Hasson O et al: Pediatric sialolithiasis, *Oral Surg Oral Med Oral Pathol Oral Radiol Endod* 90:709-712, 2000.

Ottaviani F, Capaccio P, Rivolta R et al: Salivary gland stones: US evaluation in shock wave lithotripsy, *Radiology* 204:437-441, 1997.

Williams MF: Sialolithiasis, *Otolaryngol Clin North Am* 32:819-834, 1999.

Zenk J, Bozzato A, Winter M et al: Extracorporeal shock wave lithotripsy of submandibular stones: evaluation after 10 years, *Ann Otol Rhinol Laryngol* 113:378-383, 2004.

Ziegler CM, Steveling H, Seubert M et al: Endoscopy: a minimally invasive procedure for diagnosis and treatment of diseases of the salivary glands—six years of practical experience, *Br J Oral Maxillofac Surg* 42:1-7, 2004.

Sialadenitis

Fattahi TT, Lyu PE, Van Sickels JE: Management of acute suppurative parotitis, *J Oral Maxillofac Surg* 60:446-448, 2002.

Fowler CB, Brannon RB: Subacute necrotizing sialadenitis: report of 7 cases and a review of the literature, *Oral Surg Oral Med Oral Pathol Oral Radiol Endod* 89:600-609, 2000.

Mandel L, Surattanont F: Bilateral parotid swelling: a review, *Oral Surg Oral Med Oral Pathol Oral Radiol Endod* 93:221-237, 2002.

McQuone SJ: Acute viral and bacterial infections of the salivary glands, *Otolaryngol Clin North Am* 32:793-811, 1999.

Motamed M, Laugharne D, Bradley PJ: Management of chronic parotitis: a review, *J Laryngol Otol* 117:521-526, 2003.

Nahlieli O, Bar T, Shacham R et al: Management of chronic recurrent parotitis: current therapy, *J Oral Maxillofac Surg* 62:1150-1155, 2004.

Seifert G: Aetiological and histological classification of sialadenitis, *Pathologica* 89:7-17, 1997.

Suresh L, Aguirre A: Subacute necrotizing sialadenitis: a clinicopathological study, *Oral Surg Oral Med Oral Pathol Oral Radiol Endod* 104:385-390, 2007.

Vasama J-P: Tympanic neurectomy and chronic parotitis, *Acta Otolaryngol* 120:995-998, 2000.

Werning JT, Waterhouse JP, Mooney JW: Subacute necrotizing sialadenitis, *Oral Surg Oral Med Oral Pathol* 70:756-759, 1990.

Williams HK, Connor R, Edmondson H: Chronic sclerosing sialadenitis of the submandibular and parotid glands: a report of a case and review of the literature, *Oral Surg Oral Med Oral Pathol Oral Radiol Endod* 89:720-723, 2000.

Cheilitis Glandularis

Carrington PR, Horn TD: Cheilitis glandularis: a clinical marker for both malignancy and/or severe inflammatory disease of the oral cavity, *J Am Acad Dermatol* 54:336-337, 2006.

Cohen DM, Green JG, Dickmann SL: Concurrent anomalies: cheilitis glandularis and double lip: report of a case, *Oral Surg Oral Med Oral Pathol* 66:397-399, 1988.

Doku HC, Shklar G, McCarthy PL: Cheilitis glandularis, *Oral Surg Oral Med Oral Pathol* 20:563-571, 1965.

Oliver ID, Pickett AB: Cheilitis glandularis, *Oral Surg Oral Med Oral Pathol* 49:526-529, 1980.

Stoopler ET, Carrasco L, Stanton DC et al: Cheilitis glandularis: an unusual histopathologic presentation, *Oral Surg Oral Med Oral Pathol Oral Radiol Endod* 95:312-317, 2003.

Swerlick RA, Cooper PH: Cheilitis glandularis: a re-evaluation, *J Am Acad Dermatol* 10:466-472, 1984.

Sialorrhea

Banerjee KJ, Glasson C, O'Flaherty SJ: Parotid and submandibular botulinum toxin A injections for sialorrhoea in children with cerebral palsy, *Dev Med Child Neurol* 48:883-887, 2006.

Contarino MF, Pompili M, Tittoto P et al: Botulinum toxin B ultrasound-guided injections for sialorrhea in amyotrophic lateral sclerosis and Parkinson's disease, *Parkinsonism Relat Disord* 13:299-303, 2007.

Ethunandan M, Macpherson DW: Persistent drooling: treatment by bilateral submandibular duct transposition and simultaneous sublingual gland excision, *Ann R Coll Surg Engl* 80:279-282, 1998.

Freudenreich O: Drug-induced sialorrhea, *Drugs Today* 41:411-418, 2005.

Lamey P-J, Clifford TJ, El-Karim IA et al: Personality analysis of patients complaining of sialorrhoea, *J Oral Pathol Med* 35:307-310, 2006.

Lieblich S: Episodic supersalivation (idiopathic paroxysmal sialorrhea): description of a new clinical syndrome, *Oral Surg Oral Med Oral Pathol* 68:159-161, 1989.

Mandel L, Tamari K: Sialorrhea and gastroesophageal reflux, *J Am Dent Assoc* 126:1537-1541, 1995.

Meningaud J-P, Pitak-Arnnop P, Chikhani L et al: Drooling of saliva: a review of the etiology and management options, *Oral*

Surg Oral Med Oral Pathol Oral Radiol Endod 101:48-57, 2006.

O'Dwyer TP, Conlon BJ: The surgical management of drooling–a 15 year follow-up, *Clin Otolaryngol* 22:284-287, 1997.

Shirley WP, Hill JS, Woolley AL et al: Success and complications of four-duct ligation for sialorrhea, *Int J Pediatr Otorhinolaryngol* 67:1-6, 2003.

Talmi YP, Finkelstein Y, Zohar Y: Reduction of salivary flow with transdermal scopolamine: a four-year experience, *Otolaryngol Head Neck Surg* 103:615-618, 1990.

Xerostomia

Cassolato SF, Turnbull RS: Xerostomia: clinical aspects and treatment, *Gerodontology* 20:64-77, 2003.

Epstein JB, Emerton S, Le ND et al: A double-blind crossover trial of Oral Balance gel and Biotene toothpaste versus placebo in patients with xerostomia following radiation therapy, *Oral Oncol* 35:132-137, 1999.

Fox PC: Salivary enhancement therapies, *Caries Res* 38:241-246, 2004.

Jensen SB, Pedersen AM, Reibel J et al: Xerostomia and hypofunction of the salivary glands in cancer therapy, *Support Care Cancer* 11:207-225, 2003.

Johnson JT, Ferretti GA, Nethery WJ et al: Oral pilocarpine for post-irradiation xerostomia in patients with head and neck cancer, *N Engl J Med* 329:390-395, 1993.

Kirstilä V, Lenander-Lumikari M, Söderling E et al: Effects of oral hygiene products containing lactoperoxidase, lysozyme, and lactoferrin on the composition of whole saliva and on subjective oral symptoms in patients with xerostomia, *Acta Odontol Scand* 54:391-397, 1996.

Närhi, TO, Meurman JH, Ainamo A: Xerostomia and hyposalivation. Causes, consequences and treatment in the elderly, *Drugs Aging* 15:103-116, 1999.

Nieuw Amerongen AV, Veerman ECI: Current therapies for xerostomia and salivary gland hypofunction associated with cancer therapies, *Support Care Cancer* 11:226-231, 2003.

Porter SR, Scully C, Hegarty AM: An update of the etiology and management of xerostomia, *Oral Surg Oral Med Oral Pathol Oral Radiol Endod* 97:28-46, 2004.

Scully C: Drug effects on salivary glands: dry mouth, *Oral Dis* 9:165-176, 2003.

Sreebny LM, Schwartz SS: A reference guide to drugs and dry mouth–2nd edition, *Gerodontology* 14:33-47, 1997.

Warde P, Kroll B, O'Sullivan B et al: A phase II study of Biotene in the treatment of postradiation xerostomia in patients with head and neck cancer, *Support Care Cancer* 8:203-208, 2000.

Benign Lymphoepithelial Lesion

Bridges AJ, England DM: Benign lymphoepithelial lesion: relationship to Sjögren's syndrome and evolving malignant lymphoma, *Semin Arthritis Rheum* 19:201-208, 1989.

Chaudhry AP, Cutler LS, Yamane GM et al: Light and ultrastructural features of lymphoepithelial lesions of the salivary glands in Mikulicz's disease, *J Pathol* 146:239-250, 1986.

DiGiuseppe JA, Corio RL, Westra WH: Lymphoid infiltrates of the salivary glands: pathology, biology, and clinical significance, *Curr Opin Oncol* 8:232-237, 1996.

Herbst H, Niedobitek G: Sporadic EBV-associated lymphoepithelial salivary gland carcinoma with EBV-positive low-grade myoepithelial component, *Virchows Arch* 448:648-654, 2006.

Penfold CN: Mikulicz syndrome, *J Oral Maxillofac Surg* 43:900-905, 1985.

Quintana PG, Kapadia SB, Bahler DW et al: Salivary gland lymphoid infiltrates associated with lymphoepithelial lesions: a clinicopathologic, immunophenotypic, and genotypic study, *Hum Pathol* 28:850-861, 1997.

Sato K, Kawana M, Sato Y et al: Malignant lymphoma in the head and neck associated with benign lymphoepithelial lesion of the parotid gland, *Auris Nasus Larynx* 29:209-214, 2002.

Saw D, Lau WH, Ho JHC et al: Malignant lymphoepithelial lesion of the salivary gland, *Hum Pathol* 17:914-923, 1986.

Wu DL, Shemen L, Brady T et al: Malignant lymphoepithelial lesion of the parotid gland: a case report and review of the literature, *Ear Nose Throat J* 80:803-806, 2001.

Sjögren Syndrome

Al-Hashimi I: Xerostomia secondary to Sjögren's syndrome in the elderly, *Drugs Aging* 22:887-899, 2005.

Biasi D, Caramaschi P, Ambrosetti A et al: Mucosa-associated lymphoid tissue lymphoma of the salivary glands occurring in patients affected by Sjögren's syndrome: report of 6 cases, *Acta Haematol* 105:83-88, 2001.

Daniels TE: Labial salivary gland biopsy in Sjögren's syndrome: assessment as a diagnostic criterion in 362 suspected cases, *Arthritis Rheum* 27:147-156, 1984.

Daniels TE, Fox PC: Salivary and oral components of Sjögren's syndrome, *Rheum Dis Clin North Am* 18:571-589, 1992.

Delaleu N, Jonsson R, Koller MM: Sjögren's syndrome, *Eur J Oral Sci* 113:101-113, 2005.

Fox RI: Sjögren's syndrome, *Lancet* 366:321-331, 2005.

Fox RI, Törnwall J, Maruyama T et al: Evolving concepts of diagnosis, pathogenesis, and therapy of Sjögren's syndrome, *Curr Opin Rheumatol* 10:446-456, 1998.

Friedlaender MH: Ocular manifestations of Sjögren's syndrome: keratoconjunctivitis sicca, *Rheum Dis Clin North Am* 18:591-608, 1992.

García-Carrasco M, Ramos-Casals M, Rosas J et al: Primary Sjögren syndrome: clinical and immunologic disease patterns in a cohort of 400 patients, *Medicine* 81:270-280, 2002.

Jonsson R, Moen K, Vestrheim D et al: Current issues in Sjögren's syndrome, *Oral Dis* 8:130-140, 2002.

Jordan R, Diss TC, Lench NJ et al: Immunoglobulin gene rearrangements in lymphoplasmacytic infiltrates of labial salivary glands in Sjögren's syndrome. A possible predictor of lymphoma development, *Oral Surg Oral Med Oral Pathol Oral Radiol Endod* 79:723-729, 1995.

Jordan RCK, Speight PM: Lymphoma in Sjögren's syndrome. From histopathology to molecular pathology, *Oral Surg Oral Med Oral Pathol Oral Radiol Endod* 81:308-320, 1996.

Manthorpe R, Benoni C, Jacobsson L et al: Lower frequency of focal lip sialadenitis (focus score) in smoking patients. Can tobacco diminish the salivary gland involvement as judged by histological examination and anti-SSA/Ro and anti-SSB/La antibodies in Sjögren's syndrome, *Ann Rheum Dis* 59:54-60, 2000.

Marx RE, Hartman KS, Rethman KV: A prospective study comparing incisional labial to incisional parotid biopsies in the detection and confirmation of sarcoidosis, Sjögren's disease, sialosis and lymphoma, *J Rheumatol* 15:621-629, 1988.

Pedersen AM, Reibel J, Nauntofte B: Primary Sjögren's syndrome (pSS): subjective symptoms and salivary findings, *J Oral Pathol Med* 28:303-311, 1999.

Vitali C, Bombardieri S, Jonsson R et al: Classification criteria for Sjögren's syndrome: a revised version of the European criteria proposed by the American-European Consensus Group, *Ann Rheum Dis* 61:554-558, 2002.

Vivino FB, Gala I, Hermann GA: Change in final diagnosis on second evaluation of labial minor salivary gland biopsies, *J Rheumatol* 29:938-944, 2002.

Sialadenosis

Chilla R: Sialadenosis of the salivary glands of the head: studies on the physiology and pathophysiology of parotid secretion, *Adv Otorhinolaryngol* 26:1-38, 1981.

Coleman H, Altini M, Nayler S et al: Sialadenosis: a presenting sign in bulimia, *Head Neck* 20:758-762, 1998.

Mehler PS, Wallace JA: Sialadenosis in bulimia: a new treatment, *Arch Otolaryngol Head Neck Surg* 119:787-788, 1993.

Mignogna MD, Fedele S, Lo Russo L: Anorexia/bulimia-related sialadenosis of palatal minor salivary glands, *J Oral Pathol Med* 33:441-442, 2004.

Pape SA, MacLeod RI, McLean NR et al: Sialadenosis of the salivary glands, *Br J Plast Surg* 48:419-422, 1995.

Satoh M, Yoshihara T: Clinical and ultracytochemical investigation of sialadenosis, *Acta Otolaryngol Suppl* 553:122-127, 2004.

Adenomatoid Hyperplasia

Arafat A, Brannon RB, Ellis GL: Adenomatoid hyperplasia of mucous salivary glands, *Oral Surg Oral Med Oral Pathol* 52:51-55, 1981.

Barrett AW, Speight PM: Adenomatoid hyperplasia of oral minor salivary glands, *Oral Surg Oral Med Oral Pathol Oral Radiol Endod* 79:482-487, 1995.

Buchner A, Merrell PW, Carpenter WM et al: Adenomatoid hyperplasia of minor salivary glands, *Oral Surg Oral Med Oral Pathol* 71:583-587, 1991.

Giansanti JS, Baker GO, Waldron CA: Intraoral, mucinous, minor salivary gland lesions presenting clinically as tumors, *Oral Surg Oral Med Oral Pathol* 32:918-922, 1971.

Shimoyama T, Wakabayashi M, Kato T et al: Adenomatoid hyperplasia of the palate mimicking clinically as a salivary gland tumor, *J Oral Sci* 43:135-138, 2001.

Necrotizing Sialometaplasia

Abrams AM, Melrose RJ, Howell FV: Necrotizing sialometaplasia: a disease simulating malignancy, *Cancer* 32:130-135, 1973.

Brannon RB, Fowler CB, Hartman KS: Necrotizing sialometaplasia: a clinicopathologic study of sixty-nine cases and review of the literature, *Oral Surg Oral Med Oral Pathol* 72:317-325, 1991.

Imbery TA, Edwards PA: Necrotizing sialometaplasia: literature review and case reports, *J Am Dent Assoc* 127:1087-1092, 1996.

Schöning H, Emshoff R, Kreczy A: Necrotizing sialometaplasia in two patients with bulimia and chronic vomiting, *Int J Oral Maxillofac Surg* 27:463-465, 1998.

Sneige N, Batsakis JG: Necrotizing sialometaplasia, *Ann Otol Rhinol Laryngol* 101:282-284, 1992.

Salivary Gland Tumors: General Considerations

Dardick I: *Color atlas/text of salivary gland tumor pathology*, New York, 1996, Igaku-Shoin.

Ellies M, Schaffranietz F, Arglebe C et al: Tumor of the salivary glands in childhood and adolescence, *J Oral Maxillofac Surg* 64:1049-1058, 2006.

Ellis GL, Auclair PL: *Tumors of the salivary glands*, Washington DC, 1996, Armed Forces Institute of Pathology.

Ellis GL, Auclair PL, Gnepp DR: *Surgical pathology of the salivary glands*, Philadelphia, 1991, WB Saunders.

Eneroth C-M: Salivary gland tumors in the parotid gland, submandibular gland, and the palate region, *Cancer* 27:1415-1418, 1971.

Eveson JW, Cawson RA: Salivary gland tumours: a review of 2410 cases with particular reference to histological types, site, age, and sex distribution, *J Pathol* 146:51-58, 1985.

Eveson JW, Cawson RA: Tumours of the minor (oropharyngeal) salivary glands: a demographic study of 336 cases, *J Oral Pathol* 14:500-509, 1985.

Foote FW, Frazell EL: Tumors of the major salivary glands, *Cancer* 6:1065-1113, 1953.

Neville BW, Damm DD, Weir JC et al: Labial salivary gland tumors: an analysis of 103 cases, *Cancer* 61:2113-2116, 1988.

Pires FR, Pringle GA, de Almeida OP et al: Intra-oral minor salivary gland tumors: a clinicopathological study of 546 cases, *Oral Oncol* 43:463-470, 2007.

Seifert G, Brocheriou C, Cardesa A et al: WHO international histological classification of tumours: tentative histological classification of salivary gland tumours, *Pathol Res Pract* 186:555-581, 1990.

Seifert G, Miehlke A, Haubrich J et al: *Diseases of the salivary glands. Pathology–diagnosis–treatment–facial nerve surgery*, New York, 1986, George Thieme Verlag.

Spiro RH: Salivary neoplasms: overview of a 35-year experience with 2,807 patients, *Head Neck Surg* 8:177-184, 1986.

Thackray AC, Lucas RB: *Tumors of the major salivary glands: atlas of tumor pathology*, series 2, fascicle 10, Washington, DC, 1974, Armed Forces Institute of Pathology.

Waldron CA, El-Mofty SK, Gnepp DR: Tumors of the intraoral minor salivary glands: a demographic and histologic study of 426 cases, *Oral Surg Oral Med Oral Pathol* 66:323-333, 1988.

Whatley WS, Thompson JW, Rao B: Salivary gland tumors in survivors of childhood cancer, *Otolaryngol Head Neck Surg* 134:385-388, 2006.

Yih W-Y, Kratochvil FJ, Stewart JCB: Intraoral minor salivary gland neoplasms: review of 213 cases, *J Oral Maxillofac Surg* 63:805-810, 2005.

Pleomorphic Adenoma

Chau MNY, Radden BG: A clinical-pathological study of 53 intraoral pleomorphic adenomas, *Int J Oral Maxillofac Surg* 18:158-162, 1989.

Dardick I: Myoepithelioma: definitions and diagnostic criteria, *Ultrastruct Pathol* 19:335-345, 1995.

Friedrich RE, Li L, Knop J et al: Pleomorphic adenoma of the salivary glands: analysis of 94 patients, *Anticancer Res* 25:1703-1705, 2005.

Kanazawa H, Furuya T, Watanabe T et al: Plasmacytoid myoepithelioma of the palate, *J Oral Maxillofac Surg* 57:857-860, 1999.

Myssiorek D, Ruah CB, Hybels RL: Recurrent pleomorphic adenomas of the parotid gland, *Head Neck* 12:332-336, 1990.

Noguchi S, Aihara T, Yoshino K et al: Demonstration of monoclonal origin of human parotid gland pleomorphic adenoma, *Cancer* 77:431-435, 1996.

Silva SJ, Costa GT, Brant Filho AC et al: Metachronous bilateral pleomorphic adenoma of the parotid gland, *Oral Surg Oral Med Oral Pathol Oral Radiol Endod* 101:333-338, 2006.

Sciubba JJ, Brannon R: Myoepithelioma of salivary glands: report of 23 cases, *Cancer* 47:562-572, 1982.

Stennert E, Guntinas-Lichius O, Klussman JP et al: Histopathology of pleomorphic adenoma in the parotid gland: a prospective unselected series of 100 cases, *Laryngoscope* 111:2195-2200, 2001.

Stennert E, Wittekindt C, Klussman JP et al: Recurrent pleomorphic adenoma of the parotid gland: a prospective histopathological and immunohistochemical study, *Laryngoscope* 114:158-163, 2004.

Oncocytoma and Oncocytosis

Brandwein MS, Huvos AG: Oncocytic tumors of major salivary glands: a study of 68 cases with follow-up of 44 patients, *Am J Surg Pathol* 15:514-528, 1991.

Capone RB, Ha PK, Westra WH et al: Oncocytic neoplasms of the parotid gland: a 16-year institutional review, *Otolaryngol Head Neck Surg* 126:657-662, 2002.

Damm DD, White DK, Geissler RH Jr et al: Benign solid oncocytoma of intraoral minor salivary glands, *Oral Surg Oral Med Oral Pathol* 67:84-86, 1989.

Ellis GL: "Clear cell" oncocytoma of salivary gland, *Human Pathol* 19:862-867, 1988.

Goode RK, Corio RL: Oncocytic adenocarcinoma of salivary glands, *Oral Surg Oral Med Oral Pathol* 65:61-66, 1988.

Loreti A, Sturla M, Gentileschi S et al: Diffuse hyperplastic oncocytosis of the parotid gland, *Br J Plast Surg* 55:151-152, 2002.

Ozolek JA, Bastacky SI, Myers EN et al: Immunophenotypic comparison of salivary gland oncocytoma and metastatic renal cell carcinoma, *Laryngoscope* 115:1097-1100, 2005.

Palmer TJ, Gleeson MJ, Eveson JW et al: Oncocytic adenomas and oncocytic hyperplasia of salivary glands: a clinicopathological study of 26 cases, *Histopathology* 16:487-493, 1990.

Stomeo F, Meloni F, Bozzo C et al: Bilateral oncocytoma of the parotid gland, *Acta Otolaryngol* 126:324-326, 2006.

Thompson LD, Wenig BM, Ellis GL: Oncocytomas of the submandibular gland. A series of 22 cases and a review of the literature, *Cancer* 78:2281-2287, 1996.

Warthin Tumor

Aguirre JM, Echebarría MA, Martínez-Conde R et al: Warthin tumor. A new hypothesis concerning its development, *Oral Surg Oral Med Oral Pathol Oral Radiol Endod* 85:60-63, 1998.

Batsakis JG: Carcinoma ex papillary cystadenoma lymphomatosum. Malignant Warthin's tumor, *Ann Otol Rhinol Laryngol* 96:234-235, 1987.

Dietert SE: Papillary cystadenoma lymphomatosum (Warthin's tumor) in patients in a general hospital over a 24-year period, *Am J Clin Pathol* 63:866-875, 1975.

Fantasia JE, Miller AS: Papillary cystadenoma lymphomatosum arising in minor salivary glands, *Oral Surg Oral Med Oral Pathol* 52:411-416, 1981.

Honda K, Kashima K, Daa T et al: Clonal analysis of the epithelial component of Warthin's tumor, *Hum Pathol* 31:1377-1380, 2000.

Klussmann JP, Wittekindt C, Preuss SF et al: High risk for bilateral Warthin tumor in heavy smokers—review of 185 cases, *Acta Otolaryngol* 126:1213-1217, 2006.

Kotwall CA: Smoking as an etiologic factor in the development of Warthin's tumor of the parotid gland, *Am J Surg* 164:646-647, 1992.

Martins C, Fonseca I, Roque L et al: Cytogenetic characterisation of Warthin's tumour, *Oral Oncol* 33:344-347, 1997.

Monk JS Jr, Church JS: Warthin's tumor: a high incidence and no sex predominance in central Pennsylvania, *Arch Otolaryngol Head Neck Surg* 118:477-478, 1992.

Takezawa K, Jackson C, Gnepp DR et al: Molecular characterization of Warthin tumor, *Oral Surg Oral Med Oral Pathol Oral Radiol Endod* 85:569-575, 1998.

Teymoortash A, Werner JA: Tissue that has lost its track: Warthin's tumour, *Virchows Arch* 446:585-588, 2005.

van der Wal JE, Davids JJ, van der Waal I: Extraparotid Warthin's tumours—report of 10 cases, *Br J Oral Maxillofac Surg* 31:43-44, 1993.

Zappia JJ, Sullivan MJ, McClatchey KD: Unilateral multicentric Warthin's tumors, *J Otolaryngol* 20:93-96, 1991.

Canalicular Adenoma

Daley TD, Gardner DG, Smout MS: Canalicular adenoma: not a basal cell adenoma, *Oral Surg Oral Med Oral Pathol* 57:181-188, 1984.

Fantasia JE, Neville BW: Basal cell adenomas of the minor salivary glands, *Oral Surg Oral Med Oral Pathol* 50:433-440, 1980.

Gardner DG, Daley TD: The use of the terms monomorphic adenoma, basal cell adenoma, and canalicular adenoma as applied to salivary gland tumors, *Oral Surg Oral Med Oral Pathol* 56:608-615, 1983.

Nelson JF, Jacoway JR: Monomorphic adenoma (canalicular type): report of 29 cases, *Cancer* 31:1511-1513, 1973.

Neville BW, Damm DD, Weir JC et al: Labial salivary gland tumors: an analysis of 103 cases, *Cancer* 61:2113-2116, 1988.

Rousseau A, Mock D, Dover DG et al: Multiple canalicular adenomas: a case report and review of the literature, *Oral Surg Oral Med Oral Pathol Oral Radiol Endod* 87:346-350, 1999.

Suarez P, Hammond HL, Luna MA et al: Palatal canalicular adenoma: report of 12 cases and review of the literature, *Ann Diagn Pathol* 2:224-228, 1998.

Yoon AJ, Beller DE, Woo, VL et al: Bilateral canalicular adenomas of the upper lip, *Oral Surg Oral Med Oral Pathol Oral Radiol Endod* 102:341-343, 2006.

Basal Cell Adenoma

Batsakis JG, Brannon RB: Dermal analogue tumours of major salivary glands, *J Laryngol* 95:155-164, 1981.

Ellis GL, Wiscovitch JG: Basal cell adenocarcinomas of the major salivary glands, *Oral Surg Oral Med Oral Pathol* 69:461-469, 1990.

Fonseca I, Soares J: Basal cell adenocarcinoma of minor salivary and seromucous glands of the head and neck region, *Semin Diagn Pathol* 13:128-137, 1996.

Jayakrishnan A, Elmalah I, Hussain K et al: Basal cell adenocarcinoma in minor salivary glands, *Histopathology* 42:610-614, 2003.

Luna MA, Tortoledo ME, Allen M: Salivary dermal analogue tumors arising in lymph nodes, *Cancer* 59:1165-1169, 1987.

Machado de Sousa SO, Soares de Araújo N, Corrêa L et al: Immunohistochemical aspects of basal cell adenoma and canalicular adenoma of salivary glands, *Oral Oncol* 37:365-368, 2001.

Muller S, Barnes L: Basal cell adenocarcinoma of the salivary glands: report of seven cases and review of the literature, *Cancer* 78:2471-2477, 1996.

Parashar P, Baron E, Papadimitriou JC et al: Basal cell adenocarcinoma of the oral minor salivary glands: review of the literature and presentation of two cases, *Oral Surg Oral Med Oral Pathol Oral Radiol Endod* 103:77-84, 2007.

Pogrel MA: The intraoral basal cell adenoma, *J Craniomaxillofac Surg* 15:372-375, 1987.

Zarbo RJ, Prasad AR, Regezi JA et al: Salivary gland basal cell and canalicular adenomas: immunohistochemical demonstration of myoepithelial cell participation and morphogenetic considerations, *Arch Pathol Lab Med* 124:401-405, 2000.

Salivary Papillomas

Abbey LM: Solitary intraductal papilloma of the minor salivary glands, *Oral Surg Oral Med Oral Pathol* 40:135-140, 1975.

Abrams AM, Finck FM: Sialadenoma papilliferum: a previously unreported salivary gland tumor, *Cancer* 24:1057-1063, 1969.

Brannon RB, Sciubba JJ, Giulani M: Ductal papillomas of salivary gland origin: a report of 19 cases and a review of the litterature, *Oral Surg Oral Med Oral Pathol Oral Radiol Endod* 92:68-77, 2001.

Cabov T, Macan D, Manojlovic S et al: Oral inverted ductal papilloma, *Br J Oral Maxillofac Surg* 42:75-77, 2004.

Fantasia JE, Nocco CE, Lally ET: Ultrastructure of sialadenoma papilliferum, *Arch Pathol Lab Med* 110:523-527, 1986.

Gomes APN, Sobral APV, Loducca SVL et al: Sialadenoma papilliferum: immunohistochemical study, *Int J Oral Maxillofac Surg* 33:621-624, 2004.

Hegarty DJ, Hopper C, Speight PM: Inverted ductal papilloma of minor salivary glands, *J Oral Pathol Med* 23:334-336, 1994.

Iguchi H, Yamane H, Nasako Y et al: Intraductal papilloma in the parotid duct, *Acta Otolaryngol* 122:314-317, 2002.

Maiorano E, Favia G, Ricco R: Sialadenoma papilliferum: an immunohistochemical study of five cases, *J Oral Pathol Med* 25:336-342, 1996.

Nagao T, Sugano I, Matsuzaki O et al: Intraductal papillary tumors of the major salivary glands. Case reports of benign and malignant variants, *Arch Pathol Lab Med* 124:291-295, 2000.

de Sousa SO, Sesso A, de Araújo NS et al: Inverted ductal papilloma of minor salivary gland origin: morphological aspects and cytokeratin expression, *Eur Arch Otorhinolaryngol* 252:370-373, 1995.

White DK, Miller AS, McDaniel RK et al: Inverted ductal papilloma: a distinctive lesion of minor salivary gland, *Cancer* 49:519-524, 1982.

Mucoepidermoid Carcinoma

Auclair PL, Goode RK, Ellis GL: Mucoepidermoid carcinoma of intraoral salivary glands, *Cancer* 69:2021-2030, 1992.

Batsakis JG, Luna MA: Histopathologic grading of salivary gland neoplasms. I. Mucoepidermoid carcinomas, *Ann Otol Rhinol Laryngol* 99:835-838, 1990.

Brandwein MS, Ivanov K, Wallace DI et al: Mucoepidermoid carcinoma: a clinicopathologic study of 80 patients with special reference to histological grading, *Am J Surg Pathol* 25:835-845, 2001.

Evans HL: Mucoepidermoid carcinoma of salivary glands: a study of 69 cases with special attention to histologic grading, *Am J Clin Pathol* 81:696-701, 1984.

Goode RK, Auclair PL, Ellis GL: Mucoepidermoid carcinoma of the major salivary glands: clinical and histopathologic analysis of 234 cases with evaluation of grading criteria, *Cancer* 82:1217-1224, 1998.

Guzzo M, Andreola S, Sirizzotti G et al: Mucoepidermoid carcinoma of the salivary glands: clinicopathologic review of 108 patients treated at the National Cancer Institute of Milan, *Ann Surg Oncol* 9:688-695, 2002.

Hicks J, Flaitz C: Mucoepidermoid carcinoma of salivary glands in children and adolescents: assessment of proliferation markers, *Oral Oncol* 36:454-460, 2000.

Luna MA: Salivary mucoepidermoid carcinoma: revisited, *Adv Anat Pathol* 13:293-307, 2006.

Spiro RH, Huvos AG, Berk R et al: Mucoepidermoid carcinoma of salivary gland origin: a clinicopathologic study of 367 cases, *Am J Surg* 136:461-468, 1978.

Stewart FW, Foote FW, Becker WF: Mucoepidermoid tumors of salivary glands, *Ann Surg* 122:820-844, 1945.

Védrine PO, Coffinet L, Temam S et al: Mucoepidermoid carcinoma of salivary glands in the pediatric age group: 18 clinical cases, including 11 second malignant neoplasms, *Head Neck* 28:827-833, 2006.

Whatley WS, Thompson JW, Rao B: Salivary gland tumors in survivors of childhood cancer, *Otolaryngol Head Neck Surg* 134:385-388, 2006.

Intraosseous Mucoepidermoid Carcinoma

Bouquot JE, Gnepp DR, Dardick I et al: Intraosseous salivary tissue: jawbone examples of choristomas, hamartomas, embryonic rests, and inflammatory entrapment—another histogenetic source for intraosseous adenocarcinoma, *Oral Surg Oral Med Oral Pathol Oral Radiol Endod* 90:205-217, 2000.

Brookstone MS, Huvos AG: Central salivary gland tumors of the maxilla and mandible: a clinicopathologic study of 11 cases with an analysis of the literature, *J Oral Maxillofac Surg* 50:229-236, 1992.

Browand BC, Waldron CA: Central mucoepidermoid tumors of the jaws, *Oral Surg Oral Med Oral Pathol* 40:631-643, 1975.

Inagaki M, Yuasa K, Nakayama E et al: Mucoepidermoid carcinoma in the mandible. Findings of panoramic radiography and computed tomography, *Oral Surg Oral Med Oral Pathol Oral Radiol Endod* 85:613-618, 1998.

Martínez-Madrigal F, Pineda-Daboin K, Casiraghi O et al: Salivary gland tumors of the mandible, *Ann Diagn Pathol* 4:347-353, 2000.

Pires FR, Paes de Almeida O, Lopes MA et al: Central mucoepidermoid carcinoma of the mandible: report of four cases with long-term follow-up, *Int J Oral Maxillofac Surg* 32:378-382, 2003.

Waldron CA, Koh ML: Central mucoepidermoid carcinoma of the jaws: report of four cases with analysis of the literature and discussion of the relationship to mucoepidermoid, sialodontogenic, and glandular odontogenic cysts, *J Oral Maxillofac Surg* 48:871-877, 1990.

Acinic Cell Adenocarcinoma

Batsakis JG, Luna MA, El-Naggar AK: Histopathologic grading of salivary gland neoplasms. II. Acinic cell carcinomas, *Ann Otol Rhinol Laryngol* 99:929-933, 1990.

Chen S-Y, Brannon RB, Miller AS et al: Acinic cell adenocarcinoma of minor salivary glands, *Cancer* 42:678-685, 1978.

Ellis GL, Corio RL: Acinic cell adenocarcinoma: a clinicopathologic analysis of 294 cases, *Cancer* 52:542-549, 1983.

Hamper K, Mausch H-E, Caselitz J et al: Acinic cell carcinoma of the salivary glands: the prognostic relevance of DNA cytophotometry in a retrospective study of long duration (1965-1987), *Oral Surg Oral Med Oral Pathol* 69:68-75, 1990.

Hoffman HT, Karnell LH, Robinson RA et al: National Cancer Data Base report on cancer of the head and neck: acinic cell carcinoma, *Head Neck* 21:297-309, 1999.

Lewis JE, Olsen KD, Weiland LH: Acinic cell carcinoma: clinicopathologic review, *Cancer* 67:172-179, 1991.

Michal M, Skálová A, Simpson RHW et al: Well-differentiated acinic cell carcinoma of salivary glands associated with lymphoid stroma, *Hum Pathol* 28:595-600, 1997.

Perzin KH, LiVolsi VA: Acinic cell carcinomas arising in salivary glands: a clinicopathologic study, *Cancer* 44:1434-1457, 1979.

Malignant Mixed Tumor

Auclair PL, Ellis GL: Atypical features in salivary gland mixed tumors: their relationship to malignant transformation, *Mod Pathol* 9:652-657, 1996.

Bradley PJ: "Metastasizing pleomorphic salivary adenoma" should now be considered a low-grade malignancy with a lethal potential, *Curr Opin Otolaryngol Head Neck Surg* 13:123-126, 2005.

Brandwein M, Huvos AG, Dardick I et al: Noninvasive and minimally invasive carcinoma ex mixed tumor: a clinicopathologic and ploidy study of 12 patients with major salivary tumors of low (or no?) malignant potential, *Oral Surg Oral Med Oral Pathol Oral Radiol Endod* 81:655-664, 1996.

Carson HJ, Tojo DP, Chow JM et al: Carcinosarcoma of salivary glands with unusual stromal components: report of two cases and review of the literature, *Oral Surg Oral Med Oral Pathol Oral Radiol Endod* 79:738-746, 1995.

Gnepp DR: Malignant mixed tumors of the salivary glands: a review, *Pathol Annu* 28(pt 1):279-328, 1993.

Klijanienko J, El-Naggar AK, Servois V et al: Clinically aggressive metastasizing pleomorphic adenoma: report of two cases, *Head Neck* 19:629-633, 1997.

Kwon MY, Gu M: True malignant mixed tumor (carcinosarcoma) of parotid gland with unusual mesenchymal component: a case report and review of the literature, *Arch Pathol Lab Med* 125:812-815, 2001.

Lewis JE, Olsen KD, Sebo TJ: Carcinoma ex pleomorphic adenoma: pathologic analysis of 73 cases, *Hum Pathol* 32:596-604, 2001.

LiVolsi VA, Perzin KH: Malignant mixed tumors arising in salivary glands. I. Carcinomas arising in benign mixed tumor: a clinicopathologic study, *Cancer* 39:2209-2230, 1977.

Nouraei SAR, Ferguson MS, Clarke PM et al: Metastasizing pleomorphic salivary adenoma, *Arch Otolaryngol Head Neck Surg* 132:788-793, 2006.

Nouraei SAR, Hope KL, Kelly CG et al: Carcinoma ex benign pleomorphic adenoma of the parotid gland, *Plast Reconstr Surg* 116:1206-1213, 2005.

Spiro RH, Huvos AG, Strong EW: Malignant mixed tumor of salivary origin: a clinicopathologic study of 146 cases, *Cancer* 39:388-396, 1977.

Tortoledo ME, Luna MA, Batsakis JG: Carcinomas ex pleomorphic adenoma and malignant mixed tumors, *Arch Otolaryngol* 110:172-176, 1984.

Wenig BM, Hitchcock CL, Ellis GL et al: Metastasizing mixed tumor of salivary glands. A clinicopathologic and flow cytometric analysis, *Am J Surg Pathol* 16:845-858, 1992.

Adenoid Cystic Carcinoma

Araújo VC, Loducca SVL, Sousa SOM et al: The cribriform features of adenoid cystic carcinoma and polymorphous low-grade adenocarcinoma: cytokeratin and integrin expression, *Ann Diagn Pathol* 5:330-334, 2001.

Beltran D, Faquin WC, Gallagher G et al: Selective immunohistochemical comparison of polymorphous low-grade adenocarcinoma and adenoid cystic carcinoma, *J Oral Maxillofac Surg* 64:415-423, 2006.

Bradley PJ: Adenoid cystic carcinoma of the head and neck: a review, *Curr Opin Otolaryngol Head Neck Surg* 12:127-132, 2004.

da Cruz Perez DE, de Abreu Alves F, Nobuko Nishimoto I et al: Prognostic factors in head and neck adenoid cystic carcinoma, *Oral Oncol* 42:139-146, 2006.

Darling MR, Schneider JW, Phillips VM: Polymorphous low-grade adenocarcinoma and adenoid cystic carcinoma: a review and comparison of immunohistochemical markers, *Oral Oncol* 38:641-645, 2002.

Enamorado I, Lakhani R, Korkmaz H et al: Correlation of histopathological variants, cellular DNA content, and clinical outcome in adenoid cystic carcinoma of the salivary glands, *Otolaryngol Head Neck Surg* 131:646-650, 2004.

Gurney TA, Eisele DW, Weinberg V et al: Adenoid cystic carcinoma of the major salivary glands treated with surgery and radiation, *Laryngoscope* 115:1278-1282, 2005.

Hamper K, Lazar F, Dietel M et al: Prognostic factors for adenoid cystic carcinoma of the head and neck: a retrospective evaluation of 96 cases, *J Oral Pathol Med* 19:101-107, 1990.

Jones AS, Hamilton JW, Rowley H et al: Adenoid cystic carcinoma of the head and neck, *Clin Otolaryngol* 22:434-443, 1997.

Loducca SVL, Raitz R, Araújo NS et al: Polymorphous low-grade adenocarcinoma and adenoid cystic carcinoma: distinct architectural composition revealed by collagen IV, laminin and their integrin ligands (α2β1 and α3β1), *Histopathology* 37:118-123, 2000.

Penner CR, Folpe AL, Budnick SD: C-kit expression distinguishes salivary gland adenoid cystic carcinoma from polymorphous low-grade adenocarcinoma, *Mod Pathol* 15:687-691, 2002.

Perzin KH, Gullane P, Clairmont AC: Adenoid cystic carcinomas arising in salivary glands: a correlation of histologic features and clinical course, *Cancer* 42:265-282, 1978.

Spiro RH: Distant metastasis in adenoid cystic carcinoma of salivary origin, *Am J Surg* 174:495-498, 1997.

Szanto PA, Luna MA, Tortoledo ME et al: Histologic grading of adenoid cystic carcinoma of the salivary glands, *Cancer* 54:1062-1069, 1984.

van der Wal JE, Snow GB, van der Waal I: Intraoral adenoid cystic carcinoma: the presence of perineural spread in relation to site, size, local extension, and metastatic spread in 22 cases, *Cancer* 66:2031-2033, 1990.

Woo VL, Bhuiya T, Kelsch R: Assessment of CD43 expression in adenoid cystic carcinomas, polymorphous low-grade adenocarcinomas, and monomorphic adenomas, *Oral Surg Oral Med Oral Pathol Oral Radiol Endod* 102:495-500, 2006.

Polymorphous Low-Grade Adenocarcinoma

Araújo VC, Loducca SVL, Sousa SOM et al: The cribriform features of adenoid cystic carcinoma and polymorphous low-grade adenocarcinoma: cytokeratin and integrin expression, *Ann Diagn Pathol* 5:330-334, 2001.

Araújo V, Sousa S, Jaeger M et al: Characterization of the cellular component of polymorphous low-grade adenocarcinoma by immunohistochemistry and electron microscopy, *Oral Oncol* 35:164-172, 1999.

Batsakis JG, Pinkston GR, Luna MA et al: Adenocarcinomas of the oral cavity: a clinicopathologic study of terminal duct carcinomas, *J Laryngol Otol* 97:825-835, 1983.

Beltran D, Faquin WC, Gallagher G et al: Selective immunohistochemical comparison of polymorphous low-grade adenocarcinoma and adenoid cystic carcinoma, *J Oral Maxillofac Surg* 64:415-423, 2006.

Castle JT, Thompson LDR, Frommelt RA et al: Polymorphous low grade adenocarcinoma: a clinicopathologic study of 164 cases, *Cancer* 86:207-219, 1999.

Curran AE, White DK, Damm DD et al: Polymorphous low-grade adenocarcinoma versus pleomorphic adenoma of minor salivary glands: resolution of a diagnostic dilemma by immunohistochemical analysis with glial fibrillary acidic protein, *Oral Surg Oral Med Oral Pathol Oral Radiol Endod* 91:194-199, 2001.

Darling MR, Schneider JW, Phillips VM: Polymorphous low-grade adenocarcinoma and adenoid cystic carcinoma: a review and comparison of immunohistochemical markers, *Oral Oncol* 38:641-645, 2002.

Evans HL, Luna MA: Polymorphous low-grade adenocarcinoma: a study of 40 cases with long-term follow up and an evaluation of the importance of papillary areas, *Am J Surg Pathol* 24:1319-1328, 2000.

Freedman PD, Lumerman H: Lobular carcinoma of intraoral minor salivary glands, *Oral Surg Oral Med Oral Pathol* 56:157-165, 1983.

Nagao T, Gaffey TA, Kay PA et al: Polymorphous low-grade adenocarcinoma of the major salivary glands: report of three cases in an unusual location, *Histopathology* 44:164-171, 2004.

Penner CR, Folpe AL, Budnick SD: C-kit expression distinguishes salivary gland adenoid cystic carcinoma from polymorphous low-grade adenocarcinoma, *Mod Pathol* 15:687-691, 2002.

Vincent SD, Hammond HL, Finkelstein MW: Clinical and therapeutic features of polymorphous low-grade adenocarcinoma, *Oral Surg Oral Med Oral Pathol* 77:41-47, 1994.

Woo VL, Bhuiya T, Kelsch R: Assessment of CD43 expression in adenoid cystic carcinomas, polymorphous low-grade adenocarcinomas, and monomorphic adenomas, *Oral Surg Oral Med Oral Pathol Oral Radiol Endod* 102:495-500, 2006.

Salivary Adenocarcinoma, Not Otherwise Specified

Li J, Wang BY, Nelson M et al: Salivary adenocarcinoma, not otherwise specified: a collection of orphans, *Arch Pathol Lab Med* 128:1385-1394, 2004.

Matsuba HM, Mauney M, Simpson JR et al: Adenocarcinomas of major and minor salivary gland origin: a histopathologic review of treatment failure patterns, *Laryngoscope* 98:784-788, 1988.

Spiro RH, Huvos AG, Strong EW: Adenocarcinoma of salivary origin: clinicopathologic study of 204 patients, *Am J Surg* 144:423-431, 1982.

Stene T, Koppang HS: Intraoral adenocarcinomas, *J Oral Pathol* 10:216-225, 1981.

Wahlberg P, Anderson H, Biörklund A et al: Carcinoma of the parotid and submandibular glands—a study of survival in 2465 patients, *Oral Oncol* 38:706-713, 2002.

Soft Tissue Tumors

CHAPTER OUTLINE

FIBROMA (IRRITATION FIBROMA; TRAUMATIC FIBROMA; FOCAL FIBROUS HYPERPLASIA; FIBROUS NODULE)

The **fibroma** is the most common "tumor" of the oral cavity. However, it is doubtful that it represents a true neoplasm in most instances; rather, it is a reactive hyperplasia of fibrous connective tissue in response to local irritation or trauma.

CLINICAL FEATURES

Although the irritation fibroma can occur anywhere in the mouth, the most common location is the buccal mucosa along the bite line. Presumably, this is a consequence of trauma from biting the cheek (Figs. 12-1 and 12-2). The labial mucosa, tongue, and gingiva also are common sites (Figs. 12-3 and 12-4). It is likely that many gingival fibromas represent fibrous maturation of a preexisting pyogenic granuloma. The lesion

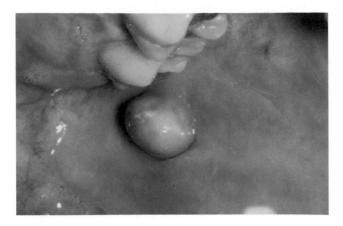

Fig. 12-1   Fibroma. Pink nodule of the posterior buccal mucosa near the level of the occlusal plane.

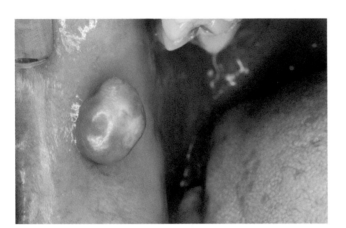

Fig. 12-2   Fibroma. Black patient with a smooth-surfaced pigmented nodule on the buccal mucosa near the commissure.

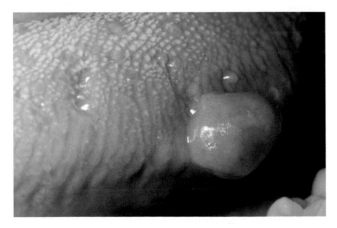

Fig. 12-3   Fibroma. Lesion on the lateral border of the tongue.

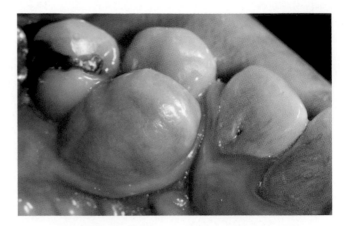

Fig. 12-4   Fibroma. Smooth-surfaced, pink nodular mass of the palatal gingiva between the cuspid and first bicuspid.

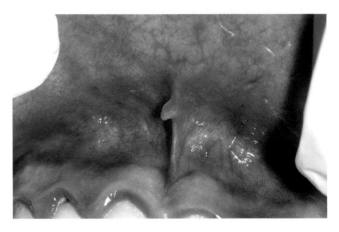

Fig. 12-5   Frenal tag. A small fingerlike projection of tissue attached to the maxillary labial frenum.

typically appears as a smooth-surfaced pink nodule that is similar in color to the surrounding mucosa. In black patients, the mass may demonstrate gray-brown pigmentation. In some cases the surface may appear white as a result of hyperkeratosis from continued irritation. Most fibromas are sessile, although some are pedunculated. They range in size from tiny lesions that are only a couple of millimeters in diameter to large masses that are several centimeters across; however, most fibromas are 1.5 cm or less in diameter. The lesion usually produces no symptoms, unless secondary traumatic ulceration of the surface has occurred. Irritation fibromas are most common in the fourth to sixth decades of life, and the male-to-female ratio is almost 1:2 for cases submitted for biopsy.

The **frenal tag** is a commonly observed type of fibrous hyperplasia, which most frequently occurs on the maxillary labial frenum. Such lesions present as small, asymptomatic, exophytic growths attached to the thin frenum surface (Fig. 12-5).

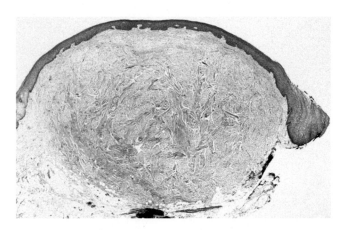

Fig. 12-6   Fibroma. Low-power view showing an exophytic nodular mass of dense fibrous connective tissue.

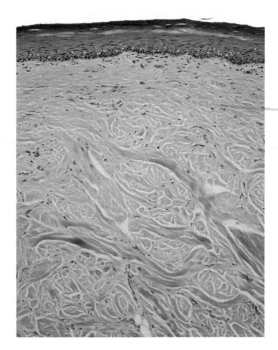

Fig. 12-7   Fibroma. Higher-power view demonstrating dense collagen beneath the epithelial surface.

HISTOPATHOLOGIC FEATURES

Microscopic examination of the irritation fibroma shows a nodular mass of fibrous connective tissue covered by stratified squamous epithelium (Figs. 12-6 and 12-7). This connective tissue is usually dense and collagenized, although in some cases it is looser in nature. The lesion is not encapsulated; the fibrous tissue instead blends gradually into the surrounding connective tissues. The collagen bundles may be arranged in a radiating, circular, or haphazard fashion. The covering epithelium often demonstrates atrophy of the rete ridges because of the underlying fibrous mass. However, the surface may exhibit hyperkeratosis from secondary trauma. Scattered inflammation may be

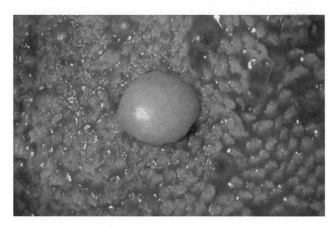

Fig. 12-8   Giant cell fibroma. Exophytic nodule on the dorsum of the tongue.

seen, most often beneath the epithelial surface. Usually this inflammation is chronic and consists mostly of lymphocytes and plasma cells.

TREATMENT AND PROGNOSIS

The irritation fibroma is treated by conservative surgical excision; recurrence is extremely rare. However, it is important to submit the excised tissue for microscopic examination because other benign or malignant tumors may mimic the clinical appearance of a fibroma.

Because frenal tags are small, innocuous growths that are easily diagnosed clinically, no treatment is usually necessary.

GIANT CELL FIBROMA

The **giant cell fibroma** is a fibrous tumor with distinctive clinicopathologic features. Unlike the traumatic fibroma, it does not appear to be associated with chronic irritation. The giant cell fibroma represents approximately 2% to 5% of all oral fibrous proliferations submitted for biopsy.

CLINICAL FEATURES

The giant cell fibroma is typically an asymptomatic sessile or pedunculated nodule, usually less than 1 cm in size (Fig. 12-8). The surface of the mass often appears papillary; therefore, the lesion may be clinically mistaken for a papilloma. Compared with the common irritation fibroma, the lesion usually occurs at a younger age. In about 60% of cases, the lesion is diagnosed during the first 3 decades of life. Some studies have suggested a slight female predilection. Approximately 50% of all cases occur on the gingiva. The mandibular gingiva is affected twice as often as the maxillary gingiva. The tongue and palate also are common sites.

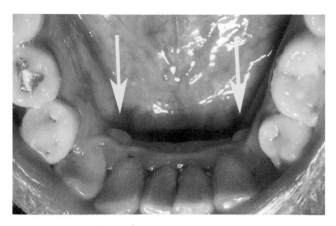

Fig. 12-9   Retrocuspid papilla. Bilateral papular lesions on the gingiva lingual to the mandibular canines *(arrows)*.

The **retrocuspid papilla** is a microscopically similar developmental lesion that occurs on the gingiva lingual to the mandibular cuspid. It is frequently bilateral and typically appears as a small, pink papule that measures less than 5 mm in diameter (Fig. 12-9). Retrocuspid papillae are quite common, having been reported in 25% to 99% of children and young adults. The prevalence in older adults drops to 6% to 19%, suggesting that the retrocuspid papilla represents a normal anatomic variation that disappears with age.

HISTOPATHOLOGIC FEATURES

Microscopic examination of the giant cell fibroma reveals a mass of vascular fibrous connective tissue, which is usually loosely arranged (Fig. 12-10). The hallmark is the presence of numerous large, stellate fibroblasts within the superficial connective tissue. These cells may contain several nuclei. Frequently, the surface of the lesion is pebbly. The covering epithelium often is thin and atrophic, although the rete ridges may appear narrow and elongated.

TREATMENT AND PROGNOSIS

The giant cell fibroma is treated by conservative surgical excision. Recurrence is rare. Because of their characteristic appearance, retrocuspid papillae should be recognized clinically and do not need to be excised.

EPULIS FISSURATUM (INFLAMMATORY FIBROUS HYPERPLASIA; DENTURE INJURY TUMOR; DENTURE EPULIS)

The **epulis fissuratum** is a tumorlike hyperplasia of fibrous connective tissue that develops in association with the flange of an ill-fitting complete or partial denture. Although the simple term *epulis* sometimes is

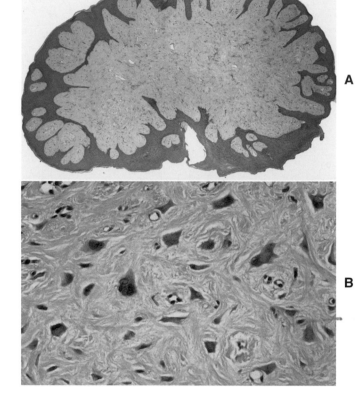

Fig. 12-10   Giant cell fibroma. A, Low-power view showing a nodular mass of fibrous connective tissue covered by stratified squamous epithelium. Note the elongation of the rete ridges. **B,** High-power view showing multiple large stellate-shaped and multinucleated fibroblasts.

used synonymously for epulis fissuratum, *epulis* is actually a generic term that can be applied to any tumor of the gingiva or alveolar mucosa. Therefore, some authors have advocated not using this term, preferring to call these lesions *inflammatory fibrous hyperplasia* or other descriptive names. However, the term *epulis fissuratum* is still widely used today and is well understood by virtually all clinicians. Other examples of epulides include the **giant cell epulis (peripheral giant cell granuloma)** (see page 520), **ossifying fibroid epulis (peripheral ossifying fibroma)** (see page 521), and **congenital epulis** (see page 537).

CLINICAL FEATURES

The epulis fissuratum typically appears as a single or multiple fold or folds of hyperplastic tissue in the alveolar vestibule (Figs. 12-11 and 12-12). Most often, there are two folds of tissue, and the flange of the associated denture fits conveniently into the fissure between the folds. The redundant tissue is usually firm and fibrous, although some lesions appear erythematous and ulcer-

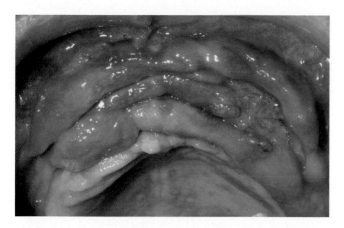

Fig. 12-11   Epulis fissuratum. Hyperplastic folds of tissue in the anterior maxillary vestibule.

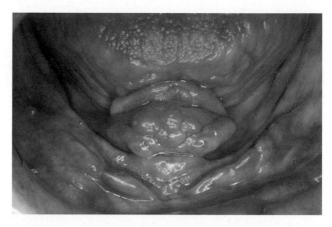

Fig. 12-13   Epulis fissuratum. Redundant folds of tissue arising in the floor of the mouth in association with a mandibular denture.

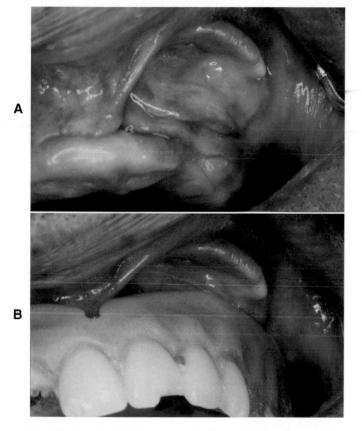

Fig. 12-12   Epulis fissuratum. A, Several folds of hyperplastic tissue in the maxillary vestibule. **B,** An ill-fitting denture fits into the fissure between two of the folds. *(Courtesy of Dr. William Bruce.)*

ated, similar to the appearance of a pyogenic granuloma. Occasional examples of epulis fissuratum demonstrate surface areas of inflammatory papillary hyperplasia (see page 512). The size of the lesion can vary from localized hyperplasias less than 1 cm in size to massive lesions that involve most of the length of the

vestibule. The epulis fissuratum usually develops on the facial aspect of the alveolar ridge, although occasional lesions are seen lingual to the mandibular alveolar ridge (Fig. 12-13).

The epulis fissuratum most often occurs in middle-aged and older adults, as would be expected with a denture-related lesion. It may occur on either the maxilla or mandible. The anterior portion of the jaws is affected much more often than the posterior areas. There is a pronounced female predilection; most studies show that two thirds to three fourths of all cases submitted for biopsy occur in women.

Another similar but less common fibrous hyperplasia, often called a **fibroepithelial polyp** or **leaflike denture fibroma,** occurs on the hard palate beneath a maxillary denture. This characteristic lesion is a flattened pink mass that is attached to the palate by a narrow stalk (Fig. 12-14). Usually, the flattened mass is closely applied to the palate and sits in a slightly cupped-out depression. However, it is easily lifted up with a probe, which demonstrates its pedunculated nature. The edge of the lesion often is serrated and resembles a leaf.

HISTOPATHOLOGIC FEATURES

Microscopic examination of the epulis fissuratum reveals hyperplasia of the fibrous connective tissue. Often multiple folds and grooves occur where the denture impinges on the tissue (Fig. 12-15). The overlying epithelium is frequently hyperparakeratotic and demonstrates irregular hyperplasia of the rete ridges. In some instances, the epithelium shows inflammatory papillary hyperplasia (see page 513) or pseudoepitheliomatous (pseudocarcinomatous) hyperplasia. Focal areas of ulceration are not unusual, especially at the

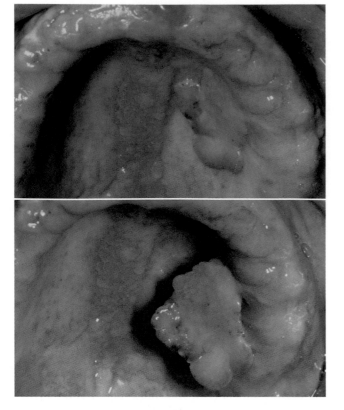

Fig. 12-14   Fibroepithelial polyp. Flattened mass of tissue arising on the hard palate beneath a maxillary denture; note its pedunculated nature. Because of its serrated edge, this lesion also is known as a *leaflike denture fibroma.* Associated inflammatory papillary hyperplasia is visible in the palatal midline.

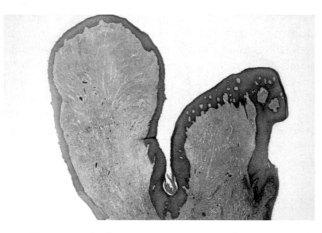

Fig. 12-15   Epulis fissuratum. Low-power photomicrograph demonstrating folds of hyperplastic fibrovascular connective tissue covered by stratified squamous epithelium.

base of the grooves between the folds. A variable chronic inflammatory infiltrate is present; sometimes, it may include eosinophils or show lymphoid follicles. If minor salivary glands are included in the specimen, then they usually show chronic sialadenitis.

In rare instances, the formation of osteoid or chondroid is observed. This unusual-appearing product, known as **osseous and chondromatous metaplasia**, is a reactive phenomenon caused by chronic irritation by the ill-fitting denture (see page 318). The irregular nature of this bone or cartilage can be microscopically disturbing, and the pathologist should not mistake it for a sarcoma.

The denture-related fibroepithelial polyp has a narrow core of dense fibrous connective tissue covered by stratified squamous epithelium. Like the epulis fissuratum, the overlying epithelium may be hyperplastic.

TREATMENT AND PROGNOSIS

The treatment of the epulis fissuratum or fibroepithelial polyp consists of surgical removal, with microscopic examination of the excised tissue. The ill-fitting denture should be remade or relined to prevent a recurrence of the lesion.

INFLAMMATORY PAPILLARY HYPERPLASIA (DENTURE PAPILLOMATOSIS)

Inflammatory papillary hyperplasia is a reactive tissue growth that usually, although not always, develops beneath a denture. Some investigators classify this lesion as part of the spectrum of denture stomatitis (see page 216). Although the exact pathogenesis is unknown, the condition most often appears to be related to the following:

- An ill-fitting denture
- Poor denture hygiene
- Wearing the denture 24 hours a day

Approximately 20% of patients who wear their dentures 24 hours a day have inflammatory papillary hyperplasia. *Candida* organisms also have been suggested as a cause, but any possible role appears uncertain.

CLINICAL FEATURES

Inflammatory papillary hyperplasia usually occurs on the hard palate beneath a denture base (Figs. 12-16 and 12-17). Early lesions may involve only the palatal vault, although advanced cases cover most of the palate. Less frequently, this hyperplasia develops on the edentulous mandibular alveolar ridge or on the surface of an epulis fissuratum. On rare occasions, the condition occurs on the palate of a patient without a denture, especially in people who habitually breathe through their mouth or have a high palatal vault. *Candida*-associated palatal papillary hyperplasia also has been

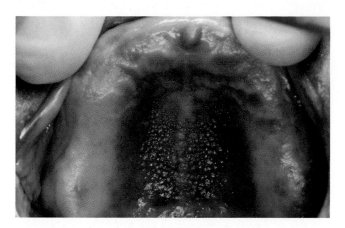

Fig. 12-16 Inflammatory papillary hyperplasia. Erythematous, pebbly appearance of the palatal vault.

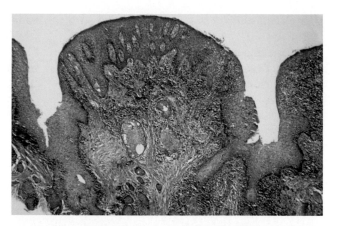

Fig. 12-18 Inflammatory papillary hyperplasia. Medium-power view showing fibrous and epithelial hyperplasia resulting in papillary surface projections. Heavy chronic inflammation is present.

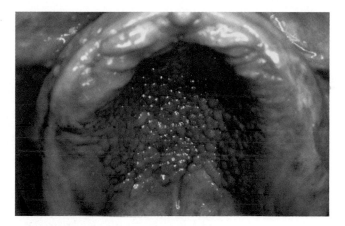

Fig. 12-17 Inflammatory papillary hyperplasia. An advanced case exhibiting more pronounced papular lesions of the hard palate.

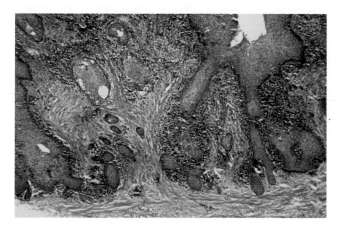

Fig. 12-19 Inflammatory papillary hyperplasia. Higher-power view showing pseudoepitheliomatous hyperplasia of the epithelium. This epithelium has a bland appearance that should not be mistaken for carcinoma.

reported in dentate patients with human immunodeficiency virus (HIV) infection.

Inflammatory papillary hyperplasia is usually asymptomatic. The mucosa is erythematous and has a pebbly or papillary surface. Many cases are associated with denture stomatitis.

HISTOPATHOLOGIC FEATURES

The mucosa in inflammatory papillary hyperplasia exhibits numerous papillary growths on the surface that are covered by hyperplastic, stratified squamous epithelium (Fig. 12-18). In advanced cases, this hyperplasia is pseudoepitheliomatous in appearance, and the pathologist should not mistake it for carcinoma (Fig. 12-19). The connective tissue can vary from loose and edematous to densely collagenized. A chronic inflammatory cell infiltrate is usually seen, which consists of lymphocytes and plasma cells. Less frequently,

polymorphonuclear leukocytes are also present. If underlying salivary glands are present, then they often show sclerosing sialadenitis.

TREATMENT AND PROGNOSIS

For very early lesions of inflammatory papillary hyperplasia, removal of the denture may allow the erythema and edema to subside, and the tissues may resume a more normal appearance. The condition also may show improvement after topical or systemic antifungal therapy. For more advanced and collagenized lesions, many clinicians prefer to excise the hyperplastic tissue before fabricating a new denture. Various surgical methods have been used, including the following:

- Partial-thickness or full-thickness surgical blade excision
- Curettage
- Electrosurgery
- Cryosurgery
- Laser surgery

After surgery, the existing denture can be lined with a temporary tissue conditioner that acts as a palatal dressing and promotes greater comfort. After healing, the patient should be encouraged to leave the new denture out at night and to keep it clean.

FIBROUS HISTIOCYTOMA

Fibrous histiocytomas are a diverse group of tumors that exhibit fibroblastic and histiocytic differentiation. Although the cell of origin is still uncertain, it may arise from the tissue histiocyte, which then assumes fibroblastic properties. Because of the variable nature of these lesions, an array of terms has been used for them, including **dermatofibroma, sclerosing hemangioma, fibroxanthoma**, and **nodular subepidermal fibrosis**. Unlike other fibrous growths discussed previously in this chapter, the fibrous histiocytoma is generally considered to represent a true neoplasm.

CLINICAL FEATURES

The fibrous histiocytoma can develop almost anywhere in the body. The most common site is the skin of the extremities, where the lesion is called a *dermatofibroma*. Tumors of the oral and perioral region are uncommon. Although oral tumors can occur at any site, the most frequent location is the buccal mucosa and vestibule. Rare intrabony lesions of the jaws have also been reported. Oral fibrous histiocytomas tend to occur in middle-aged and older adults; cutaneous examples are most frequent in young adults. The tumor is usually a painless nodular mass and can vary in size from a few millimeters to several centimeters in diameter (Fig. 12-20). Deeper tumors tend to be larger.

HISTOPATHOLOGIC FEATURES

Microscopically, the fibrous histiocytoma is characterized by a cellular proliferation of spindle-shaped fibroblastic cells with vesicular nuclei (Figs. 12-21 and 12-22). The margins of the tumor often are not sharply defined. The tumor cells are arranged in short, intersecting fascicles, known as a *storiform* pattern because of its resemblance to the irregular, whorled appearance of a straw mat. Rounded histiocyte-like cells, lipid-containing xanthoma cells, or multinucleated giant cells can be seen occasionally, as may scattered

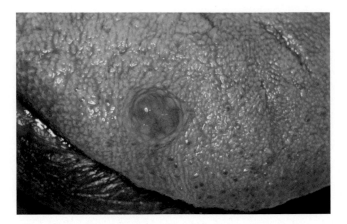

Fig. 12-20   Fibrous histiocytoma. Nodular mass on the dorsum of the tongue.

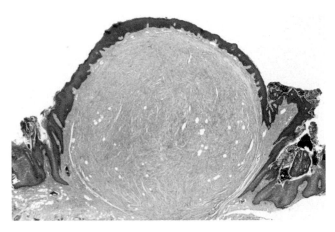

Fig. 12-21   Fibrous histiocytoma. Low-power view showing a moderately cellular nodular tumor of the tongue.

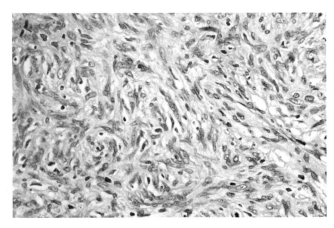

Fig. 12-22   Fibrous histiocytoma. High-power view demonstrating storiform arrangement of spindle-shaped cells with vesicular nuclei.

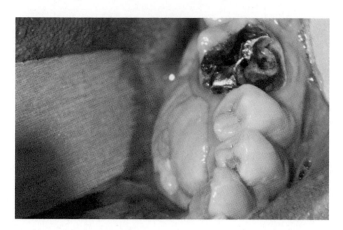

Fig. 12-23   Fibromatosis. Locally aggressive proliferation of fibrous connective tissue of the lingual mandibular gingival mucosa.

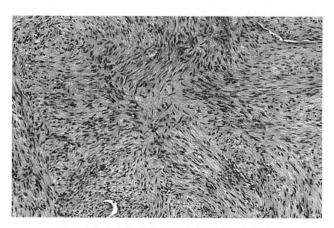

Fig. 12-24   Fibromatosis. Streaming fascicles of fibroblastic cells that demonstrate little pleomorphism.

lymphocytes. The stroma may demonstrate areas of myxoid change or focal hyalinization.

TREATMENT AND PROGNOSIS

Local surgical excision is the treatment of choice. Recurrence is uncommon, especially for superficial tumors. Larger lesions of the deeper soft tissues have a greater potential to recur.

FIBROMATOSIS

The **fibromatoses** are a broad group of fibrous proliferations that have a biologic behavior and histopathologic pattern that is intermediate between those of benign fibrous lesions and fibrosarcoma. A number of different forms of fibromatosis are recognized throughout the body, and they often are named based on their particular clinicopathologic features. In the soft tissues of the head and neck, these lesions are frequently called **juvenile aggressive fibromatoses** or **extraabdominal desmoids**. Similar lesions within the bone have been called **desmoplastic fibromas** (see page 658). Individuals with familial adenomatous polyposis and Gardner syndrome (see page 651) have a greatly increased risk for developing aggressive fibromatosis.

CLINICAL AND RADIOGRAPHIC FEATURES

Soft tissue fibromatosis of the head and neck is a firm, painless mass, which may exhibit rapid or insidious growth (Fig. 12-23). The lesion most frequently occurs in children or young adults; hence, the term **juvenile fibromatosis**. However, cases also have been seen in middle-aged adults. The most common oral site is the paramandibular soft tissue region, although the lesion

can occur almost anywhere. The tumor can grow to considerable size, resulting in significant facial disfigurement. Destruction of adjacent bone may be observed on radiographs and other imaging studies.

HISTOPATHOLOGIC FEATURES

Soft tissue fibromatosis is characterized by a cellular proliferation of spindle-shaped cells that are arranged in streaming fascicles and are associated with a variable amount of collagen (Fig. 12-24). The lesion is usually poorly circumscribed and infiltrates the adjacent tissues. Hyperchromatism and pleomorphism of the cells should not be observed.

TREATMENT AND PROGNOSIS

Because of its locally aggressive nature, the preferred treatment for soft tissue fibromatosis is wide excision that includes a generous margin of adjacent normal tissues. Adjuvant chemotherapy or radiation therapy sometimes has been used for incompletely resected or recurrent tumors. A 23% recurrence rate has been reported for oral and paraoral fibromatosis, but a higher recurrence rate has been noted for other head and neck sites. Metastasis does not occur.

MYOFIBROMA (MYOFIBROMATOSIS)

Myofibroma is a rare spindle cell neoplasm that consists of myofibroblasts (i.e., cells with both smooth muscle and fibroblastic features). Such cells are not specific for this lesion, however, because they also can be identified in other fibrous proliferations. Most myofibromas occur as solitary lesions, but some patients develop a multicentric tumor process known as **myofibromatosis**.

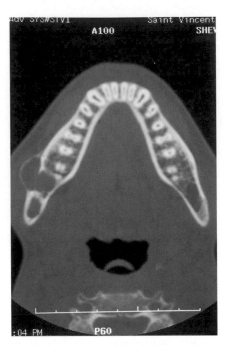

Fig. 12-25   Myofibroma. Computed tomography (CT) scan showing an expansile lytic mass of the posterior mandible on the left side of the illustration. *(Courtesy of Dr. Timothy Armanini.)*

CLINICAL AND RADIOGRAPHIC FEATURES

Although myofibromas are rare neoplasms, they demonstrate a predilection for the head and neck region. Solitary tumors develop most frequently in the first 4 decades of life, with a mean age of 22 years. The most common oral location is the mandible, followed by the tongue and buccal mucosa. The tumor is typically a painless mass that sometimes exhibits rapid enlargement. Intrabony tumors create radiolucent defects that usually tend to be poorly defined, although some may be well defined or multilocular (Fig. 12-25). Multicentric myofibromatosis primarily affects neonates and infants who may have tumors of the skin, subcutaneous tissue, muscle, bone, and viscera. The number of tumors can vary from several to more than 100.

HISTOPATHOLOGIC FEATURES

Myofibromas are composed of interlacing bundles of spindle cells with tapered or blunt-ended nuclei and eosinophilic cytoplasm (Fig. 12-26). Nodular fascicles may alternate with more cellular zones, imparting a biphasic appearance to the tumor. Scattered mitoses are not uncommon. Centrally, the lesion is often more vascular with a hemangiopericytoma-like appearance. The tumor cells are positive for smooth muscle actin and muscle-specific actin with immunohistochemistry, but they are negative for desmin.

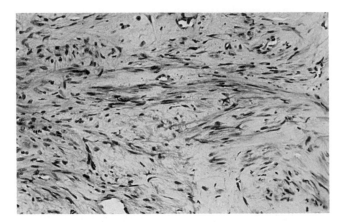

Fig. 12-26   Myofibromatosis. Proliferation of spindle-shaped cells with both fibroblastic and smooth muscle features.

TREATMENT AND PROGNOSIS

Solitary myofibromas are usually treated by surgical excision. A small percentage of tumors will recur after treatment, but typically, these can be controlled with reexcision. Multifocal tumors arising in soft tissues and bone rarely recur after surgical excision. Spontaneous regression may occur in some cases. However, myofibromatosis involving the viscera or vital organs in infants can act more aggressively and sometimes proves to be fatal within a few days after birth.

ORAL FOCAL MUCINOSIS

Oral focal mucinosis is an uncommon tumorlike mass that is believed to represent the oral counterpart of cutaneous focal mucinosis or a cutaneous myxoid cyst. The cause is unknown, although the lesion may result from overproduction of hyaluronic acid by fibroblasts.

CLINICAL FEATURES

Oral focal mucinosis is most common in young adults and shows a 2:1 female-to-male predilection. The gingiva is the most common site; two thirds to three fourths of all cases are found there. The hard palate is the second most common location. The mass rarely appears at other oral sites. The lesion usually presents as a sessile or pedunculated, painless nodular mass that is the same color as the surrounding mucosa (Fig. 12-27). The surface is typically smooth and nonulcerated, although occasional cases exhibit a lobulated appearance. The size varies from a few millimeters up to 2 cm in diameter. The patient often has been aware of the mass for many months or years before the diagnosis is made.

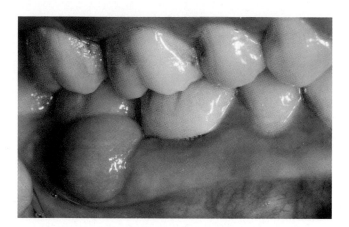

Fig. 12-27   Oral focal mucinosis. Nodular mass arising from the gingiva between the mandibular first and second molars.

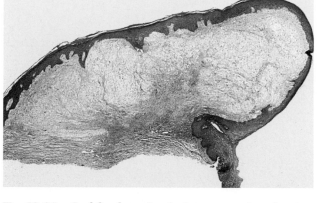

Fig. 12-28   Oral focal mucinosis. Low-power view showing a nodular mass of loose, myxomatous connective tissue.

HISTOPATHOLOGIC FEATURES

Microscopic examination of oral focal mucinosis shows a well-localized but nonencapsulated area of loose, myxomatous connective tissue surrounded by denser, normal collagenous connective tissue (Figs. 12-28 and 12-29). The lesion is usually found just beneath the surface epithelium and often causes flattening of the rete ridges. The fibroblasts within the mucinous area can be ovoid, fusiform, or stellate, and they may demonstrate delicate, fibrillar processes. Few capillaries are seen within the lesion, especially compared with the surrounding denser collagen. Similarly, no significant inflammation is observed, although a perivascular lymphocytic infiltrate often is noted within the surrounding collagenous connective tissue. No appreciable reticulin is evident within the lesion, and special stains suggest that the mucinous product is hyaluronic acid.

TREATMENT AND PROGNOSIS

Oral focal mucinosis is treated by surgical excision and does not tend to recur.

PYOGENIC GRANULOMA

The **pyogenic granuloma** is a common tumorlike growth of the oral cavity that traditionally has been considered to be nonneoplastic in nature.* Although it was originally thought to be caused by pyogenic organisms, it is now believed to be unrelated to infection.

---

*However, some pyogenic granulomas (also known as *lobular capillary hemangiomas*) currently are categorized as *vascular tumors* under the classification scheme of the International Society for the Study of Vascular Anomalies (see Box 12-2, page 539).

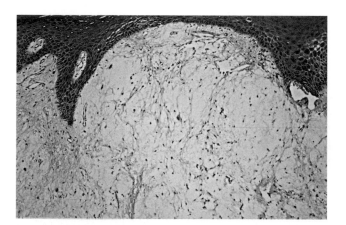

Fig. 12-29   Oral focal mucinosis. High-power view demonstrating the myxomatous change.

Instead, the pyogenic granuloma is thought to represent an exuberant tissue response to local irritation or trauma. In spite of its name, it is not a true granuloma.

CLINICAL FEATURES

The pyogenic granuloma is a smooth or lobulated mass that is usually pedunculated, although some lesions are sessile (Figs. 12-30 to 12-32). The surface is characteristically ulcerated and ranges from pink to red to purple, depending on the age of the lesion. Young pyogenic granulomas are highly vascular in appearance; older lesions tend to become more collagenized and pink. They vary from small growths only a few millimeters in size to larger lesions that may measure several centimeters in diameter. Typically, the mass is painless, although it often bleeds easily because of its extreme vascularity. Pyogenic granulomas may exhibit rapid

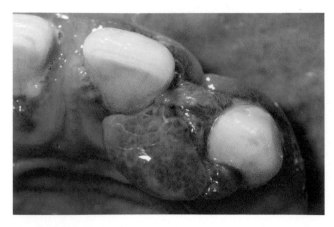

Fig. 12-30   Pyogenic granuloma. Erythematous, hemorrhagic mass arising from the maxillary anterior gingiva.

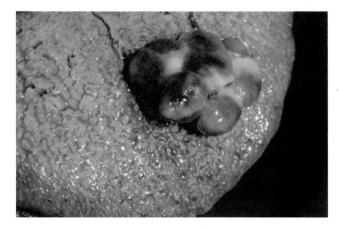

Fig. 12-31   Pyogenic granuloma. Ulcerated and lobulated mass on the dorsum of the tongue.

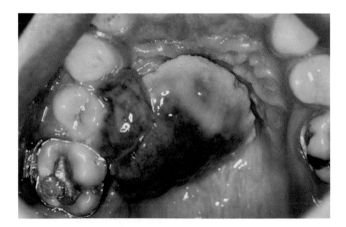

Fig. 12-32   Pyogenic granuloma. Unusually large lesion arising from the palatal gingiva in association with an orthodontic band. The patient was pregnant.

growth, which may create alarm for both the patient and the clinician, who may fear that the lesion might be malignant.

Oral pyogenic granulomas show a striking predilection for the gingiva, which accounts for 75% of all cases. Gingival irritation and inflammation that result from poor oral hygiene may be a precipitating factor in many patients. The lips, tongue, and buccal mucosa are the next most common sites. A history of trauma before the development of the lesion is not unusual, especially for extragingival pyogenic granulomas. Lesions are slightly more common on the maxillary gingiva than the mandibular gingiva; anterior areas are more frequently affected than posterior areas. These lesions are much more common on the facial aspect of the gingiva than the lingual aspect; some extend between the teeth and involve both the facial and the lingual gingiva.

Although the pyogenic granuloma can develop at any age, it is most common in children and young adults. Most studies also demonstrate a definite female predilection, possibly because of the vascular effects of female hormones. Pyogenic granulomas of the gingiva frequently develop in pregnant women, so much so that the terms *pregnancy tumor* or *granuloma gravidarum* often are used. Such lesions may begin to develop during the first trimester, and their incidence increases up through the seventh month of pregnancy. The gradual rise in development of these lesions throughout pregnancy may be related to the increasing levels of estrogen and progesterone as the pregnancy progresses. After pregnancy and the return of normal hormone levels, some of these pyogenic granulomas resolve without treatment or undergo fibrous maturation and resemble a fibroma (Fig. 12-33).

Epulis granulomatosa is a term used to describe hyperplastic growths of granulation tissue that sometimes arise in healing extraction sockets (Fig. 12-34). These lesions resemble pyogenic granulomas and usually represent a granulation tissue reaction to bony sequestra in the socket.

HISTOPATHOLOGIC FEATURES

Microscopic examination of pyogenic granulomas shows a highly vascular proliferation that resembles granulation tissue (Figs. 12-35 and 12-36). Numerous small and larger endothelium-lined channels are formed that are engorged with red blood cells. These vessels sometimes are organized in lobular aggregates, and some pathologists require this lobular arrangement for the diagnosis (*lobular capillary hemangioma*). The surface is usually ulcerated and replaced by a thick fibrinopurulent membrane. A mixed inflammatory cell infiltrate of neutrophils, plasma cells, and lymphocytes

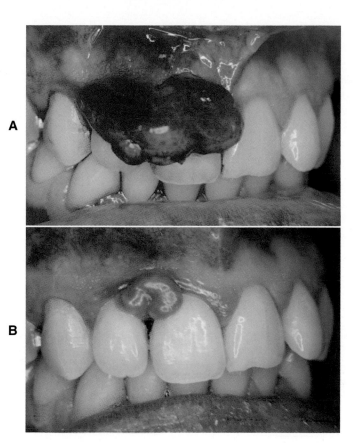

Fig. 12-33   Pyogenic granuloma. A, Large gingival mass in a pregnant woman just before childbirth. **B,** The mass has decreased in size and undergone fibrous maturation 3 months after childbirth. *(Courtesy of Dr. George Blozis.)*

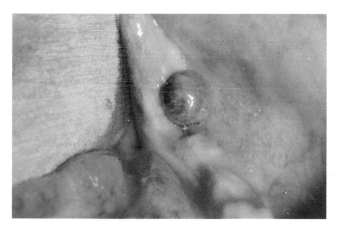

Fig. 12-34   Epulis granulomatosa. Nodular mass of granulation tissue that developed in a recent extraction site.

is evident. Neutrophils are most prevalent near the ulcerated surface; chronic inflammatory cells are found deeper in the specimen. Older lesions may have areas with a more fibrous appearance. In fact, many gingival fibromas probably represent pyogenic granulomas that have undergone fibrous maturation.

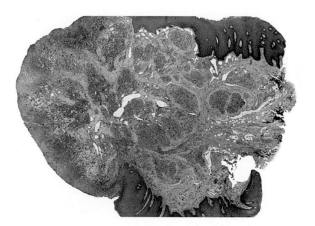

Fig. 12-35   Pyogenic granuloma. Low-power view showing an exophytic mass of granulation-like tissue with an ulcerated surface. Note the lobular endothelial proliferation in the deeper connective tissue.

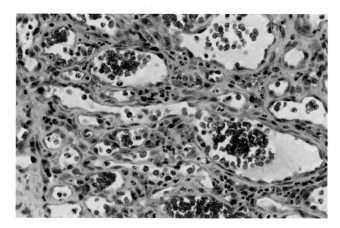

Fig. 12-36   Pyogenic granuloma. Higher-power view showing capillary blood vessels and scattered inflammation.

TREATMENT AND PROGNOSIS

The treatment of patients with pyogenic granuloma consists of conservative surgical excision, which is usually curative. The specimen should be submitted for microscopic examination to rule out other more serious diagnoses. For gingival lesions, the excision should extend down to periosteum and the adjacent teeth should be thoroughly scaled to remove any source of continuing irritation. Occasionally, the lesion recurs and reexcision is necessary. In rare instances, multiple recurrences have been noted.

For lesions that develop during pregnancy, usually treatment should be deferred unless significant functional or aesthetic problems develop. The recurrence rate is higher for pyogenic granulomas removed during pregnancy, and some lesions will resolve spontaneously after parturition.

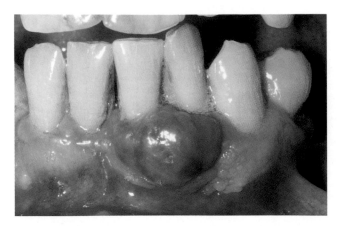

Fig. 12-37   Peripheral giant cell granuloma. Nodular blue-purple mass of the mandibular gingiva.

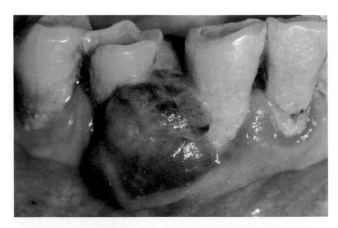

Fig. 12-38   Peripheral giant cell granuloma. Ulcerated mass of the mandibular gingiva.

PERIPHERAL GIANT CELL GRANULOMA (GIANT CELL EPULIS)

The **peripheral giant cell granuloma** is a relatively common tumorlike growth of the oral cavity. It probably does not represent a true neoplasm but rather is a reactive lesion caused by local irritation or trauma. In the past, it often was called a *peripheral giant cell reparative granuloma*, but any reparative nature appears doubtful. Some investigators believe that the giant cells show immunohistochemical features of osteoclasts, whereas other authors have suggested that the lesion is formed by cells from the mononuclear phagocyte system. The peripheral giant cell granuloma bears a close microscopic resemblance to the **central giant cell granuloma** (see page 626), and some pathologists believe that it may represent a soft tissue counterpart of this central bony lesion.

CLINICAL AND RADIOGRAPHIC FEATURES

The peripheral giant cell granuloma occurs exclusively on the gingiva or edentulous alveolar ridge, presenting as a red or red-blue nodular mass (Figs. 12-37 and 12-38). Most lesions are smaller than 2 cm in diameter, although larger ones are seen occasionally. The lesion can be sessile or pedunculated and may or may not be ulcerated. The clinical appearance is similar to the more common pyogenic granuloma of the gingiva (see page 517), although the peripheral giant cell granuloma often is more blue-purple compared with the bright red of a typical pyogenic granuloma.

Peripheral giant cell granulomas can develop at almost any age, especially during the first through sixth decades of life. The mean age in several large series ranges from 31 to 41 years. Approximately 60% of cases occur in females. It may develop in either the anterior or posterior regions of the gingiva or alveolar mucosa, and the mandible is affected slightly more often than the maxilla. Although the peripheral giant cell granuloma develops within soft tissue, "cupping" resorption of the underlying alveolar bone sometimes is seen. On occasion, it may be difficult to determine whether the mass arose as a peripheral lesion or as a central giant cell granuloma that eroded through the cortical plate into the gingival soft tissues.

HISTOPATHOLOGIC FEATURES

Microscopic examination of a peripheral giant cell granuloma shows a proliferation of multinucleated giant cells within a background of plump ovoid and spindle-shaped mesenchymal cells (Figs. 12-39 and 12-40). The giant cells may contain only a few nuclei or up to several dozen. Some of these cells may have large, vesicular nuclei; others demonstrate small, pyknotic nuclei. Mitotic figures are fairly common in the background mesenchymal cells. Abundant hemorrhage is characteristically found throughout the mass, which often results in deposits of hemosiderin pigment, especially at the periphery of the lesion.

The overlying mucosal surface is ulcerated in about 50% of cases. A zone of dense fibrous connective tissue usually separates the giant cell proliferation from the mucosal surface. Adjacent acute and chronic inflammatory cells are frequently present. Areas of reactive bone formation or dystrophic calcifications are not unusual.

TREATMENT AND PROGNOSIS

The treatment of the peripheral giant cell granuloma consists of local surgical excision down to the underlying bone. The adjacent teeth should be carefully scaled to remove any source of irritation and to minimize the risk of recurrence. Approximately 10% of lesions are reported to recur, and reexcision must be performed.

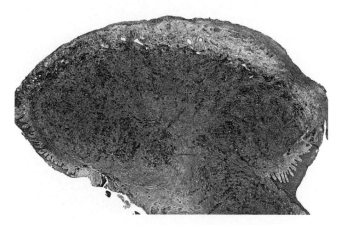

Fig. 12-39   Peripheral giant cell granuloma. Low-power view showing a nodular proliferation of multinucleated giant cells within the gingiva.

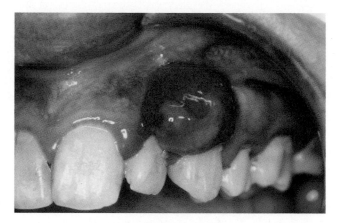

Fig. 12-41   Peripheral ossifying fibroma. Red, ulcerated mass of the maxillary gingiva. Such ulcerated lesions are easily mistaken for a pyogenic granuloma.

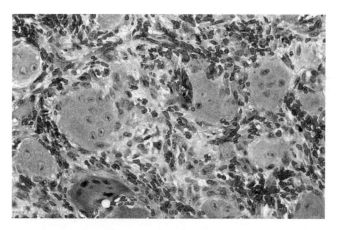

Fig. 12-40   Peripheral giant cell granuloma. High-power view showing scattered multinucleated giant cells within a hemorrhagic background of ovoid and spindle-shaped mesenchymal cells.

On rare occasions, lesions indistinguishable from peripheral giant cell granulomas have been seen in patients with hyperparathyroidism (see page 838). They apparently represent the so-called osteoclastic brown tumors associated with this endocrine disorder. However, the brown tumors of hyperparathyroidism are much more likely to be intraosseous in location and mimic a central giant cell granuloma.

PERIPHERAL OSSIFYING FIBROMA (OSSIFYING FIBROID EPULIS; PERIPHERAL FIBROMA WITH CALCIFICATION; CALCIFYING FIBROBLASTIC GRANULOMA)

The **peripheral ossifying fibroma** is a relatively common gingival growth that is considered to be reactive rather than neoplastic in nature. The pathogenesis of this lesion is uncertain. Because of their clinical and histopathologic similarities, researchers believe that some peripheral ossifying fibromas develop initially as pyogenic granulomas that undergo fibrous maturation and subsequent calcification. However, not all peripheral ossifying fibromas may develop in this manner. The mineralized product probably has its origin from cells of the periosteum or periodontal ligament.

Considerable confusion has existed over the nomenclature of this lesion, and several terms have been used to describe its variable histopathologic features. In the past, the terms *peripheral odontogenic fibroma* (see page 727) and *peripheral ossifying fibroma* often were used synonymously, but the peripheral odontogenic fibroma is now considered to be a distinct and separate entity. In addition, in spite of the similarity in names, the peripheral ossifying fibroma does not represent the soft tissue counterpart of the central ossifying fibroma (see page 646).

CLINICAL FEATURES

The peripheral ossifying fibroma occurs exclusively on the gingiva. It appears as a nodular mass, either pedunculated or sessile, that usually emanates from the interdental papilla (Figs. 12-41 and 12-42). The color ranges from red to pink, and the surface is frequently, but not always, ulcerated. The growth probably begins as an ulcerated lesion; older ones are more likely to demonstrate healing of the ulcer and an intact surface. Red, ulcerated lesions often are mistaken for pyogenic granulomas; the pink, nonulcerated ones are clinically similar to irritation fibromas. Most lesions are less than 2 cm in size, although larger ones occasionally occur. The lesion often has been present for many weeks or months before the diagnosis is made.

The peripheral ossifying fibroma is predominantly a lesion of teenagers and young adults, with peak prevalence between the ages of 10 and 19. Almost two thirds

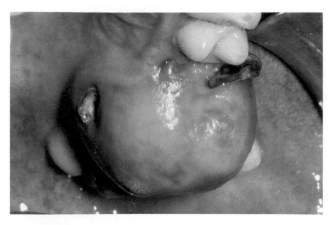

Fig. 12-42 Peripheral ossifying fibroma. Pink, nonulcerated mass arising from the maxillary gingiva. The remaining roots of the first molar are present.

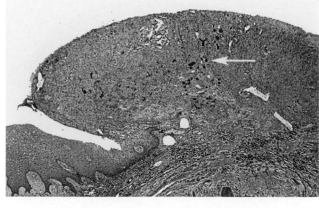

Fig. 12-43 Peripheral ossifying fibroma. Ulcerated gingival mass demonstrating focal early mineralization (*arrow*).

of all cases occur in females. There is a slight predilection for the maxillary arch, and more than 50% of all cases occur in the incisor-cuspid region. Usually, the teeth are unaffected; rarely, there can be migration and loosening of adjacent teeth.

HISTOPATHOLOGIC FEATURES

The basic microscopic pattern of the peripheral ossifying fibroma is one of a fibrous proliferation associated with the formation of a mineralized product (Figs. 12-43 and 12-44). If the epithelium is ulcerated, then the surface is covered by a fibrinopurulent membrane with a subjacent zone of granulation tissue. The deeper fibroblastic component often is cellular, especially in areas of mineralization. In some cases, the fibroblastic proliferation and associated mineralization is only a small component of a larger mass that resembles a fibroma or pyogenic granuloma.

The type of mineralized component is variable and may consist of bone, cementum-like material, or dystrophic calcifications. Frequently, a combination of products is formed. Usually, the bone is woven and trabecular in type, although older lesions may demonstrate mature lamellar bone. Trabeculae of unmineralized osteoid are not unusual. Less frequently, ovoid droplets of basophilic cementum-like material are formed. Dystrophic calcifications are characterized by multiple granules, tiny globules, or large, irregular masses of basophilic mineralized material. Such dystrophic calcifications are more common in early, ulcerated lesions; older, nonulcerated examples are more likely to demonstrate well-formed bone or cementum. In some cases, multinucleated giant cells may be found, usually in association with the mineralized product.

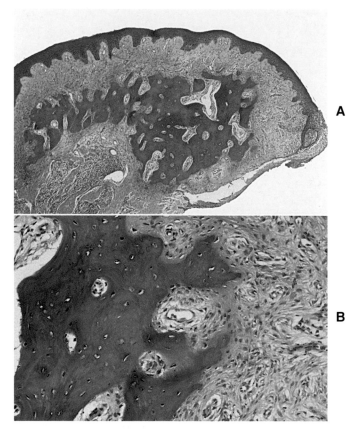

Fig. 12-44 Peripheral ossifying fibroma. A, Nonulcerated fibrous mass of the gingiva showing central bone formation. **B,** Higher-power view showing trabeculae of bone with adjacent fibrous connective tissue.

TREATMENT AND PROGNOSIS

The treatment of choice for the peripheral ossifying fibroma is local surgical excision with submission of the specimen for histopathologic examination. The mass should be excised down to periosteum because recurrence is more likely if the base of the lesion is allowed to remain. In addition, the adjacent teeth should be thoroughly scaled to eliminate any possible irritants. Periodontal surgical techniques, such as repositioned flaps or connective tissue grafts, may be necessary to repair the gingival defect in an aesthetic manner. Although excision is usually curative, a recurrence rate of 8% to 16% has been reported.

LIPOMA

The **lipoma** is a benign tumor of fat. Although it represents by far the most common mesenchymal neoplasm, most examples occur on the trunk and proximal portions of the extremities. Lipomas of the oral and maxillofacial region are much less frequent. The pathogenesis of lipomas is uncertain, but they appear to be more common in obese people. However, the metabolism of lipomas is completely independent of the normal body fat. If the caloric intake is reduced, then lipomas do not decrease in size, although normal body fat may be lost.

CLINICAL FEATURES

Oral lipomas are usually soft, smooth-surfaced nodular masses that can be sessile or pedunculated (Figs. 12-45 and 12-46). Typically, the tumor is asymptomatic and often has been noted for many months or years before diagnosis. Most are less than 3 cm in size, but occasional lesions can become much larger. Although a subtle or more obvious yellow hue often is detected clinically, deeper examples may appear pink. The buccal mucosa and buccal vestibule are the most common intraoral sites and account for 50% of all cases. Some buccal cases may not represent true tumors, but rather herniation of the buccal fat pad through the buccinator muscle, which may occur after local trauma in young children or subsequent to surgical removal of third molars in older patients. Less common sites include the tongue, floor of the mouth, and lips. Most patients are 40 years of age or older; lipomas are uncommon in children. Lipomas of the oral and maxillofacial region have shown a fairly balanced sex distribution in some studies, although one recent large series demonstrated a marked male predilection.

HISTOPATHOLOGIC FEATURES

Most oral lipomas are composed of mature fat cells that differ little in microscopic appearance from the surrounding normal fat (Figs. 12-47 and 12-48). The tumor is usually well circumscribed and may demonstrate a thin fibrous capsule. A distinct lobular arrange-

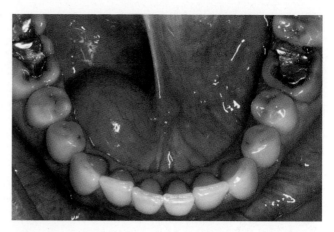

Fig. 12-45 **Lipoma.** Soft, yellow nodular mass in the floor of the mouth. *(Courtesy of Dr. Michael Tabor.)*

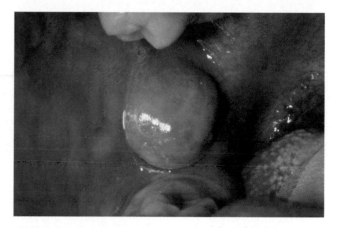

Fig. 12-46 **Lipoma.** Nodular mass of the posterior buccal mucosa.

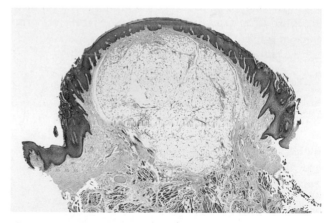

Fig. 12-47 **Lipoma.** Low-power view of a tumor of the tongue demonstrating a mass of mature adipose tissue.

ment of the cells often is seen. On rare occasions, central cartilaginous or osseous metaplasia may occur within an otherwise typical lipoma.

A number of microscopic variants have been described. The most common of these is the **fibroli-**

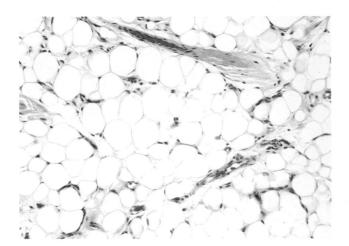

Fig. 12-48   Lipoma. High-power view showing the similarity of the tumor cells to normal fat.

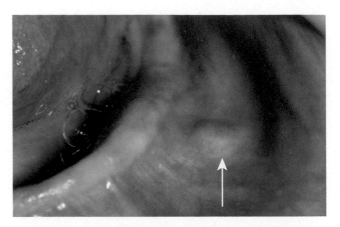

Fig. 12-49   Traumatic neuroma. Painful nodule of the mental nerve as it exits the mental foramen (*arrow*).

poma, which is characterized by a significant fibrous component intermixed with the lobules of fat cells. The remaining variants are rare.

The **angiolipoma** consists of an admixture of mature fat and numerous small blood vessels. The **spindle cell lipoma** demonstrates variable amounts of uniform-appearing spindle cells in conjunction with a more typical lipomatous component. Some spindle cell lipomas exhibit a mucoid background (*myxoid lipoma*) and may be confused with myxoid liposarcomas. **Pleomorphic lipomas** are characterized by the presence of spindle cells plus bizarre, hyperchromatic giant cells; they can be difficult to distinguish from a pleomorphic liposarcoma. **Intramuscular (infiltrating) lipomas** often are more deeply situated and have an infiltrative growth pattern that extends between skeletal muscle bundles.

TREATMENT AND PROGNOSIS

Lipomas are treated by conservative local excision, and recurrence is rare. Most microscopic variants do not affect the prognosis. Intramuscular lipomas have a higher recurrence rate because of their infiltrative growth pattern, but this variant is rare in the oral and maxillofacial region.

TRAUMATIC NEUROMA (AMPUTATION NEUROMA)

The **traumatic neuroma** is not a true neoplasm but a reactive proliferation of neural tissue after transection or other damage of a nerve bundle. After a nerve has been damaged or severed, the proximal portion attempts to regenerate and reestablish innervation of the distal segment by the growth of axons through

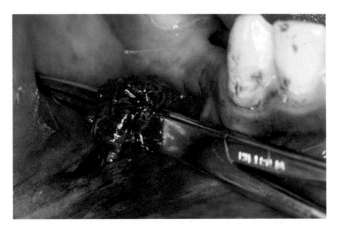

Fig. 12-50   Traumatic neuroma. Note the irregular nodular proliferation along the mental nerve that is being exposed at the time of surgery.

tubes of proliferating Schwann cells. If these regenerating elements encounter scar tissue or otherwise cannot reestablish innervation, then a tumorlike mass may develop at the site of injury.

CLINICAL AND RADIOGRAPHIC FEATURES

Traumatic neuromas of the oral mucosa are typically smooth-surfaced, nonulcerated nodules. They can develop at any location but are most common in the mental foramen area, tongue, and lower lip (Figs. 12-49 and 12-50). A history of trauma often can be elicited; some lesions arise subsequent to tooth extraction or other surgical procedures. Intraosseous traumatic neuromas may demonstrate a radiolucent defect on oral radiographs. Examples also may occur

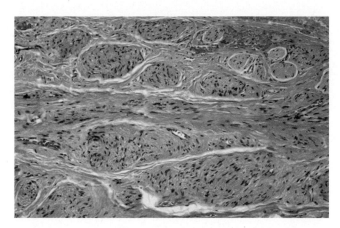

Fig. 12-51   Traumatic neuroma. Low-power view showing the haphazard arrangement of nerve bundles within the background fibrous connective tissue.

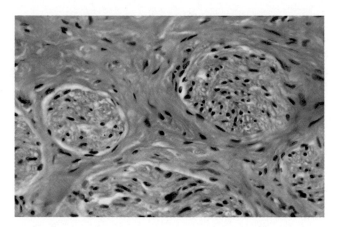

Fig. 12-52   Traumatic neuroma. High-power view showing cross-sectioned nerve bundles within dense fibrous connective tissue.

at other head and neck sites; it has been estimated that traumatic neuromas of the greater auricular nerve develop in 5% to 10% of patients undergoing surgery for pleomorphic adenomas of the parotid gland.

Traumatic neuromas can occur at any age, but they are diagnosed most often in middle-aged adults. They appear to be slightly more common in women. Many traumatic neuromas are associated with altered nerve sensations that can range from anesthesia to dysesthesia to overt pain. Although pain has been traditionally considered a hallmark of this lesion, studies indicate that only one fourth to one third of oral traumatic neuromas are painful. This pain can be intermittent or constant and ranges from mild tenderness or burning to severe radiating pain. Neuromas of the mental nerve are frequently painful, especially when impinged on by a denture or palpated.

HISTOPATHOLOGIC FEATURES

Microscopic examination of traumatic neuromas shows a haphazard proliferation of mature, myelinated and unmyelinated nerve bundles within a fibrous connective tissue stroma that ranges from densely collagenized to myxomatous in nature (Figs. 12-51 and 12-52). An associated mild chronic inflammatory cell infiltrate may be present. Traumatic neuromas with inflammation are more likely to be painful than those without significant inflammation.

TREATMENT AND PROGNOSIS

The treatment of choice for the patient with a traumatic neuroma is surgical excision, including a small portion of the involved nerve bundle. Most lesions do not recur; in some cases, however, the pain persists or returns at a later date.

PALISADED ENCAPSULATED NEUROMA (SOLITARY CIRCUMSCRIBED NEUROMA)

The **palisaded encapsulated neuroma** is a benign neural tumor with distinctive clinical and histopathologic features. Although it was first recognized only as recently as 1972, it represents one of the more common superficial nerve tumors, especially in the head and neck region. The cause is uncertain, but some authors have speculated that trauma may play an etiologic role; the tumor is generally considered to represent a reactive lesion rather than a true neoplasm.

CLINICAL FEATURES

The palisaded encapsulated neuroma shows a striking predilection for the face, which accounts for approximately 90% of reported cases. The nose and cheek are the most common specific sites. The lesion is most frequently diagnosed between the fifth and seventh decades of life, although the tumor often has been present for many months or years. It is a smooth-surfaced, painless, dome-shaped papule or nodule that is usually less than 1 cm in diameter. There is no sex predilection.

Oral palisaded encapsulated neuromas are not uncommon, although many are probably diagnosed microscopically as neurofibromas or neurilemomas. The lesion appears most frequently on the hard palate (Fig. 12-53) and maxillary labial mucosa, although it also may occur in other oral locations.

HISTOPATHOLOGIC FEATURES

Palisaded encapsulated neuromas appear well circumscribed and often encapsulated (Fig. 12-54), although this capsule may be incomplete, especially along the

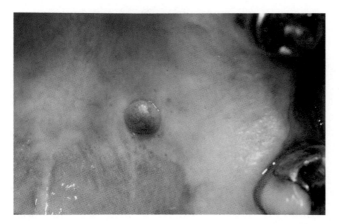

Fig. 12-53   Palisaded encapsulated neuroma. Small, painless nodule of the lateral hard palate.

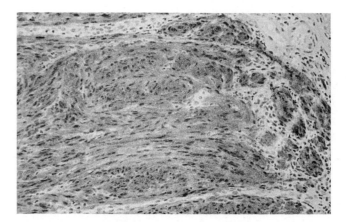

Fig. 12-55   Palisaded encapsulated neuroma. Immunohistochemical reaction demonstrating spindle-shaped cells that are strongly positive for S-100 protein.

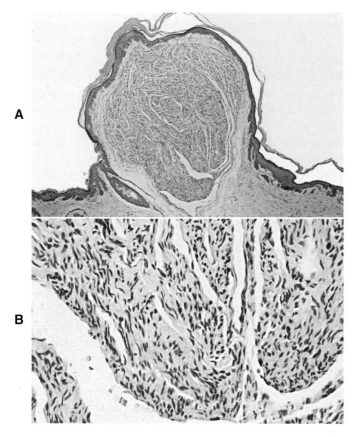

Fig. 12-54   Palisaded encapsulated neuroma. A, Low-power view showing a well-circumscribed, nodular proliferation of neural tissue. **B,** Higher-power view demonstrating spindle cells with wavy nuclei.

superficial aspect of the tumor. Some lesions have a lobulated appearance. The tumor consists of moderately cellular interlacing fascicles of spindle cells that are consistent with Schwann cells. The nuclei are characteristically wavy and pointed, with no significant pleomorphism or mitotic activity. Although the nuclei

show a similar parallel orientation within the fascicles, the more definite palisading and **Verocay bodies** typical of the **Antoni A** tissue of a neurilemoma are usually not seen. Special stains reveal the presence of numerous axons within the tumor and the cells show a positive immunohistochemical reaction for S-100 protein (Fig. 12-55). Because the tumor is not always encapsulated and the cells are usually not truly palisaded, some pathologists prefer **solitary circumscribed neuroma** as a better descriptive term for this lesion.

TREATMENT AND PROGNOSIS

The treatment for the palisaded encapsulated neuroma consists of conservative local surgical excision. Recurrence is rare. However, specific recognition of this lesion is important because it is not associated with neurofibromatosis or multiple endocrine neoplasia (MEN) type 2B.

NEURILEMOMA (SCHWANNOMA)

The **neurilemoma** is a benign neural neoplasm of Schwann cell origin. It is relatively uncommon, although 25% to 48% of all cases occur in the head and neck region. Bilateral neurilemomas of the auditory-vestibular nerve are a characteristic feature of the hereditary condition, **neurofibromatosis type II** (NF2).

CLINICAL AND RADIOGRAPHIC FEATURES

The solitary neurilemoma is a slow-growing, encapsulated tumor that typically arises in association with a nerve trunk. As it grows, it pushes the nerve aside.

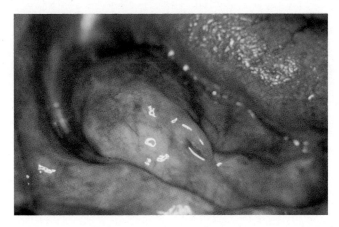

Fig. 12-56 **Neurilemoma.** Nodular mass in the floor of the mouth. (*Courtesy of Dr. Art A. Gonty.*)

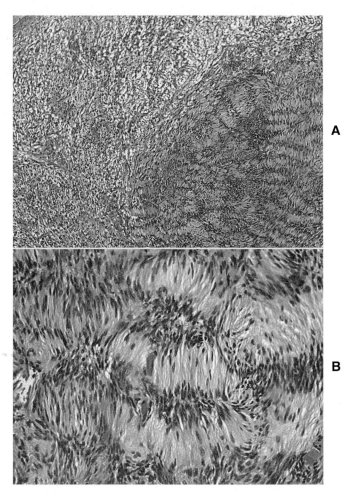

Fig. 12-57 **Neurilemoma. A,** Low-power view showing well-organized Antoni A tissue (*right*) with adjacent myxoid and less organized Antoni B tissue (*left*). **B,** The Schwann cells of the Antoni A tissue form a palisaded arrangement around acellular zones known as *Verocay bodies.*

Usually, the mass is asymptomatic, although tenderness or pain may occur in some instances. The lesion is most common in young and middle-aged adults and can range from a few millimeters to several centimeters in size.

The tongue is the most common location for oral neurilemomas, although the tumor can occur almost anywhere in the mouth (Fig. 12-56). On occasion, the tumor arises centrally within bone and may produce bony expansion. Intraosseous examples are most common in the posterior mandible and usually appear as either unilocular or multilocular radiolucencies on radiographs. Pain and paresthesia are not unusual for intrabony tumors.

NF2 is an autosomal dominant condition caused by a mutation of a tumor suppressor gene on chromosome 22, which codes for a protein known as *merlin.* In addition to bilateral neurilemomas ("acoustic neuromas") of the vestibular nerve, patients also develop neurilemomas of peripheral nerves, plus meningiomas and ependymomas of the central nervous system (CNS). Characteristic symptoms include progressive sensorineural deafness, dizziness, and tinnitus.

HISTOPATHOLOGIC FEATURES

The neurilemoma is usually an encapsulated tumor that demonstrates two microscopic patterns in varying amounts: (1) **Antoni A** and (2) **Antoni B.** Streaming fascicles of spindle-shaped Schwann cells characterize Antoni A tissue. These cells often form a palisaded arrangement around central acellular, eosinophilic areas known as **Verocay bodies** (Fig. 12-57). These Verocay bodies consist of reduplicated basement membrane and cytoplasmic processes. Antoni B tissue is less cellular and less organized; the spindle cells are randomly arranged within a loose, myxomatous stroma. Typically, neurites cannot be demonstrated within the tumor mass. The tumor cells will show a diffuse, positive immunohistochemical reaction for S-100 protein.

Degenerative changes can be seen in some older tumors (*ancient neurilemomas*). These changes consist of hemorrhage, hemosiderin deposits, inflammation, fibrosis, and nuclear atypia. However, these tumors are still benign, and the pathologist must be careful not to mistake these alterations for evidence of a sarcoma.

TREATMENT AND PROGNOSIS

The solitary neurilemoma is treated by surgical excision, and the lesion should not recur. Malignant transformation does not occur or is extremely rare.

Vestibular schwannomas in patients with NF2 are difficult to manage. Surgical removal is indicated for

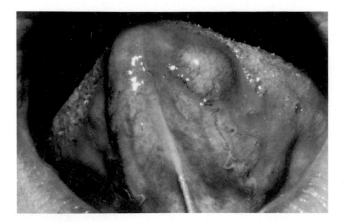

Fig. 12-58 **Neurofibroma.** Nodular mass of the anterior ventral tongue. *(Courtesy of Dr. Lindsey Douglas.)*

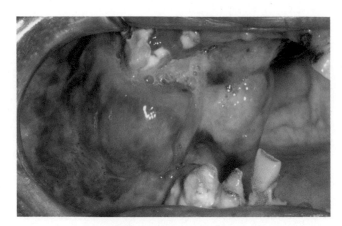

Fig. 12-59 **Neurofibroma.** Huge tumor involving the maxillary gingiva and hard palate.

large symptomatic tumors, but this almost always results in total deafness and risks facial nerve damage. Stereotactic radiosurgery may be considered for older adult or frail patients, as well as for individuals who decline traditional surgery.

NEUROFIBROMA

The **neurofibroma** is the most common type of peripheral nerve neoplasm. It arises from a mixture of cell types, including Schwann cells and perineural fibroblasts.

CLINICAL AND RADIOGRAPHIC FEATURES

Neurofibromas can arise as solitary tumors or be a component of neurofibromatosis (see page 529). Solitary tumors are most common in young adults and present as slow-growing, soft, painless lesions that vary in size from small nodules to larger masses. The skin is the most frequent location for neurofibromas, but lesions of the oral cavity are not uncommon (Figs. 12-58 and 12-59). The tongue and buccal mucosa are the most common intraoral sites. On rare occasions, the tumor can arise centrally within bone, where it may produce a well-demarcated or poorly defined unilocular or multilocular radiolucency (Fig. 12-60).

HISTOPATHOLOGIC FEATURES

The solitary neurofibroma often is well circumscribed, especially when the proliferation occurs within the perineurium of the involved nerve. Tumors that proliferate outside the perineurium may not appear well demarcated and tend to blend with the adjacent connective tissues.

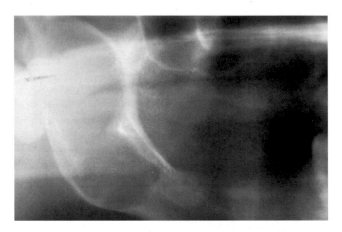

Fig. 12-60 **Neurofibroma.** Intraosseous tumor filling the right mandibular ramus. *(Courtesy of Dr. Paul Allen.)*

The tumor is composed of interlacing bundles of spindle-shaped cells that often exhibit wavy nuclei (Figs. 12-61 and 12-62). These cells are associated with delicate collagen bundles and variable amounts of myxoid matrix. Mast cells tend to be numerous and can be a helpful diagnostic feature. Sparsely distributed small axons usually can be demonstrated within the tumor tissue by using silver stains. Immunohistochemically, the tumor cells show a scattered, positive reaction for S-100 protein.

TREATMENT AND PROGNOSIS

The treatment for solitary neurofibromas is local surgical excision, and recurrence is rare. Any patient with a lesion that is diagnosed as a neurofibroma should be evaluated clinically for the possibility of **neurofibromatosis** (see next topic). Malignant transformation of solitary neurofibromas can occur, although the risk

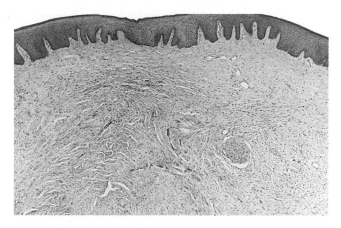

Fig. 12-61   Neurofibroma. Low-power view showing a cellular tumor mass below the epithelial surface.

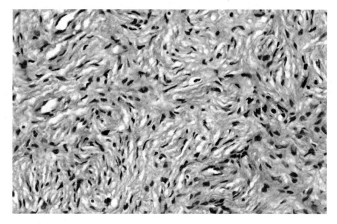

Fig. 12-62   Neurofibroma. High-power view showing spindle-shaped cells with wavy nuclei.

appears to be remote, especially compared with that in patients with neurofibromatosis.

NEUROFIBROMATOSIS TYPE I (VON RECKLINGHAUSEN'S DISEASE OF THE SKIN)

Neurofibromatosis is a relatively common hereditary condition that is estimated to occur in one of every 3000 births. At least eight forms of neurofibromatosis have been recognized, but the most common form is **neurofibromatosis type I (NF1)**, which is discussed here. This form of the disease, also known as **von Recklinghausen's disease of the skin**, accounts for 85% to 97% of cases and is inherited as an autosomal dominant trait (although 50% of all patients have no family history and apparently represent new mutations). It is caused by a variety of mutations of the *NF1* gene, which is located on chromosome region 17q11.2 and is responsible for a tumor suppressor protein product known as *neurofibromin*.

Box 12-1

Diagnostic Criteria for Neurofibromatosis Type I (NF1)

The diagnostic criteria are met if a patient has two or more of the following features:
1. Six or more *café au lait* macules more than 5 mm in greatest diameter in prepubertal persons and more than 15 mm in greatest diameter in postpubertal persons
2. Two or more neurofibromas of any type or one plexiform neurofibroma
3. Freckling in the axillary or inguinal regions
4. Optic glioma
5. Two or more Lisch nodules (iris hamartomas)
6. A distinctive osseous lesion such as sphenoid dysplasia or thinning of long bone cortex with or without pseudoarthrosis
7. A first-degree relative (parent, sibling, or offspring) with NF1, based on the previously mentioned criteria

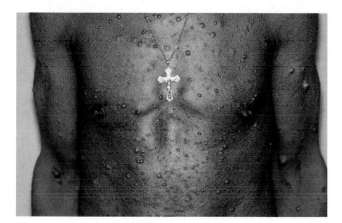

Fig. 12-63   Neurofibromatosis type I. Multiple tumors of the trunk and arms.

CLINICAL AND RADIOGRAPHIC FEATURES

The diagnostic criteria for NF1 are summarized in Box 12-1. Patients have multiple neurofibromas that can occur anywhere in the body but are most common on the skin. The clinical appearance can vary from small papules to larger soft nodules to massive baggy, pendulous masses (**elephantiasis neuromatosa**) on the skin (Figs. 12-63 and 12-64). The plexiform variant of neurofibroma, which feels like a "bag of worms," is considered pathognomonic for NF1. The tumors may be present at birth, but they often begin to appear during puberty and may continue to develop slowly throughout adulthood. Accelerated growth may be seen during

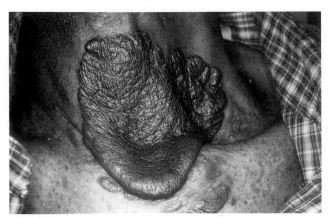

Fig. 12-64   Neurofibromatosis type I. Baggy, pendulous neurofibroma of the lower neck.

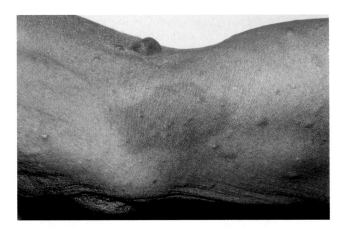

Fig. 12-65   Neurofibromatosis type I. Same patient as depicted in Fig. 12-63. Note the *café au lait* pigmentation on the arm.

pregnancy. There is a wide variability in the expression of the disease. Some patients have only a few neurofibromas; others have literally hundreds or thousands of tumors. However, two thirds of patients have relatively mild disease.

Another highly characteristic feature is the presence of *café au lait* (coffee with milk) pigmentation on the skin (Fig. 12-65). These spots are smooth-edged, yellow-tan to dark-brown macules that vary in diameter from 1 to 2 mm to several centimeters. They are usually present at birth or may develop during the first year of life. Axillary freckling (**Crowe's sign**) is also a highly suggestive sign.

Lisch nodules, translucent brown-pigmented spots on the iris, are found in nearly all affected individuals. The most common general medical problem is hypertension, which may develop secondary to coarctation of the aorta, pheochromocytoma, or renal artery steno-

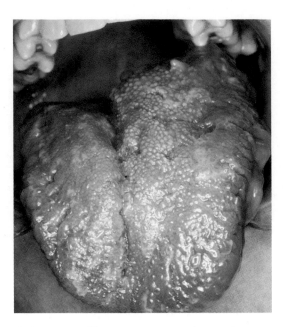

Fig. 12-66   Neurofibromatosis type I. Intraoral involvement characterized by unilateral enlargement of the tongue.

sis. Other possible abnormalities include CNS tumors, macrocephaly, mental deficiency, seizures, short stature, and scoliosis.

In the past, oral lesions were estimated to occur in 4% to 7% of cases (Fig. 12-66). However, two studies suggest that oral manifestations may occur in as many as 72% to 92% of cases, especially if a detailed clinical and radiographic examination is performed. The most common reported finding is enlargement of the fungiform papillae (in about 50% of all affected patients); however, the specificity of this finding for neurofibromatosis is unknown. Only about 25% of patients examined in these two studies exhibited actual intraoral neurofibromas. Radiographic findings may include enlargement of the mandibular foramen, enlargement or branching of the mandibular canal, increased bone density, concavity of the medial surface of the ramus, and increase in dimension of the coronoid notch.

Several unusual clinical variants of NF1 have been described. On occasion, the condition can include unilateral enlargement that mimics hemifacial hyperplasia (see page 38). In addition, several patients with NF1 have been described with associated Noonan syndrome or with central giant cell granulomas of the jaw.

TREATMENT AND PROGNOSIS

There is no specific therapy for NF1, and treatment often is directed toward prevention or management of complications. Facial neurofibromas can be removed

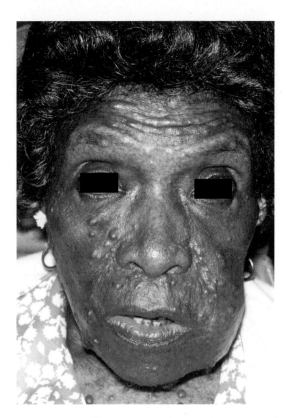

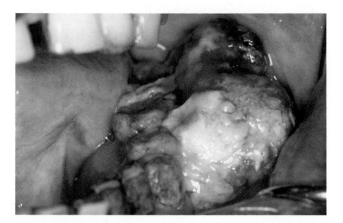

Fig. 12-68   Neurofibromatosis type I. Same patient as depicted in Fig. 12-67. Note the intraoral appearance of malignant peripheral nerve sheath tumor of the mandibular buccal vestibule. The patient eventually died of this tumor. *(From Neville BW, Hann J, Narang R et al: Oral neurofibrosarcoma associated with neurofibromatosis type I, Oral Surg Oral Med Oral Pathol 72:456-461, 1991.)*

Fig. 12-67   Neurofibromatosis type I. Malignant peripheral nerve sheath tumor of the left cheek in a patient with type I neurofibromatosis. *(From Neville BW, Hann J, Narang R et al: Oral neurofibrosarcoma associated with neurofibromatosis type I, Oral Surg Oral Med Oral Pathol 72:456-461, 1991.)*

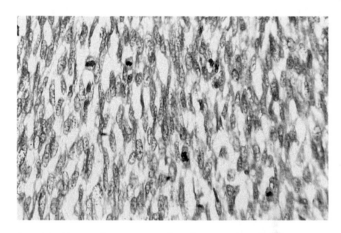

Fig. 12-69   Malignant peripheral nerve sheath tumor. High-power view of an intraoral tumor that developed in a patient with neurofibromatosis type I. There is a cellular spindle cell proliferation with numerous mitotic figures.

for cosmetic purposes. Carbon dioxide (CO_2) laser and dermabrasion have been used successfully for extensive lesions.

One of the most feared complications is the development of cancer, most often a **malignant peripheral nerve sheath tumor (neurofibrosarcoma; malignant schwannoma)**, which has been reported to occur in about 5% of cases. These tumors are most common on the trunk and extremities, although head and neck involvement is occasionally seen (Figs. 12-67 to 12-69). The prognosis for malignant peripheral nerve sheath tumors associated with neurofibromatosis is poor, with a 5-year survival rate of only 15%. Other malignancies also have been associated with neurofibromatosis, including CNS tumors, pheochromocytoma, leukemia, rhabdomyosarcoma, and Wilms' tumor. The average lifespan of individuals with NF1 is 15 years less than the general population, mostly related to vascular disease and malignant neoplasms.

In recent years, there has been considerable interest in Joseph (not John) Merrick, the so-called Elephant Man. Although Merrick once was mistakenly considered to have neurofibromatosis, it is now generally accepted that his horribly disfigured appearance was not because of neurofibromatosis, but that he most likely had a rare condition known as **Proteus syndrome**. Because patients with neurofibromatosis may fear acquiring a similar clinical appearance, they should be reassured that they have a different condition. The phrase "Elephant Man disease" is incorrect and misleading, and it should be avoided. Genetic counseling is extremely important for all patients with neurofibromatosis.

MULTIPLE ENDOCRINE NEOPLASIA TYPE 2B (MULTIPLE ENDOCRINE NEOPLASIA TYPE 3; MULTIPLE MUCOSAL NEUROMA SYNDROME)

The **multiple endocrine neoplasia (MEN) syndromes** are a group of rare conditions characterized by tumors or hyperplasias of the neuroendocrine tissues. For example, patients with MEN type 1 have benign tumors of the pancreatic islets, adrenal cortex, parathyroid glands, and pituitary gland. MEN type 2A, also known as **Sipple syndrome,** includes the development of adrenal pheochromocytomas and medullary thyroid carcinoma. In addition to pheochromocytomas and medullary thyroid carcinoma, patients with MEN type 2B have mucosal neuromas that especially involve the oral mucous membranes. Because oral manifestations are most prominent in MEN type 2B, the remainder of the discussion is limited to this condition.

Similar to the other MEN syndromes, MEN type 2B is inherited as an autosomal dominant trait. However, researchers believe that 50% of cases represent spontaneous mutations. The condition is caused by a mutation of the RET protooncogene on chromosome 10, which has been detected in 95% of affected individuals.

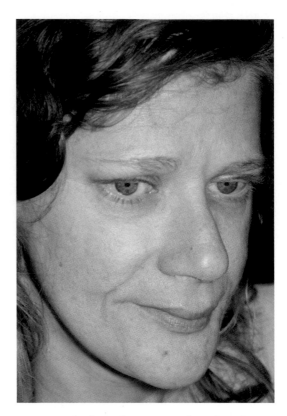

Fig. 12-70 **Multiple endocrine neoplasia (MEN) type 2B.** Note the narrow face and eversion of the upper eyelids.

CLINICAL FEATURES

Patients with MEN type 2B usually have a marfanoid body build characterized by thin, elongated limbs with muscle wasting. The face is narrow, but the lips are characteristically thick and protuberant because of the diffuse proliferation of nerve bundles. The upper eyelid sometimes is everted because of thickening of the tarsal plate (Fig. 12-70). Small, pedunculated neuromas may be observable on the conjunctiva, eyelid margin, or cornea.

Oral mucosal neuromas are usually the first sign of the condition. These neuromas appear as soft, painless papules or nodules that principally affect the lips and anterior tongue but also may be seen on the buccal mucosa, gingiva, and palate (Fig. 12-71). Bilateral neuromas of the commissural mucosa are highly characteristic.

Pheochromocytomas of the adrenal glands develop in at least 50% of all patients and become more prevalent with increasing age. These neuroendocrine tumors are frequently bilateral or multifocal. The tumor cells secrete catecholamines, which result in symptoms such as profuse sweating, intractable diarrhea, headaches, flushing, heart palpitations, and severe hypertension.

The most significant aspect of this condition is the development of medullary carcinoma of the thyroid

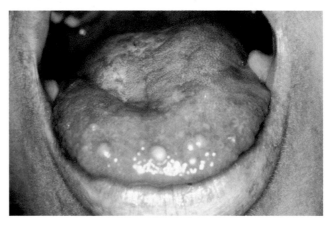

Fig. 12-71 **Multiple endocrine neoplasia (MEN) type 2B.** Multiple neuromas along the anterior margin of the tongue and bilaterally at the commissures. *(Courtesy of Dr. Emmitt Costich.)*

gland, which occurs in more than 90% of cases. This aggressive tumor arises from the parafollicular cells (C cells), which are responsible for calcitonin production. Medullary carcinoma most often is diagnosed in patients between the ages of 18 and 25, and it shows a marked propensity for metastasis. The average age at death from this neoplasm is 21 years.

LABORATORY VALUES

If medullary carcinoma of the thyroid gland is present, then serum or urinary levels of calcitonin are elevated. An increase in calcitonin levels may herald the onset of the tumor, and calcitonin also can be monitored to detect local recurrences or metastases after treatment. Pheochromocytomas may result in increased levels of urinary vanillylmandelic acid (VMA) and increased epinephrine-to-norepinephrine ratios.

HISTOPATHOLOGIC FEATURES

The mucosal neuromas are characterized by marked hyperplasia of nerve bundles in an otherwise normal or loose connective tissue background (Figs. 12-72 and 12-73). Prominent thickening of the perineurium is typically seen.

TREATMENT AND PROGNOSIS

The prognosis for patients with MEN type 2B centers on early recognition of the oral features, given the serious nature of the medullary thyroid carcinoma. Some investigators advocate prophylactic removal of the thyroid gland at an early age because medullary carcinoma is almost certain to occur. Once it has developed, this tumor often exhibits an aggressive behavior with a poor prognosis. The patient also should be observed for the development of pheochromocytomas because they may result in a life-threatening hypertensive crisis, especially if surgery with general anesthesia is performed.

MELANOTIC NEUROECTODERMAL TUMOR OF INFANCY

The **melanotic neuroectodermal tumor of infancy** is a rare pigmented neoplasm that usually occurs during the first year of life. It is generally accepted that this lesion is of neural crest origin. In the past, however, a number of tissues were suggested as possible sources of this tumor. These included odontogenic epithelium and retina, which resulted in various older terms for this entity, such as **pigmented ameloblastoma**, **retinal anlage tumor**, and **melanotic progonoma**. Because these names are inaccurate, however, they should no longer be used. *Melanotic (pigmented) neuroectodermal tumor of infancy* is the preferred term.

CLINICAL AND RADIOGRAPHIC FEATURES

Melanotic neuroectodermal tumor of infancy almost always develops in young children during the first year of life; only 9% of cases are diagnosed after the age of

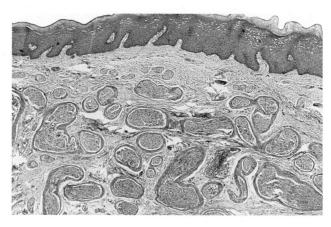

Fig. 12-72   Multiple endocrine neoplasia (MEN) type 2B. Low-power view of an oral mucosal neuroma showing marked hyperplasia of nerve bundles.

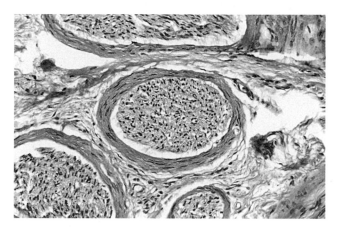

Fig. 12-73   Multiple endocrine neoplasia (MEN) type 2B. High-power view of the same neuroma as depicted in Fig. 12-72. Note the prominent thickening of the perineurium.

12 months. There is a striking predilection for the maxilla, which accounts for 61% of reported cases. Less frequently reported sites include the skull (16%), epididymis and testis (9%), mandible (6%), and brain (6%). A slight male predilection has been noted.

The lesion is most common in the anterior region of the maxilla, where it classically appears as a rapidly expanding mass that is frequently blue or black (Fig. 12-74). The tumor often destroys the underlying bone and may be associated with displacement of the developing teeth (Fig. 12-75). In some instances, there may be an associated osteogenic reaction, which exhibits a "sun ray" radiographic pattern that can be mistaken for osteosarcoma.

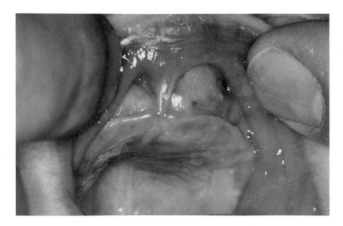

Fig. 12-74   Melanotic neuroectodermal tumor of infancy.
Infant with an expansile mass of the anterior maxilla. *(From
Steinberg B, Shuler C, Wilson S: Melanotic neuroectodermal tumor of
infancy: evidence for multicentricity, Oral Surg Oral Med Oral Pathol
66:666-669, 1988.)*

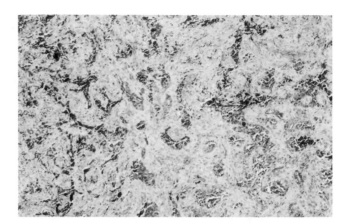

Fig. 12-76   Melanotic neuroectodermal tumor of infancy.
Low-power view showing nests of epithelioid cells within a
fibrous stroma.

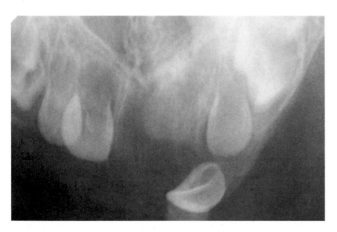

Fig. 12-75   Melanotic neuroectodermal tumor of infancy.
Radiolucent destruction of the anterior maxilla associated
with displacement of the developing teeth. *(Courtesy of Dr. Len
Morrow.)*

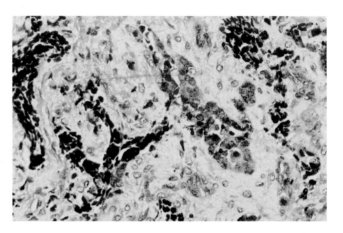

Fig. 12-77   Melanotic neuroectodermal tumor of infancy.
High-power view of a tumor nest demonstrating two cell
types: (1) small, hyperchromatic round cells and (2) larger
epithelioid cells with vesicular nuclei. Some stippled melanin
pigment is also present.

LABORATORY VALUES

High urinary levels of vanillylmandelic acid (VMA)
often are found in patients with melanotic neuroectodermal tumor of infancy. These levels may return to
normal once the tumor has been resected. This finding
supports the hypothesis of neural crest origin because
other tumors from this tissue (e.g., pheochromocytoma,
neuroblastoma) often secrete norepinephrine-like hormones that are metabolized to VMA and excreted in
the urine.

HISTOPATHOLOGIC FEATURES

The tumor consists of a biphasic population of cells that
form nests, tubules, or alveolar structures within a
dense, collagenous stroma (Figs. 12-76 and 12-77).

The alveolar and tubular structures are lined by
cuboidal epithelioid cells that demonstrate vesicular
nuclei and granules of dark-brown melanin pigment.
The second cell type is neuroblastic in appearance
and consists of small, round cells with hyperchromatic nuclei and little cytoplasm. These cells grow
in loose nests and are frequently surrounded by the
larger pigment-producing cells. Mitotic figures are
rare.

Because of the tumor's characteristic microscopic
features, immunohistochemistry usually is not essential to establish the diagnosis. However, the larger epithelioid cells typically are positive for cytokeratin and
also may express neuron-specific enolase. In addition,
the smaller cells usually are positive for neuron-specific
enolase and CD56, and sometimes they will express

other neuroendocrine markers such as glial fibrillary acidic protein and synaptophysin.

TREATMENT AND PROGNOSIS

Despite their rapid growth and potential to destroy bone, most melanotic neuroectodermal tumors of infancy are benign. The lesion is best treated by surgical removal. Some clinicians prefer simple curettage, although others advocate that a 5-mm margin of normal tissue be included with the specimen. Recurrence of the tumor has been reported in about 20% of cases. In addition, about 6% of reported cases, mostly from the brain or skull, have acted in a malignant fashion, resulting in metastasis and death. Although this estimation of 6% is probably high (because unusual malignant cases are more likely to be reported), it underscores the potentially serious nature of this tumor and the need for careful clinical evaluation and follow-up of affected patients.

PARAGANGLIOMA (CAROTID BODY TUMOR; CHEMODECTOMA; GLOMUS JUGULARE TUMOR; GLOMUS TYMPANICUM TUMOR)

The paraganglia are specialized tissues of neural crest origin that are associated with the autonomic nerves and ganglia throughout the body. Some of these cells act as chemoreceptors, such as the carotid body (located at the carotid bifurcation), which can detect changes in blood pH or oxygen tension and subsequently cause changes in respiration and heart rate. Tumors that arise from these structures are collectively known as **paragangliomas,** with the term preferably preceded by the anatomic site at which they are located. Therefore, tumors of the carotid body are appropriately known as **carotid body paragangliomas (carotid body tumors)**; those that develop in the temporal bone and middle ear are called **jugulotympanic paragangliomas.** Jugulotympanic paragangliomas also are commonly known as **glomus jugulare tumors,** although some authors prefer to reserve this term only for those examples that arise from the jugular bulb and to use the term **glomus tympanicum tumors** for those that arise in the middle ear.

CLINICAL AND RADIOGRAPHIC FEATURES

Although paragangliomas are rare, the head and neck area is the most common site for these lesions. The most common paraganglioma is the carotid body tumor, which develops at the bifurcation of the internal and external carotid arteries. This tumor usually occurs in middle-aged adults. Most often it is a slowly enlarging, painless mass of the upper lateral neck below the angle of the jaw. It is seen more frequently in patients who live at high altitudes, indicating that some cases may arise from chronic hyperplasia of the carotid body in response to lower oxygen levels. Angiography can help to localize the tumor and demonstrate its characteristic vascular nature.

Jugulotympanic paragangliomas are the second most common type of these tumors. They also are most frequent in middle-aged individuals but show a 2:1 female predilection. The most common symptoms include dizziness, tinnitus (a ringing or other noise in the ear), hearing loss, and cranial nerve palsies. Imaging studies, especially three-dimensional (3D) time-of-flight magnetic resonance angiography, can help to detect and characterize such lesions. Other less common paragangliomas of the head and neck include vagal, nasopharyngeal, laryngeal, and orbital paragangliomas.

Approximately 10% to 20% of affected patients have multifocal tumors. In 10% of all cases, there is a family history of such tumors, with an autosomal dominant pattern of inheritance that is modified by genomic imprinting. The gene responsible for familial paragangliomas has been mapped to chromosome 11q23. In genomic imprinting, the gene is transmitted in a mendelian manner, but expression of that gene is determined by the sex of the transmitting parent. Paternal transmission results in development of tumors in the offspring, even if the father is clinically unaffected. Maternal transmission does not result in development of tumors in the offspring, although these children will carry the gene and have the ability to pass it down to subsequent generations. Hereditary cases have an even greater chance of being multicentric; about one third of affected patients have more than one tumor.

HISTOPATHOLOGIC FEATURES

The paraganglioma is characterized by round or polygonal epithelioid cells that are organized into nests or *zellballen* (Fig. 12-78). The overall architecture is similar to that of the normal paraganglia, except the *zellballen* are usually larger and more irregular in shape. These nests consist primarily of chief cells, which demonstrate centrally located, vesicular nuclei and somewhat granular, eosinophilic cytoplasm. The tumor is typically vascular and may be surrounded by a thin fibrous capsule.

TREATMENT AND PROGNOSIS

The treatment of paragangliomas may include surgery, radiation therapy, or both, depending on the extent and location of the tumor. Localized carotid body para-

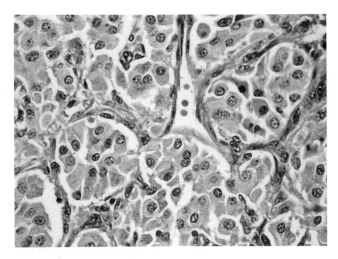

Fig. 12-78   Carotid body tumor. Nested arrangement of tumor cells.

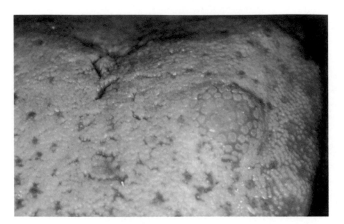

Fig. 12-79   Granular cell tumor. Submucosal nodule on the dorsum of the tongue.

gangliomas often can be treated by surgical excision with maintenance of the vascular tree. If the carotid artery is encased by tumor, it also may need to be resected, followed by vascular grafting. Radiation therapy may be used as adjunctive treatment or for unresectable carotid body tumors.

Although most carotid body paragangliomas are benign and can be controlled with surgery and radiation therapy, vascular complications can lead to considerable surgical morbidity or mortality. In addition, 6% to 9% of carotid body paragangliomas metastasize, either to regional lymph nodes or distant sites. Unfortunately, it is usually difficult to predict which tumors will act in a malignant fashion based on their microscopic features. Because such metastases may develop many years after the original diagnosis is made, long-term follow-up is important.

Because of their location near the base of the brain, jugulotympanic paragangliomas are more difficult to manage. Recent advances in both diagnostic radiology and neurosurgery have greatly improved the potential for resection of these tumors. Radiation therapy may be used in conjunction with surgery or as a primary treatment for unresectable tumors. Stereotactic radiosurgery (gamma knife treatment) has shown promise in the management of primary or recurrent glomus jugulare tumors in patients who are poor surgical candidates. This technique allows the delivery of a focused, large, single dose of radiation under stereotactic guidance. Malignant behavior has been documented in approximately 4% of jugulotympanic paragangliomas.

GRANULAR CELL TUMOR

The **granular cell tumor** is an uncommon benign soft tissue neoplasm that shows a predilection for the oral cavity. The histogenesis of this lesion has long been debated. Originally, it was believed to be of skeletal muscle origin and was called the *granular cell myoblastoma*. However, more recent investigations do not support a muscle origin but point to a derivation from Schwann cells (**granular cell schwannoma**) or neuroendocrine cells. At present, it seems best to use the noncommittal term **granular cell tumor** for this lesion.

CLINICAL FEATURES

Granular cell tumors are most common in the oral cavity and on the skin. The single most common site is the tongue, which accounts for one third to half of all reported cases. Tongue lesions most often occur on the dorsal surface. The buccal mucosa is the second most common intraoral location. The tumor most frequently occurs in the fourth to sixth decades of life and is rare in children. There is a 2:1 female predilection.

The granular cell tumor is typically an asymptomatic sessile nodule that is usually 2 cm or less in size (Figs. 12-79 and 12-80). The lesion often has been noted for many months or years, although sometimes the patient is unaware of its presence. The mass is typically pink, but occasional granular cell tumors appear yellow. The granular cell tumor is usually solitary, although multiple, separate tumors sometimes occur, especially in black patients.

HISTOPATHOLOGIC FEATURES

The granular cell tumor is composed of large, polygonal cells with abundant pale eosinophilic, granular cytoplasm and small, vesicular nuclei (Fig. 12-81). The cells are usually arranged in sheets, but they also may be found in cords and nests. The cell borders often are indistinct, which results in a syncytial appearance. The lesion is not encapsulated and sometimes appears to

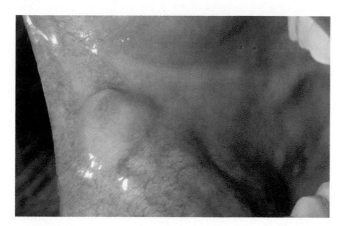

Fig. 12-80 **Granular cell tumor.** Nodular mass of the buccal mucosa near the commissure.

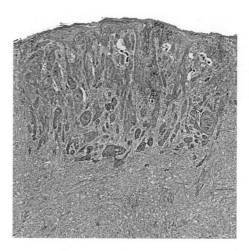

Fig. 12-82 **Granular cell tumor.** Marked pseudoepitheliomatous hyperplasia overlying a granular cell tumor. Such cases may easily be mistaken for squamous cell carcinoma.

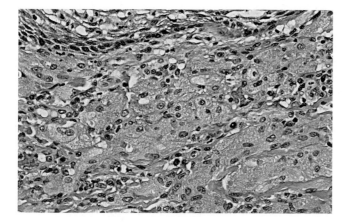

Fig. 12-81 **Granular cell tumor.** Medium-high-power view showing polygonal cells with abundant granular cytoplasm.

infiltrate the adjacent connective tissues. Often, there appears to be a transition from normal adjacent skeletal muscle fibers to granular tumor cells; this finding led earlier investigators to suggest a muscle origin for this tumor. Less frequently, one may see groups of granular cells that envelop small nerve bundles. Immunohistochemical analysis reveals positivity for S-100 protein within the cells—a finding that is supportive, but not diagnostic, of neural origin.

An unusual and significant microscopic finding is the presence of acanthosis or pseudoepitheliomatous (pseudocarcinomatous) hyperplasia of the overlying epithelium, which has been reported in up to 50% of all cases (Fig. 12-82). Although this hyperplasia is usually minor in degree, in some cases it may be so striking that it results in a mistaken diagnosis of squamous cell carcinoma and subsequent unnecessary cancer surgery. The pathologist must be aware of this possibility, especially when dealing with a superficial

biopsy sample or a specimen from the dorsum of the tongue—an unusual location for oral cancer.

TREATMENT AND PROGNOSIS

The granular cell tumor is best treated by conservative local excision, and recurrence is uncommon. Extremely rare examples of malignant granular cell tumor have been reported.

CONGENITAL EPULIS (CONGENITAL EPULIS OF THE NEWBORN; CONGENITAL GRANULAR CELL LESION)

The **congenital epulis** is an uncommon soft tissue tumor that occurs almost exclusively on the alveolar ridges of newborns. It is often known by the redundant term, **congenital epulis of the newborn.** Rare examples also have been described on the tongue; therefore, some authors prefer using the term **congenital granular cell lesion,** because not all cases present as an *epulis* on the alveolar ridge. It also has been called **gingival granular cell tumor of the newborn,** but this term should be avoided. Although it bears a light microscopic resemblance to the granular cell tumor (discussed previously), it exhibits ultrastructural and immunohistochemical differences that warrant its classification as a distinct and separate entity. However, the histogenesis of this tumor is still uncertain.

CLINICAL FEATURES

The congenital epulis typically appears as a pink-to-red, smooth-surfaced, polypoid mass on the alveolar ridge of a newborn (Fig. 12-83). Most examples are

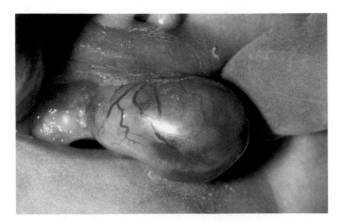

Fig. 12-83   Congenital epulis. Polypoid mass of the anterior maxillary alveolar ridge in a newborn.

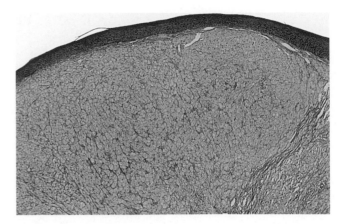

Fig. 12-84   Congenital epulis. Low-power photomicrograph showing a nodular tumor mass. Note the atrophy of the rete ridges.

2 cm or less in size, although lesions as large as 7.5 cm have been reported. On occasion, the tumor has been detected *in utero* via ultrasound examination. Multiple tumors develop in 10% of cases. A few rare examples on the tongue have been described in infants who also had alveolar tumors.

The tumor is two to three times more common on the maxillary ridge than on the mandibular ridge. It most frequently occurs lateral to the midline in the area of the developing lateral incisor and canine teeth. The congenital epulis shows a striking predilection for females, which suggests a hormonal influence in its development, although estrogen and progesterone receptors have not been detected. Nearly 90% of cases occur in females.

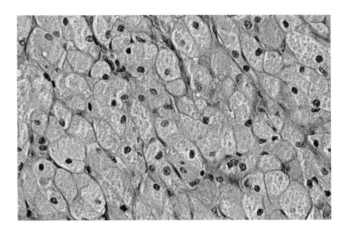

Fig. 12-85   Congenital epulis. High-power view of rounded cells with abundant granular cytoplasm.

HISTOPATHOLOGIC FEATURES

The congenital epulis is characterized by large, rounded cells with abundant granular, eosinophilic cytoplasm and round to oval, lightly basophilic nuclei (Figs. 12-84 and 12-85). In older tumors, these cells may become elongated and separated by fibrous connective tissue. In contrast to the granular cell tumor, the overlying epithelium never shows pseudoepitheliomatous hyperplasia but typically demonstrates atrophy of the rete ridges. In addition, in contradistinction to the granular cell tumor, immunohistochemical analysis shows the tumor cells to be negative for S-100 protein.

TREATMENT AND PROGNOSIS

The congenital epulis is usually treated by surgical excision. The lesion never has been reported to recur, even with incomplete removal.

After birth, the tumor appears to stop growing and may even diminish in size. Eventual complete regres-

sion has been reported in a few patients, even without treatment (Fig. 12-86).

HEMANGIOMA AND VASCULAR MALFORMATIONS

In recent years, great progress has been made in the classification and understanding of tumors and tumor-like proliferations of vascular origin. A modified classification scheme for these vascular anomalies is presented in Box 12-2.

The term **hemangioma** has traditionally been used to describe a variety of developmental vascular anomalies. Currently, hemangiomas are considered to be benign tumors of infancy that display a rapid growth phase with endothelial cell proliferation, followed by gradual involution. Most hemangiomas cannot be recognized at birth, but arise subsequently during the first 8 weeks of life. On the other hand, **vascular malfor-**

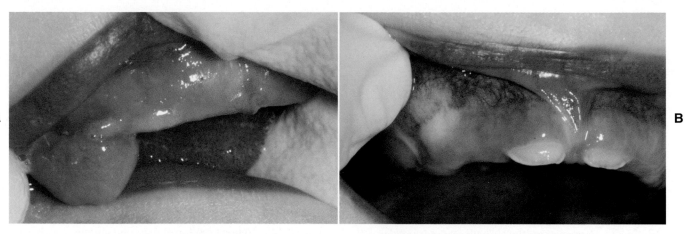

Fig. 12-86   Congenital epulis. A, Nodular mass on the maxillary alveolar ridge. Instead of being excised, the lesion was monitored clinically. **B,** Clinical appearance of the child at 1 year of age. The mass has disappeared without treatment. *(Courtesy of Dr. Erwin Turner.)*

mations are structural anomalies of blood vessels without endothelial proliferation. By definition, vascular malformations are present at birth and persist throughout life. They can be categorized according to the type of vessel involved (capillary, venous, arteriovenous) and according to hemodynamic features (low flow or high flow).

CLINICAL AND RADIOGRAPHIC FEATURES

HEMANGIOMA OF INFANCY

Hemangiomas are the most common tumors of infancy, occurring in 5% to 10% of 1-year-old children. They are much more common in females than in males (ratio: 3:1 to 5:1), and they occur more frequently in whites than in other racial groups. The most common location is the head and neck, which accounts for 60% of all cases. Eighty percent of hemangiomas occur as single lesions, but 20% of affected patients will have multiple tumors.

Fully developed hemangiomas are rarely present at birth, although a pale macule with threadlike telangiectasias may be noted on the skin. During the first few weeks of life, the tumor will demonstrate rapid development that occurs at a faster pace than the infant's overall growth. Superficial tumors of the skin appear raised and bosselated with a bright-red color ("strawberry" hemangioma) (Fig. 12-87). They are firm and rubbery to palpation, and the blood cannot be evacuated by applying pressure. Deeper tumors may appear only slightly raised with a bluish hue.

The proliferative phase usually lasts for 6 to 10 months, after which the tumor slows in growth and begins to involute. The color gradually changes to a

Box 12-2
Classification of Vascular Anomalies

VASCULAR TUMORS
Hemangiomas of Infancy
Superficial
Deep
Mixed

Congenital Hemangiomas
Noninvoluting congenital hemangioma (NICH)
Rapidly involuting congenital hemangioma (RICH)

Kaposiform Hemangioendothelioma
Tufted Angioma
Pyogenic Granuloma (lobular capillary hemangioma)

VASCULAR MALFORMATIONS
Simple
Capillary malformation
Venous malformation
Lymphatic malformation
Arteriovenous malformation

Combined Malformations

dull-purple hue and the lesion feels less firm to palpation. By age 5, most of the red color is usually gone. About half of all hemangiomas will show complete resolution by 5 years of age, with 90% resolving by age 9. After tumor regression is complete, normal skin will be restored in about 50% of patients; however, up to 40% of affected individuals will show permanent changes such as atrophy, scarring, wrinkling, or telangiectasias.

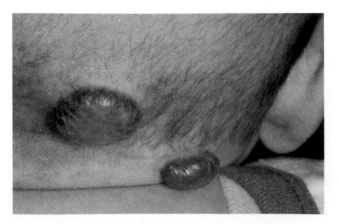

Fig. 12-87   Hemangioma. Infant with two red, nodular masses on the posterior scalp and neck ("strawberry" hemangioma).

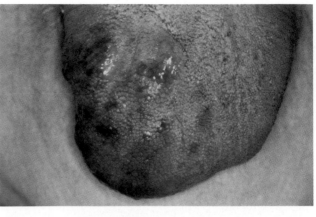

Fig. 12-88   Venous malformation. Blue-purple mass of the anterior tongue.

Complications occur in about 20% of hemangiomas. The most common problem is ulceration, which may occur with or without secondary infection. Although hemorrhage may be noted, significant blood loss does not usually occur. Hemangiomas that occur in crucial areas can be associated with significant morbidity. Periocular tumors often result in amblyopia (dimness of vision), strabismus, or astigmatism. Patients with multiple cutaneous hemangiomas or large facial hemangiomas are at increased risk for concomitant visceral hemangiomas. Tumors in the neck and laryngeal region can lead to airway obstruction.

Large, segmental cervicofacial hemangioma can be a component of a well-recognized hemangioma syndrome—**PHACE(S) syndrome.** This acronym stands for the following:

- **P**osterior fossa brain anomalies (usually Dandy-Walker malformation)
- **H**emangioma (usually cervical segmental hemangioma)
- **A**rterial anomalies
- **C**ardiac defects and **C**oarctation of the aorta
- **E**ye anomalies
- **S**ternal cleft or **S**upraumbilical raphe

Kasabach-Merritt phenomenon is a serious coagulopathy that has been associated with two rare vascular tumors known as *tufted hemangioma* and *kaposiform hemangioendothelioma*. This disorder is characterized by severe thrombocytopenia and hemorrhage because of platelet trapping within the tumor. The mortality rate is as high as 20% to 30%.

VASCULAR MALFORMATIONS

In contrast to hemangiomas, vascular malformations are present at birth and persist throughout life. Port wine stains are relatively common capillary malforma-

tions that occur in 0.3% to 1.0% of newborns. They are most common on the face, particularly along the distribution of the trigeminal nerve. In Sturge-Weber angiomatosis, associated intracranial lesions are present (see page 543). Port wine stains are typically pink or purple macular lesions that grow commensurately with the patient. As the patient gets older, the lesion often darkens and becomes nodular because of vascular ectasia.

Low-flow **venous malformations** encompass a wide spectrum of lesions, from small isolated ectasias to complex growths that involve multiple tissues and organs. They are present at birth, although they may not always be immediately apparent. Typically, venous malformations are blue and are easily compressible (Fig. 12-88). They often grow proportionately with the patient, but they may swell when dependent or with increased venous pressure. Secondary thrombosis and phlebolith formation can occur.

Arteriovenous malformations are high-flow lesions that result from persistent direct arterial and venous communication. Although they are present from birth, they may not become noticeable until later in childhood or adulthood. Because of the fast vascular flow through these lesions, a palpable thrill or bruit often is noticeable. The overlying skin typically feels warmer to touch. Presenting symptoms may include pain, bleeding, and skin ulceration.

INTRABONY VASCULAR MALFORMATIONS

Intrabony "hemangiomas" also may occur and probably represent either venous or arteriovenous malformations. In the jaws, such lesions are detected most often during the first 3 decades of life. They are slightly more common in females than in males and occur three times more often in the mandible than the maxilla. The lesion may be completely asymptomatic, although some examples are associated with pain and swelling. Mobility of teeth or bleeding from the gingival sulcus may occur. A bruit or pulsation may be apparent on auscultation and palpation.

The radiographic appearance of intrabony vascular malformations is variable. Most commonly, the lesion shows a multilocular radiolucent defect. The individual loculations may be small (honeycomb appearance) or large (soap bubble appearance). In other cases the lesion may present as an ill-defined radiolucent area or a well-defined, cystlike radiolucency (Fig. 12-89). Large malformations may cause cortical expansion, and occasionally a "sunburst" radiographic pattern is produced (Fig. 12-90). Angiography can be helpful in demonstrating the vascular nature of the lesion (Fig. 12-91).

HISTOPATHOLOGIC FEATURES

Early hemangiomas of infancy are characterized by numerous plump endothelial cells and often-indistinct vascular lumina (Figs. 12-92 and 12-93). At this stage, such lesions often are known microscopically as *juvenile* or *cellular* hemangiomas. Because of their cellular nature, these lesions also have been called **juvenile**

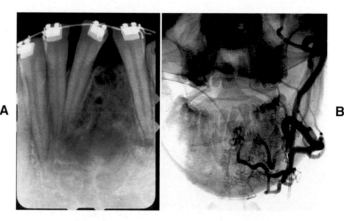

Fig. 12-91   Intrabony arteriovenous malformation. A, Periapical radiograph showing an expansile, mottled radiolucency in the mandibular incisor region. Pulsatile hemorrhage was encountered when a biopsy of this lesion was attempted. **B,** Angiogram demonstrating a vascular proliferation between the mandibular incisors. *(Courtesy of Dr. Larry Cunningham and Dr. Jason Ford.)*

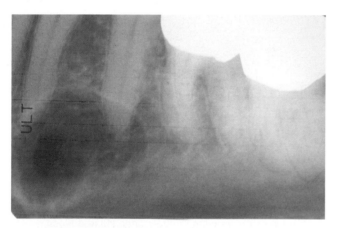

Fig. 12-89   Intrabony venous malformation. Well-circumscribed radiolucency that contains fine trabeculations.

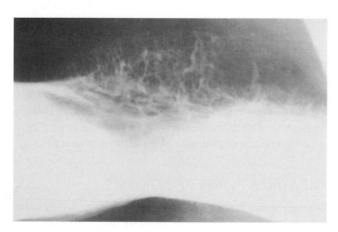

Fig. 12-90   Intrabony venous malformation. Occlusal radiograph demonstrating cortical destruction and a "sunburst" periosteal reaction resembling osteosarcoma.

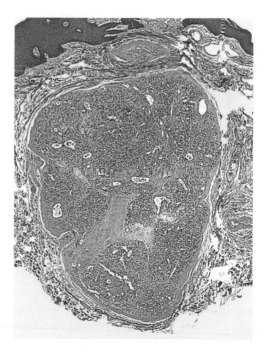

Fig. 12-92   Juvenile (cellular) hemangioma. Low-power photomicrograph showing a circumscribed cellular mass of vascular endothelial cells arranged in lobular aggregates.

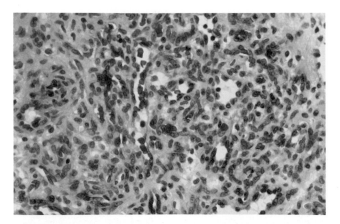

Fig. 12-93 Juvenile (cellular) hemangioma. High-power view showing a highly cellular endothelial proliferation forming occasional indistinct vascular lumina.

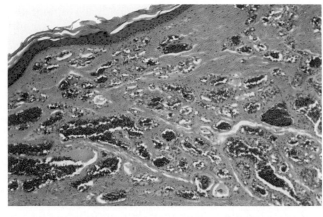

Fig. 12-95 Capillary malformation. Low-power view of a vascular proliferation forming multiple capillary blood vessels.

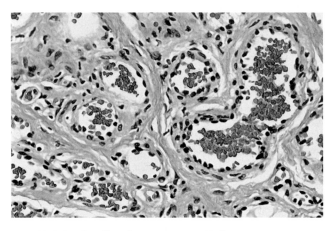

Fig. 12-94 Capillary hemangioma. High-power photomicrograph demonstrating well-formed capillary-sized vessels.

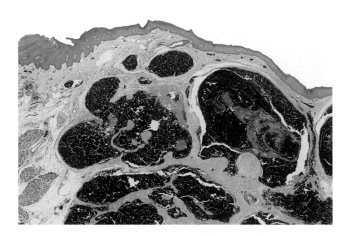

Fig. 12-96 Venous malformation. Low-power photomicrograph showing multiple large, dilated blood vessels.

hemangioendothelioma, although this term should be avoided because hemangioendothelioma also is used to designate other vascular tumors of intermediate malignant potential. As the lesion matures, the endothelial cells become flattened, and the small, capillary-sized vascular spaces become more evident (Fig. 12-94). As the hemangioma undergoes involution, the vascular spaces become less prominent and are replaced by fibrous connective tissue.

Vascular malformations do not show active endothelial cell proliferation, and the channels resemble the vessels of origin. Therefore, capillary malformations may be similar to the capillary stage of hemangioma (Fig. 12-95), whereas venous malformations may show more dilated vessels (Fig. 12-96). Because of their similar features, many vascular malformations are incorrectly categorized as *hemangiomas*. Arteriovenous malformations demonstrate a mixture of thick-walled arteries and veins, along with capillary vessels.

GLUT1 is an immunohistochemical marker that is consistently positive in the hemangioma of infancy. In contrast, this marker is negative in other developmental vascular tumors and anomalies listed in Box 12-2 (rapidly involuting congenital hemangioma [RICH], noninvoluting congenital hemangioma [NICH], tufted angioma, kaposiform hemangioendothelioma, pyogenic granuloma, and vascular malformations).

TREATMENT AND PROGNOSIS

Because most hemangiomas of infancy undergo involution, management often consists of "watchful neglect." It is important to educate parents that although rapid growth may be seen, regression will occur. Surgical resection is rarely warranted during infancy. For problematic or life-threatening hemangiomas, pharmacologic therapy may be indicated. Systemic corticosteroids may help to reduce the size of the lesion and are associated with a 70% to 90% response rate. Intralesional and topical corticosteroids also have been used for smaller localized, problematic lesions. Intravenous (IV) vincristine is currently the drug of choice for complicated tumors that are unresponsive to systemic corticosteroid therapy. Interferon α-2a is no longer widely used because of the reported risk of permanent spastic diplegia.

Flashlamp pulsed dye lasers can be effective in the treatment of port wine stains. The management of venous malformations depends on the size, location, and associated complications of the lesion. Small, stable malformations may not require treatment. Larger, problematic lesions may be treated with a combination of sclerotherapy and surgical excision. Sclerotherapy involves the injection of sclerosing agents, such as 95% ethanol, directly into the lesion to induce fibrosis. Sclerotherapy alone may be sufficient for smaller lesions; for larger lesions, subsequent surgical resection can be accomplished with less risk of bleeding after sclerotherapy.

The treatment of arteriovenous malformations is more challenging and also depends on the size of the lesion and degree of involvement of vital structures. For cases that require resection, radiographic embolization often is performed 24 to 48 hours before surgery to minimize blood loss.

Vascular malformations of the jaws are potentially dangerous lesions because of the risk of severe bleeding, which may occur spontaneously or during surgical manipulation. Needle aspiration of any undiagnosed intrabony lesion before biopsy is a wise precaution to rule out the possibility of a vascular malformation. Severe and even fatal hemorrhages have occurred after incisional biopsy or extraction of teeth in the area of such lesions.

STURGE-WEBER ANGIOMATOSIS (ENCEPHALOTRIGEMINAL ANGIOMATOSIS; STURGE-WEBER SYNDROME)

Sturge-Weber angiomatosis is a rare, nonhereditary developmental condition that is characterized by a hamartomatous vascular proliferation involving the tissues of the brain and face. It is believed to be caused by the persistence of a vascular plexus around the cephalic portion of the neural tube. This plexus develops during the sixth week of intrauterine development but normally undergoes regression during the ninth week.

CLINICAL AND RADIOGRAPHIC FEATURES

Patients with Sturge-Weber angiomatosis are born with a dermal capillary vascular malformation of the face known as a **port wine stain** or **nevus flammeus** because of its deep-purple color. This port wine stain usually has a unilateral distribution along one or more segments of the trigeminal nerve. Occasionally, patients have bilateral involvement or additional port wine lesions elsewhere on the body. Not all patients with facial port wine nevi have Sturge-Weber angiomatosis. In one study of patients with facial port wine nevi, only slightly more than 10% had Sturge-Weber angiomatosis. Only patients with involvement along the distribution of the ophthalmic branch of the trigeminal nerve were at risk for the full condition (Figs. 12-97 and 12-98).

In addition to the facial port wine nevus, affected individuals also have leptomeningeal angiomas that overlie the ipsilateral cerebral cortex. This meningeal angiomatosis is usually associated with a convulsive disorder and often results in mental retardation or contralateral hemiplegia. Imaging studies of the brain may reveal gyriform "tramline" calcifications on the affected side (Fig. 12-99). Ocular involvement may be manifested by glaucoma and vascular malformations of the conjunctiva, episclera, choroid, and retina.

Intraoral involvement in Sturge-Weber angiomatosis is common, resulting in hypervascular changes to the ipsilateral mucosa (Fig. 12-100). The gingiva may exhibit slight vascular hyperplasia or a more massive hemangiomatous proliferation that can resemble a

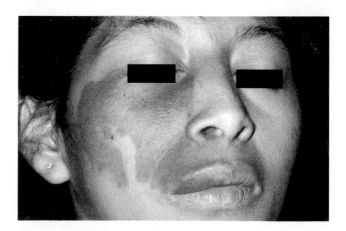

Fig. 12-97   Port wine stain. Nevus flammeus of the malar area in a patient without Sturge-Weber angiomatosis. Unless the vascular lesion includes the region innervated by the ophthalmic branch of the trigeminal nerve, usually the patient does not have central nervous system (CNS) involvement.

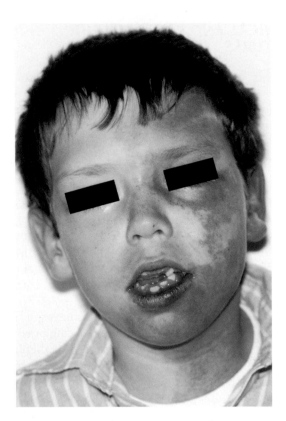

Fig. 12-98 Sturge-Weber angiomatosis. Port wine stain of the left face, including involvement along the ophthalmic branch of the trigeminal nerve. The patient also was mentally retarded and had a seizure disorder.

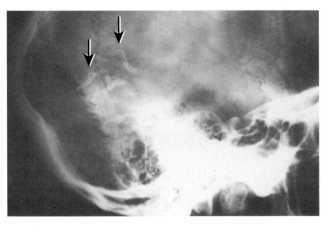

Fig. 12-99 Sturge-Weber angiomatosis. Skull film showing "tramline" calcifications *(arrows)*. *(Courtesy of Dr. Reg Munden.)*

pyogenic granuloma. Such gingival hyperplasia may be attributable to the increased vascular component, phenytoin therapy used to control the epileptic seizures, or both. Destruction of the underlying alveolar bone has been reported in rare instances.

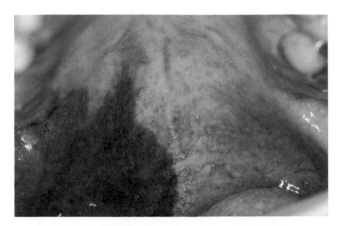

Fig. 12-100 Sturge-Weber angiomatosis. Unilateral vascular involvement of the soft palate.

HISTOPATHOLOGIC FEATURES

The port wine nevus is characterized by excessive numbers of dilated blood vessels in the middle and deep dermis. The intraoral lesions show a similar vascular dilatation. Proliferative gingival lesions may resemble a pyogenic granuloma.

TREATMENT AND PROGNOSIS

The treatment and prognosis of Sturge-Weber angiomatosis depend on the nature and severity of the possible clinical features. Usually, facial port wine nevi can be improved by using the newer flashlamp pulsed dye lasers. Cortical excision of angiomatous meningeal lesions may be necessary in some cases. Patients with intractable epilepsy and progressive mental retardation eventually may require more extensive neurosurgical treatment, including lobectomy or hemispherectomy.

Port wine nevi that affect the gingiva can make flossing and dental prophylaxis difficult. Great care must be taken when performing surgical procedures in affected areas of the mouth because severe hemorrhage may be encountered. Lasers also may be helpful in the removal of hyperplastic oral lesions.

NASOPHARYNGEAL ANGIOFIBROMA

The **nasopharyngeal angiofibroma** is a rare vascular and fibrous tumorlike lesion that occurs only in the nasopharynx. Although microscopically benign, it frequently exhibits locally destructive and aggressive behavior. It may represent a vascular malformation rather than a true neoplasm.

CLINICAL AND RADIOGRAPHIC FEATURES

Nasopharyngeal angiofibromas occur almost exclusively in males. The tumor is exceedingly rare in females—so much so that the diagnosis in a female patient should be viewed with skepticism and closely scrutinized. The lesion also shows a striking predilection for adolescents between the ages of 10 and 17 and often has been called the *juvenile nasopharyngeal angiofibroma*. However, rare examples also have been reported in slightly younger and older patients. Because of its almost exclusive occurrence in adolescent boys, a hormonal influence seems likely, although no endocrine abnormalities have been detected.

Nasal obstruction and epistaxis are common early symptoms. The lesion is currently presumed to arise in the pterygopalatine fossa and expands medially into the nasal cavity via the sphenopalatine foramen. Some cases will show extension into the paranasal sinuses, orbits, or middle cranial fossa. Invasion into the oral cavity or cheek rarely has been reported. Computed tomography (CT) scans and magnetic resonance imaging (MRI) studies are helpful adjuncts in visualizing the extent of the lesion and degree of adjacent tissue destruction. Anterior bowing of the posterior wall of the maxillary sinus is a characteristic feature (Fig. 12-101). Angiograms can be used to confirm the vascular nature of the lesion (Fig. 12-102).

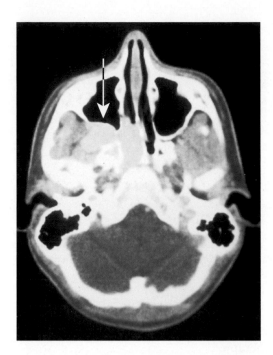

Fig. 12-101 Nasopharyngeal angiofibroma. A contrasted computed tomography (CT) scan showing a tumor of the nasopharynx and pterygopalatine fossa, with characteristic anterior bowing of the posterior wall of the right maxillary sinus (***arrow***). *(Courtesy of Dr. Pamela Van Tassel.)*

HISTOPATHOLOGIC FEATURES

The nasopharyngeal angiofibroma consists of dense fibrous connective tissue that contains numerous dilated, thin-walled blood vessels of variable size (Fig. 12-103). Typically, the vascular component is more prominent at the periphery of the tumor, especially in lesions from younger patients.

TREATMENT AND PROGNOSIS

The primary treatment of nasopharyngeal angiofibroma usually consists of surgical excision. Depending on the extent of the lesion, this may be accomplished via endoscopic surgery, lateral rhinotomy, midfacial degloving procedure, infratemporal fossa approach, or combined craniofacial resection. Preoperative embolization of the tumor is helpful in controlling blood loss. Radiation therapy is usually reserved for recurrent lesions and extensive tumors with unusual vascular supplies or intracranial extension.

The recurrence rate varies from 20% to 40% in most recent studies. Such recurrences are usually retreated with further surgery or radiation therapy. Malignant transformation into fibrosarcoma has rarely been

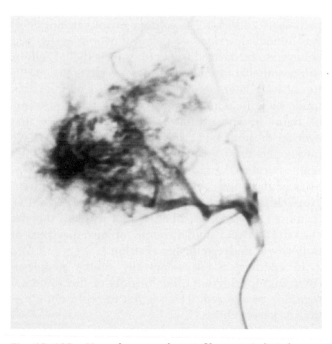

Fig. 12-102 Nasopharyngeal angiofibroma. A digital subtraction angiogram of the external carotid artery showing the intense vascular blush of the tumor. *(Courtesy of Dr. Pamela Van Tassel.)*

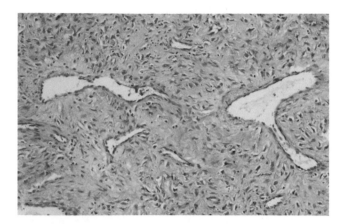

Fig. 12-103 Nasopharyngeal angiofibroma. Moderately cellular fibrous connective tissue with prominent blood vessels.

reported and is probably associated with prior radiation therapy.

HEMANGIOPERICYTOMA–SOLITARY FIBROUS TUMOR

As originally described, the **hemangiopericytoma** (HPC) was a rare neoplasm that presumably was derived from pericytes (i.e., cells with processes that encircled endothelial cells of capillaries). However, in many examples it was difficult to confirm pericytic differentiation, making diagnostic reproducibility among pathologists difficult. The **solitary fibrous tumor** (SFT) was initially described as a pleural neoplasm that was believed to be derived from either mesothelial cells or submesothelial fibroblasts. However, examples of this tumor were later identified in a number of other anatomic sites, including the head and neck region. Many of these lesions exhibit microscopic features that overlap those of HPC. In recent years, experts have questioned the concept of the HPC, suggesting that many purported examples should be reclassified as SFTs or designated by the combined name, **hemangiopericytoma–solitary fibrous tumor** (HPC-SFT). As more knowledge is gained, it appears likely that the classification and nomenclature of this spectrum of tumors will undergo further revision.

In addition, a microscopically similar neoplasm **(hemangiopericytoma-like tumor)** of the sinonasal region is recognized, which is felt to represent a distinct, separate entity.

CLINICAL FEATURES

HPC-SFTs have been reported primarily in adults and are rare in children. The tumor is usually described as a slow-growing, painless, submucosal, or deep soft

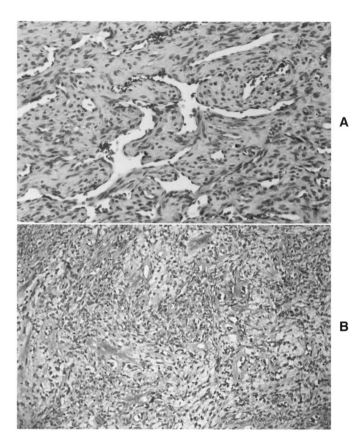

Fig. 12-104 Hemangiopericytoma–solitary fibrous tumor. A, "Staghorn" blood vessels with surrounding pericytes. **B,** Moderately cellular fibrous proliferation ("patternless pattern") with prominent vascularity, slightly myxoid areas, and scattered dense collagen bundles.

tissue mass that is easily removed from the surrounding tissues. One of the most common oral locations is the buccal mucosa, which accounts for 75% of cases reported under the designation of SFT.

Hemangiopericytoma-like tumors of the nasal cavity and paranasal sinuses primarily occur in middle-aged and older adults. Common presenting symptoms include nasal obstruction and epistaxis.

HISTOPATHOLOGIC FEATURES

HPC-SFTs are usually well-circumscribed lesions that exhibit a variable microscopic appearance. At the traditional HPC end of the spectrum, the tumor exhibits tightly packed cells that surround endothelium-lined vascular channels. The cells are haphazardly arranged and demonstrate round to ovoid nuclei and indistinct cytoplasmic borders. The blood vessels often show irregular branching, which results in a characteristic "staghorn" and "antlerlike" appearance (Fig. 12-104, A).

At the SFT end of the spectrum, the cells are more spindled and arranged in either short fascicles or in a disorganized fashion ("patternless pattern") (Fig. 12-104, *B*). The tumor often demonstrates alternating hypercellular and hypocellular zones with a variable degree or myxoid background change. Prominent hyalinized collagen bundles are characteristically observed in the hypocellular areas. Immunohistochemical studies show the lesional cells to be positive for CD34.

The identification of four or more mitoses per 10 high-power fields suggests a rapidly growing tumor that is capable of metastasis. The presence of necrosis also suggests malignancy. However, it is difficult to predict microscopically whether a particular tumor will act in a benign or malignant fashion.

Hemangiopericytoma-like tumors of the sinonasal region have a more prominent spindle cell pattern, with the cells arranged in a more orderly fashion. Mitotic figures are rare or absent. The vascular component is less intricate, and less interstitial collagen is found among the tumor cells.

TREATMENT AND PROGNOSIS

For HPC-SFTs with a benign histopathologic appearance, local excision is the treatment of choice. More extensive surgery is required for tumors with malignant characteristics. Oral examples usually behave in a benign fashion, although up to 10% of extraplural SFTs have been reported to show malignant behavior. One recent paper reported a 5-year survival rate of 86% for HPC. Therefore, long-term follow-up of all patients with this tumor spectrum is recommended.

Studies show that patients with hemangiopericytoma-like tumors of the sinonasal region have a better prognosis than do those with tumors at other sites.

LYMPHANGIOMA

Lymphangiomas are benign, hamartomatous tumors of lymphatic vessels. It is doubtful that they are true neoplasms; instead, they most likely represent developmental malformations that arise from sequestrations of lymphatic tissue that do not communicate normally with the rest of the lymphatic system.

There are three types of lymphangioma:
1. **Lymphangioma simplex (capillary lymphangioma)**, which consists of small, capillary-sized vessels
2. **Cavernous lymphangioma**, which is composed of larger, dilated lymphatic vessels
3. **Cystic lymphangioma (cystic hygroma)**, which exhibits large, macroscopic cystic spaces

However, this classification system is rather arbitrary because all three sizes of vessels often can be found within the same lesion.

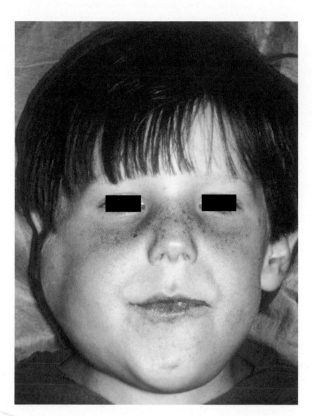

Fig. 12-105   Lymphangioma. Young boy with a cystic hygroma primarily involving the right side of the face. *(Courtesy of Dr. Frank Kendrick.)*

The subtypes are probably variants of the same pathologic process, and the size of the vessels may depend on the nature of the surrounding tissues. Cystic lymphangiomas most often occur in the neck and axilla, where the loose adjacent connective tissues allow for more expansion of the vessels. Cavernous lymphangiomas are more frequent in the mouth, where the denser surrounding connective tissue and skeletal muscle limit vessel expansion.

CLINICAL FEATURES

Lymphangiomas have a marked predilection for the head and neck, which accounts for 50% to 75% of all cases (Fig. 12-105). About half of all lesions are noted at birth, and around 90% develop by 2 years of age.

Cervical lymphangiomas are more common in the posterior triangle and are typically soft, fluctuant masses. They occur less frequently in the anterior triangle, although lesions in this location are more likely to result in respiratory difficulties or dysphagia if they grow large. Occasionally, cervical lymphangiomas extend into the mediastinum or upward into the oral cavity. Such tumors can become massive and can measure 15 cm or greater in size. Rapid tumor enlargement may occur secondary to an upper respiratory tract infection, presumably because of increased lymph

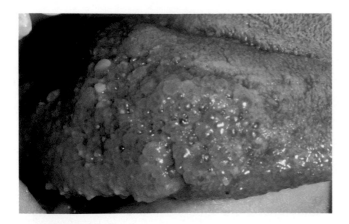

Fig. 12-106   Lymphangioma. Pebbly, vesicle-like appearance of a tumor of the right lateral tongue.

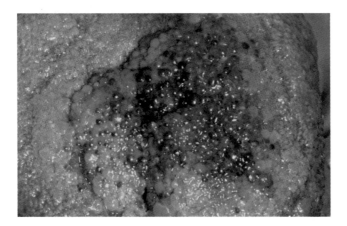

Fig. 12-107   Lymphangioma. Dorsal tongue lesion demonstrating a purple color, which can be caused by secondary hemorrhage or an associated hemangiomatous component.

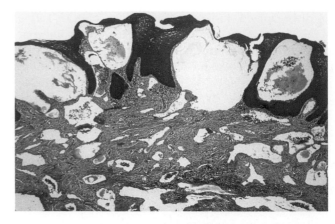

Fig. 12-108   Cavernous lymphangioma. Lesion of the tongue showing dilated lymphatic vessels beneath the epithelium and in the deeper connective tissues.

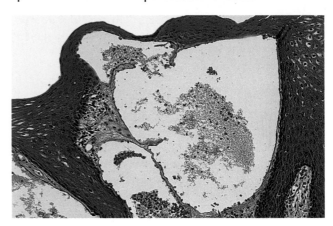

Fig. 12-109   Cavernous lymphangioma. High-power photomicrograph showing dilated, lymph-filled vessels immediately below the atrophic surface epithelium.

production, blocked lymphatic drainage, or secondary infection of the tumor.

Oral lymphangiomas may occur at various sites but are most frequent on the anterior two thirds of the tongue, where they often result in macroglossia (Figs. 12-106 and 12-107). Usually, the tumor is superficial in location and demonstrates a pebbly surface that resembles a cluster of translucent vesicles. The surface has been likened to the appearance of frog eggs or tapioca pudding. Secondary hemorrhage into the lymphatic spaces may cause some of these "vesicles" to become purple. Deeper tumors present as soft, ill-defined masses.

Small lymphangiomas less than 1 cm in size occur on the alveolar ridge in around 4% of black neonates. These lesions often occur bilaterally on the mandibular ridge and show a 2:1 male-to-female distribution. Most of these alveolar lymphangiomas apparently resolve spontaneously because they are not observed in older people.

HISTOPATHOLOGIC FEATURES

Lymphangiomas are composed of lymphatic vessels that may show marked dilatation (cavernous lymphangioma) (Figs. 12-108 and 12-109) or macroscopic cyst-like structures (cystic hygroma) (Fig. 12-110). The vessels often diffusely infiltrate the adjacent soft tissues and may demonstrate lymphoid aggregates in their walls. The lining endothelium is typically thin, and the spaces contain proteinaceous fluid and occasional lymphocytes. Some channels also may contain red blood cells, which creates uncertainty as to whether they are lymphatic or blood vessels. Although many of these likely represent secondary hemorrhage into a lymphatic vessel, some actually may be examples of mixed lymphangioma and hemangioma.

In intraoral tumors, the lymphatic vessels are characteristically located just beneath the epithelial surface and often replace the connective tissue papillae. This superficial location results in the translucent, vesicle-

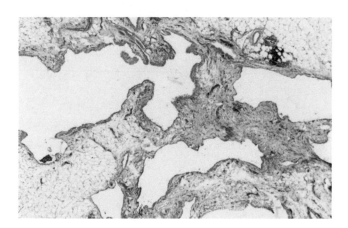

Fig. 12-110 Cystic hygroma. Lesion from the neck showing markedly dilated lymphatic vessels.

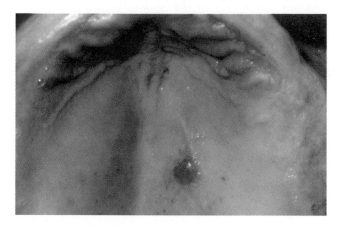

Fig. 12-111 Leiomyoma. Small, pink-red nodule on the posterior hard palate lateral to the midline.

like clinical appearance. However, extension of these vessels into the deeper connective tissue and skeletal muscle also may be seen.

TREATMENT AND PROGNOSIS

The treatment of lymphangiomas usually consists of surgical excision, although total removal may not be possible in all cases because of large size or involvement of vital structures. Recurrence is common, especially for cavernous lymphangiomas of the oral cavity, because of their infiltrative nature. Some clinicians do not recommend treatment for nonenlarging lymphangiomas of the tongue because of the difficulty in removal and high recurrence rate. Cystic lymphangiomas of the cervical region are often well circumscribed and have a lower rate of recurrence. Spontaneous regression of lymphangiomas is rare.

Unfortunately, lymphangiomas do not respond to sclerosing agents as do hemangiomas. However, some success with sclerosant therapy for unresectable lymphangiomas has been reported using OK-432, a lyophilized incubation mixture of a low-virulent strain of *Streptococcus pyogenes* with penicillin G potassium, which has lost its streptolysin S–producing ability.

The prognosis is good for most patients, although large tumors of the neck or tongue may result in airway obstruction and death. The mortality rate for cystic hygromas ranges from 2% to 5% in most series.

LEIOMYOMA

Leiomyomas are benign tumors of smooth muscle that most commonly occur in the uterus, gastrointestinal tract, and skin. Leiomyomas of the oral cavity are rare. Most of these probably have their origin from vascular smooth muscle.

The three types are as follows:
1. Solid leiomyomas
2. Vascular leiomyomas (angiomyomas or angioleiomyomas)
3. Epithelioid leiomyomas (leiomyoblastomas)

Almost all oral leiomyomas are either solid or vascular in type; angiomyomas account for nearly 75% of all oral cases.

CLINICAL AND RADIOGRAPHIC FEATURES

The oral leiomyoma can occur at any age and is usually a slow-growing, firm, mucosal nodule (Fig. 12-111). Most lesions are asymptomatic, although occasional tumors can be painful. Solid leiomyomas are typically normal in color, although angiomyomas may exhibit a bluish hue. The most common sites are the lips, tongue, palate, and cheek, which together account for 80% of cases. Extremely rare intraosseous examples may present as unilocular radiolucencies of the jaws.

HISTOPATHOLOGIC FEATURES

Solid leiomyomas are well-circumscribed tumors that consist of interlacing bundles of spindle-shaped smooth muscle cells (Figs. 12-112 and 12-113). The nuclei are elongated, pale staining, and blunt ended. Mitotic figures are uncommon. Angiomyomas also are well-circumscribed lesions that demonstrate multiple tortuous blood vessels with thickened walls caused by hyperplasia of their smooth muscle coats (Fig. 12-114). Intertwining bundles of smooth muscle may be found between the vessels, sometimes with intermixed adipose tissue. As its name implies, the epithelioid leiomyoma is composed primarily of epithelioid cells rather than spindle cells.

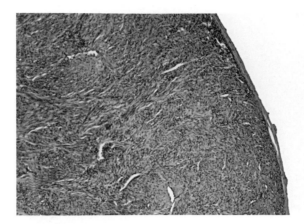

Fig. 12-112 Leiomyoma. Low-power view showing a well-circumscribed cellular mass of spindle-shaped smooth muscle cells.

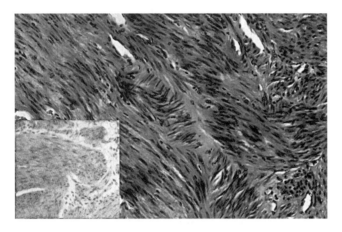

Fig. 12-113 Leiomyoma. High-power view showing spindle-shaped cells with blunt-ended nuclei. Immuno-histochemical analysis shows strong positivity for smooth muscle actin (inset).

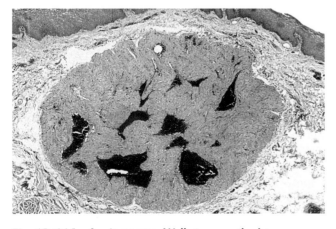

Fig. 12-114 Angiomyoma. Well-circumscribed tumor exhibiting prominent blood vessels surrounded by smooth muscle.

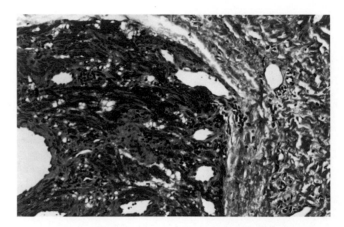

Fig. 12-115 Angiomyoma. Masson trichrome stain demonstrating bundles of smooth muscle (red) with adjacent normal collagen (blue).

Special stains and immunohistochemistry may be helpful to confirm the smooth muscle origin if the diagnosis is in doubt. The smooth muscle stains bright red with the Masson trichrome stain (Fig. 12-115). Immunohistochemical analysis usually reveals the tumor cells to be positive for vimentin, smooth muscle actin, and muscle-specific actin; desmin positivity also may be seen.

TREATMENT AND PROGNOSIS

Oral leiomyomas are treated by local surgical excision. The lesion should not recur.

RHABDOMYOMA

Benign neoplasms of skeletal muscle are called **rhabdomyomas.** The term *rhabdomyoma* also is used to describe a hamartomatous lesion of the heart that often is associated with tuberous sclerosis (see page 757). Despite the great amount of skeletal muscle throughout the body, benign skeletal muscle tumors are extremely rare. However, these extracardiac rhabdomyomas show a striking predilection for the head and neck. Rhabdomyomas of the head and neck can be subclassified into two major categories: (1) adult rhabdomyomas and (2) fetal rhabdomyomas.

CLINICAL FEATURES

ADULT RHABDOMYOMAS

Adult rhabdomyomas of the head and neck occur primarily in middle-aged and older patients, with about 70% of cases found in men. The most frequent sites are the pharynx, oral cavity, and larynx; intraoral lesions are most common in the floor of the mouth, soft palate,

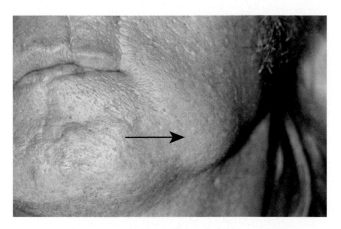

Fig. 12-116   Adult rhabdomyoma. Nodular mass *(arrow)* in the left cheek. *(Courtesy of Dr. Craig Little.)*

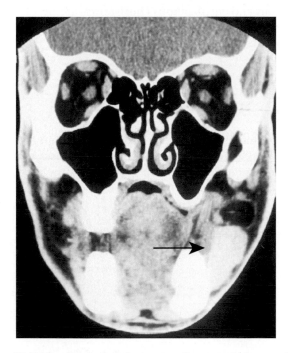

Fig. 12-117   Adult rhabdomyoma. Computed tomography (CT) scan of the same tumor depicted in Fig. 12-116. Note the mass *(arrow)* lateral to the left body of the mandible. *(Courtesy of Dr. Craig Little.)*

and base of tongue. The tumor appears as a nodule or mass that can grow to many centimeters before discovery (Figs. 12-116 and 12-117). Laryngeal and pharyngeal lesions often lead to airway obstruction. Sometimes, the tumor is multinodular in nature, with two or more discrete nodules found in the same anatomic location. Occasional cases are multicentric, with separate, distinct tumors at different sites.

FETAL RHABDOMYOMAS

Fetal rhabdomyomas usually occur in young children, although some also develop in adults. A similar male

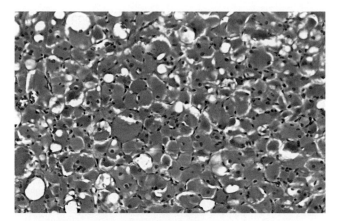

Fig. 12-118   Adult rhabdomyoma. Medium-power view showing a uniform tumor composed of rounded and polygonal cells with focal vacuolization.

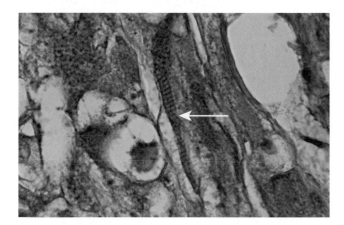

Fig. 12-119   Adult rhabdomyoma. Phosphotungstic acid hematoxylin (PTAH) stain that demonstrates focal cross striations in some cells *(arrow).*

predilection is noted. The most common locations are the face and periauricular region.

HISTOPATHOLOGIC FEATURES

ADULT RHABDOMYOMAS

The adult rhabdomyoma is composed of well-circumscribed lobules of large, polygonal cells, which exhibit abundant granular, eosinophilic cytoplasm (Fig. 12-118). These cells often demonstrate peripheral vacuolization that results in a "spider web" appearance of the cytoplasm. Focal cells with cross striations can be identified in most cases (Fig. 12-119). Although rarely necessary for the diagnosis, immunohistochemical examination will show the tumor cells to be positive for myoglobin, desmin, and muscle-specific actin.

FETAL RHABDOMYOMAS

The fetal rhabdomyoma has a less mature appearance and consists of a haphazard arrangement of spindle-shaped muscle cells that sometimes are found within a myxoid stroma. Some tumors may show considerable cellularity and mild pleomorphism, which makes them easily mistaken for rhabdomyosarcomas.

TREATMENT AND PROGNOSIS

The treatment of both variants of rhabdomyoma consists of local surgical excision. Recurrence is uncommon but has been reported in a few cases.

OSSEOUS AND CARTILAGINOUS CHORISTOMAS

A **choristoma** is a tumorlike growth of microscopically normal tissue in an abnormal location. Several different tissue types may occur in the mouth as choristomas. These include gastric mucosa, glial tissue, and tumorlike masses of sebaceous glands. However, the most frequently observed choristomas of the oral cavity are those that consist of bone, cartilage, or both. These lesions sometimes have been called **soft tissue osteomas** or **soft tissue chondromas**, but *choristoma* is a better term because they do not appear to be true neoplasms.

CLINICAL FEATURES

Osseous and cartilaginous choristomas show a striking predilection for the tongue, which accounts for 85% of cases. The most common location is the posterior tongue near the foramen cecum, although rare examples also have been reported elsewhere on the tongue and at other oral locations. The lesion is usually a firm, smooth-surfaced, sessile or pedunculated nodule between 0.5 and 2.0 cm in diameter (Fig. 12-120). Many patients are unaware of the lesion, although

some complain of gagging or dysphagia. More than 70% of osseous choristomas have been reported in women.

HISTOPATHOLOGIC FEATURES

Microscopic examination of choristomas shows a well-circumscribed mass of dense lamellar bone or mature cartilage that is surrounded by dense fibrous connective tissue (Fig. 12-121). Sometimes a combination of bone and cartilage is formed. The bone has a well-developed haversian canal system and occasionally demonstrates central fatty or hematopoietic marrow.

TREATMENT AND PROGNOSIS

Osseous and cartilaginous choristomas are best treated by local surgical excision. Recurrence has not been reported.

 ## Soft Tissue Sarcomas

Fortunately, soft tissue sarcomas are rare in the oral and maxillofacial region and account for less than 1% of the cancers in this area. Because of their relative rarity, it is beyond the scope of this book to give a complete, detailed discussion of each of these tumors. However, a review of these entities is included in the following section.

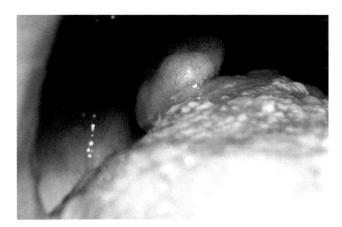

Fig. 12-120   Osseous choristoma. Hard pedunculated nodule on the posterior dorsum of the tongue. *(Courtesy of Dr. Michael Meyrowitz.)*

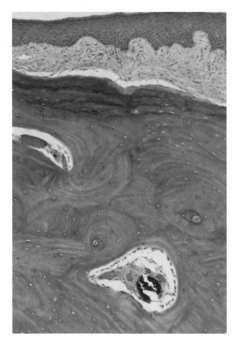

Fig. 12-121   Osseous choristoma. Mass of dense lamellar bone beneath the surface epithelium.

Over the past two decades, clinicians have seen a radical shift in the classification and nomenclature of many soft tissue sarcomas on the basis of detailed histochemical, immunohistochemical, and ultrastructural studies. Because of this, a number of previous tumor concepts have changed or are being critically reevaluated.

FIBROSARCOMA

The **fibrosarcoma** is a malignant tumor of fibroblasts. At one time, it was considered one of the most common soft tissue sarcomas. However, the diagnosis of fibrosarcoma is made much less frequently today because of the recognition and separate classification of other spindle cell lesions that have similar microscopic features. The tumor is most common in the extremities; only 10% occur in the head and neck region.

CLINICAL FEATURES

Fibrosarcomas most often present as slow-growing masses that may reach considerable size before they produce pain (Fig. 12-122). They can occur anywhere in the head and neck region. A number of cases have been reported in the nose and paranasal sinuses, where they often result in obstructive symptoms. They can occur at any age but are most common in young adults and children.

HISTOPATHOLOGIC FEATURES

Well-differentiated fibrosarcomas consist of fascicles of spindle-shaped cells that classically form a "herringbone" pattern (Fig. 12-123). The cells often show little variation in size and shape, although variable numbers of mitotic figures can usually be identified. In poorly differentiated tumors, the cells are less organized and may appear rounder or ovoid. Mild pleomorphism along with more frequent mitotic activity may be seen. Poorly differentiated tumors tend to produce less collagen than do well-differentiated tumors.

TREATMENT AND PROGNOSIS

The treatment of choice is usually surgical excision, including a wide margin of adjacent normal tissue. Recurrence is noted in about half of cases, and 5-year survival rates range from 40% to 70%.

MALIGNANT FIBROUS HISTIOCYTOMA

The **malignant fibrous histiocytoma** is considered to be a sarcoma with both fibroblastic and histiocytic features. After the introduction of this term in 1963, this tumor concept rapidly gained acceptance and became the most common soft tissue sarcoma diagnosed in adults. However, some experts today question the concept of malignant fibrous histiocytoma and now favor reclassification of the various tumors in this family into other categories, including undifferentiated pleomorphic sarcoma, liposarcoma, myxofibrosarcoma, melanoma, and anaplastic carcinoma. On the other hand, other authors still support the concept of this neoplasm. The following brief discussion reviews the traditional features of malignant fibrous histiocytoma, although it is possible that use of this term may fall further out of favor in the future.

CLINICAL FEATURES

The malignant fibrous histiocytoma is primarily considered to be a tumor of older age groups. The most common complaint is an expanding mass that may or

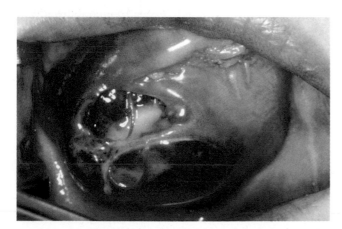

Fig. 12-122   Fibrosarcoma. Child with a large mass of the hard palate and maxillary alveolar ridge. *(Courtesy of Dr. John McDonald.)*

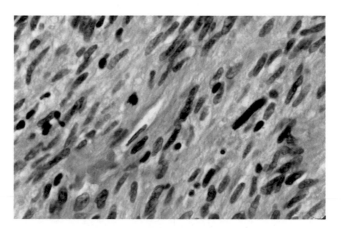

Fig. 12-123   Fibrosarcoma. Cellular mass of spindle-shaped cells demonstrating mild pleomorphism.

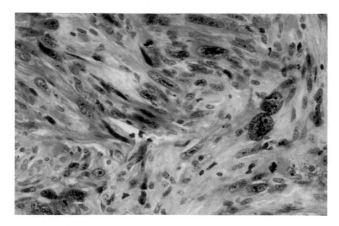

Fig. 12-124   Malignant fibrous histiocytoma. Spindle cell neoplasm demonstrating marked pleomorphism of some of the larger histiocytic cells.

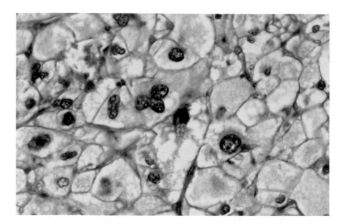

Fig. 12-125   Liposarcoma. High-power view showing vacuolated lipoblasts with pleomorphic nuclei.

may not be painful or ulcerated. Tumors of the nasal cavity and paranasal sinuses produce obstructive symptoms.

HISTOPATHOLOGIC FEATURES

Several histopathologic subtypes have been described. The storiform-pleomorphic type is the most common. This pattern is characterized by short fascicles of plump spindle cells arranged in a storiform pattern, admixed with areas of pleomorphic giant cells (Fig. 12-124). Myxoid, giant cell, inflammatory, and angiomatoid subtypes also have been recognized.

TREATMENT AND PROGNOSIS

The malignant fibrous histiocytoma is considered to be an aggressive tumor that is usually treated by radical surgical resection. Approximately 40% of patients have had local recurrences. A similar percentage has developed metastases, usually within 2 years of the initial diagnosis. The survival rate for patients with oral tumors appears to be worse than for those with tumors at other body sites.

LIPOSARCOMA

The **liposarcoma** is a malignant neoplasm of fatty origin. It currently is considered to be the most common soft tissue sarcoma and accounts for 20% of all soft tissue malignancies in adults. The most common sites are the thigh, retroperitoneum, and inguinal region. Liposarcomas of the head and neck are rare.

CLINICAL FEATURES

Liposarcomas are primarily seen in adults, with peak prevalence between the ages of 40 and 60. The tumor is typically a soft, slow-growing, ill-defined mass that

may appear normal in color or yellow. Pain or tenderness is uncommon; when present, it is usually a late feature. The neck is the most common site for liposarcomas of the head and neck region. The most frequent oral locations are the tongue and cheek.

HISTOPATHOLOGIC FEATURES

Most liposarcomas can be divided into three major categories:
1. Well-differentiated liposarcoma/atypical lipomatous tumor
2. Myxoid/round cell liposarcoma
3. Pleomorphic liposarcoma

The most common of these variants in the oral cavity is the **well-differentiated liposarcoma**, which accounts for 55% to 90% of all cases. These tumors resemble benign lipomas but demonstrate scattered lipoblasts and atypical, hyperchromatic stromal cells (Fig. 12-125).

Myxoid liposarcomas demonstrate proliferating lipoblasts within a myxoid stroma that contains a rich capillary network. The **round cell liposarcoma** is a more aggressive form of myxoid liposarcoma with less differentiated, rounded cells.

Pleomorphic liposarcomas exhibit extreme cellular pleomorphism and bizarre giant cells. **Dedifferentiated liposarcomas** are characterized by the combination of well-differentiated liposarcoma with poorly differentiated, nonlipogenic sarcomatous changes. These features may coexist in the same neoplasm, or the dedifferentiated changes may develop in a recurrent tumor or metastasis.

TREATMENT AND PROGNOSIS

Radical excision is the treatment of choice for most liposarcomas throughout the body. In spite of this, around 50% of all tumors recur. The overall 5-year survival rate ranges from 59% to 70%. There is a 10-year survival rate of approximately 50%. The histopathologic subtype is extremely important in predicting the prognosis; the outlook for pleomorphic liposarcomas is much worse than for myxoid and well-differentiated tumors.

In contrast, the prognosis for oral liposarcoma is more favorable because of the predominance of well-differentiated subtypes and because most tumors are small when diagnosed. Local recurrence has been reported in 15% to 20% of cases, but metastasis and death as a result of tumor is rare.

MALIGNANT PERIPHERAL NERVE SHEATH TUMOR (MALIGNANT SCHWANNOMA; NEUROFIBROSARCOMA; NEUROGENIC SARCOMA)

The principal malignancy of peripheral nerve origin is preferably called a **malignant peripheral nerve sheath tumor**. These tumors account for 5% of all soft tissue sarcomas, with about half of such cases occurring in patients with neurofibromatosis type I (see page 529). The lesion is most common on the proximal portions of the extremities and the trunk; only 10% to 15% of cases occur in the head and neck.

CLINICAL AND RADIOGRAPHIC FEATURES

Malignant peripheral nerve sheath tumors are most common in young adults. The mean age in patients with neurofibromatosis (29 to 36 years) is about one decade younger than in those without this condition (40 to 46 years). The tumor is an enlarging mass that sometimes exhibits rapid growth. Associated pain or a nerve deficit is common.

Oral tumors may occur anywhere, but the most common sites are the mandible, lips, and buccal mucosa (see Figs. 12-67 and 12-68, page 531). Radiographic examination of intraosseous tumors of the mandible may reveal widening of the mandibular canal or the mental foramen, with or without irregular destruction of the surrounding bone.

HISTOPATHOLOGIC FEATURES

The malignant peripheral nerve sheath tumor shows fascicles of atypical spindle-shaped cells, which often resemble the cells of fibrosarcoma (see Fig. 12-69, page 531). However, these cells are frequently more irregular in shape with wavy or comma-shaped nuclei. In addition to streaming fascicles, less cellular myxoid areas also may be present. With some tumors, there can be heterologous elements, which include skeletal

muscle differentiation (**malignant Triton tumor**), cartilage, bone, or glandular structures.

A definitive diagnosis of neural origin is often difficult, especially in the absence of neurofibromatosis. Positive immunostaining for S-100 protein is a helpful clue, but this is found in only about 50% of all cases.

TREATMENT AND PROGNOSIS

The treatment of malignant peripheral nerve sheath tumors consists primarily of radical surgical excision, possibly along with adjuvant radiation therapy and chemotherapy. The prognosis is poor, especially in patients with neurofibromatosis. One study showed the 5-year survival rate in individuals with neurofibromatosis type I to be only 16%. For other patients, the 5-year survival rate was 53%; this rate dropped to 38% at 10 years. However, another study showed an overall 5-year survival rate of 44%, which was nearly equal between both groups.

OLFACTORY NEUROBLASTOMA (ESTHESIONEUROBLASTOMA)

The **olfactory neuroblastoma** is a rare neuroectodermal neoplasm of the upper nasal vault that shows some similarities to neuroblastomas seen elsewhere in the body. Traditionally, it is believed to arise from the olfactory epithelium.

CLINICAL AND RADIOGRAPHIC FEATURES

Unlike the usual neuroblastoma, the olfactory neuroblastoma is rare in patients younger than the age of 10 years. Instead, it is more common in adults and occurs over a wide age range. The tumor arises high in the nasal cavity close to the cribriform plate. From there it may extend into the adjacent paranasal sinuses (especially the ethmoid sinus), the orbit, and the anterior cranial fossa (Fig. 12-126). The most common symptoms are nasal obstruction, anosmia, epistaxis, and pain.

HISTOPATHOLOGIC FEATURES

Olfactory neuroblastomas consist of small, round to ovoid basophilic cells that are arranged in sheets and lobules (Fig. 12-127). Rosette and pseudorosette formation and areas of delicate neurofibrillary material may be seen.

TREATMENT AND PROGNOSIS

The treatment of olfactory neuroblastoma consists of surgical excision, often with adjuvant radiation therapy. A combined craniofacial surgical approach frequently

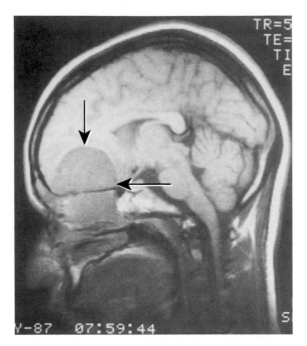

Fig. 12-126   Olfactory neuroblastoma. A T1-weighted sagittal magnetic resonance image (MRI) showing a tumor filling the superior nasal cavity and ethmoid sinus, with extension into the anterior cranial fossa *(arrows)*. *(Courtesy of Dr. Pamela Van Tassel.)*

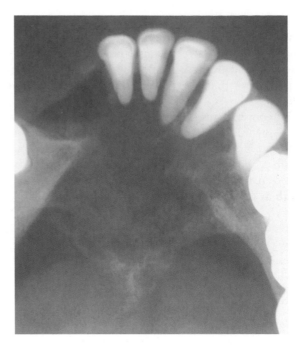

Fig. 12-128   Angiosarcoma. Occlusal radiograph showing a destructive, expansile tumor of the anterior mandible. *(Courtesy of Dr. W.C. John.)*

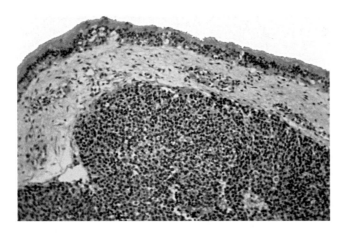

Fig. 12-127   Olfactory neuroblastoma. Sheet of small, basophilic cells adjacent to the sinonasal epithelium *(top).*

is used. Chemotherapy also has been administered, especially in advanced cases.

The prognosis depends on the stage of the disease. For patients with stage A lesions (tumor confined to the nasal cavity), the 5-year survival rate ranges from 72% to nearly 90%. The 5-year survival rate drops to 59% to 70% for stage B disease (tumor extending into the paranasal sinuses). For stage C disease (tumor extending beyond the nasal cavity and sinuses), the 5-year survival rate has improved to nearly 50% or even greater

with newer treatment regimens. Death is usually a result of local recurrence; metastasis occurs in approximately 20% to 37% of cases.

ANGIOSARCOMA

Angiosarcoma is a rare malignancy of vascular endothelium, which may arise from either blood or lymphatic vessels. More than 50% of all cases occur in the head and neck region, with the scalp and forehead being the most common sites. Oral lesions are quite rare.

The term **hemangioendothelioma** is used to describe vascular tumors with microscopic features intermediate between those of hemangiomas and angiosarcomas. Such tumors also are rare and are considered to be of intermediate malignancy.

CLINICAL FEATURES

Cutaneous angiosarcomas of the head and neck are most common in older adult patients. Early lesions often resemble a simple bruise, which may lead to a delay in diagnosis. However, the lesion continues to enlarge, which results in an elevated, nodular, or ulcerated surface. Many examples appear multifocal in nature. Oral angiosarcomas have been reported in various locations; the tongue and mandible are two of the more common sites (Fig. 12-128).

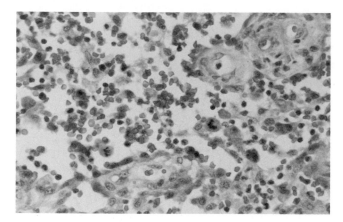

Fig. 12-129   Angiosarcoma. Sinusoidal vascular spaces lined by pleomorphic endothelial cells.

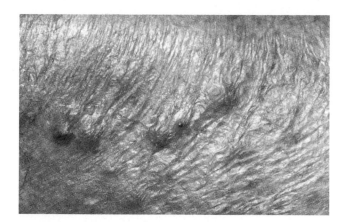

Fig. 12-130   Kaposi's sarcoma. Classic Kaposi's sarcoma in an older man presenting as multiple purple macules and plaques on the lower leg.

HISTOPATHOLOGIC FEATURES

Angiosarcoma is characterized by an infiltrative proliferation of endothelium-lined blood vessels that form an anastomosing network (Fig. 12-129). The endothelial cells appear hyperchromatic and atypical; they often tend to pile up within the vascular lumina. Increased mitotic activity may be seen. Immunohistochemical studies show the tumor cells to be positive for CD31 and factor VIII–related antigen in most cases, whereas CD34 positivity is observed less consistently.

TREATMENT AND PROGNOSIS

Treatment usually consists of radical surgical excision, radiation therapy, or both. The prognosis for angiosarcoma of the face and scalp is poor, with a reported 10-year survival rate of only 21%. However, angiosarcomas of the oral cavity and salivary glands appear to have a better outcome. One recent study showed 11 of 14 patients with oral and salivary angiosarcoma to be free of tumor on follow-up (mean follow-up period: 8.6 years).

KAPOSI'S SARCOMA

Kaposi's sarcoma is an unusual vascular neoplasm that was first described in 1872 by Moritz Kaposi, a Hungarian dermatologist. Before the advent of the acquired immunodeficiency syndrome (AIDS) epidemic, it was a rare tumor; however, beginning in the early 1980s, Kaposi's sarcoma became quite common because of its propensity to develop in individuals infected by the human immunodeficiency virus (HIV). Since the introduction of highly active antiretroviral therapy (HAART) in the mid- to late 1990s, the preva-

lence of AIDS-related Kaposi's sarcoma in the Western world has declined. Unfortunately, however, the frequency of this tumor still appears to be increasing in certain developing African nations.

Current evidence suggests that Kaposi's sarcoma is caused by human herpesvirus 8 (HHV-8; Kaposi's sarcoma–associated herpesvirus [KSHV]). The lesion most likely arises from endothelial cells, with some evidence of lymphatic origin. Four clinical presentations are recognized:

1. Classic
2. Endemic (African)
3. Iatrogenic immunosuppression associated
4. AIDS related

The first three forms are discussed here; AIDS-related Kaposi's sarcoma is covered in the section on HIV disease (see page 270).

CLINICAL FEATURES

CLASSIC TYPE

Classic (chronic) Kaposi's sarcoma is primarily a disease of late adult life, and 70% to 90% of cases occur in men. It mostly affects individuals of Italian, Jewish, or Slavic ancestry. Multiple blue-purple macules and plaques are present on the skin of the lower extremities (Fig. 12-130). These lesions grow slowly over many years and develop into painless tumor nodules. Oral lesions are rare and most frequently involve the palate. Some earlier reports suggested that patients with classic Kaposi's sarcoma had an increased prevalence of lymphoreticular malignancies, but more recent analysis has questioned any significant association.

ENDEMIC TYPE

Endemic Kaposi's sarcoma in Africa has been divided into four subtypes:

1. A **benign nodular** type, similar to classic Kaposi's sarcoma
2. An **aggressive** or infiltrative type, characterized by progressive development of locally invasive lesions that involve the underlying soft tissues and bone
3. A **florid** form, characterized by rapidly progressive and widely disseminated, aggressive lesions with frequent visceral involvement
4. A unique **lymphadenopathic** type, occurring primarily in young black children and exhibiting generalized, rapidly growing tumors of the lymph nodes, occasional visceral organ lesions, and sparse skin involvement

IATROGENIC TYPE

Iatrogenic immunosuppression-associated Kaposi's sarcoma most often occurs in recipients of organ transplants. It affects 0.5% of renal transplant patients, usually several months to a few years after the transplant. It is probably related to the loss of cellular immunity, which occurs as a result of immunosuppressive drugs. Like classic Kaposi's sarcoma, iatrogenic immunosuppression-associated cases are most common in individuals of Italian, Jewish, and Slavic ancestry; however, the disease may run a more aggressive course.

HISTOPATHOLOGIC FEATURES

Kaposi's sarcoma typically evolves through three stages:

1. Patch (macular)
2. Plaque
3. Nodular

A proliferation of miniature vessels characterizes the **patch stage**. This results in an irregular, jagged vascular network that surrounds preexisting vessels. Sometimes normal structures, such as hair follicles or preexisting blood vessels, may appear to protrude into these new vessels (promontory sign). The lesional endothelial cells have a bland appearance and may be associated with scattered lymphocytes and plasma cells.

The **plaque stage** demonstrates further proliferation of these vascular channels along with the development of a significant spindle cell component.

In the **nodular stage**, the spindle cells increase to form a nodular tumorlike mass that may resemble a fibrosarcoma or other spindle cell sarcomas (Figs. 12-131 and 12-132). However, numerous extrava-

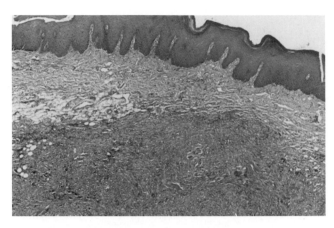

Fig. 12-131   Kaposi's sarcoma. Low-power photomicrograph showing a cellular spindle cell tumor within the connective tissue.

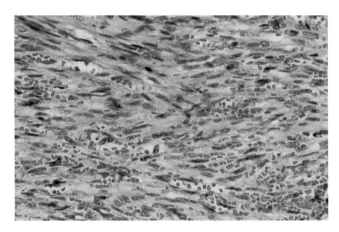

Fig. 12-132   Kaposi's sarcoma. High-power photomicrograph showing spindle cells and poorly defined vascular slits.

sated erythrocytes are present, and slitlike vascular spaces may be discerned.

TREATMENT AND PROGNOSIS

The treatment of Kaposi's sarcoma depends on the clinical subtype and stage of the disease. For skin lesions in the classic form of the disease, radiation therapy (especially electron beam) often is used. Radiation therapy for oral lesions must be approached with caution, because an unusually severe mucositis can develop. Surgical excision can be performed for the control of individual lesions of the skin or mucosa. Systemic chemotherapy, especially vinblastine, also may be helpful. Intralesional injection of chemotherapeutic agents is used to control individual lesions.

The prognosis is variable, depending on the form of the disease and the patient's immune status. The classic form of the disease is slowly progressive; only 10% to

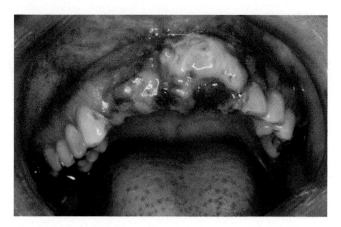

Fig. 12-133   **Leiomyosarcoma.** Ulcerated mass of the anterior maxillary alveolar ridge. *(Courtesy of Dr. Jim Weir.)*

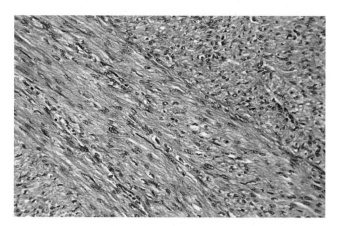

Fig. 12-134   **Leiomyosarcoma.** Medium-high-power view of a pleomorphic spindle cell proliferation.

20% of patients develop disseminated lesions. The mean survival time is 10 to 15 years, and patients often die from unrelated causes. The benign nodular, endemic African form of the disease is similar in behavior to classic non-African Kaposi's sarcoma. However, the other endemic African forms are more aggressive and the prognosis is poorer. The lymphadenopathic form runs a particularly fulminant course, usually resulting in the death of the patient within 2 to 3 years. In transplant patients, the disease also may be somewhat more aggressive, although the tumors may regress if immunosuppressive therapy is discontinued or reduced.

LEIOMYOSARCOMA

The **leiomyosarcoma** is a malignant neoplasm of smooth muscle differentiation, which accounts for 5% to 10% of all soft tissue sarcomas. The most common sites are the uterine wall and gastrointestinal tract. Leiomyosarcomas of the oral cavity are rare.

CLINICAL FEATURES

In general, leiomyosarcomas are most common in middle-aged and older adults. However, tumors in the oral and maxillofacial region occur over a wide age range without a predilection for any age group. They have been reported at various sites, but half of all oral cases occur in the jawbones. The clinical appearance is nonspecific; there is usually an enlarging mass that may or may not be painful (Fig. 12-133). Secondary ulceration of the mucosal surface may occur.

HISTOPATHOLOGIC FEATURES

The microscopic examination of a leiomyosarcoma shows fascicles of spindle-shaped cells with abundant eosinophilic cytoplasm and blunt-ended, cigar-shaped

nuclei (Fig. 12-134). Some tumors may be composed primarily of rounded epithelioid cells that have either eosinophilic or clear cytoplasm (epithelioid leiomyosarcoma). The degree of pleomorphism varies from one tumor to the next, but smooth muscle tumors with the presence of five or more mitoses per 10 high-power fields should be considered malignant. Glycogen can usually be demonstrated within the cells with a periodic acid-Schiff (PAS) stain, and the cell cytoplasm appears bright red with a Masson trichrome stain. Immunohistochemical analysis usually reveals the presence of one or more of the following myogenic markers: desmin, muscle-specific actin (HHF 35), smooth muscle myosin (SMMS), and smooth muscle actin.

TREATMENT AND PROGNOSIS

The treatment of leiomyosarcoma primarily consists of radical surgical excision, sometimes with adjunctive chemotherapy or radiation therapy. The prognosis for oral tumors is guarded, with the potential for local recurrence and distant metastasis. Although few cases are available for analysis, a 5-year survival rate of 62% has been estimated.

RHABDOMYOSARCOMA

Rhabdomyosarcoma is a malignant neoplasm that is characterized by skeletal muscle differentiation. These tumors are much more common in young children, accounting for 60% of soft tissue sarcomas in childhood. In contrast, rhabdomyosarcoma comprises only 2% to 5% of soft tissue sarcomas in adults. The most frequent site is the head and neck, which accounts for 35% of all cases. The genitourinary tract is the second most common location. Several microscopic patterns

Table **12-1** **Pediatric Rhabdomyosarcomas**

Major Types	Distribution	Five-Year Survival	Relative Prognosis
Embryonal rhabdomyosarcoma			
NOS	49%	66%	Intermediate
Botryoid	6%	95%	Excellent
Spindle	3%	88%	Excellent
Alveolar rhabdomyosarcoma	31%	53%	Poor
Undifferentiated sarcoma	3%	44%	Poor
Anaplastic rhabdomyosarcoma	2%	45%	Poor

Adapted from Hicks J, Flaitz C: Rhabdomyosarcoma of the head and neck in children, *Oral Oncol* 38:450-459, 2002.
NOS, Not otherwise specified.

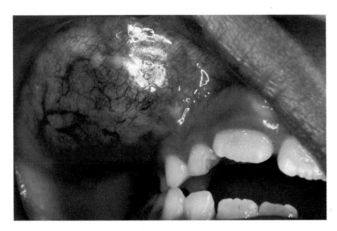

Fig. 12-135 **Embryonal rhabdomyosarcoma.** Young child with a mass of the right maxilla. *(Courtesy of Dr. Robert Achterberg.)*

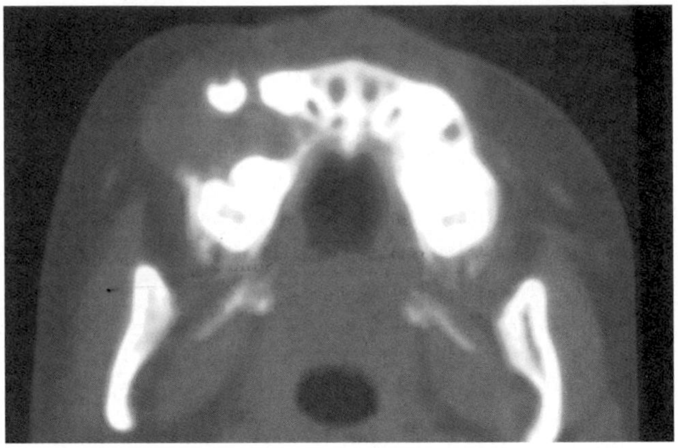

Fig. 12-136 **Embryonal rhabdomyosarcoma.** Computed tomography (CT) scan of patient from Fig. 12-135 showing expansile lytic lesion of the maxilla. *(Courtesy of Dr. Robert Achterberg.)*

of pediatric rhabdomyosarcoma are recognized (Table 12-1), although discussion here will be limited primarily to the embryonal and alveolar subtypes.

CLINICAL FEATURES

Rhabdomyosarcoma primarily occurs during the first decade of life but also may occur in teenagers and young adults. It is rare in people older than 45 years, and approximately 60% of all cases occur in males. Embryonal rhabdomyosarcomas are most common in the first 10 years of life and account for about 60% of all cases. Alveolar rhabdomyosarcomas occur most often in persons between 10 and 25 years of age; they account for 20% to 30% of all tumors. Pleomorphic rhabdomyosarcomas represent less than 5% of all cases and show a peak prevalence in patients older than 40 years of age. Most head and neck lesions are embryonal or alveolar types; pleomorphic rhabdomyosarcomas primarily occur on the extremities.

The tumor is most often a painless, infiltrative mass that may grow rapidly (Figs. 12-135 and 12-136). In the head and neck region, the face and orbit are the most frequent locations, followed by the nasal cavity. The palate is the most frequent intraoral site, and some lesions may appear to arise in the maxillary sinus and break through into the oral cavity. Some embryonal rhabdomyosarcomas that arise within a cavity, such as the vagina or oropharynx, demonstrate an exophytic, polypoid growth pattern that resembles a cluster of grapes. The term *botryoid* (grapelike) *rhabdomyosarcoma* has been used for these lesions.

HISTOPATHOLOGIC FEATURES
EMBRYONAL TYPE

The embryonal rhabdomyosarcoma resembles various stages in the embryogenesis of skeletal muscle. Poorly differentiated examples may be difficult to diagnose and consist of small round or oval cells with hyperchromatic nuclei and indistinct cytoplasm (Fig. 12-137).

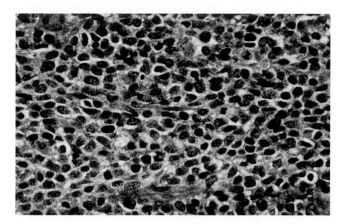

Fig. 12-137 Embryonal rhabdomyosarcoma. Medium-power view showing a sheet of small, round cells with hyperchromatic nuclei.

Alternating hypercellular and myxoid zones may be seen. Better-differentiated lesions show round to ovoid rhabdomyoblasts with distinctly eosinophilic cytoplasm and fibrillar material around the nucleus. Cross striations are rarely found. Some tumors show better-differentiated, elongated, strap-shaped rhabdomyoblasts.

The **botryoid** subtype of embryonal rhabdomyosarcoma is sparsely cellular and has a pronounced myxoid stroma. Increased cellularity, or a so-called cambium layer, is usually seen just beneath the mucosal surface.

Immunohistochemical analysis for the presence of desmin, myogenin, and muscle-specific actin can be helpful in supporting the muscular nature of the tumor. However, the intensity of the immunostaining can vary depending on the degree of rhabdomyoblastic differentiation.

ALVEOLAR TYPE

Both classic and solid variants of alveolar rhabdomyosarcoma are recognized. The classic pattern is characterized by aggregates of poorly differentiated round to oval cells separated by fibrous septa. These cells demonstrate a central loss of cohesiveness, which results in an alveolar pattern. The peripheral cells of these aggregates adhere to the septal walls in a single layer. The central cells appear to float freely within the alveolar spaces. Mitoses are common, and multinucleated giant cells also may be seen. In contrast, solid alveolar rhabdomyosarcoma demonstrates cellular fields of small round basophilic cells without fibrovascular septa.

Cytogenetic and molecular studies play an important role in the diagnosis of rhabdomyosarcoma. Two distinct translocations have been identified in alveolar rhabdomyosarcoma (PAX3-FKHR and PAX7-FKHR). Embryonal rhabdomyosarcoma is characterized by a consistent loss of heterozygosity or loss of imprinting at chromosome 11p15.

TREATMENT AND PROGNOSIS

Before 1960 the prognosis for a patient with rhabdomyosarcoma was extremely poor, with more than 90% of patients dying. With the advent of multimodal therapy during the past several decades, the prognosis has improved dramatically.

Treatment typically consists of local surgical excision followed by multiagent chemotherapy (vincristine, actinomycin D, and cyclophosphamide). Postoperative radiation therapy also is used, except for localized tumors that have been completely resected at initial surgery. The 5-year survival rate for embryonal rhabdomyosarcoma (not otherwise specified [NOS]) is around 66%, although the figures for botryoid (95%) and spindle cell variants (88%) are much better. The 5-year survival rate for alveolar rhabdomyosarcoma is only 53%, and survival drops to slightly less than 50% for anaplastic rhabdomyosarcoma and undifferentiated sarcomas.

SYNOVIAL SARCOMA

Synovial sarcoma is an uncommon malignancy that represents 5% to 10% of all soft tissue sarcomas. The tumor occurs primarily near large joints and bursae, especially in the extremities, but most authorities now agree that this lesion probably does not arise from the synovium. Although it is often para-articular in location, the tumor rarely occurs within the joint capsule. In some instances, it arises in areas without any obvious relationship to synovial structures. Synovial sarcomas of the head and neck are rare (only 4% to 9% of all cases), and many of these apparently are unrelated to joint areas.

Over 90% of synovial sarcomas exhibit a specific balanced reciprocal translocation between the X chromosome and chromosome 18: t(X;18)(p11.2;q11.2). Detection of this translocation can be helpful in making the diagnosis, evaluating tumor margins, and confirming the presence of metastatic disease.

CLINICAL FEATURES

Synovial sarcomas most frequently occur in teenagers and young adults, and there is a slight male predilection. The most common presentation is a gradually enlarging mass that often is associated with pain or tenderness. Tumors in the head and neck region are most common in the paravertebral and parapharyngeal areas. Often, they produce symptoms of dysphagia, dyspnea, or hoarseness. Oral tumors most often have been reported in the tongue and cheek.

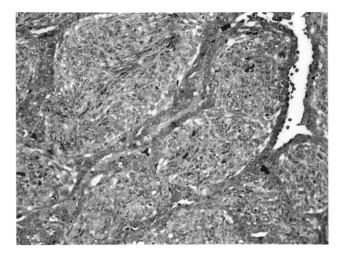

Fig. 12-138   Synovial sarcoma. Biphasic tumor consisting of spindle cells intermixed with cuboidal to columnar epithelial cells that line glandlike spaces.

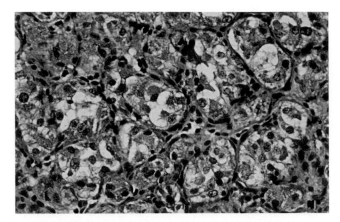

Fig. 12-139   Alveolar soft-part sarcoma. Alveolar collections of large, polygonal cells containing abundant granular cytoplasm.

HISTOPATHOLOGIC FEATURES

Classic synovial sarcoma is a biphasic tumor that consists of a combination of spindle cells and epithelial cells (Fig. 12-138). The spindle cells usually predominate and produce a pattern that is similar to fibrosarcoma. Within this spindle cell background are groups of cuboidal to columnar epithelial cells that surround glandlike spaces or form nests, cords, or whorls. Calcifications are seen in around 30% of cases.

Less frequently, the tumor is monophasic and consists primarily or entirely of spindle cells. The diagnosis of these tumors is difficult, but most lesions demonstrate at least focal positive immunostaining of spindle cells for cytokeratin or epithelial membrane antigen. Rare examples of monophasic epithelial synovial sarcomas also have been reported.

TREATMENT AND PROGNOSIS

Treatment of synovial sarcoma usually consists of radical surgical excision, possibly with adjunctive radiation therapy or chemotherapy. The prognosis is poor because the tumor has a high rate of recurrence and metastasis. The reported 5-year survival rate ranges from 36% to 64%. However, the 10-year survival rate drops to 20% to 38% because of the high rate of late metastases.

ALVEOLAR SOFT-PART SARCOMA

The **alveolar soft-part sarcoma** is a rare neoplasm of uncertain histogenesis. About 25% of all cases occur in the head and neck.

CLINICAL FEATURES

The alveolar soft-part sarcoma is usually a slow-growing, painless mass. The tumor is most common in young adults and children. In adults, the lower extremity is the most frequent location; in younger patients, the head and neck region is the most common site. The orbit and tongue are the most common head and neck locations, and the median age for lingual tumors is only 5 to 8 years. During the first 2 decades of life, the tumor shows nearly a 2:1 female predilection. However, cases that develop after the age of 30 are more common in men.

HISTOPATHOLOGIC FEATURES

Alveolar soft-part sarcomas are composed of groups of large, polygonal cells that are arranged around central alveolar spaces (Fig. 12-139). These cells have abundant granular, eosinophilic cytoplasm and one to several vesicular nuclei. Mitoses are rare. Special stains will reveal PAS-positive, diastase-resistant crystals that are highly characteristic for this tumor. Under the electron microscope, these crystals appear as rhomboid, polygonal, or rod-shaped structures with a regular latticework pattern.

Immunohistochemistry has played a limited role in the specific diagnosis of alveolar soft-part sarcoma, except to rule out other tumors with more characteristic staining patterns. However, molecular analysis of fresh tissue may be helpful in difficult cases because the tumor shows a characteristic genetic translocation, der(17)t(X;17)(p11.2;q25), which results in an *ASPL-TFE3* fusion gene. Recently, an antibody against the C-terminus of the *ASPL-TFE3* fusion protein has been created, allowing the development of a sensitive immunohistochemical marker for this tumor.

TREATMENT AND PROGNOSIS

Most patients with alveolar soft-part sarcomas are treated by radical surgical excision, possibly in conjunction with radiation therapy and chemotherapy. The prognosis is poor, often as a result of late metastasis. One study reported a 5-year survival rate of 60%, but the 20-year survival rate dropped to only 15%. Another series showed a 5-year disease-free survival of 71% for patients with localized disease, compared with only 20% for patients who presented with metastatic disease. However, the prognosis for children appears to be better than for adults. Lingual and orbital tumors have very high survival rates, possibly because of smaller tumor size at diagnosis and younger patient age.

METASTASES TO THE ORAL SOFT TISSUES

Metastatic tumors to the oral cavity are uncommon and represent approximately 1% of all oral malignancies. Such metastases can occur to bone (see page 669) or to the oral soft tissues. The mechanism by which tumors can spread to the oral cavity is poorly understood. Primary malignancies from immediately adjacent tissues might be able to spread by a lymphatic route; however, such a mechanism cannot explain metastases from tumors from lower parts of the body, which are almost certainly blood-borne and should be filtered out by the lungs. One possible explanation for blood-borne metastases to the head and neck, especially in the absence of pulmonary metastases, is **Batson's plexus**, a valveless vertebral venous plexus that might allow retrograde spread of tumor cells, bypassing filtration through the lungs.

CLINICAL FEATURES

The most common site for oral soft tissue metastases is the gingiva, which accounts for slightly more than 50% of all cases. The next most common site is the tongue, which accounts for 25% of cases. The lesion usually appears as a nodular mass that often resembles a hyperplastic or reactive growth, such as a pyogenic granuloma (Figs. 12-140 to 12-142). Occasionally, the lesion appears as a surface ulceration. Adjacent teeth may become loosened by an underlying destruction of the alveolar bone. The presence of teeth may play an important role in the preference of metastases for the gingiva. Once malignant cells reach the oral cavity, the rich vascular network of inflamed gingival tissues may serve as a fertile site for further growth.

Oral soft tissue metastases are more common in males and are seen most frequently in middle-aged and older adults. Almost any malignancy from any

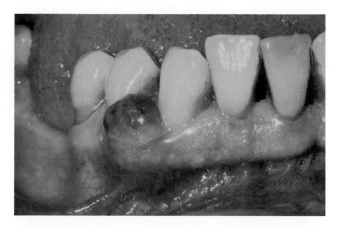

Fig. 12-140   Metastatic melanoma. Pigmented nodule of the mandibular gingiva.

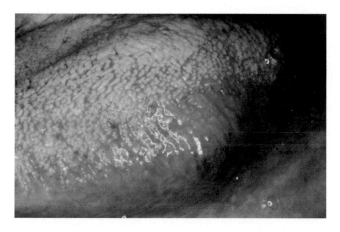

Fig. 12-141   Metastatic renal carcinoma. Nodular mass of the left lateral border of the tongue. *(Courtesy of Dr. Mark Bowden.)*

body site is capable of metastasis to the oral cavity, and a wide variety of tumors have been reported to spread to the mouth. (However, there is probably a bias in the literature toward reporting more unusual cases.) In the cases reported, lung cancer is responsible for more than one third of all oral soft tissue metastases in men, followed by renal carcinoma and melanoma. Although prostate cancer is common in men, metastases from these tumors have an affinity for bone and rarely occur in soft tissues. For women, breast cancer accounts for 25% of all cases, followed by malignancies of the genital organs, lung, bone, and kidney. It is probable that in the future we will see an increased number of metastatic lung cancers in women (today this is the most common cancer killer of women in the United States).

In most cases the primary tumor already is known when the metastatic lesion is discovered. In some cases,

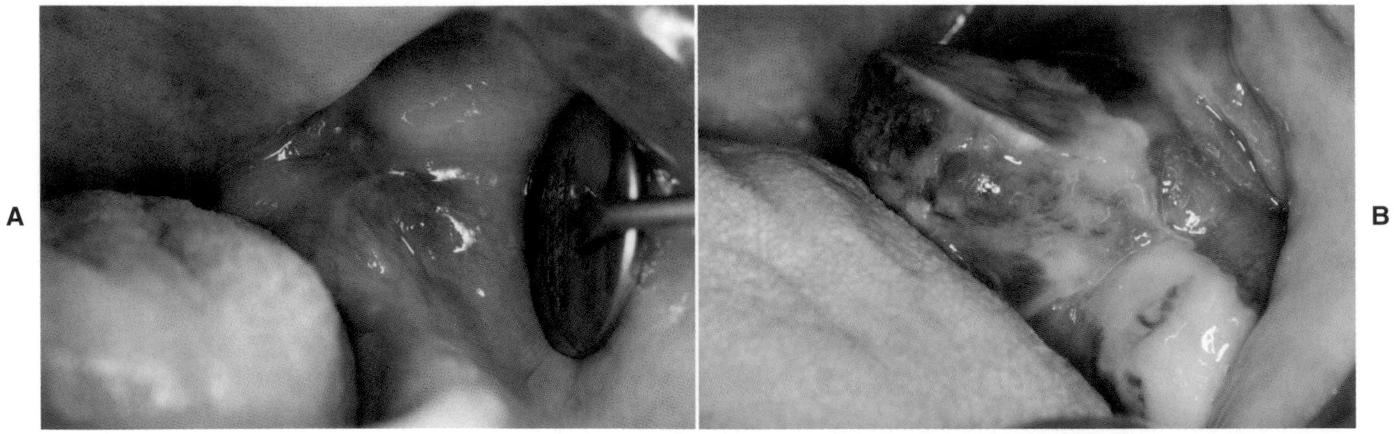

Fig. 12-142 Metastatic adenocarcinoma of the colon. A, Focal swelling of the left retromolar pad area. **B,** Same patient 4 weeks later. Note the marked enlargement of the lesion. *(Courtesy of Dr. George Blozis.)*

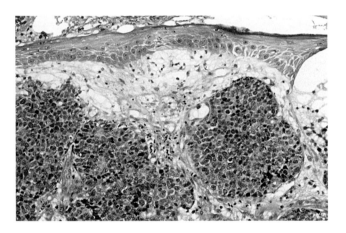

Fig. 12-143 Metastatic carcinoma of the lung. Aggregates of malignant epithelial cells below the surface epithelium.

however, the oral lesion is the first sign of the malignant disease.

HISTOPATHOLOGIC FEATURES

The microscopic appearance of the metastatic neoplasm should resemble the tumor of origin (Fig. 12-143). Most cases represent carcinomas; metastatic sarcomas to the oral region are rare.

TREATMENT AND PROGNOSIS

The prognosis for patients with metastatic tumors is generally poor because other metastatic sites also are frequently present. Management of the oral lesion is usually palliative and should be coordinated with the patient's overall treatment.

BIBLIOGRAPHY

Fibroma and Giant Cell Fibroma

Barker DS, Lucas RB: Localised fibrous overgrowth of the oral mucosa, *Br J Oral Surg* 5:86-92, 1967.

Brannon RB, Pousson RR: The retrocuspid papillae: a clinical evaluation of 51 cases, *J Dent Hyg* 77:180-184, 2003.

Buchner A, Merrell PW, Hansen LS et al: The retrocuspid papilla of the mandibular lingual gingiva, *J Periodontol* 61:586-590, 1990.

Gonsalves WC, Chi AC, Neville BW: Common oral lesions: part II. Masses and neoplasia, *Am Fam Physician* 75:509-512, 2007.

Houston GD: The giant cell fibroma: a review of 464 cases, *Oral Surg Oral Med Oral Pathol* 53:582-587, 1982.

Magnusson BC, Rasmusson LG: The giant cell fibroma: a review of 103 cases with immunohistochemical findings, *Acta Odontol Scand* 53:293-296, 1995.

Savage NW, Monsour PA: Oral fibrous hyperplasias and the giant cell fibroma, *Aust Dent J* 30:405-409, 1985.

Souza LB, Andrade ES, Miguel MC et al: Origin of stellate giant cells in oral fibrous lesions determined by immunohistochemical expression of vimentin, HHF-35, CD68 and factor XIIIa, *Pathology* 36:316-320, 2004.

Weathers DR, Callihan MD: Giant cell fibroma, *Oral Surg Oral Med Oral Pathol* 37:374-384, 1974.

Epulis Fissuratum

Buchner A, Begleiter A, Hansen LS: The predominance of epulis fissuratum in females, *Quintessence Int* 15:699-702, 1984.

Cutright DE: Osseous and chondromatous metaplasia caused by dentures, *Oral Surg Oral Med Oral Pathol* 34:625-633, 1972.

Cutright DE: The histopathologic findings in 583 cases of epulis fissuratum, *Oral Surg Oral Med Oral Pathol* 37:401-411, 1974.

Inflammatory Papillary Hyperplasia

Antonelli JR, Panno FV, Witko A: Inflammatory papillary hyperplasia: supraperiosteal excision by the blade-loop technique, *Gen Dent* 46:390-397, 1998.

Bergendal T, Heimdahl A, Isacsson G: Surgery in the treatment of denture-related inflammatory papillary hyperplasia of the palate, *Int J Oral Surg* 9:312-319, 1980.

Bhaskar SN, Beasley JD III, Cutright DE: Inflammatory papillary hyperplasia of the oral mucosa: report of 341 cases, *J Am Dent Assoc* 81:949-952, 1970.

Budtz-Jørgensen E: Oral mucosal lesions associated with the wearing of removable dentures, *J Oral Pathol* 10:65-80, 1981.

Cutright DE: Morphogenesis of inflammatory papillary hyperplasia, *J Prosthet Dent* 33:380-385, 1975.

Infante-Cossio P, Martinez-de-Fuentes R, Torres-Carranza E et al: Inflammatory papillary hyperplasia of the palate: treatment with carbon dioxide laser, followed by restoration with an implant-supported prosthesis, *Br J Oral Maxillofac Surg* 45:658-660, 2007.

Reichart PA, Schmidt-Westhausen A, Samaranayake LP et al: *Candida*-associated palatal papillary hyperplasia in HIV infection, *J Oral Pathol Med* 23:403-405, 1994.

Salonen MAM, Raustia AM, Oikarinen KS: Effect of treatment of palatal inflammatory papillary hyperplasia with local and systemic antifungal agents accompanied by renewal of complete dentures, *Acta Odontol Scand* 54:87-91, 1996.

Fibrous Histiocytoma

Alves FA, Vargas PA, Siqueira SA et al: Benign fibrous histiocytoma of the buccal mucosa: case report with immunohistochemical features, *J Oral Maxillofac Surg* 61:269-271, 2003.

Gray PB, Miller AS, Loftus MJ: Benign fibrous histiocytoma of the oral/perioral regions: report of a case and review of 17 additional cases, *J Oral Maxillofac Surg* 50:1239-1242, 1992.

Harsanyi BB, Larsson A: Xanthomatous lesions of the mandible: osseous expression of non-X histiocytosis and benign fibrous histiocytoma, *Oral Surg Oral Med Oral Pathol* 65:551-566, 1988.

Heo M-S, Cho H-J, Kwon K-J et al: Benign fibrous histiocytoma in the mandible, *Oral Surg Oral Med Oral Pathol Oral Radiol Endod* 97:276-280, 2004.

Thompson SH, Shear M: Fibrous histiocytomas of the oral and maxillofacial regions, *J Oral Pathol* 13:282-294, 1984.

Fibromatosis

Buitendijk S, van de Ven CP, Dumans TG et al: Pediatric aggressive fibromatosis: a retrospective analysis of 13 patients and review of the literature, *Cancer* 104:1090-1099, 2005.

Dormans JP, Spiegel D, Meyer J et al: Fibromatoses in childhood: the desmoid/fibromatosis complex, *Med Pediatr Oncol* 37:126-131, 2001.

Fowler CB, Hartman KS, Brannon RB: Fibromatosis of the oral and paraoral region, *Oral Surg Oral Med Oral Pathol* 77:373-386, 1994.

Gnepp DR, Henley J, Weiss S et al: Desmoid fibromatosis of the sinonasal tract and nasopharynx: a clinicopathologic study of 25 cases, *Cancer* 78:2572-2579, 1996.

Vally IM, Altini M: Fibromatoses of the oral and paraoral soft tissues and jaws: review of the literature and report of 12 new cases, *Oral Surg Oral Med Oral Pathol* 69:191-198, 1990.

Myofibroma (Myofibromatosis)

Allon I, Vered M, Buchner A et al: Central (intraosseous) myofibroma of the mandible: clinical, radiologic, and histopathologic features of a rare lesion, *Oral Surg Oral Med Oral Pathol Oral Radiol Endod* 103:e45-e53, 2007.

Foss RD, Ellis GL: Myofibromas and myofibromatosis of the oral region: a clinicopathologic analysis of 79 cases, *Oral Surg Oral Med Oral Pathol Oral Radiol Endod* 89:57-65, 2000.

Jones AC, Freedman PD, Kerpel SM: Oral myofibromas: a report of 13 cases and review of the literature, *J Oral Maxillofac Surg* 52:870-875, 1994.

Lingen MW, Mostofi RS, Solt DB: Myofibromas of the oral cavity, *Oral Surg Oral Med Oral Pathol Oral Radiol Endod* 80:297-302, 1995.

Matthews MS, Tabor MW, Thompson SH et al: Infantile myofibromatosis of the mandible, *J Oral Maxillofac Surg* 48:884-889, 1990.

Sedghizadeh PP, Allen CM, Kalmar JR et al: Solitary central myofibroma presenting in the gnathic region, *Ann Diagn Pathol* 8:284-289, 2004.

Vered M, Allon I, Buchner A et al: Clinico-pathologic correlations of myofibroblastic tumor of the oral cavity. II. Myofibroma and myofibromatosis of the oral soft tissues, *J Oral Pathol Med* 36:304-314, 2007.

Oral Focal Mucinosis

Aldred MJ, Talacko AA, Ruljancich K et al: Oral focal mucinosis: report of 15 cases and review of the literature, *Pathology* 35:393-396, 2003.

Buchner A, Merrell PW, Leider AS et al: Oral focal mucinosis, *Int J Oral Maxillofac Surg* 19:337-340, 1990.

Soda G, Baiocchini A, Bosco D et al: Oral focal mucinosis of the tongue, *Pathol Oncol Res* 4:304-307, 1998.

Tomich CE: Oral focal mucinosis: a clinicopathologic and histochemical study of eight cases, *Oral Surg Oral Med Oral Pathol* 38:714-724, 1974.

Pyogenic Granuloma

Bhaskar SN, Jacoway JR: Pyogenic granuloma—clinical features, incidence, histology, and result of treatment: report of 242 cases, *J Oral Surg* 24:391-398, 1966.

Daley TD, Nartey NO, Wysocki GP: Pregnancy tumor: an analysis, *Oral Surg Oral Med Oral Pathol* 72:196-199, 1991.

Epivatianos A, Antoniades D, Zaraboukas T et al: Pyogenic granuloma of the oral cavity: comparative study of its clinicopathological and immunohistochemical features, *Pathol Int* 55:391-397, 2005.

Kerr DA: Granuloma pyogenicum, *Oral Surg Oral Med Oral Pathol* 4:158-176, 1951.

Mills SE, Cooper PH, Fechner RE: Lobular capillary hemangioma: the underlying lesion of pyogenic granuloma: a study of 73 cases from the oral and nasal mucous membranes, *Am J Surg Pathol* 4:471-479, 1980.

Patrice SJ, Wiss K, Mulliken JB: Pyogenic granuloma (lobular capillary hemangioma): a clinicopathologic study of 178 cases, *Pediatr Dermatol* 8:267-276, 1991.

Toida M, Hasegawa T, Watanabe F et al: Lobular capillary hemangioma of the oral mucosa: clinicopathological study of 43 cases with a special reference to immunohistochemical characterization of the vascular elements, *Pathol Int* 53:1-7, 2003.

Zain RB, Khoo SP, Yeo JF: Oral pyogenic granuloma (excluding pregnancy tumor)—a clinical analysis of 304 cases, *Singapore Dent J* 20:8-10, 1995.

Peripheral Giant Cell Granuloma

Carvalho YR, Loyola AM, Gomez RS et al: Peripheral giant cell granuloma. An immunohistochemical and ultrastructural study, *Oral Dis* 1:20-25, 1995.

Flanagan AM, Tinkler SMB, Horton MA et al: The multinucleate cells in giant cell granulomas of the jaw are osteoclasts, *Cancer* 62:1139-1145, 1988.

Giansanti JS, Waldron CA: Peripheral giant cell granuloma: review of 720 cases, *J Oral Surg* 17:787-791, 1969.

Katsikeris N, Kakarantza-Angelopoulou E, Angelopoulos AP: Peripheral giant cell granuloma: clinicopathologic study of 224 new cases and review of 956 reported cases, *Int J Oral Maxillofac Surg* 17:94-99, 1988.

Motamedi MHK, Eshghyar N, Jafari SM et al: Peripheral and central giant cell granulomas of the jaws: a demographic study, *Oral Surg Oral Med Oral Pathol Oral Radiol Endod* 103: e39-e43, 2007.

Smith BR, Fowler CB, Svane TJ: Primary hyperparathyroidism presenting as a "peripheral" giant cell granuloma, *J Oral Maxillofac Surg* 46:65-69, 1988.

Peripheral Ossifying Fibroma

Buchner A, Hansen LS: The histomorphologic spectrum of peripheral ossifying fibroma, *Oral Surg Oral Med Oral Pathol* 63:452-461, 1987.

Cuisia ZE, Brannon RB: Peripheral ossifying fibroma—a clinical evaluation of 134 pediatric cases, *Pediatr Dent* 23:245-248, 2001.

Kendrick F, Waggoner WF: Managing a peripheral ossifying fibroma, *ASDC J Dent Child* 63:135-138, 1996.

Kenney JN, Kaugars GE, Abbey LM: Comparison between the peripheral ossifying fibroma and peripheral odontogenic fibroma, *J Oral Maxillofac Surg* 47:378-382, 1989.

Walters JD, Will JK, Hatfield RD et al: Excision and repair of the peripheral ossifying fibroma: a report of 3 cases, *J Periodontol* 72:939-944, 2001.

Zain RB, Fei YJ: Fibrous lesions of the gingiva: a histopathologic analysis of 204 cases, *Oral Surg Oral Med Oral Pathol* 70:466-470, 1990.

Lipoma

Bataineh AB, Mansour MJ, Abalkhail A: Oral infiltrating lipomas, *Br J Oral Maxillofac Surg* 34:520-523, 1996.

Billings SD, Henley JD, Summerlin D-J et al: Spindle cell lipoma of the oral cavity, *Am J Dermatopathol* 28:28-31, 2006.

Chen S-Y, Fantasia JE, Miller AS: Myxoid lipoma of oral soft tissue: a clinical and ultrastructural study, *Oral Surg Oral Med Oral Pathol* 57:300-307, 1984.

Darling MR, Daley TD: Intraoral chondroid lipoma: a case report and immunohistochemical investigation, *Oral Surg Oral Med Oral Pathol Oral Radiol Endod* 99:331-333, 2005.

Epivatianos A, Markopoulos AK, Papanayotou P: Benign tumors of adipose tissue of the oral cavity: a clinicopathologic study of 13 cases, *J Oral Maxillofac Surg* 58:1113-1117, 2000.

Fregnani ER, Pires FR, Falzoni R et al: Lipomas of the oral cavity: clinical findings, histological classification and proliferative activity of 46 cases, *Int J Oral Maxillofac Surg* 32:49-53, 2003.

Furlong MA, Fanburg-Smith JC, Childers ELB: Lipoma of the oral and maxillofacial region: site and subclassification of 125 cases, *Oral Surg Oral Med Oral Pathol Oral Radiol Endod* 98:441-450, 2004.

Garavaglia J, Gnepp DR: Intramuscular (infiltrating) lipoma of the tongue, *Oral Surg Oral Med Oral Pathol* 63:348-350, 1987.

Horie N, Shimoyama T, Kaneko T et al: Traumatic herniation of the buccal fat pad, *Pediatr Dent* 23:249-252, 2001.

Traumatic Neuroma

Lee EJ, Calcaterra TC, Zuckerbraun L: Traumatic neuromas of the head and neck, *Ear Nose Throat J* 77:670-676, 1998.

Peszkowski MJ, Larsson Å: Extraosseous and intraosseous oral traumatic neuromas and their association with tooth extraction, *J Oral Maxillofac Surg* 48:963-967, 1990.

Sist TC Jr, Greene GW: Traumatic neuroma of the oral cavity: report of thirty-one new cases and review of the literature, *Oral Surg Oral Med Oral Pathol* 51:394-402, 1981.

Vora AR, Loescher AR, Craig GT et al: A light microscopical study on the structure of traumatic neuromas of the human lingual nerve, *Oral Surg Oral Med Oral Pathol Oral Radiol Endod* 99:395-403, 2005.

Palisaded Encapsulated Neuroma

Chauvin PJ, Wysocki GP, Daley TD et al: Palisaded encapsulated neuroma of oral mucosa, *Oral Surg Oral Med Oral Pathol* 73:71-74, 1992.

Dakin MC, Leppard B, Theaker JM: The palisaded, encapsulated neuroma (solitary circumscribed neuroma), *Histopathology* 20:405-410, 1992.

Dover JS, From L, Lewis A: Palisaded encapsulated neuromas: a clinicopathologic study, *Arch Dermatol* 125:386-389, 1989.

Fletcher CDM: Solitary circumscribed neuroma of the skin (so-called palisaded, encapsulated neuroma): a clinicopathologic and immunohistochemical study, *Am J Surg Pathol* 13:574-580, 1989.

Magnusson B: Palisaded encapsulated neuroma (solitary circumscribed neuroma) of the oral mucosa, *Oral Surg Oral Med Oral Pathol Oral Radiol Endod* 82:302-304, 1996.

Neurilemoma and Neurofibroma

Chi AC, Carey J, Muller S: Intraosseous schwannoma of the mandible: a case report and review of the literature, *Oral Surg Oral Med Oral Pathol Oral Radiol Endod* 96:54-65, 2003.

Colreavy MP, Lacy PD, Hughes J et al: Head and neck schwannomas—a 10 year review, *J Laryngol Otol* 114:119-124, 2000.

Ellis GL, Abrams AM, Melrose RJ: Intraosseous benign neural sheath neoplasms of the jaws: report of seven new cases and review of the literature, *Oral Surg Oral Med Oral Pathol* 44:731-743, 1977.

Ferner RE: Neurofibromatosis 1 and neurofibromatosis 2: a twenty-first century perspective, *Lancet Neurol* 6:340-351, 2007.

Hanemann CO, Evans DG: News on the genetics, epidemiology, medical care and translational research of schwannomas, *J Neurol* 253:1533-1541, 2006.

Marocchio LS, Oliveira DT, Pereira MC et al: Sporadic and multiple neurofibromas in the head and neck region: a retrospective study of 33 years, *Clin Oral Invest* 11:165-169, 2007.

Muramatsu T, Hashimoto S, Inoue T et al: Melanotic schwannoma arising in the floor of the mouth, *J Oral Maxillofac Surg* 63:703-706, 2005.

Williams HK, Cannell H, Silvester K et al: Neurilemmoma of the head and neck, *Br J Oral Maxillofac Surg* 31:32-35, 1993.

Woodruff JM: The pathology and treatment of peripheral nerve tumors and tumor-like conditions, *CA Cancer J Clin* 43:290-308, 1993.

Wright BA, Jackson D: Neural tumors of the oral cavity, *Oral Surg Oral Med Oral Pathol* 49:509-522, 1980.

Neurofibromatosis Type I

D'Ambrosio JA, Langlais RP, Young RS: Jaw and skull changes in neurofibromatosis, *Oral Surg Oral Med Oral Pathol* 66:391-396, 1988.

Edwards PC, Fantasia JE, Saini T et al: Clinically aggressive central giant cell granulomas in two patients with neurofibromatosis 1, *Oral Surg Oral Med Oral Pathol Oral Radiol Endod* 102:765-772, 2006.

Ferner RE: Neurofibromatosis 1 and neurofibromatosis 2: a twenty-first century perspective, *Lancet Neurol* 6:340-351, 2007.

Lee L, Yan Y-H, Pharoah MJ: Radiographic features of the mandible in neurofibromatosis. A report of 10 cases and review of the literature, *Oral Surg Oral Med Oral Pathol Oral Radiol Endod* 81:361-367, 1996.

Neville BW, Hann J, Narang R et al: Oral neurofibrosarcoma associated with neurofibromatosis type I, *Oral Surg Oral Med Oral Pathol* 72:456-461, 1991.

Overdiek A, Feifel H, Schaper J et al: Diagnostic delay of NF1 in hemifacial hypertrophy due to plexiform neurofibromas, *Brain Dev* 28:275-280, 2006.

Rasmussen SA, Yang Q, Friedman JM: Mortality in neurofibromatosis 1: an analysis using U.S. death certificates, *Am J Hum Genet* 68:1110-1118, 2001.

Riccardi VM: *Neurofibromatosis: phenotype, natural history, and pathogenesis*, ed 2, Baltimore, 1992, Johns Hopkins University Press.

Ruggieri M: The different forms of neurofibromatosis, *Childs Nerv Syst* 15:295-308, 1999.

Shapiro SD, Abramovitch K, Van Dis ML et al: Neurofibromatosis: oral and radiographic manifestations, *Oral Surg Oral Med Oral Pathol* 58:493-498, 1984.

Yazdizadeh M, Tapia JL, Baharvand M et al: A case of neurofibromatosis-Noonan syndrome with a central giant cell granuloma, *Oral Surg Oral Med Oral Pathol Oral Radiol Endod* 98:316-320, 2004.

Multiple Endocrine Neoplasia Type 2B

Calender A, Giraud S, Schuffenecker I et al: Genetic testing in presymptomatic diagnosis of multiple endocrine neoplasia, *Horm Res* 47:199-210, 1997.

Carney JA: Familial multiple endocrine neoplasia: the first 100 years, *Am J Surg Pathol* 29:254-274, 2005.

Gorlin RJ, Cohen MM Jr, Hennekam RCM: Multiple endocrine neoplasia, type 2B (multiple mucosal neuroma syndrome, MEN type 3). In *Syndromes of the head and neck*, ed 4, pp 462-468, New York, 2001, Oxford University Press.

Kahn MA, Cote GJ, Gagel RF: RET protooncogene mutational analysis in multiple endocrine neoplasia syndrome type 2B. Case report and review of the literature, *Oral Surg Oral Med Oral Pathol Oral Radiol Endod* 82:288-294, 1996.

Lakhani VT, You YN, Wells SA: The multiple endocrine neoplasia syndromes, *Annu Rev Med* 58:253-265, 2007.

Melanotic Neuroectodermal Tumor of Infancy

Barrett AW, Morgan M, Ramsay AD et al: A clinicopathologic and immunohistochemical analysis of melanotic neuroectodermal tumor of infancy, *Oral Surg Oral Med Oral Pathol Oral Radiol Endod* 93:688-698, 2002.

Bouckaert MMR, Raubenheimer EJ: Gigantiform melanotic neuroectodermal tumor of infancy, *Oral Surg Oral Med Oral Pathol Oral Radiol Endod* 86:569-572, 1998.

Kapadia SB, Frisman DM, Hitchcock CL et al: Melanotic neuroectodermal tumor of infancy: clinicopathological, immunohistochemical, and flow cytometric study, *Am J Surg Pathol* 17:566-573, 1993.

Kruse-Lösler B, Gaertner C, Bürger H et al: Melanotic neuroectodermal tumor of infancy: systematic review of the literature and presentation of a case, *Oral Surg Oral Med Oral Pathol Oral Radiol Endod* 102:204-216, 2006.

Pettinato G, Manivel C, d'Amore ESG et al: Melanotic neuroectodermal tumor of infancy: a reexamination of a histogenetic problem based on immunohistochemical, flow cytometric, and ultrastructural study of 10 cases, *Am J Surg Pathol* 15:233-245, 1991.

Paraganglioma

Hodge KM, Byers RM, Peters LJ: Paragangliomas of the head and neck, *Arch Otolaryngol Head Neck Surg* 114:872-877, 1988.

Jordan JA, Roland PS, McManus C et al: Stereotactic radiosurgery for glomus jugulare tumors, *Laryngoscope* 110:35-38, 2000.

LaMuraglia GM, Fabian RL, Brewster DC et al: The current surgical management of carotid body paragangliomas, *J Vasc Surg* 15:1038-1045, 1992.

Pellitteri PK, Rinaldo A, Myssiorek D et al: Paragangliomas of the head and neck, *Oral Oncol* 40:563-575, 2004.

Robertson JH, Gardner G, Cocke EW Jr: Glomus jugulare tumors, *Clin Neurosurg* 41:39-61, 1994.

van den Berg, R: Imaging and management of head and neck paragangliomas, *Eur Radiol* 15:1310-1318, 2005.

Granular Cell Tumor

Brannon RB, Anand PM: Oral granular cell tumors: an analysis of 10 new pediatric and adolescent cases and a review of the literature, *J Clin Pediatr Dent* 29:69-74, 2004.

Collins BM, Jones AC: Multiple granular cell tumors of the oral cavity: report of a case and review of the literature, *J Oral Maxillofac Surg* 53:707-711, 1995.

Fliss DM, Puterman M, Zirkin H et al: Granular cell lesions in head and neck: a clinicopathological study, *J Surg Oncol* 42:154-160, 1989.

Mirchandani R, Sciubba JJ, Mir R: Granular cell lesions of the jaws and oral cavity: a clinicopathologic, immunohistochemical, and ultrastructural study, *J Oral Maxillofac Surg* 47:1248-1255, 1989.

Stewart CM, Watson RE, Eversole LR et al: Oral granular cell tumors: a clinicopathologic and immunocytochemical study, *Oral Surg Oral Med Oral Pathol* 65:427-435, 1988.

Williams HK, Williams DM: Oral granular cell tumours: a histological and immunocytochemical study, *J Oral Pathol Med* 26:164-169, 1997.

Congenital Epulis

Damm DD, Cibull ML, Geissler RH et al: Investigation into the histogenesis of congenital epulis of the newborn, *Oral Surg Oral Med Oral Pathol* 76:205-212, 1993.

Kumar P, Kim HHS, Zahtz GD et al: Obstructive congenital epulis: prenatal diagnosis and perinatal management, *Laryngoscope* 112:1935-1939, 2002.

Lack EE, Worsham GF, Callihan MD et al: Gingival granular cell tumors of the newborn (congenital "epulis"): a clinical and pathologic study of 21 patients, *Am J Surg Pathol* 5:37-46, 1981.

Loyola AM, Gatti AF, Santos Pinto D Jr et al: Alveolar and extra-alveolar granular cell lesions of the newborn: report of case and review of literature, *Oral Surg Oral Med Oral Pathol Oral Radiol Endod* 84:668-671, 1997.

O'Brien FV, Pielou WD: Congenital epulis: its natural history, *Arch Dis Child* 46:559-560, 1971.

Hemangioma and Vascular Malformations

Adams DM, Lucky AW: Cervicofacial vascular anomalies. I. Hemangiomas and other benign vascular tumors, *Semin Pediatr Surg* 15:124-132, 2006.

Bunel K, Sindet-Pederson S: Central hemangioma of the mandible, *Oral Surg Oral Med Oral Pathol* 75:565-570, 1993.

Chang MW: Updated classification of hemangiomas and other vascular anomalies, *Lymphat Res Biol* 1:259-265, 2003.

Drolet BA, Esterly NB, Frieden IJ: Hemangiomas in children, *N Engl J Med* 341:173-181, 1999.

Elluru RG, Azizkhan RG: Cervicofacial vascular anomalies. II. Vascular malformations, *Semin Pediatr Surg* 15:133-139, 2006.

Ethunandan M, Mellor TK: Haemangiomas and vascular malformations of the maxillofacial region—a review, *Br J Oral Maxillofac Surg* 44:263-272, 2006.

Fishman SJ, Mulliken JB: Hemangiomas and vascular malformations of infancy and childhood, *Pediatr Clin North Am* 40:1177-1200, 1993.

Kaposi's Sarcoma

Brenner B, Weissmann-Brenner A, Rakowsky E et al: Classical Kaposi sarcoma. Prognostic factor analysis of 248 patients, *Cancer* 95:1982-1987, 2002.

Cohen A, Wolf DG, Guttman-Yassky et al: Kaposi's sarcoma-associated herpesvirus: clinical, diagnostic, and epidemiological aspects, *Crit Rev Clin Lab Sci* 42:101-153, 2005.

Ficarra G, Berson AM, Silverman S Jr et al: Kaposi's sarcoma of the oral cavity: a study of 134 patients with a review of the pathogenesis, epidemiology, clinical aspects, and treatment, *Oral Surg Oral Med Oral Pathol* 66:543-550, 1988.

Flaitz CM, Jin Y-T, Hicks MJ et al: Kaposi's sarcoma-associated herpesvirus-like DNA sequences (KSHV/HHV-8) in oral AIDS-Kaposi's sarcoma: a PCR and clinicopathologic study, *Oral Surg Oral Med Oral Pathol Oral Radiol Endod* 83:259-264, 1997.

Fossati S, Boneschi V, Ferrucci S et al: Human immunodeficiency virus negative Kaposi sarcoma and lymphoproliferative disorders, *Cancer* 85:1611-1615, 1999.

Friedman-Kien AE, Saltzman BR: Clinical manifestations of classical, endemic African, and epidemic AIDS-associated Kaposi's sarcoma, *J Am Acad Dermatol* 22:1237-1250, 1990.

Lager I, Altini M, Coleman H et al: Oral Kaposi's sarcoma: a clinicopathologic study from South Africa, *Oral Surg Oral Med Oral Pathol Oral Radiol Endod* 96:701-710, 2003.

Stein ME, Spencer D, Ruff P et al: Endemic African Kaposi's sarcoma: clinical and therapeutic implications. 10-year experience in the Johannesburg Hospital (1980-1990), *Oncology* 51:63-69, 1994.

Tappero JW, Conant MA, Wolfe SF et al: Kaposi's sarcoma. Epidemiology, pathogenesis, histology, clinical spectrum, staging criteria and therapy, *J Am Acad Dermatol* 28:371-395, 1993.

Leiomyosarcoma

Dry SM, Jorgensen JL, Fletcher CDM: Leiomyosarcomas of the oral cavity: an unusual topographic subset easily mistaken for nonmesenchymal tumours, *Histopathology* 36:210-220, 2000.

Freedman PD, Jones AC, Kerpel SM: Epithelioid leiomyosarcoma of the oral cavity: report of two cases and review of the literature, *J Oral Maxillofac Surg* 51:928-932, 1993.

Nikitakis NG, Lopes MA, Bailey JS et al: Oral leiomyosarcoma: review of the literature and report of two cases with assessment of the prognostic and diagnostic significance of immunohistochemical and molecular markers, *Oral Oncol* 38:201-208, 2002.

Sedghizadeh PP, Angiero F, Allen CM et al: Post-irradiation leiomyosarcoma of the maxilla: report of a case in a patient with prior radiation treatment for retinoblastoma, *Oral Surg Oral Med Oral Pathol Oral Radiol Endod* 97:726-731, 2004.

Vilos GA, Rapidis AD, Lagogiannis GD et al: Leiomyosarcomas of the oral tissues: clinicopathologic analysis of 50 cases, *J Oral Maxillofac Surg* 63:1461-1477, 2005.

Rhabdomyosarcoma

Bras J, Batsakis JG, Luna MA: Rhabdomyosarcoma of the oral soft tissues, *Oral Surg Oral Med Oral Pathol* 64:585-596, 1987.

Dagher R, Helman L: Rhabdomyosarcoma: an overview, *Oncologist* 4:34-44, 1999.

Hicks J, Flaitz C: Rhabdomyosarcoma of the head and neck in children, *Oral Oncol* 38:450-459, 2002.

Kaste SC, Hopkins KP, Bowman LC: Dental abnormalities in long-term survivors of head and neck rhabdomyosarcoma, *Med Pediatr Oncol* 25:96-101, 1995.

Nakhleh RE, Swanson PE, Dehner LP: Juvenile (embryonal and alveolar) rhabdomyosarcoma of the head and neck in adults: a clinical, pathologic, and immunohistochemical study of 12 cases, *Cancer* 67:1019-1024, 1991.

Parham DM, Ellison DA: Rhabdomyosarcomas in adults and children. An update, *Arch Pathol Lab Med* 130:1454-1465, 2006.

Walterhouse DO, Pappo AS, Baker KS et al: Rhabdomyosarcoma of the parotid region occurring in childhood and adolescence. A report from the Intergroup Rhabdomyosarcoma Study Group, *Cancer* 92:3135-3146, 2001.

Synovial Sarcoma

Bukachevsky RP, Pincus RL, Shechtman FG et al: Synovial sarcoma of the head and neck, *Head Neck* 14:44-48, 1992.

Ferrari A, Gronchi A, Casanova M et al: Synovial sarcoma: a retrospective analysis of 271 patients of all ages treated at a single institution, *Cancer* 101:627-634, 2004.

Fisher C: Synovial sarcoma, *Ann Diagn Pathol* 2:401-421, 1988.

Meer S, Coleman H, Altini M: Oral synovial sarcoma: a report of 2 cases and a review of the literature, *Oral Surg Oral Med Oral Pathol Oral Radiol Endod* 96:306-315, 2003.

Shmookler BM, Enzinger FM, Brannon RB: Orofacial synovial sarcoma: a clinicopathologic study of 11 new cases and review of the literature, *Cancer* 50:269-276, 1982.

Alveolar Soft-Part Sarcoma

do Nascimento Souza KC, Faria PR, Costa IM et al: Oral alveolar soft-part sarcoma: review of literature and case report with immunohistochemistry study for prognostic markers, *Oral Surg Oral Med Oral Pathol Oral Radiol Endod* 99:64-70, 2005.

Fanburg-Smith JC, Miettinen M, Folpe AL et al: Lingual alveolar soft part sarcoma; 14 cases: novel clinical and morphological observations, *Histopathology* 45:526-537, 2004.

Folpe AL, Deyrup AT: Alveolar soft-part sarcoma: a review and update, *J Clin Pathol* 59:1127-1132, 2006.

Lieberman PH, Brennan MF, Kimmel M et al: Alveolar soft-part sarcoma: a clinico-pathologic study of half a century, *Cancer* 63:1-13, 1989.

Ordóñez NG: Alveolar soft part sarcoma: a review and update, *Adv Anat Pathol* 6:125-139, 1999.

Metastases to the Oral Soft Tissues

Allen CM, Neville B, Damm DD et al: Leiomyosarcoma metastatic to the oral region: report of three cases, *Oral Surg Oral Med Oral Pathol* 76:752-756, 1993.

Hirshberg A, Buchner A: Metastatic tumours to the oral region. An overview, *Eur J Cancer B Oral Oncol* 31B:355-360, 1995.

Hirshberg A, Leibovich P, Buchner A: Metastases to the oral mucosa: analysis of 157 cases, *J Oral Pathol Med* 22:385-390, 1993.

Lim S-Y, Kim S-A, Ahn S-G et al: Metastatic tumours to the jaws and oral soft tissues: a retrospective analysis of 41 Korean patients, *Int J Oral Maxillofac Surg* 35:412-415, 2006.

van der Waal RIF, Buter J, van der Wall I: Oral metastases: report of 24 cases, *Br J Oral Maxillofac Surg* 41:3-6, 2003.

Zachariades N: Neoplasms metastatic to the mouth, jaws and surrounding tissues, *J Craniomaxillofac Surg* 17:283-290, 1989.

13

Hematologic Disorders

LYMPHOID HYPERPLASIA

The lymphoid tissue of the body plays an important role in the recognition and processing of foreign antigens, such as viruses, fungi, and bacteria. In addition, the lymphoid tissue has a protective function through a variety of direct and indirect mechanisms. In responding to antigenic challenges, lymphoid cells proliferate, thus increasing their numbers, to combat the offending agent more effectively. This proliferation results in enlargement of the lymphoid tissue, which is seen clinically as **lymphoid hyperplasia**.

CLINICAL FEATURES

Lymphoid hyperplasia may affect the lymph nodes, the lymphoid tissue of Waldeyer's ring, or the aggregates of lymphoid tissue that are normally scattered throughout the oral cavity, particularly in the oropharynx, the soft palate, the lateral tongue, and the floor of the mouth. When lymphoid hyperplasia affects the lymph nodes, usually the site that the lymph node drains can be identified as a source of active or recent infection. In the head and neck region, the anterior cervical chain of lymph nodes is most commonly involved, although any lymph node in the area may be affected.

With acute infections, the lymphadenopathy appears as enlarged, tender, relatively soft, freely movable nodules. Chronic inflammatory conditions produce enlarged, rubbery firm, nontender, freely movable nodes. Sometimes these chronic hyperplastic lymph nodes may be difficult to distinguish clinically from lymphoma, and a history of a preceding inflammatory process and lack of progressive enlargement are helpful clues that are consistent with a reactive process. Another condition, however, that should be considered in the differential diagnosis of multiple, persistently enlarged, nontender lymph nodes is human immunodeficiency virus (HIV) infection (see page 271).

Tonsillar size is variable from one person to the next, but lymphoid tissue is normally more prominent in younger individuals, usually reaching its peak early during the second decade of life and gradually diminishing thereafter. Some patients have such large tonsils that it seems as if they would occlude the airway (so-called kissing tonsils). Often, however, these patients have no symptoms and are unaware of a problem. As long as the large tonsils are symmetrical and

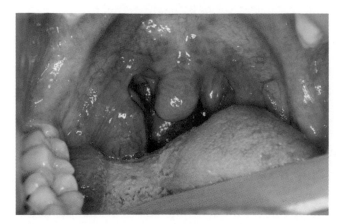

Fig. 13-1 **Lymphoid hyperplasia.** The large tonsil observed in this patient represents a benign hyperplasia of the lymphoid cells. If significant asymmetry is observed, further investigation may be warranted to rule out the possibility of lymphoma.

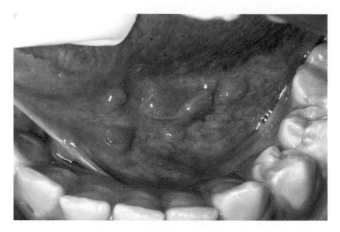

Fig. 13-3 **Lymphoid hyperplasia.** Multiple prominent lymphoid aggregates in the floor of the mouth.

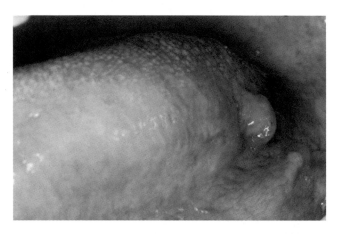

Fig. 13-2 **Lymphoid hyperplasia.** The smooth-surfaced papule of the posterior lateral tongue represents an enlarged lymphoid aggregate. The lesion exhibits a lighter color as a result of the accumulation of lymphocytes, which are white blood cells. *(Courtesy of Dr. Dean White.)*

asymptomatic (Fig. 13-1), it is likely that they are normal for that particular patient. Tonsillar asymmetry is a potentially serious sign that should be evaluated further to rule out the presence of a metastatic tumor or lymphoma.

Hyperplastic intraoral lymphoid aggregates appear as discrete, nontender, submucosal swellings, usually less than 1 cm in diameter, which may appear normal or dark pink in color if the aggregate is deeper; they may have a creamy yellow-orange hue if the collection of lymphocytes is closer to the surface (Figs. 13-2 and 13-3). Lymphoid hyperplasia commonly involves the posterior lateral tongue, where it may appear somewhat ominous. The enlargement is usually bilaterally symmetrical, however, which helps to distinguish the

condition from a malignancy. The buccal lymph node may also become hyperplastic and appear as a non-tender, solitary, freely movable nodule, usually less than 1 cm in diameter, within the substance of the cheek. Infrequently, a more diffuse lymphoid hyperplasia involves the posterior hard palate, producing a slowly growing, nontender, boggy swelling with an intact mucosal surface and little color change. These palatal lesions may be clinically impossible to distinguish from extranodal lymphoma and would, there-fore, necessitate biopsy.

HISTOPATHOLOGIC FEATURES

The microscopic features of lymphoid hyperplasia include sheets of small, well-differentiated lympho-cytes with numerous interspersed, sharply demarcated collections of reactive lymphoblasts called **germinal centers.** The cells that comprise the germinal centers are primarily transformed B lymphocytes that may demonstrate numerous mitoses. Macrophages can also be identified by the presence of phagocytized material **(tingible bodies)** in their cytoplasm as they engulf nuclear debris from the proliferating lymphocytes. In some instances, immunohistochemical studies and clonality assays must be performed to rule out the pos-sibility of follicular lymphoma.

TREATMENT AND PROGNOSIS

Once the diagnosis of lymphoid hyperplasia is con-firmed, no treatment is usually required because it is a completely benign process. For those patients with palatal lymphoid hyperplasia that may interfere with a dental prosthesis, complete excision of the lesion is recommended.

Table **13-1**   **Comparison of the Most Commonly Encountered Inherited Bleeding Disorders**

Type	Defect	Inheritance	Findings
Hemophilia A (classic hemophilia)	Factor VIII deficiency	X-linked recessive	Abnormal PTT
Hemophilia B (Christmas disease)	Factor IX deficiency	X-linked recessive	Abnormal PTT
von Willebrand's disease	Abnormal von Willebrand's factor, abnormal platelets	Autosomal dominant	Abnormal BT, abnormal PTT

PTT, Partial thromboplastin time; BT, bleeding time.

HEMOPHILIA

Hemophilia (*hemo* = blood; *philia* = loving) represents a variety of bleeding disorders associated with a genetic deficiency of any one of the clotting factors of the blood (Table 13-1). This condition was common in certain European royal families, many of whom carried an X-linked hereditary deficiency of either factor VIII or factor IX. Consequently, as a result of inbreeding, a significant proportion of the male members of these families had hemophilia. In the days before blood transfusions and clotting factor replacement therapy, many of these patients died as a direct result of, or from the complications of, uncontrolled hemorrhage. It is not known whether these people had factor VIII or factor IX deficiency, because all of the affected individuals died before the definitive diagnostic studies were developed to determine precisely which deficiency was present. Because **hemophilia A** (factor VIII deficiency) is the most significant and widely recognized form of hemophilia and accounts for 80% to 85% of the bleeding diatheses associated with a specific clotting factor deficiency, most of this discussion centers on that entity. Its estimated prevalence in the United States is 1 in 10,000 persons (or 1 in 5000 males).

As previously mentioned, a deficiency of factor IX or **hemophilia B (Christmas disease)** also may be encountered. Hemophilia B is similar to hemophilia A in its presentation, being transmitted in an X-linked fashion. Hemophilia B is much less common than hemophilia A, occurring with a prevalence of 1 in 60,000 (or 1 in 30,000 males). The term *Christmas disease* was obtained from the surname of the first person, a Canadian boy, who was identified as having hemophilia B in 1952.

Another clotting disorder that is sometimes seen, **von Willebrand's disease**, is the result of a genetic deficiency of a plasma glycoprotein called **von Willebrand's factor**. This glycoprotein aids in the adhesion of platelets at a site of bleeding, and it also binds to factor VIII, acting as a transport molecule. Von Willebrand's disease is a genetically heterogeneous condition, with several subtypes currently identified, and it may be transmitted in an autosomal dominant or recessive pattern. It is the most common of the inherited bleeding disorders, affecting an estimated 1 in 800 to 1000 persons. However, many cases of von Willebrand's disease are mild and may be clinically insignificant.

CLINICAL FEATURES

Hemophilia A is an X-linked disorder. Females typically carry the trait, but it is expressed primarily in males. Approximately 1 in 5000 males is born with this genetic disease, with about 30% of the cases representing new mutations. Failure of normal hemostasis after circumcision is typically one of the first signs that a bleeding disorder is present.

The severity of the bleeding disorder depends on the extent of the clotting factor deficiency. Hemophilia A is a heterogeneous disorder that is caused by any one of a variety of mutations associated with the gene for factor VIII. Because the mutations occur at different sites in the factor VIII gene (more than 900 different mutations have been identified), a clinical spectrum of deficiency of factor VIII is seen. This results in varying degrees of disease expression, with those mutations affecting more significant or larger portions of the factor VIII gene causing more severe clinical disease. Not all patients have an absolute lack of the particular clotting factor; rather, the deficiency may be a percentage of the normal value in a given patient. For example, a patient with only 25% of normal factor VIII levels may be able to function normally under most circumstances; one with less than 5% commonly manifests a marked tendency to bruise with only minor trauma.

In infants, oral lacerations and ecchymoses that involve the lips and tongue are a frequent occurrence as a result of the common falls and bumps experienced by this age group. If not treated appropriately, then such lacerations may result in significant blood loss in more severely affected patients. Sometimes deep hemorrhage occurs during normal activity and may involve

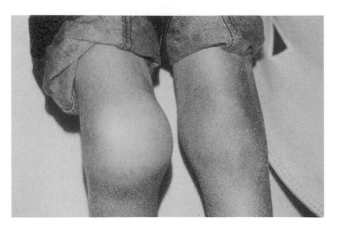

Fig. 13-4   Hemophilia. The enlargement of the knees of this patient with factor VIII deficiency is due to repeated episodes of bleeding into the joints (hemarthrosis). Inflammation and scarring have resulted.

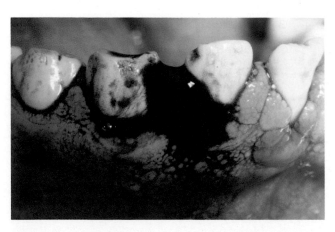

Fig. 13-5   Hemophilia. Hemorrhage in a patient with factor IX deficiency occurred after routine periodontal curettage.

the muscles, soft tissues, and weight-bearing joints **(hemarthrosis),** especially the knees (Fig. 13-4). The result of such uncontrolled bleeding is the formation of scar tissue as the body removes the extravasated blood. This often causes a crippling deformity of the knee joints secondary to arthritis and ankylosis. Sometimes the tissue hemorrhage results in the formation of a tumorlike mass, which has been called **pseudotumor of hemophilia.** Such lesions have been reported in the oral regions.

An increased coagulation time (delay in blood clotting), of course, is the hallmark feature of this group of conditions. Uncontrollable or delayed hemorrhage may result from any laceration; this includes surgical incisions, dental extractions, and periodontal curettage (Fig. 13-5). Measurements of the platelet count, bleeding time, prothrombin time (PT), and partial thromboplastin time (PTT) should be ordered as screening tests for any patient with a possible bleeding disorder.

TREATMENT AND PROGNOSIS

The treatment of clotting factor deficiencies essentially consists of replacement therapy with the appropriate clotting factor. Whether treatment is instituted depends on the severity of the clotting factor deficiency.

Patients who have greater than 25% of normal values of factor VIII may function normally. For patients with mild hemophilia (5% to 40% of normal levels of factor VIII), no special treatment is typically required for normal activities. If surgery is to be performed, then clotting factor replacement therapy may be indicated.

For patients with severe deficiencies (<1% of normal levels of factor VIII), injections with the clotting factor must be performed as soon as a hemorrhagic episode

occurs to prevent such complications as the crippling joint deformities of the knees.

The use of aspirin is strictly contraindicated because of its adverse effect on blood platelet function. Severe hemorrhage may result if these patients use aspirin-containing medications.

Genetic counseling should be provided to these patients and their families to help them understand the mechanism of inheritance. Using molecular techniques, women who are carriers can be confirmed. In addition, affected male fetuses can now be identified, and the severity of the factor VIII mutation can be assessed.

Optimal dental care is strongly encouraged for these patients to prevent oral problems that might require surgery. If oral or periodontal surgery is necessary, then consultation with the patient's physician is mandatory. The patient is usually prepared for the procedure by the administration of clotting factor just before the surgery. With an extensive surgical procedure, additional doses of clotting factor may be needed subsequently. In addition, epsilon-aminocaproic acid (EACA), an antifibrinolytic agent that inhibits clot degradation, should be given 1 day before the surgery and continued for 7 to 10 days afterward. Alternative therapy for patients who have levels of factor VIII greater than 5% of normal is desmopressin, which can be given just before surgery. This drug causes the release of bound factor VIII, producing a temporary increase in the plasma levels of the clotting factor. Desmopressin may also be used to manage most patients affected by type 1 von Willebrand's disease, which represents approximately 70% to 80% of the cases of that disorder.

Although it saved many lives, clotting factor replacement therapy has also resulted in a tragic complication for many of these patients. Cryoprecipitation, the traditional method of concentrating clotting factors from the serum, also resulted in the concentration of several viruses, including the hepatitis viruses and human immunodeficiency virus (HIV). Currently more than 40% of hemophilia A and B patients in the United States are estimated to be infected with hepatitis C virus. In addition, as many as 80% to 90% of hemophiliac patients treated with multiple doses of factor VIII cryoprecipitate were infected with HIV. The methods of preparing the clotting factors have been modified to eliminate the risk of acquiring HIV from the preparation; however, many hemophiliac patients who were infected developed acquired immunodeficiency syndrome (AIDS). Recombinant DNA technology now provides a source of factor VIII that is manufactured by inserting the human factor VIII gene into bacteria that then synthesize the protein. Therefore, this product can now be manufactured without contamination by any viral organisms, and young people affected by hemophilia have minimal risk of contracting these infections.

Other problems must occasionally be confronted, however. Approximately 6% of patients with hemophilia A may develop antibodies directed against factor VIII, and this is a very serious complication. Because the antibodies react with the factor VIII molecule, the result is an inhibition of the activity of the clotting factor, and these patients are once more faced with the prospect of uncontrolled bleeding. Patients with factor IX deficiency can develop similar inhibitory antibodies to factor IX, but this appears to occur much less frequently. Attempts to induce immune tolerance may help some individuals, although more immediate care has generally centered on bypassing the factor VIII–related portion of the clotting cascade by administration of recombinant factor VIIa. Research has shown this approach to be effective, although costly.

PLASMINOGEN DEFICIENCY (LIGNEOUS CONJUNCTIVITIS; HYPOPLASMINOGENEMIA)

Plasminogen deficiency is a rare autosomal recessive condition that is caused by any one of several mutations of the gene responsible for the production of plasminogen, the precursor to plasmin. In the clotting cascade, factors are activated that lead to the development of a clot; however, simultaneously serum proteins such as plasminogen are converted to plasmin, which is responsible for degrading the clot. Without the formation of plasmin, the clot tends to grow and persist despite having performed its original hemostatic function. The result of plasminogen deficiency is a buildup of fibrin, deposited as irregular plaques and nodules that primarily affect mucosal surfaces. Involvement of

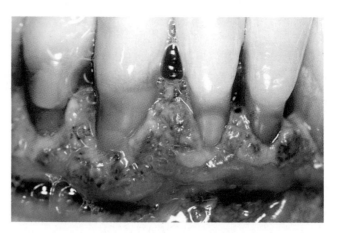

Fig. 13-6 Plasminogen deficiency. The ulcerated plaques and papules seen on the gingiva of this patient with plasminogen deficiency represent accumulations of fibrin. *(Courtesy of Dr. Kenneth Rasenberger.)*

the conjunctival mucosa is characterized by the formation of thick, firm plaques, for which the term *ligneous conjunctivitis* has been used (*ligneous* means "woodlike"). Even though this condition was initially described in the nineteenth century, it was during the late 1990s that an explanation for the majority of these cases was provided. Similar lesions have been produced in mice that have been genetically manipulated to create knock-out mutations of the plasminogen gene.

CLINICAL FEATURES

The most striking aspect of plasminogen deficiency is the development of thick, creamy yellow to erythematous, firm plaques and nodules involving primarily the conjunctival mucosa of the upper eyelid. Typically the condition is detected during the first decade of life, but lesions can develop later as well. Even though this is an autosomal recessive condition, there is a tendency for the disease to present more often in women, although the reason for this is unknown.

In addition to the conjunctival lesions, other mucosal surfaces can be affected, including the oral mucosa, laryngeal mucosa, and vaginal mucosa. In a recent series of 50 patients with this condition, ocular lesions were documented in 80%, gingival lesions in 34%, respiratory tract lesions in 16%, and vaginal lesions in 8%. Laryngeal mucosal involvement often includes the vocal cords, which will typically cause a raspy, hoarse voice.

Oral lesions of plasminogen deficiency primarily involve the gingivae, presenting as patchy ulcerated papules and nodules with a very irregular surface (Fig. 13-6). These lesions may be few in number or distributed diffusely in all quadrants, and they tend to wax and wane in severity.

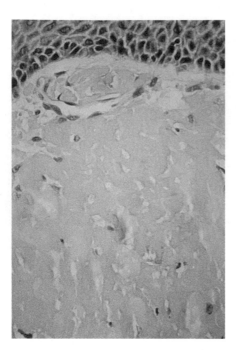

Fig. 13-7   Plasminogen deficiency. This high-power photomicrograph shows attenuated surface epithelium and a collection of relatively acellular eosinophilic material that superficially resembles amyloid.

HISTOPATHOLOGIC FEATURES

The microscopic features of the lesions associated with this condition can be very confusing for the pathologist who is not familiar with the disease. The accumulation of fibrin appears as diffuse sheets of acellular eosinophilic material that bears a close resemblance to amyloid (Fig. 13-7). Special stains for amyloid (such as Congo red) are negative, however, because this material represents fibrin. Confirmation that the eosinophilic material is fibrin can be done using the Fraser-Lendrum histochemical staining method. Variable numbers of inflammatory cells are seen, and granulation tissue is usually seen adjacent to the fibrin deposits.

TREATMENT AND PROGNOSIS

Treatment of plasminogen deficiency remains a problem. Damage to the mucosal tissues, including surgical trauma, should be minimized to reduce the likelihood of fibrin accumulation. Careful, thorough oral hygiene practices should be encouraged to diminish the effect of local inflammation. Sporadic reports describe resolution of the conjunctival lesions with either topical or systemic plasminogen; however, this agent is not available commercially. Some patients have experienced spontaneous regression of their lesions over time. Currently topical heparin combined with prednisone may be the most reasonable approach until replacement plasminogen is marketed or gene therapy is feasible. Interestingly, these patients do not have any unusual problems with intravascular thrombus formation, and their lifespan does not appear to be shortened.

ANEMIA

Anemia is a general term for either a decrease in the volume of red blood cells (hematocrit) or in the concentration of hemoglobin. This problem can result from a number of factors, including a decreased production of erythrocytes or an increased destruction or loss of erythrocytes. Laboratory studies, such as the red blood cell (RBC) count, hematocrit, hemoglobin concentration, mean corpuscular volume (MCV), mean corpuscular hemoglobin (MCH), and mean corpuscular hemoglobin concentration (MCHC), can help indicate the probable cause of the anemia.

Rather than being a disease itself, anemia is often a sign of an underlying disease, such as renal failure, liver disease, chronic inflammatory conditions, malignancies, or vitamin or mineral deficiencies. The diverse causes and complexity of the problem of anemia are presented in Box 13-1.

CLINICAL FEATURES

The symptoms of anemia are typically related to the reduced oxygen-carrying capacity of the blood, which is a result of the reduced numbers of erythrocytes. Symptoms such as tiredness, headache, or lightheadedness are often present.

Pallor of the mucous membranes may be observed in severe cases of anemia. The palpebral conjunctiva is often the site where this paleness is most easily appreciated, but the oral mucosa may show similar signs.

TREATMENT AND PROGNOSIS

The treatment of anemia depends on determining the underlying cause of the anemia and correcting that problem, if possible.

SICKLE CELL ANEMIA

Sickle cell anemia is one of the more severe genetic disorders of hemoglobin synthesis (**hemoglobinopathies**). Because of the mutational substitution of a thymine molecule for an adenine in DNA, the codon is altered to code for the amino acid valine rather than glutamic acid in the β-globin chain of hemoglobin. This results in a hemoglobin molecule that, in the deoxygenated state, is prone to molecular aggregation and

Box 13-1

Causes of Anemia

ANEMIAS WITH DISTURBED IRON METABOLISM

- Iron deficiency anemia
- Sideroblastic anemias

MEGALOBLASTIC ANEMIAS

- Cobalamin (B$_{12}$) deficiency (pernicious anemia)
- Folic acid deficiency

ANEMIA ASSOCIATED WITH CHRONIC DISORDERS

- Anemia of chronic infection (infective endocarditis, tuberculosis, osteomyelitis, lung abscess, pyelonephritis)
- Anemia of inflammatory connective tissue disorders (rheumatoid arthritis, lupus erythematosus, sarcoidosis, temporal arteritis, regional enteritis)
- Anemia associated with malignancy
  - Secondary to chronic bleeding
  - Myelophthisic anemia
- Anemia of uremia
- Anemia of endocrine failure
- Anemia of liver disease

HEMOLYTIC ANEMIAS

- Extrinsic causes
  - Splenomegaly
  - Red cell antibodies
  - Trauma in the circulation
  - Direct toxic effects (various microorganisms, copper salts, venom of certain snakes)
- Membrane abnormalities
  - Spur cell anemia
  - Paroxysmal nocturnal hemoglobinuria
  - Hereditary spherocytosis
  - Hereditary elliptocytosis
- Disorders of the interior of the red cell
  - Defects in the Embden-Meyerhof pathway
  - Defects in the hexose monophosphate shunt

DISORDERS OF HEMOGLOBIN

- Sickle cell anemia
- Thalassemias

---

polymerization. Consequently, the red blood cells of patients with sickle cell anemia have a marked tendency to undergo deformation from the normal biconcave disk shape to a rigid-and-curved (sickle) shape. Because the genes for hemoglobin synthesis are codominant, if only one allele is affected, then only 40% to 50% of that patient's hemoglobin will be abnormal. Such a patient is simply a carrier and is said to have **sickle cell trait**, a condition that has no significant clinical manifestations in most everyday circumstances. Some sick-

ling may be precipitated under certain conditions, however, particularly with low-oxygen tensions associated with exercise or high altitudes.

This abnormal gene has persisted in the human race perhaps because it confers a degree of resistance to the malarial organism. As a result, the gene is seen most frequently in populations, such as African, Mediterranean, and Asian, who reside in areas where malaria is endemic. In the United States, nearly 2.5 million people (approximately 8% of the black population) carry this trait.

Unfortunately, in patients who inherit two alleles that code for sickle hemoglobin, the red blood cells contain primarily sickle hemoglobin, which results in the condition called **sickle cell disease**. In the United States, about 1 of every 350 to 400 blacks is born with this disease. Such patients are often susceptible to the problems associated with abnormal red blood cell morphology. The sickled erythrocytes are more fragile than normal and they tend to block the capillaries because of their shape and adherence properties. As a result, these patients have a chronic hemolytic anemia and many difficulties related to reduced blood flow to organs and tissues, which produces ischemia, infarction, and tissue death.

CLINICAL AND RADIOGRAPHIC FEATURES

Virtually any tissue or organ may be affected in sickle cell disease. The clinical spectrum of involvement can vary tremendously, with approximately one third of patients exhibiting severe manifestations. Perhaps the most dramatic sign of this disease is the **sickle cell crisis**, a situation in which the sickling of the erythrocytes becomes severe. Hypoxia, infection, hypothermia, or dehydration may precipitate a crisis; however, for most crises there is no identifiable predisposing factor. Patients who experience a crisis suffer extreme pain from ischemia and infarction of the affected tissue. The long bones, lungs, and abdomen are among the most commonly affected sites, and each episode lasts 3 to 10 days. Pulmonary involvement, known as **acute chest syndrome**, is particularly serious, and one large study indicated that this is frequently precipitated by fat embolism or community-acquired pneumonia. Some patients may experience such crises monthly; others may go for 1 year or longer without problems. Often fever accompanies the crisis; therefore, infection must be considered in the differential diagnosis.

Patients with sickle cell disease are susceptible to infections, especially those caused by *Streptococcus pneumoniae*, probably because of the destruction of the spleen at an early age by repeated infarctions. Such infections are the most common cause of death among

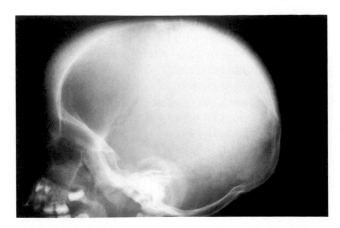

Fig. 13-8   Sickle cell anemia. Lateral skull radiograph reveals an altered trabecular pattern, including a slight degree of "hair-on-end" appearance of the cranial bones. *(Courtesy of Dr. Reg Munden.)*

children affected by sickle cell disease in the United States.

Other problems include delayed growth and development in most patients. Impaired kidney function and ocular abnormalities develop secondary to the damage caused by vaso-occlusive episodes in the capillary networks of those organs. If the patient lives long enough, then renal failure may eventually develop. In addition, approximately 5% to 8% of these patients will experience central nervous system (CNS) damage in the form of a stroke, which occurs at an average age of about 8 years.

The oral radiographic features of sickle cell disease are relatively nonspecific. They consist of a reduced trabecular pattern of the mandible because of increased hematopoiesis occurring in the marrow spaces. Occasionally, a "hair-on-end" appearance is seen on the skull radiograph, although this is less prominent than that seen in thalassemia (Fig. 13-8). Other oral problems that have been reported include an increased prevalence of osteomyelitis of the mandible, prolonged paresthesia of the mandibular nerve, and asymptomatic pulpal necrosis.

HISTOPATHOLOGIC FEATURES

In homozygous sickle cell disease, a peripheral blood smear shows a peculiar curved distortion of the erythrocytes, resembling a sickle or boomerang shape.

TREATMENT AND PROGNOSIS

The patient experiencing a sickle cell crisis should be managed with supportive care, including fluids, rest, and appropriate analgesic therapy (usually narcotic

preparations). It is important, but often difficult, to rule out the possibility of infection.

All 50 states now screen for this hemoglobin disorder as part of their newborn infant health care system to identify affected individuals as soon as possible so that appropriate therapy can be instituted. For children with a diagnosis of sickle cell disease, continuous prophylactic penicillin therapy is indicated until at least 5 years of age. In addition, the child should be given polyvalent pneumococcal vaccinations. Situations that might precipitate a crisis, such as strenuous exercise, dehydration, or exposure to cold, should be avoided. For adults with relatively severe disease, hydroxyurea has been approved for treatment. This drug increases the fetal form of hemoglobin (hemoglobin F), which may inhibit polymerization of hemoglobin S and may also reduce the adherence of erythrocytes to the vessel walls. Unfortunately, hydroxyurea has a number of potential side effects and should be used judiciously. Bone marrow transplantation is curative, but this is a procedure with multiple potential complications and is used primarily for severely affected patients having a histocompatibility antigen (HLA)-matched donor sibling. Only about 1% of sickle cell anemia patients currently meet these criteria.

When surgery is necessary, local anesthesia, if possible, is usually preferred. If general anesthesia is indicated, then precautions should be taken to avoid conditions that might induce a crisis, such as hypoxia, vascular stasis, acidosis, infection, reduced body temperature, or dehydration.

For patients who have either the sickle cell trait or the disease, genetic counseling is appropriate. DNA diagnostic techniques have been used for several years to assess whether a fetus is affected by sickle cell disease, permitting consideration of termination of the pregnancy. Molecular evaluation of the DNA from a single cell obtained from an embryo that was fertilized *in vitro* has allowed selection of a nonaffected embryo for uterine implantation. For parents who are carriers of the sickle cell trait, this is one method to ensure that their offspring do not have sickle cell disease.

Although the mortality rate for sickle cell disease in developed countries has improved dramatically over the past few years, the prognosis is variable because of the wide spectrum of disease activity. Those who are severely affected, however, often are quite disabled because of the many complications of the disease and have a decreased life span.

THALASSEMIA

Thalassemia represents a group of disorders of hemoglobin synthesis that are characterized by reduced synthesis of either the α-globin or β-globin chains of the hemoglobin molecule. As in those with sickle cell trait, people who carry the trait for one of the forms of thalassemia seem to be more resistant to infection by the malarial organism; an increased frequency of these genes is seen in Mediterranean, African, Indian, and Southeast Asian populations. Because the original cases were reported from the region of the Mediterranean Sea, the name *thalassemia* was given, derived from the Greek word *thalassa*, meaning "sea." The thalassemias are considered to be among the most common inherited conditions that affect humans.

An understanding of the structure and synthesis of hemoglobin is helpful in explaining the pathophysiology of these conditions. The hemoglobin molecule is a tetramer that is composed of two α chains and two β chains; if one of the chains is not being made in adequate quantities, then the normal amount of hemoglobin cannot be made. Furthermore, the excess globin chains accumulate within the erythrocyte, further compromising the structure and function of the cell. These abnormal erythrocytes are recognized by the spleen and selected for destruction **(hemolysis)**. In addition, there is evidence of ineffective erythropoiesis caused by premature cell death of erythrocyte precursors in the bone marrow because of activation of apoptotic mechanisms. The net result is that the patient has hypochromic, microcytic anemia.

Because two genes code for the β chain and four genes code for the α chain, the degree of clinical severity in these conditions can vary considerably. The severity depends on which specific genetic alteration is present and whether it is heterozygous or homozygous. In the heterozygous state, an adequate amount of normal hemoglobin can be made and the affected patient experiences few signs or symptoms. In the homozygous state, however, the problems are often severe or even fatal. In addition, variations in the severity of the clinical presentation may be a reflection of the specific alteration in the genetic code, because more than 200 different mutations have been documented for β-thalassemia alone.

CLINICAL AND RADIOGRAPHIC FEATURES

β-THALASSEMIA

If only one defective gene for the β-globin molecule is inherited **(thalassemia minor)**, no significant clinical manifestations are usually present.

When two defective genes for the β-globin molecule are inherited, the patient is affected with **thalassemia major**, also called **Cooley's anemia** or **Mediterranean anemia**. The disease is usually detected during the first year of life because a severe microcytic, hypochromic anemia develops when fetal hemoglobin synthesis ceases after 3 to 4 months of age. The red blood cells that are produced are extremely fragile and survive for only a few days in the peripheral circulation.

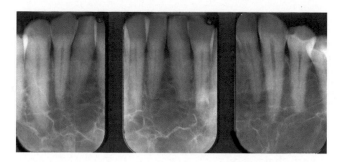

Fig. 13-9   Thalassemia. Periapical radiographs of the anterior mandible showing reduced trabeculation because of increased hematopoiesis. *(Courtesy of Dr. José Luis Tapia.)*

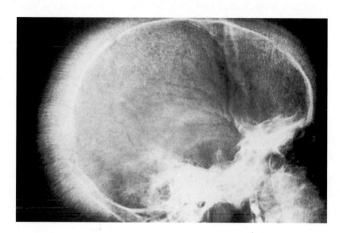

Fig. 13-10   Thalassemia. Lateral skull radiograph depicting the characteristic "hair-on-end" appearance in a patient with thalassemia.

In an attempt to maintain adequate oxygenation, the rate of hematopoiesis (despite being ineffective) is greatly increased (up to 30 times normal), resulting in massive bone marrow hyperplasia, as well as hepatosplenomegaly and lymphadenopathy because of extramedullary hematopoiesis. The bone marrow hyperplasia may affect the jaws especially, producing an altered trabecular pattern and marked, painless enlargement of the mandible and maxilla (Fig. 13-9). This results in a characteristic "chipmunk" facies and causes reduced size or obliteration of the paranasal sinuses. Frontal bossing is also present, and a skull radiograph may show a prominent "hair-on-end" appearance of the calvaria (Fig. 13-10). Generalized maturational delay of the patient is typically seen. Delayed development of the dentition also has been described, with the teeth showing a mean delay of approximately 1 year compared with a matched population.

Without therapy, tissue hypoxia worsens and serious bacterial infections with pneumococcal organisms often develop. Eventually, high-output cardiac failure occurs; many patients die by 1 year of age as a result of infection or heart problems.

α-THALASSEMIA

Because four α-globin genes may be affected, **α-thalassemia** has a broader spectrum of involvement than does β-thalassemia.

With the alteration of only one gene, no disease can be detected. With the inheritance of two altered genes, the condition is known as **α-thalassemia trait**. These patients have a mild degree of anemia and microcytosis that is usually not clinically significant. With three altered genes, the term **hemoglobin H (HbH) disease** is applied. Patients have problems with hemolytic anemia and splenomegaly. For patients with severe hemolysis, splenectomy may be indicated.

The homozygous state, in which all four genes are abnormal, causes severe generalized fetal edema, a condition that has been termed **hydrops fetalis**. Hydrops fetalis is not specific for α-thalassemia and can be seen as a manifestation of other diseases, such as severe Rh incompatibility. Infants with α-thalassemia who are affected by this problem typically die within a few hours of birth.

TREATMENT AND PROGNOSIS

Thalassemia major is treated today primarily by means of blood transfusions. These should be administered every 2 to 3 weeks to simulate the normal hematologic state. Unfortunately, with repeated blood transfusions, iron overload inevitably develops because of the constant infusion of exogenous red blood cells. This is a serious problem, and often death is due to **hemochromatosis**, an abnormal deposition of iron throughout the tissues of the body. The heart, liver, and endocrine glands are particularly affected by the toxic accumulation of iron. To combat this problem, an iron-chelating agent, deferoxamine (also known as *desferrioxamine*), must be given. If such therapy is used steadfastly, patients with β-thalassemia may have a relatively normal life span; however, problems may arise with patient compliance because this medication must be infused parenterally over several hours for at least 250 nights each year. Hematopoietic stem cell transplantation has also been used with considerable success for individuals who are relatively young, have little organ damage, and have an HLA-matched donor.

Clinicians can now identify α-thalassemia, with its attendant hydrops fetalis (historically considered a fatal condition), *in utero* by molecular testing, and the fetus can be given intrauterine umbilical vein transfusions. An 80% survival rate has been reported for these infants, although they will require either lifelong transfusion therapy or hematopoietic stem cell transplantation.

For patients who have developed an abnormal facial appearance caused by thalassemia, surgical correction can be performed in many cases. Prevention of thalassemia also is desirable, either by screening for carriers of the genetic trait or by prenatal diagnosis.

APLASTIC ANEMIA

Aplastic anemia is a rare, life-threatening hematologic disorder that is characterized by failure of the hematopoietic precursor cells in the bone marrow to produce adequate numbers of all types of blood cells. A significant amount of evidence supports the concept that most cases of aplastic anemia represent an immune-mediated disease caused by cytotoxic T lymphocytes that target differentiating hematopoietic cells in the marrow. As a result, the hematopoietic stem cells do not seem to undergo normal maturation despite normal or increased levels of cytokines, such as granulocyte-macrophage colony-stimulating factor (GM-CSF), which normally induce the production and maturation of several types of white blood cells.

Although the underlying trigger for the immune-mediated destruction of the hematopoietic cells is unknown, some cases of aplastic anemia are associated with exposure to certain environmental toxins (e.g., benzene), treatment with certain drugs (especially the antibiotic chloramphenicol), or infection with certain viruses (particularly non-A, non-B, non-C, non-G hepatitis). It is possible that the abnormal immune response is perhaps initiated by such exogenous stimuli in certain instances. A few genetic disorders, such as **Fanconi's anemia** and **dyskeratosis congenita** (see page 746), also are associated with an increased frequency of aplastic anemia.

CLINICAL FEATURES

Because all of the formed elements of the blood are decreased in patients with aplastic anemia, the initial symptoms may be related to any one or several of the deficiencies. The erythrocyte deficiency produces signs and symptoms related to a decreased oxygen-carrying capacity of the blood; therefore, patients may experience fatigue, lightheadedness, tachycardia, or weakness. The platelet deficiency (thrombocytopenia) is seen as a marked tendency for bruising and bleeding, which affects a variety of sites. Retinal and cerebral hemorrhages are some of the more devastating manifestations of this bleeding tendency. Deficiency of white blood cells (neutropenia, leukopenia, or granulo-

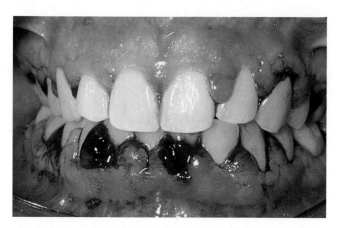

Fig. 13-11   Aplastic anemia. Diffuse gingival hyperplasia with sulcular hemorrhage.

cytopenia) is the most significant complication of this disease, predisposing the patient to bacterial and fungal infections that often are the cause of death.

The oral findings related to thrombocytopenia include gingival hemorrhage (Fig. 13-11), oral mucosal petechiae, purpura, and ecchymoses. The oral mucosa may appear pale because of the decreased numbers of red blood cells. Oral ulcerations associated with infection, particularly those that involve the gingival tissues, may be present. Minimal erythema is usually associated with the periphery of the ulcers. Gingival hyperplasia has also been reported in association with aplastic anemia.

HISTOPATHOLOGIC FEATURES

A bone marrow biopsy specimen usually demonstrates a relatively acellular marrow with extensive fatty infiltration. The histopathologic features of an oral ulceration in a patient with aplastic anemia show numerous microorganisms in addition to a remarkable lack of inflammatory cells in the ulcer bed.

DIAGNOSIS

The diagnosis of aplastic anemia is usually established by laboratory studies. A pancytopenia is characterized by at least two of the following findings:
- Fewer than 500 granulocytes/μL
- Fewer than 20,000 platelets/μL
- Fewer than 20,000 reticulocytes/μL

TREATMENT AND PROGNOSIS

The course for patients with aplastic anemia is unpredictable. For the milder forms of the disease, spontaneous recovery of the marrow may occur in some instances; progression to severe aplastic anemia may

be seen in others. Generally, in severe cases, the chances of spontaneous recovery are slim. If a particular environmental toxin or drug is associated with the process, then withdrawal of the offending agent may sometimes result in recovery.

The treatment is initially supportive. Appropriate antibiotics are given for the infections that develop, and transfusions of packed red blood cells or platelets are administered for symptomatic treatment of anemia and bleeding problems, respectively.

Definitive therapy for aplastic anemia is to replace the defective marrow with normal marrow, either by bone marrow transplantation or peripheral blood stem cell transplantation from a matched donor. Patients must be carefully selected; patients younger than 40 years of age and those with an HLA-matched donor (usually a sibling) have the best prognosis, but unfortunately only about 30% of patients meet these criteria.

For those patients who would not be a good prospect for bone marrow transplantation because of their advanced age or no matched donor, immunosuppressive therapy is recommended. Antithymocyte globulin (in the United States) or antilymphocyte globulin (in Europe) combined with cyclosporine produces a response in the majority of these patients. Compared with treatment results from only 25 years ago, the prognosis for this condition has markedly improved. In the past, for patients with severe aplastic anemia treated with only antibiotics and transfusions, the mortality rate was greater than 80% in the first year after the diagnosis. Currently, an overall long-term survival of 75% of these patients can be achieved with either bone marrow transplant or immunosuppressive therapy. However, even if the disease is controlled, then these patients remain at risk for recurrent marrow aplasia and are at increased risk for acute leukemia.

NEUTROPENIA

Neutropenia refers to a decrease in the number of the circulating neutrophils below 1500/mm^3 in an adult. It is often associated with an increased susceptibility of the patient to bacterial infections. Clinicians must be aware of this disorder because infection of the oral mucosa may be the initial sign of the disease. Interestingly, several ethnic groups, including patients of African and Middle Eastern background, will consistently have neutrophil counts that would qualify as neutropenia (as low as 1200/mm^3), yet these individuals are otherwise healthy. This finding has been termed **benign ethnic neutropenia**, and it appears to have no effect on the health of the patient because neutrophil counts respond to bacterial challenge.

A decrease in neutrophils may be precipitated by several mechanisms, most of which involve decreased production or increased destruction of these important inflammatory cells. When infections are noted in infancy and neutropenia is detected, the problem is usually the result of a congenital or genetic abnormality, such as **Schwachman-Diamond syndrome, dyskeratosis congenita** (see page 746), **cartilage-hair syndrome,** or **severe congenital neutropenia.** If the neutropenia is detected later in life, it usually represents one of the acquired forms. Many acquired neutropenias have an unknown cause; however, others are clearly associated with various causes. A decreased production of neutrophils and the other formed elements of the blood may result from the destruction of the bone marrow by malignancies, such as leukemia (see page 587), or by metabolic diseases, such as Gaucher disease (see page 818), and osteopetrosis (see page 615).

Many drugs may affect neutrophil production, either through direct toxic effects on the bone marrow progenitor cells or by unknown idiosyncratic mechanisms. These drugs include the following:

- Anticancer chemotherapeutic agents (e.g., nitrogen mustard, busulfan, chlorambucil, cyclophosphamide)
- Antibiotics (e.g., penicillins and sulfonamides)
- Phenothiazines
- Tranquilizers
- Diuretics

Nutritional deficiencies of vitamin B_{12} or folate, which may be a consequence of malabsorption syndromes, can inhibit neutrophil production.

A variety of viral and bacterial infections not only may reduce production of neutrophils but also seem to increase their destruction, typically at the sites of infection. Viral infections that have been implicated include the following:

- Hepatitis A and B
- Rubella
- Measles
- Respiratory syncytial virus
- Varicella
- Human immunodeficiency virus (HIV)

Numerous bacterial infections, such as typhoid, tuberculosis, brucellosis, and tularemia, may also cause neutropenia. The increased destruction of neutrophils by an autoimmune mechanism also occurs in such disorders as systemic lupus erythematosus (SLE), in which autoantibodies directed against the neutrophil are produced.

CLINICAL FEATURES

Most patients with neutropenia have some form of bacterial infection rather than a viral or fungal infection, particularly if the other elements of the immune system (lymphocytes, plasma cells, and monocytes) are still intact. *Staphylococcus aureus* and gram-negative organisms seem to cause the most problems for patients with neutropenia. The suppuration and abscess formation normally associated with such infections may be markedly reduced because of the lack of neutrophils. The most common sites of infection include the middle ear, the oral cavity, and the perirectal area. When neutrophil counts drop below 500/mm³, however, pulmonary infections often develop.

The oral lesions of neutropenia consist of ulcerations that usually involve the gingival mucosa, probably because of the heavy bacterial colonization of this area and the chronic trauma that it receives. These ulcers characteristically lack an erythematous periphery, although this finding has been variable. Premature periodontal bone loss with exfoliation of the deciduous dentition has been described.

HISTOPATHOLOGIC FEATURES

A biopsy specimen of a neutropenic ulceration usually shows a reduced number or the absence of neutrophils. Bacterial invasion of the host tissue may be apparent in some instances.

TREATMENT AND PROGNOSIS

Infections related to neutropenia are managed with appropriate antibiotic therapy. The patient should be encouraged to maintain optimal oral hygiene to decrease the bacterial load in the oral cavity. Studies using recombinant human granulocyte colony-stimulating factor (G-CSF), a cytokine that promotes the growth and differentiation of neutrophils, have shown remarkable results. Patients with severe neutropenia have a significant increase in neutrophil counts and resolution of infections after treatment with this agent. Patients who do not respond to G-CSF may have to be considered for hematopoietic stem cell transplantation, depending on the severity of the neutropenia and subsequent infections.

AGRANULOCYTOSIS

Agranulocytosis is a condition in which the cells of the granulocytic series, particularly neutrophils, are absent. As in other disorders of the formed elements of the blood, agranulocytosis may occur as a result of decreased production or increased destruction or use of these cells. Although some cases are idiopathic, most are induced by exposure to one of several drugs. Some drugs, such as the anticancer chemotherapeutic agents, induce agranulocytosis by inhibiting the normal mitotic division and maturation of the hematopoietic stem cells. In other instances, the drugs trigger an immunologic reaction that results in the destruction of granulocytes. Rarely, agranulocytosis may be a congenital syndrome **(congenital agranulocytosis, Kostmann syndrome)** that results from a decreased level of the cytokine granulocyte colony-stimulating factor (G-CSF).

CLINICAL FEATURES

Agranulocytosis typically develops within a few days after a person ingests the offending drug. Because of the lack of granulocytes (especially neutrophils), bacterial infections often develop and patients may show signs and symptoms of malaise, sore throat, swelling, fever, chills, bone pain, pneumonia, and shock. The erythrocyte and platelet counts are usually normal or only slightly depressed.

Oral lesions are common and include necrotizing, deep, punched-out ulcerations of the buccal mucosa, tongue, and palate. The gingivae are especially susceptible to infection, often resembling the pattern of necrotizing ulcerative gingivitis (NUG) (see page 157).

HISTOPATHOLOGIC FEATURES

Microscopic examination of a biopsy specimen from one of the oral ulcerations in agranulocytosis characteristically shows abundant bacterial organisms, both on the surface and within the tissue. The host inflammatory response is relatively sparse, with few granulocytes, particularly neutrophils, seen in the ulcer bed.

TREATMENT AND PROGNOSIS

If the clinician believes that a particular drug has caused the agranulocytosis, the medication should be discontinued as soon as is reasonably possible. In many instances, the granulocyte count returns to normal within 10 to 14 days after cessation of the offending agent. For patients who have agranulocytosis secondary to cancer chemotherapy, oral hygiene should be meticulous to foster an immaculate oral environment. In addition, the use of chlorhexidine-containing mouth rinses seems to reduce the severity of the oral lesions. Active infections are treated with appropriate antibiotic medications.

If the agranulocytosis is related to cancer treatment, the white blood cell count usually returns to normal after a period of weeks. For patients whose granulocyte counts do not recover, administration of G-CSF or granulocyte-macrophage colony-stimulating factor (GM-CSF) may be beneficial. The overall mortality rate for this condition in the past was 20% to 30%, although cytokine therapy and the newer broad-spectrum antibiotics have improved the outlook for these patients.

CYCLIC NEUTROPENIA (CYCLIC HEMATOPOIESIS)

Cyclic neutropenia is a rare idiopathic hematologic disorder that is characterized by regular periodic reductions in the neutrophil population of the affected patient. The underlying cause seems to be a mutation of the neutrophil elastase *(ELA2)* gene, resulting in arrested development of neutrophils at the promyelocyte stage within the marrow. This mutation is also associated with premature apoptosis of these myeloid precursor cells. The best estimated frequency of this disease in the population is about 1 in 1 million. Although an autosomal dominant pattern of inheritance has been described in a few cases, most examples of cyclic neutropenia are isolated.

Symptoms usually begin in childhood and tend to correlate with the neutrophil counts. When the neutrophil count is at its nadir (i.e., lowest point), the patient experiences problems with infection. As the neutrophil count rises toward normal, the signs and symptoms abate. Very low neutrophil counts usually are present for 3 to 6 days, and blood monocyte and eosinophil levels are typically increased when the neutrophil count is depressed. Even when the neutrophil count is at its peak, the levels are often less than normal.

CLINICAL AND RADIOGRAPHIC FEATURES

The signs and symptoms of cyclic neutropenia occur in rather uniformly spaced episodes, which usually have a 21-day cycle. Patients typically complain of recurrent episodes of fever, anorexia, cervical lymphadenopathy, malaise, pharyngitis, and oral mucosal ulcerations. Other gastrointestinal mucosal areas, including the colon, rectum, and anus, may be affected by recurrent ulcerations.

The oral ulcerations develop on any oral mucosal surface that is exposed to even minor trauma, particularly the lips, tongue, buccal mucosa, and oropharynx (Fig. 13-12). An erythematous halo is variably present at the periphery of the ulcers. The gingiva is the most severely affected region of the oral cavity. Severe periodontal bone loss with marked gingival recession and tooth mobility are also characteristic (Fig. 13-13).

DIAGNOSIS

The diagnosis of cyclic neutropenia should be established by sequential complete blood counts (typically two to three times per week for 8 weeks) to determine whether cycling of the neutrophil levels occurs. The neutrophil count should be less than 500/mm^3 for 3 to 5 days during each of at least three successive cycles to make this diagnosis.

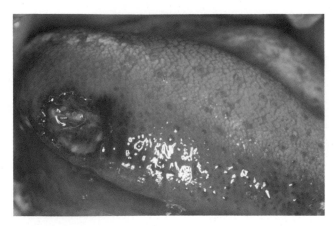

Fig. 13-12 Cyclic neutropenia. Ulceration of the lateral tongue is typical of the lesions associated with cyclic neutropenia. *(From Allen CM, Camisa C: Diseases of the mouth and lips. In Sams WM, Lynch P, editors: Principles and practice of dermatology, ed 2, New York, 1996, Churchill Livingstone.)*

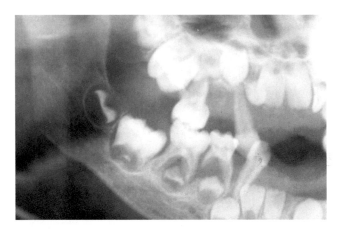

Fig. 13-13 Cyclic neutropenia. Cyclic neutropenia is one of several conditions that may produce premature bone loss, as shown in the interradicular regions of the mandibular deciduous molar teeth.

HISTOPATHOLOGIC FEATURES

The histopathologic features of cyclic neutropenia are similar to those of the other neutropenic and granulocytopenic ulcerations if the biopsy is performed during the nadir of the neutrophil count.

TREATMENT AND PROGNOSIS

Supportive care for the patient with cyclic neutropenia includes antibiotic therapy for significant infections that might occur while the neutrophil count is at its lowest. Unfortunately, this approach cannot be considered a permanent treatment. Other methods that have been used with marginal success include splenectomy, corticosteroid therapy, and nutritional supplementation. Studies have shown that administration of the cytokine granulocyte colony-stimulating factor (G-CSF) several times weekly seems to correct the lack of production of neutrophils. This treatment results in a decrease in the time of neutropenia from 5 days to 1 day, which improves the clinical course of the disease. The cycles are reduced from 18 to 21 days to 11 to 13 days, and the severity of mucositis and infection are reduced.

Supportive care in the form of optimal oral hygiene should be maintained to reduce the number and severity of oral infections and improve the prognosis of the periodontal structures. Fortunately, for many of these patients, the severity of symptoms related to cyclic neutropenia seems to diminish after the second decade of life, despite the fact that the cycling of the neutrophils continues.

THROMBOCYTOPENIA

Thrombocytopenia is a hematologic disorder that is characterized by a markedly decreased number of circulating blood platelets (formed elements derived from megakaryocyte precursors in the bone marrow). Platelets are necessary for hemostasis and clot formation. A platelet count of 200,000 to 400,000/mm^3 is considered normal. The decrease in platelets may be the result of the following:
- Reduced production
- Increased destruction
- Sequestration in the spleen

REDUCED PLATELET PRODUCTION

Reduced production of platelets may be the result of various causes, such as infiltration of the bone marrow by malignant cells or the toxic effects of cancer chemotherapeutic drugs. In such instances, decreases in the other formed elements of the blood are also seen.

INCREASED PLATELET DESTRUCTION

Increased destruction of platelets may be caused by an immunologic reaction, which is often precipitated by any one of more than 100 different drugs; heparin is one of the most common offending agents. This type of reaction is typically idiosyncratic and, therefore, not related to the dose of the drug. Similarly, autoantibodies directed against platelets, specifically certain surface glycoproteins, may on rare occasions be induced by viral infection or vaccination. In addition, certain systemic diseases may have thrombocytopenia as a component, such as systemic lupus erythematosus and HIV infection. Increased destruction may also occur by nonimmunologic means because of increased consumption of platelets associated with abnormal blood clot formation. This occurs in patients with conditions such as **thrombotic thrombocytopenic purpura (TTP)**.

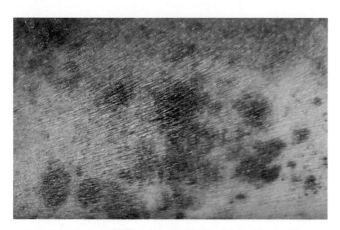

Fig. 13-14   Thrombocytopenia. The bruising (purpura) seen on this patient's forearm is a result of reduced platelet count secondary to myelodysplasia, a preleukemic bone marrow disorder.

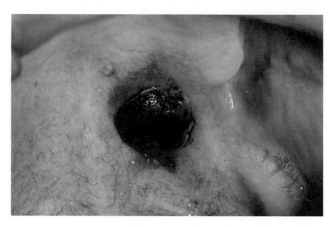

Fig. 13-15   Thrombocytopenia. This dark palatal lesion represents a hematoma caused by a lack of normal coagulation, characteristic of thrombocytopenia.

SEQUESTRATION IN THE SPLEEN

Under normal conditions, one third of the platelet population is sequestered in the spleen. Consequently, conditions that cause splenomegaly (e.g., portal hypertension secondary to liver disease, splenic enlargement secondary to tumor infiltration, splenomegaly associated with Gaucher disease) also cause larger numbers of platelets to be taken out of circulation. Regardless of the cause, the result for the patient is a bleeding problem because normal numbers of platelets are not available for proper hemostasis.

CLINICAL FEATURES

Clinical evidence of thrombocytopenia is not usually seen until the platelet levels drop below 100,000/mm^3. The severity of involvement is directly related to the extent of platelet reduction. The condition often is initially detected because of the presence of oral lesions. Minor traumatic events are continuously inflicted on the oral mucosa during chewing and swallowing of food. The small capillaries that are damaged during this process are normally sealed off with microscopic thrombi. In a patient with thrombocytopenia, however, the thrombi do not form properly. This results in a leakage of blood from the small vessels. Clinically, this usually produces pinpoint hemorrhagic lesions known as **petechiae**. If a larger quantity of blood is extravasated, then an **ecchymosis** or bruise results (Fig. 13-14). With even larger amounts of extravasated blood, a **hematoma** (*hemat* = blood; *oma* = tumor) will develop (Fig. 13-15). Spontaneous gingival hemorrhage often occurs in these patients, as does bleeding from sites of minor trauma.

Similar hemorrhagic events occur throughout the body. With severe thrombocytopenia (<10,000 plate-lets/mm^3), massive bleeding from the gastrointestinal or urinary tract may be fatal. Epistaxis is often present in these patients, and hemoptosis indicates significant pulmonary hemorrhage. Intracranial hemorrhage is also a potentially fatal complication of severe thrombocytopenia.

Special types of thrombocytopenia include **idiopathic (immune) thrombocytopenic purpura (ITP)** and TTP. ITP usually occurs during childhood, classically after a nonspecific viral infection. The symptoms of thrombocytopenia appear quickly and may be severe. Most cases, however, resolve spontaneously within 4 to 6 weeks, and 90% of patients recover by 3 to 6 months.

TTP is a serious disorder of coagulation and is thought to be caused by some form of endothelial damage that appears to trigger the formation of numerous thrombi within the small blood vessels of the body.

HISTOPATHOLOGIC FEATURES

Gingival biopsy may be performed for diagnostic purposes in patients with suspected TTP. Approximately 30% to 40% of such biopsy specimens show the presence of fibrin deposits in the small vessels. These deposits are more readily appreciated after staining the tissue section using the periodic acid-Schiff (PAS) method.

TREATMENT AND PROGNOSIS

If the clinician believes the thrombocytopenia to be drug-related, the drug should be discontinued immediately. In most instances, the platelet count returns to normal after several days. Platelet transfusions and corticosteroid therapy may be necessary if life-threatening hemorrhage occurs. As mentioned earlier, ITP often resolves spontaneously, but those cases that are more severe may require corticosteroid therapy or intravenous immunoglobulin (IVIG) therapy. For some forms of thrombocytopenia, such as TTP, the patient's prognosis is relatively guarded. In the past, the condition was almost uniformly fatal, although the outlook has improved since therapy with plasmapheresis or plasma exchange transfusions became available. More than 70% of these patients now survive with proper treatment.

POLYCYTHEMIA VERA (PRIMARY POLYCYTHEMIA; POLYCYTHEMIA RUBRA VERA; PRIMARY ACQUIRED ERYTHROCYTOSIS)

Polycythemia vera is a rare idiopathic hematologic disorder that is best thought of as an increase in the mass of the red blood cells. Uncontrolled production of platelets and granulocytes, however, is often seen concurrently, and most authorities feel that this condition represents a relatively nonaggressive myeloproliferative disorder. Researchers believe the overproduction is related to the abnormal behavior of a single progenitor marrow stem cell, which begins multiplying without regard to the normal regulatory hormones, such as erythropoietin. This gives rise to a group or clone of unregulated cells that then produce the excess numbers of these formed elements of the blood at two to three times the normal rate. These cells generally function in a normal fashion.

CLINICAL FEATURES

Polycythemia vera typically affects older adults. The median age at diagnosis is 60 years. Only 5% of cases are diagnosed before the age of 40 years. No sex predilection is seen, and the annual incidence estimates of the condition have ranged widely, from 0.2 to 28.0 cases per million population. Recent evidence suggests that an acquired mutation of one of the tyrosine kinase genes, Janus kinase 2 (JAK2), may play a significant role in the development of this disorder, because more than 95% of patients with polycythemia vera have been shown to have this mutation.

The initial symptoms of the disease are nonspecific and include the following:
- Headache
- Weakness
- Dizziness
- Drowsiness
- Visual disturbances

- Sweating
- Weight loss
- Dyspnea
- Epigastric pain

A ruddy complexion may be evident on physical examination. One relatively characteristic complaint, described in about 40% of affected patients, is that of generalized pruritus (itching), particularly after bathing, without evidence of a rash.

The problems caused by thrombus formation, which would be expected with the increased viscosity of the blood and the increased platelet numbers, include transient ischemic attacks, cerebrovascular accidents, and myocardial infarctions. Hypertension and splenomegaly are also common.

A peculiar peripheral vascular event called **erythromelalgia** affects the hands and feet. Patients experience a painful burning sensation accompanied by erythema and warmth. This may eventually lead to thrombotic occlusion of the vessels that supply the digits. Digital gangrene and necrosis may result. Erythromelalgia is probably caused by excessive platelets, and its onset seems to be precipitated by exercise, standing, or warm temperatures.

Strangely enough, these patients may also have problems with excess hemorrhage. Epistaxis and ecchymoses are often a problem, and gingival hemorrhage has been described.

TREATMENT AND PROGNOSIS

With the initial diagnosis of polycythemia vera, an immediate attempt is made to reduce the red blood cell mass. The first treatment is usually phlebotomy, with as much as 500 mL of blood removed daily. If thrombotic events are an immediate problem, then treatment with low-dose aspirin should be started. To control the platelet levels, anagrelide hydrochloride, a selective inhibitor of megakaryocyte maturation and platelet production, may be prescribed. Antihistamines are used to help control the symptoms of pruritus.

Long-term management may include intermittent phlebotomy, although myelosuppressive therapy has also been advocated. Each has disadvantages. An increased risk of thrombosis is associated with phlebotomy, and an increased risk of leukemia is associated with some chemotherapeutic drugs. Hydroxyurea is one chemotherapeutic agent that may not pose an increased risk of leukemia, however, because it acts as an antimetabolite and does not appear to have any mutagenic properties. Nevertheless, in 2% to 10% of patients with polycythemia vera, acute leukemia ultimately develops.

Overall, the prognosis is fair; patients with polycythemia vera survive an average of 10 to 12 years after the diagnosis, if treated. Given the fact that the median age at diagnosis is 60 years, the majority of affected patients do not seem to have a markedly higher death rate compared with their unaffected peers.

LEUKEMIA

Leukemia represents several types of malignancies of hematopoietic stem cell derivation. The disease begins with the malignant transformation of one of the stem cells, which initially proliferates in the bone marrow and eventually overflows into the peripheral blood of the affected patient. Problems arise when the leukemic cells crowd out the normal defense cell and erythrocyte precursors. In the United States, approximately 2.5% of all cancers are leukemia, and 3.9% of deaths from cancer can be attributed to this disease.

Leukemias are usually classified according to their histogenesis and clinical behavior. Therefore, the broad categories would be **acute** or **chronic** (referring to the clinical course) and **myeloid** or **lymphocytic/lymphoblastic** (referring to the histogenetic origin). Myeloid leukemias can differentiate along several different pathways; thus they produce malignant cells that usually show features of granulocytes or monocytes, and less frequently, erythrocytes or megakaryocytes.

Acute leukemias, if untreated, run an aggressive course and often result in the death of the patient within a few months. Chronic leukemias tend to follow a more indolent course, although the end result is the same. One of the greatest successes in cancer treatment has been achieved in acute lymphoblastic leukemia of childhood, a condition that used to be uniformly fatal but now is often capable of being controlled.

Leukemias are probably the result of a combination of environmental and genetic factors. Certain syndromes are associated with an increased risk. These genetic disorders include the following:

- Down syndrome
- Bloom syndrome
- Neurofibromatosis type I
- Schwachman syndrome
- Ataxia-telangiectasia syndrome
- Klinefelter syndrome
- Fanconi's anemia
- Wiskott-Aldrich syndrome

In addition, certain types of leukemia show specific chromosomal abnormalities. The first chromosomal abnormality to be detected was found in patients with **chronic myeloid leukemia**, and this malignancy was characterized by a genetic alteration called the **Philadelphia chromosome**. This abnormality represents a translocation of the chromosomal material between the long arms of chromosomes 22 and 9. This rearrangement of the genetic material occurs in such a fashion as to fuse the breakpoint cluster region (*bcr*) gene with the Abelson (*c-abl*) oncogene, producing an entirely new gene: *bcr-abl*. This gene is continuously transcribed, and the resulting protein product, a tyrosine kinase, causes the uncontrolled proliferation of the leukemic cells. Identifying such pathogenetic mechanisms has opened up an entirely new field of chemotherapy that targets specific molecular mechanisms of carcinogenesis. A variety of other genetic alterations in the bone marrow stem cells has been associated with the **myelodysplasia syndromes**, a group of disorders that appear to represent early stages in the evolution of **acute myeloid leukemia**. As the genetic alterations accumulate in the stem cells, the chances of the patient developing leukemia increase.

Some environmental agents are associated with an increased risk of leukemia, but their overall contribution to the leukemia problem is thought to be less than 5%. Exposure to pesticides, benzene, and benzene-like chemicals has been associated with an increased risk of developing leukemia. Ionizing radiation has also been implicated; this was documented by the increased frequency of chronic myeloid leukemia in the survivors of the atomic bomb blasts at Hiroshima and Nagasaki during World War II. Viruses have also been shown to produce leukemia, although this is not a common finding. The most thoroughly studied is the retrovirus known as *human T-cell leukemia/lymphoma virus type 1* (HTLV-1), which is transmitted by contaminated blood from infected to uninfected individuals. This virus can cause a relatively rare form of malignancy of T lymphocytes, which may present as a leukemia or non-Hodgkin's lymphoma (see page 595). Most cases have been identified in parts of the Caribbean, central Africa, and southwestern Japan.

As knowledge about this group of diseases increases, the fact that the leukemias are diverse and complex cannot be overlooked. For example, eight distinct subtypes of acute myeloid leukemia have now been identified, and each subtype has a different treatment approach and prognosis. Because of the complexity of this area, the discussion is limited to those aspects of leukemia that are more directly related to the oral or head and neck region.

CLINICAL FEATURES

If all types of leukemia are considered, this condition occurs at a rate of 13 cases per 100,000 population annually. Slightly more males than females are affected. The myeloid leukemias generally affect an adult population; **acute myeloid leukemia** affects a broader age range, which includes children. **Chronic myeloid leukemia** shows a peak incidence during the third and fourth decades of life. **Acute lymphoblastic**

leukemia, in contrast, occurs predominantly in children and represents one of the more common childhood malignancies. **Chronic lymphocytic leukemia**, the most common type of leukemia, primarily affects older adults.

Many of the clinical signs and symptoms of leukemia are related to the marked reduction in the numbers of normal white and red blood cells, a phenomenon that results from the crowding out of the normal hematopoietic stem cells by the malignant proliferation (**myelophthisic anemia**). Because of the reduced red blood cell count and subsequent reduction in oxygen-carrying capacity of the blood, patients complain of fatigue, easy tiring, and dyspnea on mild exertion. The malignant cells may also infiltrate other organs and often cause splenomegaly, hepatomegaly, and lymphadenopathy.

Leukemic patients may also complain of easy bruising and bleeding, problems that are caused by a lack of blood platelets (**thrombocytopenia**), the result of megakaryocytes being crowded out of the marrow. Petechial hemorrhages of the posterior hard palate and the soft palate may be observed, and these may be accompanied by spontaneous gingival hemorrhage, especially with platelet counts less than 10,000 to 20,000/mm³. Because disturbances in stem cell differentiation accompany the myelodysplasia syndromes, thrombocytopenia is often present in these patients, and gingival hemorrhage has been reported in this setting. Serious hemorrhagic complications may result from bleeding into the central nervous system or the lungs.

A fever associated with infection may be the initial sign of the leukemic process. Perirectal infections, pneumonia, urinary tract infections, and septicemia are common infectious complications. The microorganisms that are typically involved include gram-negative bacteria, gram-positive cocci, and certain *Candida* species.

Ulceration of the oral mucosa is often present as a result of the impaired ability of the host to combat the normal microbial flora. Usually, the gingival mucosa is the most severely affected because of the abundant bacteria normally present around the teeth. The neutropenic ulcers that are produced are typically deep, punched-out lesions with a gray-white necrotic base. Oral candidiasis is often a complication of leukemia, involving the oral mucosa diffusely. Herpetic infections are the most common viral lesions, and these may involve any area of the oral mucosa rather than being confined to the keratinized mucosa, as in immunocompetent patients.

Occasionally, the leukemic cells infiltrate the oral soft tissues and produce a diffuse, boggy, nontender swelling that may or may not be ulcerated. This occurs most frequently with the myelomonocytic types of leu-

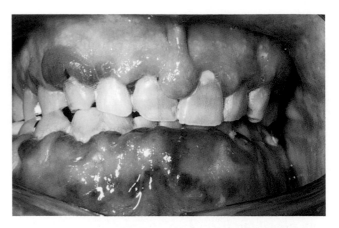

Fig. 13-16 Leukemia. Diffuse gingival enlargement, as depicted in this photograph, may occur in leukemic patients, particularly in those with monocytic leukemia. This older man had a history of myelodysplasia for several years before the development of leukemia.

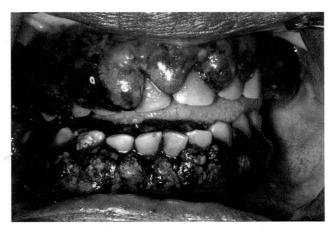

Fig. 13-17 Leukemia. Extensive hemorrhagic enlargement of the maxillary and mandibular gingivae. *(Courtesy of Dr. Michael Tabor.)*

kemia, and it may result in diffuse gingival enlargement (Figs. 13-16 and 13-17) or a prominent tumorlike growth (Fig. 13-18). The tumorlike collection of leukemic cells is known as **granulocytic sarcoma** or **extramedullary myeloid tumor**, and historically the term *chloroma* has been used because it is often greenish (*chlor* = green; *oma* = tumor) on fresh-cut sections. Other oral manifestations include infiltration of the periapical tissues, simulating periapical inflammatory disease both clinically and radiographically.

HISTOPATHOLOGIC FEATURES

Microscopic examination of leukemia-affected tissue shows diffuse infiltration and destruction of the normal host tissue by sheets of poorly differentiated cells with either myelomonocytic characteristics or lymphoid features.

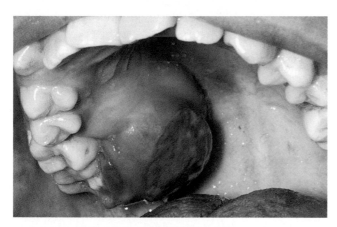

Fig. 13-18 Leukemia. The ulcerated soft tissue nodule of the hard palate represents leukemic cells that have proliferated in this area.

DIAGNOSIS

The diagnosis is usually established by confirming the presence of poorly differentiated leukemic cells in the peripheral blood and bone marrow. Bone marrow biopsy is normally performed in conjunction with the peripheral blood studies because some patients may go through an aleukemic phase in which the atypical cells are absent from the circulation. Classifying the type of leukemia requires establishing the immunophenotype by using immunohistochemical markers to identify cell surface antigens expressed by the tumor cells. Immunohistochemical confirmation of certain characteristic enzymes (e.g., myeloperoxidase, lysozyme) is necessary to identify and classify the myeloid leukemias. In addition, cytogenetic and molecular characterization of the lesional cells is typically necessary. In many cases, the results of these various studies will be significant because the patient's prognosis is directly affected.

TREATMENT AND PROGNOSIS

The treatment of a patient with leukemia consists of various forms of chemotherapy; the type of leukemia dictates the chemotherapeutic regimen. In most cases the purpose of chemotherapy is to destroy as many of the atypical cells as possible in a short time, thus inducing a remission. For this reason, this technique has been termed **induction chemotherapy**. Usually, this phase of chemotherapy requires high doses of toxic chemotherapeutic agents; often, the patient experiences a number of unpleasant side effects during treatment. Once remission has been induced, this state must be maintained. This is the purpose of **maintenance chemotherapy**, which typically requires lower doses of chemotherapeutic drugs given over a longer period.

If the bcr-abl fusion is identified in the leukemic cells of a patient with chronic myeloid leukemia, then treatment with a tyrosine kinase inhibitor is appropriate. The first tyrosine kinase inhibitor to be developed and marketed was imatinib mesylate, and a significant proportion of patients will respond dramatically to this therapy. Imatinib must be taken continuously, because relapses develop quickly if the drug is stopped. Other tyrosine kinase inhibitors are currently being investigated as well.

Newer treatments for chronic lymphocytic leukemia include monoclonal antibodies directed against cell surface antigens, such as CD20, a B-lymphocyte antigen. Rituximab is one such agent that is now being investigated in the treatment of hematologic malignancies of B-cell differentiation.

Drug therapy may be combined with radiation therapy to the CNS because the chemotherapeutic drugs often do not cross the blood-brain barrier effectively. Therefore, the leukemic cells may survive in this site and cause a relapse of the leukemia. Direct intrathecal infusion of the chemotherapeutic agent may be performed to circumvent the problem of the blood-brain barrier. If this strategy succeeds in inducing a remission, then a bone marrow transplant may be considered as a therapeutic option, particularly for the types of leukemia that tend to relapse. This option often is reserved for patients younger than 45 years of age because the success rate is less favorable in older patients.

Supportive care is often necessary if these patients are to survive their leukemia. For patients with bleeding problems, transfusions with platelets may be necessary. If severe anemia is present, packed red blood cells may be required. Infections, of course, should be evaluated with respect to the causative organism, and appropriate antibiotics must be prescribed. Support must be maintained from an oral perspective because many of these patients experience infections of the oral mucosa during the course of their disease. Optimal oral hygiene should be encouraged, and aggressive investigation of any oral complaint should be performed as soon as possible to prevent potentially serious oral infectious complications.

The prognosis of a particular patient depends on a number of variables, including the type of leukemia, the age of the patient, and the cytogenetic alterations associated with the disease. In children with **acute lymphoblastic leukemia**, more than 80% of these patients are now considered to be cured after appropriate treatment. In an adult with the same diagnosis, even though the rate of initial remission induction is 80%, the 5-year survival rate is generally much lower in most reported series.

Patients younger than 60 years of age with **acute myeloid leukemia** have a 5-year survival rate of approximately 40% today. This form of leukemia in a patient older than 60 years, however, has a much poorer prognosis, with less than a 10% chance of survival seen in that population. Similarly, patients with a previous history of myelodysplasia have an unfavorable prognosis.

Even though an indolent period is experienced with **chronic myeloid leukemia**, eventually the neoplastic cells undergo a process known as **blast transformation**, in which they become less differentiated, proliferate wildly, and cause the patient's death within 3 to 6 months. In the past, the 5-year survival rate for chronic myeloid leukemia was in the 20% range. Today, most centers are reporting 5-year survival rates of approximately 80%, a dramatic improvement presumably because of the effect of tyrosine kinase inhibitor therapy. Additional factors that may play a role in improved survival include diagnosis of the disease at an earlier stage and the availability of better supportive care. Attempts to control chronic myeloid leukemia by bone marrow transplantation from an HLA-matched donor have resulted in 5-year survival rates of 60% to 70% in younger patients with this disease. This may be an option for those patients who do not respond to tyrosine kinase inhibitor therapy.

Chronic lymphocytic leukemia is considered to be incurable, but its course is highly variable and depends on the stage of the disease. Patients with limited disease have an average survival time of more than 10 years. Those with more advanced disease survive an average of only 2 years.

LANGERHANS CELL HISTIOCYTOSIS (HISTIOCYTOSIS X; LANGERHANS CELL DISEASE; IDIOPATHIC HISTIOCYTOSIS; EOSINOPHILIC GRANULOMA; LANGERHANS CELL GRANULOMA; LANGERHANS CELL GRANULOMATOSIS)

The term *histiocytosis X* was introduced as a collective designation for a spectrum of clinicopathologic disorders characterized by proliferation of histiocyte-like cells that are accompanied by varying numbers of eosinophils, lymphocytes, plasma cells, and multinucleated giant cells. The distinctive histiocytic cells present in this lesion have been identified as Langerhans cells, and the condition is now designated as **Langerhans cell histiocytosis**. Langerhans cells are dendritic mononuclear cells normally found in the epidermis, mucosa, lymph nodes, and bone marrow. These cells process and present antigens to T lymphocytes. For many years, researchers have debated whether Langer-

hans cell histiocytosis represents a nonneoplastic condition or a true neoplasm. Studies examining the clonality of the lesional cells of this condition have shown this to be a monoclonal proliferation, a finding that is more consistent with a neoplastic process.

CLINICAL AND RADIOGRAPHIC FEATURES

The clinicopathologic spectrum traditionally considered under the designation of Langerhans cell histiocytosis includes the following:

- Monostotic or polyostotic eosinophilic granuloma of bone—solitary or multiple bone lesions without visceral involvement
- Chronic disseminated histiocytosis—a disease involving bone, skin, and viscera (**Hand-Schüller-Christian disease**)
- Acute disseminated histiocytosis—a disease with prominent cutaneous, visceral, and bone marrow involvement occurring mainly in infants (**Letterer-Siwe disease**)

It is difficult to categorize many patients into one of these classic designations because of overlapping clinical features. The often-cited Hand-Schüller-Christian triad—bone lesions, exophthalmos, and diabetes insipidus—is present in only a few patients with chronic disseminated disease. It is widely believed that the traditional designations of Hand-Schüller-Christian and Letterer-Siwe disease serve no useful purpose and should be discontinued. Many cases reported as Letterer-Siwe disease in the older literature probably included obscure infections, immunodeficiency syndromes, and malignant histiocytic lesions. Pulmonary Langerhans cell histiocytosis has also been described, but this probably is unrelated to the condition that affects the jaws. Patients who develop pulmonary Langerhans cell histiocytosis are usually adults with a history of smoking, and clonality studies suggest that this is probably a reactive process.

Although Langerhans cell histiocytosis may be encountered in patients over a wide age range, more than 50% of all cases are seen in patients younger than age 15. Although some series have reported a male predilection, overall the sexes appear to be equally affected. Bone lesions, either solitary or multiple, are the most common clinical presentation. Lesions may be found in almost any bone, but the skull, ribs, vertebrae, and mandible are among the most frequent sites. Children younger than age 10 most often have skull and femoral lesions; patients older than age 20 more often have lesions in the ribs, shoulder girdle, and mandible. Adult patients with solitary or multiple bone lesions may have lymphadenopathy but usually do not have significant visceral involvement.

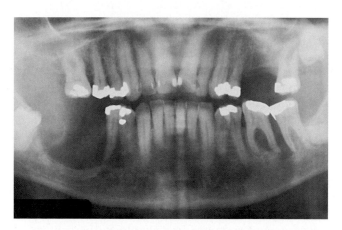

Fig. 13-19   Langerhans cell histiocytosis. Severe bone loss in the mandibular molar regions that resembles advanced periodontitis. *(Courtesy of Dr. James White.)*

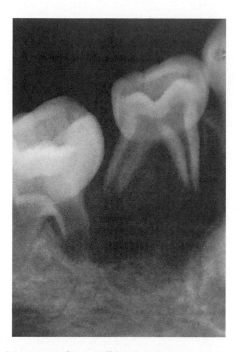

Fig. 13-20   Langerhans cell histiocytosis. Periapical radiograph showing marked bone loss involving the mandibular teeth in a young girl, resulting in a "floating-in-air" appearance of the teeth.

The jaws are affected in 10% to 20% of all cases. Dull pain and tenderness often accompany bone lesions. Radiographically, the lesions often appear as sharply punched-out radiolucencies without a corticated rim, but occasionally an ill-defined radiolucency is seen. Bone involvement in the mandible usually occurs in the posterior areas, and a characteristic "scooped out" appearance may be evident when the superficial alveolar bone is destroyed. The resulting bone destruction and loosening of the teeth clinically may resemble severe periodontitis (Fig. 13-19). Extensive alveolar involvement causes the teeth to appear as if they are "floating in air" (Fig. 13-20).

Ulcerative or proliferative mucosal lesions or a proliferative gingival mass may develop if the disease breaks out of bone (Fig. 13-21). Occasionally, this process may involve only the oral soft tissues. Lesions also can occur within the body of the mandible or maxilla, where they may simulate a periapical inflammatory condition.

HISTOPATHOLOGIC FEATURES

The bone lesions of patients with Langerhans cell histiocytosis show a diffuse infiltration of large, pale-staining mononuclear cells that resemble histiocytes. These cells have indistinct cytoplasmic borders and rounded or indented vesicular nuclei. Varying numbers of eosinophils are typically interspersed among the histiocyte-like cells (Fig. 13-22). Plasma cells, lymphocytes, and multinucleated giant cells are often seen, and areas of necrosis and hemorrhage may be present.

The identification of lesional Langerhans cells is necessary to confirm the diagnosis. Because Langerhans cells cannot be differentiated from other histiocytes by routine histologic staining, additional diagnostic

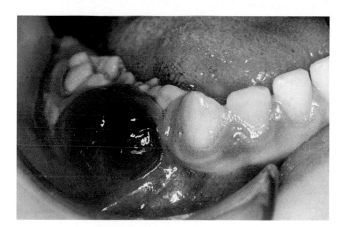

Fig. 13-21   Langerhans cell histiocytosis. Clinical photograph of the same patient shown in Fig. 13-20. The lesion has broken out of bone and produced this soft tissue mass.

methods are required. Electron microscopic evaluation of lesional tissue has been the gold standard for many years because, ultrastructurally, Langerhans cells contain rod-shaped cytoplasmic structures known as **Birbeck granules**, which differentiate them from other mononuclear phagocytes (Fig. 13-23). Most laboratories now rely on immunohistochemical procedures to identify the lesional Langerhans cells because of their immunoreactivity with antibodies directed against

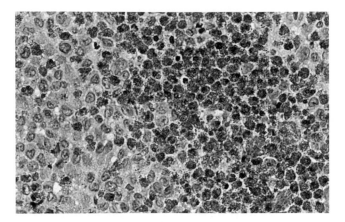

Fig. 13-22   Langerhans cell histiocytosis. There is a diffuse infiltrate of pale-staining Langerhans cells intermixed with numerous red granular eosinophils.

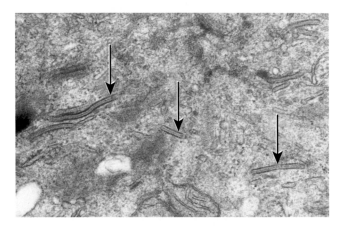

Fig. 13-23   Langerhans cell histiocytosis. Electron micrograph showing rod-shaped Birbeck bodies (*black arrows*) in the cytoplasm of a Langerhans cell. (*Courtesy of Richard Geissler.*)

either CD-1a or CD-207, the latter marker being even more specific for Langerhans cells. To a lesser extent, the lesional cells have S-100 protein immunoreactivity, and they also may show affinity for peanut agglutinin (PNA).

TREATMENT AND PROGNOSIS

Accessible bone lesions, such as those in the maxilla and mandible, are usually treated by curettage. Low doses of radiation may be used for less accessible bone lesions, although the potential for induction of malignancy secondary to this treatment is a concern in younger patients. Intralesional injection with corticosteroid agents has also been reported to be effective in some patients with localized bone lesions. Infrequently,

the apparent spontaneous regression of localized Langerhans cell histiocytosis has been reported. The prognosis for bone lesions in the absence of significant visceral involvement is generally good; however, progression or dissemination of the disease may occur, particularly for patients who have three or more bones affected.

Chronic disseminated disease is often associated with considerable morbidity, but few patients die as a result of the disease. Because of the relative rarity of disseminated cases, the ideal treatment has yet to be identified. Single-agent chemotherapy using prednisolone, etoposide, vincristine, or cyclosporine has produced a good response in a significant percentage of such patients, although recurrence is typically seen in over half of the cases. A combination of vincristine and prednisone seems to reduce this risk of recurrence. The acute disseminated form of the disease seen in infants and young children may not respond to these more conservative approaches, and multiple chemotherapeutic agents are given in that situation. Diffuse involvement with compromise of multiple organs is associated with a poor prognosis and is often fatal. In general, the prognosis is poorer for patients in whom the first sign of the disease develops at a very young age and somewhat better for patients who are older at the time of onset.

HODGKIN'S LYMPHOMA (HODGKIN'S DISEASE)

Hodgkin's lymphoma represents a malignant lymphoproliferative disorder, although for many years the exact nature of the process was poorly understood. The difficulty in comprehending the character of the condition is reflected in the relatively noncommittal term *Hodgkin's disease*, which was used for decades and still may be heard today. Perhaps one reason why Hodgkin's lymphoma was not easily understood is that, unlike most malignancies, the neoplastic cells (**Reed-Sternberg cells**) make up only about 1% to 3% of the cells in the enlarged lymph nodes that characterize this condition. Current evidence regarding the histogenesis of the Reed-Sternberg cell points to a B-lymphocyte origin. Certainly, the disease can cause death if appropriate therapy is not instituted, although the treatment of this malignancy is one of the few major success stories in cancer therapy during the past 20 years. In the United States, Hodgkin's lymphoma is about one sixth as common as non-Hodgkin's lymphoma; approximately 8000 cases are diagnosed annually. Although the cause of this disease is unknown, epidemiologic and molecular studies have linked Epstein-Barr virus (EBV) infection to a significant percentage of these lesions.

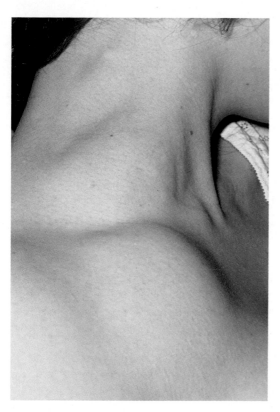

Fig. 13-24 Hodgkin's lymphoma. The prominent supraclavicular and cervical masses represent Hodgkin's lymphoma.

CLINICAL FEATURES

Hodgkin's lymphoma almost always begins in the lymph nodes, and any lymph node group is susceptible. The most common sites of initial presentation are the cervical and supraclavicular nodes (70% to 75%) or the axillary and mediastinal nodes (5% to 10% each). The disease initially appears less than 5% of the time in the abdominal and inguinal lymph nodes.

Overall, a male predilection is observed, and a bimodal pattern is noted with respect to the patient's age at diagnosis. One peak is observed between 15 and 35 years of age; another peak is seen after the age of 50.

The usual presenting sign is the identification by the patient of a persistently enlarging, nontender, discrete mass or masses in one lymph node region (Fig. 13-24). In the early stages, the involved lymph nodes are often rather movable; as the condition progresses, the nodes become more matted and fixed to the surrounding tissues. If it is untreated, then the condition spreads to other lymph node groups and eventually involves the spleen and other extralymphatic tissues, such as bone, liver, and lung. Oral involvement has been reported, but it is rare. In about 30% of patients with Hodgkin's disease, other systemic signs and symptoms may be present, such as weight loss, fever, night sweats, and generalized pruritus (itching). The absence of these systemic signs and symptoms is considered to be better in terms of the patient's prognosis, and this information is used in staging the disease. Patients who have no systemic signs are assigned to category A and those with systemic signs to category B.

The staging of Hodgkin's lymphoma is important for planning treatment and estimating the prognosis for a given patient. The staging procedure typically includes confirmation of the pathologic diagnosis, careful history and physical examination, abdominal and thoracic computed tomography (CT) scans or magnetic resonance imaging (MRI) studies, chest radiographs, and routine hematologic studies (e.g., complete blood count, serum chemistries, erythrocyte sedimentation rate). Evaluation of the extent of disease involvement using positron emission tomography (PET) scans is becoming part of the standard protocol, particularly at large institutions. Lymphangiography, gallium scan, bone marrow biopsy, exploratory laparotomy, and splenectomy may be necessary if the information that they would provide might have an effect on staging or treatment. A summary of the staging system for Hodgkin's lymphoma is presented in Table 13-2.

HISTOPATHOLOGIC FEATURES

Hodgkin's lymphoma is recognized to comprise two main forms, (1) nodular lymphocyte-predominant Hodgkin's lymphoma and (2) classical Hodgkin's lymphoma, the latter of which is divided into five subtypes. Although this group of diseases has certain features in common, current immunohistochemical and molecular biologic techniques have allowed distinctions to be made among the various types. The common features include effacement of the normal nodal architecture by a diffuse, often mixed, infiltrate of inflammatory cells that is interspersed with large, atypical neoplastic lymphoid cells. In the case of classical Hodgkin's lymphoma, this atypical cell is known as a **Reed-Sternberg cell** (Fig. 13-25). The Reed-Sternberg cell is typically binucleated ("owl-eye" nuclei), although it may be multinucleated ("pennies on a plate"), with prominent nucleoli. The malignant cell in nodular lymphocyte-predominant Hodgkin's lymphoma is the "popcorn cell," which is so-named because of the resemblance of the nucleus to a kernel of popped corn. The pathologist must see one of these types of distinctive atypical cells to make a diagnosis of Hodgkin's lymphoma, although their presence does not automatically imply that diagnosis, because similar cells may be seen in certain viral infections, especially infectious mononucleosis. To summarize, Hodgkin's lymphoma is currently classified in the following manner:

Table **13-2** **Ann Arbor System for Classification of Hodgkin's Lymphoma**

Stage	Defining Features
I	Involvement of a single lymph node region (I) or a single extralymphatic organ or site (I$_E$)
II	Involvement of two or more lymph node regions on the same side of the diaphragm (II) or one or more lymph node regions with an extralymphatic site (II$_E$)
III	Involvement of lymph node regions on both sides of the diaphragm (III), possibly with an extralymphatic organ or site (III$_E$), the spleen (III$_S$), or both (III$_{SE}$)
IV	Diffuse or disseminated involvement of one or more extralymphatic organs (identified by symbols), with or without associated lymph node involvement
	A: Absence of systemic signs
	B: Presence of fever, night sweats, and/or unexplained loss of 10% or more of body weight during the 6-month period before diagnosis

Adapted from DeVita VT, Hubbard SM: Hodgkin's disease, *N Engl J Med* 328:560-565, 1993.

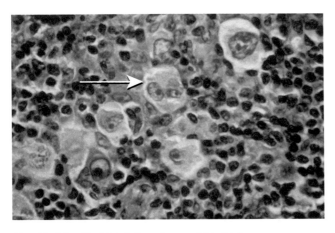

Fig. 13-25 **Hodgkin's lymphoma.** This high-power photomicrograph shows the characteristic Reed-Sternberg cell (*arrow*) of Hodgkin's lymphoma, identified by its "owl-eye" nucleus.

- Nodular lymphocyte–predominant Hodgkin's lymphoma, or
- Classical Hodgkin's lymphoma (comprising five histopathologic subtypes):
  1. Lymphocyte rich
  2. Nodular sclerosis
  3. Mixed cellularity
  4. Lymphocyte depletion
  5. Unclassifiable

These names describe the most prominent histopathologic feature of each type, and specific epidemiologic and prognostic characteristics are associated with each type.

Nodular lymphocyte-predominant Hodgkin's lymphoma constitutes 4% to 5% of all cases of Hodgkin's lymphoma in the United States. In the past, this form was probably combined with the lymphocyte-rich subtype, but the presence of the characteristic popcorn cells is a significant clue to the diagnosis.

Lymphocyte-rich classical Hodgkin's lymphoma represents about 6% of all cases. Sheets of small lymphocytes with few Reed-Sternberg cells characterize this form.

The **nodular sclerosis** subtype makes up 60% to 80% of cases and occurs more frequently in females during the second decade of life. This type gets its name from the broad fibrotic bands that extend from the lymph node capsule into the lesional tissue. Reed-Sternberg cells in the nodular sclerosis form appear to reside in clear spaces and, therefore, are referred to as *lacunar cells.*

The **mixed cellularity** form accounts for about 15% to 30% of the cases and is characterized by a mixture of small lymphocytes, plasma cells, eosinophils, and histiocytes with abundant Reed-Sternberg cells.

The **lymphocyte depletion** subtype, the most aggressive type, makes up less than 1% of the cases in recent reports. Before modern immunohistochemical techniques, many examples of large cell lymphoma or anaplastic T-cell lymphoma were undoubtedly included in this category. In this form of Hodgkin's lymphoma, numerous bizarre giant Reed-Sternberg cells are present, with few lymphocytes.

Occasionally, examples of Hodgkin's lymphoma are encountered that really do not fit the criteria for any of the known subtypes, and these are designated as **unclassifiable**.

TREATMENT AND PROGNOSIS

The treatment of Hodgkin's lymphoma depends on the stage of involvement. Patients who had limited disease (stages I and II) often were managed by local radiation therapy alone. Recent treatment trends, however, combine less extensive radiotherapy fields with milder multiagent chemotherapy regimens to maximize disease control and minimize long-term complications of therapy. Patients with stage III or IV disease require chemotherapy; radiation therapy is used conjointly if significant mediastinal involvement or residual disease is detected. For many years a regimen known as **MOPP** (mechlorethamine, Oncovin, procarbazine, prednisone) was widely used to treat Hodgkin's lymphoma. Because significant long-term side effects can be associated with this chemotherapy, another regimen known as **ABVD** (Adriamycin, bleomycin, vinblastine, dacarbazine [DTIC]) is now used most often, particularly for early and intermediate stage disease, because it has fewer complications.

Before modern cancer therapy was developed for Hodgkin's lymphoma, the 5-year survival rate was only 5%. The prognosis for this disease is fairly good today; the best treatment results occur in those who present in the early stages. Patients with stage I and II disease often have an 80% to 90% relapse-free 10-year survival rate; those with stage III and IV disease have a 55% to 75% 10-year survival rate.

The histopathologic subtype also influences the response to therapy. Patients with the lymphocyte-predominant and nodular sclerosis forms have the best prognosis, whereas those with the mixed cellularity form have a less favorable prognosis. In the past, researchers believed that the lymphocyte depletion form had a poor prognosis. However, with newer immunohistochemical studies, clinicians now realize that many of these cases were misdiagnosed; therefore, the available data are probably not reliable. In most instances, however, the stage of disease now plays a more important role in determining the patient's prognosis than does the histopathologic subtype.

After 15 years posttreatment, patient mortality is due more often to the complications of therapy: either secondary malignancy or cardiovascular disease. Currently, research is focused on the development of treatment regimens that continue to have a superior cure rate, while simultaneously decreasing the risk of treatment-related complications.

NON-HODGKIN'S LYMPHOMA

The **non-Hodgkin's lymphomas** include a diverse and complex group of malignancies of lymphoreticular histogenesis and differentiation. In most instances, they initially arise within lymph nodes and tend to grow as solid masses. This is in contrast to lymphocytic leukemias (see page 587), which begin in the bone marrow and are characterized by a large proportion of malignant cells that circulate in the peripheral blood. The non-Hodgkin's lymphomas most commonly originate from cells of the B-lymphocyte series, with an estimated 85% of European and American lymphoid neoplasms having this derivation. Tumors with a T-

lymphocyte derivation are less common, whereas true histiocyte-derived lymphomas are even rarer.

The microscopic appearance of the lesional cells was used in the past to classify the tumors as either *lymphocytic* or *histiocytic*. With the development of modern immunologic techniques, however, it is now known that many of the lesions that had been classified as *histiocytic* were in fact neoplasms composed of transformed B lymphocytes. In the early 1980s, a group of American pathologists devised a classification scheme, known as the *Working Formulation for Clinical Use*, which may still be referred to in the United States. Based on this classification, lymphomas were broadly grouped into three categories:
1. Low grade
2. Intermediate grade
3. High grade

Unfortunately, the Working Formulation has been shown to be somewhat limited in its utility and accuracy. Many lesions that have been recently defined are not included in this classification. For these reasons, an international study group in the early 1990s devised a new method of categorizing the lymphomas, known as the REAL (*revised European-American lymphoma*) *classification*. With this system, a combination of histopathologic features, immunologic cell surface markers, and gene rearrangement studies are used to organize this group of neoplasms. Recently the World Health Organization (WHO) revised its lymphoma classification system to conform to a slightly modified version of the REAL classification (Box 13-2). The latter two classifications appear to be more precise than the Working Formulation, and currently most pathologists in the United States categorize lymphomas according to the modified REAL system, although some of the more sophisticated molecular studies may not be available at smaller laboratories.

More than 58,000 cases of non-Hodgkin's lymphoma are diagnosed in the United States annually; approximately one third of this number will die of the disease each year. For reasons that are currently unclear, the incidence of this malignancy seems to be rising in the United States. The prevalence of lymphoma is increased in patients who have immunologic problems, such as congenital immunodeficiencies (e.g., Bloom syndrome, Wiskott-Aldrich syndrome, common variable immunodeficiency), AIDS, organ transplantation, and autoimmune disease (e.g., Sjögren syndrome, systemic lupus erythematosus, rheumatoid arthritis).

Viruses may play a role in the pathogenesis of at least some of these lesions. For example, Epstein-Barr virus (EBV) has been implicated, but not proven, to be an etiopathogenic agent in Burkitt's lymphoma (see page 600), a type of high-grade, small, noncleaved B-cell lymphoma. In addition, EBV may be related to lympho-

Classification of Hematopoietic and Lymphoid Neoplasms, Modified from the REAL/WHO Classification

B-CELL NEOPLASMS

I. Precursor B-cell neoplasm: precursor B-acute lymphoblastic leukemia/lymphoblastic lymphoma (LBL)
II. Peripheral (mature) B-cell neoplasms
   A. B-cell chronic lymphocytic leukemia/small lymphocytic lymphoma
   B. B-cell prolymphocytic leukemia
   C. Lymphoplasmacytic lymphoma/immunocytoma
   D. Mantle cell lymphoma
   E. Follicular lymphoma
   F. Extranodal marginal zone B-cell lymphoma of mucosa-associated lymphatic tissue (MALT) type
   G. Nodal marginal zone B-cell lymphoma (± monocytoid B-cells)
   H. Splenic marginal zone lymphoma (± villous lymphocytes)
   I. Hairy cell leukemia
   J. Plasmacytoma/plasma cell myeloma
   K. Diffuse large B-cell lymphoma
   L. Burkitt lymphoma

T-CELL AND PUTATIVE NK-CELL NEOPLASMS

I. Precursor T-cell neoplasm: precursor T-acute lymphoblastic leukemia/LBL
II. Peripheral (mature) T-cell and NK-cell neoplasms
   A. T-cell chronic lymphocytic leukemia/prolymphocytic leukemia
   B. T-cell granular lymphocytic leukemia
   C. Mycosis fungoides/Sézary syndrome
   D. Peripheral T-cell lymphoma, not otherwise characterized
   E. Hepatosplenic gamma/delta T-cell lymphoma
   F. Subcutaneous panniculitis-like T-cell lymphoma
   G. Angioimmunoblastic T-cell lymphoma
   H. Extranodal T-/NK-cell lymphoma, nasal type
   I. Enteropathy-type intestinal T-cell lymphoma
   J. Adult T-cell lymphoma/leukemia (human T-lymphotrophic virus [HTLV] 1+)
   K. Anaplastic large cell lymphoma, primary systemic type
   L. Anaplastic large cell lymphoma, primary cutaneous type
   M. Aggressive NK-cell leukemia

REAL, Revised European-American Lymphoma; *WHO,* World Health Organization; *NK,* natural killer.

mas developing in the setting of immunosuppression after solid organ or bone marrow transplant (resulting in the condition known as **posttransplant lymphoproliferative disorder**) or in association with AIDS (see page 272). Human herpesvirus 8 (HHV-8) has not only been associated with Kaposi's sarcoma but also with primary body cavity lymphoma and some cases of plasmablastic lymphoma. A blood-borne human retrovirus called *human T-cell leukemia/lymphoma virus type I* (HTLV-1) has been shown to cause an aggressive form of peripheral T-cell lymphoma among certain populations in the Caribbean, central Africa, and southwest Japan.

Even bacteria have been shown to induce the formation of so-called **mucosa-associated lymphoid tissue** (MALT) **lymphoma** of the stomach. Antibiotic treatment of *Helicobacter pylori* infection of the stomach lining often results in complete regression of this low-grade lymphoma.

CLINICAL AND RADIOGRAPHIC FEATURES

Non-Hodgkin's lymphoma occurs primarily in adults, although children may be affected, particularly by the more aggressive intermediate- and high-grade lympho-

mas. The condition most commonly develops in the lymph nodes, but so-called extranodal lymphomas are also found. In the United States, approximately 20% to 40% of lymphomas develop in an extranodal site, but in Asian countries such as Korea and Japan, nearly half of all lymphomas are extranodal.

With a nodal presentation, the patient usually is aware of a nontender mass that has been slowly enlarging for months. The lesion typically involves a local lymph node collection, such as the cervical, axillary, or inguinal nodes; one or two freely movable nodules are noticed initially. As the malignancy progresses, the nodes become more numerous and are fixed to adjacent structures or matted together (Fig. 13-26). Gradually, the process involves other lymph node groups, and invasion of adjoining normal tissues occurs.

In the oral cavity, lymphoma usually appears as extranodal disease. Although the oral lesions of lymphoma are often a component of more widely disseminated disease, at times the lymphoma begins in the oral tissues and has not spread to other sites. The malignancy may develop in the oral soft tissues or centrally within the jaws. Soft tissue lesions appear as nontender, diffuse swellings; they most commonly affect the buccal vestibule, posterior hard palate, or gingiva (Figs. 13-27

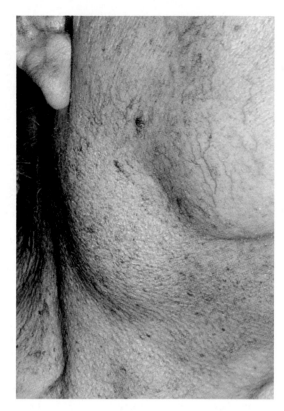

Fig. 13-26   Non-Hodgkin's lymphoma. The matted, nontender lymph node enlargement in the lateral cervical region represents a common presentation of lymphoma.

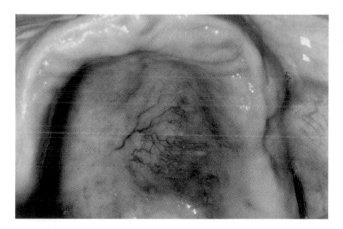

Fig. 13-27   Non-Hodgkin's lymphoma. One of the frequent locations of extranodal lymphoma in the head and neck area is the palate, where the tumor appears as a nontender, boggy swelling. Note the overlying telangiectatic blood vessels, a feature often seen with malignancy.

and 13-28). Such swellings characteristically have a boggy consistency. The lesion may appear erythematous or purplish, and it may or may not be ulcerated. Patients who wear a denture that contacts the lesional site often complain that their denture does not fit because it feels too tight.

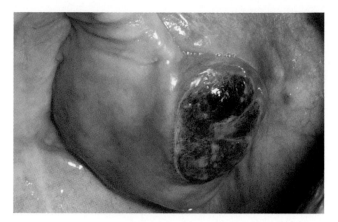

Fig. 13-28   Non-Hodgkin's lymphoma. Ulcerated mass of the left posterior maxilla.

Lymphoma of bone may cause vague pain or discomfort, which might be mistaken for a toothache. The patient may complain of paresthesia, particularly with a mandibular lesion (so-called numb chin syndrome). Radiographs usually show an ill-defined or ragged radiolucency, although in the early stages, the radiographic changes may be subtle or nonexistent. If untreated, then the process typically causes expansion of the bone, eventually perforating the cortical plate and producing a soft tissue swelling. Such lesions have been mistaken for a dental abscess, although a significant amount of pain is not present in most cases.

Clinical staging to determine the extent to which the disease has spread is an important factor in assessing the prognosis for a particular patient. The staging evaluation should include a history, physical examination, complete blood count, liver function studies, routine chest radiographs, CT scans of the pelvic and abdominal regions, lymphangiography, and bone marrow biopsy. The staging system for Hodgkin's lymphoma (see Table 13-2) has been widely adopted for use with the non-Hodgkin's lymphomas.

HISTOPATHOLOGIC FEATURES

Non-Hodgkin's lymphomas are histopathologically characterized by a proliferation of lymphocytic-appearing cells that may show varying degrees of differentiation, depending on the type of lymphoma. Low-grade lesions consist of well-differentiated small lymphocytes. High-grade lesions tend to be composed of less differentiated cells. All lymphomas grow as infiltrative, broad sheets of relatively uniform neoplastic cells that usually show little or no evidence of lesional tissue necrosis (Figs. 13-29 and 13-30). In some lesions, particularly those of B-lymphocyte origin, a vague semblance of germinal center formation may be seen (i.e., a *nodular* or *follicular* pattern). Other lymphomas show

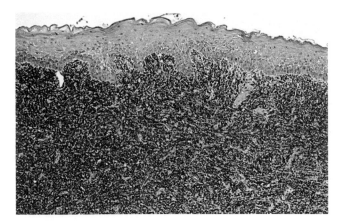

Fig. 13-29 Non-Hodgkin's lymphoma. This low-power photomicrograph shows a diffuse infiltration of the subepithelial connective tissue by lymphoma.

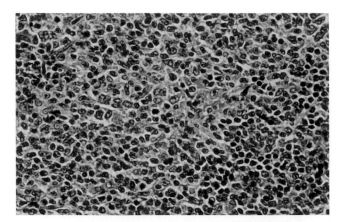

Fig. 13-30 Non-Hodgkin's lymphoma. This high-power photomicrograph shows lesional cells of lymphoma, consisting of a population of poorly differentiated cells of the lymphocytic series with minimal cytoplasm.

no evidence of such differentiation, and this pattern is termed *diffuse*. If the lymphoma arises in a lymph node, then the tumor destroys the normal architecture of the node. An extranodal lymphoma destroys the normal adjacent host tissue by infiltrating throughout the area. In the oral cavity, diffuse large B-cell lymphoma, which is considered to be a high-grade lymphoma, is the most common diagnosis, comprising approximately 60% of the cases.

Standard of care demands that appropriate immunohistochemical and cytogenetic studies be performed for a tumor diagnosed as lymphoma. In general, these studies can become quite involved and, therefore, are beyond the scope of this text.

TREATMENT AND PROGNOSIS

The treatment of a patient with non-Hodgkin's lymphoma is based on several factors, including the stage and grade of the lymphoma, the overall health of the patient, and the patient's pertinent past medical history. The patient's health must be considered because many of the chemotherapeutic regimens are quite debilitating. Surgical management is not usually indicated.

Low-grade lymphomas are perhaps the most controversial in terms of treatment. Some authorities recommend no particular treatment because these tumors are slow growing and tend to recur despite chemotherapy. Given the fact that low-grade lymphomas arise in older adults and the median survival without treatment is 8 to 10 years, many clinicians opt for a "watch and wait" strategy, treating the patient only if symptoms develop. Unfortunately, approximately 40% of low-grade lymphomas eventually transform to a high-grade lymphoma, leading to the patient's demise. Because these low-grade lymphomas have been con-

sidered "incurable," new treatments are being investigated. Most of these lesions are of B-cell differentiation, so treatment strategies using monoclonal antibodies directed against CD20, a B-cell surface antigen, are now being evaluated. Rituximab is one of the agents being examined in clinical trials.

For the **intermediate-grade** and **high-grade** lymphomas, the treatment of localized disease consists of radiation plus chemotherapy. With more advanced and disseminated disease, chemotherapy alone usually is implemented. Multiagent chemotherapy is used routinely, and new combinations are being evaluated continuously. Unfortunately, although the response rate of many lesions is good and much progress has been made in this area, the cure rate is not high. For intermediate-grade lesions, a failure rate of 30% to 50% can be expected. High-grade lymphomas are associated with a 60% mortality rate at 5 years after diagnosis and treatment.

MYCOSIS FUNGOIDES (CUTANEOUS T-CELL LYMPHOMA)

From its name, one might think that **mycosis fungoides** is a fungal infection. The early dermatologists who first recognized mycosis fungoides knew that this was not the case; however, they still thought the disease resembled a fungal condition. Thus this term has persisted. This condition, in fact, represents a lymphoma that is derived from T lymphocytes, specifically the T-helper (CD4+) lymphocyte. With modern diagnostic techniques, clinicians now know that there are several types of cutaneous lymphomas, each having specific T-lymphocyte or B-lymphocyte differentiation patterns. Even though mycosis fungoides is the most common of these cutaneous lymphomas, it is still a relatively rare

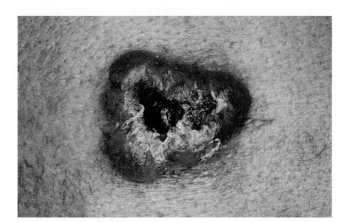

Fig. 13-31   Mycosis fungoides. In the tumor stage of the disease, patients with mycosis fungoides have ulcerated nodules of the skin. *(From Damm DD, White DK, Cibull ML et al: Mycosis fungoides: initial diagnosis via palatal biopsy with discussion of diagnostic advantages of plastic embedding,* Oral Surg Oral Med Oral Pathol 58:413-419, 1984.)

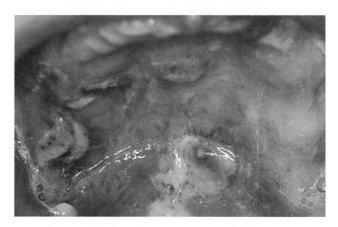

Fig. 13-32   Mycosis fungoides. The ulcerated palatal lesions represent a rare example of oral mucosal involvement by mycosis fungoides.

malignancy; only about 400 new cases are diagnosed in the United States annually. This condition exhibits a peculiar property called **epidermotropism** (i.e., a propensity to invade the epidermis of the skin). Oral involvement, although infrequent, may also be present.

CLINICAL FEATURES

Mycosis fungoides is a condition that usually affects middle-aged adult men; there is a 2:1 male-to-female ratio and a mean age at diagnosis of 55 to 60 years. The disease progresses through three stages, usually over the course of several years.

The first stage, known as the **eczematous (erythematous) stage**, is often mistaken for psoriasis of the skin because of the well-demarcated, scaly, erythematous patches that characterize these lesions. Patients may complain of pruritus. With time, the erythematous patches evolve into slightly elevated, red lesions **(plaque stage)**. These plaques tend to grow and become distinct papules and nodules. At this time, the disease has entered the **tumor stage** (Fig. 13-31). Visceral involvement is also seen at this point.

Approximately 35 cases of mycosis fungoides with oral involvement have been reported. The most commonly affected sites are the tongue, hard and soft palates, and gingiva (Fig. 13-32). The buccal mucosa, tonsils, lips, sinuses, and nasopharynx may also be affected. The oral lesions present as erythematous, indurated plaques or nodules that are typically ulcerated. Generally, these lesions appear late in the course of the disease and develop after the cutaneous lesions.

Sézary syndrome is an aggressive expression of mycosis fungoides that essentially represents a derma-

topathic T-cell leukemia. The patient has a generalized exfoliative erythroderma, as well as lymphadenopathy, hepatomegaly, and splenomegaly. The lung, kidneys, and CNS can also be involved. This condition follows a fulminant course and typically results in the patient's death within a short period of time; the median survival for this form of the disease is 2 to 3 years.

HISTOPATHOLOGIC FEATURES

ECZEMATOUS STAGE

The early stages of mycosis fungoides may be difficult to diagnose histopathologically because of the subtle changes that characterize the initial lesions. A psoriasiform pattern of epithelial alteration is seen, with parakeratin production and elongation of the epithelial rete ridges. Scattered, slightly atypical lymphocytic cells may be seen in the connective tissue papillae, but such features are often mistaken for an inflammatory process.

PLAQUE STAGE

With the development of the plaque stage, a more readily identifiable microscopic pattern emerges. Examination of the surface epithelium reveals infiltration by atypical lymphocytic cells, which are sometimes referred to as *mycosis cells* or *Sézary cells*. These atypical lymphocytes classically form small intraepithelial aggregates termed *Pautrier's microabscesses* (Fig. 13-33). The lesional cells have an extremely unusual nucleus because of the marked infolding of the nuclear membrane, which results in what is termed a *cerebriform nucleus*. This feature can best be appreciated when viewed in special semithin, plastic-embedded microscopic sections (Fig. 13-34). The diagnosis of mycosis

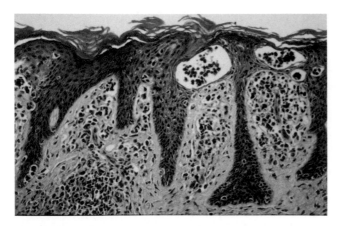

Fig. 13-33   Mycosis fungoides. This medium-power photomicrograph of a cutaneous lesion of mycosis fungoides shows infiltration of the epithelium by the malignant infiltrate that forms Pautrier's microabscesses.

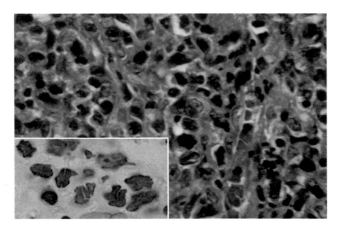

Fig. 13-34   Mycosis fungoides. This high-power photomicrograph of an oral biopsy specimen reveals the atypical, malignant lymphoid cells of mycosis fungoides that exhibit a cerebriform morphology *(inset).*

fungoides can be confirmed by demonstrating positivity for CD4 (a cell surface marker for T-helper cells) in the lesional cell population. In addition, T-cell receptor gene rearrangement analysis should identify a monoclonal population of T lymphocytes. A mixed infiltrate of eosinophils, histiocytes, and plasma cells may be observed in the subepithelial connective tissue.

TUMOR STAGE

As the condition progresses to the tumor stage, the diffuse infiltration of the dermis and epidermis by atypical lymphocytic cells makes it easier to identify as a malignant process. Other types of lymphoma would enter into the histopathologic differential diagnosis.

Immunohistochemical studies demonstrating a T-helper phenotype, combined with the T-cell receptor gene rearrangement studies, would help to distinguish the malignant infiltrate from other lymphomas and establish the diagnosis of mycosis fungoides. Examination of the peripheral blood of a patient with Sézary syndrome shows circulating atypical lymphoid cells.

TREATMENT AND PROGNOSIS

Topical nitrogen mustard, topical carmustine, superpotent topical corticosteroids, electron beam therapy, or photochemotherapy (**PUVA** [8-methoxy-**p**soralen + **u**ltraviolet **A**]) are effective in controlling mycosis fungoides during the early stages. Ultimately, the topical forms of therapy fail, and aggressive chemotherapy is necessary, particularly if there is visceral involvement. Newer agents that may be added to the chemotherapy regimen include monoclonal antibodies directed against the cell surface marker CD52, certain retinoid compounds, and specific interferon compounds. Another new agent that may be used for advanced disease is known as *denileukin diftitox,* which is derived from diphtheria toxin and targets the interleukin-2 receptor on the neoplastic lymphocytes. If Sézary syndrome develops, then extracorporeal photopheresis or chemotherapy is used as a treatment modality. Extracorporeal photopheresis involves the ingestion of the photoactive drug 8-methoxypsoralen, followed by the removal of a portion of the patient's blood and a separation of red and white blood cells. The red blood cells are returned to the patient immediately. The white blood cells are irradiated outside the body (extracorporeal) with ultraviolet A. These altered white cells are then infused back into the patient. Their altered state may help generate an immunologic response to the patient's own abnormal lymphocytes.

Although mycosis fungoides is not considered to be curable, the disease is usually slowly progressive. As a result, there is a median survival time of 8 to 10 years, and patients may die of causes unrelated to their lymphoma. Once the disease progresses beyond the cutaneous involvement, the course becomes much worse. The patient usually dies of organ failure or sepsis within 1 year.

BURKITT'S LYMPHOMA

Burkitt's lymphoma is a malignancy of B-lymphocyte origin that represents an undifferentiated lymphoma. It was named after the missionary doctor, Denis Burkitt, who first documented the process. In the original report, this type of lymphoma was described in young African children, and it seemed to have a predilection for the jaws. Because it was seen frequently in sub-Saharan Africa, the term **African Burkitt's lymphoma** has been applied to the disease. In addition, there is increased prevalence in other areas of the world, such as northeastern Brazil, and some investigators now refer to such tumors arising in these areas of increased prevalence as **endemic Burkitt's lymphoma.** Researchers believe this malignancy is related pathogenetically to Epstein-Barr virus (EBV), because more than 90% of the tumor cells, particularly in the African type, show expression of EBV nuclear antigen, and affected patients have elevated antibody titers to EBV. Characteristic cytogenetic chromosomal translocations, which may also be responsible for neoplastic transformation, have also been described. Tumors with a similar histomorphology, commonly referred to as **sporadic** or **American Burkitt's lymphoma,** have been observed in other countries where the neoplasm is usually first detected as an abdominal mass. Some HIV-related lymphomas may also have the microscopic features of Burkitt's lymphoma, and these lesions have been designated **immunodeficiency-associated Burkitt's lymphoma.** Similar tumors have been reported in other immunodeficiency settings, such as in patients who have received allografts or have a congenital immunodeficiency syndrome.

CLINICAL AND RADIOGRAPHIC FEATURES

As many as 50% to 70% of the cases of endemic Burkitt's lymphoma present in the jaws. The malignancy usually affects children (peak prevalence, about 7 years of age) who live in Central Africa, and a male predilection is usually reported. The posterior segments of the jaws are more commonly affected, and the maxilla is involved more commonly than the mandible (a 2:1 ratio). Sometimes all four quadrants of the jaws show tumor involvement.

The tendency for jaw involvement seems to be age related; nearly 90% of 3-year-old patients have jaw lesions, in contrast to only 25% of patients older than age 15. Sporadic Burkitt's lymphoma tends to affect patients over a greater age range than is noted for the African tumor. Although the abdominal region is typically affected, jaw lesions have been reported in sporadic Burkitt's lymphoma (Fig. 13-35).

The growth of the tumor mass may produce facial swelling and proptosis. Pain, tenderness, and paresthesia are usually minimal, although marked tooth mobility may be present because of the aggressive destruction of the alveolar bone. Premature exfoliation of deciduous teeth and enlargement of the gingiva or alveolar process may also be seen.

The radiographic features are consistent with a malignant process and include a radiolucent destruction of the bone with ragged, ill-defined margins (Fig. 13-36). This process may begin as several smaller sites, which eventually enlarge and coalesce. Patchy loss of

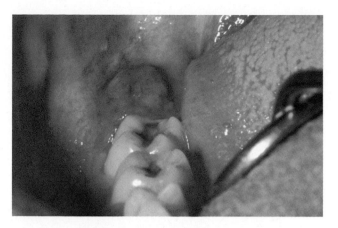

Fig. 13-35 Burkitt's lymphoma. This patient had documented American Burkitt's lymphoma involving the abdominal region. The retromolar swelling represents oral involvement with the malignancy.

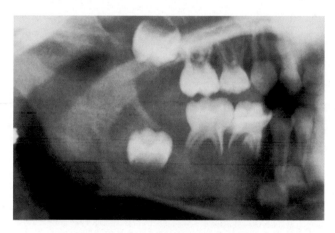

Fig. 13-36 Burkitt's lymphoma. This 4-year-old child had evidence of bone destruction with tooth mobility in all four quadrants of his jaws. Note the patchy, ill-defined loss of bone. *(Courtesy of Dr. Gregory Anderson.)*

the lamina dura has been mentioned as an early sign of Burkitt's lymphoma.

HISTOPATHOLOGIC FEATURES

Burkitt's lymphoma histopathologically represents an undifferentiated, small, noncleaved B-cell lymphoma. The lesion invades as broad sheets of tumor cells that exhibit round nuclei with minimal cytoplasm. Each tumor nucleus often has several prominent nucleoli, and numerous mitoses are seen. Immunohistochemical studies using markers that identify proliferating cells (e.g., Ki-67) typically indicate that almost 100% of the tumor cells are in the process of replicating. On viewing the lesion on low-power magnification, a classic "starry-sky" pattern is often appreciated—a phenomenon that is caused by the presence of

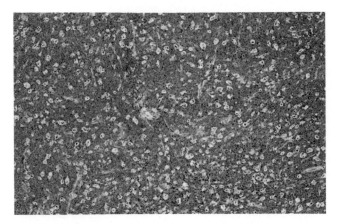

Fig. 13-37 Burkitt's lymphoma. This low-power photomicrograph shows the classic "starry-sky" appearance, a pattern caused by interspersed histiocytic cells with abundant cytoplasm ("stars") set against a background of malignant, darkly staining lymphoma cells ("night sky").

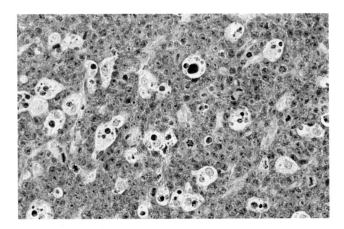

Fig. 13-38 Burkitt's lymphoma. This high-power photomicrograph demonstrates the undifferentiated, small, dark lesional cells with numerous histiocytes.

macrophages within the tumor tissue (Fig. 13-37). These macrophages have abundant cytoplasm, which microscopically appears less intensely stained in comparison with the surrounding process. Thus these cells tend to stand out as "stars" set against the "night sky" of deeply hyperchromatic neoplastic lymphoid cells (Fig. 13-38).

Because the histopathologic features of Burkitt's lymphoma can appear similar to some cases of diffuse large B-cell lymphoma, standard of care now dictates that, in addition to immunohistochemical studies, molecular genetic analysis of the tumor tissue should be performed. This distinction is important because these two malignancies are treated differently. Burkitt's lymphoma is characterized by one of several specific translocations, the most common being t(8;14), that results in overexpression of the oncogene *c-myc*, an event that presumably drives the neoplastic proliferation.

TREATMENT AND PROGNOSIS

Burkitt's lymphoma is an aggressive malignancy that usually results in the death of the patient within 4 to 6 months after diagnosis if it is not treated. Treatment generally consists of an intensive chemotherapeutic regimen, which emphasizes the use of high doses of cyclophosphamide. More than 90% of the patients respond to this treatment.

The prognosis for Burkitt's lymphoma in the past was poor, with a median survival time of only $10\frac{1}{2}$ months. More recent trials with more intensive, multi-agent chemotherapeutic protocols have shown an 85% to 95% event-free (no evidence of recurrence) survival rate 3 to 5 years after treatment for patients with stage I or II disease. Even for advanced stage (III and IV) Burkitt's lymphoma, the event-free survival has improved to 75% to 85%.

EXTRANODAL NK/T-CELL LYMPHOMA, NASAL-TYPE (ANGIOCENTRIC T-CELL LYMPHOMA; MIDLINE LETHAL GRANULOMA; IDIOPATHIC MIDLINE DESTRUCTIVE DISEASE; POLYMORPHIC RETICULOSIS; MIDLINE MALIGNANT RETICULOSIS; ANGIOCENTRIC IMMUNOPROLIFERATIVE LESION)

Also known as **angiocentric T-cell lymphoma, extranodal NK/T-cell lymphoma, nasal-type** is a rare process that is characterized clinically by aggressive, nonrelenting destruction of the midline structures of the palate and nasal fossa. For many decades, the nature of this process has been controversial, a fact that can readily be appreciated by the wide variety of terms by which it has been called. In actuality, many of the cases reported as "midline lethal granuloma" in the past represented a wide variety of immunologic (e.g., Wegener's granulomatosis) and infectious (e.g., tertiary syphilis) diseases. The term **midline lethal granuloma** should be used only as a descriptive designation of a destructive midline condition, and thorough diagnostic evaluation, including biopsy and culture, is necessary to make a definitive diagnosis. Once the other causes of midline destruction have been eliminated, the consensus among most investigators is that this disorder should be classified as a *natural killer (NK) T-cell lymphoma*, based on modern cytogenetic, immunologic, and molecular studies. The difficulty in distinguishing among these destructive disorders can be appreciated by the fact that **lymphomatoid granulo-**

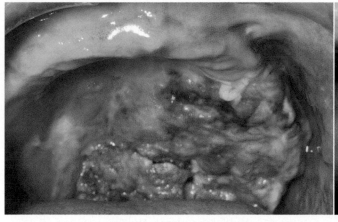
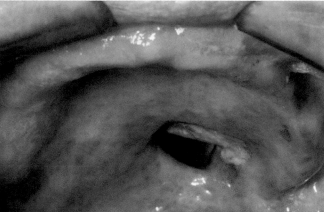

A

B

Fig. 13-39   Extranodal NK/T-cell lymphoma, nasal-type. A, This 62-year-old man had a destructive palatal lesion that proved to be a T-cell lymphoma, and evaluation showed cervical lymph node involvement as well. **B,** Resolution of the lesion 1 month later, after multiagent chemotherapy.

matosis, which until recently was considered part of this T-cell lymphoma spectrum, has now been determined to be an Epstein-Barr virus (EBV)-driven proliferation of B lymphocytes.

Even though extranodal NK/T-cell lymphoma often does not have the classic histopathologic features of lymphoma microscopically, it behaves in a malignant fashion and responds to the same treatments to which lymphomas respond. For reasons that are unclear, this condition is seen with greater frequency in Asian, Guatemalan, and Peruvian populations.

CLINICAL FEATURES

Extranodal NK/T-cell lymphoma is typically observed in adults. The initial signs and symptoms are often localized to the nasal region and include nasal stuffiness or epistaxis. Pain may accompany the nasal symptoms. Swelling of the soft palate or posterior hard palate may precede the formation of a deep, necrotic ulceration, which usually occupies a midline position. This ulceration enlarges and destroys the palatal tissues, which typically creates an oronasal fistula (Fig. 13-39). Secondary infection may complicate the course of the disease, and life-threatening hemorrhage is a potential problem in some instances.

HISTOPATHOLOGIC FEATURES

Histopathologic examination of one of these lesions shows a mixed infiltrate of a variety of inflammatory cells, often arranged around blood vessels (angiocentric) (Fig. 13-40). The lesional process appears to invade and destroy the normal tissue in the area. Necrosis is often present in some areas of the lesion, presumably

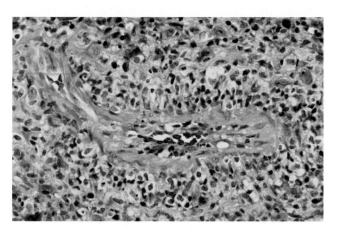

Fig. 13-40   Extranodal NK/T-cell lymphoma, nasal-type. This medium-power photomicrograph shows atypical lymphoid cells infiltrating the wall and filling the lumen of a blood vessel. Such a pattern is termed *angiocentric* (i.e., around blood vessels).

secondary to infiltration of the blood vessels by the tumor cells. Large, angular, lymphocytic cells with an atypical appearance are usually identified as a component of the cellular infiltrate. Immunohistochemical evaluation of this infiltrate often shows that the large atypical cells mark with antibodies directed against T-lymphocyte antigens. Molecular genetic studies typically show monoclonal gene rearrangements of the T-lymphocyte receptor, consistent with a lymphoreticular malignancy.

TREATMENT AND PROGNOSIS

Without treatment, extranodal NK/T-cell lymphoma is a relentlessly progressive, highly destructive process that ultimately leads to the patient's death by secondary infection, massive hemorrhage, or infiltration of vital structures in the area. Lesions that are localized usually respond to radiation therapy, a feature that is similar to that of T-cell lymphomas of other sites. Approximately 4500 cGy is required to control the disease, and many of these patients show no evidence of recurrence or dissemination of the lesion. Five-year survival rates in some series have been reported to be as high as 85%. For patients with more disseminated disease, combination chemotherapy is indicated, and a less favorable prognosis can be expected, with 30% to 50% 5-year survival generally reported.

MULTIPLE MYELOMA

Multiple myeloma is a relatively uncommon malignancy of plasma cell origin that often appears to have a multicentric origin within bone. The cause of the condition is unknown, although sometimes a plasmacytoma (see page 606) may evolve into multiple myeloma. This disease makes up about 1% of all malignancies and 10% to 15% of hematologic malignancies. If metastatic disease is excluded, then multiple myeloma accounts for nearly 50% of all malignancies that involve the bone. Nearly 20,000 cases are diagnosed annually in the United States.

The abnormal plasma cells that compose this tumor are typically monoclonal. The abnormal cells probably arise from a single malignant precursor that has undergone uncontrolled mitotic division and has spread throughout the body. Because the neoplasm develops from a single cell, all the daughter cells that comprise the lesional tissue have the same genetic makeup and produce the same proteins. These proteins are the immunoglobulin components that the plasma cell would normally produce, although in the case of this malignant tumor the immunoglobulins are not normal or functional. The signs and symptoms of this disease result from the uncontrolled proliferation of the tumor cells and the uncontrolled manufacture of their protein products.

CLINICAL AND RADIOGRAPHIC FEATURES

Multiple myeloma is typically a disease of adults, with men being affected slightly more often than women. The median age at diagnosis is between 60 and 70 years, and it is rarely diagnosed before age 40. For reasons that are not understood, the disease occurs twice as frequently in blacks as whites, making this the most common hematologic malignancy among black persons in the United States.

Bone pain, particularly in the lumbar spine, is the most characteristic presenting symptom. Some patients

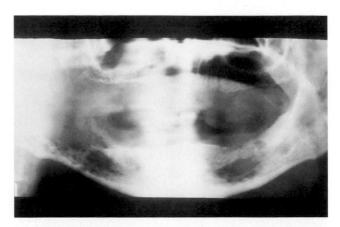

Fig. 13-41   Multiple myeloma. Multiple myeloma affecting the mandible. The disease produced several radiolucencies with ragged, ill-defined margins. *(Courtesy of Dr. Joseph Finelli.)*

experience pathologic fractures caused by tumor destruction of bone. They may also complain of fatigue as a consequence of myelophthisic anemia. Petechial hemorrhages of the skin and oral mucosa may be seen if platelet production has been affected. Fever may be present as a result of neutropenia with increased susceptibility to infection. Metastatic calcifications may involve the soft tissues and are thought to be caused by hypercalcemia secondary to tumor-related osteolysis.

Radiographically, multiple well-defined, punched-out radiolucencies or ragged radiolucent lesions may be seen in multiple myeloma (Fig. 13-41). These may be especially evident on a skull film. Although any bone may be affected, the jaws have been reported to be involved in as many as 30% of cases. The radiolucent areas of the bone contain the abnormal plasma cell proliferations that characterize multiple myeloma.

Renal failure may be a presenting sign in these patients because the kidneys become overburdened with the excess circulating light chain proteins of the tumor cells. These light chain products, which are found in the urine of 30% to 50% of patients with multiple myeloma, are called **Bence Jones proteins**, after the British physician who first described them in detail.

Approximately 15% of patients with multiple myeloma show deposition of amyloid (see page 822) in various soft tissues of the body, and this may be the initial manifestation of the disease. Amyloid deposits are due to the accumulation of the abnormal light chain proteins. Sites that are classically affected include the oral mucosa, particularly the tongue. The tongue may show diffuse enlargement and firmness or may have more of a nodular appearance. Sometimes the nodules are ulcerated. Another area that is commonly affected is the periorbital skin, with the amyloid

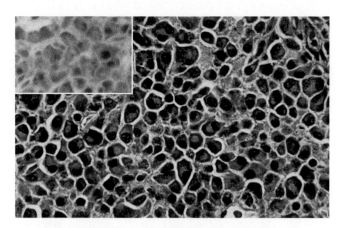

Fig. 13-42   Multiple myeloma. This high-power photomicrograph reveals sheets of malignant plasma cells with eccentric nuclei and stippled nuclear chromatin. Immunohistochemical studies (*inset*) show a uniform reaction of the lesional cells for antibodies directed against kappa light chains, indicating a monoclonal neoplastic proliferation.

deposits appearing as waxy, firm, plaquelike lesions (see Fig. 17-7 on page 823).

HISTOPATHOLOGIC FEATURES

Histopathologic examination of the lesional tissue in multiple myeloma shows diffuse, monotonous sheets of neoplastic, variably differentiated, plasmacytoid cells that invade and replace the normal host tissue (Fig. 13-42). Mitotic activity may be seen with some frequency. The monoclonality of the plasma cell population can be demonstrated using antibodies directed against the lambda and kappa light chain components of the immunoglobulin molecule. In a neoplastic proliferation of plasma cells, virtually all of the lesional cells will mark with only one of these antibodies. In contrast, a reactive plasma cell infiltrate will show a mixture of lambda- and kappa-producing plasma cells. Occasionally, deposition of amyloid may be observed in association with the neoplastic cells. Like other types of amyloid, this material appears homogeneous, eosinophilic, and relatively acellular. It stains metachromatically with crystal violet and shows an affinity for Congo red, demonstrating apple-green birefringence on viewing with polarized light. A biopsy specimen of bone marrow from a patient with multiple myeloma should show at least 10% atypical plasma cells making up the marrow cell population.

DIAGNOSIS

Although the histopathologic and radiographic findings strongly suggest a diagnosis of multiple myeloma, screening of the serum or urine by protein electrophoresis should be performed. If an abnormality is detected, then this should be confirmed by protein immunoelectrophoresis, which is a more sensitive test, as an additional parameter to establish the diagnosis. The serum and urine protein immunoelectrophoresis should show the presence of myeloma protein (M-protein). This represents the massive overproduction of one abnormal immunoglobulin by the neoplastic clone of plasma cells, thus this feature is termed **monoclonal gammopathy**. This monoclonal protein consists of two heavy chain polypeptides of the same immunoglobulin (Ig) class (IgA, IgG, IgM, IgD, or IgE) and one of two light chain polypeptides of the same class (kappa or lambda). Occasionally, the neoplastic cells produce only the light chain component.

TREATMENT AND PROGNOSIS

The goals of treatment related to multiple myeloma include not only controlling the malignancy but also making the patient comfortable and prolonging the patient's survival. Initial attempts to control multiple myeloma generally consist of chemotherapy. An alkylating agent, such as melphalan or cyclophosphamide, is often used in conjunction with prednisone, and approximately 60% of patients will respond initially to this regimen. However, virtually all patients eventually experience relapse of their disease. More aggressive chemotherapeutic regimens and bone marrow transplantation, either autologous or allogeneic, may be considered in otherwise healthy patients under the age of 55 to 65 years, but these individuals comprise a minority of multiple myeloma patients. Addition of thalidomide to the treatment protocol may improve survival; however, ongoing studies are evaluating the effect of this drug. Radiation therapy is useful only as palliative treatment for painful bone lesions. Any one of several bisphosphonate medications (clodronate, pamidronate, or zoledronic acid) can be prescribed to reduce the possibility of myeloma-related fracture with its attendant pain, but these medications do not appear to increase survival. A small percentage of these patients may experience the complication of bisphosphonate-related osteonecrosis of the jaws (see page 299).

The prognosis is considered poor, but younger patients tend to fare better than older ones. Pretreatment serologic studies examining the levels of β_2-microglobulin and albumin should be performed. With lower levels of β_2-microglobulin (<3.5 mg/L) and higher levels of albumin (>35 g/L), the median survival is approximately 5 years. In contrast, when serum β_2-microglobulin levels are >5.5 mg/L, the 5-year survival rate falls to about $2\frac{1}{2}$ years. A median survival time of about 3 to 4 years can be expected after the onset of symptoms. In the past, a 10% 5-year survival rate was typical; the prognosis today has improved only slightly. Most hematology and oncology centers report a 5-year survival rate of 25%. With aggressive chemotherapy and bone marrow transplantation, the 5-year survival rate may be improved to as high as 50%; however, only a small percentage of multiple myeloma patients can reasonably tolerate this treatment. This approach seems to hold the most promise for control of this aggressive disease, however, and some centers have indicated that as many as 20% of their patients may survive for longer than 10 years.

PLASMACYTOMA

The **plasmacytoma** is a unifocal, monoclonal, neoplastic proliferation of plasma cells that usually arises within bone. Infrequently, it is seen in soft tissue, in which case, the term **extramedullary plasmacytoma** is used. Some investigators believe that this lesion represents the least aggressive part of a spectrum of plasma cell neoplasms that extends to **multiple myeloma**. Therefore, the plasmacytoma is important because it may ultimately give rise to the more serious problem of multiple myeloma.

CLINICAL AND RADIOGRAPHIC FEATURES

The plasmacytoma usually is detected in an adult male, with an average age at diagnosis of 55 years. The male-to-female ratio is 3:1. Most of the lesions present centrally within a single bone, and the spine is the most commonly involved site. About one third of the cases are reported in that location. The initial symptoms often relate to swelling or bone pain; occasionally, however, this lesion is detected on routine radiographic examination. The extramedullary plasmacytoma appears as a relatively nondescript, well-circumscribed, nontender soft tissue mass. An even stronger male predilection is seen with this lesion, approaching a 6:1 male-to-female ratio. Approximately 80% to 90% of extramedullary plasmacytomas develop in the head and neck region, and such lesions have been reported in the tonsils, the nasopharynx, the paranasal sinuses, the nose, and the parotid gland.

Radiographically, the lesion may be seen as a well-defined, unilocular radiolucency with no evidence of sclerotic borders or as a ragged radiolucency similar to the appearance of multiple myeloma (Fig. 13-43). No other lesions should be identifiable by a skeletal survey or careful physical examination, however.

HISTOPATHOLOGIC FEATURES

The histopathologic features of the plasmacytoma are identical to those of multiple myeloma. Sheets of plasma cells show varying degrees of differentiation.

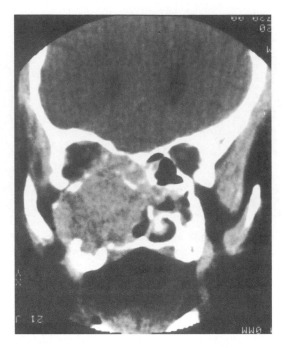

Fig. 13-43   Plasmacytoma. This computed tomography (CT) scan depicts a solitary plasmacytoma involving the left maxillary sinus and nasal cavity.

Immunohistochemical studies demonstrate that these plasma cells are monoclonal. As many as 25% to 50% of these patients also show a monoclonal gammopathy on evaluation by serum protein immunoelectrophoresis, although the amount of abnormal protein is much less than that seen with multiple myeloma. Solitary plasmacytoma also differs from multiple myeloma in that no evidence of plasma cell infiltration should be seen by a random bone marrow biopsy, and the patient should not show signs of anemia, hypercalcemia, or renal failure. Immunohistochemically, extramedullary plasmacytoma appears to differ from its intrabony counterparts in that it shows a marked decrease or lack of immunoreactivity for antibodies directed against cyclin D1 and CD56.

TREATMENT AND PROGNOSIS

Plasmacytomas are usually treated with radiation therapy, and typically a dose of at least 4000 cGy is delivered to the tumor site. A few lesions have been surgically excised with good results, although this is not the preferred treatment in most instances. Unfortunately, when patients with plasmacytoma of bone are observed on a long-term basis, most will eventually develop multiple myeloma. About 50% show evidence of disseminated disease within 2 to 3 years. However, one third of these patients will not have symptoms of multiple myeloma for as long as 10 years. Extramedullary plasmacytoma seems to have a much better prognosis, with only 30% of these patients showing progression to multiple myeloma and 70% having a 10-year disease-free period after treatment.

BIBLIOGRAPHY

Lymphoid Hyperplasia
Bradley G, Main JHP, Birt BD et al: Benign lymphoid hyperplasia of the palate, *J Oral Pathol* 16:18-26, 1987.

Harsany DL, Ross J, Fee WE: Follicular lymphoid hyperplasia of the hard palate simulating lymphoma, *Otolaryngol Head Neck Surg* 88:349-356, 1980.

Kolokotronis A, Dimitrakopoulos I, Asimaki A: Follicular lymphoid hyperplasia of the palate: report of a case and review of the literature, *Oral Surg Oral Med Oral Pathol Oral Radiol Endod* 96:172-175, 2003.

Menasce LP, Shanks JH, Banerjee SS et al: Follicular lymphoid hyperplasia of the hard palate and oral mucosa: report of three cases and a review of the literature, *Histopathology* 39:353-358, 2001.

Napier SS, Newlands C: Benign lymphoid hyperplasia of the palate: report of two cases and immunohistochemical profile, *J Oral Pathol Med* 19:221-225, 1990.

Wright J, Dunsworth A: Follicular lymphoid hyperplasia of the hard palate: a benign lymphoproliferative process, *Oral Surg Oral Med Oral Pathol* 55:162-168, 1983.

Hemophilia
Blanco-Carrion J, Liñares-Gonzalez A, Batalla-Vazquez P et al: Morbidity and economic complications following mucogingival surgery in a hemophiliac HIV-infected patient: a case report, *J Periodontol* 75:1413-1416, 2004.

Cahill MR, Colvin BT: Haemophilia, *Postgrad Med J* 73:201-206, 1997.

Dunn AL, Abshire TC: Recent advances in the management of the child who has hemophilia, *Hematol Oncol Clin North Am* 18:1249-1276, 2004.

Federici AB: Clinical diagnosis of von Willebrand disease, *Haemophilia* 10(suppl 4):169-176, 2004.

Federici AB, Berntorp E, Lee CA: The 80th anniversary of von Willebrand's disease: history, management and research, *Haemophilia* 12:563-572, 2006.

Heiland M, Weber M, Schmelzle R: Life-threatening bleeding after dental extraction in a hemophilia A patient with inhibitors to factor VIII: a case report, *J Oral Maxillofac Surg* 61:1350-1353, 2003.

Izumi Y, Taniguchi T, Maruyama Y et al: Effective periodontal treatment in a patient with type IIA von Willebrand's disease: report of a case, *J Periodontol* 70:548-553, 1999.

Kitchens CS: Approach to the bleeding patient, *Hematol Oncol Clin North Am* 6:983-989, 1992.

Laguna P, Klukowska A: Management of oral bleedings with recombinant factor VIIa in children with haemophilia A and inhibitor, *Haemophilia* 11:2-4, 2005.

Lee CA, Lillicrap D, Astermark J: Inhibitor development in hemophiliacs: the roles of genetic versus environmental factors, *Semin Thromb Hemost* 32(suppl 2):10-14, 2006.

Lofqvist T, Nilsson IM, Berntorp E et al: Haemophilia prophylaxis in young patients—a long-term follow-up, *J Intern Med* 241:395-400, 1997.

Mannucci PM: Treatment of von Willebrand's disease, *N Engl J Med* 351:683-694, 2004.

Morimoto Y, Yoshioka A, Shima M et al: Intraoral hemostasis using a recombinant activated factor VII preparation in a hemophilia A patient with inhibitor, *J Oral Maxillofac Surg* 61:1095-1097, 2003.

Pruthi RK: Hemophilia: a practical approach to genetic testing, *Mayo Clin Proc* 80:1485-1499, 2005.

Sutor AH: Desmopressin (DDAVP) in bleeding disorders of childhood, *Semin Thromb Hemost* 24:555-566, 1998.

Plasminogen Deficiency
Drew AF, Kaufman AH, Kombrinck KW et al: Ligneous conjunctivitis in plasminogen-deficient mice, *Blood* 91:1616-1624, 1998.

Gokbuget AY, Mutlu S, Scully C et al: Amyloidaceous ulcerated gingival hyperplasia: a newly described entity related to ligneous conjunctivitis, *J Oral Pathol Med* 26:100-104, 1997.

Schott D, Dempfle C-E, Beck P et al: Therapy with a purified plasminogen concentrate in an infant with ligneous conjunctivitis and homozygous plasminogen deficiency, *N Engl J Med* 339:1679-1686, 1998.

Schuster V, Seregard S: Ligneous conjunctivitis, *Surv Ophthalmol* 48:369-388, 2003.

Scully C, Gokbuget AY, Allen C et al: Oral lesions indicative of plasminogen deficiency (hypoplasminogenemia), *Oral Surg Oral Med Oral Pathol Oral Radiol Endod* 91:334-337, 2001.

Tefs K, Gueorguieva M, Klammt J et al: Molecular and clinical spectrum of type I plasminogen deficiency: a series of 50 patients, *Blood* 108:3021-3026, 2006.

Watts P, Suresh P, Mezer E et al: Effective treatment of ligneous conjunctivitis with topical plasminogen, *Am J Ophthalmol* 133:451-455, 2002.

Anemia
Beddall A: Anaemias, *Practitioner* 234:713-715, 1990.

Brown RG: Determining the cause of anemia: general approach, with emphasis on microcytic hypochromic anemias, *Postgrad Med* 89:161-170, 1991.

Groopman JE, Itri LM: Chemotherapy-induced anemia in adults: incidence and treatment, *J Natl Cancer Inst* 91:1616-1634, 1999.

Hoggarth K: Macrocytic anaemias, *Practitioner* 237:331-335, 1993.

Hoggarth K: Microcytic anaemias, *Practitioner* 237:338-341, 1993.

Means RT: Advances in the anemia of chronic disease, *Int J Hematol* 70:7-12, 1999.

Provan D: Mechanisms and management of iron deficiency anaemia, *Br J Haematol* 105(suppl 1):19-26, 1999.

Remuzzi G, Ingelfinger JR: Correction of anemia—payoffs and problems, *N Engl J Med* 355:2144-2146, 2006.

Tefferi A: Anemia in adults: a contemporary approach to diagnosis, *Mayo Clin Proc* 78:1274-1280, 2003.

Sickle Cell Anemia
Ashley-Koch A, Yang Q, Olney RS: Sickle hemoglobin (HbS) allele and sickle cell disease: a human genome epidemiology review, *Am J Epidemiol* 151:839-845, 2000.

Brosco JP, Seider MI, Dunn AC: Universal newborn screening and adverse medical outcomes: a historical note, *Ment Retard Dev Disabil Res Rev* 12:262-269, 2006.

Crowley JJ, Sarnaik S: Imaging of sickle cell disease, *Pediatr Radiol* 29:646-661, 1999.

Kelleher M, Bishop K, Briggs P: Oral complications associated with sickle cell anemia. A review and case report, *Oral Surg Oral Med Oral Pathol Oral Radiol Endod* 82:225-228, 1996.

Mehta SR, Afenyi-Annan A, Byrns PJ et al: Opportunities to improve outcomes in sickle cell disease, *Am Fam Physician* 74:303-310, 313-314, 2006.

Okpala IE: New therapies for sickle cell disease, *Hematol Oncol Clin North Am* 19:975-987, 2005.

Steinberg MH: Management of sickle cell disease, *N Engl J Med* 340:1021-1030, 1999.

Stuart MJ, Nagel RL: Sickle-cell disease, *Lancet* 364:1343-1360, 2004.

Vichinsky EP, Neumayr LD, Earles AN et al: Causes and outcomes of the acute chest syndrome in sickle cell disease, *N Engl J Med* 342:1855-1865, 2000.

Xu K, Shi ZM, Veeck LL et al: First unaffected pregnancy using preimplantation genetic diagnosis for sickle cell anemia, *JAMA* 281:1701-1706, 1999.

Thalassemia

Cannell H: The development of oral and facial signs in beta-thalassaemia major, *Br Dent J* 164:50-51, 1988.

Clarke GM, Higgins TN: Laboratory investigation of hemoglobinopathies and thalassemias: review and update, *Clin Chem* 46:1284-1290, 2000.

Drew SJ, Sachs SA: Management of the thalassemia-induced skeletal facial deformity, *J Oral Maxillofac Surg* 55:1331-1339, 1997.

Hazza'a AM, Al-Jamal G: Dental development in subjects with thalassemia major, *J Contemp Dent Pract* 7:63-70, 2006.

Hazza'a AM, Al-Jamal G: Radiographic features of the jaws and teeth in thalassemia major, *Dentomaxillofac Radiol* 35:283-288, 2006.

Joshi D-D, Nickerson HJ, McManus MJ: Hydrops fetalis caused by homozygous α-thalassemia and Rh antigen alloimmunization: report of a survivor and literature review, *Clin Med Res* 2:228-232, 2004.

Olivieri NF: The beta-thalassemias, *N Engl J Med* 341:99-109, 1999.

Richer J, Chudley AE: The hemoglobinopathies and malaria, *Clin Genet* 68:332-336, 2005.

Riggs DR: The thalassemia syndromes, *Q Rev Med* 86:559-564, 1993.

Rund D, Rachmilewitz E: β-thalassemia, *N Engl J Med* 353:1135-1146, 2005.

Schrier SL, Angelucci E: New strategies in the treatment of the thalassemias, *Annu Rev Med* 56:157-171, 2005.

Tyler PA, Madani G, Chaudhuri R et al: The radiological appearances of thalassaemia, *Clin Radiol* 61:40-52, 2006.

Aplastic Anemia

Bacigalupo A, Brand R, Oneto R et al: Treatment of acquired severe aplastic anemia: bone marrow transplantation compared with immunosuppressive therapy—the European Group for Blood and Marrow Transplantation experience, *Semin Hematol* 37:69-80, 2000.

Ball SE: The modern management of severe aplastic anaemia, *Br J Haematol* 110:41-53, 2000.

Brodsky RA, Jones RJ: Aplastic anemia, *Lancet* 365:1647-1656, 2005.

Fonseca R, Tefferi A: Practical aspects in the diagnosis and management of aplastic anemia, *Am J Med Sci* 313:159-169, 1997.

Horowitz MM: Current status of allogeneic bone marrow transplantation in acquired aplastic anemia, *Semin Hematol* 37:30-42, 2000.

Keohane EM: Acquired aplastic anemia, *Clin Lab Sci* 17:165-171, 2004.

Luker J, Scully C, Oakhill A: Gingival swelling as a manifestation of aplastic anemia, *Oral Surg Oral Med Oral Pathol* 71:55-56, 1991.

Marsh JCW: Hematopoietic growth factors in the pathogenesis and for the treatment of aplastic anemia, *Semin Hematol* 37:81-90, 2000.

Schrezenmeier H, Raghavachar A, Heimpel H: Granulocyte-macrophage colony-stimulating factor in the sera of patients with aplastic anemia, *Clin Investig* 71:102-108, 1993.

Sepúlveda E, Brethauer U, Rojas J et al: Oral manifestations of aplastic anemia in children, *J Am Dent Assoc* 137:474-478, 2006.

Socie G, Henry-Amar M, Bacigalupo A et al: Malignant tumors occurring after treatment of aplastic anemia, *N Engl J Med* 329:1152-1157, 1993.

Young NS: Acquired aplastic anemia, *Ann Intern Med* 136:534-546, 2002.

Young NS, Calado RT, Scheinberg P: Current concepts in the pathophysiology and treatment of aplastic anemia, *Blood* 108:2509-2519, 2006.

Neutropenia

Alexander SW, Pizzo PA: Current considerations in the management of fever and neutropenia, *Curr Clin Top Infect Dis* 19:160-180, 1999.

Ancliff PJ: Congenital neutropenia, *Blood Rev* 17:209-216, 2003.

Boxer LA, Hutchinson R, Emerson S: Recombinant human granulocyte-colony-stimulating factor in the treatment of patients with neutropenia, *Clin Immunol Immunopathol* 62:S39-S46, 1992.

Dale DC: Immune and idiopathic neutropenia, *Curr Opin Hematol* 5:33-36, 1998.

Haddy TB, Rana SR, Castro O: Benign ethnic neutropenia: what is a normal absolute neutrophil count? *J Lab Clin Med* 133:15-22, 1999.

Hakki SS, Aprikyan AAG, Yildirim S et al: Periodontal status in two siblings with severe congenital neutropenia: diagnosis and mutational analysis of the cases, *J Periodontol* 76:837-844, 2005.

James RM, Kinsey SE: The investigation and management of chronic neutropenia in children, *Arch Dis Child* 91:852-858, 2006.

Vandendries ER, Drews RE: Drug-associated disease: hematologic dysfunction, *Crit Care Clin* 22:347-355, 2006.

Welte K, Zeidler C, Dale DC: Severe congenital neutropenia, *Semin Hematol* 43:189-195, 2006.

Zaromb A, Chamberlain D, Schoor R et al: Periodontitis as a manifestation of chronic benign neutropenia, *J Periodontol* 77:1921-1926, 2006.

Agranulocytosis

Bergman OJ: Oral infections in haematological patients, *Dan Med Bull* 39:15-29, 1992.

Carey PJ: Drug-induced myelosuppression: diagnosis and management, *Drug Safety* 26:691-706, 2003.

Deas DE, Mackey SA, McDonnell HT: Systemic disease and periodontitis: manifestations of neutrophil dysfunction, *Periodontol 2000* 32:82-104, 2003.

Glasser L, Duncan BR, Corrigan JJ: Measurement of serum granulocyte-colony-stimulating factor in a patient with congenital agranulocytosis (Kostmann's syndrome), *Am J Dis Child* 145:925-928, 1991.

Kuipers EJ, Vellenga E, de Wolf JTM et al: Sulfasalazine-induced agranulocytosis treated with granulocyte-macrophage colony stimulating factor, *J Rheumatol* 19:621-622, 1992.

Pisciotta AV: Drug-induced agranulocytosis: peripheral destruction of polymorphonuclear leukocytes and their marrow precursors, *Blood Rev* 4:226-237, 1990.

Salama A, Mueller-Eckhardt C: Immune-mediated blood cell dyscrasias related to drugs, *Semin Hematol* 29:54-63, 1992.

Cyclic Neutropenia

Aprikyan AAG, Liles WC, Boxer LA et al: Mutant elastase in pathogenesis of cyclic and severe congenital neutropenia, *J Pediatr Hematol Oncol* 24:784-786, 2002.

Baer PN, Iacono VJ: Cyclic neutropenia: report of a case with a 15-year follow-up, *Periodontal Clin Investig* 16:14-19, 1994.

Boxer LA, Hutchinson R, Emerson S: Recombinant human granulocyte-colony-stimulating factor in the treatment of patients with neutropenia, *Clin Immunol Immunopathol* 62:S39-S46, 1992.

Dale DC, Bolyard AA, Aprikyan A: Cyclic neutropenia, *Semin Hematol* 39:89-94, 2002.

Haurie C, Dale DC, Mackey MC: Cyclical neutropenia and other periodic hematological disorders: a review of mechanisms and mathematical models, *Blood* 92:2629-2640, 1998.

Kinane D: Blood and lymphoreticular disorders, *Periodontol 2000* 21:84-93, 1999.

Nakai Y, Ishihara C, Ogata S et al: Oral manifestations of cyclic neutropenia in a Japanese child: case report with a 5-year follow-up, *Pediatr Dent* 25:383-388, 2003.

Pernu HE, Pajari UH, Lanning M: The importance of regular dental treatment in patients with cyclic neutropenia. Follow-up of 2 cases, *J Periodontol* 67:454-459, 1996.

Thrombocytopenia

Bolton-Maggs PHB: Idiopathic thrombocytopenic purpura, *Arch Dis Child* 83:220-222, 2000.

Chong BH: Clinical aspects of thrombocytopenias, *Aust Fam Physician* 23:1463-1464, 1468-1470, 1473, 1994.

George JN: Thrombotic thrombocytopenic purpura, *N Engl J Med* 354:1927-1935, 2006.

Lusher JM: Screening and diagnosis of coagulation disorders, *Am J Obstet Gynecol* 175:778-783, 1996.

Medeiros D, Buchanan GR: Idiopathic thrombocytopenic purpura: beyond consensus, *Curr Opin Pediatr* 12:4-9, 2000.

Murrin RJA, Murray JA: Thrombotic thrombocytopenic purpura: aetiology, pathophysiology and treatment, *Blood Rev* 20:51-60, 2006.

Rogers GM: Overview of platelet physiology and laboratory evaluation of platelet function, *Clin Obstet Gynecol* 42:349-359, 1999.

Thompson CC, Tacke RB, Woolley LH et al: Purpuric oral and cutaneous lesions in a case of drug-induced thrombocytopenia, *J Am Dent Assoc* 105:465-467, 1982.

Wazny LD, Ariano RE: Evaluation and management of drug-induced thrombocytopenia in the acutely ill patient, *Pharmacotherapy* 20:292-307, 2000.

Polycythemia Vera

Campbell PJ, Green AR: The myeloproliferative disorders, *N Engl J Med* 355:2452-2466, 2006.

Cao M, Olsen RJ, Zu Y: Polycythemia vera: new clinicopathologic perspectives, *Arch Pathol Lab Med* 130:1126-1132, 2006.

Johansson P: Epidemiology of the myeloproliferative disorders polycythemia vera and essential thrombocythemia, *Semin Thromb Hemost* 32:171-173, 2006.

Lengfelder E, Merx K, Hehlmann R: Diagnosis and therapy of polycythemia vera, *Semin Thromb Hemost* 32:267-275, 2006.

Silver RT: Treatment of polycythemia vera, *Semin Thromb Hemost* 32:437-442, 2006.

Tefferi A, Spivak JL: Polycythemia vera: scientific advances and current practice, *Semin Hematol* 42:206-220, 2005.

Leukemia

Abbott BL: Recent advances in chronic lymphocytic leukemia, *Cancer Invest* 24:302-309, 2006.

Amin KS, Ehsan A, McGuff HS et al: Minimally differentiated acute myelogenous leukemia (AML-M0) granulocytic sarcoma presenting in the oral cavity, *Oral Oncol* 38:516-519, 2002.

Barrett AP: Gingival lesions in leukemia: a classification, *J Periodontol* 55:585-588, 1984.

Bhatia S, Robison LL: Epidemiology of leukemia and lymphoma, *Curr Opin Hematol* 6:201-204, 1999.

Chapple ILC, Saxby MS, Murray JA: Gingival hemorrhage, myelodysplastic syndromes, and acute myeloid leukemia. A case report, *J Periodontol* 70:1247-1253, 1999.

Estey E, Döhner H: Acute myeloid leukaemia, *Lancet* 368:1894-1907, 2006.

Faderl S, Talpaz M, Estrov Z et al: Chronic myelogenous leukemia: biology and therapy, *Ann Intern Med* 131:207-219, 1999.

Farhi DC, Rosenthal NS: Acute lymphoblastic leukemia, *Clin Lab Med* 20:17-28, 2000.

Heaney ML, Golde DW: Myelodysplasia, *N Engl J Med* 340:1649-1660, 1999.

Hollsberg P, Hailer DA: Pathogenesis of diseases induced by human lymphotropic virus type I infection, *N Engl J Med* 328:1173-1182, 1993.

Keating MJ: Chronic lymphocytic leukemia, *Semin Oncol* 26(suppl 14):107-114, 1999.

Krause JR: Morphology and classification of acute myeloid leukemias, *Clin Lab Med* 20:1-16, 2000.

Larson RA: Management of acute lymphoblastic leukemia in older patients, *Semin Hematol* 43:126-133, 2006.

Lowenberg B, Downing JR, Burnett A: Acute myeloid leukemia, *N Engl J Med* 341:1051-1062, 1999.

Menasce LP, Banerjee SS, Beckett E et al: Extra-medullary myeloid tumour (granulocytic sarcoma) is often misdiagnosed: a study of 26 cases, *Histopathology* 34:391-398, 1999.

Peterson DE, Gerad H, Williams LT: An unusual instance of leukemic infiltrate: diagnosis and management of periapical tooth involvement, *Cancer* 51:1716-1719, 1983.

Pui C-H, Evans WE: Treatment of acute lymphoblastic leukemia, *N Engl J Med* 354:166-178, 2006.

Quintás-Cardama A, Cortes JE: Chronic myeloid leukemia: diagnosis and treatment, *Mayo Clin Proc* 81:973-988, 2006.

Rhee D, Myssiorek D, Zahtz G et al: Recurrent attacks of facial nerve palsy as the presenting sign of leukemic relapse, *Laryngoscope* 112:235-237, 2002.

Shanafelt TD, Byrd JC, Call TG et al: Narrative review: initial management of newly diagnosed, early-stage chronic lymphocytic leukemia, *Ann Intern Med* 145:435-447, 2006.

Sollecito TP, Draznin J, Parisi E et al: Leukemic gingival infiltrate as an indicator of chemotherapeutic failure following monoclonal antibody therapy: a case report, *Spec Care Dentist* 23:108-110, 2003.

Stoopler ET, Pinto A, Alawi F et al: Granulocytic sarcoma: an atypical presentation in the oral cavity, *Spec Care Dentist* 24:65-69, 2004.

Vibhute P, Carneiro E, Genden E et al: Palatal enlargement in chronic lymphocytic leukemia, *AJNR Am J Neuroradiol* 27:1649-1650, 2006.

Vural F, Ozcan MA, Ozsan GH et al: Gingival involvement in a patient with CD56⁺ chronic myelomonocytic leukemia, *Leuk Lymphoma* 45:415-418, 2004.

Weirda WG, Kipps TJ: Chronic lymphocytic leukemia, *Curr Opin Hematol* 6:253-261, 1999.

Yee KWL, O'Brien SM: Chronic lymphocytic leukemia: diagnosis and treatment, *Mayo Clin Proc* 81:1105-1129, 2006.

Langerhans Cell Histiocytosis

Azouz EM, Saigal G, Rodriguez MM et al: Langerhans' cell histiocytosis: pathology, imaging and treatment of skeletal involvement, *Pediatr Radiol* 35:103-115, 2005.

Bartnick A, Friedrich RE, Roeser K et al: Oral Langerhans cell histiocytosis, *J Craniomaxillofac Surg* 30:91-96, 2002.

Cleveland DB, Goldberg KM, Greenspan JS et al: Langerhans' cell histiocytosis. Report of three cases with unusual oral soft tissue involvement, *Oral Surg Oral Med Oral Pathol Oral Radiol Endod* 82:541-548, 1996.

Dagenais M, Pharoah MJ, Sikorski PA: The radiographic characteristics of histiocytosis X: a study of 29 cases that involve the jaws, *Oral Surg Oral Med Oral Pathol* 74:230-236, 1992.

Eckardt A, Schultze A: Maxillofacial manifestations of Langerhans cell histiocytosis: a clinical and therapeutic analysis of 10 patients, *Oral Oncol* 39:687-694, 2003.

Hartman KH: A review of 114 cases of histiocytosis X, *Oral Surg Oral Med Oral Pathol* 49:38-54, 1980.

Hicks J, Flaitz CM: Langerhans cell histiocytosis: current insights in a molecular age with emphasis on clinical oral and maxillofacial pathology practice, *Oral Surg Oral Med Oral Pathol Oral Radiol Endod* 100:S42-S66, 2005.

Howarth DM, Gilchrist GS, Mullan BP et al: Langerhans cell histiocytosis: diagnosis, natural history, management, and outcome, *Cancer* 85:2278-2290, 1999.

Key SJ, O'Brien CJ, Silvester KC et al: Eosinophilic granuloma: resolution of maxillofacial bony lesions following minimal intervention. Report of three cases and a review of the literature, *J Craniomaxillofac Surg* 32:170-175, 2004.

Manfredi M, Corradi D, Vescovi P: Langerhans-cell histiocytosis: a clinical case without bone involvement, *J Periodontol* 76:143-147, 2005.

Mitomi T, Tomizawa, Noda T: Tooth development included in the multifocal jaw lesions of Langerhans cell histiocytosis, *Int J Paediatr Dent* 15:123-126, 2005.

Muzzi L, Prato GPP, Ficarra G: Langerhans' cell histiocytosis diagnosed through periodontal lesions: a case report, *J Periodontol* 73:1528-1533, 2002.

Putters TF, de Visscher JGAM, van Veen A et al: Intralesional infiltration of corticosteroids in the treatment of localized Langerhans' cell histiocytosis of the mandible. Report of known cases and three new cases, *Int J Oral Maxillofac Surg* 34:571-575, 2005.

Scolozzi P, Lombardi T, Monnier P et al: Multisystem Langerhans' cell histiocytosis (Hand-Schüller-Christian disease) in an adult: a case report and review of the literature, *Eur Arch Otorhinolaryngol* 261:326-330, 2004.

Yousem SA, Colby TV, Chen Y-Y et al: Pulmonary Langerhans' cell histiocytosis. Molecular analysis of clonality, *Am J Surg Pathol* 25:630-636, 2001.

Hodgkin's Lymphoma

Advani RH, Horning SJ: Treatment of early-stage Hodgkin's disease, *Semin Hematol* 36:270-281, 1999.

Aisenberg AC: Problems in Hodgkin's disease management, *Blood* 93:761-779, 1999.

Ansell SM, Armitage JO: Management of Hodgkin lymphoma, *Mayo Clin Proc* 81:419-426, 2006.

Connors JM: State-of-the-art therapeutics: Hodgkin's lymphoma, *J Clin Oncol* 23:6400-6408, 2005.

Diehl V, Josting A: Hodgkin's disease, *Cancer J Sci Am* 6(suppl 2): S150-S158, 2000.

Harris NL: Hodgkin's disease: classification and differential diagnosis, *Mod Pathol* 12:159-176, 1999.

Herrin HK: The oral implications of Hodgkin's disease, *Gen Dent* 47:572-575, 1999.

Jaffe ES: Introduction: Hodgkin's lymphoma—pathology, pathogenesis, and treatment, *Semin Hematol* 36:217-219, 1999.

Küppers R, Hansmann M-L: The Hodgkin and Reed/Sternberg cell, *Int J Biochem Cell Biol* 37:511-517, 2005.

Küppers R, Yahalom J, Josting A: Advances in biology, diagnostics, and treatment of Hodgkin's disease, *Biol Blood Marrow Transplant* 12:66-76, 2006.

Re D, Küppers R, Diehl V: Molecular pathogenesis of Hodgkin's lymphoma, *J Clin Oncol* 23:6379-6386, 2005.

Yencha MW: Primary parotid gland Hodgkin's lymphoma, *Ann Otol Rhinol Laryngol* 111:338-342, 2002.

Non-Hodgkin's Lymphoma

Ando M, Matsuzaki M, Murofushi T: Mucosa-associated lymphoid tissue lymphoma presented as diffuse swelling of the parotid gland, *Am J Otolaryngol* 26:285-288, 2005.

Armitage JO: Staging non-Hodgkin lymphoma, *CA Cancer J Clin* 55:368-376, 2005.

Chan JKC, Banks PM, Cleary ML et al: A revised European-American classification of lymphoid neoplasms proposed by the International Lymphoma Study Group, *Am J Clin Pathol* 103:543-560, 1995.

Chang C-C, Rowe JJ, Hawkins P et al: Mantle cell lymphoma of the hard palate: a case report and review of the differential diagnosis based on the histomorphology and immunophenotyping pattern, *Oral Surg Oral Med Oral Pathol Oral Radiol Endod* 96:316-320, 2003.

Cheson BD: What is new in lymphoma? *CA Cancer J Clin* 54:260-272, 2004.

Evans LS, Hancock BW: Non-Hodgkin lymphoma, *Lancet* 362:139-146, 2003.

Folk GS, Abbondanzo SL, Childers EL et al: Plasmablastic lymphoma: a clinicopathologic correlation, *Ann Diagn Pathol* 10:8-12, 2006.

Hennessy BT, Hanrahan EO, Daly PA: Non-Hodgkin lymphoma: an update, *Lancet Oncol* 5:341-353, 2004.

Isaacson PG, Du M-Q: MALT lymphoma: from morphology to molecules, *Nature Rev Cancer* 4:644-653, 2004.

Kolokotronis A, Konstantinou N, Christakis I et al: Localized B-cell non-Hodgkin's lymphoma of the oral cavity and maxillofacial region: a clinical study, *Oral Surg Oral Med Oral Pathol Oral Radiol Endod* 99:303-310, 2005.

Krause JR, Shahidi-Asl M: Molecular pathology in the diagnosis and treatment of non-Hodgkin's lymphomas, *J Cell Mol Med* 7:494-512, 2003.

Knowles DM: Immunodeficiency-associated lymphoproliferative disorders, *Mod Pathol* 12:200-217, 1999.

Lu P: Staging and classification of lymphoma, *Semin Nucl Med* 35:160-165, 2005.

Mealey BL, Tunder GS, Pemble CW: Primary extranodal malignant lymphoma affecting the periodontium, *J Periodontol* 73:937-941, 2002.

Mishima K, Matsuoka H, Yamada E et al: Application of the polymerase chain reaction for the diagnosis of malignant lymphoma of the nasal and oral cavities, *J Oral Pathol Med* 27:43-47, 1998.

Mounter PJ, Lennard AL: Management of non-Hodgkin's lymphomas, *Postgrad Med J* 75:2-6, 1999.

Ostrowski ML, Unni KK, Banks PM et al: Malignant lymphoma of bone, *Cancer* 58:2646-2655, 1986.

Rizvi MA, Evens AM, Tallman MS et al: T-cell non-Hodgkin lymphoma, *Blood* 107:1255-1264, 2006.

Sandlund JT, Downing JR, Crist WM: Non-Hodgkin's lymphoma in childhood, *N Engl J Med* 334:1238-1248, 1996.

Shine NP, Blake SP, O'Leary G: Extranodal lymphoma: clinical presentation and diagnostic pitfalls, *Hosp Med* 66:341-345, 2005.

Solomides CC, Miller AS, Christman RA et al: Lymphomas of the oral cavity: histology, immunologic type, and incidence of Epstein-Barr virus infection, *Hum Pathol* 33:153-157, 2002.

Tomich CE, Shafer WG: Lymphoproliferative disease of the hard palate: a clinicopathologic entity, *Oral Surg Oral Med Oral Pathol* 39:754-768, 1975.

Van der Waal RIF, Huijgens PC, van der Valk P et al: Characteristics of 40 primary extranodal non-Hodgkin lymphomas of the oral cavity in perspective of the new WHO classification and the International Prognostic Index, *Int J Oral Maxillofac Surg* 34:391-395, 2005.

Vega F, Lin P, Medeiros J: Extranodal lymphomas of the head and neck, *Ann Diagn Pathol* 9:340-350, 2005.

Mycosis Fungoides

Abel EA, Wood GS, Hoppe RT: Mycosis fungoides: clinical and histologic features, staging evaluation, and approach to treatment, *CA Cancer J Clin* 43:93-115, 1993.

Berti E, Tomasini D, Vermeer MH et al: Primary cutaneous CD8-positive epidermotropic cytotoxic T cell lymphomas: a distinct clinicopathological entity with an aggressive clinical behavior, *Am J Pathol* 155:483-492, 1999.

Chua M S-T, Veness MJ: Mycosis fungoides involving the oral cavity, *Australas Radiol* 46:336-339, 2002.

Damm DD, White DK, Cibull ML et al: Mycosis fungoides: initial diagnosis via palatal biopsy with discussion of diagnostic advantages of plastic embedding, *Oral Surg Oral Med Oral Pathol* 58:413-419, 1984.

Hata T, Aikoh T, Hirokawa M et al: Mycosis fungoides with involvement of the oral mucosa, *Int J Oral Maxillofac Surg* 27:127-128, 1998.

Kerl H, Cerroni L: Primary cutaneous B-cell lymphomas: then and now, *J Cutan Pathol* 33(suppl 1):1-5, 2006.

Kim EJ, Hess S, Richardson SK et al: Immunopathogenesis and therapy of cutaneous T cell lymphoma, *J Clin Invest* 115:798-812, 2005.

Kim YH, Hoppe RT: Mycosis fungoides and the Sézary syndrome, *Semin Oncol* 26:276-289, 1999.

Scarisbrick JJ: Staging and management of cutaneous T-cell lymphoma, *Clin Exp Dermatol* 31:181-186, 2006.

Sirois DA, Miller AS, Harwick RD et al: Oral manifestations of cutaneous T-cell lymphoma: a report of eight cases, *Oral Surg Oral Med Oral Pathol* 75:700-705, 1993.

Wain EM, Setterfield J, Judge MR et al: Mycosis fungoides involving the oral mucosa in a child, *Clin Exp Dermatol* 28:499-501, 2003.

Wright JM, Balciunas BA, Muus JH: Mycosis fungoides with oral manifestations: report of a case and review of the literature, *Oral Surg Oral Med Oral Pathol* 51:24-31, 1981.

Zackheim HS: Cutaneous T cell lymphoma: update of treatment, *Dermatology* 199:102-105, 1999.

Zic J, Arzubiaga C, Salhaney KE et al: Extracorporeal photopheresis for the treatment of cutaneous T-cell lymphoma, *J Am Acad Dermatol* 27:729-736, 1992.

Burkitt's Lymphoma

Cairo MS, Sposto R, Perkins SL et al: Burkitt's and Burkitt-like lymphoma in children and adolescents: review of the Children's Cancer Group experience, *Br J Haematol* 120:660-670, 2003.

Dave SS, Fu K, Wright GW et al: Molecular diagnosis of Burkitt's lymphoma, *N Engl J Med* 354:2431-2442, 2006.

Ferry JA: Burkitt's lymphoma: clinicopathologic features and differential diagnosis, *Oncologist* 11:375-383, 2006.

Hummel M, Bentink S, Berger H et al: A biologic definition of Burkitt's lymphoma from transcriptional and genomic profiling, *N Engl J Med* 354:2419-2430, 2006.

Sandlund JT, Downing JR, Crist WM: Non-Hodgkin's lymphoma in childhood, *N Engl J Med* 334:1238-1248, 1996.

Tsui SHC, Wong MH, Lam WY: Burkitt's lymphoma presenting as mandibular swelling—report of a case and review of publications, *Br J Oral Maxillofac Surg* 38:8-11, 2000.

Uğar DA, Bozkaya S, Karaca İ et al: Childhood craniofacial Burkitt's lymphoma presenting as maxillary swelling: report of a case and review of literature, *J Dent Child* 73:45-50, 2006.

Extranodal NK/T-Cell Lymphoma, Nasal Type

Al-Hakeem DA, Fedele S, Carlos R et al: Extranodal NK/T-cell lymphoma, nasal type, *Oral Oncol* 43:4-14, 2007.

Batsakis JG, Luna MA: Midfacial necrotizing lesions, *Semin Diagn Pathol* 4:90-116, 1987.

Koom WS, Chung EJ, Yang W-I et al: Angiocentric T-cell and NK/T-cell lymphomas: radiotherapeutic viewpoints, *Int J Radiat Oncol Biol Phys* 59:1127-1137, 2004.

Lee PY, Freeman NJ, Khorsand J et al: Angiocentric T-cell lymphoma presenting as lethal midline granuloma, *Int J Dermatol* 36:419-427, 1997.

Mosqueda-Taylor A, Meneses-Garcia A, Zarate-Osorno A et al: Angiocentric lymphomas of the palate: clinico-pathological considerations in 12 cases, *J Oral Pathol Med* 26:93-97, 1997.

Pagano L, Gallamini A, Fianchi L et al: NK/T-cell lymphomas "nasal type": an Italian multicentric retrospective survey, *Ann Oncol* 17:794-800, 2006.

Patel V, Mahajan S, Kharkar V et al: Nasal extranodal NK/T-cell lymphoma presenting as a perforating palatal ulcer: a diagnostic challenge, *Indian J Dermatol Venereol Leprol* 72:218-221, 2006.

Vidal RW, Devaney K, Ferlito A et al: Sinonasal malignant lymphomas: a distinct clinicopathological category, *Ann Otol Rhinol Laryngol* 108:411-419, 1999.

Wu SM, Min Y, Ostrzega N et al: Lymphomatoid granulomatosis: a rare mimicker of vasculitis, *J Rheumatol* 32:2242-2245, 2005.

Yong W, Zheng W, Zhu J et al: Midline NK/T-cell lymphoma nasal-type: treatment outcome, the effect of L-asparaginase based regimen, and prognostic factors, *Hematol Oncol* 24:28-32, 2006.

Multiple Myeloma

Baldini L, Radaelli F, Chiorboli O et al: No correlation between response and survival in patients with multiple myeloma treated with vincristine, melphalan, cyclophosphamide, and prednisone, *Cancer* 68:62-67, 1991.

Denz U, Haas PS, Wäsch R et al: State of the art therapy in multiple myeloma and future perspectives, *Eur J Cancer* 42:1591-1600, 2006.

Dimopoulos MA, Moulopoulos A, Smith T et al: Risk of disease progression in asymptomatic multiple myeloma, *Am J Med* 94:57-61, 1993.

George ED, Sadovsky R: Multiple myeloma: recognition and management, *Am Fam Physician* 59:1885-1894, 1999.

Hogan MC, Lee A, Solberg LA et al: Unusual presentation of multiple myeloma with unilateral visual loss and numb chin syndrome in a young adult, *Am J Hematol* 70:55-59, 2002.

Kyle RA, Rajkumar SV: Treatment of multiple myeloma: an emphasis on new developments, *Ann Med* 38:111-115, 2006.

Lebowitz RA, Morris L: Plasma cell dyscrasias and amyloidosis, *Otolaryngol Clin North Am* 36:747-764, 2003.

Ludwig H: Advances in biology and treatment of multiple myeloma, *Ann Oncol* (suppl 2):ii106-ii112, 2005.

Palumbo A, Bertola A, Musto P et al: Oral melphalan, prednisone, and thalidomide for newly diagnosed patients with myeloma, *Cancer* 104:1428-1433, 2005.

Riedel DA, Pottern LM: The epidemiology of multiple myeloma, *Hematol Oncol Clin North Am* 6:225-247, 1992.

Smith A, Wisloff F, Samson D: Guidelines on the diagnosis and management of multiple myeloma 2005, *Br J Haematol* 132:410-451, 2005.

Plasmacytoma

Dimopoulos MA, Kiamouris C, Moulopoulos LA: Solitary plasmacytoma of bone and extramedullary plasmacytoma, *Hematol Oncol Clin North Am* 13:1249-1257, 1999.

González J, Elizondo J, Trull JM et al: Plasma-cell tumours of the condyle, *Br J Oral Maxillofac Surg* 29:274-276, 1991.

Kremer M, Ott G, Nathrath M et al: Primary extramedullary plasmacytoma and multiple myeloma: phenotypic differences revealed by immunohistochemical analysis, *J Pathol* 205:92-101, 2005.

Majumdar S, Raghavan U, Jones NS: Solitary plasmacytoma and extramedullary plasmacytoma of the paranasal sinuses and soft palate, *J Laryngol Otol* 116:962-965, 2002.

Meis JM, Butler JJ, Osborne BM et al: Solitary plasmacytomas of bone and extramedullary plasmacytomas: a clinicopathologic and immunohistochemical study, *Cancer* 59:1475-1485, 1987.

Nofsinger YC, Mirza N, Rowan PT et al: Head and neck manifestations of plasma cell neoplasms, *Laryngoscope* 107:741-746, 1997.

Rothfield RE, Johnson JT, Slavrides A: Extramedullary plasmacytoma of the parotid, *Head Neck* 12:352-354, 1990.

14

Bone Pathology*

Revised by ANGELA C. CHI

CHAPTER OUTLINE

OSTEOGENESIS IMPERFECTA

Osteogenesis imperfecta comprises a heterogeneous group of heritable disorders characterized by impairment of collagen maturation. Except on rare occasions, the disorder arises from heterozygosity for mutations in one of two genes that guide the formation of type I collagen: the *COL1A1* gene on chromosome 17 and the *COL1A2* gene on chromosome 7. Collagen forms a major portion of bone, dentin, sclerae, ligaments, and skin; osteogenesis imperfecta demonstrates a variety of changes that involve these sites. Several different forms of osteogenesis imperfecta are seen, and they represent the most common type of inherited bone disease. Abnormal collagenous maturation results in bone with a thin cortex, fine trabeculation, and diffuse osteoporosis. Upon fracture, healing will occur but may be associated with exuberant callus formation.

CLINICAL AND RADIOGRAPHIC FEATURES

Osteogenesis imperfecta is a rare disorder that affects 1 in 8000 individuals, with many being stillborn or dying shortly after birth. Both autosomal dominant and recessive hereditary patterns occur, and many cases are sporadic. The severity of the disease varies widely, even in affected members of a single family. In addition to bone fragility, some affected individuals also have

---

*Dr. Charles A. Waldron wrote the original version of this chapter in the first edition of this book.

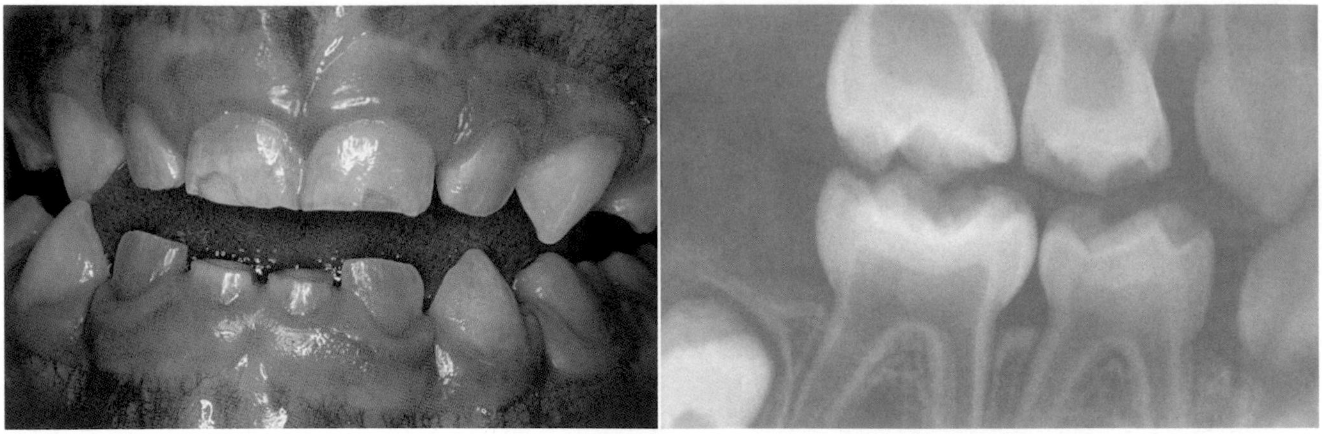

Fig. 14-1 Osteogenesis imperfecta. A, Opalescent dentin in a patient with osteogenesis imperfecta. **B,** Bite-wing radiograph of the same patient showing shell teeth with thin dentin and enamel of normal thickness. *(Courtesy of Dr. Tom Ison.)*

blue sclera, altered teeth, hypoacusis (hearing loss), long bone and spine deformities, and joint hyperextensibility.

The radiographic hallmarks of osteogenesis imperfecta include osteopenia, bowing, angulation or deformity of the long bones, multiple fractures, and wormian bones in the skull. Wormian bones consist of 10 or more sutural bones that are 6×4 mm in diameter or larger and arranged in a mosaic pattern. Wormian bones are not specific and can be seen in other processes, such as cleidocranial dysplasia.

Several distinctive findings are noted in the oral cavity. Dental alterations that appear clinically and radiographically identical to dentinogenesis imperfecta (see page 106) are occasionally noted (Fig. 14-1, A). In affected patients, both dentitions are involved and demonstrate blue to brown translucence. Radiographs typically reveal premature pulpal obliteration, although shell teeth rarely may be seen (Fig. 14-1, B). Although the altered teeth closely resemble dentinogenesis imperfecta, the two diseases are the result of different mutations and should be considered as separate processes. Such dental defects in association with the systemic bone disease should be termed **opalescent teeth**, reserving the diagnosis of dentinogenesis imperfecta for those patients with alterations isolated to the teeth.

In addition, patients with osteogenesis imperfecta demonstrate an increased prevalence of Class III malocclusion that is caused by maxillary hypoplasia, with or without mandibular hyperplasia. On rare occasions, panoramic radiographs may reveal multifocal radiolucencies, mixed radiolucencies, or radiopacities that resemble those seen in florid cemento-osseous dysplasia. When predominantly radiopaque, these areas are sensitive to inflammation and undergo sequestration easily. In these patients, marked coarseness also is noted in the remainder of the skeleton.

Four major types of osteogenesis imperfecta are recognized, each having several subtypes.

TYPE I OSTEOGENESIS IMPERFECTA

Type I is the most common and mildest form. Affected patients have mild to moderately severe bone fragility. Fractures are present at birth in about 10% of cases, but there is great variability in frequency and age of onset of fractures, with 10% of patients not demonstrating fractures. Most fractures occur during the preschool years and are less common after puberty. Hearing loss commonly develops before age 30, and most older patients have hearing deficits. Hypermobile joints and easy bruising because of capillary fragility are not rare. Some affected patients have normal teeth, but others show opalescent dentin. The sclerae are distinctly blue at all ages and aid in classification. Osteogenesis imperfecta type I is inherited as an autosomal dominant trait.

TYPE II OSTEOGENESIS IMPERFECTA

Osteogenesis imperfecta type II is the most severe form and exhibits extreme bone fragility and frequent fractures, which may occur during delivery. Many patients are stillborn, and 90% die before 4 weeks of age. Blue sclerae are present (Fig. 14-2). Opalescent teeth may be present. Both autosomal recessive and dominant patterns may occur, and many cases appear to be sporadic.

TYPE III OSTEOGENESIS IMPERFECTA

Type III is the most severe form noted in individuals beyond the perinatal period and demonstrates moderately severe to severe bone fragility. The sclerae are

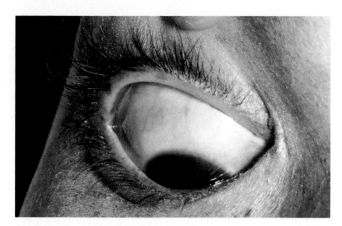

Fig. 14-2   Osteogenesis imperfecta. Blue sclera in a patient with osteogenesis imperfecta.

normal or pale blue or gray at birth; if discoloration is present, then it fades as the child grows older. Ligamentous laxity and hearing loss are common. Fractures may be present at birth, but there is a low mortality in infancy. Although one third survive into adulthood, the majority of affected individuals die during childhood, usually from cardiopulmonary complications caused by kyphoscoliosis. Some patients have opalescent dentin, whereas others have normal teeth. Both autosomal dominant and recessive hereditary patterns are noted.

TYPE IV OSTEOGENESIS IMPERFECTA

Type IV is associated with mild to moderately severe bone fragility. The sclerae may be pale blue in early childhood, but the blue color fades later in life. Fractures are present at birth in about 50% of these patients. The frequency of fractures decreases after puberty, and some individuals never experience bone fracture at any time. Some of these patients have opalescent dentin; others have normal teeth. This variant appears to be inherited as an autosomal dominant trait.

HISTOPATHOLOGIC FEATURES

On histopathologic examination, cortical bone appears attenuated. Osteoblasts are present, but bone matrix production is reduced markedly. The bone architecture remains immature throughout life, and there is a failure of woven bone to become transformed to lamellar bone.

Histopathologically, teeth from affected patients can exhibit abnormalities of dentin similar to those described for patients with dentinogenesis imperfecta (see page 108). These microscopic findings tend to be most pronounced in teeth that clinically appear opal-

escent. However, mild dentinal abnormalities may be found even in teeth that appear normal clinically and radiographically.

TREATMENT AND PROGNOSIS

There is no cure for osteogenesis imperfecta; thus symptomatic improvement is the primary goal of currently available treatment options. Management of the fractures may be a major problem. The mainstays of treatment are physiotherapy, rehabilitation, and orthopedic surgery. Medical treatment with intravenous (IV) or oral bisphosphonates can provide clinical benefits, including decreased pain, reduced risk of fracture, and improved mobility. However, the long-term consequences of bisphosphonate therapy—particularly when administered to a pediatric patient population—are currently unknown; therefore, bisphosphonates are generally reserved for moderately to severely affected patients. Patients with opalescent dentin usually show severe attrition of their teeth, leading to tooth loss. Treatment of the dentition is similar to that used for dentinogenesis imperfecta (see page 108), but use of implants is questionable because of the deficient quality of the supporting bone.

In patients with significant malocclusion, orthognathic surgery may be performed. Alternatively, osteodistraction may be a consideration to reduce the risk of atypical fractures from conventional orthognathic procedures (e.g., Le Fort I osteotomy). The potential for associated medical problems makes presurgical planning paramount. Although the risks are highly variable, occasional patients have associated bleeding disorders, cardiac malformations, and an increased potential for hyperthermia. Intubation may be difficult because of kyphoscoliosis and ease of fracture of the mandible and cervical vertebrae.

The prognosis varies from relatively good to very poor. Some patients have little to no disability, whereas others have severe crippling as a result of the fractures. In severe forms, death occurs *in utero*, during delivery, or early in childhood.

OSTEOPETROSIS (ALBERS-SCHÖNBERG DISEASE; MARBLE BONE DISEASE)

Osteopetrosis is a group of rare hereditary skeletal disorders characterized by a marked increase in bone density resulting from a defect in remodeling caused by failure of normal osteoclast function. The number of osteoclasts present is often increased; however, because of their failure to function normally, bone is not resorbed. Defective osteoclastic bone resorption, combined with continued bone formation and endochondral ossification, results in thickening of cortical bone and sclerosis of the cancellous bone.

Although genetic defects have yet to be identified in a substantial percentage of patients with osteopetrosis, mutations discovered thus far have been found to cause defects in key elements necessary for osteoclast function, including the H^+-ATPase proton pump, chloride channel, and carbonic anhydrase II. These proteins are necessary for acidification of resorption lacunae, regulation of ionic charge across the osteoclast cell membrane, and subsequent resorption of the bone matrix.

Although a number of types have been identified, these pathoses group into two major clinical patterns: (1) **infantile** and (2) **adult osteopetrosis.** The infantile form has an estimated incidence of 1:200,000 to 1:300,000, and the adult form has an estimated incidence of 1 in 100,000 to 1:500,000. The clinical severity of the disease varies widely, even within the same pattern of osteopetrosis.

CLINICAL AND RADIOGRAPHIC FEATURES

INFANTILE OSTEOPETROSIS

Patients discovered with osteopetrosis at birth or in early infancy usually have severe disease that is termed **malignant osteopetrosis.** In most cases, infantile osteopetrosis is inherited as an autosomal recessive trait and leads to a diffusely sclerotic skeleton. Marrow failure, frequent fractures, and evidence of cranial nerve compression are common.

The initial signs of infantile osteopetrosis often are normocytic anemia with hepatosplenomegaly resulting from compensatory extramedullary hematopoiesis. Increased susceptibility to infection is common as a result of granulocytopenia. Facial deformity develops in many of the children, manifesting as a broad face, hypertelorism, snub nose, and frontal bossing. Tooth eruption almost always is delayed. Failure of resorption and remodeling of the skull bones produces narrowing of the skull foramina that press on the various cranial nerves and results in optic nerve atrophy and blindness, deafness, and facial paralysis. In spite of the dense bone, pathologic fractures are common. Osteomyelitis of the jaws is a common complication of tooth extraction (Fig. 14-3).

Radiographically, there is a widespread increase in skeletal density with defects in metaphyseal remodeling. The radiographic distinction between cortical and cancellous bone is lost (Fig. 14-4). In dental radiographs, the roots of the teeth often are difficult to visualize because of the density of the surrounding bone.

Less severe variants of infantile osteopetrosis exist and have been termed **intermediate osteopetrosis.**

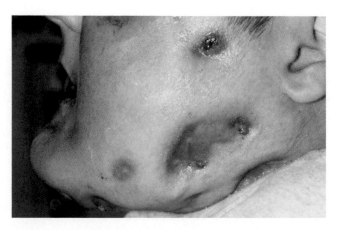

Fig. 14-3   Osteopetrosis. This 24-year-old white man has the infantile form of osteopetrosis. He has mandibular osteomyelitis, and multiple draining fistulae are present on his face. *(Courtesy of Dr. Dan Sarasin.)*

Affected patients often are asymptomatic at birth but frequently exhibit fractures by the end of the first decade. Marrow failure and hepatosplenomegaly are rare.

In some cases, patients show radiographic evidence of diffuse sclerosis and associated marrow failure but resolve without specific therapy. This pattern has been termed **transient osteopetrosis.** and most affected patients return to normalcy with no known sequelae.

ADULT OSTEOPETROSIS

Adult osteopetrosis is usually discovered later in life and exhibits less severe manifestations. In most patients, this pattern is inherited as an autosomal dominant trait and has been termed **benign osteopetrosis.** The axial skeleton usually reveals significant sclerosis, whereas the long bones demonstrate little or no defects. Approximately 40% of affected patients are asymptomatic, and marrow failure is rare. Occasionally, the diagnosis is discovered initially on review of dental radiographs that reveal a diffuse increased radiopacity of the medullary portions of the bone. In symptomatic patients, bone pain is frequent.

Two major variants of adult osteopetrosis are seen. In one form, cranial nerve compression is common, although fractures occur rarely. In contrast, the second pattern demonstrates frequent fractures, but nerve compression is uncommon. When the mandible is involved, fracture and osteomyelitis after tooth extraction are significant complications.

Although distinctly uncommon, other causes of widespread osteosclerosis exist and should be considered during evaluation of patients with osteopetrosis. Such diseases include autosomal dominant osteosclerosis (endosteal hyperostosis, Worth type), sclerosteosis, and Van Buchem disease.

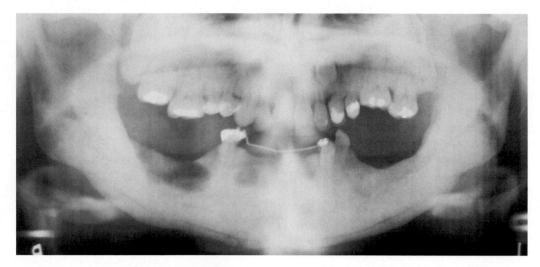

Fig. 14-4   Osteopetrosis. Extensive mandibular involvement is apparent in this radiograph of a 31-year-old woman. She received a diagnosis of osteopetrosis as a child. There is a history of multiple fractures and osteomyelitis of the jaws. *(Courtesy of Dr. Dan Sarasin.)*

HISTOPATHOLOGIC FEATURES

Several patterns of abnormal endosteal bone formation have been described. These include the following:

- Tortuous lamellar trabeculae replacing the cancellous portion of the bone
- Globular amorphous bone deposition in the marrow spaces (Fig. 14-5)
- Osteophytic bone formation

Numerous osteoclasts may be seen, but there is no evidence that they function because Howship's lacunae are not visible.

TREATMENT AND PROGNOSIS

Because of the mild severity of the disease, adult osteopetrosis is usually associated with long-term survival. In contrast, the prognosis of infantile osteopetrosis without therapy is typically poor, with most affected patients dying during the first decade of life. Bone marrow transplantation is the only hope for permanent cure. However, an appropriately matched donor is available for only about half of affected patients, and successful engraftment occurs in only approximately 45% of those receiving bone marrow transplantation.

Because of the unavailability or risk of bone marrow transplantation, search for other therapies is ongoing. Interferon gamma-1b, often in combination with calcitriol, has been shown to reduce bone mass, decrease the prevalence of infections, and lower the frequency of nerve compression. Other therapeutic avenues include administration of corticosteroids (to increase circulating red blood cells and platelets), parathormone, macrophage colony stimulating factor, and

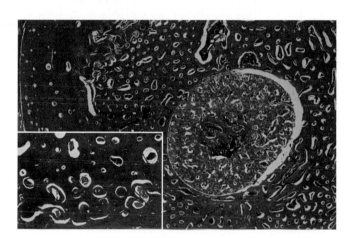

Fig. 14-5   Osteopetrosis. Low-power photomicrograph showing sclerotic bone that is replacing the normal cancellous bone. The *inset* shows a nodular pattern of the dense bone obliterating the marrow spaces.

erythropoietin. Limiting calcium intake also has been suggested.

Additional therapy consists of supportive measures, such as transfusions and antibiotics for the complications. Osteomyelitis of the jaws requires rapid intervention to minimize osseous destruction. Affected patients should receive early diagnosis, appropriate drainage and surgical débridement, bacterial culture with sensitivity, appropriate antibiotic therapy, and reconstruction if necessary. The infection often requires prolonged antibiotic therapy, with fluoroquinolones and lincomycin often being most effective. Hyperbaric oxygen is useful in promoting healing of recalcitrant cases.

CLEIDOCRANIAL DYSPLASIA

Best known for its dental and clavicular abnormalities, **cleidocranial dysplasia** is a disorder of bone caused by a defect in the *CBFA1* gene (also known as the *RUNX2* gene) of chromosome 6p21. This gene normally guides osteoblastic differentiation and appropriate bone formation. This condition initially was thought to involve only membranous bones (e.g., clavicles, skull, flat bones), but it is now known to affect endochondral ossification and to represent a generalized disorder of skeletal structures. Recent evidence suggests that the *CBFA1* gene additionally plays an important role in odontogenesis via participation in odontoblast differentiation, enamel organ formation, and dental lamina proliferation. Disruption of these functions might explain the distinct dental anomalies found in patients with this disorder. The disease has an estimated prevalence of 1:1,000,000 and shows an autosomal dominant inheritance pattern, but as many as 40% of cases appear to represent spontaneous mutations. This condition formerly was known as *cleidocranial dysostosis*.

CLINICAL AND RADIOGRAPHIC FEATURES

The bone defects in patients with cleidocranial dysplasia chiefly involve the clavicles and skull, although a wide variety of anomalies may be found in other bones. The clavicles are absent, either unilaterally or bilaterally, in about 10% of all cases. More commonly, the clavicles show varying degrees of hypoplasia and malformation.

The muscles associated with the abnormal clavicles are underdeveloped. The patient's neck appears long; the shoulders are narrow and show marked drooping. The absence or hypoplasia of the clavicles leads to an unusual mobility of the patient's shoulders. In some instances, the patient can approximate the shoulders in front of the chest (Fig. 14-6). Although the clavicular defects result in variations of the associated muscles, function is remarkably good.

The appearance of the patient affected by cleidocranial dysplasia often is diagnostic. The patients tend to be of short stature and have large heads with pronounced frontal and parietal bossing. Ocular hypertelorism and a broad base of the nose with a depressed nasal bridge often are noted. On skull radiographs, the sutures and fontanels show delayed closure or may remain open throughout the patient's life. Secondary centers of ossification appear in the suture lines, and many wormian bones may be seen. Abnormal development of the temporal bone and eustachian tube may lead to conductive or sensorineural hearing loss.

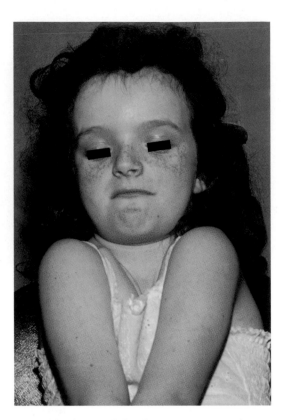

Fig. 14-6   Cleidocranial dysplasia. Patient can almost approximate her shoulders in front of her chest. *(Courtesy of Dr. William Bruce.)*

The gnathic and dental manifestations are distinctive and may lead to the initial diagnosis. The patients often have a narrow, high-arched palate, and there is an increased prevalence of cleft palate. Prolonged retention of deciduous teeth and delay or complete failure of eruption of permanent teeth are characteristic features. There may be abnormal spacing in the mandibular incisor area because of widening of the alveolar bone. On review of dental radiographs, the most dramatic finding is the presence of numerous unerupted permanent and supernumerary teeth, many of which frequently exhibit distorted crown and root shapes (Fig. 14-7). The number of supernumerary teeth can be impressive, with reports of some patients demonstrating more than 60 such teeth.

In addition to the dental alterations, review of panoramic radiographs reveals an increased prevalence of a number of additional osseous malformations. The mandible often demonstrates coarse trabeculation with areas of increased density. The mandibular rami are often narrow with nearly parallel-sided anterior and posterior borders, and the coronoid processes may be slender and pointed with a distal curvature. In some cases the mandibular symphysis remains patent. The

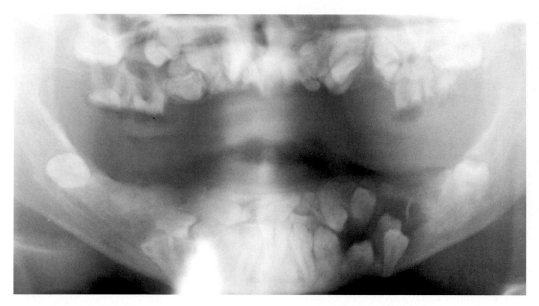

Fig. 14-7   Cleidocranial dysplasia. Panoramic radiograph showing multiple unerupted teeth. *(Courtesy of Dr. John R. Cramer.)*

maxilla often is associated with a thin zygomatic arch and small or absent maxillary sinuses.

Although young patients typically exhibit a relatively normal jaw relationship, as the individuals age, a short lower face height, acute gonial angle, anterior inclination of the mandible, and mandibular prognathism develop. Clinicians believe that these changes may be from inadequate vertical growth of the maxilla and hypoplastic alveolar ridge development caused by delay or lack of eruption of the permanent teeth.

Computed tomography (CT) studies have demonstrated a decreased thickness of the masseter muscle in some patients. This finding may be related to hypoplasia of the zygomatic arch resulting in hypofunction of the attached masseter muscle.

HISTOPATHOLOGIC FEATURES

The reason for failure of permanent tooth eruption in patients with cleidocranial dysplasia is not understood well. Microscopic studies of unerupted permanent teeth have shown that these teeth lack secondary cementum. However, a recent histomorphometric study demonstrated no statistically significant difference in the percentage of root surface covered by cementum between teeth extracted from a patient with cleidocranial dysplasia and teeth from control patients. Some investigators alternatively have proposed that insufficient alveolar bone resorption is the reason for impaired tooth eruption; this theory is based on obser-vations of decreased osteoclasts in the alveolar bone of heterozygous *CBFA1* knockout mice.

TREATMENT AND PROGNOSIS

No treatment exists for the skull, clavicular, and other bone anomalies associated with cleidocranial dysplasia. Most patients function well without any significant problems. It is not unusual for an affected individual to be unaware of the disease until some professional calls it to his or her attention.

Treatment of the dental problems associated with the disease, however, may be a major problem. Therapeutic options include full-mouth extractions with denture construction, autotransplantation of selected impacted teeth followed by prosthetic restoration, or removal of primary and supernumerary teeth followed by exposure of permanent teeth that are subsequently extruded orthodontically. The latter mode of therapy appears to be the treatment of choice; if performed before adulthood, then it can prevent the short lower face height and mandibular prognathism.

FOCAL OSTEOPOROTIC MARROW DEFECT

The **focal osteoporotic marrow defect** is an area of hematopoietic marrow that is sufficient in size to produce an area of radiolucency that may be confused with an intraosseous neoplasm. The area does not

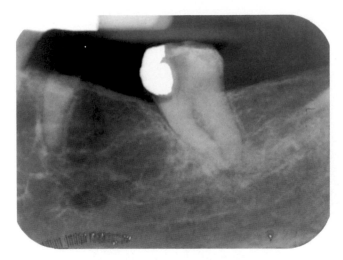

Fig. 14-8 Focal osteoporotic marrow defect.
Circumscribed radiolucency with central trabeculations in the extraction site of a mandibular molar. *(Courtesy of Dr. R. Sidney Jones.)*

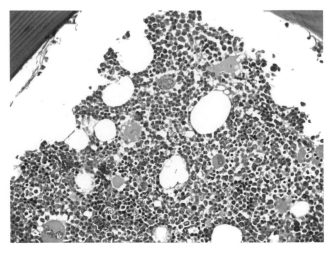

Fig. 14-9 Focal osteoporotic marrow defect.
Photomicrograph showing normal hematopoietic bone marrow.

represent a pathologic process, but its radiographic features may be confused with a variety of pathoses. The pathogenesis of this condition is unknown. Various theories include the following:

- Aberrant bone regeneration after tooth extraction
- Persistence of fetal marrow
- Marrow hyperplasia in response to increased demand for erythrocytes

CLINICAL AND RADIOGRAPHIC FEATURES

The focal osteoporotic marrow defect is typically asymptomatic and detected as an incidental finding on a radiographic examination. The area appears as a radiolucent lesion, varying in size from several millimeters to several centimeters in diameter. In many instances, when discovered in panoramic radiographs, the area appears radiolucent and somewhat circumscribed; however, on review of more highly detailed periapical radiographs, the defect typically exhibits ill-defined borders and fine central trabeculations (Fig. 14-8). More than 75% of all cases are discovered in adult women. About 70% occur in the posterior mandible, most often in edentulous areas. No expansion of the jaw is noted clinically.

HISTOPATHOLOGIC FEATURES

Microscopically, the defects contain cellular hematopoietic and/or fatty marrow. Lymphoid aggregates may be present. Bone trabeculae included in the biopsy specimen show no evidence of abnormal osteoblastic or osteoclastic activity (Fig. 14-9).

TREATMENT AND PROGNOSIS

The radiographic findings, although often suggestive of the diagnosis, are not specific and may simulate those of a variety of other diseases. Incisional biopsy, therefore, often is necessary to establish the diagnosis.

Once the diagnosis is established, no further treatment is needed. The prognosis is excellent, and no association between focal osteoporotic marrow defects and anemia or other hematologic disorders has been established.

IDIOPATHIC OSTEOSCLEROSIS

Idiopathic osteosclerosis refers to a focal area of increased radiodensity that is of unknown cause and cannot be attributed to any inflammatory, dysplastic, neoplastic, or systemic disorder. Idiopathic osteosclerosis also has been termed *dense bone island, bone eburnation, bone whorl, bone scar, enostosis,* and *focal periapical osteopetrosis.* These sclerotic areas are not restricted to the jaws, and radiographically similar lesions may be found in other bones.

Similar radiopaque foci may develop in the periapical areas of teeth with nonvital or significantly inflamed pulps; these lesions most likely represent a response to a low-grade inflammatory stimulus. Such reactive foci should be designated as **condensing osteitis** or **focal chronic sclerosing osteomyelitis** (see page 147) and should not be included under the designation of *idio-*

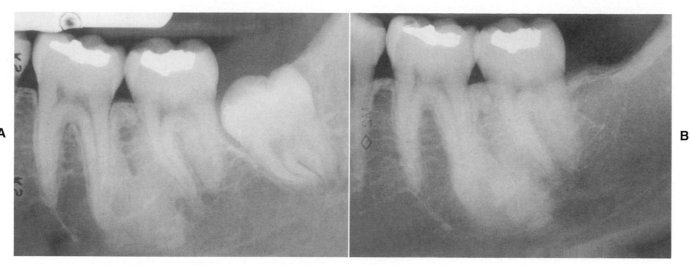

Fig. 14-10   **Idiopathic osteosclerosis. A,** An asymptomatic area of bone sclerosis is seen between and apical to the roots of the first and second mandibular molars. **B,** No appreciable change can be seen on this radiograph taken 10 years later. *(Courtesy of Dr. Michael Quinn.)*

pathic osteosclerosis. Because past studies did not distinguish the idiopathic lesions from those of inflammatory origin, confusion in terminology has resulted.

CLINICAL AND RADIOGRAPHIC FEATURES

Although previous studies often are difficult to interpret because of differences in diagnostic criteria, the prevalence appears to be approximately 5%, with some investigators suggesting a slightly increased frequency in blacks and Asians. No significant sex predilection is seen.

On review of several studies with long-term follow-up, a pattern has emerged. Although exceptions can be seen, most areas of idiopathic osteosclerosis arise in the late first or early second decade. Once noted, the lesions may remain static, but many reveal a slow increase in size. In almost all cases, once the patient reaches full maturity, all enlargement ceases and the sclerotic area stabilizes. In a smaller percentage, the lesion diminishes or undergoes complete regression. The peak prevalence of osteosclerosis occurs in the third decade, with the attainment of peak bone mass seen in the fourth decade.

Idiopathic osteosclerosis is invariably asymptomatic, not associated with detectable cortical expansion, and is typically detected during a routine radiographic examination. About 90% of examples are seen in the mandible, most often in the first molar area. The second premolar and second molar areas also are common sites. In most cases, only one focus of sclerotic bone is present. A small number of patients have two or even three separate areas of involvement. For patients with multiple areas of involvement, the possibility of multiple osteomas within the setting of Gardner syndrome (see page 651) should be excluded.

Radiographically, the lesions are characterized by a well-defined, rounded, or elliptic radiodense mass. Although the majority is uniformly radiopaque, occasional large lesions demonstrate a nonhomogeneous mixture of increased and reduced radiopacity. This is most likely because of variation in the three-dimensional (3D) shape of the lesion and is unrelated to differences in the mineral content of the mass. The lesions vary from 3.0 mm to more than 2.0 cm in greatest extent. A radiolucent rim does not surround the radiodense area. Most examples of idiopathic osteosclerosis are associated with a root apex. In a lesser number of cases, the sclerotic area may extend into or be located only in the interradicular area (Fig. 14-10). In about 20% of cases, the sclerotic area is located in the jaw, with no apparent relationship to a tooth. Rarely, the sclerotic bone may surround all or portions of an impacted tooth. Root resorption and movement of teeth have been noted but are uncommon.

HISTOPATHOLOGIC FEATURES

In the few microscopic studies that have been reported, the lesion consists of dense lamellar bone with scant fibrofatty marrow. Inflammatory cells are inconspicuous or absent.

DIAGNOSIS

Usually a diagnosis of idiopathic osteosclerosis may be made with confidence, based on history, clinical features, and radiographic findings. Biopsy is considered only if associated symptoms or significant cortical expansion is present. Although idiopathic osteosclerosis demonstrates radiographic and histopathologic similarities with a compact osteoma (see page 650), the lack of cortical expansion and failure of continued growth rule against a neoplastic process. Differentiation from condensing osteitis may be difficult; however, in the absence of a deep restoration or caries, a periapical radiodense area associated with a vital tooth is likely to represent idiopathic osteosclerosis.

TREATMENT AND PROGNOSIS

If the lesion is discovered during adolescence, periodic radiographs appear prudent until the area stabilizes. After that point, no treatment is indicated for idiopathic osteosclerosis, because there is little or no tendency for the lesions to progress or change in adulthood.

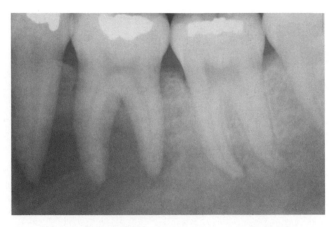

Fig. 14-11   Massive osteolysis. Periapical radiograph showing an ill-defined radiolucency associated with vital mandibular teeth. Note the loss of lamina dura. *(Courtesy of Dr. John R. Cramer.)*

MASSIVE OSTEOLYSIS (GORHAM DISEASE; GORHAM-STOUT SYNDROME; VANISHING BONE DISEASE; PHANTOM BONE DISEASE)

Massive osteolysis is a rare disease that is characterized by spontaneous and usually progressive destruction of one or more bones. The destroyed bone initially is replaced by a vascular proliferation. The affected area does not regenerate or repair itself; eventually, the site of destruction fills with dense fibrous tissue.

The cause of massive osteolysis is unknown. There is no evidence of any underlying metabolic or endocrine imbalance. Hyperactivity of osteoclasts initially was proposed to be the major pathogenetic mechanism underlying this disease. However, many investigators also believe that massive osteolysis is primarily related to a proliferation of blood or lymphatic vessels that is occasionally multicentric and has been termed **angiomatosis** of bone.

CLINICAL AND RADIOGRAPHIC FEATURES

Although massive osteolysis has been documented in patients up to 70 years of age, most affected patients are children and young adults. About 50% of all patients report an episode of trauma before the diagnosis, but this is often trivial in nature. Lesions have occurred in almost any bone or combination of bones. The most commonly involved sites are the pelvis, humeral head, humeral shaft, and axial skeleton. Generally, the results of laboratory studies are completely within normal limits.

In approximately 30% of affected patients, maxillofacial involvement is noted, with the mandible being affected most frequently. Simultaneous involvement of the maxilla and mandible may occur. Signs and symptoms include mobile teeth, pain, malocclusion, deviation of the mandible, and clinically obvious deformity. Obstructive sleep apnea syndrome has been noted secondary to posterior mandibular displacement after extensive osteolysis. Pathologic fracture of the mandible may occur. Temporomandibular joint (TMJ) involvement may be confused with other conditions that can cause TMJ dysfunction.

Radiographically, the earliest changes consist of intramedullary radiolucent foci of varying size with indistinct margins (Fig. 14-11). These coalesce to become larger and involve the cortical bone. Eventually, large portions of the involved bone disappear (Fig. 14-12). As the process proceeds, newly involved areas often demonstrate loss of the lamina dura and thinning of the cortical plates before development of obvious radiolucency. In some cases the bone destruction may mimic periodontitis or periapical inflammatory disease.

HISTOPATHOLOGIC FEATURES

The microscopic findings in massive osteolysis contrast sharply with the striking clinical and radiographic findings. In the early stages of disease, specimens removed from the radiolucent defects consist of a nonspecific vascular proliferation intermixed with fibrous connective and a chronic inflammatory infiltrate of lymphocytes and plasma cells. The vascular proliferation varies in intensity and is characterized by thin-walled channels that may be capillary or cavernous in nature

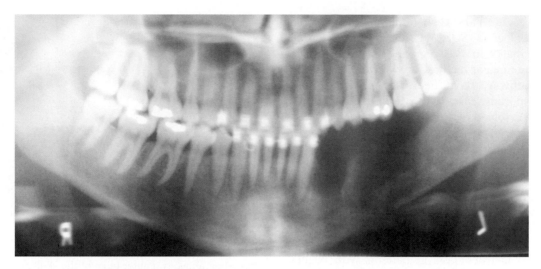

Fig. 14-12   Massive osteolysis. Panoramic radiograph of the same patient shown in Fig. 14-11, showing extensive bone loss and a pathologic fracture of the left mandible. This destruction occurred over an 8-month period. *(Courtesy of Dr. John R. Cramer.)*

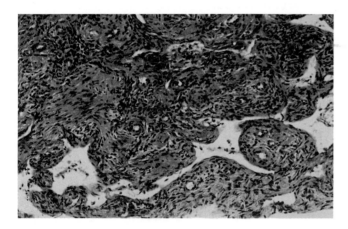

Fig. 14-13   Massive osteolysis. Biopsy specimen from the same patient shown in Figs. 14-11 and 14-12. The loose, highly vascular connective tissue shows a diffuse chronic inflammatory cell infiltrate.

(Fig. 14-13). Osteoclastic reaction in the adjacent bone fragments is usually not conspicuous.

In the later stages, tissue from the area of bone loss is more collagenized. Evidence of repair by new bone formation is not seen.

TREATMENT AND PROGNOSIS

The clinical course of massive osteolysis is variable and impossible to predict. In most cases, bone destruction progresses over months to a few years and results in the total loss of the affected bone or bones. Some patients, however, experience a spontaneous arrest of the process without complete loss of the affected bone. The prognosis varies from slight to severe disability.

Mortality from massive osteolysis is relatively uncommon and usually the result of severe chest cage involvement or destruction of vertebral bodies with spinal cord compression.

Treatment is not particularly satisfactory. Previous reported therapies include estrogens, magnesium, calcium, vitamin D, fluoride, calcitonin, alpha-2b interferon, and chemotherapeutic agents (e.g., cisplatin, actinomycin D, etoposide). Surgical intervention has met with limited success. When surgical removal is combined with bone grafting, the newly placed bone often undergoes osteolysis. Radiation therapy is the most successful and widely accepted mode of therapy, but failures may occur. In addition, this therapy places the patient at risk for postirradiation sarcoma. In a limited number of patients, stabilization of disease after bisphosphonate therapy has been reported, although longer-term studies on a greater number of patients are needed to assess this proposed treatment modality. The effectiveness of any therapeutic intervention is difficult to evaluate, not only because the disease is so rare but also because the condition may arrest spontaneously in some patients.

PAGET'S DISEASE OF BONE (OSTEITIS DEFORMANS)

Paget's disease of bone is a condition characterized by abnormal and anarchic resorption and deposition of bone, resulting in distortion and weakening of the affected bones. The cause of Paget's disease is unknown, but inflammatory, genetic, and endocrine factors may be contributing agents. In some studies, 15% to 40% of affected patients have a positive family history of the disease. In recent years, recurrent mutations in the sequestosome 1 gene (*SQSTM1*) (also known as *p62*), which participates in the regulation of osteoclastic activity via the nuclear factor-κB (NF-κB) transcription activation pathway, have been identified in both familial and sporadic cases of the disease. Mutations in another gene involved in the NF-κB signaling pathway, the valosin-containing protein (*VCP*) gene, have been found in patients with a rare hereditary syndrome that includes Paget's disease of bone, inclusion body myopathy, and frontotemporal dementia. In addition, the possibility that Paget's disease is the result of a slow virus infection has received considerable attention, but a viral cause remains unproven. Inclusion bodies identified as nucleocapsids from a paramyxovirus have been detected in osteoclasts in patients with Paget's disease, but a cause-and-effect relationship has not been established.

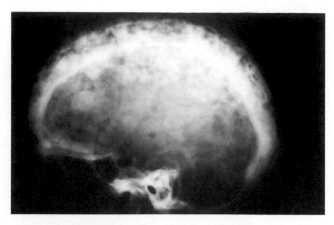

Fig. 14-14 Paget's disease. Lateral skull film shows marked enlargement of the cranium with new bone formation above the outer table of the skull and a patchy, dense, "cotton wool" appearance. *(Courtesy of Dr. Reg Munden.)*

CLINICAL AND RADIOGRAPHIC FEATURES

Paget's disease is relatively common, although there is a marked geographic variance in its prevalence. It is more common in Britain than in the United States, whereas it is rare in Africa and Asia. The disease principally affects older adults and is rarely encountered in patients younger than 40 years of age. Men are affected more often than women, and whites are affected more frequently than blacks. Reviews have estimated that 1 in 100 to 150 individuals older than 45 years of age have Paget's disease. Subclinical disease is not rare, and an increased number of cases are being seen as the population ages. Asymptomatic disease often is discovered in radiographs taken for unrelated reasons or from an unexpected elevation in serum alkaline phosphatase. The frequency increases with age, and the true prevalence (including undiscovered subclinical disease) probably ranges from 1% in the fifth decade to 10% in the tenth decade.

Although the disease may be **monostotic** (i.e., limited to one bone), most cases of Paget's disease are **polyostotic** (i.e., more than one bone is affected). Symptoms vary, and some patients may remain relatively asymptomatic. Bone pain, which may be quite severe, is a common complaint. In addition, pagetic bone often forms near joints and promotes osteoarthritic changes, with associated joint pain and limited mobility.

The lumbar vertebrae, pelvis, skull, and femur are the most commonly affected bones. Affected bones become thickened, enlarged, and weakened. Involvement of weight-bearing bones often leads to a bowing deformity, resulting in what is described as a simian (monkeylike) stance. Paget's disease affecting the skull generally leads to a progressive increase in the circumference of the head.

Jaw involvement is present in approximately 17% of patients diagnosed with Paget's disease. Maxillary disease, which is far more common than mandibular involvement, results in enlargement of the middle third of the face. In extreme cases, the alteration results in a lionlike facial deformity (**leontiasis ossea**). Nasal obstruction, enlarged turbinates, obliterated sinuses, and deviated septum may develop secondary to maxillary involvement. The alveolar ridges tend to remain symmetrical but become grossly enlarged. If the patient is dentulous, then the enlargement causes spacing of the teeth. Edentulous patients may complain that their dentures no longer fit because of the increased alveolar size.

Radiographically, the early stages of Paget's disease reveal a decreased radiodensity of the bone and alteration of the trabecular pattern. Particularly in the skull, large circumscribed areas of radiolucency may be present (**osteoporosis circumscripta**). During the osteoblastic phase of the disease, patchy areas of sclerotic bone are formed, which tend to become confluent. The patchy sclerotic areas often are described as having a "cotton wool" appearance (Figs. 14-14 and 14-15). On radiographic examination, the teeth often demonstrate extensive hypercementosis.

On initial discovery of Paget's disease, bone scintigraphy should be performed to evaluate fully the extent of involvement. When the mandible is affected, the bone scan may demonstrate marked uptake throughout the entire mandible from condyle to condyle, a feature that has been termed *black beard* or *Lincoln's sign.*

Radiographic findings of Paget's disease may resemble those of cemento-osseous dysplasia (see page 640).

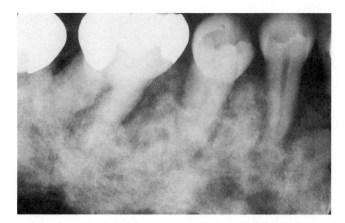

Fig. 14-15   Paget's disease. Periapical film showing the "cotton wool" appearance of the bone.

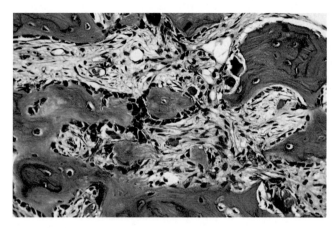

Fig. 14-16   Paget's disease. Prominent osteoblastic and osteoclastic activity surround the bone trabeculae. Note the resting and reversal lines.

Patients with presumed cemento-osseous dysplasia who demonstrate clinical expansion of the jaws should be evaluated further to rule out Paget's disease.

HISTOPATHOLOGIC FEATURES

Microscopic examination shows an apparent uncontrolled alternating resorption and formation of bone. In the active resorptive stages, numerous osteoclasts surround bone trabeculae and show evidence of resorptive activity. Simultaneously, osteoblastic activity is seen with formation of osteoid rims around bone trabeculae. A highly vascular fibrous connective tissue replaces the marrow. A characteristic microscopic feature is the presence of basophilic reversal lines in the bone. These lines indicate the junction between alternating resorptive and formative phases of the bone and result in a "jigsaw puzzle," or "mosaic," appearance of the bone (Fig. 14-16). In the less active phases, large masses of dense bone showing prominent reversal lines are present.

DIAGNOSIS

Patients with Paget's disease show high elevations in serum alkaline phosphatase levels but usually have normal blood calcium and phosphorus levels. Although serum bone-specific alkaline phosphatase is considered the most sensitive marker of bone formation, it is not widely available; thus total serum alkaline phosphatase is typically used in routine clinical practice. However, because serum alkaline phosphatase also may be elevated in other conditions, such as cholelithiasis, other laboratory studies are indicated to confirm the diagnosis. Urinary hydroxyproline levels often are markedly elevated, although it is recognized that hydroxyproline often breaks down before excretion, making it a less precise method for measurement of bone resorption. Newer and more sensitive markers of bone resorption are N-telopeptides, C-telopeptides, and pyridinoline cross-link assays. The clinical and radiographic features, combined with supportive laboratory findings, are typically sufficient for diagnosis. Histopathologic examination can be confirmatory but often is unnecessary for a strong presumptive diagnosis.

TREATMENT AND PROGNOSIS

Although Paget's disease is chronic and slowly progressive, it is seldom the cause of death. In patients with more limited involvement and no symptoms, treatment often is not required. In asymptomatic patients, systemic therapy is usually not initiated unless the alkaline phosphatase is more than 25% to 50% above normal. When symptomatic, bone pain is noted most frequently and often may be controlled by acetaminophen or nonsteroidal antiinflammatory drugs (NSAIDs). Neurologic complications, such as deafness or visual disturbances, may result from bony encroachment on cranial nerves passing through skull foramina.

Pharmacologic antiresorptive therapy is recommended for patients with the following signs or symptoms: considerable bone pain, headache related to skull involvement, deafness or visual disturbances because of narrowing of the skull foramina, back pain because of pagetic radiculopathy or arthropathy, bone fractures, and hypercalcemia resulting from immobilization. Use of parathyroid hormone (PTH) antagonists, such as calcitonin and bisphosphonates, can reduce bone turnover and improve the biochemical abnormalities. For several decades, the mainstays of therapy were calcitonin and the bisphosphonate etidronate. However, these agents have been largely supplanted by the newer bisphosphonates, alendronate and risedronate, which provide enhanced control of bone turnover. Bisphosphonates are typically administered orally for a period of 2 to 6 months. Intravenous pamidronate can be an alternative for those patients who cannot tolerate oral bisphosphonates because of gastrointestinal irritation or who require treatment before surgery in an area of pagetic bone. A recently reported regimen of notable efficacy is single-infusion therapy with the potent bisphosphonate, zoledronic acid. In mild cases, a single infusion of a bisphosphonate often is associated with yearlong remissions. Patients with more severe disease usually require higher doses or more frequent courses of a particular bisphosphonate. The goal of therapy is to achieve midrange normal levels of serum alkaline phosphatase, with retreatment occurring when values rise 25% higher than normal. Plicamycin, a cytotoxic antibiotic, is known to inhibit osteoclastic activity, but its use is restricted to patients with severe disease that is refractory to calcitonin and bisphosphonate medications.

Case reports of osteonecrosis of the jaw as a complication of bisphosphonate therapy for Paget's disease of bone have raised some safety concerns. Long-term data are needed to fully assess the potential risks and benefits of bisphosphonate therapy; thus the merits of aggressive preventive or prolonged maintenance therapy remain uncertain at this time.

Edentulous patients may require new and larger dentures periodically to compensate for progressive enlargement of the alveolar processes. Dental complications include difficulties in extraction of teeth exhibiting significant hypercementosis. During active disease, pagetoid bone is extremely vascular with multiple arteriovenous shunts. Oral surgical procedures during this time can result in extensive hemorrhage. During the later sclerotic phase, the bone is hypersensitive to inflammation and can develop osteomyelitis with minimal provocation. In one recent report, long-term correction of maxillary deformity was achieved by removal, reshaping, and reinsertion of the maxillomalar complex in a patient who had received no prior medical treatment for his disease.

Development of a malignant bone tumor, usually an osteosarcoma, is a recognized complication of Paget's disease. Osteosarcoma in adults older than 40 years is quite uncommon in individuals who do not have Paget's disease. The frequency of bone sarcoma complicating Paget's disease ranges from 0.9% to 13.0% in various studies. The true frequency is probably in the range of 1% or less. Most of the osteosarcomas develop in the pelvis and long bones of the lower extremities. The skull and jaws are very rare sites for sarcomas associated with Paget's disease. Clinical signs and symptoms that should raise suspicion of possible underlying malignancy include the development of constant and worsening bone pain, a new mass, or sudden fracture. Osteosarcoma in Paget's disease is very aggressive and associated with a poor prognosis. Although survival rates generally have improved over the last several decades for patients with nonpagetoid osteosarcoma, no significant improvement in survival has been observed among patients with Paget's-related osteosarcoma. Benign and malignant giant cell tumors (see page 629) also may develop in bones affected by Paget's disease. Most of these occur in the craniofacial skeleton.

CENTRAL GIANT CELL GRANULOMA (GIANT CELL LESION; GIANT CELL TUMOR)

The **giant cell granuloma** is considered widely to be a nonneoplastic lesion. Although formerly designated as *giant cell reparative granuloma*, there is little evidence that the lesion represents a reparative response. Some lesions demonstrate aggressive behavior similar to that of a neoplasm. Most oral and maxillofacial pathologists have dropped the term *reparative*; today, these lesions are designated as **giant cell granuloma** or by the more noncommittal term, **giant cell lesion**. Whether or not true **giant cell tumors** occur in the jaws is uncertain and controversial. (This topic is discussed later in the chapter.) Likewise, it is not certain whether some reported cases of extragnathic giant cell granulomas actually represent true giant cell tumors.

CLINICAL AND RADIOGRAPHIC FEATURES

Giant cell granulomas may be encountered in patients ranging from 2 to 80 years of age, although more than 60% of all cases occur before age 30. Although the sex ratio varies in different reviews, a majority of giant cell granulomas are noted in females, and approximately 70% arise in the mandible. Lesions are more common in the anterior portions of the jaws, and mandibular lesions frequently cross the midline.

Most giant cell granulomas of the jaws are asymptomatic and first come to attention during a routine radiographic examination or as a result of painless expansion of the affected bone. A minority of cases, however, may be associated with pain, paresthesia, or perforation of the cortical bone plate, occasionally resulting in ulceration of the mucosal surface by the underlying lesion (Fig. 14-17).

Based on the clinical and radiographic features, several groups of investigators have suggested that central giant cell lesions of the jaws may be divided into two categories:

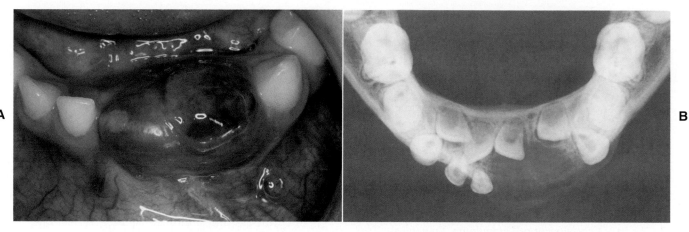

A

B

Fig. 14-17 Central giant cell granuloma. A, A blue-purple mass is present on the anterior alveolar ridge of this 4-year-old white boy. **B,** The occlusal radiograph shows a radiolucent lesion with cortical expansion.

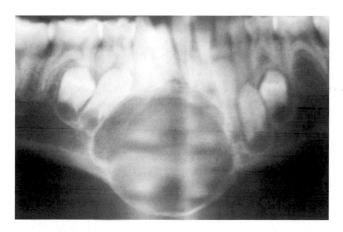

Fig. 14-18 Central giant cell granuloma. Panoramic radiograph showing a large, expansile radiolucent lesion in the anterior mandible. *(Courtesy of Dr. Gregory R. Erena.)*

1. **Nonaggressive lesions** make up most cases, exhibit few or no symptoms, demonstrate slow growth, and do not show cortical perforation or root resorption of teeth involved in the lesion.
2. **Aggressive lesions** are characterized by pain, rapid growth, cortical perforation, and root resorption. They show a marked tendency to recur after treatment, compared with the non-aggressive types.

Radiographically, central giant cell lesions appear as radiolucent defects, which may be unilocular or multilocular. The defect is usually well delineated, but the margins are generally noncorticated. The lesion may vary from an incidental radiographic finding of 5×5 mm to a destructive lesion greater than 10 cm in size (Fig. 14-18). The radiographic findings are not specifically diagnostic. Small unilocular lesions may be confused with periapical granulomas or cysts (Fig.

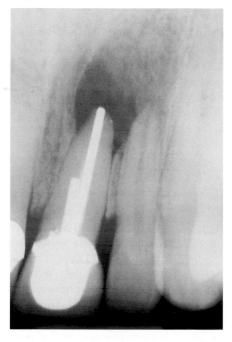

Fig. 14-19 Central giant cell granuloma. The periapical radiograph shows a radiolucent area involving the apex of an endodontically treated tooth. This was considered preoperatively to represent a periapical granuloma or periapical cyst.

14-19). Multilocular giant cell lesions cannot be distinguished radiographically from ameloblastomas or other multilocular lesions.

Areas histopathologically identical to giant cell granuloma have been noted in aneurysmal bone cysts (see page 634) and intermixed with central odontogenic fibromas (see page 727). Because giant cell granulomas are also histopathologically identical to brown tumors, hyperparathyroidism (see page 838) should

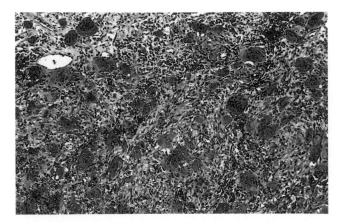

Fig. 14-20 Central giant cell granuloma. Numerous multinucleated giant cells within a background of plump proliferating mesenchymal cells. Note extensive red blood cell extravasation.

be ruled out in all instances. In addition, multifocal involvement in childhood suggests cherubism (see next section) and warrants further investigation. Most giant cell granulomas are single lesions; rarely, multifocal involvement is seen in patients who demonstrate no evidence of an associated disease, such as hyperparathyroidism or cherubism.

HISTOPATHOLOGIC FEATURES

Giant cell lesions of the jaw show a variety of features. Common to all is the presence of few to many multinucleated giant cells in a background of ovoid to spindle-shaped mesenchymal cells and round monocyte-macrophages (Fig. 14-20). There is evidence that these giant cells represent osteoclasts, although others suggest the cells may be aligned more closely with macrophages. The spindle-shaped cells appear to be fibroblast related. It has been proposed that the spindle cell component is the proliferating cell population and recruits monocyte-macrophage precursors, inducing them to differentiate into osteoclastic giant cells by activation of the receptor activator of the nuclear factor-κB (RANK)/RANK ligand signaling pathway. The giant cells may be aggregated focally in the lesional tissue or may be present diffusely throughout the lesion. These cells vary considerably in size and shape from case to case. Some are small and irregular in shape and contain only a few nuclei. In other cases, the giant cells are large and round and contain 20 or more nuclei.

In some cases the stroma is loosely arranged and edematous; in other cases it may be quite cellular. Areas of erythrocyte extravasation and hemosiderin deposition often are prominent. Older lesions may show considerable fibrosis of the stroma. Foci of osteoid

and newly formed bone are occasionally present within the lesion. Correlation of the histopathologic features with clinical behavior remains debatable, but lesions showing large, uniformly distributed giant cells and a predominantly cellular stroma appear more likely to be clinically aggressive with a greater tendency to recur after surgical treatment.

TREATMENT AND PROGNOSIS

Central giant cell lesions of the jaws are usually treated by thorough curettage. In reports of large series of cases, recurrence rates range from 11% to 50% or greater. Most studies indicate a recurrence rate of about 15% to 20%. Those lesions considered on clinical and radiologic grounds to be potentially aggressive show a higher frequency of recurrence. Many investigators have noted a propensity for recurrence among lesions in younger patients. Recurrent lesions often respond to further curettage, although some aggressive lesions require more radical surgery for cure.

In patients with aggressive tumors, three alternatives to surgery–(1) corticosteroids, (2) calcitonin, and (3) interferon alfa-2a–are being investigated. Several investigators have reported small numbers of patients, some of which exhibited remarkable response to these interventions. Weekly injections directly into the tumor with triamcinolone acetonide for approximately 6 weeks have been used successfully. Calcitonin typically is administered daily for approximately 12 months as an intradermal injection or nasal spray. Several cases of large lesions resolving with systemic administration of salmon calcitonin have been reported, although a recent randomized, double-blind, controlled clinical trial performed on a limited number of patients found no significant difference between the calcitonin-treated and placebo patient groups. Interferon alfa-2a, alone or in combination with surgery, also has been reported to result in resolution of large lesions. The response of central giant cell lesions to interferon alfa-2a has been proposed to be the result of this drug's antiangiogenic properties, although speculation about the vascular nature of these lesions has not been proven. Clinicians should be aware of the potential side effects of interferon alfa-2a therapy, which can include flulike symptoms (e.g., fever, malaise, nausea, joint pain, weakness) and in rare cases more serious complications, including pancreatitis and drug-induced lupus erythematosus. The previously discussed medical therapeutic approaches provide possible alternatives for large lesions that if treated surgically would result in significant deformity. Evaluation of greater numbers of patients with appropriate controls is necessary to compare these therapeutic approaches to surgery adequately.

In spite of the reported recurrence rate, the long-term prognosis of giant cell granulomas is good and metastases do not develop.

GIANT CELL TUMOR

The question of whether true **giant cell tumors,** which most often occur in the epiphyses of long tubular bones, occur in the jaws has been argued for many years and still is unresolved. Although most central giant cell lesions can be distinguished histopathologically from the long bone tumors, a number of jaw lesions are indistinguishable microscopically from the typical giant cell tumor of long bone (Fig. 14-21). Despite the histopathologic similarity, these jaw lesions appear to have a biologically different behavior from long bone lesions, which have higher recurrence rates after curettage and show malignant change in up to 10% of cases. One case of metastasis from a mandibular tumor, however, has been reported. It has been suggested that giant cell granulomas of the jaws and giant cell tumors of the extragnathic skeleton are not distinct and separate entities; rather, they represent a continuum of a single disease process modified by the age of the patients, the locations of the lesions, and possibly other factors that are not yet understood.

CHERUBISM

Cherubism is a rare developmental jaw condition that is generally inherited as an autosomal dominant trait with high penetrance but variable expressivity. Several investigators have reported a higher disease penetrance in males than in females. Sporadic cases also can occur and are thought to represent spontaneous mutations. In two reports published simultaneously by laboratories on different continents, the gene for cherubism was mapped to chromosome 4p16. Mutations subsequently were identified in the *SH3BP2* gene within this locus. The protein encoded by this gene is believed to function in signal transduction pathways and to increase the activity of osteoclasts and osteoblasts during normal tooth eruption. It has been suggested that mutations in the *SH3BP2* gene may lead to pathologic activation of osteoclasts and disruption of jaw morphogenesis. However, the molecular pathogenesis of cherubism remains poorly understood.

The name *cherubism* was applied to this condition because the facial appearance is similar to that of the plump-cheeked little angels (cherubs) depicted in Renaissance paintings. Although cherubism also has been called *familial fibrous dysplasia*, this term should be avoided because cherubism has no relationship to fibrous dysplasia of bone (see page 635).

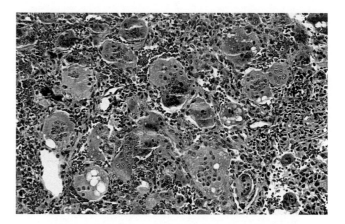

Fig. 14-21   Giant cell tumor. This photomicrograph shows large giant cells that are distributed in a cellular mesenchymal tissue. This specimen was from an aggressive lesion that had destroyed most of the maxilla.

CLINICAL AND RADIOGRAPHIC FEATURES

Although some examples of cherubism may develop as early as 1 year of age, the disease usually occurs between the ages of 2 and 5 years. In mild cases the diagnosis may not be made until the patient reaches 10 to 12 years of age. The clinical alterations typically progress until puberty, then stabilize and slowly regress.

The cherublike facies arises from bilateral involvement of the posterior mandible that produces angelic chubby cheeks (Fig. 14-22). In addition, there is an "eyes upturned to heaven" appearance that is due to a wide rim of exposed sclerae noted below the iris. This latter feature is due to involvement of the infraorbital rim and orbital floor that tilts the eyeballs upward, as well as to stretching of the upper facial skin that pulls the lower lid downward. On occasion, affected patients also reveal marked cervical lymphadenopathy.

The mandibular lesions typically appear as a painless, bilateral expansion of the posterior mandible that tends to involve the angles and ascending rami. The bony expansion is usually bilaterally symmetrical; in severe cases, most of the mandible is involved. Milder maxillary involvement occurs in the tuberosity areas; in severe cases, the entire maxilla can be affected.

Extensive bone involvement causes a marked widening and distortion of the alveolar ridges. In addition to the aesthetic and psychologic effect, the enlargements may cause tooth displacement or failure of eruption, impair mastication, create speech difficulties, or

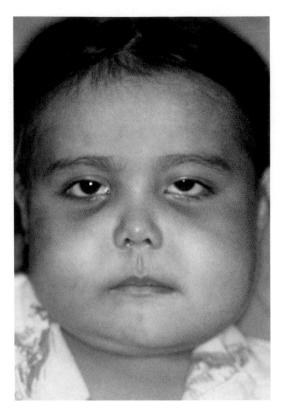

Fig. 14-22   Cherubism. This young girl shows the typical cherubic facies resulting from bilateral expansile mandibular and maxillary lesions. (*Courtesy of Dr. Román Carlos.*)

rarely lead to loss of normal vision or hearing. Although there have been rare reports of unilateral cherubism, it is difficult to accept these as examples of this disease unless there is a strong family history.

Radiographically, the lesions are typically multilocular, expansile radiolucencies (Fig. 14-23). The appearance is virtually diagnostic as a result of their bilateral location. Less commonly, the lesions appear as unilocular radiolucencies. Although cherubism typically involves only the jaws, involvement also has been reported rarely in other bones such as the ribs and humerus.

No unusual biochemical findings have been reported in patients with cherubism. If laboratory results do not suggest the diagnosis of hyperparathyroidism, then most children with multiple symmetrical giant cell granulomas represent examples of cherubism. However, multiple giant cell lesions may be seen in association with other conditions, including Ramon syndrome, Jaffe-Campanacci syndrome, and a Noonan-like syndrome. It has been suggested that the bony lesions of cherubism represent a phenotypic picture common to a number of disease processes that arise from multiple, distinct, initiating pathogenetic events.

HISTOPATHOLOGIC FEATURES

The microscopic findings of cherubism are essentially similar to those of isolated giant cell granulomas, and they seldom permit a specific diagnosis of cherubism in the absence of clinical and radiologic information. The lesional tissue consists of vascular fibrous tissue containing variable numbers of multinucleated giant cells. The giant cells tend to be small and usually aggregated focally (Fig. 14-24). Like the giant cells in central giant cell granulomas, the giant cells in cherubism express markers suggestive of osteoclastic origin. Foci of extravasated blood are commonly present. The stroma in cherubism often tends to be more loosely arranged than that seen in giant cell granulomas. In some cases, cherubism reveals eosinophilic, cufflike deposits surrounding small blood vessels throughout the lesion. The eosinophilic cuffing appears to be specific for cherubism. However, these deposits are not present in many cases, and their absence does not exclude a diagnosis of cherubism. In older, resolving lesions of cherubism, the tissue becomes more fibrous, the number of giant cells decreases, and new bone formation is seen.

TREATMENT AND PROGNOSIS

The prognosis in any given case is unpredictable. In most instances the lesions tend to show varying degrees of remission and involution after puberty (see Fig. 14-23). By the fourth decade, the facial features of most patients approach normalcy. In spite of the typical scenario, some patients demonstrate very mild alterations, whereas others reveal grotesque changes that often are very slow to resolve. In occasional patients, the deformity can persist.

The question of whether to treat or simply observe a patient with cherubism is difficult. Excellent results have been obtained in some cases by early surgical intervention with curettage of the lesions. Conversely, early surgical intervention sometimes has been followed by rapid regrowth of the lesions and worsening deformity. A course limited only to observation may result in extreme and sometimes grotesque facial deformity, with associated psychologic problems and functional deformity that may necessitate extensive surgery. Several investigators have suggested the use of calcitonin in severe cases, but such therapy awaits further study. Radiation therapy is contraindicated because of the risk of development of postirradiation sarcoma. The optimal therapy for cherubism has not been determined.

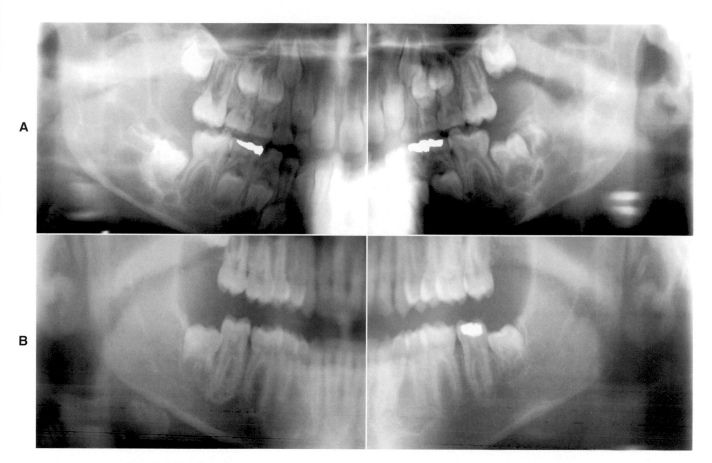

Fig. 14-23 **Cherubism. A,** Panoramic radiograph of a 7-year-old white boy. Bilateral multilocular radiolucencies can be seen in the posterior mandible. **B,** Same patient 6 years later. The lesions in the mandibular rami demonstrate significant resolution, but areas of involvement are still present in the body of the mandible. *(Courtesy of Dr. John R. Cramer.)*

SIMPLE BONE CYST (TRAUMATIC BONE CYST; HEMORRHAGIC BONE CYST; SOLITARY BONE CYST; IDIOPATHIC BONE CAVITY)

The **simple bone cyst** is a benign, empty, or fluid-containing cavity within bone that is devoid of an epithelial lining. The lesion is undoubtedly more common in the jaws than the literature would indicate. The cause and pathogenesis are uncertain and controversial. Several theories have been proposed, but none of them explains all of the clinical and pathologic features of this disease.

The **trauma-hemorrhage theory** has many advocates, as evidenced by the widely used designation **traumatic bone cyst**. This theory suggests that trauma to the bone that is insufficient to cause a fracture results in an intraosseous hematoma. If the hematoma does not undergo organization and repair, it may liquefy and result in a cystic defect. Some affected patients may recall an episode of trauma to the affected area, but this anecdotal information is of uncertain significance

and has not been subjected to detailed, controlled analysis.

Although the trauma-hemorrhage theory appears to be accepted widely in the dental literature, it has little support in the orthopedic literature to explain similar cysts most commonly found in the metaphysis or diaphysis of the proximal humerus and femur in young patients. In addition, it cannot explain gnathic simple bone cysts that have demonstrated progressive enlargement over several years and, on surgical investigation, fail to reveal any evidence of continued hemorrhage. Other etiologic theories include inability of interstitial fluid to exit the bone because of inadequate venous drainage, local disturbance in bone growth, ischemic marrow necrosis, and localized alteration in bone metabolism resulting in osteolysis.

CLINICAL AND RADIOGRAPHIC FEATURES

Simple bone cysts have been reported in almost every bone of the body, but the vast majority involves the long bones. Simple bone cysts within the jaws are common

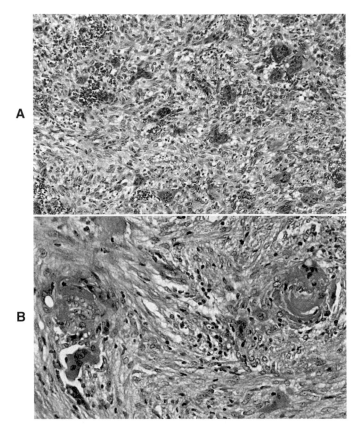

Fig. 14-24   **Cherubism. A,** Photomicrograph showing scattered giant cells within a background of cellular, hemorrhagic mesenchymal tissue. **B,** High-power view showing perivascular eosinophilic cuffing.

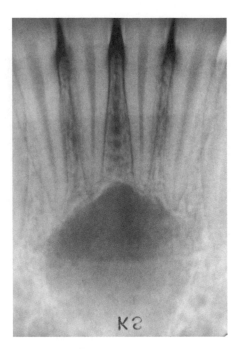

Fig. 14-25   **Simple bone cyst.** Periapical radiograph showing a radiolucent area in the apical region of the anterior mandible. The incisor teeth responded normally to vitality testing, and no restorations are present.

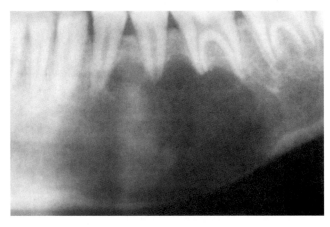

Fig. 14-26   **Simple bone cyst.** Panoramic film showing a large simple bone cyst of the mandible in a 12-year-old girl. The scalloping superior aspect of the cyst between the roots of the teeth is highly suggestive of, but not diagnostic for, a simple bone cyst. *(Courtesy of Dr. Lon Doles.)*

and most frequently encountered in patients between 10 and 20 years of age. The lesion is rare in children younger than age 5 and is seldom seen in patients older than age 35. Simple bone cysts of the jaws are essentially restricted to the mandible, although there have been reports of the lesion in the maxilla. Bilateral simple bone cysts of the mandible are occasionally encountered. About 60% of cases occur in males.

The simple bone cyst usually produces no symptoms and is discovered only when radiographs are taken for some other reason. About 20% of patients, however, have a painless swelling of the affected area. Pain and paresthesia may be noted in a few cases. Although any area of the mandible may be involved, simple bone cysts are more common in the premolar and molar areas.

Radiographically, the lesion most frequently appears as a well-delineated radiolucent defect. In some areas, the margins of the defect are sharply defined; in other areas, the margins are ill defined. The defect may range from 1 to 10 cm in diameter. When several teeth are involved in the lesion, the radiolucent defect often shows domelike projections that scallop upward between the roots. This feature is highly suggestive but not diagnostic of a simple bone cyst (Figs. 14-25 and 14-26). In many cases, a cone-shaped outline (pointed at one or both ends in the anterior-posterior direction) may be noted, particularly when the lesion is large. Oval, irregular, or rounded borders are possible as well. Teeth that appear to be involved in the lesion are generally vital and do not show root resorption.

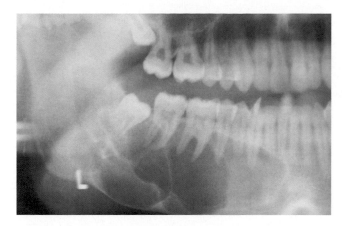

Fig. 14-27   **Simple bone cyst.** Panoramic film showing a large multilocular simple bone cyst of the mandible in a 16-year-old white adolescent. *(Courtesy of Dr. Amy Bogardus.)*

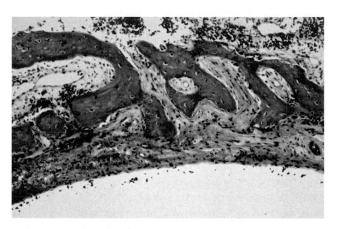

Fig. 14-28   **Simple bone cyst.** Photomicrograph of the bony wall of a simple bone cyst. A thin, vascular connective tissue membrane is adjacent to the bone, and no epithelial lining is identified.

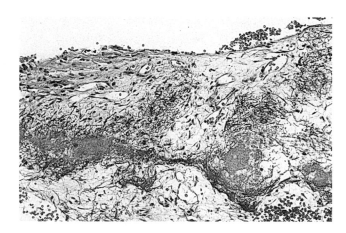

Fig. 14-29   **Simple bone cyst.** Loose vascular connective tissue exhibiting areas of basophilic lacelike calcification in the wall of a simple bone cyst.

Although not characteristic, a simple bone cyst may appear as a multilocular radiolucency associated with cortical expansion and slow enlargement. When expansion is present, an occlusal radiograph typically demonstrates a thin shell of cortical bone that exhibits no further reactive changes. Extensive lesions involving a substantial portion of the body and ascending ramus are occasionally encountered (Fig. 14-27).

Similar simple cysts may be associated with lesions of cemento-osseous dysplasia and other fibro-osseous proliferations. These typically occur in older patients and are discussed later (see page 643).

HISTOPATHOLOGIC FEATURES

The walls of the defect may be lined by a thin band of vascular fibrous connective tissue or demonstrate a thickened myxofibromatous proliferation that often is intermixed with trabeculae of cellular and reactive bone. This lining may exhibit areas of vascularity, fibrin, erythrocytes, and occasional giant cells adjacent to the bone surface (Fig. 14-28). Stringy lacelike dystrophic calcifications occasionally are noted (Fig. 14-29). There is never any evidence of an epithelial lining. The bony surface next to the cavity often shows resorptive areas (Howship's lacunae) indicative of past osteoclastic activity.

DIAGNOSIS

The radiographic features of the simple bone cyst, although often suggestive of the diagnosis, are not diagnostic and may be confused with a wide variety of odontogenic and nonodontogenic radiolucent jaw lesions. Surgical exploration is necessary to establish the diagnosis.

Because little to no tissue often is obtained at the time of surgery, the diagnosis of simple bone cyst is primarily based on the clinical and radiographic features, together with the surgical findings. In about one third of cases, the lytic defect will be found to be an empty cavity with smooth, shiny bony walls. In about two thirds of cases, the cavity will contain small amounts of serosanguineous fluid. The mandibular neurovascular bundle may be seen lying free in the cavity.

TREATMENT AND PROGNOSIS

Although the treatment of simple bone cysts of the long bones often is more aggressive and includes intralesional steroid injections or thorough surgical curettage, simple surgical exploration to establish the diagnosis is usually sufficient therapy for gnathic lesions. Even though the bony walls of the cavity at surgical exploration often appear smooth and shiny, it is wise to curette them and submit the small amount of tissue obtained for microscopic examination to rule out more serious diseases. Rarely, on microscopic examination, a lesion considered to be a simple bone cyst at surgical exploration will prove to be a thin-walled lesion, such as an odontogenic keratocyst or cystic ameloblastoma. When a thickened myxofibromatous wall is encountered, curettage and submission of this material appears prudent. After surgical exploration with or without curettage of the bony walls, obliteration of the defect by new bone formation is generally rapid. Even large defects may show normal radiographic findings within 6 months after exploration. Recurrence or persistence of the lesion is most unusual, but it has been reported. Periodic radiographic examination should be continued until complete resolution has been confirmed. The prognosis is excellent, however.

ANEURYSMAL BONE CYST

Aneurysmal bone cyst is an intraosseous accumulation of variable-sized, blood-filled spaces surrounded by cellular fibrous connective tissue that often is admixed with trabeculae of reactive woven bone. The cause and pathogenesis of the aneurysmal bone cyst are poorly understood. Several investigators have proposed that aneurysmal bone cyst arises from a traumatic event, vascular malformation, or neoplasm that disrupts the normal osseous hemodynamics and leads to an enlarging, hemorrhagic extravasation. As a corollary of this theory, others have suggested that aneurysmal bone cyst and giant cell granuloma are closely related. An aneurysmal bone cyst may form when an area of hemorrhage maintains connection with the disrupted feeding vessels; subsequently, giant cell granuloma-like areas can develop after loss of connection with the original vascular source.

Some authors have presented large series of cases involving the extragnathic skeleton and claim that none of their cases has shown evidence of a preexisting lesion. Others have reported similar large series and contend that a preexisting lesion may be evident in one third of cases. It is likely that the aneurysmal bone cyst may occur either as a primary lesion or as a result of disrupted vascular dynamics in a preexisting intrabony lesion.

Cytogenetic analysis has demonstrated the presence of various chromosomal abnormalities in some cases, particularly those involving 17p11-13 and 16q22. However, the significance of these chromosomal abnormalities in the molecular pathogenesis of the aneurysmal bone cyst remains unclear.

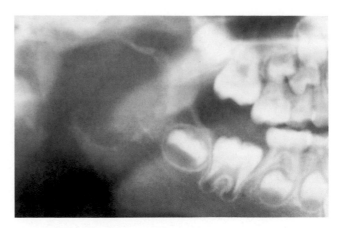

Fig. 14-30   Aneurysmal bone cyst. A large radiolucent lesion involves most of the ascending ramus in a 5-year-old white boy. *(Courtesy of Dr. Samuel McKenna.)*

CLINICAL AND RADIOGRAPHIC FEATURES

Aneurysmal bone cysts are located most commonly in the shaft of a long bone or in the vertebral column in patients younger than age 30. Gnathic aneurysmal bone cysts are uncommon, with approximately 2% reported from the jaws. Within the jaws, a wide age range is noted; however, most cases arise in children and young adults, with an approximate mean age of 20 years. No significant sex predilection is noted. A mandibular predominance is noted, and the vast majority arises in the posterior segments of the jaws.

The most common clinical manifestation is a swelling that has usually developed rapidly. Pain often is reported; paresthesia, compressibility, and crepitus are rarely seen. On occasion, malocclusion, mobility, migration, or resorption of involved teeth may be present. Maxillary lesions often bulge into the adjacent sinus; nasal obstruction, nasal bleeding, proptosis, and diplopia are noted uncommonly.

Radiographic study shows a unilocular or multilocular radiolucent lesion often associated with marked cortical expansion and thinning (Fig. 14-30). The radiographic borders are variable and may be well defined or diffuse. Frequently, a ballooning or "blow-out" distention of the contour of the affected bone is described. Uncommonly, small radiopaque foci, thought to be small trabeculae of reactive bone, are noted within the radiolucency.

At the time of surgery, intact periosteum and a thin shell of bone are typically found covering the lesion. Cortical perforation may occur, but spread into the adjacent soft tissue has not been documented. When the periosteum and bony shell are removed, dark venous blood frequently wells up and venouslike

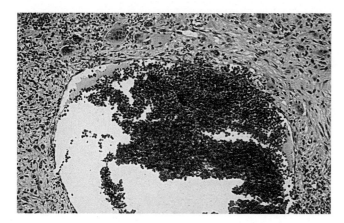

Fig. 14-31   Aneurysmal bone cyst. Photomicrograph showing a blood-filled space surrounded by fibroblastic connective tissue. Scattered multinucleated giant cells are seen adjacent to the vascular space.

bleeding may be encountered. The appearance at surgery has been likened to that of a "blood-soaked sponge."

HISTOPATHOLOGIC FEATURES

Microscopically, the aneurysmal bone cyst is characterized by spaces of varying size, filled with unclotted blood surrounded by cellular fibroblastic tissue containing multinucleated giant cells and trabeculae of osteoid and woven bone. On occasion, the wall contains an unusual lacelike pattern of calcification that is uncommon in other intraosseous lesions. The blood-filled spaces are not lined by endothelium (Fig. 14-31). In approximately 20% of the cases, aneurysmal bone cyst is associated with another pathosis, most commonly a fibro-osseous lesion or giant cell granuloma.

TREATMENT AND PROGNOSIS

Aneurysmal bone cysts of the jaws are usually treated by curettage or enucleation, sometimes supplemented with cryosurgery. The vascularity of gnathic lesions is typically low flow, and removal of the bulk of the lesion is usually sufficient to control the bleeding. Rare cases require more extensive surgical resection. In most instances, the surgical defect heals within 6 months to 1 year and does not necessitate bone grafting. Irradiation is contraindicated.

The reported recurrence rates are variable and have been as low as 8% and as high as 60%. Most recurrent examples arise from inadequate or subtotal removal on initial therapy. On occasion, recurrence may be related to incomplete removal of a coexisting lesion such as an osteoblastoma or ossifying fibroma. Overall, in spite of recurrences, the long-term prognosis appears favorable.

Fibro-Osseous Lesions of the Jaws

Fibro-osseous lesions are a diverse group of processes that are characterized by replacement of normal bone by fibrous tissue containing a newly formed mineralized product. The designation *fibro-osseous lesion* is not a specific diagnosis and describes only a process. Fibro-osseous lesions of the jaws include developmental (hamartomatous) lesions, reactive or dysplastic processes, and neoplasms.

The pathologic features on a biopsy specimen may be very similar in lesions of diverse cause, behavior, and prognosis. Clinical, radiographic, and histopathologic correlation is usually most beneficial in establishing a specific diagnosis. Commonly included among the fibro-osseous lesions of the jaws are the following:
- Fibrous dysplasia
- Cemento-osseous dysplasia
  - Focal cemento-osseous dysplasia
  - Periapical cemento-osseous dysplasia
  - Florid cemento-osseous dysplasia
- Ossifying fibroma

Although these processes have been grouped under the encompassing heading of benign fibro-osseous lesions, a more specific diagnosis often is critical because the treatment of these pathoses varies from none to surgical recontouring to complete removal. Although many examples can be diagnosed from the clinical and radiographic features, others require knowledge of the histopathologic, clinical, and radiographic features for an appropriate diagnosis.

FIBROUS DYSPLASIA

Fibrous dysplasia is a developmental tumorlike condition that is characterized by replacement of normal bone by an excessive proliferation of cellular fibrous connective tissue intermixed with irregular bony trabeculae. Although considerable confusion has existed regarding the nature of fibrous dysplasia, much has been learned about the genetics of this group of disorders, and this knowledge makes the wide variety of clinical patterns more understandable.

Fibrous dysplasia is a sporadic condition that results from a postzygotic mutation in the *GNAS1* (guanine nucleotide–binding protein, α-stimulating activity polypeptide 1) gene. Clinically, fibrous dysplasia may manifest as a localized process involving only one bone, as a condition involving multiple bones, or as multiple bone lesions in conjunction with cutaneous and endocrine abnormalities. The clinical severity of the condition presumably depends on the point in time during fetal or postnatal life that the mutation of *GNAS1* occurs.

If the mutation occurs in one of the undifferentiated stem cells during early embryologic life, the osteoblasts, melanocytes, and endocrine cells that represent the progeny of that mutated cell all will carry that mutation and express the mutated gene. The clinical presentation of multiple bone lesions, cutaneous pigmentation, and endocrine disturbances would result. Skeletal progenitor cells at later stages of embryonic development are assumed to migrate and differentiate as part of the process of normal skeletal formation. If the mutation occurs during this later period, then the progeny of the mutated cell will disperse and participate in the formation of the skeleton resulting in multiple bone lesions of fibrous dysplasia. Finally, if the mutation occurs during postnatal life, then the progeny of that mutated cell are essentially confined to one site, resulting in fibrous dysplasia affecting a single bone.

CLINICAL AND RADIOGRAPHIC FEATURES

MONOSTOTIC FIBROUS DYSPLASIA OF THE JAWS

When the disease is limited to a single bone, it is termed **monostotic fibrous dysplasia**. This type accounts for about 80% to 85% of all cases, with the jaws being among the most commonly affected sites. Although the postnatal mutation of *GNAS1* may occur during infancy, childhood, or adulthood, most examples of monostotic fibrous dysplasia are diagnosed during the second decade of life. Males and females are affected with about equal frequency. A painless swelling of the affected area is the most common feature (Fig. 14-32). Growth is generally slow, and the patient or parents are often unable to recall when the lesion was noted first. Occasionally, however, the growth may be fairly rapid. The maxilla is involved more often than the mandible.

Although mandibular lesions are truly monostotic, maxillary lesions often involve adjacent bones (e.g., zygoma, sphenoid, occipital) and are not strictly monostotic. The designation of **craniofacial fibrous dysplasia** is appropriate for these lesions. Teeth involved in the lesion usually remain firm but may be displaced by the bony mass.

The chief radiographic feature is a fine "ground-glass" opacification that results from superimposition of a myriad of poorly calcified bone trabeculae arranged in a disorganized pattern. Radiographically, the lesions

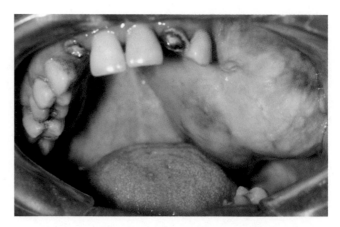

Fig. 14-32 Fibrous dysplasia. Expansile mass of the left maxilla in a 45-year-old woman. This lesion was known to have been present for at least 20 years.

of fibrous dysplasia are not well demarcated. The margins blend imperceptibly into the adjacent normal bone so that the limits of the lesion may be difficult to define (Figs. 14-33 to 14-35). In the earlier stages, the lesion may be largely radiolucent or mottled.

Involvement of the mandible often results not only in expansion of the lingual and buccal plates but also bulging of the lower border. Superior displacement of the inferior alveolar canal is not uncommon. Periapical radiographs of the involved dentition often demonstrate narrowing of the periodontal ligament space with an ill-defined lamina dura that blends with the abnormal bone pattern.

When the maxilla is involved, the lesional tissue displaces the sinus floor superiorly and commonly obliterates the maxillary sinus. Imaging studies in cases with maxillary involvement may show increased density of the base of the skull involving the occiput, sphenoid, roof of the orbit, and frontal bones (Fig. 14-36). This is said to be the most characteristic radiographic feature of fibrous dysplasia of the skull.

POLYOSTOTIC FIBROUS DYSPLASIA; JAFFE-LICHTENSTEIN SYNDROME; McCUNE-ALBRIGHT SYNDROME

Involvement of two or more bones is termed **polyostotic fibrous dysplasia**, a relatively uncommon condition. The number of involved bones varies from a few to 75% of the entire skeleton. When seen with *café au lait* (coffee with milk) pigmentation, the process is termed **Jaffe-Lichtenstein syndrome**. Polyostotic fibrous dysplasia also may be combined with *café au lait* pigmentation and multiple endocrinopathies, such as sexual precocity, pituitary adenoma, or hyperthyroidism. This pattern is known as the **McCune-Albright syndrome**. Another rare disorder associated with

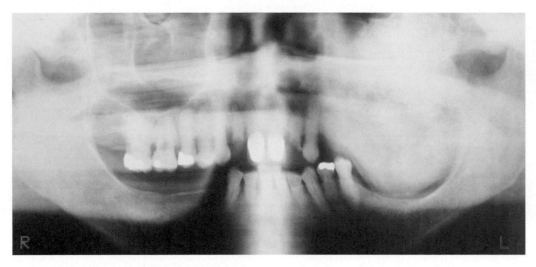

Fig. 14-33 Fibrous dysplasia. Panoramic radiograph of the patient shown in Fig. 14-32. A diffuse "ground-glass" radiopacity is evident. *(Courtesy of Dr. Richard Brock.)*

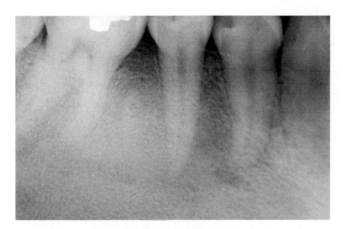

Fig. 14-34 Fibrous dysplasia. Periapical radiograph showing a diffuse "ground-glass" radiographic appearance.

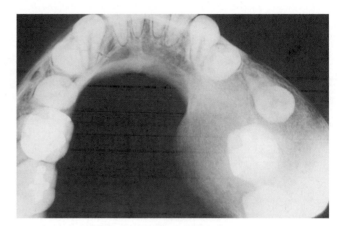

Fig. 14-35 Fibrous dysplasia. Occlusal radiograph showing localized expansion of the mandible and the "ground-glass" radiographic appearance. The margins of the lesion are not well defined and blend into the adjacent bone. *(From Waldron CA, Giansanti JS: Benign fibro-osseous lesions of the jaws: a clinical-radiologic-histologic review of 65 cases. I. Fibrous dysplasia of the jaws, Oral Surg Oral Med Oral Pathol 35:190-201, 1973.)*

fibrous dysplasia is **Mazabraud syndrome**, characterized by fibrous dysplasia in combination with intramuscular myxomas.

Although the skull and jaws may be affected with resultant facial asymmetry, the clinical picture in patients with polyostotic fibrous dysplasia is usually dominated by symptoms related to the long bone lesions (Fig. 14-37). Pathologic fracture with resulting pain and deformity is frequently noted. Leg length discrepancy is very common as a result of involvement of the upper portion of the femur (hockey stick deformity).

Hypophosphatemia caused by renal phosphate wasting is another fairly common finding among patients with polyostotic fibrous dysplasia. The mechanism for this finding appears to be related to the renal influences of circulating fibroblast growth factor 23 (FGF23), which is produced and released by affected bone.

When present, the *café au lait* pigmentation consists of well-defined, generally unilateral tan macules on the trunk and thighs. These pigmented lesions may be congenital, and pigmented oral mucosal macules also may be present. The margins of the *café au lait* spots are typically very irregular, resembling a map of the coastline of Maine (Fig. 14-38). This is in contrast to the *café au lait* spots of neurofibromatosis (see page 529), which have smooth borders (like the coast of California).

In McCune-Albright syndrome, sexual precocity is the most common endocrine manifestation of the

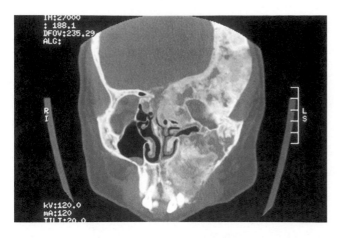

Fig. 14-36   Fibrous dysplasia. Computed tomography (CT) image showing extensive involvement of the maxilla and skull.

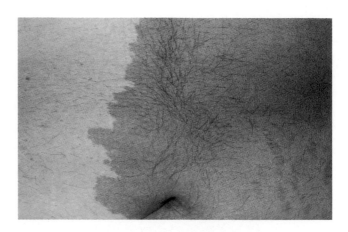

Fig. 14-38   Polyostotic fibrous dysplasia. Jaffe-Lichtenstein syndrome. *Café au lait* pigmentation of the abdomen. This is the same patient as shown in Fig. 14-37.

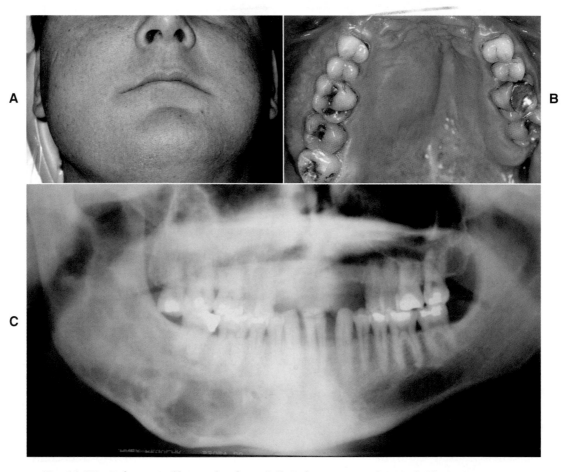

Fig. 14-37   Polyostotic fibrous dysplasia. Jaffe-Lichtenstein syndrome. **A,** Young man exhibiting enlargement of the right maxilla and mandible. **B,** Intraoral photograph showing unilateral maxillary expansion. **C,** Panoramic radiograph showing ill-defined lesions of the right side of both jaws.

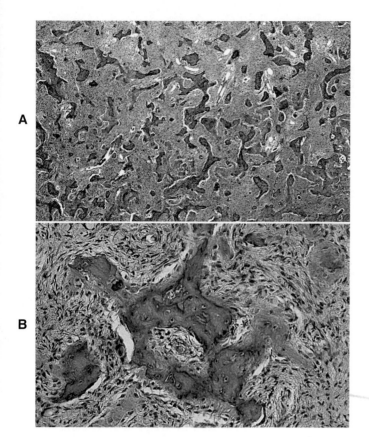

Fig. 14-39   **Fibrous dysplasia. A,** Irregularly shaped trabeculae of woven bone in a fibrous stroma. **B,** Medium-power view showing peripheral osteoid without osteoblastic rimming.

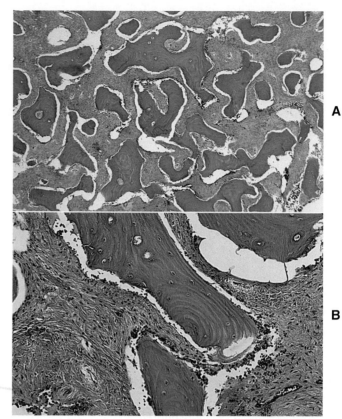

Fig. 14-40   **Mature fibrous dysplasia. A,** This long-standing lesion shows separate, broad trabeculae of bone within fibrous connective tissue. **B,** Note the lamellar maturation of the bone.

syndrome, particularly in females. Menstrual bleeding may occur during the first few months of life. Breast development and pubic hair may be apparent within the first few years of life in affected girls.

HISTOPATHOLOGIC FEATURES

The typical microscopic findings of fibrous dysplasia consist of irregularly shaped trabeculae of immature (woven) bone in a cellular, loosely arranged fibrous stroma. The bone trabeculae are not connected to each other. They often assume curvilinear shapes, which have been likened to Chinese script writing. The bone trabeculae are considered to arise by metaplasia and are not surrounded by plump appositional osteoblasts (Fig. 14-39). Tiny calcified spherules may be seen rarely but are never numerous. In contrast to ossifying fibroma and cemento-osseous dysplasia, fibrous dysplasia typically demonstrates a rather monotonous pattern throughout the lesion rather than being a haphazard mixture of woven bone, lamellar bone, and spheroid particles. The lesional bone fuses directly to

normal bone at the periphery of the lesion so that no capsule or line of demarcation is present. Although fibrous dysplasia of the long bones does not undergo maturation, jaw and skull lesions tend to be more ossified than their counterparts in the rest of the skeleton. This is particularly true in specimens from older patients.

Serial biopsy specimens in some cases have shown that histopathologically classic fibrous dysplasia of the jaws undergoes progressive maturation to a lesion consisting of lamellar bone in a moderately cellular connective tissue stroma (Fig. 14-40). The bone trabeculae in these mature lesions tend to run parallel to one another.

TREATMENT AND PROGNOSIS

Clinical management of fibrous dysplasia of the jaws may present a major problem. Although smaller lesions, particularly in the mandible, may be surgically resected in their entirety without too much difficulty, the diffuse nature and large size of many lesions, particularly those of the maxilla, preclude removal without extensive surgery. In many cases, the disease tends to stabilize and essentially stops enlarging when skeletal maturation is reached. Some lesions, however, continue to grow, although generally slowly, in adult patients.

Some patients with minimal cosmetic or functional deformity may not require or desire surgical treatment. Cosmetic deformity with associated psychologic problems or functional deformity may dictate surgical intervention in the younger patient. Such a procedure usually entails surgical reduction of the lesion to an acceptable contour without attempts to remove the entire lesion. The cosmetic result is usually good, but regrowth of the lesion occurs over time.

The prevalence of regrowth after surgical reduction is difficult to determine, but it has been estimated that between 25% and 50% of patients show some regrowth after surgical shave-down of the lesion. The regrowth is more common in younger patients, and many surgeons believe that surgical intervention should be delayed for as long as possible.

In a few studies, patients with primarily polyostotic disease have been effectively managed with bisphosphonate therapy, such as intravenous pamidronate and oral alendronate. Bisphosphonates have been shown to provide pain relief and improve skeletal strength. However, further studies are needed for adequate assessment of the risks and benefits of bisphosphonate therapy.

Malignant change, usually development of an osteosarcoma, has been rarely associated with fibrous dysplasia. Most examples have been found in patients who had received radiation therapy for fibrous dysplasia, but a few examples of spontaneous sarcomatous changes have been reported. Radiation therapy for fibrous dysplasia is contraindicated because it carries the risk for development of postirradiation bone sarcoma. It also has been suggested that patients with Mazabraud syndrome may have a slightly increased risk of sarcoma development, even in the absence of radiation exposure.

CEMENTO-OSSEOUS DYSPLASIAS (OSSEOUS DYSPLASIA)

Cemento-osseous dysplasia occurs in the tooth-bearing areas of the jaws and is probably the most common fibro-osseous lesion encountered in clinical practice. In spite of its frequency, the associated nomenclature and diagnostic criteria remain an area of debate. Because the pathologic features share many similarities with fibrous dysplasia and ossifying fibroma, correct diagnosis can be problematic but is critical to appropriate management.

Because cemento-osseous dysplasia arises in close approximation to the periodontal ligament and exhibits histopathologic similarities with the structure, some investigators have suggested these lesions are of periodontal ligament origin. Others believe cemento-osseous dysplasia represents a defect in extraligamentary bone remodeling that may be triggered by local factors and possibly correlated to an underlying hormonal imbalance.

Based on the clinical and radiographic features, it is convenient to separate cemento-osseous dysplasias into three groups: (1) **focal**, (2) **periapical**, and (3) **florid**. Although the focal pattern is somewhat different from the other two forms, it is likely that these categories may represent variants of the same pathologic process.

CLINICAL AND RADIOGRAPHIC FEATURES

FOCAL CEMENTO-OSSEOUS DYSPLASIA

Focal cemento-osseous dysplasia exhibits single site of involvement. The concept of focal cemento-osseous dysplasia was not clarified until the mid 1990s. Before that time, most cases were misdiagnosed as a variant of ossifying fibroma.

An examination of this pattern reveals slightly different epidemiology from the other two variants. About 90% of cases of focal cemento-osseous dysplasia occur in females, with an approximate mean age of 38 years and a predilection for the third to sixth decades. In contrast to the periapical and florid variants, a higher percentage of cases have been reported in whites. However, this apparent white predilection may be the result of a population bias in one of the major reported case series.

Focal cemento-osseous dysplasia may occur in any area of the jaws, but the posterior mandible is the predominant site. The disease is typically asymptomatic and is detected only on a radiographic examination. Most lesions are smaller than 1.5 cm in diameter.

Radiographically, the lesion varies from completely radiolucent to densely radiopaque with a thin peripheral radiolucent rim. Most commonly, however, there is a mixed radiolucent and radiopaque pattern (Fig. 14-41). The lesion tends to be well defined, but the borders are usually slightly irregular. Lesions occur in dentulous and edentulous areas, with many examples noted in extraction sites. Occasionally, an apparently focal lesion may represent an early stage in the transition to multifocal involvement and, as would be expected, this is seen most frequently in black females.

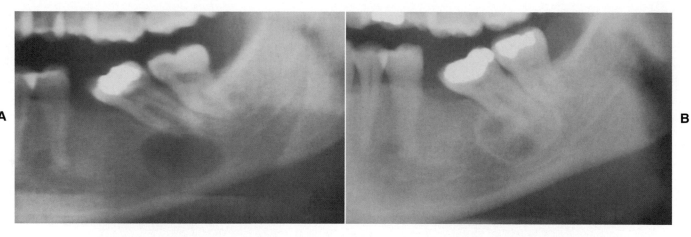

Fig. 14-41   Focal cemento-osseous dysplasia. A, A radiolucent area involves the edentulous first molar area and the apical area of the second molar. **B,** Radiograph of the same patient taken 9 years later showing a mixed radiolucent and radiopaque pattern.

PERIAPICAL CEMENTO-OSSEOUS DYSPLASIA (OSSEOUS DYSPLASIA; CEMENTAL DYSPLASIA; CEMENTOMAS)

Periapical cemento-osseous dysplasia predominantly involves the periapical region of the anterior mandible. Solitary lesions may occur, but multiple foci are present more frequently. There is a marked predilection for female patients (ranging from 10:1 to 14:1), and approximately 70% of cases affect blacks. Most patients are diagnosed initially between the ages of 30 and 50, with the diagnosis almost never made in individuals younger than age 20. Teeth associated with the lesions are almost invariably vital and seldom have restorations.

Periapical cemento-osseous dysplasia is an asymptomatic condition that is discovered when radiographs are taken for other purposes. Early lesions appear as circumscribed areas of radiolucency involving the apical area of a tooth. At this stage the lesion cannot be differentiated radiographically from a periapical granuloma or periapical cyst (Fig. 14-42). With time, adjacent lesions often fuse to form a linear pattern of radiolucency that envelops the apices of several teeth (Fig. 14-43).

Serial radiographic studies reveal that the lesions tend to "mature" over time to create a mixed radiolucent and radiopaque appearance (Fig. 14-44). In the end stage, the lesions show a circumscribed dense calcification surrounded by a narrow radiolucent rim. However, the periodontal ligament is intact, and fusion to the tooth is not seen. Individual lesions seldom exceed 1.0 cm in diameter. Each lesion is self-limiting and does not typically expand the cortex. Progressive growth seldom, if ever, occurs.

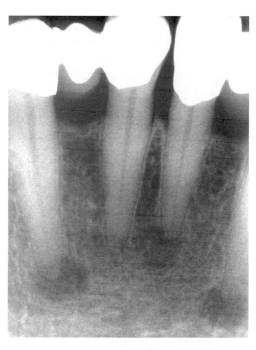

Fig. 14-42   Periapical cemento-osseous dysplasia. Periapical radiograph showing multiple radiolucent lesions at the apices of the anterior mandibular teeth. *(Courtesy of Dr. Aaron Carner.)*

FLORID CEMENTO-OSSEOUS DYSPLASIA

Florid cemento-osseous dysplasia appears with multifocal involvement not limited to the anterior mandible. Although many cases demonstrate multifocal lesions only in the posterior portions of the jaws, many patients also reveal synchronous involvement of the anterior mandible (Fig. 14-45). Like the periapical pattern, this form predominantly involves black women (in some

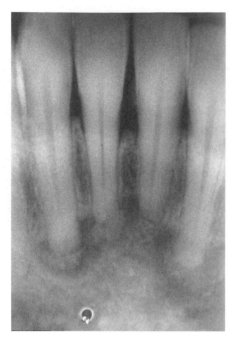

Fig. 14-43 Periapical cemento-osseous dysplasia. Later-stage lesions exhibiting significant mineralization.

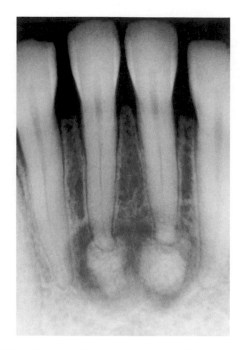

Fig. 14-44 Periapical cemento-osseous dysplasia. Later-stage lesions exhibiting significant mineralization.

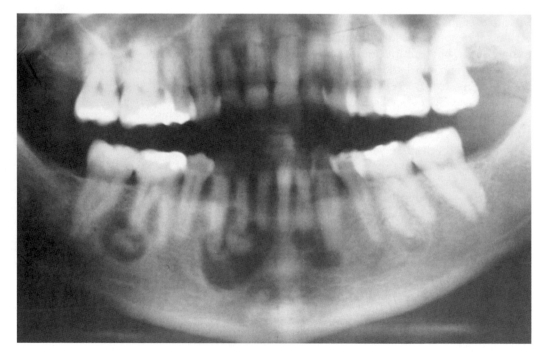

Fig. 14-45 Florid cemento-osseous dysplasia. Multiple mixed radiolucent and radiopaque lesions involving the anterior and posterior regions of the mandible.

series, more than 90% of patients), with a marked predilection for middle-aged to older adults. An intermediate frequency among East Asian populations also has been described.

The lesions show a marked tendency for bilateral and often quite symmetrical involvement, and it is not unusual to encounter extensive lesions in all four pos-

terior quadrants. The disease may be completely asymptomatic and, in such cases, is discovered only when radiographs are taken for some other purpose. In other instances, the patient may complain of dull pain, and an alveolar sinus tract may be present, exposing yellowish, avascular bone to the oral cavity (Fig. 14-46). Although rarely prominent, some degree of expansion may be noted in one or more of the involved areas.

Radiographically, the lesions typically demonstrate an identical pattern of maturation noted in the other two forms. Initially, the lesions are predominantly radiolucent but with time become mixed, then predominantly radiopaque with only a thin peripheral radiolucent rim (Fig. 14-47). On occasion, a lesion can become almost totally radiopaque and blend with the adjacent normal-appearing bone. Although it is most common for the radiopacities to remain separated from adjacent teeth with an intervening intact periodontal ligament space, in some cases fusion of cemento-osseous material directly on the tooth root surface may be observed in end-stage lesions. Such a process may result in thickened root apices surrounded by radiolucency (or a "hypercementosis-like" appearance).

Both dentulous and edentulous areas may be affected, and involvement appears to be unrelated to the presence or absence of teeth. More sharply defined radiolucent areas, which on surgical exploration prove to be simple bone cysts (see page 631), may be intermixed with the other lesional elements. The cysts may be single or multiple and, in some cases, represent a sizable portion of the lesion. It has been suggested that these simple bone cysts arise from obstruction to drainage of the normal interstitial fluid by the fibro-osseous proliferation.

HISTOPATHOLOGIC FEATURES

All three patterns of cemento-osseous dysplasia demonstrate similar histopathologic features. The tissue consists of fragments of cellular mesenchymal tissue composed of spindle-shaped fibroblasts and collagen fibers with numerous small blood vessels (Fig. 14-48). Free hemorrhage is typically noted interspersed throughout the lesion.

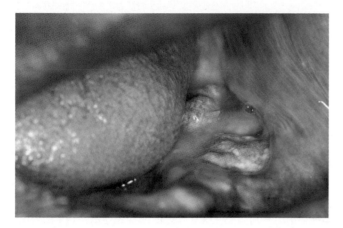

Fig. 14-46   Florid cemento-osseous dysplasia. Yellowish, avascular cementum-like material is beginning to exfoliate through the oral mucosa.

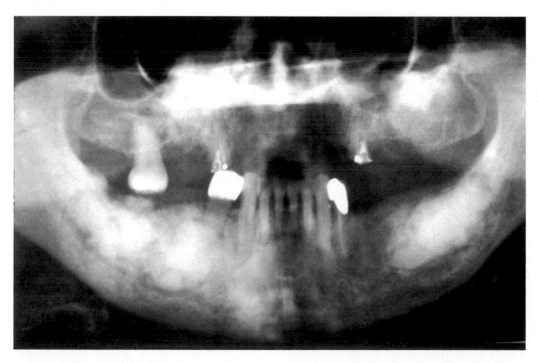

Fig. 14-47   Florid cemento-osseous dysplasia. Multifocal radiopaque lesions of the posterior areas of the jaws. *(Courtesy of Dr. Solomon Israel.)*

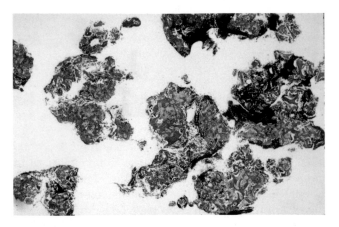

Fig. 14-48 Cemento-osseous dysplasia. Low-power photomicrograph showing fragments of cellular fibrous connective tissue containing scattered trabeculae of bone.

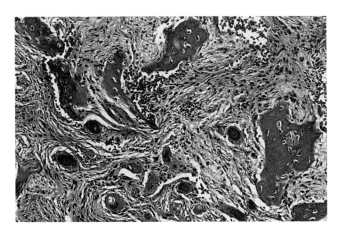

Fig. 14-49 Cemento-osseous dysplasia. High-power photomicrograph showing spicules of bone and cementum-like hard tissue within moderately cellular fibrous connective tissue. Note the hemorrhage around the bony trabeculae.

Within this fibrous connective tissue background is a mixture of woven bone, lamellar bone, and cementum-like particles (Fig. 14-49). The proportion of each mineralized material varies from lesion to lesion and from area to area in individual sites of involvement. As the lesions mature and become more sclerotic, the ratio of fibrous connective tissue to mineralized material decreases. With maturation, the bone trabeculae become thick curvilinear structures that have been said to resemble the shape of ginger roots. With progression to the final radiopaque stage, individual trabeculae fuse and form lobular masses composed of sheets or fused globules of relatively acellular and disorganized cemento-osseous material (Fig. 14-50).

DIAGNOSIS

In most instances of periapical or florid cemento-osseous dysplasia, the distinctive clinical and radiographic patterns (e.g., a black female patient with

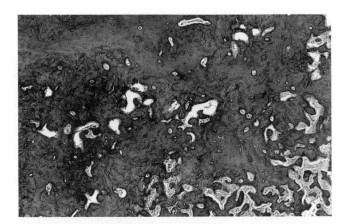

Fig. 14-50 Cemento-osseous dysplasia. Late-stage lesion showing a sclerotic mass of cemento-osseous material.

multiquadrant involvement or multiple lesions involving vital lower incisor teeth) allow a strong presumptive diagnosis without the necessity of biopsy. The features of focal cemento-osseous dysplasia are less specific and often mandate surgical investigation. Even on histopathologic review, distinguishing focal cemento-osseous dysplasia from ossifying fibroma often can be difficult. The findings at surgery are very helpful in discriminating between these two lesions. Before the final sclerotic stage, cemento-osseous dysplasia consists of easily fragmented and gritty tissue that can be curetted easily from the defect but does not separate cleanly from the adjacent normal bone. In contrast, ossifying fibromas tend to separate cleanly from the bone and are removed in one or several large masses.

Several histopathologic features also can help to confirm the impression obtained from the surgical and gross descriptions. Although cemento-osseous dysplasia and ossifying fibroma demonstrate a mixture of bone and cementum-like particles, the trabeculae in ossifying fibroma tend to be more delicate and often demonstrate osteoblastic rimming. The cementum-like particles in cemento-osseous dysplasia are irregularly shaped and often exhibit retraction from the adjacent stroma, whereas those in ossifying fibroma are more ovoid and often demonstrate brush borders in intimate association with the adjacent stroma. Although ossifying fibroma can exhibit hemorrhage along the margins of the specimen, cemento-osseous dysplasia typically reveals free hemorrhage throughout the lesion and a sinusoidal vascularity in close association with the bony trabeculae.

TREATMENT AND PROGNOSIS

The various forms of cemento-osseous dysplasia do not appear neoplastic; therefore, they generally do not require removal. However, these lesions can cause significant clinical problems for some patients. During the predominantly radiolucent phase, the lesions cause few problems. Once significant sclerosis is present, the lesions of cemento-osseous dysplasia tend to be hypovascular and prone to necrosis with minimal provocation. For the asymptomatic patient, the best management consists of regular recall examinations with prophylaxis and reinforcement of good home hygiene care to control periodontal disease and prevent tooth loss.

Because the onset of symptoms is usually associated with exposure of the sclerotic masses to the oral cavity, biopsy or elective extraction of teeth should be avoided. In other instances, symptoms begin after exposure of the sclerotic masses to the oral cavity as a result of progressive alveolar atrophy under a denture. Affected patients should be encouraged to retain their teeth to prevent development of symptoms later.

Management of the symptomatic patient is more difficult. At this stage, there is an inflammatory component to the disease and the process is basically a chronic osteomyelitis involving dysplastic bone and cementum. Antibiotics may be indicated but often are not effective. Sequestration of the sclerotic cementum-like masses occurs slowly and is followed by healing. Saucerization of dead bone may speed healing. Although a single case of a malignant fibrous histiocytoma arising within a focus of florid cemento-osseous dysplasia has been reported, such neoplastic transformation appears unique, and the prognosis for patients with cemento-osseous dysplasia is good.

When simple bone cysts arise within foci of cemento-osseous dysplasia, surgical exploration is necessary to establish the diagnosis. These simple bone cysts often do not heal as rapidly as those noted in a younger patient who does not have cemento-osseous dysplasia. In some cases the cysts persist or enlarge after surgical intervention; when they fill in, the bone retains an abnormal radiographic appearance. To assist healing, the cyst and the surrounding fibro-osseous proliferation are usually curetted thoroughly.

FAMILIAL GIGANTIFORM CEMENTOMA

Although the term *gigantiform cementoma* has been used in the past as a synonym for florid cemento-osseous dysplasia, most authorities now restrict use of this term to an uncommon hereditary disorder that is significantly different from conventional cemento-osseous dysplasia. **Familial gigantiform cementoma** is a disorder of gnathic bone that ultimately leads to the formation of massive sclerotic masses of disorganized mineralized material.

CLINICAL AND RADIOGRAPHIC FINDINGS

Familial gigantiform cementoma is an autosomal dominant disorder that demonstrates high penetrance and variable expressivity. Although the majority of reported cases have occurred in whites, well-documented examples have been seen in African blacks. No sexual predilection has been observed.

Most affected patients begin to develop radiographic alterations during the first decade of life. By adolescence, clinically obvious alterations are typically noted and are followed by a rapid and expansive growth pattern (Fig. 14-51). The osseous pathosis appears limited to the jaws and typically demonstrates multifocal involvement of both the maxilla and the mandible. Although the course is variable, the gnathic enlargement in most patients results in significant facial deformity, as well as impaction, malposition, and malocclusion of the involved dentition. If not treated, then the osseous enlargement eventually ceases during the fifth decade.

Radiographically, the initial features resemble those seen in cemento-osseous dysplasia, appearing as multiple radiolucencies in the periapical regions. With progression, the affected sites expand to replace much of the normal bone within the involved quadrant and develop a mixed radiolucent and radiopaque pattern. With further maturation, the lesions become predominantly radiopaque but often maintain a thin radiolucent rim.

As noted in cemento-osseous dysplasia, the affected bone during the final radiopaque stage is very sensitive to inflammatory stimuli and becomes necrotic with minimal provocation. Before therapy, some investigators have reported elevated serum alkaline phosphatase that subsequently declines after surgical removal of the osseous proliferations. Anemia also has been reported in a number of affected females in different kindreds. In one family, all affected females demonstrated multifocal polypoid adenomas of the uterus that were associated with chronic hemorrhage and thought responsible for the anemia. A gynecologic examination appears prudent in all affected females, especially those with anemia. In two kindreds, bone fragility and tendency for long bone fractures were noted. It is not clear whether such patients might fall within a spectrum that also includes cases reported as osteogenesis imperfecta with associated fibro-osseous lesions of the jaws.

Sporadic cases with clinical and radiographic features similar to those of familial gigantiform cementoma also have been reported. It is possible that these cases may represent spontaneous mutations. Some of these nonfamilial cases have been termed *multiple (cemento-) ossifying fibromas* or *bilateral ossifying fibromas*.

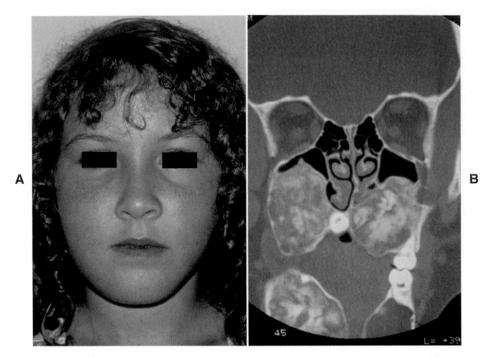

Fig. 14-51   Familial gigantiform cementoma. Young woman with massive lesions involving all four quadrants of the jaws. (**A** *from Abdelsayed RA, Eversole LR, Singh BS et al: Gigantiform cementoma: clinicopathologic presentation of 3 cases,* Oral Surg Oral Med Oral Pathol Oral Radiol Endod 91:438-444, 2001; **B** *courtesy of Dr. Rafik Abdelsayed.*)

Whether such cases are best considered multiple cemento-ossifying fibromas, sporadic cases of familial gigantiform cementoma, or unusual progressive forms of cemento-osseous dysplasia remains unclear. Future insights into the genetic basis and molecular pathogenesis of this problematic spectrum of diseases may improve the understanding and appropriate classification of such cases.

HISTOPATHOLOGIC FEATURES

Histopathologically, familial gigantiform cementoma shows the same spectrum of changes seen in florid cemento-osseous dysplasia, and the two cannot be distinguished microscopically.

TREATMENT AND PROGNOSIS

Before the final sclerotic stage, attempts to improve aesthetics by shave-down surgical procedures have not been successful because the dysplastic tissue rapidly regrows. Once the lesions are predominantly radiopaque, partial removal may lead to sequestration of the remaining affected bone. Therefore, extensive resection of the altered bone and reconstruction of the facial skeleton and associated soft tissues have been recommended and can produce acceptable functional and aesthetic results. The extent of the required surgi-

cal procedures often is greater for patients who are treated during the later stages of the disease.

OSSIFYING FIBROMA (CEMENTIFYING FIBROMA; CEMENTO-OSSIFYING FIBROMA)

Although it can resemble focal cemento-osseous dysplasia radiographically and, to a lesser extent, histopathologically, **ossifying fibroma** is a true neoplasm with a significant growth potential. Before the refining of the concept of focal cemento-osseous dysplasia in the mid 1990s, ossifying fibroma was thought to be a common neoplasm. In reality, true ossifying fibromas are relatively rare, with many previously reported examples actually being focal cemento-osseous dysplasia.

The neoplasm is composed of fibrous tissue that contains a variable mixture of bony trabeculae, cementum-like spherules, or both. Although the lesions do contain a variety of mineralized structures, most authorities agree the same progenitor cell produces the different materials. It has been suggested that the origin of these tumors is odontogenic or from periodontal ligament, but microscopically identical neoplasms with cementum-like differentiation also have been reported in the orbital, frontal, ethmoid, sphenoid, and temporal bones, leaving these prior theories of origin open to

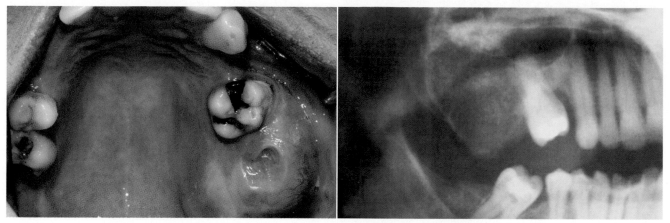

Fig. 14-52   Ossifying fibroma. A, Enlargement of the posterior maxilla caused by a large ossifying fibroma. **B,** Note the mixed radiolucent and radiopaque lesion expanding the posterior maxilla.

question. Today, many authorities prefer to designate the cementum-like material present in ossifying fibromas as a variation of bone. The designations ossifying fibroma, cemento-ossifying fibroma, and cementifying fibroma are all appropriate for this tumor and continue to be used by many. In spite of this, however, it is agreed that these are the same lesion and are classified best as osteogenic neoplasms. In this section, all of these variations are combined under the term *ossifying fibroma*.

Recently, mutations in the tumor suppressor gene *HRPT2* were identified in patients with a rare condition known as *hyperparathyroidism-jaw tumor syndrome*, which is characterized by parathyroid adenoma or carcinoma, ossifying fibromas of the jaws, renal cysts, and Wilms' tumors. This discovery led to the subsequent finding of *HRPT2* gene mutations in two sporadic cases of ossifying fibroma of the jaws. The function of the *HRPT2* protein product (known as *parafibromin*) and the mechanism by which mutations in this gene lead to tumor formation are not well understood.

CLINICAL AND RADIOGRAPHIC FEATURES

The epidemiology of ossifying fibroma is unclear because many previous reports confused focal cemento-osseous dysplasia with true ossifying fibromas. It appears ossifying fibromas occur across a wide age range, with the greatest number of cases encountered during the third and fourth decades of life. There is a definite female predilection, with the mandible involved far more often than the maxilla. The mandibular premolar and molar area is the most common site.

Small lesions seldom cause any symptoms and are detected only on radiographic examination. Larger tumors result in a painless swelling of the involved bone (Fig. 14-52); they may cause obvious facial asymmetry, which on occasion reaches grotesque size. Pain and paresthesia are rarely associated with an ossifying fibroma.

Radiographically, the lesion most often is well defined and unilocular. Some examples show a sclerotic border. Depending on the amount of calcified material produced in the tumor, it may appear completely radiolucent; more often, varying degrees of radiopacity are noted. True ossifying fibromas that become largely radiopaque with only a thin radiolucent periphery are uncommon; many reported examples with this radiographic pattern likely represent end-stage focal cemento-osseous dysplasia. Root divergence or resorption of roots of teeth associated with the tumor may be seen. Large ossifying fibromas of the mandible often demonstrate a characteristic downward bowing of the inferior cortex of the mandible.

HISTOPATHOLOGIC FEATURES

At surgical exploration, the lesion is well demarcated from the surrounding bone, thus permitting relatively easy separation of the tumor from its bony bed. A few ossifying fibromas will show, grossly and microscopically, a fibrous capsule surrounding the tumor. Most are not encapsulated but are well demarcated grossly and microscopically from the surrounding bone.

On gross examination, the tumor is usually submitted in one mass or as a few large pieces (Fig. 14-53). Ossifying fibromas consist of fibrous tissue that exhibits varying degrees of cellularity and contains mineralized

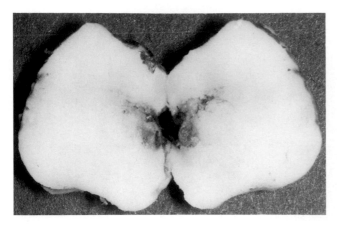

Fig. 14-53 Ossifying fibroma. Gross specimen showing a well-circumscribed tumor that shelled out in one piece.

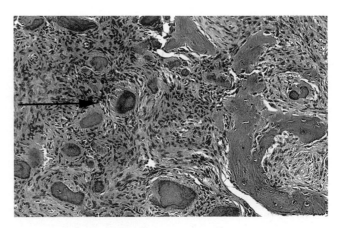

Fig. 14-55 Ossifying fibroma. High-power photomicrograph showing a mixture of woven bone and cementum-like material. Note the spherules demonstrating peripheral brush borders (*arrow*).

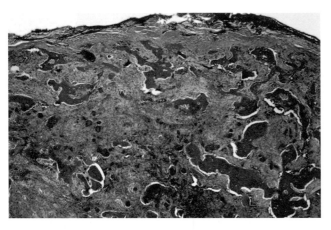

Fig. 14-54 Ossifying fibroma. This low-magnification photomicrograph shows a well-circumscribed solid tumor mass. Trabeculae of bone and droplets of cementum-like material can be seen forming within a background of cellular fibrous connective tissue.

material (Fig. 14-54). The hard tissue portion may be in the form of trabeculae of osteoid and bone or basophilic and poorly cellular spherules that resemble cementum. Admixtures of the two types are typical. The bony trabeculae vary in size and frequently demonstrate a mixture of woven and lamellar patterns. Peripheral osteoid and osteoblastic rimming are usually present. The spherules of cementum-like material often demonstrate peripheral brush borders that blend into the adjacent connective tissue (Fig. 14-55). Significant intralesional hemorrhage is unusual. Variation in the types of mineralized material produced may be helpful in distinguishing ossifying fibroma from fibrous dysplasia, which has a more uniform pattern of osseous differentiation.

TREATMENT AND PROGNOSIS

The circumscribed nature of the ossifying fibroma generally permits enucleation of the tumor with relative ease. Some examples, however, which have grown large and destroyed considerable bone, may necessitate surgical resection and bone grafting. The prognosis, however, is very good, and recurrence after removal of the tumor is rarely encountered. There is no evidence that ossifying fibromas ever undergo malignant change.

JUVENILE OSSIFYING FIBROMA (JUVENILE ACTIVE OSSIFYING FIBROMA; JUVENILE AGGRESSIVE OSSIFYING FIBROMA)

The **juvenile ossifying fibroma** is a controversial lesion that has been distinguished from the larger group of ossifying fibromas on the basis of the age of the patients, most common sites of involvement, and clinical behavior. Two different neoplasms have been reported under the term, and disagreement exists over the spectrum of what should be accepted as juvenile ossifying fibromas. Although the two forms demonstrate different histopathologic and clinical features, several investigators have chosen to compromise and accept two patterns of juvenile ossifying fibroma: (1) **trabecular** and (2) **psammomatoid**. Among lesions involving the craniofacial skeleton, the number of psammomatoid cases reported exceeds the number of trabecular cases reported by a ratio of approximately 4:1.

A recent study of three cases of the psammomatoid variant arising in the orbit of adolescent boys demon-

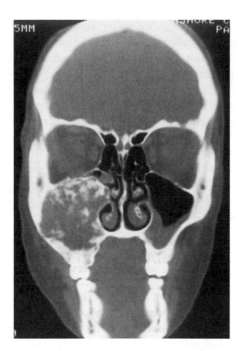

Fig. 14-56   Juvenile ossifying fibroma. Computed tomography (CT) scan showing a large tumor involving the left maxilla and maxillary sinus of a 12-year-old girl. Clinically, the tumor was growing rapidly.

strated the presence of nonrandom chromosomal breakpoints at Xq26 and 2q33 resulting in (X;2) translocation. Although no similar studies have been reported with respect to the trabecular variant, it is possible that future insights into the cytogenetic abnormalities of these two variants may aid in defining them as distinct entities.

CLINICAL AND RADIOGRAPHIC FEATURES

In most instances, the neoplasms often grow rapidly, are well-circumscribed, and lack continuity with the adjacent normal bone. The lesions are circumscribed radiolucencies that in some cases contain central radiopacities (Fig. 14-56). In some cases "ground glass" opacification may be observed. Those present within a sinus may appear radiodense and often create a clouding that may be confused with sinusitis.

The age at diagnosis varies, with reported cases occurring in patients from younger than 6 months to older than 70 years of age. Although both patterns reveal similar radiographic features and growth patterns, the trabecular form is diagnosed initially in younger patients. The mean age of trabecular juvenile ossifying fibromas is approximately 11 years, whereas the mean age of patients diagnosed with the psammomatoid variant approaches 22 years. Both forms exhibit a slight male predilection and occur in either jaw but reveal a maxillary predominance. Although many of these tumors are initially discovered on routine radiographic examination, cortical expansion may result in clinically detectable facial enlargement. The psammomatoid variant frequently appears outside the jaws, with more than 70% arising in the orbital and frontal bones and paranasal sinuses.

Complications secondary to the neoplasm are typically the result of impingement on neighboring structures. With persistent growth, lesions arising in the paranasal sinuses penetrate the orbital, nasal, and cranial cavities. Nasal obstruction, exophthalmos, or proptosis may be seen. Rarely, temporary or permanent blindness occurs.

Intracranial extension has been discovered in neoplasms arising adjacent to the cribriform plates. Because of the circumscribed growth pattern of the tumor, the frontal lobe is typically elevated without any associated neurologic signs. Rarely, intracranial extension has resulted in meningitis, with one report of a maxillary tumor leading to convulsions and death from pneumococcal meningitis.

In some cases of the psammomatoid variant, development of an aneurysmal bone cyst has been reported. Such cystic changes tend to occur in younger patients in the first and second decades of life and have been associated with large maxillary lesions exhibiting aggressive behavior.

HISTOPATHOLOGIC FEATURES

Both patterns are typically nonencapsulated but well demarcated from the surrounding bone. The tumor consists of cellular fibrous connective tissue that exhibits areas that are loose and other zones that are so cellular that the cytoplasm of individual cells is hard to discern because of nuclear crowding. Myxomatous foci are not rare and often are associated with pseudocystic degeneration. Mitotic figures can be found but are not numerous. Areas of hemorrhage and small clusters of multinucleated giant cells are usually seen.

The mineralized component in the two patterns is very different. The trabecular variant shows irregular strands of highly cellular osteoid encasing plump and irregular osteocytes (Fig. 14-57). These strands often are lined by plump osteoblasts and in other areas by multinucleated osteoclasts. In contrast, the psammomatoid pattern forms concentric lamellated and spherical ossicles that vary in shape and typically have basophilic centers with peripheral eosinophilic osteoid rims (Fig. 14-58). A peripheral brush border blending into the surrounding stroma is noted in many of the ossicles. Occasionally, individual ossicles undergo remodeling and form crescentic shapes.

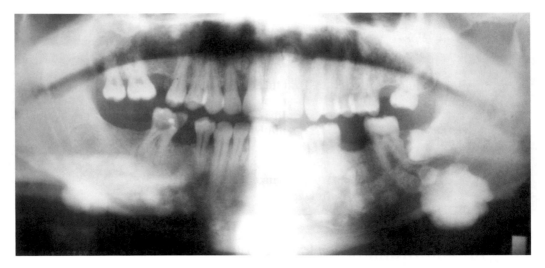

Fig. 14-61   Gardner syndrome. Panoramic radiograph showing multiple osteomas of the mandible.

CLINICAL AND RADIOGRAPHIC FEATURES

The reported prevalence of Gardner syndrome varies from 1:8300 to 1:16,000 live births. The associated colonic polyps typically develop during the second decade; because these are adenomatous, they ultimately transform into adenocarcinoma. In addition, detection of extracolonic polyps is not rare in the small intestine or stomach, with a small percentage exhibiting carcinomatous transformation.

Up to 90% of patients with Gardner syndrome demonstrate skeletal abnormalities, the most common of which are osteomas. Although the osteomas may affect any part of the skeleton, the most commonly involved areas are the skull, paranasal sinuses, and the mandible. When gnathic lesions are seen, they often occur in the region of the mandibular angles and are frequently associated with prominent facial deformity (Fig. 14-61). The osteomas are usually noted during puberty and precede the development of, or any symptoms from, the bowel polyps (Fig. 14-62). Most patients demonstrate between three and six osseous lesions. The osteomas appear as areas of increased radiodensity that vary from slight thickenings to large masses. On occasion, large osteomas of the mandible or condyle will limit the mandibular opening. Dental abnormalities include an increased prevalence of odontomas, supernumerary teeth, and impacted teeth. Although up to 20% of affected patients demonstrate supernumerary teeth, the frequency of extra teeth is not nearly as high as that noted in cleidocranial dysplasia.

Most patients show one or several epidermoid cysts of the skin (Fig. 14-63). Desmoid tumors (locally aggressive fibrous neoplasms) of the soft tissue arise in

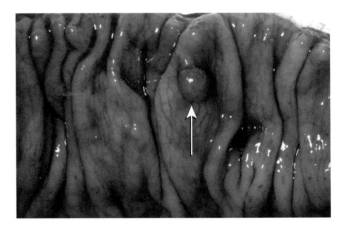

Fig. 14-62   Gardner syndrome. A segment of resected large bowel showing polyp formation (*arrow*).

approximately 10% of affected patients. These lesions are three times more frequent in females and often develop in the abdominal scar that forms after colectomy.

Although lesser known, an increased prevalence of thyroid carcinoma also is noted, with females demonstrating a 100-fold increase. In addition, pigmented lesions of the ocular fundus are evident in nearly 90% of affected patients. Identification of this ocular abnormality is useful when evaluating patients for the syndrome.

HISTOPATHOLOGIC FEATURES

Histopathologically, the osteomas are generally of the compact type. An individual lesion cannot be differentiated microscopically from a solitary osteoma.

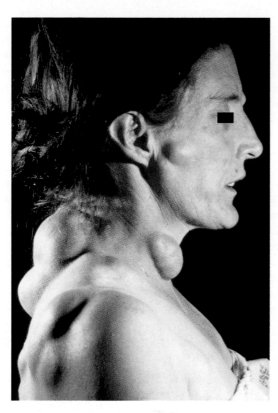

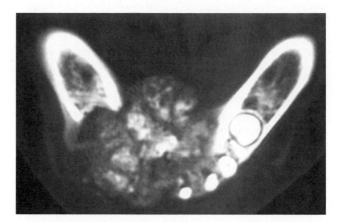

Fig. 14-64   Osteoblastoma. Computed tomography (CT) image showing a large, destructive radiolucent and radiopaque lesion of the mandible. *(Courtesy of Dr. Ed Marshall.)*

Fig. 14-63   Gardner syndrome. This patient has multiple, large epidermoid cysts. *(Courtesy of Dr. William Welton.)*

TREATMENT AND PROGNOSIS

The major problem for patients with Gardner syndrome is the high rate of malignant transformation of bowel polyps into invasive adenocarcinoma. By age 30, about 50% of patients with Gardner syndrome will develop colorectal carcinoma. The frequency of malignant change approaches 100% in older patients.

Prophylactic colectomy is usually recommended. Removal of jaw osteomas and epidermoid cysts for cosmetic reasons sometimes may be indicated, but the long-term prognosis depends on the behavior of the bowel adenocarcinomas.

OSTEOBLASTOMA AND OSTEOID OSTEOMA

Osteoblastoma and **osteoid osteoma** are closely related benign bone tumors that arise from osteoblasts. There is general agreement that the histopathologic features of these two lesions are identical, but it has been shown that the tumor nidus in osteoid osteomas contains a concentration of peripheral nerves not seen in other fibro-osseous neoplasms. In addition, the tumor produces prostaglandins that result in significant pain that is relieved by prostaglandin inhibitors such as aspirin. Classically, the distinction depends on the size of the lesion, with osteoid osteoma being smaller than 2 cm and osteoblastoma being larger than 2 cm. Some authors prefer to classify both of these lesions as *osteoblastomas.*

The features of the cementoblastoma closely resemble those present in the osteoblastoma. A number of noted authorities in orthopedic pathology consider cementoblastoma and osteoblastoma to be identical lesions and prefer to designate both as *osteoblastomas.* Because of significant radiographic and histopathologic similarities, the primary difference between an osteoblastoma and a cementoblastoma depends on whether the lesion is fused to a tooth or not, and this ability is most likely because of the final histodifferentiation of the tumor cells. Because of these similarities, cementoblastoma is presented in the next section of this chapter rather than in Chapter 15.

CLINICAL AND RADIOGRAPHIC FEATURES

OSTEOBLASTOMA

Osteoblastomas are rarely encountered and represent less than 1% of all bone tumors. The most frequently affected bones are the vertebral column, sacrum, calvarium, long bones, and the small bones of the hands and feet. For those developing within the jaws, there is a slight mandibular predilection, with most examples arising in the posterior regions. Approximately 85% of gnathic osteoblastomas occur before age 30, and there is a slight female predominance among reported cases.

Most osteoblastomas are between 2 and 4 cm, but they may be as large as 10 cm. Pain, tenderness, and swelling are common presenting features. In contrast to the osteoid osteoma, aspirin usually does not relieve the pain associated with an osteoblastoma. In many cases, pain may be misinterpreted as evidence of odontogenic infection. Lesions adjacent to teeth may lead to tooth mobility, root resorption, or tooth displacement. Radiographically, the osteoblastoma may appear as a well-defined or ill-defined radiolucent lesion often with patchy areas of mineralization (Fig. 14-64). Other lesions demonstrate considerable mineralization. Although frequently noted in osteoid osteomas, reactive sclerosis surrounding the lesion is not a constant feature. Most osteoblastomas arise within medullary bone; however, in some instances, an osteoblastoma may present as a bony outgrowth projecting from the periosteum without evidence of a more central destructive process. Such lesions are termed *periosteal osteoblastomas.*

A small group of osteoblastomas (**aggressive osteoblastomas**) is characterized by more atypical histopathologic features and locally aggressive behavior. These tumors usually occur in older patients, with most being older than 30 years of age. A variety of bones, including the mandible, may be involved. Aggressive osteoblastomas tend to be larger than conventional osteoblastomas and typically measure greater than 4 cm in diameter. Pain is a common symptom and may be severe. Radiographically, these lesions show the features of conventional osteoblastomas but tend to be larger.

OSTEOID OSTEOMA

Osteoid osteomas occur most often in the femur, tibia, and phalanges. They are very rare in the jaws. Pain is the most common presenting symptom. It is usually nocturnal in nature and alleviated by salicylates. However, nocturnal pain relieved by aspirin has been documented more often among extragnathic lesions than jaw lesions. Radiographically, the osteoid osteoma appears as a well-circumscribed radiolucent defect, usually less than 1 cm in diameter, with a surrounding zone of reactive sclerosis of varying thickness. A small radiopaque nidus may be present, resulting in a target-like appearance radiographically (Fig. 14-65).

HISTOPATHOLOGIC FEATURES

The lesions reveal mineralized material that demonstrates prominent reversal lines. The material may be present in large sheets or irregular trabeculae. At the periphery of the large masses and surrounding the trabeculae are scattered multinucleated osteoclast-like cells and numerous osteoblasts that have ample cytoplasm and hyperchromatic nuclei (Fig. 14-66). The supporting stroma consists of loose fibrous connective tissue that contains scattered dilated vascular channels. Focal areas of hemorrhage are not rare, and osteoblastomas occasionally exhibit a central zone of increased vascularity.

Microscopically, aggressive osteoblastomas are characterized by the presence of large (epithelioid) osteoblasts with increased mitotic activity and nontrabecular sheets or lacelike areas of osteoid production. On occasion, osteoblastomas may demonstrate a rich cellularity that has led to erroneous diagnoses of osteosarcoma. Differentiation between some osteoblastomas and low-grade osteosarcomas may be very difficult. Some low-grade osteosarcomas may closely resemble the microscopic appearance of osteoblastomas, and some lesions may have microscopic features intermediate between osteoblastoma and osteosarcoma.

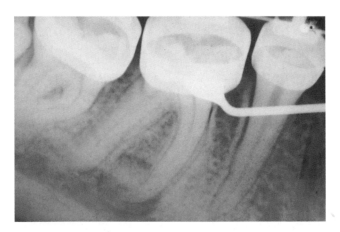

Fig. 14-65 Osteoid osteoma. A circumscribed, mixed radiolucent and radiopaque lesion near the apex of mesial root of mandibular first molar. The patient had dull, nocturnal pain that was relieved by aspirin. *(Courtesy of Dr. Ellen Eisenberg.)*

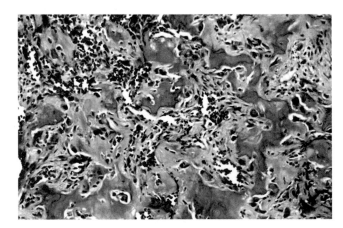

Fig. 14-66 Osteoblastoma. High-power photomicrograph showing irregular bony trabeculae with prominent osteoblastic rimming and osteoclasts.

TREATMENT AND PROGNOSIS

Most cases of osteoid osteoma and osteoblastoma are treated by local excision or curettage. The prognosis is good, and some lesions will regress even after incomplete excision. A small number of lesions will recur; in rare instances, an osteoblastoma may undergo transformation into an osteosarcoma. Although about 50% of aggressive osteoblastomas will recur, metastasis or death from the tumor has not been reported.

CEMENTOBLASTOMA (TRUE CEMENTOMA)

Cementoblastoma is an odontogenic neoplasm of cementoblasts, and many authorities believe this neoplasm represents the only true neoplasm of cementum.

CLINICAL AND RADIOGRAPHIC FEATURES

Cementoblastomas are rare neoplasms, representing less than 1% of all odontogenic tumors. Greater than 75% arise in the mandible, with 90% arising in the molar and premolar region. Almost 50% involve the first permanent molar. Impacted or unerupted teeth rarely may be affected as well. Cementoblastomas rarely affect deciduous teeth. There is no significant sex predilection. The neoplasm occurs predominantly in children and young adults, with about 50% arising before the age of 20 years and 75% occurring before the age of 30 years. Pain and swelling are present in approximately two thirds of reported patients. Although most investigators consider the cementoblastoma to represent a rather innocuous neoplasm, signs of locally aggressive behavior may be observed, including bony expansion, cortical erosion, displacement of adjacent teeth, envelopment of multiple adjacent teeth, maxillary sinus involvement, and infiltration into the pulp chamber and root canals.

Radiographically, the tumor appears as a radiopaque mass that is fused to one or more tooth roots and is surrounded by a thin radiolucent rim (Fig. 14-67). The outline of the root or roots of the involved tooth is usually obscured as a result of root resorption and fusion of the tumor with the tooth.

HISTOPATHOLOGIC FEATURES

The histopathologic presentation of cementoblastoma closely resembles that of osteoblastoma, with the primary distinguishing feature being tumor fusion with the involved tooth (Fig. 14-68). The majority of the tumor consists of sheets and thick trabeculae of mineralized material with irregularly placed lacunae and prominent basophilic reversal lines. Cellular fibrovascular tissue is present between the mineralized trabeculae. Multinucleated giant cells often are present, and prominent blastlike cells frequently line the mineralized trabeculae (Fig. 14-69). The periphery of the lesion, corresponding to the radiolucent zone seen on the radiograph, is composed of uncalcified matrix, which often is arranged in radiating columns. In few instances, the lesion may infiltrate the pulp chamber and root canals of the involved tooth.

TREATMENT AND PROGNOSIS

Treatment of a cementoblastoma usually consists of surgical extraction of the tooth together with the attached calcified mass. Surgical excision of the mass

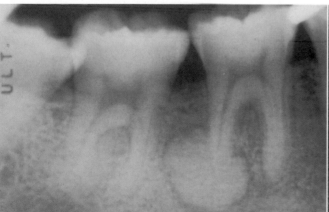 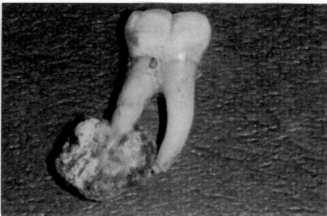

Fig. 14-67 **Cementoblastoma. A,** A densely mineralized mass is seen at the apex of the distal root of the first molar. The root is partially resorbed. **B,** The surgical specimen shows that the mass is attached to the root. *(Courtesy of Dr. John Wright.)*

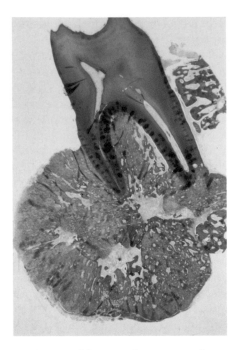

Fig. 14-68 Cementoblastoma. Low-power photomicrograph showing the tumor attached to the roots of the tooth.

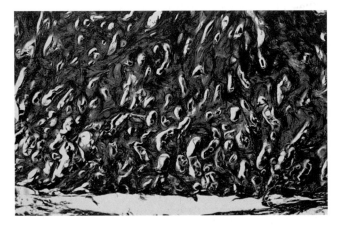

Fig. 14-69 Cementoblastoma. Mineralized tissue containing numerous plump cementoblasts.

with root amputation and endodontic treatment of the involved tooth may be considered. In the past, this tumor has been considered to exhibit a very low recurrence rate, although a recently reported series of a large number of cases suggests recurrences may be more common than previously thought, with an overall recurrence rate as high as 22%. Completeness of removal is most closely related to recurrence. Total removal of the mass and the associated tooth minimizes but does not completely eliminate the chance of recurrence. Progressive growth of the tumor after extraction of the involved tooth and incomplete removal of the mass has been documented.

CHONDROMA

Chondromas are benign tumors composed of mature hyaline cartilage. Chondromas are one of the more common bone tumors and are located most often in the short tubular bones of the hands and feet. However, a diagnosis of chondroma in the jaws, facial bones, and base of the skull should be viewed with great skepticism because many so-called benign chondromas of the craniofacial complex have recurred and acted in a malignant manner. No major series has reported enchondromas arising in the craniofacial bones. In spite of this, individual reports and small series of gnathic chondromas can be found, with most examples thought to arise from vestigial cartilaginous rests. Such rests are located in the anterior maxilla, symphysis, coronoid process, and condyle.

CLINICAL AND RADIOGRAPHIC FEATURES

Chondromas usually arise in the third and fourth decades without a significant sex predilection. Most gnathic examples have been found in the condyle or anterior maxilla of adult patients. When arising in the jaw, most chondromas are painless and slowly growing tumors. Tooth mobility and root resorption are noted occasionally. Radiographically, chondromas typically appear as radiolucencies with central areas of radiopacity.

In most cases, chondromas arise in a single site. Multiple and widespread involvement with a tendency to be unilateral is termed **Ollier disease.** In another presentation, termed **Maffucci syndrome**, skeletal chondromatosis is seen in association with soft tissue angiomas.

HISTOPATHOLOGIC FEATURES

Histopathologically, a chondroma appears as a circumscribed mass of mature hyaline cartilage that typically demonstrates well-formed lacunae containing small chondrocytes with pale cytoplasm and small, round nuclei. On occasion, the microscopic distinction between a benign chondroma and a low-grade chondrosarcoma of the jaws is difficult (see page 664).

TREATMENT AND PROGNOSIS

It is wise to consider any lesion diagnosed as chondroma of the jaws to represent a potential chondrosarcoma. Treatment is directed toward total surgical removal of the tumor. Condylar examples are usually treated by condylectomy.

CHONDROMYXOID FIBROMA

The **chondromyxoid fibroma** is an uncommon benign neoplasm accounting for less than 1% of all primary bone tumors. It is located most commonly in the metaphyseal region of the long bones. Chondromyxoid fibromas rarely involve the jaws. Cytogenetic analysis in several cases has demonstrated the presence of nonrandom, clonal abnormalities of chromosome 6, where a number of candidate genes important in cartilage development are located. Further characterization of these chromosomal abnormalities may aid in differentiating chondromyxoid fibroma from chondrosarcoma, a distinction that at times can be difficult.

CLINICAL AND RADIOGRAPHIC FEATURES

Chondromyxoid fibromas of the jaws have been encountered in patients ranging in age from 10 to 67 years. The mean age of occurrence is approximately 30 years, with the majority discovered in the second and third decades. There is no sex predilection. Of the reported cases in the jaws, about three quarters occurred in the mandible. In about one fourth, pain was an initial symptom, and swelling was noted in approximately three fourths. Some cases have been asymptomatic, being detected only on a radiographic examination.

Radiographically, the lesion is a circumscribed radiolucent defect with sclerotic or scalloped margins. Central radiopacities sometimes are present within the lesion. On initial presentation, the size of reported chondromyxoid fibromas varied from 1.0 to 6.5 cm.

HISTOPATHOLOGIC FEATURES

The tumor consists of lobulated areas of spindle-shaped or stellate cells with abundant myxoid or chondroid intercellular substance. The lobules characteristically are separated by zones of a more cellular tissue composed of spindle-shaped or round cells with varying numbers of multinucleated giant cells (Fig. 14-70).

Large pleomorphic cells that may cause confusion with chondrosarcoma may be seen. Focal areas of calcification and spicules of residual bone also may be present within the tumor.

TREATMENT AND PROGNOSIS

Although the chondromyxoid fibroma is a benign tumor, approximately 25% of cases in the long bones recur after curettage. Some orthopedic surgeons rec-

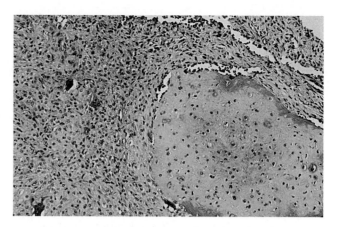

Fig. 14-70 **Chondromyxoid fibroma.** Myxoid connective tissue with scattered giant cells and foci of cartilaginous differentiation.

ommend block excision as the initial treatment. Generally, chondromyxoid fibromas of the jaws have been small and treated by curettage; recurrence is uncommon. Because of the lobular growth and associated scalloped margins, larger gnathic lesions appear to justify resection in an attempt to prevent recurrence. Radiation therapy is contraindicated because of the risk of inducing malignant transformation or osteoradionecrosis.

Distinguishing between a chondromyxoid fibroma and myxoid chondrosarcoma histopathologically may be difficult. Examples of both underdiagnosis and overdiagnosis, with resultant improper treatment, have been described.

SYNOVIAL CHONDROMATOSIS (CHONDROMETAPLASIA)

Synovial chondromatosis is a rare, benign, nonneoplastic arthropathy characterized by the metaplastic development of cartilaginous nodules within the synovial membrane. The exact cause is unknown. In many cases an association with other joint conditions (e.g., inflammatory joint disease, noninflammatory arthropathy, joint overuse or other trauma) has been described, and thus the development of synovial chondromatosis appears to represent a secondary reactive phenomenon. Less commonly, no identifiable etiologic factors are identified, and such cases have been designated as *primary synovial chondromatosis.*

The process typically proceeds through three stages. In the first stage, foci of metaplastic cartilage arise in the synovial lining. With time, these foci increase in size and begin to detach, with cartilaginous material present in both the synovial membrane and the joint.

In the final stage, metaplastic cartilage is found only in the joint.

CLINICAL AND RADIOGRAPHIC FEATURES

The disease most commonly affects large joints, such as the knee, elbow, hip, and shoulder. The number of reported cases involving the temporomandibular joint (TMJ) is less than 100. In recent years, there has been an increase in reported cases, possibly because of improved imaging techniques and increased awareness of the disease. The condition is usually limited to one joint.

Synovial chondromatosis of the TMJ occurs across a wide age range, but most affected patients are middle-aged. In contrast to the findings in other joints, there is a predilection for females. Periarticular swelling, pain, crepitus, and limitation of joint motion are usually present. These features are common to a number of pathoses involving the TMJ and are not diagnostic for synovial chondromatosis. In rare instances, the disease may produce no symptoms. The process is usually limited to the joint, although extraarticular extension and even intracranial extension have been reported in a few more aggressive cases.

Radiographically, the most common feature is the presence of **loose bodies** in the joint. These consist of rounded, irregularly shaped, and variably sized radiopaque structures in the region of the joint. Other features include irregularity of the joint space, widened joint space, and irregularity of the condylar head.

These findings, however, are not diagnostic of synovial chondromatosis and may be seen in other degenerative joint diseases. The absence of loose bodies does not preclude a diagnosis of synovial chondromatosis. Computed tomography (CT) scans and magnetic resonance imaging (MRI) have been advocated as more sensitive diagnostic imaging procedures.

HISTOPATHOLOGIC FEATURES

Nodules of cartilage are present within the synovium and lie loose in the joint space. As many as 100 nodules may be present. These cartilaginous nodules often become calcified and may ossify. The cartilage may appear atypical with hyperchromatic and binucleated chondrocytes, particularly in primary lesions (Fig. 14-71). In another clinical situation, these features would suggest a diagnosis of chondrosarcoma, but these changes are not considered significant in synovial chondromatosis.

TREATMENT AND PROGNOSIS

For patients with synovial chondromatosis, the involved synovium and all loose bodies are removed surgically. Some surgeons advocate total synovectomy to prevent

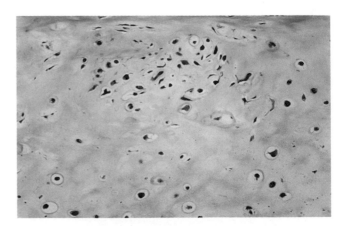

Fig. 14-71 Synovial chondromatosis. Photomicrograph from one of many nodules removed at the time of synovectomy. The cartilage shows some degree of atypia, and in a different clinical setting this histopathology could be interpreted to represent a low-grade chondrosarcoma.

recurrence. Meniscectomy may be necessary if the disc cannot be repaired. A few cases of erosion of the glenoid fossa and cranial extension of the process have been reported. Surgery is performed most commonly via open arthrotomy, although arthroscopy may be used for biopsy and occasionally for treatment of limited disease with loose bodies less than 3 mm in diameter. A wider approach is typically necessary for the rare cases with extensive extraarticular involvement.

The prognosis is good, with an overall low frequency of recurrence after surgical excision. However, some investigators have noted that the less common primary lesions may exhibit more aggressive behavior with a higher recurrence rate, even after synovectomy. Thus periodic follow-up examinations would appear to be prudent. Malignant transformation of synovial chondromatosis of the TMJ has not been noted. Most patients experience improved joint function and pain relief after surgery.

DESMOPLASTIC FIBROMA

The **desmoplastic fibroma** of bone is an uncommon tumor of fibroblastic origin. It is thought to be the osseous counterpart of the soft tissue fibromatosis (desmoid tumor) (see page 515). In a few cases, desmoplastic fibroma-like lesions of the jaws have been reported in association with tuberous sclerosis.

CLINICAL AND RADIOGRAPHIC FEATURES

Most examples of desmoplastic fibroma of bone are discovered in patients younger than 30 years of age. The age range of reported gnathic examples is from 10

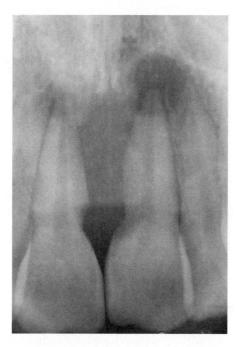

Fig. 14-72 **Desmoplastic fibroma.** Ill-defined, destructive radiolucency of the anterior maxilla. *(Courtesy of Dr. H.T. Daniel.)*

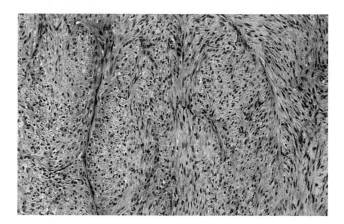

Fig. 14-73 **Desmoplastic fibroma.** The tumor consists of a cellular proliferation of fibroblasts arranged in interlacing fascicles.

months to 59 years, with a mean of approximately 16 years. There is no significant sex predilection. The most common locations are the mandible, femur, pelvic bones, radius, and tibia. Of the reported cases involving the jaws, 84% have occurred in the mandible, most often in the molar angle-ascending ramus area.

Although some tumors are associated with limited opening, with or without malocclusion, a painless swelling of the affected area is the most common initial complaint. Tooth mobility, proptosis, concurrent infection, and dysesthesia have been reported infrequently. Radiographically, the lesion appears as a multilocular or occasionally unilocular radiolucent area. The margins may be well defined or ill defined (Fig. 14-72). The bone is expanded, and the cortex is thinned; cortical reaction mimicking the appearance of an osteosarcoma is rare. If the lesion erodes through the cortex, then an accompanying soft tissue mass will be present. When this occurs, it may be difficult to determine whether the lesion is a desmoplastic fibroma of bone with soft tissue extension or a soft tissue fibromatosis with secondary extension into bone. Adjacent teeth may exhibit displacement and root resorption.

HISTOPATHOLOGIC FINDINGS

The tumor is composed of small elongated fibroblasts and abundant collagen fibers (Fig. 14-73). The degree of cellularity may vary from area to area in a given

lesion, and the cellular areas may show plumper fibroblasts and less collagen. The fibroblasts are not atypical, however, and mitoses are essentially absent. Bone spicules may be present at the interface between the tumor and adjacent bone but are never an integral part of the lesion.

Some authors have recommended that diagnostic biopsies be sampled generously from the center rather than the periphery of the lesion, because reactive bone at the periphery may be mistaken for osteoid production, which may lead to a mistaken diagnosis of a benign fibro-osseous lesion or osteosarcoma.

TREATMENT AND PROGNOSIS

Although the desmoplastic fibroma is considered to be a benign tumor, it often behaves in a locally aggressive fashion, with extensive bone destruction and soft tissue extension; therefore, radical surgery may be required to control the disease. Some surgeons prefer curettage, whereas others prefer wide local excision or resection with a wide margin. Curettage may be adequate for localized lesions without cortical perforation or soft tissue extension, but segmental resection is preferred for lesions exhibiting rapid growth, an ill-defined radiographic appearance, cortical perforation, or soft tissue extension. The recurrence rate for lesions treated by curettage alone is approximately 70%, compared with approximately 20% for those treated by resection. Given these high recurrence rates, patients should be monitored postoperatively for a minimum of 3 years. Although metastases do not occur and the long-term prognosis is good, the lesion may be associated with considerable morbidity.

It may be very difficult to distinguish desmoplastic fibroma of bone from well-differentiated fibrosarcoma.

Some authorities suggest that all desmoplastic fibromas of bone be considered potentially malignant.

OSTEOSARCOMA (OSTEOGENIC SARCOMA)

Osteosarcoma is a malignancy of mesenchymal cells that have the ability to produce osteoid or immature bone. Excluding hematopoietic neoplasms, osteosarcoma is the most common type of malignancy to originate within bone. The majority of osteosarcomas demonstrate intramedullary origin, but a small number may be juxtacortical (discussed in the following section) or rarely, extraskeletal.

CLINICAL AND RADIOGRAPHIC FEATURES

Extragnathic osteosarcoma demonstrates a bimodal age distribution. Most arise in patients between the ages of 10 and 20 years, with a lesser number diagnosed in adults older than age 50. The initial peak occurs during the period of greatest bone growth; accordingly, most of these osteosarcomas arise in the distal femoral and proximal tibial metaphyses. In older patients, the axial skeleton and flat bones are involved most frequently; Paget's disease and previous irradiation are associated with an increased prevalence.

Osteosarcomas of the jaws are uncommon and represent 6% to 8% of all osteosarcomas. These gnathic tumors have been diagnosed in patients ranging from young children to older adults, but they occur most often in the third and fourth decades of life. The mean age for patients with osteosarcoma of the jaw is about 33 years, which is 10 to 15 years older than the mean age for osteosarcomas of the long bones. As is seen in extragnathic locations, a slight male predominance is noted.

The maxilla and mandible are involved with about equal frequency. Mandibular tumors arise more frequently in the posterior body and horizontal ramus rather than the ascending ramus. Maxillary lesions are discovered more commonly in the inferior portion (alveolar ridge, sinus floor, palate) than the superior aspects (zygoma, orbital rim).

Swelling and pain are the most common symptoms (Fig. 14-74). Loosening of teeth, paresthesia, and nasal obstruction (in the case of maxillary tumors) also may be noted. Some patients report symptoms for relatively long periods before diagnosis, which indicates that some osteosarcomas of the jaws grow rather slowly (Fig. 14-75).

The radiographic findings vary from dense sclerosis to a mixed sclerotic and radiolucent lesion to an entirely radiolucent process. The peripheral border of the lesion is usually ill defined and indistinct, making it difficult to determine the extent of the tumor radiographically. In some cases, an extensive osteosarcoma may show only minimal and subtle radiographic change with only slight variation in the trabecular pattern. Occasionally, there is resorption of the roots of teeth involved by the tumor. This feature is often described as "spiking" resorption as a result of the tapered narrowing of the root. The "classic" sunburst or sun ray appearance caused by osteophytic bone production on the surface of the lesion is noted in about 25% of jaw osteosarcomas. Often this is appreciated best on an occlusal projection (Fig. 14-76). In few cases a triangular elevation of the periosteum, referred to as *Codman's triangle*, may be observed.

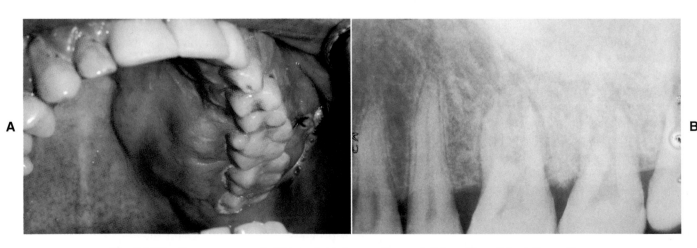

Fig. 14-74 **Osteosarcoma. A,** This patient shows a firm, painful swelling of the left maxilla of recent onset. **B,** The periapical radiograph shows a dense sclerotic change in the bone pattern. *(Courtesy of Dr. Len Morrow.)*

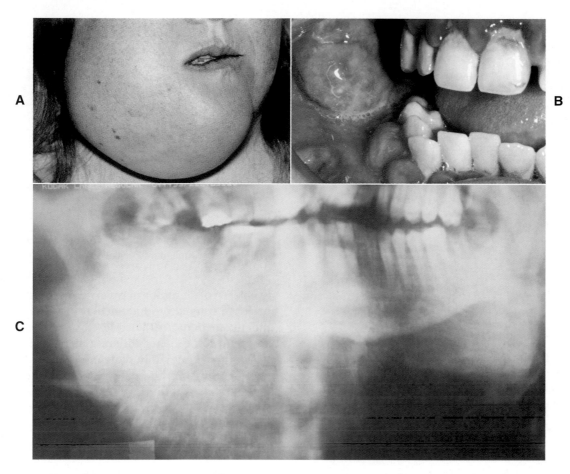

Fig. 14-75   Osteosarcoma. A, This massive tumor had been present for many months before the patient sought treatment. **B,** Intraoral photograph of the tumor mass. **C,** The panoramic radiograph shows a "sunburst" pattern of trabeculation within the tumor.

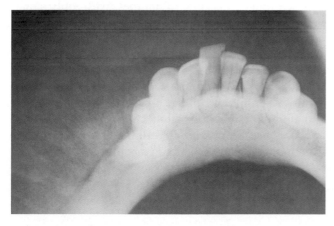

Fig. 14-76   Osteosarcoma. Occlusal radiograph demonstrating prominent exophytic tumor bone production on the buccal surface of the mandible, resulting in the "sunburst" pattern. *(Courtesy of Dr. Lewis Gilbert.)*

An important early radiographic change in patients with osteosarcoma consists of a symmetrical widening of the periodontal ligament space around a tooth or several teeth. This is the result of tumor infiltration along the periodontal ligament space (Fig. 14-77). Widening of the periodontal ligament space is not specific for osteosarcoma and may be seen associated with other malignancies. This radiographic finding, when accompanied by pain or discomfort and other minimal radiographic changes, may be of great importance in the early diagnosis of jaw osteosarcomas.

Although periapical, occlusal, and panoramic radiographs often lead to the initial diagnosis, CT scans are excellent for demonstrating the degree of intramedullary extension, tumor calcification, cortical involvement, and soft tissue involvement. These scans prove invaluable for determining the extent of surgery.

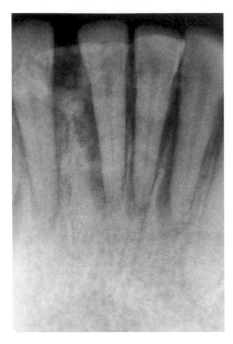

Fig. 14-77   Osteosarcoma. This 26-year-old woman had a 6-cm painful tumor of the anterior mandible. The periapical radiograph shows widening of the periodontal ligament spaces and a mottled radiopacity superimposed on the teeth. *(Courtesy of Dr. Charles Ferguson.)*

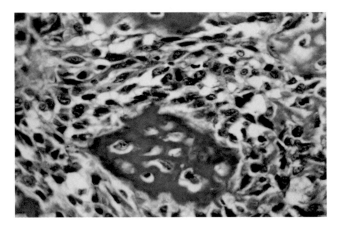

Fig. 14-78   Osteosarcoma. Anaplastic tumor cells forming cellular disorganized bone.

HISTOPATHOLOGIC FEATURES

Osteosarcomas of the jaws display considerable histopathologic variability. The essential microscopic criterion is the direct production of osteoid by malignant mesenchymal cells (Fig. 14-78). In addition to osteoid, the cells of the tumor may produce chondroid material and fibrous connective tissue. The tumor cells may vary from relatively uniform round or spindle-shaped cells to highly pleomorphic cells with bizarre nuclear and cytoplasmic shapes. The amount of matrix material

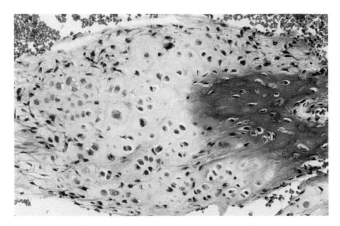

Fig. 14-79   Osteosarcoma. This tumor produced a combination of malignant cartilage and bone.

produced in the tumor may vary considerably. In some instances, osteoid production may be very minimal and difficult to demonstrate. Most osteosarcomas of the jaws tend to be better differentiated than osteosarcomas of the extragnathic skeleton.

Depending on the relative amounts of osteoid, cartilage, or collagen fibers produced by the tumor, many pathologists subclassify osteosarcomas into the following types:
- Osteoblastic
- Chondroblastic
- Fibroblastic

These histopathologic subtypes, however, do not have any great bearing on the prognosis. Other less commonly encountered histopathologic variations include malignant fibrous histiocytoma-like, small cell, epithelioid, telangiectatic, and giant cell–rich.

Chondroblastic osteosarcomas constitute a substantial proportion of all osteosarcomas of the jaws. Some examples may be composed almost entirely of malignant cartilage growing in lobules with only small foci of direct osteoid production by tumor cells being identified (Fig. 14-79). Such lesions, however, should be classified as osteosarcomas rather than chondrosarcomas.

Low-grade, well-differentiated osteosarcomas may show only minimal cellular atypia of the lesional cells and abundant bone formation. On microscopic examination, these lesions may be difficult to differentiate from benign bone lesions, such as fibrous dysplasia or ossifying fibroma.

TREATMENT AND PROGNOSIS

Many past and present investigators believe osteosarcoma of the jaws is less aggressive than those occurring in the long bones. Most gnathic osteosarcomas are low-grade, and metastases are seen less frequently. Despite these findings, many current clinicopathologic studies fail to support this contention and suggest that osteosarcomas of the jaws are aggressive neoplasms. The most important prognostic indicator is the ability to achieve initial complete surgical removal, a feat that is much more difficult to achieve in the jaws than the long bones. In particular, maxillary lesions often are more difficult to resect completely than mandibular lesions. The aggressiveness of gnathic osteosarcoma remains an area of controversy that is difficult to resolve because of the rarity of the neoplasm and the lack of consistently applied diagnostic criteria.

Multicenter investigations of different therapies to osteosarcoma of long bones have led to an improved prognosis that now appears superior to that associated with gnathic neoplasms. These protocols involve neoadjuvant (preoperative) chemotherapy followed by radical surgical excision with careful pathologic examination of the specimen to evaluate the chemotherapeutic effects on the tumor. Adjuvant (postoperative) chemotherapy is used and may be modified if poor histopathologic response to the neoadjuvant regimen is noted. Some investigators have demonstrated 4-year survival rates exceeding 80% with this approach. Limited numbers of patients with jaw osteosarcomas have been treated with these protocols, and superior results have been claimed compared with surgical treatment alone. In addition, a systematic literature review of 201 patients with craniofacial osteosarcoma demonstrated that patients treated with chemotherapy exhibited an improved long-term survival regardless of the ability to achieve complete surgical removal.

In spite of the improved prognosis in patients receiving chemotherapy, radical surgical excision remains the mainstay of therapy. Because the tumor may extend for some distance beyond the apparent clinical and radiographic margins, local recurrence after surgery is a major problem. Local uncontrolled disease is more often the cause of death for patients with jaw osteosarcoma than are the effects of distant metastases. Most deaths from uncontrolled local disease occur within 2 years of the initial treatment. Jaw osteosarcomas have less tendency to metastasize than do osteosarcomas of long bones. Although regional lymph nodes may be infrequently involved, metastases most often affect the lungs and brain. When comparing mandibular and maxillary osteosarcomas, metastasis is noted more frequently from mandibular neoplasms, whereas local recurrence is associated more frequently with maxillary tumors.

The prognosis remains serious. Various studies indicate a 30% to 70% survival rate. Survival rates of up to 80% have been reported for patients receiving initial radical surgery, the best hope for permanent cure. Additional prospective investigations of gnathic osteo-

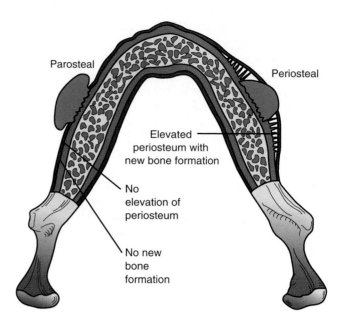

Fig. 14-80   Peripheral (juxtacortical) osteosarcoma. Illustration comparing different types of peripheral osteosarcoma. Parosteal osteosarcoma presents as a lobulated nodule without a peripheral periosteal reaction. Periosteal osteosarcoma presents as a sessile mass associated with significant periosteal new bone formation.

sarcoma treated by neoadjuvant chemotherapy followed by surgical removal and adjuvant chemotherapy are necessary in an attempt to confirm the most appropriate approach.

PERIPHERAL (JUXTACORTICAL) OSTEOSARCOMA

In contrast to the usual forms of intramedullary osteosarcoma, several varieties originate adjacent to the cortex of the bone, initially grow outward from the surface, and do not involve the underlying medullary cavity. The terminology used for these lesions by different authors is somewhat confusing. These **peripheral (juxtacortical) osteosarcomas** usually occur in the long bones, but examples involving the jaws have been reported.

The **parosteal** type of osteosarcoma is a lobulated nodule attached to the cortex by a short stalk (Fig. 14-80). There is no elevation of the periosteum and no peripheral periosteal reaction. Histopathologically, the exophytic mass demonstrates a spindle cell fibroblast-like proliferation that contains well-developed trabeculae of bone. With time, the trabeculae often coalesce and form a large mass of solid bone. Parosteal osteosarcoma is a low-grade sarcoma that has a small risk of recurrence and metastasis if treated by radical excision. With inadequate surgery, the tumor may eventually develop into a higher-grade osteosarcoma, with a resultant poor prognosis.

The **periosteal** form of osteosarcoma is a sessile lesion that arises within the cortex and elevates the overlying periosteum, which provokes the production of significant peripheral periosteal new bone formation (see Fig. 14-80). Often the leading edge of the tumor mass perforates the surface of the periosteum and extends into the surrounding soft tissue. Histopathologically, the tumor demonstrates primitive sarcomatous cells within a tumor that demonstrates significant chondroblastic differentiation. Close inspection will reveal foci of tumor osteoid and immature bone formation. Radical surgical excision with wide margins is the therapy of choice. Although the prognosis is better than that associated with intramedullary tumors, periosteal osteosarcoma has a poorer outcome than the parosteal variant. In reviews of patients with periosteal osteosarcomas, approximately 25% died from metastatic disease.

POSTIRRADIATION BONE SARCOMA

Sarcoma arising in a bone that has been previously subjected to radiation therapy is a well-recognized phenomenon. The jaws are situated closely to tissues that commonly receive therapeutic radiation and are a common site for postirradiation bone sarcomas. Postirradiation sarcomas may develop as early as 3 years after radiation, but the average latent period is about 14 years. The frequency of development of sarcoma is related to radiation dose. Postirradiation sarcoma develops in about 0.2% of patients receiving 7000 cGy; there is no increased prevalence of sarcoma for those receiving less than 1000 cGy.

Osteosarcoma is the most common type of postirradiation sarcoma, accounting for 50% of all cases. About 40% of postirradiation sarcomas are **fibrosarcomas**, with **chondrosarcomas** and other histopathologic types making up the rest. Postirradiation bone sarcomas have no distinctive histopathologic features that allow them to be distinguished from other bone sarcomas of the same type that arise *de novo.*

The prognosis for postirradiation sarcomas is about the same as for *de novo* tumors of the same type.

CHONDROSARCOMA

Chondrosarcoma is a malignant tumor characterized by the formation of cartilage, but not bone, by the tumor cells. Chondrosarcomas comprise about 10% of all primary tumors of the skeleton but are considered by most authorities to involve the jaws only rarely. Chondrosarcoma is about half as common as osteosarcoma and about twice as common as Ewing sarcoma.

Approximately 1% to 3% of all chondrosarcomas arise in the head and neck area, and such lesions comprise only 0.1% of all head and neck malignancies. Some institutions report a somewhat greater frequency of chondrosarcomas in the jaws. This may be the result of differing criteria used by the pathologists for distinguishing chondroblastic osteosarcomas from chondrosarcomas.

CLINICAL AND RADIOGRAPHIC FINDINGS

In extragnathic bones, chondrosarcoma is primarily a neoplasm of adulthood, with peak prevalence in the sixth and seventh decades of life. Although chondrosarcoma arises across a wide age range, the majority of affected patients are older than 50 years of age; tumors arising in patients younger than age 45 are uncommon. No significant sex or race predilection is noted. The most frequently involved bones are the ileum, femur, and humerus. Involvement of the head and neck is seen infrequently.

When occurring in the head and neck, chondrosarcomas arise most frequently in the maxilla; less common sites of involvement are the mandibular body, ramus, nasal septum, and paranasal sinuses. Although chondrosarcomas most often develop in osseous locations, approximately one third of head and neck lesions are extraosseous and originate in either laryngotracheal cartilage or soft tissue. Because of the rarity of chondrosarcoma, large series of jaw and facial bone lesions are uncommon. In one of the larger series, the Mayo Clinic reviewed 56 patients with chondrosarcoma of the jaws and facial bones, and a pattern of occurrence similar to the extragnathic bones was observed. In this series the peak prevalence was noted in the seventh decade, but the age at initial diagnosis had a wide range, with approximately 20% noted in patients younger than 20 years of age. The mean patient age at the time of diagnosis was 41.6 years. No sex or race predilection was noted. Involvement of the maxilla and maxillary sinus outnumbered those in the mandible by 4 to 1.

In a recent review of 400 head and neck chondrosarcomas from the American College of Surgeons' National Cancer Database, the age distribution for patients with conventional-type tumors was similar to that previously reported by the Mayo Clinic series. However, review of prior publications presents a conflicting picture in which the mean age is variable and often reveals a peak prevalence as early as the third decade. Some investigators have suggested that such conflicting results may be the result of difficulty in performing literature reviews that may contain chondroblastic osteosarcomas intermixed with true chondrosarcomas.

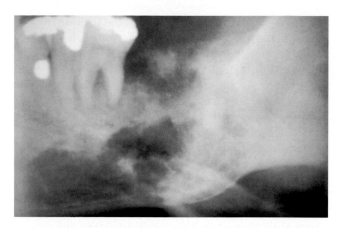

Fig. 14-81   Chondrosarcoma. Ill-defined radiolucent lesion of posterior mandible containing radiopaque foci. (*Courtesy of Dr. Ben B. Henry.*)

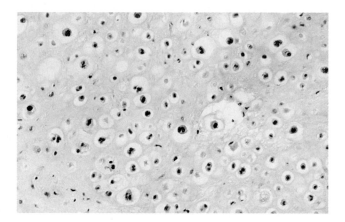

Fig. 14-82   Chondrosarcoma. This grade II chondrosarcoma shows a variation in size of chondrocyte nuclei. Occasional double nuclei are seen in the lacunae.

A painless mass or swelling is the most common presenting sign. This may be associated with separation or loosening of teeth. In contrast to osteosarcoma, pain is an unusual complaint. Maxillary tumors may cause nasal obstruction, congestion, epistaxis, photophobia, or visual loss.

Radiographically, the tumor usually shows features suggestive of a malignancy, consisting of a radiolucent process with poorly defined borders. The radiolucent area often contains scattered and variable amounts of radiopaque foci, which are caused by calcification or ossification of the cartilage matrix (Fig. 14-81). Some chondrosarcomas show extensive calcification and radiographically appear as a densely calcified mass with irregular peripheral margins. Penetration of the cortex can result in a sunburst pattern similar to that seen in some osteosarcomas.

Chondrosarcomas often demonstrate extensive infiltration between the osseous trabeculae of the pre-existing bone without causing appreciable resorption. In such cases the extent of the tumor is difficult to determine by radiographic examination. Root resorption or symmetrical widening of the periodontal ligament space of the teeth involved by the tumor also may be noted. Chondrosarcomas may grow in a lobular pattern with minimal or no foci of calcification. In such instances, the lesion can appear as a multilocular radiolucency and mimic a benign process.

HISTOPATHOLOGIC FEATURES

Chondrosarcomas are composed of cartilage showing varying degrees of maturation and cellularity. In most cases, typical lacunar formation within the chondroid matrix is visible, although this feature may be scarce in poorly differentiated tumors. The tumor often shows a lobular growth pattern, with tumor lobules separated by thin fibrous connective tissue septa. The central areas of the lobules demonstrate the greatest degree of maturation. The peripheral areas consist of immature cartilage and mesenchymal tissue consisting of round or spindle-shaped cells. Calcification or ossification may occur within the chondroid matrix. Neoplastic cartilage may be replaced by bone in a manner similar to normal endochondral ossification.

Chondrosarcomas may be divided into three histopathologic grades of malignancy. This grading system correlates well with the rate of tumor growth and prognosis for chondrosarcomas of the extragnathic skeleton.

GRADES

Grade I chondrosarcomas closely mimic the appearance of a **chondroma**, composed of chondroid matrix and chondroblasts that show only subtle variation from the appearance of normal cartilage. The distinction between benign and well-differentiated malignant cartilaginous tumors is notoriously difficult. Many believe that a tumor should be considered malignant when large, plump chondroblasts and binucleated chondrocytes are present, even in only scattered microscopic fields. Calcification or ossification of the cartilaginous matrix often is prominent, and mitoses are rare.

Grade II chondrosarcomas show a greater proportion of moderately sized nuclei and increased cellularity, particularly about the periphery of the lobules. The cartilaginous matrix tends to be more myxoid, with a less prominent hyaline matrix. The mitotic rate, however, is low (Fig. 14-82).

Grade III chondrosarcomas are highly cellular and may show a prominent spindle cell proliferation. Mitoses may be prominent. Easily recognizable cartilaginous matrix containing cells within lacunae may be scarce.

Chondrosarcomas of the jaws are predominantly of the histopathologic grades I and II. Grade III tumors are very uncommon. In the 56 cases reviewed by the Mayo Clinic, more than 75% were grade I, with the remainder being grade II; no grade III chondrosarcomas were noted in this series.

VARIANTS

Several uncommon microscopic variants of chondrosarcoma are also recognized.

The **clear cell chondrosarcoma** shows cells with abundant clear cytoplasm; this may lead to problems in differentiation from a metastatic clear cell carcinoma. The clear cell chondrosarcoma is considered to be a low-grade lesion.

Dedifferentiated chondrosarcoma is a high-grade malignancy that shows an admixture of well-differentiated chondrosarcoma and a malignant mesenchymal tumor resembling fibrosarcoma. If these variants occur in the jaws, then they are exceedingly rare.

Myxoid chondrosarcoma classically is described as a soft tissue tumor, although intraosseous lesions have been reported within the head and neck and elsewhere. This variant is characterized by a proliferation of cells with clear, vacuolated, or eosinophilic cytoplasm within a background of mucoid material.

Mesenchymal chondrosarcoma is discussed in the next section.

TREATMENT AND PROGNOSIS

The prognosis for chondrosarcoma is related to the size, location, and grade of the lesion. The most important factor is the location of the tumor because this has the greatest influence on the ability to achieve complete resection. The most effective treatment for chondrosarcoma is radical surgical excision. Radiation and chemotherapy are less effective when compared with osteosarcoma and are primarily used for unresectable high-grade chondrosarcomas.

Although aggressive tumors are occasionally seen, gnathic chondrosarcomas are usually slowly growing neoplasms with a lower potential for metastasis than osteosarcoma. Local recurrence leads to death by direct extension of the tumor into vital structures of the head and neck. Maxillary and antral tumors often are located centrally, obtain a larger size before diagnosis, occur adjacent to the central nervous system (CNS), and create more difficulty in surgical eradication; therefore, they are less amenable to cure. In the National Cancer Database series of 400 head and neck chondrosarcomas, only approximately 12% of patients had regional or distant metastasis at the time of diagnosis, with a tendency for metastasis in higher-grade and sinonasal lesions. The overall 5- and 10-year disease-specific survival rates in this series were 87.2% and 70.6%, respectively. Survival was greater for patients with conventional chondrosarcoma than for those with the myxoid or mesenchymal variants. In the Mayo Clinic review, no distant metastases occurred in the 56 reported patients; the 5-, 10-, and 15-year survivals were 67.6%, 53.7%, and 43.9%, respectively. As is obvious from these data, the importance of 5-year survival is minimal because recurrence often is a late sequela. Patients must be followed for their lifetime. Although these two large series suggest that the prognosis of gnathic and craniofacial chondrosarcoma is better than that associated with osteosarcoma, previous studies have suggested that the prognosis of chondrosarcoma is worse. This disagreement may be related to differences in the diagnostic categorization of many cartilage-producing tumors (chondrosarcoma versus chondroblastic osteosarcoma).

MESENCHYMAL CHONDROSARCOMA

The **mesenchymal chondrosarcoma,** an uncommon and distinctive tumor of bone and soft tissue, shows a biphasic histopathologic pattern. This aggressive form of chondrosarcoma represents only 3% to 9% of all chondrosarcomas.

CLINICAL AND RADIOGRAPHIC FEATURES

In contrast to other types of chondrosarcoma, the mesenchymal variant is unusual in that it most frequently affects individuals in the second or third decade of life and the jaws are among the most frequently involved bones (25% to 30%). Other commonly affected sites are the ribs, shoulder, pelvic girdle, and vertebrae. About one third to one fourth of all examples arise in the soft tissues rather than in bone.

Swelling and pain, often of fairly short duration, are the most common symptoms. Radiographically, the tumor demonstrates a radiolucency with infiltrative margins (Fig. 14-83). Stippled calcification may be present within the radiolucent area.

HISTOPATHOLOGIC FEATURES

Microscopically, the mesenchymal chondrosarcoma reveals sheets or patternless masses of small, undifferentiated spindle or round cells surrounding discrete nodules of cartilage (Fig. 14-84). The chondroid tissue is well differentiated, and its degree of cellularity and atypia may vary from that of a benign chondroma to a low-grade chondrosarcoma. The noncartilaginous component of the tumor is difficult to differentiate

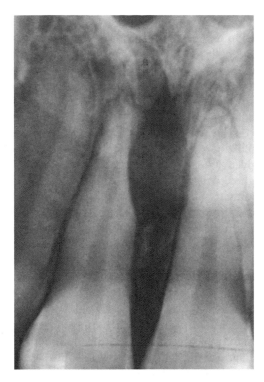

Fig. 14-83 Mesenchymal chondrosarcoma. Periapical radiograph showing a radiolucent lesion between the roots of the central incisors in a 29-year-old woman. The roots of the incisors show resorption. At surgery, the lesion was considerably larger than indicated on the radiograph. *(Courtesy of Dr. Gary Baker.)*

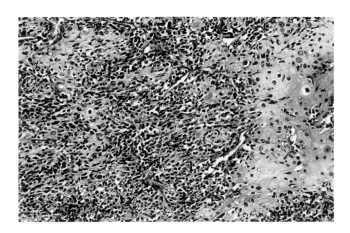

Fig. 14-84 Mesenchymal chondrosarcoma. Medium-power photomicrograph showing sheets of small basophilic cells with focal areas of cartilaginous differentiation *(right).*

from, and may be confused with, a variety of small cell tumors of bone, such as Ewing sarcoma, lymphoma, and metastatic small cell carcinoma. In some cases a prominent, branching vascular pattern is present in the soft tissue component of a mesenchymal chondrosarcoma. If cartilaginous foci are sparse, then the tumor may be misdiagnosed as a hemangiopericytoma.

TREATMENT AND PROGNOSIS

Surgical excision with wide margins is the most appropriate therapy. Radiation and chemotherapy have not prolonged survival in a predictable manner. Local recurrence and metastasis are not rare. When metastasis occurs, hematogenous spread is seen more frequently than lymphatic involvement, with the lung being a favored site for metastatic deposits. Recurrent or metastatic disease may be discovered as long as 20 years after initial therapy. The 10-year survival rate is approximately 28%.

EWING SARCOMA

Ewing sarcoma is a distinctive primary malignant tumor of bone that is composed of small, undifferentiated round cells of uncertain histogenesis. Recent studies have provided data showing that most cases of Ewing sarcoma exhibit features consistent with neuroectodermal origin. In 85% to 90% of the cases, the tumor cells demonstrate a reciprocal translocation between chromosomes 11 and 22 [t(11;22) (q24;q12)]. Ewing sarcoma constitutes 6% to 8% of all primary malignant bone tumors and represents the third most common osseous neoplasm after osteosarcoma and chondrosarcoma. In addition, extraskeletal examples have been well documented.

CLINICAL AND RADIOGRAPHIC FEATURES

The peak prevalence of Ewing sarcoma is in the second decade of life, with approximately 80% of patients being younger than 20 years of age at the time of diagnosis and 50% of these tumors being detected in the second decade. A slight male predominance is noted. The vast majority of affected patients are white, with blacks almost never developing this tumor. The long bones, pelvis, and ribs are affected most frequently, but almost any bone can be affected. Jaw involvement is uncommon, with only 1% to 2% occurring in the gnathic or craniofacial bones.

Pain, often associated with swelling, is the most common symptom. It is usually intermittent and varies from dull to severe. Fever, leukocytosis, and an elevated erythrocyte sedimentation rate also may be present and may lead to an erroneous diagnosis of osteomyelitis. The tumor commonly penetrates the cortex, resulting in a soft tissue mass overlying the affected area of the bone (Fig. 14-85). Jaw involvement is more common in the mandible than the maxilla. Paresthesia and loosening of teeth are common findings in Ewing sarcomas of the jaws.

Melrose RJ, Abrams AM, Mills BG: Florid osseous dysplasia, a clinico-pathologic study of thirty-four cases, *Oral Surg Oral Med Oral Pathol* 41:62-82, 1976.

Schneider LC, Dolinsky HB, Grodjesk JE et al: Malignant spindle cell tumor arising in the mandible of a patient with florid osseous dysplasia, *Oral Surg Oral Med Oral Pathol Oral Radiol Endod* 88:69-73, 1999.

Schneider LC, Mesa ML: Differences between florid osseous dysplasia and diffuse sclerosing osteomyelitis, *Oral Surg Oral Med Oral Pathol* 70:308-312, 1990.

Su L, Weathers DR, Waldron CA: Distinguishing features of focal cemento-osseous dysplasias and cemento-ossifying fibromas. I. A pathologic spectrum of 316 cases, *Oral Surg Oral Med Oral Pathol Oral Radiol Endod* 84:301-309, 1997.

Summerlin DJ, Tomich CE: Focal cemento-osseous dysplasia: a clinicopathologic study of 221 cases, *Oral Surg Oral Med Oral Pathol* 78:611-620, 1994.

Waldron CA: Fibro-osseous lesions of the jaws, *J Oral Maxillofac Surg* 43:249-262, 1985.

Familial Gigantiform Cementoma

Abdelsayed RA, Eversole LR, Singh BS et al: Gigantiform cementoma: clinicopathologic presentation of 3 cases, *Oral Surg Oral Med Oral Pathol Oral Radiol Endod* 91:438-444, 2001.

Cannon JS, Keller EE, Dahlin DC: Gigantiform cementoma: report of two cases (mother and son), *J Oral Surg* 38:65-70, 1980.

Coleman H, Altini M, Kieser J et al: Familial florid cemento-osseous dysplasia—a case report and review of the literature, *J Dent Assoc S Afr* 51:766-770, 1996.

Finical SJ, Kane WJ, Clay RP et al: Familial gigantiform cementoma, *Plast Reconstr Surg* 103:949-954, 1999.

Rossbach HC, Letson D, Lacson A et al: Familial gigantiform cementoma with brittle bone disease, pathologic fractures, and osteosarcoma: a possible explanation of an ancient mystery, *Pediatr Blood Cancer* 44:390-396, 2005.

Toffanin A, Benetti R, Manconi R: Familial florid cemento-osseous dysplasia: a case report, *J Oral Maxillofac Surg* 58:1440-1446, 2000.

Young SK, Markowitz NR, Sullivan S et al: Familial gigantiform cementoma: classification and presentation of a large pedigree, *Oral Surg Oral Med Oral Pathol* 68:740-747, 1989.

Ossifying Fibroma

Eversole LR, Leider AS, Nelson K: Ossifying fibroma: a clinico-pathologic study of 64 cases, *Oral Surg Oral Med Oral Pathol* 60:505-511, 1985.

MacDonald-Jankowski DS: Cemento-ossifying fibromas in the jaws of Hong Kong Chinese, *Dentomaxillofac Radiol* 27:298-304, 1998.

Pimenta FJ, Silveira LFG, Tavares GC et al: HRPT2 gene alterations in ossifying fibroma of the jaws, *Oral Oncol* 42:735-739, 2006.

Slootweg PJ: Maxillofacial fibro-osseous lesions: classification and differential diagnosis, *Semin Diagn Pathol* 13:104-112, 1996.

Su L, Weathers DR, Waldron CA: Distinguishing features of focal cemento-osseous dysplasias and cemento-ossifying fibromas. I. A pathologic spectrum of 316 cases, *Oral Surg Oral Med Oral Pathol Oral Radiol Endod* 84:301-309, 1997.

Waldron CA, Giansanti JS: Benign fibro-osseous lesions of the jaws. II. Benign fibro-osseous lesions of periodontal ligament origin, *Oral Surg Oral Med Oral Pathol* 35:340-350, 1973.

Juvenile Ossifying Fibroma

El-Mofty S: Psammomatoid and trabecular juvenile ossifying fibroma of the craniofacial skeleton: two distinct clinico-pathologic entities, *Oral Surg Oral Med Oral Pathol Oral Radiol Endod* 93:296-304, 2002.

Johnson LC, Yousefi M, Vinh TN et al: Juvenile active ossifying fibroma: its nature, dynamics and origin, *Acta Otolaryngol Suppl* 488:1-40, 1991.

Makek MS: So-called "fibroosseous lesions" of tumorous origin: biology confronts terminology, *J Craniomaxillofac Surg* 15:154-168, 1987.

Margo C, Ragsdale BD, Perman KI et al: Psammomatoid (juvenile) ossifying fibroma of the orbit, *Ophthalmology* 92:150-159, 1985.

Slootweg PJ, Panders AK, Koopmans R et al: Juvenile ossifying fibroma. An analysis of 33 cases with emphasis on histopathological aspects, *J Oral Pathol Med* 23:385-388, 1994.

Williams HK, Mangham C, Speight PM: Juvenile ossifying fibroma. An analysis of eight cases and a comparison with other fibro-osseous lesions, *J Oral Pathol Med* 29:13-18, 2000.

Osteoma

Cutilli BJ, Quinn PD: Traumatically induced peripheral osteoma: report of case, *Oral Surg Oral Med Oral Pathol* 73:667-669, 1992.

Johann AC, de Freitas JB, de Aguiar MC et al: Peripheral osteoma of the mandible: case report and review of the literature, *J Craniomaxillofac Surg* 33:276-281, 2005.

Kondoh T, Seto K, Kobayashi K: Osteoma of the mandibular condyle: report of a case with a review of the literature, *J Oral Maxillofac Surg* 56:972-979, 1998.

Ortakoglu K, Gunaydin Y, Aydintug YS et al: Osteoma of the mandibular condyle: report of a case with 5-year follow-up, *Mil Med* 170:117-120, 2005.

Richards HE, Strider JW Jr, Short SG et al: Large peripheral osteoma arising from the genial tubercle area, *Oral Surg Oral Med Oral Pathol* 61:268-271, 1986.

Schneider LC, Dolinski HB, Grodjesk JE: Solitary peripheral osteoma of the jaws: report of a case and review of the literature, *Oral Surg Oral Med Oral Pathol* 38:452-455, 1980.

Woldenberg Y, Nash M, Bodner L: Peripheral osteoma of the maxillofacial region. Diagnosis and management: a study of 14 cases, *Med Oral Patol Oral Cir Bucal* 10(suppl 2):E139-E142, 2005.

Yassin OM, Bataineh AB, Mansour MJ: An unusual osteoma of the mandible, *J Clin Pediatr Dent* 21:337-340, 1997.

Gardner Syndrome

Baykul T, Heybeli N, Oyar O et al: Multiple huge osteomas of the mandible causing disfigurement related with Gardner's syndrome: case report, *Auris Nasus Larynx* 30:447-451, 2003.

Bilkay U, Erdem O, Ozek C et al: Benign osteoma with Gardner syndrome: review of the literature and report of a case, *J Craniofac Surg* 15:506-509, 2004.

Butler J, Healy C, Toner M et al: Gardner syndrome—review and report of a case, *Oral Oncol Extra* 41:89-92, 2005.

Chimenos-Küstner E, Pascual M, Blanco I et al: Hereditary familial polyposis and Gardner's syndrome: contribution of the odontostomatology examination in its diagnosis and a case description, *Med Oral Patol Oral Cir Bucal* 10:402-409, 2005.

Fotiadis C, Tsekouras DK, Antonakis P et al: A case report and review of the literature, *World J Gastroenterol* 11:5408-5411, 2005.

Galiatsatos P, Foulkes WD: Familial adenomatous polyposis, *Am J Gastroenterol* 101:385-398, 2006.

Gorlin RJ, Cohen MM Jr, Hennekam RCM: Gardner syndrome. In *Syndromes of the head and neck*, ed 4, pp 437-444, New York, 2001, Oxford University Press.

Ida M, Nakamura T, Utsunomiya J: Osteomatous changes and tooth abnormalities found in the jaws of patients with adenomatosis coli, *Oral Surg Oral Med Oral Pathol* 52:2-11, 1981.

Lew D, DeWitt A, Hicks RJ et al: Osteomas of the condyle associated with Gardner's syndrome causing limited mandibular movement, *J Oral Maxillofac Surg* 57:1004-1009, 1999.

Sondergaard JO, Bulows S, Jarvinen H et al: Dental anomalies in familial adenomatous polyposis, *Acta Odontol Scand* 45:61-63, 1987.

Thacker NS, Evans DGR, Horner K et al: Florid oral manifestations in an atypical familial adenomatous polyposis family with late presentation of colorectal polyps, *J Oral Pathol Med* 25:459-462, 1996.

Osteoblastoma

Ahmed MS, Nwoku AL: Benign osteoblastoma of the mandibular ramus: review of the literature and report of a case, *J Oral Maxillofac Surg* 58:1310-1317, 2000.

Angiero F, Mellone P, Baldi A et al: Osteoblastoma of the jaws: report of two cases and review of the literature, *In Vivo* 20:665-670, 2006.

Capodiferro S, Maiorano E, Giardina C et al: Osteoblastoma of the mandible: clinicopathologic study of four cases and literature review, *Head Neck* 27:616-625, 2005.

Dorfman HD, Weiss SW: Borderline osteoblastic tumors: problems in differential diagnosis of aggressive osteoblastoma and low grade osteosarcoma, *Semin Diagn Pathol* 1:215-245, 1984.

Eisenbud L, Kahn L, Friedman E: Benign osteoblastoma of the mandible: fifteen year follow-up showing spontaneous regression after biopsy, *J Oral Maxillofac Surg* 45:53-57, 1987.

Jones AC, Prihoda TJ, Kacher JE et al: Osteoblastoma of the maxilla and mandible: a report of 24 cases, review of the literature, and discussion of its relationship to osteoid osteoma of the jaws, *Oral Surg Oral Med Oral Pathol Oral Radiol Endod* 102:639-650, 2006.

O'Connell JX, Nanthakumar SS, Nielsen GP et al: Osteoid osteoma: the uniquely innervated bone tumor, *Mod Pathol* 11:175-180, 1998.

Peters TED, Oliver DR, McDonald JS: Benign osteoblastoma of the mandible: report of a case, *J Oral Maxillofac Surg* 53:1347-1349, 1995.

Rawal YB, Angiero F, Allen CM et al: Gnathic osteoblastoma: clinicopathologic review of seven cases with long-term follow-up, *Oral Oncol* 42:123-130, 2006.

Unni KK: *Dahlin's bone tumors: general aspects and data on 11,087 cases*, ed 5, pp 131-142, 1996, Philadelphia, Lippincott-Raven.

Cementoblastoma

Biggs JT, Benenati FW: Surgically treating a benign cementoblastoma while retaining the involved tooth, *J Am Dent Assoc* 126:1288-1290, 1995.

Brannon RB, Fowler CB, Carpenter WM et al: Cementoblastoma: an innocuous neoplasm? A clinicopathologic study of 44 cases and review of the literature with special emphasis on recurrence, *Oral Surg Oral Med Oral Pathol Oral Radiol Endod* 93:311-320, 2002.

Jelic JS, Loftus MJ, Miller AS et al: Benign cementoblastoma: report of an unusual case and analysis of 14 additional cases, *J Oral Maxillofac Surg* 51:1033-1037, 1993.

Ohki K, Kumamoto H, Nitta Y et al: Benign cementoblastoma involving multiple maxillary teeth: report of a case with a review of the literature, *Oral Surg Oral Med Oral Pathol Oral Radiol Endod* 97:53-58, 2004.

Pacifici L, Tallarico M, Bartoli A et al: Benign cementoblastoma: a clinical case of conservative surgical treatment of the involved tooth, *Minerva Stomatol* 53:685-691, 2004.

Slootweg PJ: Cementoblastoma and osteoblastoma: a comparison of histologic features, *J Oral Pathol Med* 21:385-389, 1992.

Ulmansky M, Hjørting-Hansen E, Praetorius F et al: Benign cementoblastoma. A review and five new cases, *Oral Surg Oral Med Oral Pathol* 77:48-55, 1994.

Chondroma

Dorfman HD, Czerniak B: *Bone tumors*, pp 253-285, St Louis, 1998, Mosby.

Hyams VJ, Batsakis JG, Michaels L: *Tumors of the upper respiratory tract and ear, atlas of tumor pathology*, series 2, fascicle 25, pp 163-164, Washington, DC, 1988, Armed Forces Institute of Pathology.

Lazow SK, Pihlstrom RT, Solomon MP: Condylar chondroma: report of a case, *J Oral Maxillofac Surg* 56:373-378, 1998.

Unni KK: *Dahlin's bone tumors. General aspects and data on 11,087 cases*, ed 5, pp 25-35, Philadelphia, 1996, Lippincott-Raven.

Chondromyxoid Fibroma

Chow LTC, Lin J, Yip KMH et al: Chondromyxoid fibroma-like osteosarcoma: a distinct variant of low-grade osteosarcoma, *Histopathology* 29:429-436, 1996.

Damm DD, White DK, Geissler RH et al: Chondromyxoid fibroma of the maxilla: electron microscopic findings and review of the literature, *Oral Surg Oral Med Oral Pathol* 59:176-183, 1985.

Hammad HM, Hammond HL, Kurago ZB et al: Chondromyxoid fibroma of the jaws: case report and review of the literature, *Oral Surg Oral Med Oral Pathol Oral Radiol Endod* 85:293-300, 1998.

Macan D, Cabov T, Uglesic V et al: Chondromyxoid fibroma of the mandible, *Br J Oral Maxillofac Surg* 41:261-263, 2003.

Müller S, Whitaker SB, Weathers DR: Chondromyxoid fibroma of the mandible: diagnostic image cytometry findings and review of the literature, *Oral Surg Oral Med Oral Pathol* 73:465-468, 1992.

Smith CA, Magenis RE, Himoe E et al: Chondromyxoid fibroma of the nasal cavity with an interstitial insertion between chromosomes 6 and 19, *Cancer Genet Cytogenet* 171:97-100, 2006.

Tallini G, Dorfman H, Brys P et al: Correlation between clinicopathological features and karyotype in 100 cartilaginous and chordoid tumours. A report from the Chromosomes and Morphology (CHAMP) Collaborative Study Group, *J Pathol* 196:194-203, 2002.

Wu CT, Inwards CY, O'Laughlin S et al: Chondromyxoid fibroma of bone: a clinicopathologic review of 278 cases, *Hum Pathol* 29:438-446, 1998.

Synovial Chondromatosis

Ardekian L, Faquin W, Troulis MJ et al: Synovial chondromatosis of the temporomandibular joint: report and analysis of eleven cases, *J Oral Maxillofac Surg* 63:941-947, 2005.

Deahl ST, Ruprecht A: Asymptomatic, radiographically detected chondrometaplasia in the temporomandibular joint, *Oral Surg Oral Med Oral Pathol* 72:371-374, 1991.

Holmlund AB, Eriksson L, Reinholt FP: Synovial chondromatosis of the temporomandibular joint: clinical, surgical and histological aspects, *Int J Oral Maxillofac Surg* 32:143-147, 2003.

Karlis V, Glickman RS, Zaslow M: Synovial chondromatosis of the temporomandibular joint with intracranial extension, *Oral Surg Oral Med Oral Pathol Oral Radiol Endod* 86:664-666, 1998.

Lustman J, Zeltzer R: Synovial chondromatosis of the temporomandibular joint: review of the literature and case report, *Int J Oral Maxillofac Surg* 18:90-94, 1989.

Miyamoto H, Sakashita H, Wilson DF et al: Synovial chondromatosis of the temporomandibular joint, *Br J Oral Maxillofac Surg* 38:205-208, 2000.

Petito AR, Bennett J, Assael LA et al: Synovial chondromatosis of the temporomandibular joint: varying presentation in 4 cases, *Oral Surg Oral Med Oral Pathol Oral Radiol Endod* 90:758-764, 2000.

Von Lindern JJ, Theuerkauf I, Niederhagen B et al: Synovial chondromatosis of the temporomandibular joint: clinical, diagnostic, and histomorphologic findings, *Oral Surg Oral Med Oral Pathol Oral Radiol Endod* 94:31-38, 2002.

Yu Q, Yang Y, Wang P et al: CT features of synovial chondromatosis in the temporomandibular joint, *Oral Surg Oral Med Oral Pathol Oral Radiol Endod* 97:524-528, 2004.

Desmoplastic Fibroma

Bakaeen G, Rajab LD: Desmoplastic fibroma of the mandible: report of a case, *Int J Paediatr Dent* 9:117-121, 1999.

Bertoni F, Present D, Marchetti C et al: Desmoplastic fibroma of the jaw: the experience of the Istituto Beretta, *Oral Surg Oral Med Oral Pathol* 61:179-184, 1986.

Fletcher CDM, Uni KK, Mertens F: *WHO classification of tumors: pathology and genetics of tumors of soft tissue and bone*, p 288, Lyon, France, 2002, IARC Press.

Freedman PD, Cardo VA, Kerpel SM et al: Desmoplastic fibroma (fibromatosis) of the jaw-bones: report of a case and review of the literature, *Oral Surg Oral Med Oral Pathol* 46:386-395, 1978.

Said-Al-Naief N, Fernandes R, Louis P et al: Desmoplastic fibroma of the jaw: a case report and review of literature, *Oral Surg Oral Med Oral Pathol Oral Radiol Endod* 101:82-94, 2006.

Templeton K, Glass N, Young SK: Desmoplastic fibroma of the mandible in a child: report of a case, *Oral Surg Oral Med Oral Pathol Oral Radiol Endod* 84:620-623, 1997.

Vargas-Gonzalez R, San Martin-Brieke W, Gil-Orduna C et al: Desmoplastic fibroma-like tumor of maxillofacial region associated with tuberous sclerosis, *Pathol Oncol Res* 10:237-239, 2004.

Osteosarcoma

August M, Magennis P, Dewitt D: Osteogenic sarcoma of the jaws: factors influencing prognosis, *Int J Oral Maxillofac Surg* 26:198-204, 1997.

Bennett JH, Thomas G, Evans AW et al: Osteosarcoma of the jaws: a 30-year retrospective review, *Oral Surg Oral Med Oral Pathol Oral Radiol Endod* 90:323-333, 2000.

Canadian Society of Otolaryngology-Head and Neck Surgery Oncology Study Group: Osteogenic sarcoma of the mandible and maxilla: a Canadian review (1980-2000), *J Otolaryngol* 33:139-144, 2004.

Fernandes R, Nikitakis NG, Pazoki A et al: Osteogenic sarcoma of the jaw: a 10-year experience, *J Oral Maxillofac Surg* 65:1286-1291, 2007.

Garrington GE, Scofield HH, Cornyn J et al: Osteosarcoma of the jaws: analysis of 56 cases, *Cancer* 20:377-391, 1967.

Givol N, Buchner A, Taicher S et al: Radiological features of osteogenic sarcoma of the jaws. A comparative study of different radiographic modalities, *Dentomaxillofac Radiol* 27:313-320, 1998.

Huvos AG, Woodard HQ, Cahan WG et al: Postradiation sarcoma of bone and soft tissues: a clinicopathologic study of 66 patients, *Cancer* 55:1244-1255, 1985.

Lewis M, Perl A, Som PM et al: Osteogenic sarcoma of the jaw. A clinicopathologic review of 12 patients, *Arch Otolaryngol Head Neck Surg* 123:169-174, 1997.

Nakayama E, Sugiura K, Ishibashi H et al: The clinical and diagnostic imaging findings of osteosarcoma of the jaw, *Dentomaxillofac Radiol* 34:182-188, 2005.

Nakayama E, Sugiura K, Kobayashi I et al: The association between the computed tomography findings, histologic features, and outcome of osteosarcoma of the jaw, *J Oral Maxillofac Surg* 63:311-318, 2005.

Oda D, Bavisotto LM, Schmidt RA et al: Head and neck osteosarcoma at the University of Washington, *Head Neck* 19:513-523, 1997.

Ogunlewe MO, Ajayi OF, Adeyemo WL et al: Osteogenic sarcoma of the jaw bones: a single institution experience over a 21-year period, *Oral Surg Oral Med Oral Pathol Oral Radiol Endod* 101:76-81, 2006.

Patel SG, Meyers P, Huvos AG et al: Improved outcomes in patients with osteogenic sarcoma of the head and neck, *Cancer* 95:1495-1503, 2002.

Patel SG, See ACH, Williamson PA et al: Radiation-induced sarcoma of the head and neck, *Head Neck* 21:346-354, 1999.

Piattelli A, Favia GF: Periosteal osteosarcoma of the jaws: report of 2 cases, *J Periodontol* 71:325-329, 2000.

Rosen G, Caparros B, Huvos AG: Preoperative chemotherapy for osteogenic sarcoma: selection of postoperative chemotherapy based upon the response of the primary tumor to preoperative chemotherapy, *Cancer* 49:1221-1230, 1982.

Slootweg PJ, Müller H: Osteosarcoma of the jawbones, *J Maxillofac Surg* 13:158-166, 1985.

Smeele LE, Kostense PJ, van der Waal I et al: Effect of chemotherapy on survival of craniofacial osteosarcoma: a systematic review of 201 patients, *J Clin Oncol* 15:363-367, 1997.

Tanzawa H, Uchiyama S, Sato K: Statistical observation of osteosarcoma of the maxillofacial region in Japan, *Oral Surg Oral Med Oral Pathol Oral Radiol Endod* 2:444-448, 1991.

van Es RJJ, Keus RB, van der Waal I et al: Osteosarcoma of the jaw bones. Long-term follow up of 48 cases, *Int J Oral Maxillofac Surg* 26:191-197, 1997.

Chondrosarcoma

Aziz SR, Miremadi AR, McCabe JC: Mesenchymal chondrosarcoma of the maxilla with diffuse metastasis: case report and literature review, *J Oral Maxillofac Surg* 60:931-935, 2002.

Garrington GE, Collett WK: Chondrosarcoma. I. A selected literature review, *J Oral Pathol* 17:1-11, 1988.

Garrington GE, Collett WK: Chondrosarcoma. II. Chondrosarcoma of the jaws: analysis of 37 cases, *J Oral Pathol* 17:12-20, 1988.

Koch BB, Karnell LH, Hoffman HT et al: National Cancer Database report on chondrosarcoma of the head and neck, *Head Neck* 22:408-425, 2000.

Lockhart R, Menard P, Martin JP et al: Mesenchymal chondrosarcoma of the jaws: report of four cases, *Int J Oral Maxillofac Surg* 27:358-362, 1998.

Nakashima Y, Unni KK, Shives TC et al: Mesenchymal chondrosarcoma of bone and soft tissue: a review of 111 cases, *Cancer* 57:2444-2453, 1985.

Saito K, Unni KK, Wollan PC et al: Chondrosarcoma of the jaw and facial bones, *Cancer* 76:1550-1558, 1995.

Vencio EF, Reeve CM, Unni KK et al: Mesenchymal chondrosarcoma of the jaw bones. Clinicopathologic study of 19 cases, *Cancer* 82:2350-2355, 1998.

Ewing Sarcoma

Arafat A, Ellis G, Adrian JC: Ewing's sarcoma of the jaws, *Oral Surg Oral Med Oral Pathol* 55:589-596, 1983.

Berk R, Heller A, Heller D et al: Ewing's sarcoma of the mandible: a case report, *Oral Surg Oral Med Oral Pathol Oral Radiol Endod* 79:159-162, 1995.

Daw NC, Mahmoud HH, Meyer WH et al: Bone sarcomas of the head and neck in children: the St. Jude Children's Research Hospital experience, *Cancer* 88:2172-2180, 2000.

de Alava E, Gerald WL: Molecular biology of the Ewing's sarcoma/primitive neuroectodermal tumor family, *J Clin Oncol* 18:204-213, 2000.

Fiorillo A, Tranfa F, Canale G et al: Primary Ewing's sarcoma of the maxilla, a rare and curable localization: report of two new cases, successfully treated by radiotherapy and systemic chemotherapy, *Cancer Lett* 103:177-182, 1996.

Infante-Cassio P, Gutierrez-Perez JL, Garcia-Perla A et al: Primary Ewing's sarcoma of the maxilla and zygoma: report of a case, *J Oral Maxillofac Surg* 63:1539-1542, 2005.

Kissane JM, Askin FB, Foulkes M et al: Ewing's sarcoma of bone: clinicopathologic aspects of 303 cases from the intergroup Ewing's sarcoma study, *Hum Pathol* 14:773-779, 1983.

La TH, Meyers PA, Wexler LH et al: Radiation therapy for Ewing's sarcoma: results from Memorial Sloan-Kettering in the modern era, *Int J Radiat Oncol Biol Phys* 2:544-550, 2006.

Schultze-Mosgau S, Thorwarth M, Wehrhan F et al: Ewing sarcoma of the mandible in a child: interdisciplinary treatment concepts and surgical reconstruction, *J Craniofac Surg* 16:1140-1146, 2005.

Vaccani JP, Forte V, de Jong Al et al: Ewing's sarcoma of the head and neck in children, *Int J Pediatr Otorhinolaryngol* 48:209-216, 1999.

Wexler LH, Kacker A, Piro JD et al: Combined modality treatment of Ewing's sarcoma of the maxilla, *Head Neck* 25:168-172, 2003.

Metastatic Tumors to the Jaws

Bouquot JE, Weiland LH, Kurland LT: Metastasis to and from the upper aero-digestive tract in the population of Rochester, Minnesota, 1935-1984, *Head Neck* 11:212-218, 1989.

Clausen F, Poulson H: Metastatic carcinoma of the jaws, *Acta Pathol Microbiol Scand* 57:361-374, 1963.

D'Silva NJ, Summerlin DJ, Cordell KG et al: Metastatic tumors in the jaws: a retrospective study of 114 cases, *J Am Dent Assoc* 137:1667-1672, 2006.

Hashimoto N, Kurihara K, Yamasaki H et al: Pathologic characteristics of metastatic carcinoma in the human mandible, *J Oral Pathol* 16:362-367, 1987.

O'Carroll MK, Krolls SO, Mosca NG: Metastatic carcinoma to the mandible: report of two cases, *Oral Surg Oral Med Oral Pathol* 76:368-374, 1993.

Zachariades N: Neoplasms metastatic to the mouth, jaws and surrounding tissues, *J Craniomaxillofac Surg* 17:283-290, 1989.

15

Odontogenic Cysts and Tumors[*]

CHAPTER OUTLINE

Odontogenic cysts and tumors constitute an important aspect of oral and maxillofacial pathology. Odontogenic cysts are encountered relatively commonly in dental practice. Odontogenic tumors, by contrast, are uncommon lesions. Even in the specialized oral and maxillofacial pathology laboratory, fewer than 1% of all specimens received are odontogenic tumors.

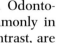

Odontogenic Cysts

With rare exceptions, epithelium-lined cysts in bone are seen only in the jaws. Other than a few cysts that may result from the inclusion of epithelium along embryonic lines of fusion, most jaw cysts are lined by epithelium that is derived from odontogenic epithelium. These are referred to as **odontogenic cysts**. (Non-odontogenic jaw cysts are discussed in Chapter 1.)

Odontogenic cysts are subclassified as developmental or inflammatory in origin. The inciting factors that initiate the formation of **developmental cysts** are

*Dr. Charles A. Waldron wrote the original version of this chapter in the first edition of this book.

Classification of Odontogenic Cysts

DEVELOPMENTAL

• Dentigerous cyst
• Eruption cyst
• Odontogenic keratocyst*
• Orthokeratinized odontogenic cyst
• Gingival (alveolar) cyst of the newborn
• Gingival cyst of the adult
• Lateral periodontal cyst
• Calcifying odontogenic cyst†
• Glandular odontogenic cyst

INFLAMMATORY

• Periapical (radicular) cyst
• Residual periapical (radicular) cyst
• Buccal bifurcation cyst

---

*Although the odontogenic keratocyst is included with the odontogenic tumors in the 2005 World Health Organization (WHO) classification ("keratocystic odontogenic tumor"), the authors prefer to classify it as an odontogenic cyst.
†The term *calcifying odontogenic cyst* includes both nonneoplastic cysts and true neoplasms. Although the calcifying odontogenic cyst Is included with odontogenic tumors in the 2005 WHO classification, it is discussed with the odontogenic cysts in this chapter.

unknown, but these lesions do not appear to be the result of an inflammatory reaction. **Inflammatory cysts** are the result of inflammation. Box 15-1 presents categories of odontogenic cysts modified from the 2005 World Health Organization (WHO) classification. (The periapical cyst is discussed in Chapter 3.)

DENTIGEROUS CYST (FOLLICULAR CYST)

The **dentigerous cyst** is defined as a cyst that originates by the separation of the follicle from around the crown of an unerupted tooth. This is the most common type of developmental odontogenic cyst, making up about 20% of all epithelium-lined cysts of the jaws. The dentigerous cyst encloses the crown of an unerupted tooth and is attached to the tooth at the cemento-enamel junction (Fig. 15-1). The pathogenesis of this cyst is uncertain, but apparently it develops by accumulation of fluid between the reduced enamel epithelium and the tooth crown.

Although most dentigerous cysts are considered to be developmental in origin, there are some examples that appear to have an inflammatory pathogenesis. For example, it has been suggested that, on occasion, a dentigerous cyst may develop around the crown of an unerupted permanent tooth as a result of periapical inflammation from an overlying primary tooth. Another

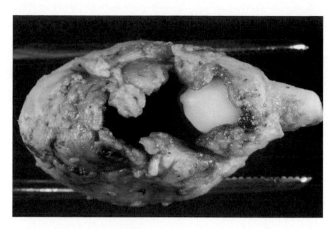

Fig. 15-1   Dentigerous cyst. Gross specimen of a dentigerous cyst involving a maxillary canine tooth. The cyst has been cut open to show the cyst-to-crown relationship.

scenario involves a partially erupted mandibular third molar that develops an inflamed cystlike lesion along the distal or buccal aspect. Although many such lesions probably are due to inflammation associated with recurrent pericoronitis, these lesions are usually diagnosed as examples of dentigerous cyst, especially because it is impossible to determine histopathologically whether the inflammatory component is primary or secondary in nature. The term **paradental cyst** sometimes has been applied to these lesions, but the use of this term in the literature is confusing because it also has been used to describe examples of what is known as the *buccal bifurcation cyst*.

CLINICAL AND RADIOGRAPHIC FEATURES

Although dentigerous cysts may occur in association with any unerupted tooth, most often they involve mandibular third molars. Other relatively frequent sites include maxillary canines, maxillary third molars, and mandibular second premolars. Dentigerous cysts rarely involve unerupted deciduous teeth. Occasionally, they are associated with supernumerary teeth or odontomas.

Although dentigerous cysts may be encountered in patients across a wide age range, they are discovered most frequently in patients between 10 and 30 years of age. There is a slight male predilection, and the prevalence is higher for whites than for blacks. Small dentigerous cysts are usually completely asymptomatic and are discovered only on a routine radiographic examination or when films are taken to determine the reason for the failure of a tooth to erupt. Dentigerous cysts can grow to a considerable size, and large cysts may be associated with a painless expansion of the bone in the involved area. Extensive lesions may result

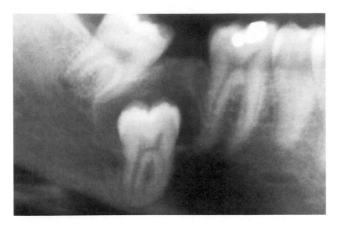

Fig. 15-2 Dentigerous cyst. Central type showing the crown projecting into the cystic cavity. *(Courtesy of Dr. Stephen E. Irwin.)*

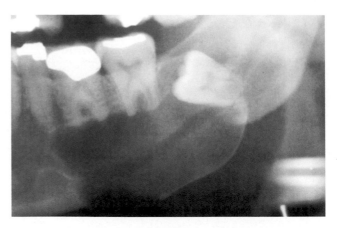

Fig. 15-3 Dentigerous cyst. Lateral variety showing a large cyst along the mesial root of the unerupted molar. This cyst exhibited mucous cell prosoplasia. *(Courtesy of Dr. John R. Cramer.)*

in facial asymmetry. Large dentigerous cysts are uncommon, and most lesions that are considered to be large dentigerous cysts on radiographic examination will prove to be odontogenic keratocysts or ameloblastomas. Dentigerous cysts may become infected and be associated with pain and swelling. Such infections may arise in a dentigerous cyst that is associated with a partially erupted tooth or by extension from a periapical or periodontal lesion that affects an adjacent tooth.

Radiographically, the dentigerous cyst typically shows a unilocular radiolucent area that is associated with the crown of an unerupted tooth. The radiolucency usually has a well-defined and often sclerotic border, but an infected cyst may show ill-defined borders. A large dentigerous cyst may give the impression of a multilocular process because of the persistence of bone trabeculae within the radiolucency. Dentigerous cysts, however, are grossly and histopathologically unilocular processes and probably never are truly multilocular lesions.

The cyst-to-crown relationship shows several radiographic variations. In the **central** variety, which is the most common, the cyst surrounds the crown of the tooth and the crown projects into the cyst (Fig. 15-2). The **lateral** variety is usually associated with mesioangular impacted mandibular third molars that are partially erupted. The cyst grows laterally along the root surface and partially surrounds the crown (Fig. 15-3). In the **circumferential** variant, the cyst surrounds the crown and extends for some distance along the root so that a significant portion of the root appears to lie within the cyst (Fig. 15-4). Rarely, a third molar may be displaced to the lower border of the mandible or higher up into the ascending ramus. Maxillary anterior teeth may be displaced into the floor of the nose, and

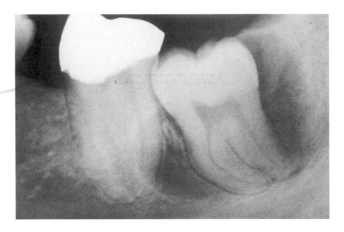

Fig. 15-4 Dentigerous cyst. Circumferential variety showing cyst extension along the mesial and distal roots of the unerupted tooth. *(Courtesy of Dr. Richard Marks.)*

other maxillary teeth may be moved through the maxillary sinus to the floor of the orbit. Dentigerous cysts may displace the involved tooth for a considerable distance. Root resorption of adjacent erupted teeth can occur.

Radiographic distinction between a small dentigerous cyst and an enlarged follicle about the crown of an unerupted tooth is difficult and may be largely an academic exercise (Fig. 15-5). For the lesion to be considered a dentigerous cyst, some investigators believe that the radiolucent space surrounding the tooth crown should be at least 3 to 4 mm in diameter. Radiographic findings are not diagnostic for a dentigerous cyst, however, because odontogenic keratocysts, unilocular ameloblastomas, and many other odontogenic and nonodontogenic tumors may have radiographic features that are essentially identical to those of a dentigerous cyst.

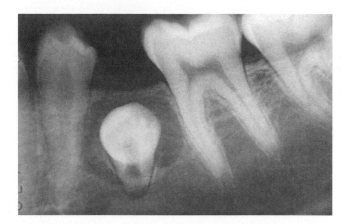

Fig. 15-5 Dentigerous cyst or enlarged follicle. Radiolucent lesion involving the crown of an unerupted mandibular premolar. Distinction between a dentigerous cyst and an enlarged follicle for a lesion of this size by radiographic and even histopathologic means is difficult, if not impossible. *(Courtesy of Dr. Wally Austelle.)*

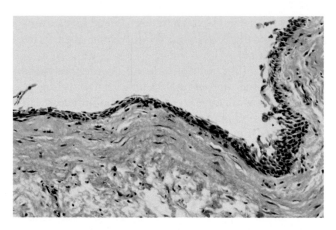

Fig. 15-6 Dentigerous cyst. This noninflamed dentigerous cyst shows a thin, nonkeratinized epithelial lining.

HISTOPATHOLOGIC FEATURES

The histopathologic features of dentigerous cysts vary, depending on whether the cyst is inflamed or not inflamed. In the **noninflamed dentigerous cyst**, the fibrous connective tissue wall is loosely arranged and contains considerable glycosaminoglycan ground substance. Small islands or cords of inactive-appearing odontogenic epithelial rests may be present in the fibrous wall. Occasionally these rests may be numerous, and at times pathologists who are not familiar with oral lesions have misinterpreted this finding as ameloblastoma. The epithelial lining consists of two to four layers of flattened nonkeratinizing cells, and the epithelium and connective tissue interface is flat (Fig. 15-6).

In the fairly common **inflamed dentigerous cyst**, the fibrous wall is more collagenized, with a variable infiltration of chronic inflammatory cells. The epithelial lining may show varying amounts of hyperplasia with the development of rete ridges and more definite squamous features (Fig. 15-7). A keratinized surface is sometimes seen, but these changes must be differentiated from those observed in the odontogenic keratocyst. Focal areas of mucous cells may be found in the epithelial lining of dentigerous cysts (Fig. 15-8). Rarely, ciliated columnar cells are present. Small nests of sebaceous cells rarely may be noted within the fibrous cyst wall. These mucous, ciliated, and sebaceous elements are believed to represent the multipotentiality of the odontogenic epithelial lining in a dentigerous cyst.

Gross examination of the wall of a dentigerous cyst may reveal one or several areas of nodular thickening

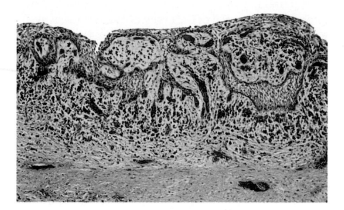

Fig. 15-7 Dentigerous cyst. This inflamed dentigerous cyst shows a thicker epithelial lining with hyperplastic rete ridges. The fibrous cyst capsule shows a diffuse chronic inflammatory infiltrate.

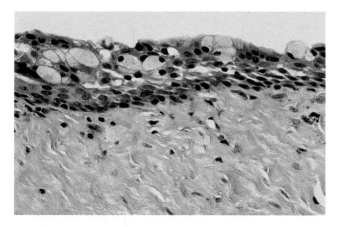

Fig. 15-8 Dentigerous cyst. Scattered mucous cells can be seen within the epithelial lining.

on the luminal surface. These areas must be examined microscopically to rule out the presence of early neoplastic change.

Because a thin layer of reduced enamel epithelium normally lines the dental follicle surrounding the crown of an unerupted tooth, it can be difficult to distinguish a small dentigerous cyst from simply a normal or enlarged dental follicle based on microscopic features alone. Again, this distinction often represents largely an academic exercise; the most important consideration is ensuring that the lesion does not represent a more significant pathologic process (e.g., odontogenic keratocyst or ameloblastoma).

TREATMENT AND PROGNOSIS

The usual treatment for a dentigerous cyst is careful enucleation of the cyst together with removal of the unerupted tooth. If eruption of the involved tooth is considered feasible, then the tooth may be left in place after partial removal of the cyst wall. Patients may need orthodontic treatment to assist eruption. Large dentigerous cysts also may be treated by marsupialization. This permits decompression of the cyst, with a resulting reduction in the size of the bone defect. The cyst can then be excised at a later date, with a less extensive surgical procedure.

The prognosis for most dentigerous cysts is excellent, and recurrence seldom is noted after complete removal of the cyst. However, several potential complications must be considered. Much has been written about the possibility that the lining of a dentigerous cyst might undergo neoplastic transformation to an **ameloblastoma**. Although undoubtedly this can occur, the frequency of such neoplastic transformation is low. Rarely, a **squamous cell carcinoma** may arise in the lining of a dentigerous cyst (see page 700). It is likely that some **intraosseous mucoepidermoid carcinomas** (see page 490) develop from mucous cells in the lining of a dentigerous cyst.

ERUPTION CYST (ERUPTION HEMATOMA)

The **eruption cyst** is the soft tissue analogue of the dentigerous cyst. The cyst develops as a result of separation of the dental follicle from around the crown of an erupting tooth that is within the soft tissues overlying the alveolar bone. One example of eruption cysts developing in a child who was taking cyclosporin A has been described. Presumably the cysts developed because of collagen deposition in the gingival connective tissue that resulted in a thicker, less penetrable, pericoronal roof.

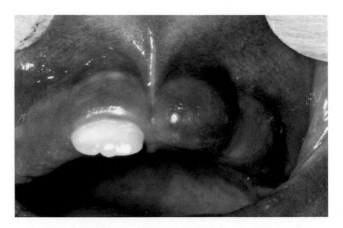

Fig. 15-9   Eruption cyst. This soft gingival swelling contains considerable blood and can also be designated as an eruption hematoma.

CLINICAL FEATURES

The eruption cyst appears as a soft, often translucent swelling in the gingival mucosa overlying the crown of an erupting deciduous or permanent tooth. Most examples are seen in children younger than age 10. Although the cyst may occur with any erupting tooth, the lesion is most commonly associated with the deciduous mandibular central incisors, the first permanent molars, and the deciduous maxillary incisors. Surface trauma may result in a considerable amount of blood in the cystic fluid, which imparts a blue to purple-brown color. Such lesions sometimes are referred to as **eruption hematomas** (Fig. 15-9).

HISTOPATHOLOGIC FEATURES

Intact eruption cysts seldom are submitted to the oral and maxillofacial pathology laboratory, and most examples consist of the excised roof of the cyst, which has been removed to facilitate tooth eruption. These show surface oral epithelium on the superior aspect. The underlying lamina propria shows a variable inflammatory cell infiltrate. The deep portion of the specimen, which represents the roof of the cyst, shows a thin layer of nonkeratinizing squamous epithelium (Fig. 15-10).

TREATMENT AND PROGNOSIS

Treatment may not be required because the cyst usually ruptures spontaneously, permitting the tooth to erupt. If this does not occur, then simple excision of the roof of the cyst generally permits speedy eruption of the tooth.

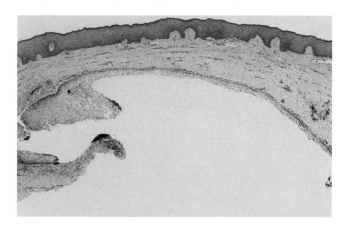

Fig. 15-10   **Eruption cyst.** A cystic epithelial cavity can be seen below the mucosal surface.

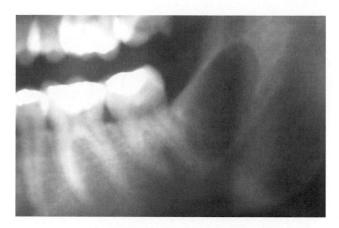

Fig. 15-11   **Primordial cyst.** This patient gave no history of extraction of the third molar. A cyst is located in the third molar area. The cyst was excised, and histopathologic examination revealed an odontogenic keratocyst.

PRIMORDIAL CYST

The concept and meaning of the term **primordial cyst** often have been controversial and confusing. In the older classification of cysts widely used in the United States, the primordial cyst was considered to originate from cystic degeneration of the enamel organ epithelium before the development of dental hard tissue. Therefore, the primordial cyst occurs in place of a tooth.

In the mid 1950s, oral pathologists in Europe introduced the term **odontogenic keratocyst** to denote a cyst with specific histopathologic features and clinical behavior, which was believed to arise from the dental lamina (i.e., the dental primordium). Subsequently, this concept was widely accepted, and the terms *odontogenic keratocyst* and *primordial cyst* were used synonymously. The 1972 WHO classification used the designation *primordial cyst* as the preferred term for this lesion. The 1992 WHO classification, however, listed *odontogenic keratocyst* as the preferred designation.

Whether there is a primordial cyst that is not microscopically an odontogenic keratocyst is still unsettled. Many believe that all primordial cysts are odontogenic keratocysts, although some recognize the existence of a primordial cyst that does not have the histopathologic features of the odontogenic keratocyst. If such a lesion exists, then it must be exceedingly rare. Reference to this lesion is almost nonexistent in the current literature, and no reported series include a significant number of cases. In the authors' experience, a cyst clinically considered to represent a primordial cyst, in the older meaning of the term, almost always is an odontogenic keratocyst after microscopic study (Fig. 15-11).

ODONTOGENIC KERATOCYST

The **odontogenic keratocyst** is a distinctive form of developmental odontogenic cyst that deserves special consideration because of its specific histopathologic features and clinical behavior. There is general agreement that the odontogenic keratocyst arises from cell rests of the dental lamina. This cyst shows a different growth mechanism and biologic behavior from the more common dentigerous cyst and radicular cyst. Most authors believe that dentigerous and radicular cysts continue to enlarge as a result of increased osmotic pressure within the lumen of the cyst. This mechanism does not appear to hold true for odontogenic keratocysts, and their growth may be related to unknown factors inherent in the epithelium itself or enzymatic activity in the fibrous wall. Several investigators have suggested that odontogenic keratocysts be regarded as benign cystic neoplasms rather than cysts, and in the latest WHO classification of odontogenic tumors, these lesions have been given the name "**keratocystic odontogenic tumor.**" The arguments to support this change in nomenclature largely rely on a few studies that have shown certain molecular genetic alterations that are also present in some neoplasms. Unfortunately, these studies have not examined other cystic lesions of the jaws; therefore, it is currently unknown whether these alterations are unique to the odontogenic keratocyst. Most oral and maxillofacial pathologists do not feel that sufficient evidence exists to justify renaming this widely recognized lesion, with the likely result of causing widespread confusion among the professional community.

Although there are wide variations in the reported frequency of odontogenic keratocysts compared with that of other types of odontogenic cysts, several studies

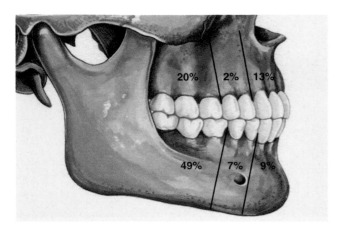

Fig. 15-12 Odontogenic keratocyst. Relative distribution of odontogenic keratocysts in the jaws.

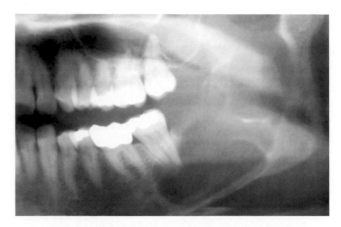

Fig. 15-13 Odontogenic keratocyst. Large, multilocular cyst involving most of the ascending ramus. *(Courtesy of Dr. S.C. Roddy.)*

that include large series of cysts indicate that odontogenic keratocysts make up 3% to 11% of all odontogenic cysts.

CLINICAL AND RADIOGRAPHIC FEATURES

Odontogenic keratocysts may be found in patients who range in age from infancy to old age, but about 60% of all cases are diagnosed in people between 10 and 40 years of age. There is a slight male predilection. The mandible is involved in 60% to 80% of cases, with a marked tendency to involve the posterior body and ascending ramus (Fig. 15-12).

Small odontogenic keratocysts are usually asymptomatic and discovered only during the course of a radiographic examination. Larger odontogenic keratocysts may be associated with pain, swelling, or drainage. Some extremely large cysts, however, may cause no symptoms.

Odontogenic keratocysts tend to grow in an anteroposterior direction within the medullary cavity of the bone without causing obvious bone expansion. This feature may be useful in differential clinical and radiographic diagnosis because dentigerous and radicular cysts of comparable size are usually associated with bony expansion. Multiple odontogenic keratocysts may be present, and such patients should be evaluated for other manifestations of the **nevoid basal cell carcinoma (Gorlin) syndrome** (see page 688).

Odontogenic keratocysts demonstrate a well-defined radiolucent area with smooth and often corticated margins. Large lesions, particularly in the posterior body and ascending ramus of the mandible, may appear multilocular (Fig. 15-13). An unerupted tooth is involved in the lesion in 25% to 40% of cases; in such instances, the radiographic features suggest

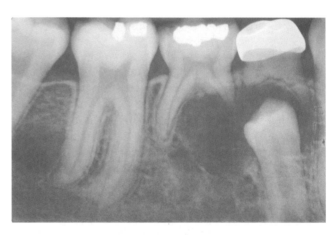

Fig. 15-14 Odontogenic keratocyst. This cyst involves the crown of an unerupted premolar. Radiographically, this lesion cannot be differentiated from a dentigerous cyst.

the diagnosis of dentigerous cyst (Figs. 15-14 and 15-15). In these cases, the cyst has presumably arisen from dental lamina rests near an unerupted tooth and has grown to envelop the unerupted tooth. Resorption of the roots of erupted teeth adjacent to odontogenic keratocysts is less common than that noted with dentigerous and radicular cysts.

The diagnosis of odontogenic keratocyst is based on the histopathologic features. The radiographic findings, although often highly suggestive, are not diagnostic. The radiographic findings in an odontogenic keratocyst may simulate those of a dentigerous cyst, a radicular cyst, a residual cyst, a lateral periodontal cyst (Fig. 15-16), or the so-called globulomaxillary cyst (which is no longer considered to be a true entity). Odontogenic keratocysts of the anterior midline maxillary region can mimic nasopalatine duct cysts. For unknown reasons, this particular subset of keratocyst usually occurs in older individuals with a mean age of

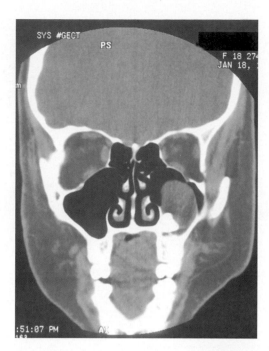

Fig. 15-15   Odontogenic keratocyst. Computed tomography (CT) scan showing a large cyst involving the crown of an unerupted maxillary third molar. The cyst largely fills the maxillary sinus. *(Courtesy of Dr. E.B. Bass.)*

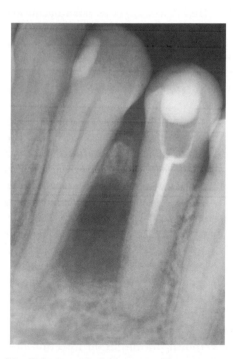

Fig. 15-16   Odontogenic keratocyst. This cyst cannot be radiographically differentiated from a lateral periodontal cyst. *(Courtesy of Dr. Keith Lemmerman.)*

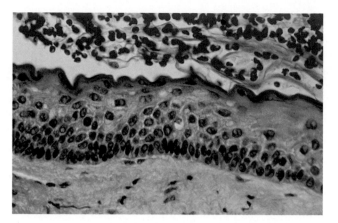

Fig. 15-17   Odontogenic keratocyst. The epithelial lining is 6 to 8 cells thick, with a hyperchromatic and palisaded basal cell layer. Note the corrugated parakeratotic surface.

nearly 70 years. Rare examples of peripheral odontogenic keratocysts within the gingival soft tissues have been reported.

HISTOPATHOLOGIC FEATURES

The odontogenic keratocyst typically shows a thin, friable wall, which is often difficult to enucleate from the bone in one piece. The cystic lumen may contain a clear liquid that is similar to a transudate of serum, or it may be filled with a cheesy material that, on microscopic examination, consists of keratinaceous debris. Microscopically, the thin fibrous wall is essentially devoid of any inflammatory infiltrate. The epithelial lining is composed of a uniform layer of stratified squamous epithelium, usually six to eight cells in thickness. The epithelium and connective tissue interface is usually flat, and rete ridge formation is inconspicuous. Detachment of portions of the cyst-lining epithelium from the fibrous wall is commonly observed. The luminal surface shows flattened parakeratotic epithelial cells, which exhibit a wavy or corrugated appearance (Fig. 15-17). The basal epithelial layer is composed of a palisaded layer of cuboidal or columnar epithelial cells, which are often hyperchromatic. Small satellite cysts, cords, or islands of odontogenic epithelium may be seen within the fibrous wall. These structures have been present in 7% to 26% of cases in various reported series. In rare instances, cartilage has been observed in the wall of an odontogenic keratocyst.

In the presence of inflammatory changes, the typical features of the odontogenic keratocyst may be altered. The parakeratinized luminal surface may disappear, and the epithelium may proliferate to form rete ridges with the loss of the characteristic palisaded basal layer (Fig. 15-18). When these changes involve most of the cyst lining, the diagnosis of odontogenic keratocyst

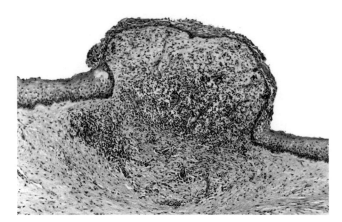

Fig. 15-18   Odontogenic keratocyst. The characteristic microscopic features have been lost in the central area of this portion of the cystic lining because of the heavy chronic inflammatory cell infiltrate.

cannot be confirmed unless other sections show the typical features described earlier.

Some investigators recognize a microscopic orthokeratotic variant and include this lesion as a subtype of the odontogenic keratocyst. However, these cysts do not demonstrate a hyperchromatic and palisaded basal cell layer, which is so characteristic of true odontogenic keratocysts. In addition, the clinical behavior of these orthokeratinized cysts differs markedly from that of the typical parakeratinized cysts described in this section. The authors believe that it is more logical to discuss these orthokeratinizing cysts separately (see following section).

TREATMENT AND PROGNOSIS

Although the presence of an odontogenic keratocyst may be suspected on clinical or radiographic grounds, histopathologic confirmation is required for the diagnosis. Consequently, most odontogenic keratocysts are treated similarly to other odontogenic cysts, that is, by enucleation and curettage. Complete removal of the cyst in one piece is often difficult because of the thin, friable nature of the cyst wall. In contrast to other odontogenic cysts, odontogenic keratocysts often tend to recur after treatment. Whether this is due to fragments of the original cyst that were not removed at the time of the operation or a "new" cyst that has developed from dental lamina rests in the general area of the original cyst cannot be determined with certainty.

The reported frequency of recurrence in various studies ranges from 5% to 62%. This wide variation may be related to the total number of cases studied, the length of follow-up periods, and the inclusion or exclusion of orthokeratinized cysts in the study group. Several reports that include large numbers of cases

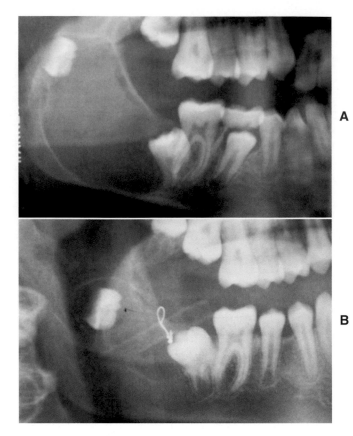

Fig. 15-19   Decompression of an odontogenic keratocyst. A, Large unilocular radiolucency associated with the right mandibular third molar. **B,** Six months after insertion of a polyethylene drainage tube to allow decompression, the cyst has shrunk and the third molar has migrated downward and forward. *(Courtesy of Dr. Tom Szakal.)*

indicate a recurrence rate of approximately 30%. Recurrence is encountered more often in mandibular odontogenic keratocysts, particularly those in the posterior body and ascending ramus. Multiple recurrences are not unusual. Although many odontogenic keratocysts recur within 5 years of the original surgery, a significant number of recurrences may not be manifested until 10 or more years after the original surgical procedure. Long-term clinical and radiographic follow-up, therefore, is necessary.

Many surgeons recommend peripheral ostectomy of the bony cavity with a bone bur to reduce the frequency of recurrence. Others advocate chemical cauterization of the bony cavity with Carnoy's solution after cyst removal. Intraluminal injection of Carnoy's solution also has been used to free the cyst from the bony wall, thereby allowing easier removal with a lower recurrence rate. After cystotomy and incisional biopsy, some surgeons have treated large odontogenic keratocysts by insertion of a polyethylene drainage tube to allow decompression and subsequent reduction in size of the cystic cavity (Fig. 15-19). Such decompression treatment results in thickening of the cyst lining, allowing easier removal with an apparently lower recurrence rate.

Other than the tendency for recurrences, the overall prognosis for most odontogenic keratocysts is good. Occasionally, a locally aggressive odontogenic keratocyst cannot be controlled without local resection and bone grafting. In extremely rare instances, keratocysts have been seen to extend up into the skull base region. A few examples of carcinoma arising in an odontogenic keratocyst have been reported, but the propensity for an odontogenic keratocyst to undergo malignant alteration is no greater and is possibly less than that for other types of odontogenic cysts. Patients with odontogenic keratocysts should be evaluated for manifestations of the nevoid basal cell carcinoma syndrome (see page 688), particularly if the patient is in the first or second decade of life or if multiple keratocysts are identified.

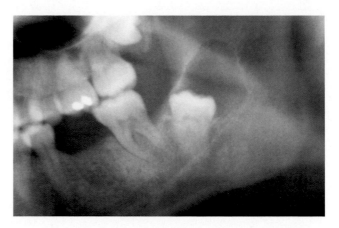

Fig. 15-20   Orthokeratinized odontogenic cyst. Small unilocular radiolucency associated with the impacted mandibular left third molar. *(Courtesy of Dr. Tom McDonald.)*

ORTHOKERATINIZED ODONTOGENIC CYST

The designation **orthokeratinized odontogenic cyst** does not denote a specific clinical type of odontogenic cyst but refers only to an odontogenic cyst that microscopically has an orthokeratinized epithelial lining. Although such lesions were originally called the *orthokeratinized variant of odontogenic keratocyst*, it is generally accepted that they are clinicopathologically different from the more common parakeratinized odontogenic keratocyst and should be placed into a different category. Orthokeratinized odontogenic cysts represent 7% to 17% of all keratinizing jaw cysts.

CLINICAL AND RADIOGRAPHIC FEATURES

Orthokeratinized odontogenic cysts occur predominantly in young adults and show a 2:1 male-to-female ratio. The lesion occurs twice as frequently in the mandible than the maxilla, with a tendency to involve the posterior areas of the jaws. They have no clinical or radiographic features that differentiate them from other inflammatory or developmental odontogenic cysts. The lesion usually appears as a unilocular radiolucency, but occasional examples have been multilocular. About two thirds of orthokeratinized odontogenic cysts are encountered in a lesion that appears clinically and radiographically to represent a dentigerous cyst; they most often involve an unerupted mandibular third molar tooth (Figs. 15-20 and 15-21). The size can vary from less than 1 cm to large lesions greater than 7 cm in diameter.

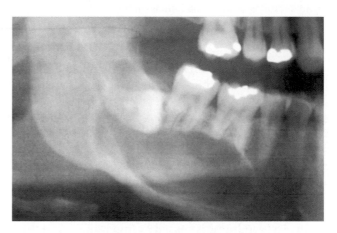

Fig. 15-21   Orthokeratinized odontogenic cyst. A large cyst involving a horizontally impacted lower third molar. *(Courtesy of Dr. Carroll Gallagher.)*

HISTOPATHOLOGIC FEATURES

The cyst lining is composed of stratified squamous epithelium, which shows an orthokeratotic surface of varying thickness. Keratohyaline granules may be prominent in the superficial epithelial layer subjacent to the orthokeratin. The epithelial lining may be relatively thin, and a prominent palisaded basal layer, characteristic of the odontogenic keratocyst, is not present (Fig. 15-22).

TREATMENT AND PROGNOSIS

Enucleation with curettage is the usual treatment for orthokeratinized odontogenic cysts. Recurrence has rarely been noted, and the reported frequency is around 2%, which is in marked contrast with the 30% or higher recurrence rate associated with odontogenic keratocysts. It has been suggested that cysts with an orthokeratinized surface may be at slightly greater risk

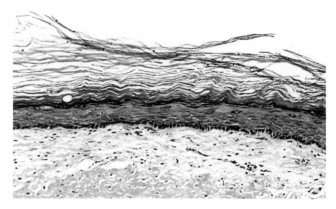

Fig. 15-22   Orthokeratinized odontogenic cyst.
Microscopic features showing a thin epithelial lining. The basal epithelial layer does not demonstrate palisading. Keratohyaline granules are present, and a thick layer of orthokeratin is seen on the luminal surface.

for malignant transformation, but evidence for this is scant. Orthokeratinized odontogenic cysts have not been associated with nevoid basal cell carcinoma syndrome.

NEVOID BASAL CELL CARCINOMA SYNDROME (GORLIN SYNDROME)

Nevoid basal cell carcinoma syndrome (Gorlin syndrome) is an autosomal dominant inherited condition that exhibits high penetrance and variable expressivity. The syndrome is caused by mutations in **patched (PTCH)**, a tumor suppressor gene that has been mapped to chromosome 9q22.3-q31. Approximately 35% to 50% of affected patients represent new mutations. The chief components are multiple basal cell carcinomas of the skin, odontogenic keratocysts, intracranial calcification, and rib and vertebral anomalies. Many other anomalies have been reported in these patients and probably also represent manifestations of the syndrome. The prevalence of Gorlin syndrome is estimated to be about 1 in 60,000.

CLINICAL AND RADIOGRAPHIC FEATURES

There is great variability in the expressivity of nevoid basal cell carcinoma syndrome, and no single component is present in all patients. The most common and significant features are summarized in Box 15-2. The patient often has a characteristic facies, with frontal and temporoparietal bossing, which results in an increased cranial circumference (>60 cm in adults). The eyes may appear widely separated, and many patients have true mild ocular hypertelorism. Mild

---

Box 15-2

Major Clinical Features of the Nevoid Basal Cell Carcinoma Syndrome

50% OR GREATER FREQUENCY
- Multiple basal cell carcinomas
- Odontogenic keratocysts
- Epidermal cysts of the skin
- Palmar/plantar pits
- Calcified falx cerebri
- Enlarged head circumference
- Rib anomalies (splayed, fused, partially missing, bifid)
- Mild ocular hypertelorism
- Spina bifida occulta of cervical or thoracic vertebrae

15% TO 49% FREQUENCY
- Calcified ovarian fibromas
- Short fourth metacarpals
- Kyphoscoliosis or other vertebral anomalies
- Pectus excavatum or carinatum
- Strabismus (exotropia)

LESS THAN 15% FREQUENCY (BUT NOT RANDOM)
- Medulloblastoma
- Meningioma
- Lymphomesenteric cysts
- Cardiac fibroma
- Fetal rhabdomyoma
- Marfanoid build
- Cleft lip and/or palate
- Hypogonadism In males
- Mental retardation

From Gorlin RJ: Nevoid basal-cell carcinoma syndrome, *Medicine* 66:98-113, 1987.

---

mandibular prognathism is also commonly present (Fig. 15-23).

Basal cell carcinomas of the skin are a major component of the syndrome. Even though the microscopic appearance of the syndromic basal cell carcinomas is identical to that of nonsyndromic basal cell carcinoma, the syndromic lesions generally have a much less aggressive biologic behavior. The basal cell carcinomas usually begin to appear at puberty or in the second and third decades of life, although they can develop in young children. The tumors may vary from flesh-colored papules to ulcerating plaques. They often appear on skin that is not exposed to sunlight, but they are most commonly located in the midface area (Fig. 15-24). The number of skin tumors may vary from only a few to many hundreds. Blacks with the syndrome tend to develop basal cell carcinomas less frequently than whites (40% versus 90%), and they have fewer of these lesions, probably because of protective skin pigmentation.

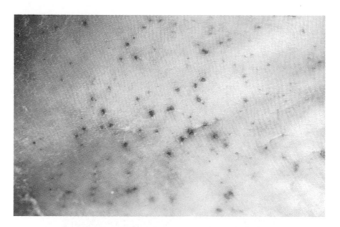

Fig. 15-25   Nevoid basal cell carcinoma syndrome. Plantar pits.

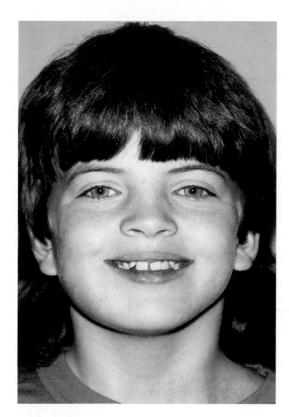

Fig. 15-23   Nevoid basal cell carcinoma syndrome. This 11-year-old girl shows hypertelorism and mandibular swelling. *(Courtesy of Dr. Richard DeChamplain.)*

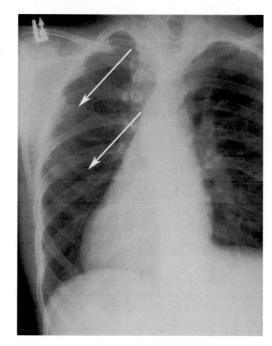

Fig. 15-26   Nevoid basal cell carcinoma syndrome. Chest film showing presence of bifid ribs *(arrows)*.

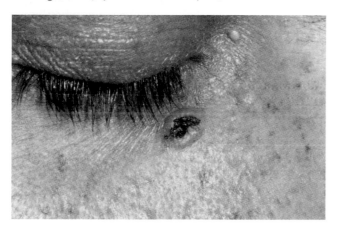

Fig. 15-24   Nevoid basal call carcinoma syndrome. An ulcerating basal cell carcinoma is present on the upper face.

Palmar and plantar pits are present in about 65% to 80% of patients (Fig. 15-25). These punctate lesions represent a localized retardation of the maturation of basal epithelial cells, resulting in a focally depressed area as the result of a markedly thinned keratin layer. Basal cell carcinomas rarely may develop at the base of the pits.

Ovarian fibromas have been reported in 15% to 25% of women with this syndrome. A number of other tumors also have been reported to occur with lesser frequency. These include medulloblastoma within the first 2 years of life, meningioma, cardiac fibroma, and fetal rhabdomyoma.

Skeletal anomalies are present in 60% to 75% of patients with this syndrome. The most common anomaly is a bifid rib or splayed ribs (Fig. 15-26). This anomaly may involve several ribs and may be bilateral. Kyphoscoliosis has been observed in about 30% to 40% of patients, and a number of other anomalies, such as spina bifida occulta and shortened metacarpals, seem to occur with unusual frequency. A distinctive lamellar calcification of the falx cerebri, noted on an anteroposterior skull radiograph or computed tomography (CT) image, is a common finding and is present in most affected patients (Fig. 15-27).

Jaw cysts are one of the most constant features of the syndrome and are present in at least 75% of the patients. The cysts are odontogenic keratocysts, although there are some differences between the cysts in patients with nevoid basal cell carcinoma syndrome and in those with isolated keratocysts. The cysts are frequently multiple; some patients have had as many as ten separate cysts. The patient's age when the first keratocyst is removed is significantly younger in those affected by

this syndrome than in those with isolated keratocysts. For most patients with this syndrome, their first keratocyst is removed before age 19. About one third of patients with nevoid basal cell carcinoma syndrome have only a solitary cyst at the time of the initial presentation, but in most cases additional cysts will develop over periods ranging from 1 to 20 years.

Radiographically, the cysts in patients with nevoid basal cell carcinoma syndrome do not differ significantly from isolated keratocysts. The cysts in patients with this syndrome are often associated with the crowns of unerupted teeth; on radiographs they may mimic dentigerous cysts (Fig. 15-28).

HISTOPATHOLOGIC FEATURES

The cysts in the nevoid basal cell carcinoma syndrome histopathologically are invariably odontogenic keratocysts. The keratocysts in patients with this syndrome tend to have more satellite cysts, solid islands of epithelial proliferation, and odontogenic epithelial rests within the fibrous capsule than do isolated keratocysts (Fig. 15-29). Foci of calcification also appear to be more common. These features, however, are not diagnostic for nevoid basal cell carcinoma syndrome because they may be seen in isolated keratocysts. Odontogenic keratocysts associated with this syndrome have been shown to demonstrate overexpression of p53 and cyclin D1 (bcl-1) oncoproteins when compared with nonsyndrome keratocysts.

The basal cell tumors of the skin cannot be distinguished from ordinary basal cell carcinomas. They exhibit a wide spectrum of histopathologic findings, from superficial basal cell lesions to aggressive, noduloulcerative basal cell carcinomas.

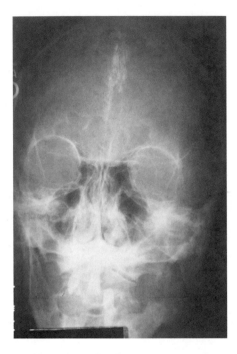

Fig. 15-27   Nevoid basal cell carcinoma syndrome. Anteroposterior skull film showing calcification of the falx cerebri. *(Courtesy of Dr. Ramesh Narang.)*

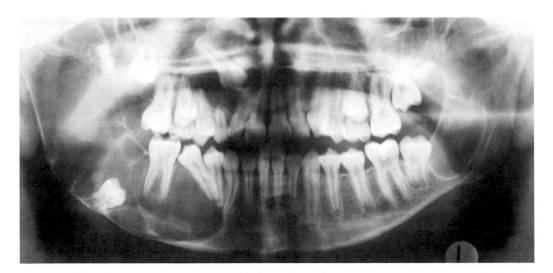

Fig. 15-28   Nevoid basal cell carcinoma syndrome. Large cysts are present in the right and left mandibular molar regions, together with a smaller cyst involving the right maxillary canine in the same patient shown in **Fig. 15-23.** *(Courtesy of Dr. Richard DeChamplain.)*

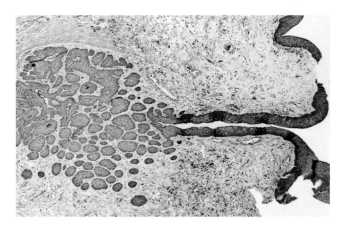

Fig. 15-29   Nevoid basal cell carcinoma syndrome. Odontogenic keratocyst showing numerous odontogenic epithelial rests in the cyst wall.

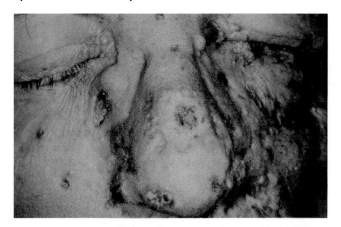

Fig. 15-30   Nevoid basal cell carcinoma syndrome. This 52-year-old man had more than 100 basal cell carcinomas removed from his face over a 30-year period. Several basal cell carcinomas are present in this photograph. The lesion at the inner canthus of the left eye was deeply invasive and was eventually fatal as a result of brain invasion.

TREATMENT AND PROGNOSIS

Most of the anomalies in nevoid basal cell carcinoma syndrome are minor and usually not life threatening. The prognosis generally depends on the behavior of the skin tumors. In a few cases, aggressive basal cell carcinomas have caused the death of the patient as a result of tumor invasion of the brain or other vital structures (Figs. 15-30 and 15-31). Because the development of the basal cell carcinomas seems to be triggered by ultraviolet (UV) light exposure, patients should take appropriate precautions to avoid sunlight. For the same reason, radiation therapy should be avoided if at all possible. The jaw cysts are treated by enucleation, but in many patients additional cysts will continue to develop. Varying degrees of jaw deformity may result from the operations for multiple cysts. Infection of the cysts in patients with this syndrome is also relatively common. Some investigators have suggested that

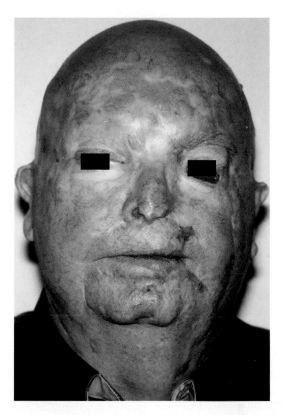

Fig. 15-31   Nevoid basal cell carcinoma syndrome. Facial deformity secondary to multiple surgical procedures to remove basal cell carcinomas.

affected children should have magnetic resonance imaging (MRI) studies every 6 months until 7 years of age to monitor for the development of medulloblastoma. Genetic counseling is appropriate for affected individuals.

GINGIVAL (ALVEOLAR) CYST OF THE NEWBORN

Gingival cysts of the newborn are small, superficial, keratin-filled cysts that are found on the alveolar mucosa of infants. These cysts arise from remnants of the dental lamina. They are common lesions, having been reported in up to half of all newborns. However, because they disappear spontaneously by rupture into the oral cavity, the lesions seldom are noticed or sampled for biopsy. Similar inclusion cysts (e.g., **Epstein's pearls** and **Bohn's nodules**) are also found in the midline of the palate or laterally on the hard and soft palate (see page 26).

CLINICAL FEATURES

Gingival cysts of the newborn appear as small, usually multiple whitish papules on the mucosa overlying the alveolar processes of neonates (Fig. 15-32). The individual cysts are usually no more than 2 to 3 mm in

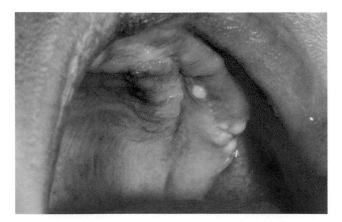

Fig. 15-32 Gingival cyst of the newborn. Multiple whitish papules on the alveolar ridge of a newborn infant.

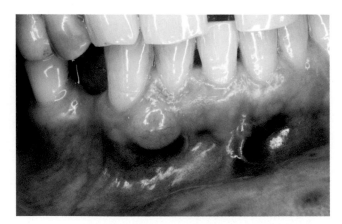

Fig. 15-33 Gingival cyst of the adult. Tense, fluid-filled swelling on the facial gingiva.

diameter. The maxillary alveolus is more commonly involved than the mandibular.

HISTOPATHOLOGIC FEATURES

Examination of an intact gingival cyst of the newborn shows a thin, flattened epithelial lining with a parakeratotic luminal surface. The lumen contains keratinaceous debris.

TREATMENT AND PROGNOSIS

No treatment is indicated for gingival cysts of the newborn because the lesions spontaneously involute as a result of the rupture of the cysts and resultant contact with the oral mucosal surface. The lesions are rarely seen after 3 months of age.

GINGIVAL CYST OF THE ADULT

The **gingival cyst of the adult** is an uncommon lesion. It is considered to represent the soft tissue counterpart of the **lateral periodontal cyst** (see next topic), being derived from rests of the dental lamina (rests of Serres). The diagnosis of gingival cyst of the adult should be restricted to lesions with the same histopathologic features as those of the lateral periodontal cyst. On rare occasions, a cyst may develop in the gingiva at the site of a gingival graft; however, such lesions probably represent *epithelial inclusion cysts* that are a result of the surgical procedure.

CLINICAL FEATURES

Like the lateral periodontal cyst, the gingival cyst of the adult shows a striking predilection to occur in the mandibular canine and premolar area (60% to 75% of cases). Gingival cysts of the adult are most commonly found

in patients in the fifth and sixth decades of life. They are almost invariably located on the facial gingiva or alveolar mucosa. Maxillary gingival cysts are usually found in the incisor, canine, and premolar areas.

Clinically, the cysts appear as painless, domelike swellings, usually less than 0.5 cm in diameter, although rarely they may be somewhat larger (Fig. 15-33). They are often bluish or blue-gray. In some instances, the cyst may cause a superficial "cupping out" of the alveolar bone, which is usually not detected on a radiograph but is apparent when the cyst is excised. If more bone is missing, one could argue that the lesion may be a lateral periodontal cyst that has eroded the cortical bone rather than a gingival cyst that originated in the mucosa.

HISTOPATHOLOGIC FEATURES

The histopathologic features of the gingival cyst of the adult are similar to those of the lateral periodontal cyst, consisting of a thin, flattened epithelial lining with or without focal plaques that contain clear cells (Figs. 15-34 and 15-35). Small nests of these glycogen-rich clear cells, which represent rests of the dental lamina, also may be seen in the surrounding connective tissue. Sometimes the cystic lining is so thin that it is easily mistaken for the endothelial lining of a dilated blood vessel.

TREATMENT AND PROGNOSIS

The gingival cyst of the adult responds well to simple surgical excision. The prognosis is excellent.

LATERAL PERIODONTAL CYST (BOTRYOID ODONTOGENIC CYST)

The **lateral periodontal cyst** is an uncommon type of developmental odontogenic cyst that typically occurs along the lateral root surface of a tooth. It is believed

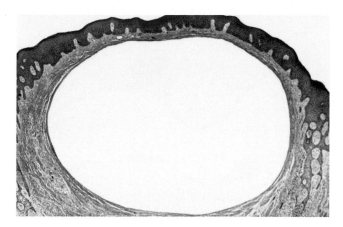

Fig. 15-34   Gingival cyst of the adult. Low-power photomicrograph showing a thin-walled cyst in the gingival soft tissue.

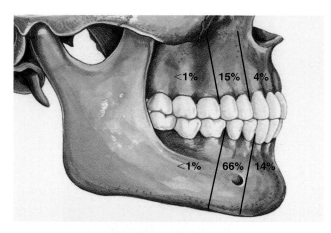

Fig. 15-36   Lateral periodontal cyst. Relative distribution of lateral periodontal cysts in the jaws.

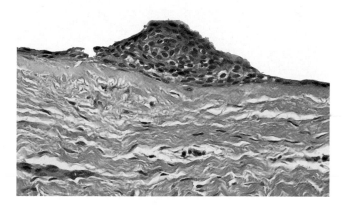

Fig. 15-35   Gingival cyst of the adult. High-power photomicrograph showing a plaquelike thickening of the epithelial lining.

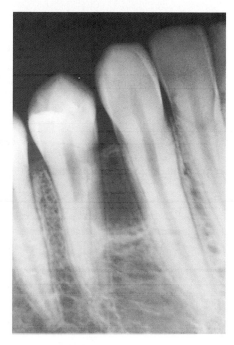

Fig. 15-37   Lateral periodontal cyst. Radiolucent lesion between the roots of a vital mandibular canine and first premolar.

to arise from rests of the dental lamina, and it represents the intrabony counterpart of the gingival cyst of the adult. The lateral periodontal cyst accounts for less than 2% of all epithelium-lined jaw cysts.

In the past, the term *lateral periodontal cyst* was used to describe any cyst that developed along the lateral root surface, including lateral radicular cysts (see page 131) and odontogenic keratocysts (see page 683). However, the lateral periodontal cyst has distinctive clinical and microscopic features that distinguish it from other lesions that sometimes develop in the same location.

CLINICAL AND RADIOGRAPHIC FEATURES

The lateral periodontal cyst is most often an asymptomatic lesion that is detected only during a radiographic examination. It most frequently occurs in patients in the fifth through the seventh decades of life; rarely does it occur in someone younger than age 30. Around 75% to 80% of cases occur in the mandibular premolar-canine-lateral incisor area. Maxillary examples also usually involve this same tooth region (Fig. 15-36).

Radiographically, the cyst appears as a well-circumscribed radiolucent area located laterally to the root or roots of vital teeth. Most such cysts are less than 1.0 cm in greatest diameter (Figs. 15-37 and 15-38).

Occasionally, the lesion may have a polycystic appearance; such examples have been termed **botryoid odontogenic cysts**. Grossly and microscopically, they show a grapelike cluster of small individual cysts (Fig. 15-39). These lesions are generally considered to

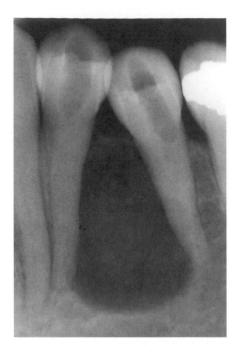

Fig. 15-38   Lateral periodontal cyst. A larger lesion causing root divergence.

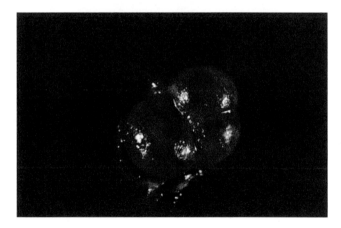

Fig. 15-39   Lateral periodontal cyst. Gross specimen of a botryoid variant. Microscopically, this grapelike cluster revealed three separate cavities.

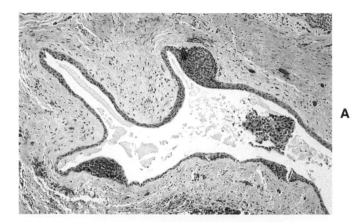

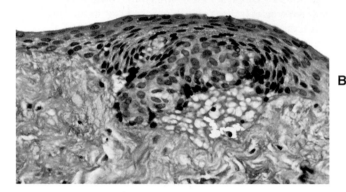

Fig. 15-40   Lateral periodontal cyst. A, This photomicrograph shows a thin epithelial lining with focal nodular thickenings. **B,** These thickenings often show a swirling appearance of the cells.

represent a variant of the lateral periodontal cyst, possibly the result of cystic degeneration and subsequent fusion of adjacent foci of dental lamina rests. The botryoid variant often shows a multilocular radiographic appearance, but it also may appear unilocular.

The radiographic features of the lateral periodontal cyst are not diagnostic; an odontogenic keratocyst that develops between the roots of adjacent teeth may show identical radiographic findings. An inflammatory radicular cyst that occurs laterally to a root in relation to an accessory foramen or a cyst that arises from periodontal inflammation also may simulate a lateral periodontal cyst radiographically (see page 132). In one study of 46 cases of cystic lesions in the lateral periodontal region, only 13 met the histopathologic criteria for the lateral periodontal cyst; 8 were odontogenic keratocysts, 20 were inflammatory cysts, and 5 were of undetermined origin.

HISTOPATHOLOGIC FEATURES

The lateral periodontal cyst has a thin, generally noninflamed, fibrous wall, with an epithelial lining that is only one to three cells thick in most areas. This epithelium usually consists of flattened squamous cells, but sometimes the cells are cuboidal in shape. Foci of glycogen-rich clear cells may be interspersed among the lining epithelial cells. Some cysts show focal nodular thickenings of the lining epithelium, which are composed chiefly of clear cells (Fig. 15-40). Clear cell epithelial rests sometimes are seen within the fibrous wall. Rarely, botryoid odontogenic cysts exhibit focal areas that histopathologically are suggestive of the glandular odontogenic cyst (see page 697).

TREATMENT AND PROGNOSIS

Conservative enucleation of the lateral periodontal cyst is the treatment of choice. Usually, this can be accomplished without damage to the adjacent teeth. Recurrence is unusual, although it has been reported with the botryoid variant, presumably because of its polycystic nature. An exceedingly rare case of squamous cell carcinoma, which apparently originated in a lateral periodontal cyst, also has been reported.

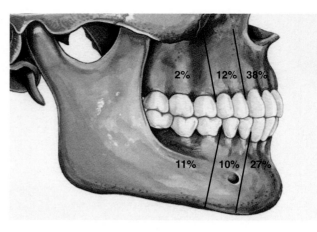

Fig. 15-41   Calcifying odontogenic cyst. Relative distribution of calcifying odontogenic cysts in the jaws.

CALCIFYING ODONTOGENIC CYST (GORLIN CYST; DENTINOGENIC GHOST CELL TUMOR; CALCIFYING CYSTIC ODONTOGENIC TUMOR; CALCIFYING GHOST CELL ODONTOGENIC CYST)

The **calcifying odontogenic cyst** is an uncommon lesion that demonstrates considerable histopathologic diversity and variable clinical behavior. Although it is widely considered to represent a cyst, some investigators prefer to classify it as a neoplasm. Some calcifying odontogenic cysts appear to represent nonneoplastic cysts; other members of this group, variously designated as **dentinogenic ghost cell tumors** or **epithelial odontogenic ghost cell tumors**, have no cystic features, may be infiltrative or even malignant, and are regarded as neoplasms.

In addition, the calcifying odontogenic cyst may be associated with other recognized odontogenic tumors, most commonly **odontomas**. However, **adenomatoid odontogenic tumors** and **ameloblastomas** have also been associated with calcifying odontogenic cysts. The WHO classification of odontogenic tumors groups the calcifying odontogenic cyst with all its variants as an odontogenic tumor rather than an odontogenic cyst. Given the innocuous clinical behavior of this lesion, the widely recognized historic categorization of the lesion as a cyst, and the cystic nature of the majority of these lesions, the change in terminology does not seem practical.

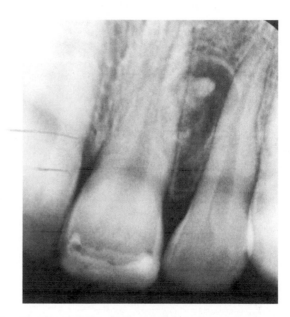

Fig. 15-42   Calcifying odontogenic cyst. Maxillary radiolucent lesion containing calcified structures.

CLINICAL AND RADIOGRAPHIC FEATURES

The calcifying odontogenic cyst is predominantly an intraosseous lesion, although 13% to 30% of cases in reported series have appeared as peripheral (extraosseous) lesions. Both the intraosseous and extraosseous forms occur with about equal frequency in the maxilla and mandible. About 65% of cases are found in the incisor and canine areas (Fig. 15-41). Patients may range in age from infant to elder. The mean age is 33 years, and most cases are diagnosed in the second and third decades of life. Calcifying odontogenic cysts that are associated with odontomas tend to occur in younger patients, with a mean age of 17 years. The rare neoplastic variants of the calcifying odontogenic cyst appear to occur in older patients; because of the paucity of reported cases, however, this may not be significant.

The central calcifying odontogenic cyst is usually a unilocular, well-defined radiolucency, although the lesion may occasionally appear multilocular. Radiopaque structures within the lesion, either irregular calcifications or toothlike densities, are present in about one third to one half of cases (Fig. 15-42). In approximately one third of cases, the radiolucent lesion is associated with an unerupted tooth, most often a canine. Most calcifying odontogenic cysts are between

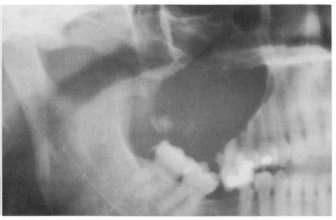

Fig. 15-43   Calcifying odontogenic cyst. A, Expansion of the posterior maxillary alveolus caused by a large calcifying odontogenic cyst. **B,** Panoramic radiograph of the same patient showing a large radiolucency in the posterior maxilla. A small calcified structure is seen in the lower portion of the cyst. *(Courtesy of Dr. Tom Brock.)*

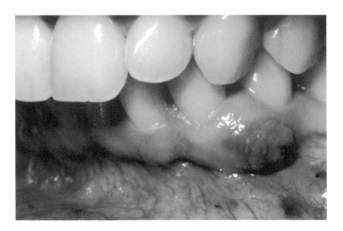

Fig. 15-44   Peripheral calcifying odontogenic cyst. Nodular mass of the mandibular facial gingiva.

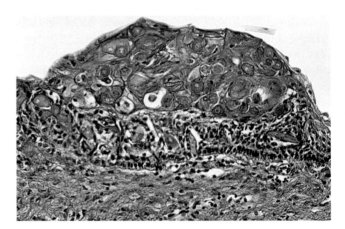

Fig. 15-45   Calcifying odontogenic cyst. The cyst lining shows ameloblastoma-like epithelial cells, with a columnar basal layer. Large eosinophilic ghost cells are present within the epithelial lining.

2.0 and 4.0 cm in greatest diameter, but lesions as large as 12.0 cm have been noted. Root resorption or divergence of adjacent teeth is seen with some frequency (Fig. 15-43).

Extraosseous calcifying odontogenic cysts are localized sessile or pedunculated gingival masses with no distinctive clinical features (Fig. 15-44). They can resemble common gingival fibromas, gingival cysts, or peripheral giant cell granulomas.

HISTOPATHOLOGIC FEATURES

The cystic (nonneoplastic) forms comprise 86% to 98% of all calcifying odontogenic cysts in various reported series. These may occur both intraosseously and extraosseously. Most commonly, a well-defined cystic lesion is found with a fibrous capsule and a lining of odontogenic epithelium of 4 to 10 cells in thickness.

The basal cells of the epithelial lining may be cuboidal or columnar and are similar to ameloblasts. The overlying layer of loosely arranged epithelium may resemble the stellate reticulum of an ameloblastoma.

The most characteristic histopathologic feature of the calcifying odontogenic cyst is the presence of variable numbers of "ghost cells" within the epithelial component. These eosinophilic ghost cells are altered epithelial cells that are characterized by the loss of nuclei with preservation of the basic cell outline (Fig. 15-45).

The nature of the ghost cell change is controversial. Some believe that this change represents coagulative necrosis or accumulation of enamel protein; others contend it is a form of normal or aberrant keratinization of odontogenic epithelium. Masses of ghost cells

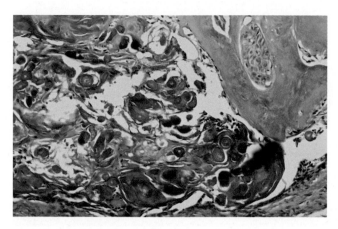

Fig. 15-46   Calcifying odontogenic cyst. Eosinophilic dentinoid material is present adjacent to a sheet of ghost cells.

may fuse to form large sheets of amorphous, acellular material. Calcification within the ghost cells is common. This first appears as fine basophilic granules that may increase in size and number to form extensive masses of calcified material. Areas of an eosinophilic matrix material that are considered by some authors to represent dysplastic dentin (dentinoid) also may be present adjacent to the epithelial component. This is believed to be the result of an inductive effect by the odontogenic epithelium on the adjacent mesenchymal tissue (Fig. 15-46).

Several variants of the cystic type of calcifying odontogenic cyst are seen. In some cases, the epithelial lining proliferates into the lumen so that the lumen is largely filled with masses of ghost cells and dystrophic calcifications. Multiple daughter cysts may be present within the fibrous wall, and a foreign body reaction to herniated ghost cells may be conspicuous.

In another variant, unifocal or multifocal epithelial proliferation of the cyst lining into the lumen may resemble ameloblastoma. These proliferations are intermixed with varying numbers of ghost cells. These epithelial proliferations superficially resemble, but do not meet, the strict histopathologic criteria for ameloblastoma.

About 20% of cystic calcifying odontogenic cysts are associated with odontomas. This variant is usually a unicystic lesion that shows the features of a calcifying odontogenic cyst together with those of a small complex or compound odontoma.

Neoplastic (solid) calcifying odontogenic cysts are uncommon, accounting for 2% to 16% of all calcifying odontogenic cysts in reported series. These may occur intraosseously or extraosseously.

The **extraosseous** forms of the solid variant appear to be more common. These show varying-sized islands of odontogenic epithelium in a fibrous stroma. The epithelial islands show peripheral palisaded columnar cells and central stellate reticulum, which resemble ameloblastoma. Nests of ghost cells, however, are present within the epithelium, and juxtaepithelial dentinoid is commonly present. These features differentiate this lesion from the peripheral ameloblastoma.

The rare **intraosseous** variant is a solid tumor that consists of ameloblastoma-like strands and islands of odontogenic epithelium in a mature fibrous connective tissue stroma. Variable numbers of ghost cells and juxtaepithelial dentinoid are present.

A small number of aggressive or malignant epithelial odontogenic ghost cell tumors (**odontogenic ghost cell carcinoma**) have been reported. These lesions have cellular pleomorphism and mitotic activity with invasion of the surrounding tissues.

TREATMENT AND PROGNOSIS

The prognosis for a patient with a calcifying odontogenic cyst is good; only a few recurrences after simple enucleation have been reported. The peripheral neoplastic calcifying odontogenic cyst appears to have the same prognosis as a peripheral ameloblastoma, with a minimal chance of recurrence after simple surgical excision.

When a calcifying odontogenic cyst is associated with some other recognized odontogenic tumor, such as an ameloblastoma, the treatment and prognosis are likely to be the same as for the associated tumor. Although few cases have been reported, odontogenic ghost cell carcinomas appear to have an unpredictable behavior. Recurrences are common, and a few patients have died from either uncontrolled local disease or metastases. An overall 5-year survival rate of 73% has been calculated for reported cases.

GLANDULAR ODONTOGENIC CYST (SIALO-ODONTOGENIC CYST)

The **glandular odontogenic cyst** is a rare type of developmental odontogenic cyst that can show aggressive behavior. Although it is generally accepted as being of odontogenic origin, it also shows glandular or salivary features that presumably are an indication of the pluripotentiality of odontogenic epithelium.

CLINICAL AND RADIOGRAPHIC FEATURES

The glandular odontogenic cyst occurs most commonly in middle-aged adults, with a mean age of 48 years at the time of diagnosis; rarely does it occur before the age of 20. Nearly 75% of reported cases have occurred in the mandible. The cyst has a strong predilection for

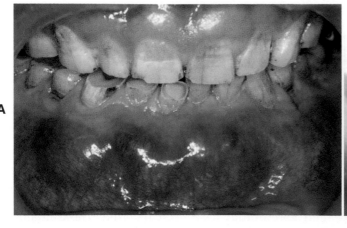

Fig. 15-47   Glandular odontogenic cyst. A, Expansile lesion of the anterior mandible. **B,** The panoramic radiograph shows a large multilocular radiolucency. *(Courtesy of Dr. Cheng-Chung Lin.)*

the anterior region of the jaws, and many mandibular lesions will cross the midline.

The size of the cyst can vary from small lesions less than 1 cm in diameter to large destructive lesions that may involve most of the jaw. Small cysts may be asymptomatic; however, large cysts often produce clinical expansion, which sometimes can be associated with pain or paresthesia (Fig. 15-47).

Radiographically, the lesion presents as either a unilocular or multilocular radiolucency. The margins of the radiolucency are usually well defined with a sclerotic rim.

HISTOPATHOLOGIC FEATURES

The glandular odontogenic cyst is lined by squamous epithelium of varying thickness. The interface between the epithelium and the fibrous connective tissue wall is generally flat. The fibrous cyst wall is usually devoid of any inflammatory cell infiltrate. The superficial epithelial cells that line the cyst cavity tend to be cuboidal to columnar, resulting in an uneven hobnail and sometimes papillary surface (Fig. 15-48). Occasionally, cilia may be noted. Pools of mucicarminophilic material are often present within the epithelium. Cuboidal cells usually line these pools. Mucous cells may or may not be present within the epithelium. In focal areas, the epithelial lining cells may form spherical nodules, similar to those seen in lateral periodontal cysts.

There is some histopathologic overlap between the features of the glandular odontogenic cyst and those of some intraosseous, low-grade, predominantly cystic mucoepidermoid carcinomas (see page 490). In selected microscopic fields, the microscopic features may be identical. Examination of multiple sections, however, usually permits the differentiation of these lesions.

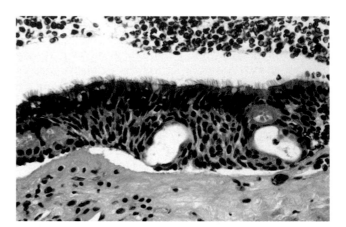

Fig. 15-48   Glandular odontogenic cyst. The cyst is lined by stratified squamous epithelium that exhibits surface columnar cells with cilia. Small microcysts and clusters of mucous cells are present.

TREATMENT AND PROGNOSIS

Most cases of glandular odontogenic cyst have been treated by enucleation or curettage. However, this cyst shows a propensity for recurrence, which is observed in approximately 30% of all cases. Recurrence appears to be more common among the lesions that present in a multilocular fashion. Because of its potentially aggressive nature and tendency for recurrence, some authors have advocated *en bloc* resection, particularly for multilocular lesions.

BUCCAL BIFURCATION CYST

The **buccal bifurcation cyst** is an uncommon inflammatory odontogenic cyst that characteristically develops on the buccal aspect of the mandibular first permanent molar. The pathogenesis of this cyst is uncertain. Some of these lesions have been associated with teeth that demonstrate buccal enamel extensions into the bifurcation area (see page 93). Such extensions may predispose these teeth to buccal pocket formation, which could then enlarge to form a cyst in response to pericoronitis. It has been speculated that when the tooth erupts, an inflammatory response may occur in the surrounding follicular tissues that stimulates cyst formation.

The term **paradental cyst** sometimes has been used synonymously for the buccal bifurcation cyst. Such lesions typically occur distal or buccal of partially erupted mandibular third molars with a history of pericoronitis. The pathogenesis of the so-called paradental cyst also is uncertain. However, the distinction of paradental cysts from secondarily inflamed dentigerous cysts is difficult, if not impossible, in many instances (see page 679).

CLINICAL AND RADIOGRAPHIC FEATURES

The buccal bifurcation cyst typically occurs in children from 5 to 13 years of age. The patient has slight-to-moderate tenderness on the buccal aspect of the mandibular first molar, which may be in the process of erupting. The patient often notes associated clinical swelling and a foul-tasting discharge. Periodontal probing usually reveals pocket formation on the buccal aspect of the involved tooth. Around one third of patients have been reported to have bilateral involvement of the first molars.

Radiographs typically show a well-circumscribed unilocular radiolucency involving the buccal bifurcation and root area of the involved tooth (Fig. 15-49). The average size of the lucent defect is 1.2 cm, but the lesion may be as large as 2.5 cm in diameter. An occlusal radiograph is most helpful in demonstrating the buccal location of the lesion. The root apices of the molar are characteristically tipped toward the lingual mandibular cortex (Fig. 15-50). Many cases are associated with proliferative periostitis (see page 148) of the overlying buccal cortex, which is characterized by a single or multiple layers of reactive bone formation.

HISTOPATHOLOGIC FEATURES

The microscopic features are nonspecific and show a cyst that is lined by nonkeratinizing stratified squamous epithelium with areas of hyperplasia. A prominent chronic inflammatory cell infiltrate is present in the surrounding connective tissue wall.

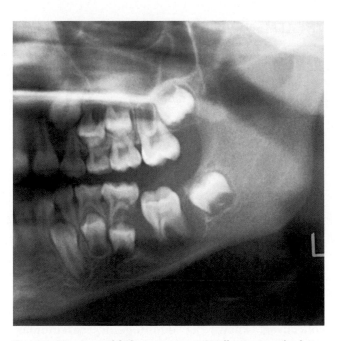

Fig. 15-49   Buccal bifurcation cyst. Well-circumscribed unilocular radiolucency superimposed on the roots of the mandibular first permanent molar. *(Courtesy of Dr. Michael Pharoah.)*

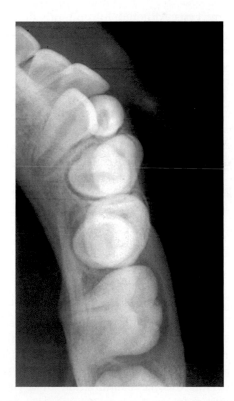

Fig. 15-50   Buccal bifurcation cyst. Occlusal radiograph of the lesion shown in Fig. 15-49. Note the lingual displacement of the roots of the first permanent molar. *(Courtesy of Dr. Michael Pharoah.)*

TREATMENT AND PROGNOSIS

The buccal bifurcation cyst is usually treated by enucleation; extraction of the associated tooth is unnecessary. Within 1 year of surgery, there is usually complete healing with normalization of periodontal probing depths and radiographic evidence of bone fill. One report described three cases that resolved without surgery—either with no treatment at all or by daily irrigation of the buccal pocket with saline and hydrogen peroxide.

CARCINOMA ARISING IN ODONTOGENIC CYSTS

Carcinoma arising within bone is a rare lesion that is essentially limited to the jaws. Because the putative source of the epithelium giving rise to the carcinoma is odontogenic, these intraosseous jaw carcinomas are collectively known as **odontogenic carcinomas**. Odontogenic carcinomas may arise in an ameloblastoma, rarely from other odontogenic tumors, *de novo* (without evidence of a preexisting lesion), or from the epithelial lining of odontogenic cysts. Some intraosseous mucoepidermoid carcinomas (see page 490) also may arise from mucous cells lining a dentigerous cyst.

Most intraosseous carcinomas apparently arise in odontogenic cysts. Although infrequently documented in the literature, carcinomatous transformation of the lining of an odontogenic cyst may be more common than is generally appreciated. Several studies have shown that 1% to 2% of all oral cavity carcinomas seen in some oral and maxillofacial pathology services may originate from odontogenic cysts. The pathogenesis of carcinomas arising in odontogenic cysts is unknown. Occasionally, areas within the lining of odontogenic cysts histopathologically demonstrate varying degrees of epithelial dysplasia, and such changes likely give rise to the carcinoma.

CLINICAL AND RADIOGRAPHIC FEATURES

Although carcinomas arising in cysts may be seen in patients across a wide age range, they are encountered most often in older patients. The mean reported age is 57 to 61 years. This lesion is about twice as common in men as in women. Pain and swelling are the most common complaints. However, many patients have no symptoms, and the diagnosis of carcinoma is made only after microscopic examination of a presumed odontogenic cyst.

Radiographic findings may mimic those of any odontogenic cyst, although the margins of the radiolucent defect are usually irregular and ragged. Computed

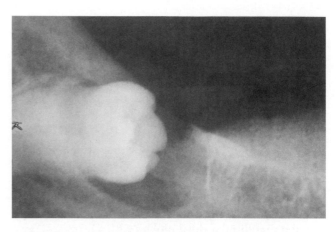

Fig. 15-51 **Carcinoma arising in a dentigerous cyst.** Radiolucent lesion surrounding the crown of an impacted third molar in a 56-year-old woman. This was clinically considered to be a dentigerous cyst. *(Courtesy of Dr. Richard Ziegler.)*

tomography of the lesion may demonstrate a destructive pattern that is not appreciated on viewing plain radiographs. A lesion considered to be a **residual periapical cyst** is apparently the most common type associated with carcinomatous transformation, although routine periapical cysts can also exhibit malignant change. In about 25% of reported cases, the carcinoma appeared to have arisen in a **dentigerous cyst** (Fig. 15-51). In one patient, the carcinoma appeared to originate in a **lateral periodontal cyst**.

A few examples of carcinoma arising in an **odontogenic keratocyst** also have been documented (Fig. 15-52). However, some reported examples do not appear to have arisen in true parakeratinized odontogenic keratocysts, but rather in **orthokeratinized odontogenic cysts**.

HISTOPATHOLOGIC FEATURES

Most carcinomas arising in cysts have histopathologically been **well-differentiated squamous cell carcinomas**. It is sometimes possible to identify a transition from a normal-appearing cyst lining to invasive squamous cell carcinoma (Figs. 15-53 and 15-54).

TREATMENT AND PROGNOSIS

The treatment of patients with carcinomas arising in cysts has varied from local block excision to radical resection, with or without radiation or adjunctive chemotherapy. The prognosis is difficult to evaluate because most reports consist of isolated cases; often the follow-up is inadequate. Several larger studies indicate an approximate 50% 5-year survival rate after

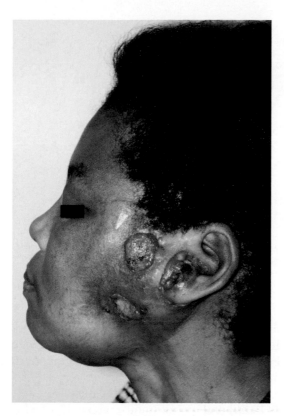

Fig. 15-52   Carcinoma arising in a cyst. There is a massive carcinoma of the mandible, with extension into the parotid gland, the face, and the base of the brain. Nineteen years previously, a large odontogenic keratocyst with areas of epithelial dysplasia had been removed from the ascending ramus. The patient had suffered multiple recurrences, with eventual change into invasive carcinoma.

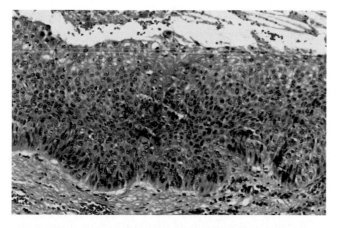

Fig. 15-53   Carcinoma arising in a cyst. High-power view of a dentigerous cyst from a 53-year-old man. The lining demonstrates full-thickness epithelial dysplasia.

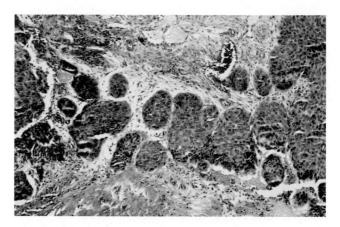

Fig. 15-54   Carcinoma arising in a cyst. Same case as Fig. 15-53 showing islands of invasive epithelial cells in the cyst wall.

treatment. Metastases to regional lymph nodes have been demonstrated in a few cases.

Before a given lesion can be accepted as an example of primary intraosseous carcinoma, the possibility that the tumor represents metastatic spread from an intraoral or extraoral site must be ruled out by appropriate studies.

Odontogenic Tumors

Odontogenic tumors comprise a complex group of lesions of diverse histopathologic types and clinical behavior. Some of these lesions are true neoplasms and may rarely exhibit malignant behavior. Others may represent tumorlike malformations (hamartomas).

Odontogenic tumors, like normal odontogenesis, demonstrate varying inductive interactions between odontogenic epithelium and odontogenic ectomesenchyme. This ectomesenchyme was formerly referred to as *mesenchyme* because it was thought to be derived from the mesodermal layer of the embryo. It is now accepted that this tissue differentiates from the ectodermal layer in the cephalic portion of the embryo. **Tumors of odontogenic epithelium** are composed only of odontogenic epithelium without any participation of odontogenic ectomesenchyme.

Other odontogenic neoplasms, sometimes referred to as **mixed odontogenic tumors**, are composed of odontogenic epithelium and ectomesenchymal elements. Dental hard tissue may or may not be formed in these lesions.

A third group, **tumors of odontogenic ectomesenchyme**, is composed principally of ectomesenchymal elements. Although odontogenic epithelium may be

Classification of Odontogenic Tumors

I. Tumors of odontogenic epithelium
   A. Ameloblastoma
      1. Malignant ameloblastoma
      2. Ameloblastic carcinoma
   B. Clear cell odontogenic carcinoma
   C. Adenomatoid odontogenic tumor
   D. Calcifying epithelial odontogenic tumor
   E. Squamous odontogenic tumor
II. Mixed odontogenic tumors
   A. Ameloblastic fibroma
   B. Ameloblastic fibro-odontoma
   C. Ameloblastic fibrosarcoma
   D. Odontoameloblastoma
   E. Compound odontoma
   F. Complex odontoma
III. Tumors of odontogenic ectomesenchyme
   A. Odontogenic fibroma
   B. Granular cell odontogenic tumor
   C. Odontogenic myxoma
   D. Cementoblastoma

included within these lesions, it does not appear to play any essential role in their pathogenesis.

Box 15-3 presents categories of odontogenic tumors modified from the 2005 WHO classification.

Tumors of Odontogenic Epithelium

Epithelial odontogenic tumors are composed of odontogenic epithelium without participation of odontogenic ectomesenchyme. Several distinctly different tumors are included in the group; ameloblastoma is the most important and common of them.

AMELOBLASTOMA

The **ameloblastoma** is the most common clinically significant odontogenic tumor. Its relative frequency equals the combined frequency of all other odontogenic tumors, excluding odontomas. Ameloblastomas are tumors of odontogenic epithelial origin. Theoretically, they may arise from rests of dental lamina, from a developing enamel organ, from the epithelial lining of an odontogenic cyst, or from the basal cells of the oral mucosa. Ameloblastomas are slow-growing, locally invasive tumors that run a benign course in most cases. They occur in three different clinicoradiographic situ-

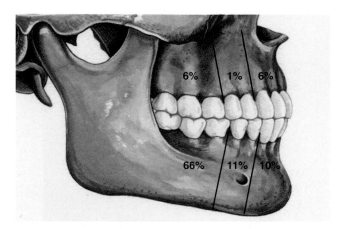

Fig. 15-55 Ameloblastoma. Relative distribution of ameloblastomas in the jaws.

ations, which deserve separate consideration because of differing therapeutic considerations and prognosis:
1. Conventional solid or multicystic (about 86% of all cases)
2. Unicystic (about 13% of all cases)
3. Peripheral (extraosseous) (about 1% of all cases)

CONVENTIONAL SOLID OR MULTICYSTIC INTRAOSSEOUS AMELOBLASTOMA

CLINICAL AND RADIOGRAPHIC FEATURES

Conventional solid or **multicystic intraosseous ameloblastoma** is encountered in patients across a wide age range. It is rare in children younger than age 10 and relatively uncommon in the 10- to 19-year-old group. The tumor shows an approximately equal prevalence in the third to seventh decades of life. There is no significant sex predilection. Some studies indicate a greater frequency in blacks; others show no racial predilection. About 80% to 85% of conventional ameloblastomas occur in the mandible, most often in the molar-ascending ramus area. About 15% to 20% of ameloblastomas occur in the maxilla, usually in the posterior regions (Fig. 15-55). The tumor is often asymptomatic, and smaller lesions are detected only during a radiographic examination. A painless swelling or expansion of the jaw is the usual clinical presentation (Figs. 15-56 and 15-57). If untreated, then the lesion may grow slowly to massive or grotesque proportions (Fig. 15-58). Pain and paresthesia are uncommon, even with large tumors.

The most typical radiographic feature is that of a multilocular radiolucent lesion. The lesion is often described as having a "soap bubble" appearance (when

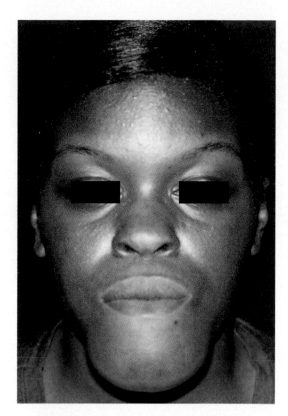

Fig. 15-56 **Ameloblastoma.** Large expansile mass of the anterior mandible. *(Courtesy of Dr. Michael Tabor.)*

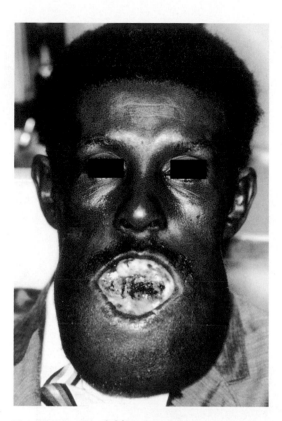

Fig. 15-58 **Ameloblastoma.** Massive tumor of the anterior mandible. *(Courtesy of Dr. Ronald Baughman.)*

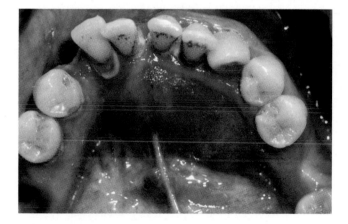

Fig. 15-57 **Ameloblastoma.** Prominent expansion of the lingual alveolus caused by a large ameloblastoma of the mandibular symphysis. The radiograph of the patient is shown in Fig. 15-61.

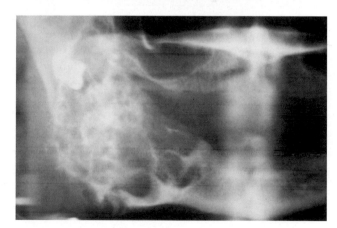

Fig. 15-59 **Ameloblastoma.** Large multilocular lesion involving the mandibular angle and ascending ramus. The large loculations show the "soap bubble" appearance. An unerupted third molar has been displaced high into the ramus.

the radiolucent loculations are large) or as being "honeycombed" (when the loculations are small) (Figs. 15-59 to 15-61). Buccal and lingual cortical expansion is frequently present. Resorption of the roots of teeth adjacent to the tumor is common. In many cases an unerupted tooth, most often a mandibular third molar, is associated with the radiolucent defect. Solid amelo-

blastomas may radiographically appear as unilocular radiolucent defects, which may resemble almost any type of cystic lesion (Fig. 15-62). The margins of these radiolucent lesions, however, often show irregular scalloping. Although the radiographic features, particularly of the typical multilocular defect, may be highly suggestive of ameloblastoma, a variety of odontogenic and

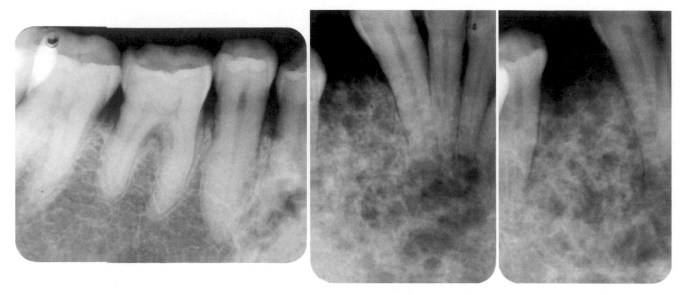

Fig. 15-60   Ameloblastoma. Periapical films showing the "honeycombed" appearance. *(Courtesy of Dr. John Hann.)*

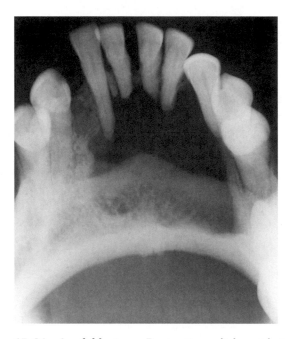

Fig. 15-61   Ameloblastoma. Destructive radiolucent lesion associated with root resorption of the anterior teeth. *(Courtesy of Dr. Richard Brock.)*

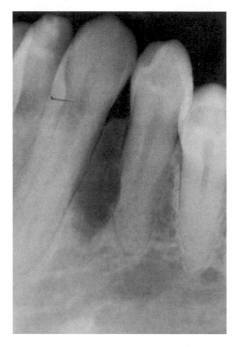

Fig. 15-62   Ameloblastoma. This small unilocular radiolucency lesion could easily be mistaken for a lateral periodontal cyst. *(Courtesy of Dr. Tony Traynham.)*

nonodontogenic lesions may show similar radiographic features (see Appendix).

One form of ameloblastoma that does not have these characteristic features is the desmoplastic ameloblastoma, a variant that Eversole and colleagues documented initially in the literature in 1984. The desmoplastic ameloblastoma has a marked predilection to occur in the anterior regions of the jaws,

particularly the maxilla. Radiographically, this type seldom suggests the diagnosis of ameloblastoma and usually resembles a fibro-osseous lesion because of its mixed radiolucent and radiopaque appearance (Fig. 15-63). This mixed radiographic appearance is due to osseous metaplasia within the dense fibrous septa that characterize the lesion, not because the tumor itself is producing a mineralized product.

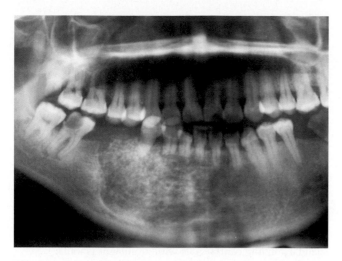

Fig. 15-63   Desmoplastic ameloblastoma. Large mixed radiolucent and radiopaque lesion of the anterior and right body of the mandible. *(Courtesy of Dr. Román Carlos.)*

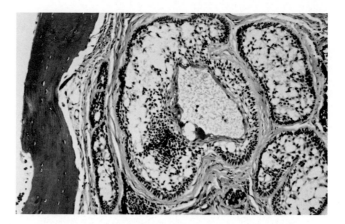

Fig. 15-64   Ameloblastoma (follicular pattern). Multiple islands of odontogenic epithelium demonstrating peripheral columnar differentiation with reverse polarization. The central zones resemble stellate reticulum and exhibit foci of cystic degeneration.

HISTOPATHOLOGIC FEATURES

Conventional solid or multicystic intraosseous ameloblastomas show a remarkable tendency to undergo cystic change; grossly, most tumors have varying combinations of cystic and solid features. The cysts may be seen only at the microscopic level or may be present as multiple large cysts that include most of the tumor. Several microscopic subtypes of conventional ameloblastoma are recognized, but these microscopic patterns generally have little bearing on the behavior of the tumor. Large tumors often show a combination of microscopic patterns.

The **follicular** and **plexiform** patterns are the most common. Less common histopathologic patterns include the **acanthomatous, granular cell, desmoplastic,** and **basal cell** types.

FOLLICULAR PATTERN

The follicular histopathologic pattern is the most common and recognizable. Islands of epithelium resemble enamel organ epithelium in a mature fibrous connective tissue stroma. The epithelial nests consist of a core of loosely arranged angular cells resembling the stellate reticulum of an enamel organ. A single layer of tall columnar ameloblast-like cells surrounds this central core. The nuclei of these cells are located at the opposite pole to the basement membrane (**reversed polarity**). In other areas, the peripheral cells may be more cuboidal and resemble basal cells. Cyst formation is common and may vary from microcysts, which form within the epithelial islands, to large macroscopic cysts, which may be several centimeters in diameter (Figs. 15-64 and 15-65).

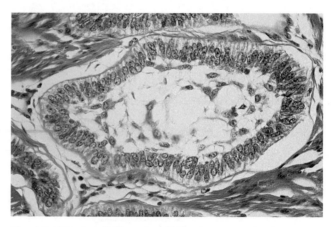

Fig. 15-65   Ameloblastoma (follicular pattern). This high-power photomicrograph highlights the peripheral columnar cells exhibiting reverse polarization.

PLEXIFORM PATTERN

The plexiform type of ameloblastoma consists of long, anastomosing cords or larger sheets of odontogenic epithelium. The cords or sheets of epithelium are bounded by columnar or cuboidal ameloblast-like cells surrounding more loosely arranged epithelial cells. The supporting stroma tends to be loosely arranged and vascular. Cyst formation is relatively uncommon in this variety. When it occurs, it is more often associated with stromal degeneration rather than cystic change within the epithelium (Fig. 15-66).

ACANTHOMATOUS PATTERN

When extensive squamous metaplasia, often associated with keratin formation, occurs in the central portions of the epithelial islands of a follicular ameloblastoma, the term **acanthomatous ameloblas-**

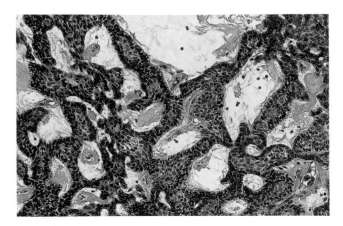

Fig. 15-66   Ameloblastoma (plexiform pattern).
Anastomosing cords of odontogenic epithelium.

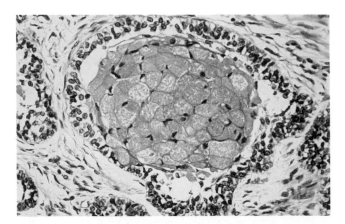

Fig. 15-68   Ameloblastoma (granular cell variant). Tumor island exhibiting central cells with prominent granular cytoplasm.

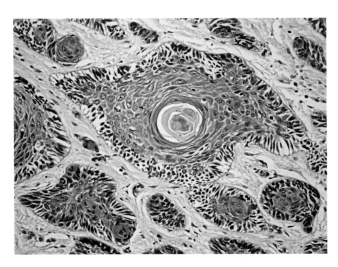

Fig. 15-67   Ameloblastoma (acanthomatous pattern). Islands of ameloblastoma demonstrating central squamous differentiation.

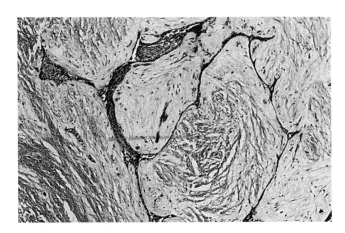

Fig. 15-69   Ameloblastoma (desmoplastic variant). Thin cords of ameloblastic epithelium within a dense fibrous connective tissue stroma.

toma is sometimes applied. This change does not indicate a more aggressive course for the lesion; histopathologically, however, such a lesion may be confused with squamous cell carcinoma or squamous odontogenic tumor (Fig. 15-67).

GRANULAR CELL PATTERN

Ameloblastomas may sometimes show transformation of groups of lesional epithelial cells to granular cells. These cells have abundant cytoplasm filled with eosinophilic granules that resemble lysosomes ultrastructurally and histochemically. Although originally considered to represent an aging or degenerative change in longstanding lesions, this variant has been seen in young patients and in clinically aggressive tumors. When this granular cell change is extensive in an ameloblastoma, the designation of **granular cell ameloblastoma** is appropriate (Fig. 15-68).

DESMOPLASTIC PATTERN

This type of ameloblastoma contains small islands and cords of odontogenic epithelium in a densely collagenized stroma. Immunohistochemical studies have shown increased production of the cytokine known as *transforming growth factor-β* (TGF-β) in association with this lesion, suggesting that this may be responsible for the desmoplasia. Peripheral columnar ameloblast-like cells are inconspicuous about the epithelial islands (Fig. 15-69).

BASAL CELL PATTERN

The basal cell variant of ameloblastoma is the least common type. These lesions are composed of nests of uniform basaloid cells, and they histopathologically are very similar to basal cell carcinoma of the skin. No stellate reticulum is present in the central portions of the nests. The peripheral cells about the nests tend to be cuboidal rather than columnar (Fig. 15-70).

TREATMENT AND PROGNOSIS

Patients with conventional solid or multicystic intraosseous ameloblastomas have been treated by a variety of means. These range from simple enucleation and curettage to *en bloc* resection (Fig. 15-71). The optimal method of treatment has been the subject of controversy for many years. The conventional ameloblastoma tends to infiltrate between intact cancellous bone trabeculae at the periphery of the lesion before bone resorption becomes radiographically evident. Therefore, the actual margin of the tumor often extends beyond its apparent radiographic or clinical margin. Attempts to remove the tumor by curettage often leave

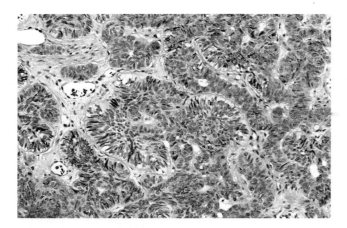

Fig. 15-70   Ameloblastoma (basal cell variant). Islands of hyperchromatic basaloid cells with peripheral palisading.

small islands of tumor within the bone, which later manifest as recurrences. Recurrence rates of 50% to 90% have been reported in various studies after curettage. Recurrence often takes many years to become clinically manifest, and 5-year disease-free periods do not indicate a cure.

Marginal resection is the most widely used treatment, but recurrence rates of up to 15% have been reported after marginal or block resection. Some surgeons advocate a more conservative approach to treatment by planning surgery after careful evaluation of computed tomography (CT) scans of the tumor. Removal of the tumor, followed by peripheral ostectomy, often reduces the need for extensive reconstructive surgery. Some tumors may not be amenable to this approach because of their size or growth pattern.

Other surgeons advocate that the margin of the resection should be at least 1.0 to 1.5 cm past the radiographic limits of the tumor. Ameloblastomas of the posterior maxilla are particularly dangerous because of the difficulty of obtaining an adequate surgical margin around the tumor. Orbital invasion by maxillary ameloblastomas occasionally has been described. Although some studies suggest that the ameloblastoma may be radiosensitive, radiation therapy has seldom been used as a treatment modality because of the intraosseous location of the tumor and the potential for secondary radiation-induced malignancy developing in a relatively young patient population.

The conventional ameloblastoma is a persistent, infiltrative neoplasm that may kill the patient by progressive spread to involve vital structures. Most of these tumors, however, are not life-threatening lesions. Rarely, an ameloblastoma exhibits frank malignant behavior. These are discussed separately.

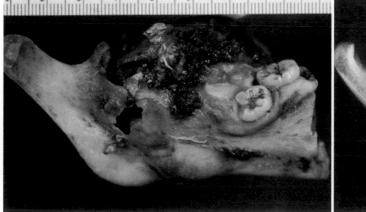
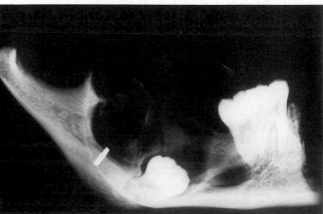

Fig. 15-71   Ameloblastoma. A, Gross photograph of a mandibular resection specimen. **B,** The radiograph of the specimen shows a large radiolucent defect associated with an inferiorly displaced third molar. *(Courtesy of Dr. Mary Richardson.)*

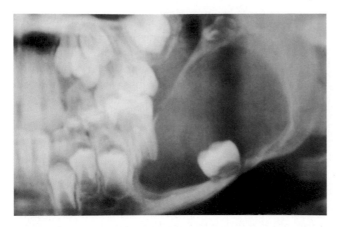

Fig. 15-72 Unicystic ameloblastoma. A large radiolucency in a 7-year-old boy with displacement of the developing second molar to the inferior border of the mandible. This was believed to be a large dentigerous cyst. *(Courtesy of Dr. Larry Chewning.)*

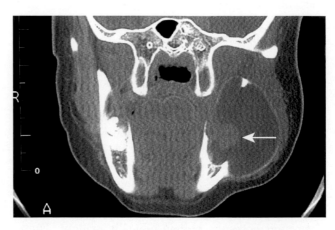

Fig. 15-73 Unicystic ameloblastoma (intraluminal plexiform type). Coronal computed tomography (CT) image that shows a large cystic lesion with an intraluminal mass arising from the cyst wall *(arrow).*

UNICYSTIC AMELOBLASTOMA

The **unicystic ameloblastoma** has for several decades been given separate consideration based on its clinical, radiographic, and pathologic features. Although its response to treatment in reports from the 1970s and 1980s suggested that this lesion might behave in a less aggressive fashion, recent reports have disputed this concept. Unicystic ameloblastomas account for 10% to 46% of all intraosseous ameloblastomas in various studies. Whether the unicystic ameloblastoma originates *de novo* as a neoplasm or whether it is the result of neoplastic transformation of nonneoplastic cyst epithelium has been long debated. Both mechanisms probably occur, but proof of which is involved in an individual patient is virtually impossible to obtain.

CLINICAL AND RADIOGRAPHIC FEATURES

Unicystic ameloblastomas are most often seen in younger patients, with about 50% of all such tumors diagnosed during the second decade of life. The average age in one large series was 23 years. More than 90% of unicystic ameloblastomas are found in the mandible, usually in the posterior regions. The lesion is often asymptomatic, although large lesions may cause a painless swelling of the jaws.

In many patients, this lesion typically appears as a circumscribed radiolucency that surrounds the crown of an unerupted mandibular third molar (Figs. 15-72 and 15-73), clinically resembling a dentigerous cyst. Other tumors simply appear as sharply defined radiolucent areas and are usually considered to be a primordial, radicular, or residual cyst, depending on the relationship of the lesion to teeth in the area. In some instances, the radiolucent area may have scalloped margins but is still a unicystic ameloblastoma. Whether a unicystic ameloblastoma can have a truly multilocular radiographic presentation is arguable.

The surgical findings may also suggest that the lesion in question is a cyst, and the diagnosis of ameloblastoma is made only after microscopic study of the specimen.

HISTOPATHOLOGIC FEATURES

Three histopathologic variants of unicystic ameloblastoma have been described. In the first type (**luminal unicystic ameloblastoma**), the tumor is confined to the luminal surface of the cyst. The lesion consists of a fibrous cyst wall with a lining that consists totally or partially of ameloblastic epithelium. This demonstrates a basal layer of columnar or cuboidal cells with hyperchromatic nuclei that show reverse polarity and basilar cytoplasmic vacuolization (Fig. 15-74). The overlying epithelial cells are loosely cohesive and resemble stellate reticulum. This finding does not seem to be related to inflammatory edema.

In the second microscopic variant, one or more nodules of ameloblastoma project from the cystic lining into the lumen of the cyst. This type is called an **intraluminal unicystic ameloblastoma**. These nodules may be relatively small or largely fill the cystic lumen. In some cases, the nodule of tumor that projects into the lumen demonstrates an edematous, plexiform pattern that resembles the plexiform pattern seen in conventional ameloblastomas (Fig. 15-75). These

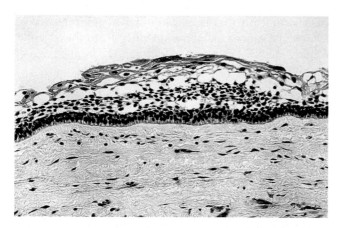

Fig. 15-74   Unicystic ameloblastoma (luminal type). The cyst is lined by ameloblastic epithelium showing a hyperchromatic, polarized basal layer. The overlying epithelial cells are loosely cohesive and resemble stellate reticulum.

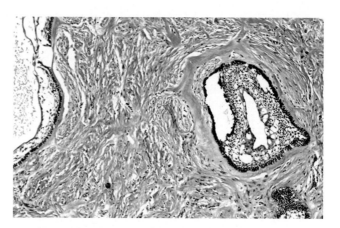

Fig. 15-76   Unicystic ameloblastoma (mural type). The epithelial lining of the cystic component can be seen on the left edge of the photomicrograph. Islands of follicular ameloblastoma are infiltrating into the fibrous connective tissue wall on the right.

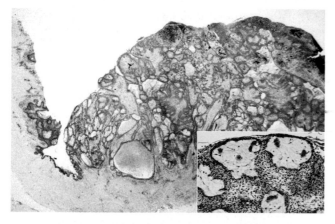

Fig. 15-75   Unicystic ameloblastoma (intraluminal plexiform type). Photomicrograph of the intraluminal mass arising from the cyst wall in the same patient shown in Fig. 15-72. The *inset* shows the intraluminal mass at higher magnification.

lesions are sometimes referred to as **plexiform unicystic ameloblastomas.** The intraluminal cellular proliferation does not always meet the strict histopathologic criteria for ameloblastoma, and this may be secondary to inflammation that nearly always accompanies this pattern. Typical ameloblastoma, however, may be found in other, less inflamed parts of the specimen.

In the third variant, known as **mural unicystic ameloblastoma,** the fibrous wall of the cyst is infiltrated by typical follicular or plexiform ameloblastoma. The extent and depth of the ameloblastic infiltration may vary considerably. With any presumed unicystic ameloblastoma, multiple sections through many levels

of the specimen are necessary to rule out the possibility of mural invasion of tumor cells (Fig. 15-76).

TREATMENT AND PROGNOSIS

The clinical and radiographic findings in most cases of unicystic ameloblastoma suggest that the lesion is an odontogenic cyst. These tumors are usually treated as cysts by enucleation. The diagnosis of ameloblastoma is made only after microscopic examination of the presumed cyst. If the ameloblastic elements are confined to the lumen of the cyst with or without intraluminal tumor extension, then the cyst enucleation has probably been adequate treatment. The patient, however, should be kept under long-term follow-up. If the specimen shows extension of the tumor into the fibrous cyst wall for any appreciable distance, then subsequent management of the patient is more controversial. Some surgeons believe that local resection of the area is indicated as a prophylactic measure; others prefer to keep the patient under close radiographic observation and delay further treatment until there is evidence of recurrence.

Recurrence rates of 10% to 20% were described after enucleation and curettage of unicystic ameloblastomas in many of the earlier series of cases. This range is considerably less than the 50% to 90% recurrence rates noted after curettage of conventional solid and multicystic intraosseous ameloblastomas. One recent series of unicystic ameloblastomas reported recurrence rates after conservative excision of 50% at one institution and 80% at another. A systematic review of the literature before 2005 determined that 30% of these lesions recurred after enucleation. These findings suggest that this lesion may not be as innocuous as previously thought. Alternatively, it is possible that some of those tumors that are designated as "unicystic" may, in fact, have a more characteristic invasive component that has not been detected histopathologically because it is essentially impossible to examine these lesions in every 360-degree plane of section.

PERIPHERAL (EXTRAOSSEOUS) AMELOBLASTOMA

The **peripheral ameloblastoma** is uncommon and accounts for about 1% to 10% of all ameloblastomas. This tumor probably arises from rests of dental lamina beneath the oral mucosa or from the basal epithelial cells of the surface epithelium. Histopathologically, these lesions have the same features as the intraosseous form of the tumor.

CLINICAL FEATURES

The peripheral ameloblastoma is usually a painless, nonulcerated sessile or pedunculated gingival or alveolar mucosal lesion. The clinical features are nonspecific, and most lesions are clinically considered to represent a fibroma or pyogenic granuloma. Most examples are smaller than 1.5 cm, but larger lesions have been reported (Fig. 15-77). The tumor has been found in patients across a wide age range, but most are seen in middle-aged persons, with an average reported age of 52 years.

Peripheral ameloblastomas are most commonly found on the posterior gingival and alveolar mucosa, and they are somewhat more common in mandibular than in maxillary areas. In some cases, the superficial alveolar bone becomes slightly eroded, but significant bone involvement does not occur. A few examples of a microscopically identical lesion have been reported in the buccal mucosa at some distance from the alveolar or gingival soft tissues.

HISTOPATHOLOGIC FEATURES

Peripheral ameloblastomas have islands of ameloblastic epithelium that occupy the lamina propria underneath the surface epithelium (Fig. 15-78). The proliferating epithelium may show any of the features described for the intraosseous ameloblastoma; plexiform or follicular patterns are the most common. Connection of the tumor with the basal layer of the surface epithelium is seen in about 50% of cases. Whether this represents origin of the tumor from the basal layer of the epithelium or merging of the tumor with the surface epithelium has not been ascertained.

Basal cell carcinomas of the oral mucosa have been reported, but most of these would be designated best as peripheral ameloblastomas. A **peripheral odontogenic fibroma** may be confused microscopically with a peripheral ameloblastoma, particularly if a prominent epithelial component is present in the former. The presence of dysplastic dentin or cementum-like elements in the peripheral odontogenic fibroma and the lack of peripheral columnar epithelial cells showing reverse polarity of their nuclei should serve to distinguish the two lesions.

TREATMENT AND PROGNOSIS

Unlike the intraosseous ameloblastoma, the peripheral ameloblastoma shows an innocuous clinical behavior. Patients respond well to local surgical excision. Although local recurrence has been noted in 15% to 20% of cases, further local excision almost always results in a cure. Several examples of malignant change

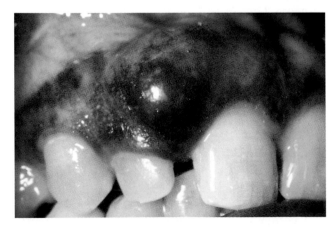

Fig. 15-77   Peripheral ameloblastoma. Sessile gingival mass. *(Courtesy of Dr. Dean K. White.)*

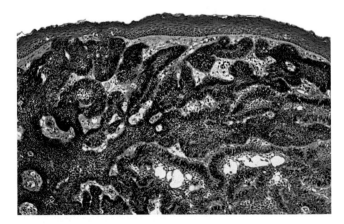

Fig. 15-78   Peripheral ameloblastoma. Interconnecting cords of ameloblastic epithelium filling the lamina propria.

in a peripheral ameloblastoma have been reported, but this is rare.

MALIGNANT AMELOBLASTOMA AND AMELOBLASTIC CARCINOMA

Rarely, an ameloblastoma exhibits frank malignant behavior with development of metastases. The frequency of malignant behavior in ameloblastomas is difficult to determine but probably occurs in far less than 1% of all ameloblastomas.

The terminology for these lesions is somewhat controversial. The term *malignant ameloblastoma* should be used for a tumor that shows the histopathologic features of ameloblastoma, both in the primary tumor and in the metastatic deposits. The term *ameloblastic carcinoma* should be reserved for an ameloblastoma that has cytologic features of malignancy in the primary tumor, in a recurrence, or in any metastatic deposit. These lesions may follow a markedly aggressive local course, but metastases do not necessarily occur.

CLINICAL AND RADIOGRAPHIC FEATURES

Malignant ameloblastomas have been observed in patients who range in age from 4 to 75 years (mean age, 30 years). For patients with documented metastases, the interval between the initial treatment of the ameloblastoma and first evidence of metastasis varies from 1 to 30 years. In nearly one third of cases, metastases do not become apparent until 10 years after treatment of the primary tumor. Ameloblastic carcinomas, in contrast, tend to develop later in life, with the mean age at diagnosis typically being in the sixth decade of life.

Metastases from ameloblastomas are most often found in the lungs. These have sometimes been regarded as aspiration or implant metastases. However, the peripheral location of some of these lung metastases suggests that they must have occurred by blood or lymphatic routes rather than aspiration.

Cervical lymph nodes are the second most common site for metastasis of an ameloblastoma. Spread to vertebrae, other bones, and viscera has also occasionally been confirmed.

The radiographic findings of malignant ameloblastomas may be essentially the same as those in typical nonmetastasizing ameloblastomas. Ameloblastic carcinomas are often more aggressive lesions, with ill-defined margins and cortical destruction (Fig. 15-79).

HISTOPATHOLOGIC FEATURES

With malignant ameloblastomas, the primary jaw tumor and the metastatic deposits show no microscopic features that differ from those of ameloblastomas with a completely benign local course. With ameloblastic carcinomas, the metastatic deposits or primary tumor shows the microscopic pattern of ameloblastoma in addition to cytologic features of malignancy. These include an increased nuclear-to-cytoplasmic ratio, nuclear hyperchromatism, and the presence of mitoses (Fig. 15-80). Necrosis in tumor islands and areas of dystrophic calcification may also be present.

A 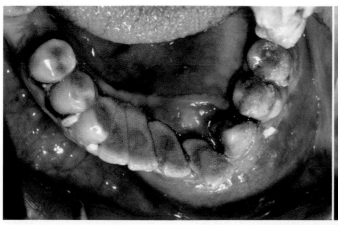   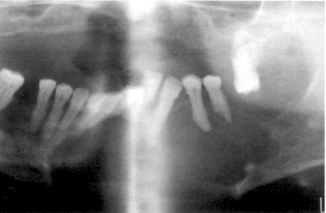 **B**

Fig. 15-79 **Ameloblastic carcinoma. A,** Rapidly growing tumor showing prominent labial expansion of the mandible in the incisor and premolar area. **B,** The panoramic radiograph shows irregular destruction of the mandible. *(From Neville BW, Damm DD, White DK: Color atlas of clinical oral pathology, ed 2, Hamilton, 1999, BC Decker.)*

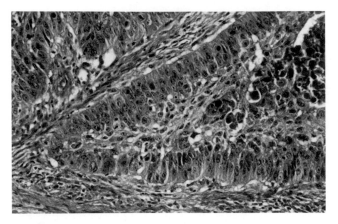

Fig. 15-80   Ameloblastic carcinoma. Ameloblastic epithelium demonstrating hyperchromatism, pleomorphism, and numerous mitotic figures.

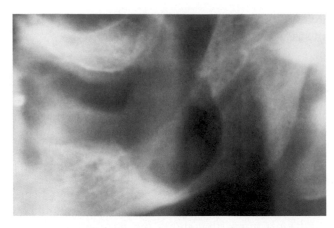

Fig. 15-81   Clear cell odontogenic carcinoma. Unilocular radiolucent defect.

TREATMENT AND PROGNOSIS

The prognosis of patients with malignant ameloblastomas appears to be poor, but the paucity of documented cases with long-term follow-up does not permit accurate assumptions to be made. About 50% of the patients with documented metastases and long-term follow-up have died of their disease. Lesions designated as *ameloblastic carcinoma* have demonstrated a uniformly aggressive clinical course, with perforation of the cortical plates of the jaw and extension of the tumor into adjacent soft tissues.

CLEAR CELL ODONTOGENIC CARCINOMA (CLEAR CELL ODONTOGENIC TUMOR)

Clear cell odontogenic carcinoma is a rare jaw tumor that was first described in 1985. To date, approximately 50 examples have been documented. The tumor appears to be of odontogenic origin, but its histogenesis is uncertain. Histochemical and ultrastructural studies show that the clear cells, which are the prominent feature of this neoplasm, have similarities to glycogen-rich presecretory ameloblasts.

CLINICAL AND RADIOGRAPHIC FEATURES

The clear cell odontogenic carcinoma exhibits a variable clinical pattern. A wide age range (from 14 to 89 years of age) has been described, but most cases are diagnosed in patients older than age 50. More than 80% of the lesions develop in the mandible. Some patients complain of pain and bony swelling; others are relatively symptom free. Approximately 60% of patients

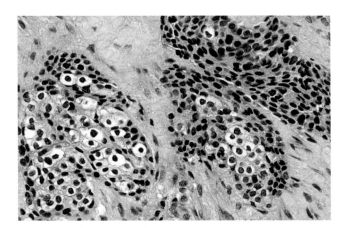

Fig. 15-82   Clear cell odontogenic carcinoma. Hyperchromatic epithelial nests including clusters of cells with abundant clear cytoplasm.

will have evidence of soft tissue involvement by the tumor at the time of diagnosis because the lesion perforates bone.

Radiographically, the lesions appear as unilocular or multilocular radiolucencies. The margins of the radiolucency are often somewhat ill defined or irregular (Fig. 15-81).

HISTOPATHOLOGIC FEATURES

Three histopathologic patterns have been described for clear cell odontogenic carcinoma. The biphasic pattern consists of varying-sized nests of epithelial cells, with a clear or faintly eosinophilic cytoplasm admixed with more eosinophilic polygonal epithelial cells (Fig. 15-82). The second pattern is more monophasic, characterized by only clear cells that are arranged in nests

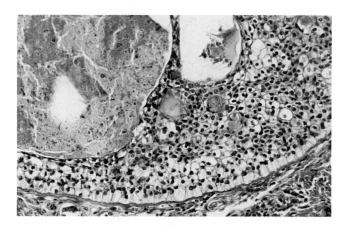

Fig. 15-83   Clear cell odontogenic carcinoma. Tumor island demonstrating cells with a clear cytoplasm. Note the peripheral columnar differentiation.

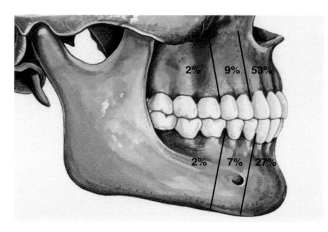

Fig. 15-84   Adenomatoid odontogenic tumor. Relative distribution of adenomatoid odontogenic tumor in the jaws.

and cords. Thin strands of hyalinized connective tissue often separate the clear cell nests. The third pattern has a resemblance to ameloblastoma in that the peripheral cells of the clear cell islands may infrequently demonstrate palisading (Fig. 15-83). Often the lesional cells do not exhibit a significant degree of nuclear or cytologic pleomorphism. Furthermore, mitoses are generally sparse and necrosis is not a prominent feature. The clear cells contain small amounts of glycogen, but mucin stains are negative. In some cases, islands more typical of ameloblastoma are interspersed among the other tumor elements.

Clear cell odontogenic carcinoma may be difficult to distinguish from intraosseous mucoepidermoid carcinoma with a prominent clear cell component, although the negative mucin stains are consistent with the former. A clear cell variant of the calcifying epithelial odontogenic tumor may also present problems in the differential diagnosis, but amyloid stains should be negative in the case of clear cell odontogenic tumor. A metastatic clear cell neoplasm, such as a renal cell carcinoma, clear cell breast carcinoma, or clear cell melanoma, may also need to be ruled out before the diagnosis of clear cell odontogenic carcinoma can be established.

TREATMENT AND PROGNOSIS

Clear cell odontogenic carcinomas largely demonstrate an aggressive clinical course, with invasion of contiguous structures and a tendency to recur. Most patients require fairly radical surgery. Metastatic involvement of regional lymph nodes has been documented in 25% of these patients, and pulmonary metastases have been described as well.

ADENOMATOID ODONTOGENIC TUMOR

The **adenomatoid odontogenic tumor** represents 3% to 7% of all odontogenic tumors, and more than 750 examples have been reported in the literature. Although this lesion was formerly considered to be a variant of the ameloblastoma and was designated as "adenoameloblastoma," its clinical features and biologic behavior indicate that it is a separate entity. Although there is evidence that the tumor cells are derived from enamel organ epithelium, investigators have also suggested that the lesion arises from remnants of dental lamina.

CLINICAL AND RADIOGRAPHIC FEATURES

Adenomatoid odontogenic tumors are largely limited to younger patients, and two thirds of all cases are diagnosed when patients are 10 to 19 years of age. This tumor is definitely uncommon in a patient older than age 30. It has a striking tendency to occur in the anterior portions of the jaws and is found twice as often in the maxilla as in the mandible (Fig. 15-84). Females are affected about twice as often as males.

Most adenomatoid odontogenic tumors are relatively small. They seldom exceed 3 cm in greatest diameter, although a few large lesions have been reported. Peripheral (extraosseous) forms of the tumor are also encountered but are rare. These usually appear as small, sessile masses on the facial gingiva of the maxilla. Clinically, these lesions cannot be differentiated from the common gingival fibrous lesions.

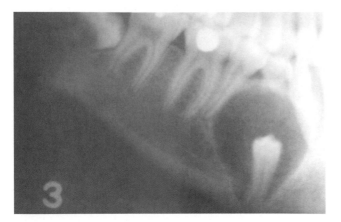

Fig. 15-85   Adenomatoid odontogenic tumor. Radiolucent lesion involving an unerupted mandibular first premolar. In contrast to the usual dentigerous cyst, the radiolucency extends almost to the apex of the tooth. (*Courtesy of Dr. Tony Traynham.*)

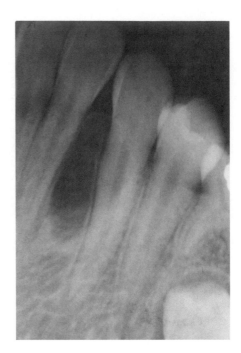

Fig. 15-86   Adenomatoid odontogenic tumor. A small radiolucency is present between the roots of the lateral incisor and canine. (*Courtesy of Dr. Ramesh Narang.*)

Adenomatoid odontogenic tumors are frequently asymptomatic and are discovered during the course of a routine radiographic examination or when films are made to determine why a tooth has not erupted. Larger lesions cause a painless expansion of the bone.

In about 75% of cases, the tumor appears as a circumscribed, unilocular radiolucency that involves the crown of an unerupted tooth, most often a canine. This follicular type of adenomatoid odontogenic tumor may be impossible to differentiate radiographically from the more common dentigerous cyst. The radiolucency associated with the follicular type of adenomatoid odontogenic tumor sometimes extends apically along the root past the cementoenamel junction. This feature may help to distinguish an adenomatoid odontogenic tumor from a dentigerous cyst (Fig. 15-85).

Less often the adenomatoid odontogenic tumor is a well-delineated unilocular radiolucency that is not related to an unerupted tooth, but rather is located between the roots of erupted teeth (extrafollicular type) (Fig. 15-86).

The lesion may appear completely radiolucent; often, however, it contains fine (snowflake) calcifications (Fig. 15-87). This feature may be helpful in differentiating the adenomatoid odontogenic tumor from a dentigerous cyst.

HISTOPATHOLOGIC FEATURES

The adenomatoid odontogenic tumor is a well-defined lesion that is usually surrounded by a thick, fibrous capsule. When the lesion is bisected, the central portion

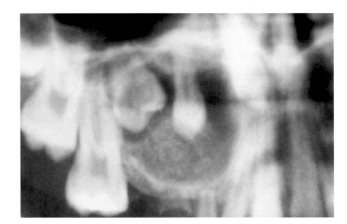

Fig. 15-87   Adenomatoid odontogenic tumor. Well-defined pericoronal radiolucency enveloping the maxillary right first bicuspid. Note the prominent snowflake calcifications. (*Courtesy of Dr. William Dobbins.*)

of the tumor may be essentially solid or may show varying degrees of cystic change (Fig. 15-88).

Microscopically, the tumor is composed of spindle-shaped epithelial cells that form sheets, strands, or whorled masses of cells in a scant fibrous stroma. The epithelial cells may form rosettelike structures about a central space, which may be empty or contain small

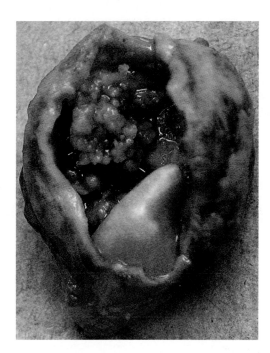

Fig. 15-88 **Adenomatoid odontogenic tumor.** A well-circumscribed cystlike mass can be seen enveloping the crown of a maxillary cuspid. Note the intraluminal vegetations, which represent nodular tumor growth.

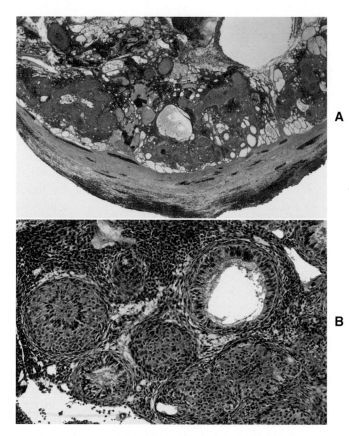

Fig. 15-89 **Adenomatoid odontogenic tumor. A,** Low-power view demonstrating a thick capsule surrounding the tumor. **B,** Higher magnification showing the ductlike epithelial structures. The nuclei of the columnar calls are polarized away from the central spaces.

amounts of eosinophilic material. This material may stain for amyloid.

The tubular or ductlike structures, which are the characteristic feature of the adenomatoid odontogenic tumor, may be prominent, scanty, or even absent in a given lesion. These consist of a central space surrounded by a layer of columnar or cuboidal epithelial cells. The nuclei of these cells tend to be polarized away from the central space. The mechanism of formation of these tubular structures is not entirely clear but is likely the result of the secretory activity of the tumor cells, which appear to be preameloblasts. In any event, these structures are not true ducts, and no glandular elements are present in the tumor (Fig. 15-89).

Small foci of calcification may also be scattered throughout the tumor. These have been interpreted as abortive enamel formation. Some adenomatoid odontogenic tumors contain larger areas of matrix material or calcification. This material has been interpreted as dentinoid or cementum.

Some lesions also have another pattern, particularly at the periphery of the tumor adjacent to the capsule. This consists of narrow, often anastomosing cords of epithelium in an eosinophilic, loosely arranged matrix.

The histopathologic features of this lesion are distinctive and should not be confused with any other odontogenic tumor. Interestingly, some adenomatoid odontogenic tumors have been described with focal areas that resemble calcifying epithelial odontogenic tumor, odontoma, or calcifying odontogenic cyst. These lesions appear to behave as a routine adenomatoid odontogenic tumor, however. The chief problem relates to mistaking this tumor for an ameloblastoma by a pathologist who is not familiar with this lesion. This error can lead to unnecessary radical surgery.

TREATMENT AND PROGNOSIS

The adenomatoid odontogenic tumor is completely benign; because of its capsule, it enucleates easily from the bone. Aggressive behavior has not been documented, and recurrence after enucleation seldom, if ever, occurs.

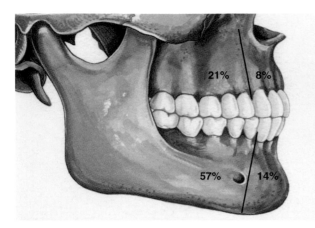

Fig. 15-90   Calcifying epithelial odontogenic tumor. Relative distribution of calcifying epithelial odontogenic tumor in the jaws.

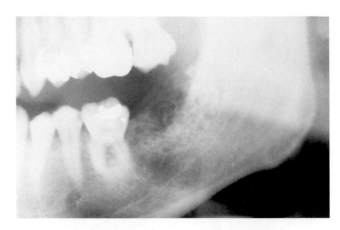

Fig. 15-91   Calcifying epithelial odontogenic tumor. Honeycombed multilocular radiolucency containing fine calcifications.

CALCIFYING EPITHELIAL ODONTOGENIC TUMOR (PINDBORG TUMOR)

The **calcifying epithelial odontogenic tumor**, also widely known as the **Pindborg tumor**, is an uncommon lesion that accounts for less than 1% of all odontogenic tumors. Approximately 200 cases have been reported to date. Although the tumor is clearly of odontogenic origin, its histogenesis is uncertain. The tumor cells bear a close morphologic resemblance to the cells of the stratum intermedium of the enamel organ; however, some investigators have recently suggested that the tumor arises from dental lamina remnants based on its anatomic distribution in the jaws.

CLINICAL AND RADIOGRAPHIC FEATURES

Although the calcifying epithelial odontogenic tumor has been found in patients across a wide age range and in many parts of the jaw, it is most often encountered in patients between 30 and 50 years of age. There is no sex predilection. About two thirds of all reported cases have been found in the mandible, most often in the posterior areas (Fig. 15-90). A painless, slow-growing swelling is the most common presenting sign.

Radiographically, the tumor exhibits either a unilocular or a multilocular radiolucent defect (Fig. 15-91), with the unilocular pattern encountered more commonly in the maxilla. The margins of the lytic defect are often scalloped and usually relatively well defined. However, approximately 20% of cases have an ill-defined periphery, and an additional 20% exhibit a corticated border. The lesion may be entirely

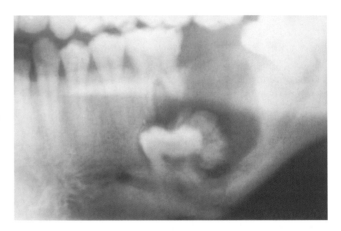

Fig. 15-92   Calcifying epithelial odontogenic tumor. Prominent calcification around the crown of an impacted second molar that is involved in the tumor. *(Courtesy of Dr. Harold Peacock.)*

radiolucent, but the defect usually contains calcified structures of varying size and density. The tumor is frequently associated with an impacted tooth, most often a mandibular molar. Calcifications are usually scattered within the tumor. Although some authors have suggested that these are often most prominent around the crown of the impacted tooth (Fig. 15-92), a recent review identified this feature in only 12% of published cases with adequate radiographic documentation. Similarly, the description of a "driven-snow" pattern of the calcifications appears to be much less common than previously believed.

A few cases of peripheral (extraosseous) calcifying epithelial odontogenic tumor have been reported. These appear as nonspecific, sessile gingival masses, most often on the anterior gingiva. Some of these have

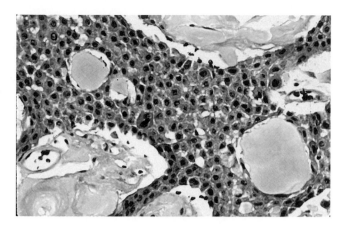

Fig. 15-93   Calcifying epithelial odontogenic tumor.
Sheets of polyhedral tumor cells with prominent eosinophilic cytoplasm and intercellular bridging. Pools of amorphous eosinophilic amyloid are present.

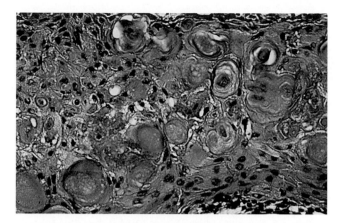

Fig. 15-94   Calcifying epithelial odontogenic tumor.
Multiple concentric Liesegang ring calcifications.

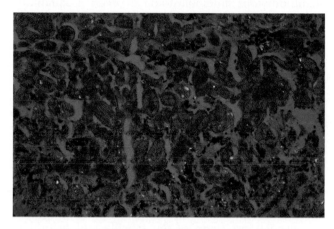

Fig. 15-95   Calcifying epithelial odontogenic tumor. With Congo red staining, the pools of amyloid exhibit an apple-green birefringence when viewed with polarized light.

been associated with cupped-out erosion of the underlying bone.

HISTOPATHOLOGIC FEATURES

The calcifying epithelial odontogenic tumor has discrete islands, strands, or sheets of polyhedral epithelial cells in a fibrous stroma (Fig. 15-93). The cellular outlines of the epithelial cells are distinct, and intercellular bridges may be noted. The nuclei show considerable variation, and giant nuclei may be seen. Some tumors show considerable nuclear pleomorphism, but this feature is not considered to indicate malignancy. Large areas of amorphous, eosinophilic, hyalinized (amyloid-like) extracellular material are also often present. The tumor islands frequently enclose masses of this hyaline material; this results in a cribriform appearance. Calcifications, which are a distinctive feature of the tumor, develop within the amyloid-like material and form concentric rings (Liesegang ring calcifications) (Fig. 15-94). These tend to fuse and form large, complex masses.

Several microscopic variations may be encountered. Some tumors consist of large sheets of epithelial cells with minimal production of amyloid-like material and calcifications. Others show large diffuse masses of amyloid-like material that contain only small nests or islands of epithelium. A clear cell variant has been described, in which clear cells constitute a significant portion of the epithelial component, and this tumor also has been reported to have a cystic growth pattern.

The amyloid-like material in the Pindborg tumor has been extensively investigated by histochemical, immunohistochemical, and biochemical methods, as well as by electron microscopy. The material generally stains as amyloid (i.e., positive staining results with Congo red or thioflavine T). After Congo red staining, the amyloid will exhibit apple-green birefringence when viewed with polarized light (Fig. 15-95). A recent report has identified this material as a unique protein that is produced by this tumor, and both the protein structure and the DNA sequence of the responsible gene have been described.

TREATMENT AND PROGNOSIS

Although it was originally believed that the calcifying epithelial odontogenic tumor had about the same biologic behavior as the ameloblastoma, accumulating experience indicates that it tends to be less aggressive. Conservative local resection to include a narrow rim of surrounding bone appears to be the treatment of choice, although lesions in the posterior maxilla should probably be treated more aggressively. A recurrence rate of about 15% has been reported; tumors treated by curettage have the highest frequency of recurrence. The overall prognosis appears good, although rare examples of malignant or borderline malignant calcifying epithelial odontogenic tumor have been reported, with documented metastasis to regional lymph nodes and lung.

SQUAMOUS ODONTOGENIC TUMOR

Squamous odontogenic tumor is a rare benign odontogenic neoplasm that was first described in 1975 and is now recognized as a distinct entity. Fewer than 50 examples have been reported to date. Most of these have been located within bone, although a few peripheral examples have been described. Before 1975, this lesion was probably believed to represent an atypical acanthomatous ameloblastoma or even a squamous cell carcinoma. The squamous odontogenic tumor may arise from neoplastic transformation of dental lamina rests or perhaps the epithelial rests of Malassez. The tumor appears to originate within the periodontal ligament that is associated with the lateral root surface of an erupted tooth.

CLINICAL AND RADIOGRAPHIC FEATURES

Squamous odontogenic tumors have been found in patients whose ages ranged from 8 to 74 years (average age, 38). They are randomly distributed throughout the alveolar processes of the maxilla and mandible, with no site of predilection. A few patients have had multiple squamous odontogenic tumors that involved several quadrants of the mouth; one family with three affected siblings who each had multiple lesions has been reported. There is no apparent sex predilection. A painless or mildly painful gingival swelling, often associated with mobility of the associated teeth, is the most common complaint. About 25% of reported patients have had no symptoms, and their lesions were detected during a radiographic examination.

The radiographic findings are not specific or diagnostic and consist of a triangular radiolucent defect lateral to the root or roots of the teeth (Fig. 15-96). In some instances, this suggests vertical periodontal bone loss. The radiolucent area may be somewhat ill defined or may show a well-defined, sclerotic margin. Most examples are relatively small lesions that seldom exceed 1.5 cm in greatest diameter.

HISTOPATHOLOGIC FEATURES

The microscopic findings of squamous odontogenic tumor are distinctive and consist of varying-shaped islands of bland-appearing squamous epithelium in a

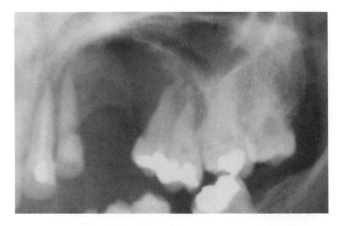

Fig. 15-96 **Squamous odontogenic tumor.** Lucent defect extending along the roots of the lateral incisor and first premolar teeth. *(Courtesy of Dr. Ed McGaha.)*

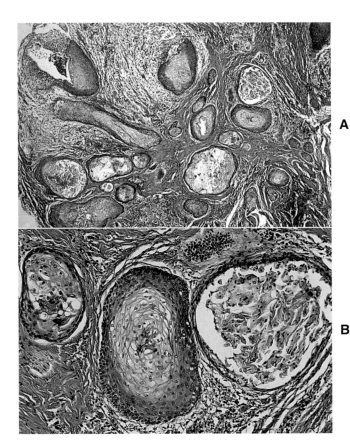

A

B

Fig. 15-97 **Squamous odontogenic tumor. A,** Low-power photomicrograph showing islands of bland-appearing squamous epithelium in a fibrous stroma. **B,** Higher-power photomicrograph showing bland appearance of the epithelium with microcyst formation.

mature fibrous connective tissue stroma. The peripheral cells of the epithelial islands do not show the characteristic polarization seen in ameloblastomas (Fig. 15-97). Microcystic vacuolization and individual cell keratinization within the epithelial islands are common features. Small microcysts are sometimes observed within the epithelial islands. Laminated calcified bodies and globular eosinophilic structures, which do not stain for amyloid, are present within the epithelium in some cases. The former probably represents dystrophic calcifications; the nature of the latter is unknown.

Islands of epithelium that closely resemble those of the squamous odontogenic tumor have been observed within the fibrous walls of dentigerous and radicular cysts. These have been designated as *squamous odontogenic tumorlike proliferations* in odontogenic cysts. These islands do not appear to have any significance relative to the behavior of the cyst, and evaluation of the clinical, radiographic, and histopathologic features should permit differentiation from a squamous odontogenic tumor.

In published reports, some squamous odontogenic tumors have been misdiagnosed initially as ameloblastomas, resulting in unnecessary radical surgery.

TREATMENT AND PROGNOSIS

Conservative local excision or curettage appears to be effective for patients with squamous odontogenic tumors, and most reported cases have not recurred after local excision. A few instances of recurrence have been reported, but these have responded well to further local excision. Maxillary squamous odontogenic tumors may be somewhat more aggressive than mandibular lesions, with a greater tendency to invade adjacent structures. This may be because of the porous, spongy nature of the maxillary bone. The multicentric lesions have typically exhibited a less aggressive, almost hamartomatous behavior when compared with solitary lesions. A well-documented example of apparent malignant transformation of squamous odontogenic tumor has been reported.

Mixed Odontogenic Tumors

The group of mixed odontogenic tumors, composed of proliferating odontogenic epithelium in a cellular ectomesenchyme resembling the dental papilla, poses problems in classification. Some of these lesions show varying degrees of inductive effect by the epithelium on the mesenchyme, leading to the formation of varying amounts of enamel and dentin. Some of these lesions (the common odontomas) are clearly nonneoplastic developmental anomalies; others appear to be true neoplasms. The nature of others is uncertain.

In some instances, the histopathologic findings alone cannot distinguish between the neoplastic lesions and the developmental anomalies. Clinical and radio-

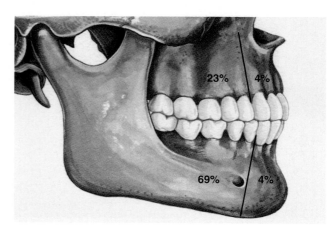

Fig. 15-98   **Ameloblastic fibroma.** Relative distribution of ameloblastic fibroma in the jaws.

graphic features often are of considerable assistance in making this distinction.

AMELOBLASTIC FIBROMA

The **ameloblastic fibroma** is considered to be a true mixed tumor in which the epithelial and mesenchymal tissues are both neoplastic. It is an uncommon tumor, but the data regarding its frequency are difficult to evaluate because (particularly in earlier reports) some lesions that were diagnosed as ameloblastic fibroma may actually have represented the early developing stage of an odontoma.

CLINICAL AND RADIOGRAPHIC FEATURES

Ameloblastic fibromas tend to occur in younger patients; most lesions are diagnosed in the first two decades of life. This lesion, however, is occasionally encountered in middle-aged patients. The tumor is slightly more common in males than in females. Small ameloblastic fibromas are asymptomatic; larger tumors are associated with swelling of the jaws. The posterior mandible is the most common site; about 70% of all cases are located in this area (Fig. 15-98). Convincing examples of this tumor arising within the gingival soft tissue have only recently been described, but this appears to represent a rare phenomenon.

Radiographically, either a unilocular or multilocular radiolucent lesion is seen, with the smaller lesions tending to be unilocular. The radiographic margins tend to be well defined, and they may be sclerotic. An unerupted tooth is associated with the lesion in about 75% of cases (Fig. 15-99). The ameloblastic fibroma may grow to a large size, and cases that involve a

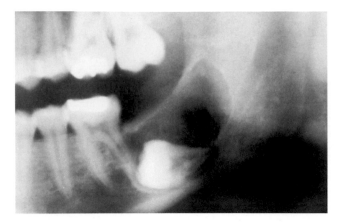

Fig. 15-99   Ameloblastic fibroma. Well-defined radiolucent defect associated with an unerupted second molar. *(Courtesy of Dr. Robert Lauer.)*

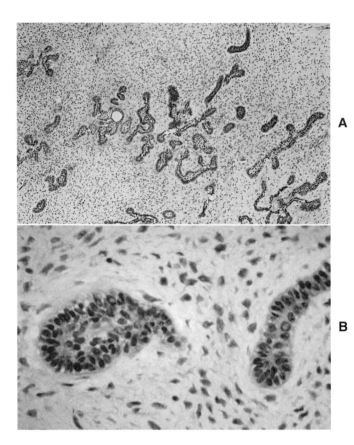

Fig. 15-100   Ameloblastic fibroma. A, Long, narrow cords of odontogenic epithelium supported by richly cellular, primitive connective tissue. **B,** Basophilic epithelial islands with peripheral nuclear palisading.

considerable portion of the body and ascending ramus of the mandible have been reported.

HISTOPATHOLOGIC FEATURES

The ameloblastic fibroma appears as a solid, soft tissue mass with a smooth outer surface. A definite capsule may or may not be present. Microscopically, the tumor is composed of a cell-rich mesenchymal tissue resembling the primitive dental papilla admixed with proliferating odontogenic epithelium. The latter may have one of two patterns, both of which are usually present in any given case. The most common epithelial pattern consists of long, narrow cords of odontogenic epithelium, often in an anastomosing arrangement. These cords are usually only two cells in thickness and are composed of cuboidal or columnar cells (Fig. 15-100). In the other pattern, the epithelial cells form small, discrete islands that resemble the follicular stage of the developing enamel organ. These show peripheral columnar cells, which surround a mass of loosely arranged epithelial cells that resemble stellate reticulum. In contrast to the follicular type of ameloblastoma, these follicular islands in the ameloblastic fibroma seldom demonstrate microcyst formation.

The mesenchymal portion of the ameloblastic fibroma consists of plump stellate and ovoid cells in a loose matrix, which closely resembles the developing dental papilla. Collagen formation is generally inconspicuous. Juxtaepithelial hyalinization of the mesenchymal portion of the tumor is sometimes seen, and occasionally diffuse areas of hyalinized acellular lesional tissue are evident.

In recent years, a few examples of ameloblastic fibroma occurring in conjunction with calcifying odontogenic cyst have been reported.

TREATMENT AND PROGNOSIS

The proper management of ameloblastic fibroma has been an ongoing topic of debate. Although initially it was believed that the ameloblastic fibroma was an innocuous lesion that seldom recurred after simple local excision or curettage, subsequent reports seemed to indicate a substantial risk of recurrence after conservative therapy. The highest recurrence rate (43.5%) was recorded in a series of cases from the Armed Forces Institute of Pathology, and it could be argued that this was a biased sample of larger lesions that were inherently more difficult to manage. In other series of cases, from 0% to 18% of ameloblastic fibromas were reported to recur after conservative removal and an adequate follow-up period. Based on these data, recent recommendations have emphasized conservative initial therapy for ameloblastic fibroma. More aggressive surgical excision should probably be reserved for recurrent lesions. Approximately 45% of the cases of the rare ameloblastic fibrosarcoma develop in the setting of a recurrent ameloblastic fibroma.

AMELOBLASTIC FIBRO-ODONTOMA

The **ameloblastic fibro-odontoma** is defined as a tumor with the general features of an ameloblastic fibroma but that also contains enamel and dentin. Some investigators believe that the ameloblastic fibroodontoma is only a stage in the development of an odontoma and do not consider it to be a separate entity. Certainly the histopathologic features of a developing odontoma may overlap somewhat with ameloblastic fibro-odontoma. There are well-documented examples, however, of this tumor exhibiting progressive growth and causing considerable deformity and bone destruction. Such lesions appear to be true neoplasms. However, distinguishing between a developing odontoma and an ameloblastic fibro-odontoma may be difficult based on histopathologic grounds alone.

CLINICAL AND RADIOGRAPHIC FEATURES

The ameloblastic fibro-odontoma is usually encountered in children with an average age of 10 years. It is rarely encountered in adults. Like the **ameloblastic fibroma**, ameloblastic fibro-odontomas occur more frequently in the posterior regions of the jaws (Fig. 15-101). There is no significant sex predilection. The lesion is commonly asymptomatic and is discovered when radiographs are taken to determine the reason for failure of a tooth to erupt. Large examples may be associated with a painless swelling of the affected bone.

Radiographically, the tumor shows a well-circumscribed unilocular or, rarely, multilocular radiolucent defect that contains a variable amount of calcified material with the radiodensity of tooth structure. The calcified material within the lesion may appear as multiple, small radiopacities or as a solid conglomerate mass (Fig. 15-102). In most instances, an unerupted tooth is present at the margin of the lesion, or the crown of the unerupted tooth may be included within the defect. Some ameloblastic fibro-odontomas contain only a minimal amount of calcifying enamel and dentin matrix and appear radiographically as radiolucent lesions (Fig. 15-103). These cannot be differentiated from the wide variety of unilocular radiolucencies that may involve the jaws. At the other extreme, some ameloblastic fibro-odontomas appear as largely calcified masses with only a narrow rim of radiolucency about the periphery of the lesion.

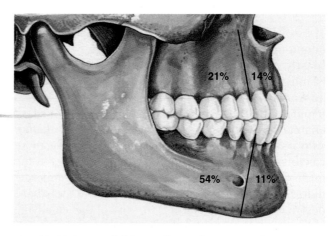

Fig. 15-101   Ameloblastic fibro-odontoma. Relative distribution of ameloblastic fibro-odontoma in the jaws.

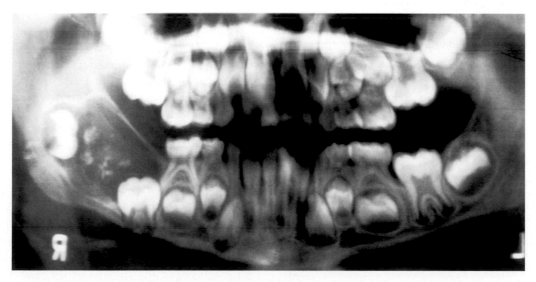

Fig. 15-102   Ameloblastic fibro-odontoma. Radiolucent defect in the ramus containing small calcifications having the radiodensity of tooth structure.

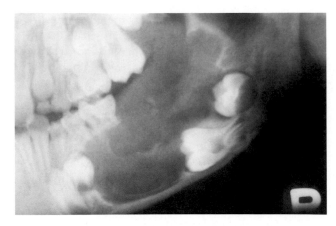

Fig. 15-103   Ameloblastic fibro-odontoma. Radiolucent defect involving several unerupted teeth. Little calcified material is present in the radiolucent defect.

HISTOPATHOLOGIC FEATURES

The soft tissue component of the ameloblastic fibro-odontoma is microscopically identical to the **ameloblastic fibroma** and has narrow cords and small islands of odontogenic epithelium in a loose primitive-appearing connective tissue that resembles the dental papilla. The calcifying element consists of foci of enamel and dentin matrix formation in close relationship to the epithelial structures (Fig. 15-104). The more calcified lesions show mature dental structures in the form of rudimentary small teeth or conglomerate masses of enamel and dentin. Some researchers have designated a similar tumor in which the calcifying component consists only of dentin matrix and dentinoid material as **ameloblastic fibro-dentinoma**. It is questionable whether this lesion represents a separate entity, and it is probably best considered as only a variant of the ameloblastic fibro-odontoma.

TREATMENT AND PROGNOSIS

A patient with an ameloblastic fibro-odontoma is generally treated by conservative curettage, and the lesion usually separates easily from its bony bed. The tumor is well circumscribed and does not invade the surrounding bone.

The prognosis is excellent, and recurrence after conservative removal is unusual. Development of an ameloblastic fibrosarcoma after curettage of an ameloblastic fibro-odontoma has been reported, but this is exceedingly rare.

AMELOBLASTIC FIBROSARCOMA (AMELOBLASTIC SARCOMA)

The rare **ameloblastic fibrosarcoma** is considered to be the malignant counterpart of the ameloblastic fibroma, and slightly more than 60 cases have been

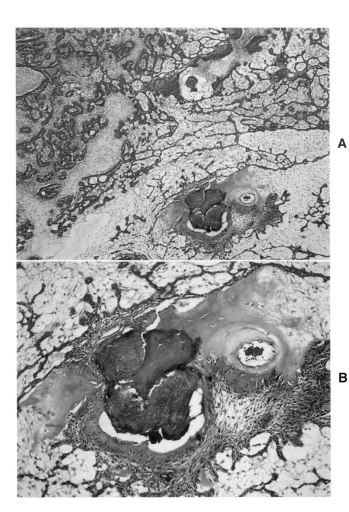

Fig. 15-104   Ameloblastic fibro-odontoma. A, The soft tissue component of the tumor is indistinguishable from an ameloblastic fibroma. **B,** Formation of disorganized tooth structure can be seen.

documented in the literature. Interestingly, in most cases, only the mesenchymal portion of the lesion shows features of malignancy; the epithelial component remains rather bland. These tumors may apparently arise *de novo*, although in approximately half of known cases, the malignant lesion represents a recurrence of a tumor previously diagnosed as an ameloblastic fibroma or an ameloblastic fibro-odontoma.

CLINICAL AND RADIOGRAPHIC FEATURES

Ameloblastic fibrosarcomas occur about 1.5 times as often in males as in females. The lesion tends to occur in younger patients (mean reported age, 27.5 years). Although either the maxilla or the mandible may be involved, about 80% of cases have occurred in the mandible. Pain and swelling associated with rapid clinical growth are the common complaints.

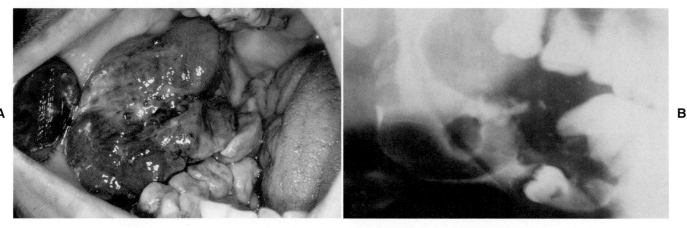

Fig. 15-105   Ameloblastic fibrosarcoma. A, A 21-year-old woman complained of facial asymmetry and recent increase in size of a mandibular mass that had been present for some years. **B,** Radiograph of the same patient. Note the lytic destruction of the posterior mandible. *(Courtesy of Dr. Sam McKenna.)*

Radiographically, the ameloblastic fibrosarcoma shows an ill-defined destructive radiolucent lesion that suggests a malignant process (Fig. 15-105).

HISTOPATHOLOGIC FEATURES

Ameloblastic fibrosarcomas contain an epithelial component similar to that seen in the ameloblastic fibroma, although it is frequently less prominent than that present in the typical ameloblastic fibroma. The epithelial component appears histopathologically benign and does not demonstrate any cytologic atypia. The mesenchymal portion of the tumor, however, is highly cellular and shows hyperchromatic and often-bizarre pleomorphic cells (Fig. 15-106). Mitoses are usually prominent. In some cases with multiple recurrences, the epithelial component becomes progressively less conspicuous so that the tumor eventually shows only a poorly differentiated fibrosarcoma.

In a few instances, dysplastic dentin or small amounts of enamel may be formed. Some have called such lesions **ameloblastic dentinosarcomas** or **ameloblastic fibro-odontosarcomas**. This additional subclassification, however, appears unnecessary. Another rare event that actually may be overrepresented in the literature is concurrent malignant transformation of both the epithelial and mesenchymal elements of an ameloblastic fibroma, resulting in an **ameloblastic carcinosarcoma**.

TREATMENT AND PROGNOSIS

Once the diagnosis of ameloblastic fibrosarcoma has been confirmed, radical surgical excision appears to be the treatment of choice. Curettage or local excision is

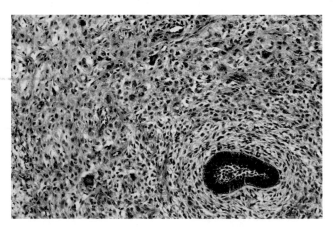

Fig. 15-106   Ameloblastic fibrosarcoma. The cellular mesenchymal tissue shows hyperchromatism and atypical cells. A small island of ameloblastic epithelium is present.

usually followed by rapid local recurrence. The tumor is locally aggressive and infiltrates adjacent bone and soft tissues.

The long-term prognosis is difficult to ascertain because of the few reported cases with adequate follow-up, with the best estimates suggesting that 20% of these patients will succumb to their tumor. Most deaths have resulted from uncontrolled local disease, and metastatic tumor has been documented in only 3 of 53 evaluable cases.

ODONTOAMELOBLASTOMA

The **odontoameloblastoma** is an extremely rare odontogenic tumor that contains an ameloblastomatous component and odontoma-like elements. Fewer than 20 cases have been reported with sufficient documentation to support this diagnosis. This tumor was formerly called *ameloblastic odontoma* and was confused with the more common (though still relatively rare) lesion currently designated as **ameloblastic fibro-odontoma**. Because the clinical behavior of these two tumors is quite different, they should be distinguished from one another. This neoplasm is also frequently confused with an odontoma that is in its early stages of development.

CLINICAL AND RADIOGRAPHIC FEATURES

Because of the rarity of odontoameloblastomas, little reliable information is available. The lesion appears to occur more often in younger patients, and either jaw can be affected. Pain, delayed eruption of teeth, and expansion of the affected bone may be noted.

Radiographically, the tumor shows a radiolucent, destructive process that contains calcified structures. These have the radiodensity of tooth structure and may resemble miniature teeth or occur as larger masses of calcified material similar to a complex odontoma.

HISTOPATHOLOGIC FEATURES

The histopathologic features of the odontoameloblastoma are complex. The proliferating epithelial portion of the tumor has features of an **ameloblastoma**, most often of the plexiform or follicular pattern. The ameloblastic component is intermingled with immature or more mature dental tissue in the form of developing rudimentary teeth, which is similar to the appearance of a **compound odontoma**, or conglomerate masses of enamel, dentin, and cementum, as seen in a **complex odontoma**.

TREATMENT AND PROGNOSIS

Multiple recurrences of odontoameloblastomas have been reported after local curettage, and it appears that this tumor has the same biologic potential as the ameloblastoma. It is probably wise to treat a patient with this lesion in the same manner as one with an ameloblastoma. However, there are no valid data on the long-term prognosis.

ODONTOMA

Odontomas are the most common types of odontogenic tumors. Their prevalence exceeds that of all other odontogenic tumors combined. Odontomas are considered to be developmental anomalies **(hamartomas)**, rather than true neoplasms. When fully developed, odontomas consist chiefly of enamel and dentin, with variable amounts of pulp and cementum. In their earlier developmental stages, varying amounts of proliferating odontogenic epithelium and mesenchyme are present.

Odontomas are further subdivided into compound and complex types. The **compound odontoma** is composed of multiple, small toothlike structures. The **complex odontoma** consists of a conglomerate mass of enamel and dentin, which bears no anatomic resemblance to a tooth. In most series, compound odontomas are more frequently diagnosed than complex, and it is possible that some compound odontomas are not submitted for microscopic examination because the clinician is comfortable with the clinical and radiographic diagnosis. Occasionally, these lesions may show features of both compound and complex odontoma.

CLINICAL AND RADIOGRAPHIC FEATURES

Most odontomas are detected during the first two decades of life, and the mean age at the time of diagnosis is 14 years. The majority of these lesions are completely asymptomatic, being discovered on a routine radiographic examination or when films are taken to determine the reason for failure of a tooth to erupt. Odontomas are typically relatively small and seldom exceed the size of a tooth in the area where they are located. However, large odontomas up to 6 cm or more in diameter are occasionally seen. These large odontomas can cause expansion of the jaw.

Odontomas occur somewhat more frequently in the maxilla than in the mandible. Although compound and complex odontomas may be found in any site, the compound type is more often seen in the anterior maxilla; complex odontomas occur more often in the molar regions of either jaw. Occasionally, an odontoma will develop completely within the gingival soft tissues.

Radiographically, the **compound odontoma** appears as a collection of toothlike structures of varying size and shape surrounded by a narrow radiolucent zone (Figs. 15-107 and 15-108). The **complex odontoma** appears as a calcified mass with the radiodensity of tooth structure, which is also surrounded by a narrow radiolucent rim. An unerupted tooth is frequently associated with the odontoma, and the odontoma prevents eruption of the tooth (Fig. 15-109). Some small odontomas are present between the roots of erupted teeth and are not associated with disturbance in eruption. The radiographic findings are usually diagnostic, and the compound odontoma is seldom confused with any other lesion. A developing odontoma may show little evidence of calcification and appear as a circumscribed radiolucent lesion. A complex odontoma, however, may be radiographically confused with an osteoma or some other highly calcified bone lesion.

HISTOPATHOLOGIC FEATURES

The compound odontoma consists of multiple structures resembling small, single-rooted teeth, contained in a loose fibrous matrix (Fig. 15-110). The mature enamel caps of the toothlike structures are lost during decalcification for preparation of the microscopic section, but varying amounts of enamel matrix are often present. Pulp tissue may be seen in the coronal and root portions of the toothlike structures. In patients with developing odontomas, structures that resemble tooth germs are present.

Complex odontomas consist largely of mature tubular dentin. This dentin encloses clefts or hollow circular structures that contained the mature enamel

that was removed during decalcification. The spaces may contain small amounts of enamel matrix or immature enamel (Fig. 15-111). Small islands of eosinophilic-staining epithelial ghost cells are present in about 20% of complex odontomas. These may represent remnants of odontogenic epithelium that have undergone keratinization and cell death from the local anoxia. A thin layer of cementum is often present about the periphery of the mass. Occasionally, a dentigerous cyst may arise from the epithelial lining of the fibrous capsule of a complex odontoma.

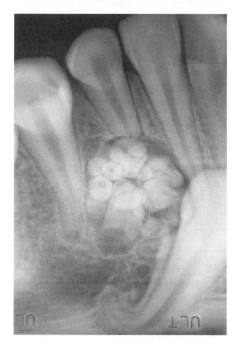

Fig. 15-108 Compound odontoma. Multiple toothlets preventing the eruption of the mandibular cuspid. *(Courtesy of Dr. Brent Bernard.)*

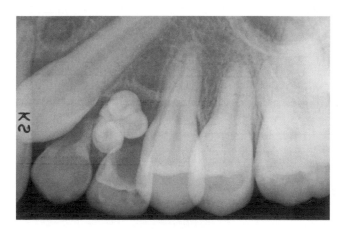

Fig. 15-107 Compound odontoma. A small cluster of toothlike structures is preventing the eruption of the maxillary canine. *(Courtesy of Dr. Robert J. Powers.)*

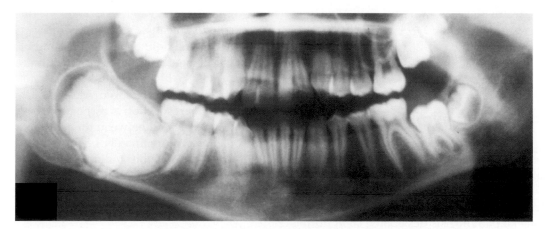

Fig. 15-109   Complex odontoma. A large radiopaque mass is overlying the crown of the mandibular right second molar, which has been displaced to the inferior border of the mandible.

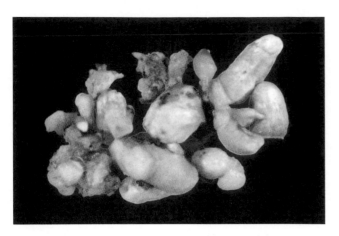

Fig. 15-110   Compound odontoma. Surgical specimen consisting of more than 20 malformed toothlike structures.

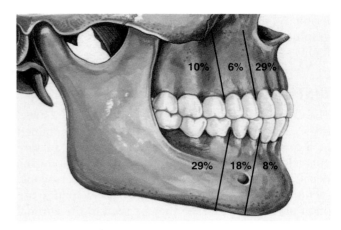

Fig. 15-112   Odontogenic fibroma. Relative distribution of odontogenic fibroma in the jaws.

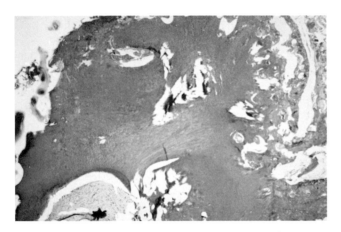

Fig. 15-111   Complex odontoma. This decalcified section shows a disorganized mass of dentin intermixed with small pools of enamel matrix.

TREATMENT AND PROGNOSIS

Odontomas are treated by simple local excision, and the prognosis is excellent.

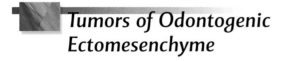

Tumors of Odontogenic Ectomesenchyme

CENTRAL ODONTOGENIC FIBROMA

The **central odontogenic fibroma** is an uncommon and somewhat controversial lesion. Approximately 70 examples have been reported. Formerly, some oral and maxillofacial pathologists designated solid fibrous masses that were almost always associated with the crown of an unerupted tooth as *odontogenic fibromas*. Most oral and maxillofacial pathologists today consider

such lesions to represent only hyperplastic dental follicles, and these should not be considered to be neoplasms.

CLINICAL AND RADIOGRAPHIC FEATURES

Odontogenic fibromas have been reported in patients whose ages ranged from 4 to 80 years (mean age, 40 years). Of those cases reported in the literature, a 2.2:1.0 female-to-male ratio has been noted, indicating a strong female predilection. About 45% of reported cases have occurred in the maxilla; most maxillary lesions are located anterior to the first molar tooth (Fig. 15-112). In the mandible, however, about half of the tumors are located posterior to the first molar. One third of odontogenic fibromas are associated with an unerupted tooth. Smaller odontogenic fibromas are usually completely asymptomatic; larger lesions may be associated with localized bony expansion or loosening of teeth.

Radiographically, smaller odontogenic fibromas tend to be well-defined, unilocular, radiolucent lesions often associated with the periradicular area of erupted teeth (Fig. 15-113). Larger lesions tend to be multilocular radiolucencies. Many lesions have a sclerotic border. Root resorption of associated teeth is common, and lesions located between the teeth often cause root divergence. Approximately 12% of central odontogenic fibromas will exhibit radiopaque flecks within the lesion.

HISTOPATHOLOGIC FEATURES

Lesions reported as central odontogenic fibroma have shown considerable histopathologic diversity; this has led some authors to describe two separate types,

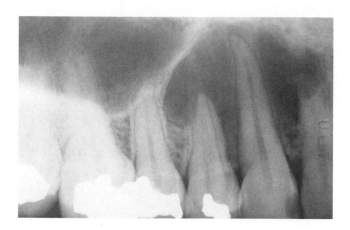

Fig. 15-113 Odontogenic fibroma. Apical radiolucent lesion in the incisor and premolar area. *(Courtesy of Dr. Robert Provencher, Jr.)*

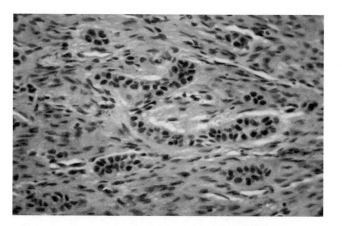

Fig. 15-115 Odontogenic fibroma (World Health Organization [WHO] type). A cellular fibroblastic lesion containing narrow cords of odontogenic epithelium.

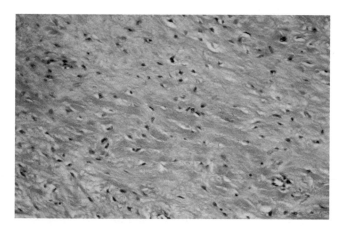

Fig. 15-114 Odontogenic fibroma (simple type). Scattered fibroblasts within a collagenous background. No epithelial rests were found on multiple sections from this tumor.

although this concept has been questioned. The so-called **simple odontogenic fibroma** is composed of stellate fibroblasts, often arranged in a whorled pattern with fine collagen fibrils and considerable ground substance (Fig. 15-114). Small foci of odontogenic epithelial rests may or may not be present. Occasional foci of dystrophic calcification may be seen. Some investigators have suggested that this lesion actually belongs with the spectrum of odontogenic myxoma and should be designated as a **myxofibroma**. A more collagenized odontogenic fibroma needs to be differentiated from a desmoplastic fibroma, which is a more aggressive lesion. The desmoplastic fibroma, however, does not have an epithelial component.

The **central odontogenic fibroma, World Health Organization (WHO) type,** has a more complex pattern, which often consists of a fairly cellular fibrous connective tissue with collagen fibers arranged in interlacing bundles. Odontogenic epithelium in the form of long strands or isolated nests is present throughout the lesion and may be a prominent component (Fig. 15-115). The fibrous component may vary from myxoid to densely hyalinized. Calcifications composed of cementum-like material or dentinoid are present in some cases.

Twelve examples of central odontogenic fibroma associated with a **giant cell granuloma**-like component have been reported since 1992 (Fig. 15-116). It seems unlikely that this process represents a "collision" tumor with synchronous occurrence of an odontogenic fibroma and a giant cell granuloma. Several of these lesions have recurred, and the recurrences typically exhibit both components. Whether the odontogenic fibroma somehow induced a giant cell response in these patients or whether this is a distinct biphasic lesion remains to be clarified.

TREATMENT AND PROGNOSIS

Odontogenic fibromas are usually treated by enucleation and vigorous curettage. Although the tumor does not have a definite capsule, it appears to have a limited growth potential, particularly in the anterior regions of the jaws. A few recurrences have been documented, but the prognosis is very good.

PERIPHERAL ODONTOGENIC FIBROMA

The relatively uncommon **peripheral odontogenic fibroma** is considered to represent the soft tissue counterpart of the **central (intraosseous) odontogenic fibroma**. In the past, some authors have designated clinically and histopathologically similar lesions as **odontogenic epithelial hamartoma** or as **peripheral**

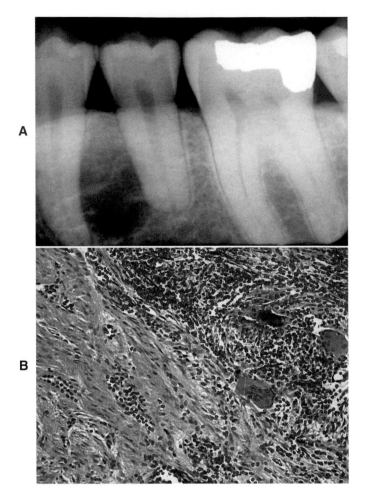

Fig. 15-116   **Odontogenic fibroma (WHO type) with associated giant cell granuloma. A,** Unilocular radiolucency between the left mandibular bicuspids. **B,** Microscopic examination reveals two distinct patterns. On the left, one can see cords of odontogenic epithelium within a fibrous background, consistent with odontogenic fibroma (WHO type). Typical features of central giant cell granuloma are present on the right side of the field.

fibroameloblastic dentinoma. It is likely that all of these terms refer to the same lesion, and peripheral odontogenic fibroma seems to be the most appropriate designation. A few series of this lesion have been reported in the past 2 decades, bringing the total number of cases in the literature to approximately 175.

CLINICAL AND RADIOGRAPHIC FEATURES

The peripheral odontogenic fibroma appears as a firm, slow-growing, and usually sessile gingival mass covered by normal-appearing mucosa (Fig. 15-117). Rarely, multifocal or diffuse lesions have been described. Clinically, the peripheral odontogenic fibroma cannot be distinguished from the much more common fibrous

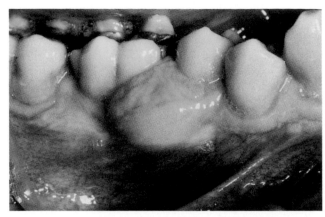

Fig. 15-117   **Peripheral odontogenic fibroma.** This sessile gingival mass cannot be clinically distinguished from the common peripheral ossifying fibroma. *(Courtesy of Dr. Jerry Stovall.)*

gingival lesions (see Chapter 12). The lesion is most often encountered on the facial gingiva of the mandible. Most lesions are between 0.5 and 1.5 cm in diameter, and they infrequently cause displacement of the teeth. Peripheral odontogenic fibromas have been recorded in patients across a wide age range, with most identified from the second to the seventh decades of life.

Radiographic studies demonstrate a soft tissue mass, which in some cases has shown areas of calcification. The lesion, however, does not involve the underlying bone.

HISTOPATHOLOGIC FEATURES

The peripheral odontogenic fibroma shows similar histopathologic features to the central odontogenic fibroma (WHO type). The tumor consists of interwoven fascicles of cellular fibrous connective tissue, which may be interspersed with areas of less cellular, myxoid connective tissue. A granular cell change has been rarely identified in the connective tissue component, and giant cell granuloma–like areas have been described in a few lesions. Islands or strands of odontogenic epithelium are scattered throughout the connective tissue. These may be prominent or scarce. The epithelial cells may show vacuolization. Dysplastic dentin, amorphous ovoid cementum-like calcifications, and trabeculae of osteoid may also be present.

TREATMENT AND PROGNOSIS

The peripheral odontogenic fibroma is treated by local surgical excision, and the prognosis is excellent. Recurrence of this lesion has been documented, however, so the patient and clinician should be aware of this possibility.

GRANULAR CELL ODONTOGENIC TUMOR (GRANULAR CELL ODONTOGENIC FIBROMA)

The rare **granular cell odontogenic tumor** was initially reported as "granular cell ameloblastic fibroma." Subsequently, it was designated as **granular cell odontogenic fibroma**, but the noncommittal term **granular cell odontogenic tumor** is probably more appropriate, given the controversial nature of the lesion. Approximately 30 cases of this unusual tumor have been reported.

CLINICAL AND RADIOGRAPHIC FEATURES

Patients with granular cell odontogenic tumors have all been adults at the time of diagnosis, with more than half being older than 40 years of age. More than 70% of the cases have developed in women. The tumor occurs primarily in the mandible and most often in the premolar and molar region. Some lesions are completely asymptomatic; others present as a painless, localized expansion of the affected area. A few cases of granular cell odontogenic tumor have been described in the gingival soft tissues as well.

Radiographically, the lesion appears as a well-demarcated radiolucency, which may be unilocular or multilocular and occasionally shows small calcifications (Fig. 15-118).

HISTOPATHOLOGIC FEATURES

The granular cell odontogenic tumor is composed of large eosinophilic granular cells, which closely resemble the granular cells seen in the soft tissue granular cell tumor (see page 536) or the granular cells seen in the granular cell variant of the ameloblastoma (see page 709). Narrow cords or small islands of odontogenic epithelium are scattered among the granular cells (Fig. 15-119). Small cementum-like or dystrophic calcifications associated with the granular cells have been seen in some lesions.

The nature of the granular cells is controversial. Ultrastructural studies reveal the features of mesenchymal cells, and bodies consistent with lysosomal structures have been identified within the lesional cell cytoplasm. Immunohistochemically, the granular cells in the granular cell odontogenic tumor do not react with antibodies directed against S-100 protein, in contrast to the positive S-100 reactivity of the granular cell tumor.

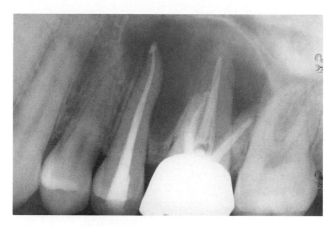

Fig. 15-118   Granular cell odontogenic tumor. Radiolucent lesion involving the apical area of endodontically treated maxillary teeth. *(Courtesy of Dr. Steve Ferry.)*

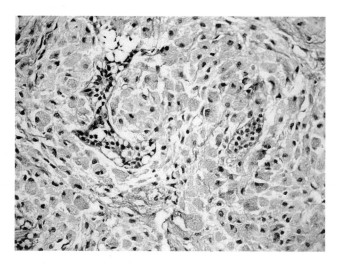

Fig. 15-119   Granular cell odontogenic tumor. Sheet of large granular mesenchymal cells with small nests of odontogenic epithelium.

TREATMENT AND PROGNOSIS

The granular cell odontogenic fibroma appears to be completely benign in the overwhelming majority of instances and responds well to curettage. Only one recurrence has been documented, and a solitary example of a malignant central granular cell odontogenic fibroma has been reported.

ODONTOGENIC MYXOMA

Myxomas of the jaws are believed to arise from odontogenic ectomesenchyme. They bear a close microscopic resemblance to the mesenchymal portion of a developing tooth. Formerly, some investigators made a distinction between **odontogenic myxomas** (derived from odontogenic mesenchyme) and **osteogenic**

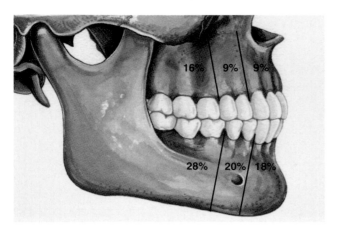

Fig. 15-120 Odontogenic myxoma. Relative distribution of odontogenic myxoma in the jaws.

myxomas (presumably derived from primitive bone tissue). However, most authorities in orthopedic pathologic practice do not accept that myxomas occur in the extragnathic skeleton, and all myxomas of the jaws are currently considered to be of odontogenic origin.

CLINICAL AND RADIOGRAPHIC FEATURES

Myxomas are predominantly found in young adults but may occur across a wide age group. The average age for patients with myxomas is 25 to 30 years. There is no sex predilection. The tumor may be found in almost any area of the jaws, and the mandible is involved more commonly than the maxilla (Fig. 15-120). Smaller lesions may be asymptomatic and are discovered only during a radiographic examination. Larger lesions are often associated with a painless expansion of the involved bone. In some instances, clinical growth of the tumor may be rapid; this is probably related to the accumulation of myxoid ground substance in the tumor.

Radiographically, the myxoma appears as a unilocular or multilocular radiolucency that may displace or cause resorption of teeth in the area of the tumor (Fig. 15-121). The margins of the radiolucency are often irregular or scalloped. The radiolucent defect may contain thin, wispy trabeculae of residual bone, which are often arranged at right angles to one another (Fig. 15-122). Large myxomas of the mandible may show a "soap bubble" radiolucent pattern, which is indistinguishable from that seen in ameloblastomas (Fig. 15-123).

HISTOPATHOLOGIC FEATURES

At the time of surgery or gross examination of the specimen, the gelatinous, loose structure of the myxoma is obvious (Fig. 15-124). Microscopically, the tumor is

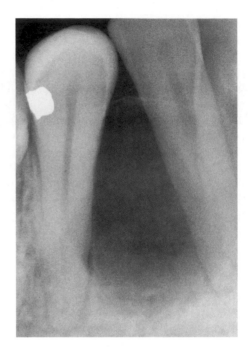

Fig. 15-121 Odontogenic myxoma. Unilocular radiolucency between the right mandibular lateral incisor and cuspid.

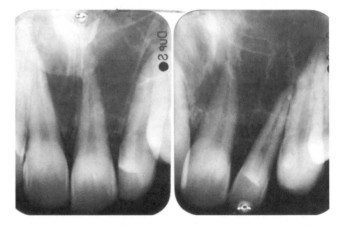

Fig. 15-122 Odontogenic myxoma. Radiolucent lesion of anterior maxilla showing fine residual bone trabeculae arranged at right angles to one another ("stepladder" pattern).

composed of haphazardly arranged stellate, spindle-shaped, and round cells in an abundant, loose myxoid stroma that contains only a few collagen fibrils (Fig. 15-125). Histochemical study shows that the ground substance is composed of glycosaminoglycans, chiefly hyaluronic acid and chondroitin sulfate. Immunohistochemically, the myxoma cells show diffuse immunoreactivity with antibodies directed against vimentin, with focal reactivity for muscle-specific actin. Small islands of inactive-appearing odontogenic epithelial rests may

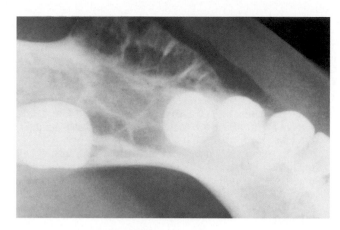

Fig. 15-123 Odontogenic myxoma. Occlusal view of a large myxoma showing buccal expansion and "soap bubble" radiolucency similar to that seen in an ameloblastoma. *(Courtesy of Dr. Mike Rohrer.)*

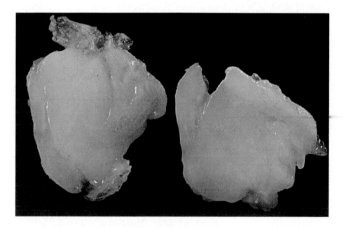

Fig. 15-124 Odontogenic myxoma. Gross specimen of case shown in Fig. 15-121, demonstrating a white gelatinous mass.

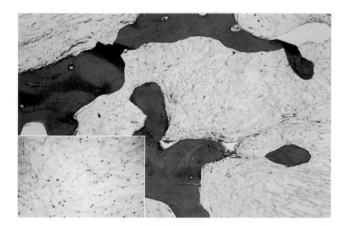

Fig. 15-125 Odontogenic myxoma. A loose, myxomatous tumor can be seen filling the marrow spaces between the bony trabeculae. The *inset* shows stellate-shaped cells and fine collagen fibrils.

be scattered throughout the myxoid ground substance. These epithelial rests are not required for the diagnosis and are not obvious in most cases. In some patients, the tumor may have a greater tendency to form collagen fibers; such lesions are sometimes designated as **fibromyxomas** or **myxofibromas**. There is no evidence that the more collagenized variants deserve separate consideration, although some investigators have suggested that these may represent part of a spectrum that includes the central odontogenic fibroma at the other endpoint.

A myxoma may be microscopically confused with other myxoid jaw neoplasms, such as the rare chondromyxoid fibroma (see page 657) or the myxoid neurofibroma (see page 528). Chondromyxoid fibroma should have areas of cartilaginous differentiation, whereas myxoid neurofibromas tend to have scattered lesional cells that are positive for antibodies directed against S-100 protein. Myxoid change in an enlarged dental follicle or the dental papilla of a developing tooth may be microscopically similar to a myxoma. Evaluation of the clinical and radiographic features, however, will prevent overdiagnosis of these lesions as myxomas.

TREATMENT AND PROGNOSIS

Small myxomas are generally treated by curettage, but careful periodic reevaluation is necessary for at least 5 years. For larger lesions, more extensive resection may be required because myxomas are not encapsulated and tend to infiltrate the surrounding bone. Complete removal of a large tumor by curettage is often difficult to accomplish, and lesions of the posterior maxilla, in particular, should be treated more aggressively in most instances. Recurrence rates from various studies average approximately 25%. In spite of local recurrences, the overall prognosis is good, and metastases do not occur.

In rare cases the myxoma microscopically shows marked cellularity and cellular atypism. Some have designated these lesions as *myxosarcomas* or *malignant odontogenic myxoma.* They appear to have a more aggressive local course than do the usual myxomas. Death because of involvement of vital structures by the tumor has been described, but distant metastases have not been reported.

CEMENTOBLASTOMA (TRUE CEMENTOMA)

Many oral and maxillofacial pathologists consider the **cementoblastoma** to represent an odontogenic tumor. However, other pathologists have pointed out that the histopathologic features of cementoblastomas of the jaws are identical to those of a bone tumor, osteoblastoma, seen both in the jaws and extragnathic skeleton. Cementoblastomas are discussed in Chapter 14 (see page 655).

BIBLIOGRAPHY

Odontogenic Cysts and Tumors—General References and Classification

Barnes L, Eveson JW, Reichart P et al, editors: *World Health Organization classification of tumours: pathology and genetics of head and neck tumours,* Lyon, France, 2005, IARC Press.

Jones AV, Craig GT, Franklin CD: Range and demographics of odontogenic cysts diagnosed in a UK population over a 30-year period, *J Oral Pathol Med* 35:500-507, 2006.

Kramer IRH, Pindborg JJ, Shear M: *Histological typing of odontogenic tumors,* ed 2, 1992, New York, Springer-Verlag.

Kramer IRH, Pindborg JJ, Shear M: The World Health Organization histological typing of odontogenic tumours: introducing the second edition, *Eur J Cancer B Oral Oncol* 29B:169-171, 1993.

Kreidler JF, Raubenheimer EJ, van Heerden WFP: A retrospective analysis of 367 cystic lesions of the jaw—the Ulm experience, *J Craniomaxillofac Surg* 21:339-341, 1993.

Nakamura T, Ishida J, Nakano Y et al: A study of cysts in the oral region: cysts of the jaws, *J Nihon Univ Sch Dent* 37:33-40, 1995.

Neville BW, Damm DD, Allen CM: Odontogenic cysts and tumors. In Gnepp D: *Diagnostic surgical pathology of the head and neck,* Philadelphia, 2001, WB Saunders.

Philipsen HP, Reichart PA: The development and fate of epithelial residues after completion of the human odontogenesis with special reference to the origins of epithelial odontogenic neoplasms, hamartomas and cysts, *Oral Biosci Med* 1:171-179, 2004.

Shear M: Developmental odontogenic cysts. An update, *J Oral Pathol Med* 23:1-11, 1994.

Shear M, Speight P: *Cysts of the oral and maxillofacial regions,* ed 4, Oxford, 2007, Blackwell.

Dentigerous Cyst

Ackermann G, Cohen MA, Altini M: The paradental cyst: a clinicopathologic study of 50 cases, *Oral Surg Oral Med Oral Pathol* 64:308-312, 1987.

Adelsperger J, Campbell JH, Coates DB et al: Early soft tissue pathosis associated with impacted third molars without pericoronal radiolucency, *Oral Surg Oral Med Oral Pathol Oral Radiol Endod* 89:402-406, 2000.

Benn A, Altini M: Dentigerous cysts of inflammatory origin: a clinicopathologic study, *Oral Surg Oral Med Oral Pathol Oral Radiol Endod* 81:203-209, 1996.

Clauser C, Zuccati G, Barone R et al: Simplified surgical-orthodontic treatment of a dentigerous cyst, *J Clin Orthod* 28:103-106, 1994.

Craig GT: The paradental cyst: a specific inflammatory odontogenic cyst, *Br Dent J* 141:9-14, 1976.

Curran AE, Damm DD, Drummond JF: Pathologically significant pericoronal lesions in adults: histopathologic evaluation, *J Oral Maxillofac Surg* 60:613-617, 2002.

Daley TD, Wysocki GP: The small dentigerous cyst: a diagnostic dilemma, *Oral Surg Oral Med Oral Pathol Oral Radiol Endod* 79:77-81, 1995.

Delbem AC, Cunha RF, Afonso RL et al: Dentigerous cysts in primary dentition: report of 2 cases, *Pediatr Dent* 28:269-272, 2006.

Gorlin RJ: Potentialities of oral epithelium manifest by mandibular dentigerous cysts, *Oral Surg Oral Med Oral Pathol* 10:271-284, 1957.

Kusukawa J, Irie K, Morimatsu M et al: Dentigerous cyst associated with a deciduous tooth: a case report, *Oral Surg Oral Med Oral Pathol* 73:415-418, 1992.

Lustmann L, Bodner L: Dentigerous cysts associated with supernumerary teeth, *Int J Oral Maxillofac Surg* 17:100-102, 1988.

Motamedi MHK, Talesh KT: Management of extensive dentigerous cysts, *Br Dent J* 198:203-206, 2005.

Takeda Y, Oikawa Y, Furuya I et al: Mucous and ciliated cell metaplasia in epithelial linings of odontogenic inflammatory and developmental cysts, *J Oral Sci* 47:77-81, 2005.

Ziccardi VB, Eggleston TI, Schneider RE: Using fenestration technique to treat a large dentigerous cyst, *J Am Dent Assoc* 128:201-205, 1997.

Eruption Cyst

Aguiló L, Cibrián R, Bagán JV et al: Eruption cysts: retrospective clinical study of 36 cases, *ASDC J Dent Child* 65:102-106, 1998.

Bodner L, Goldstein J, Sarnat H: Eruption cysts: a clinical report of 24 new cases, *J Clin Pediatr Dent* 28:183-186, 2004.

Clark CA: A survey of eruption cysts in the newborn, *Oral Surg Oral Med Oral Pathol* 15:917, 1962.

Kuczek A, Beikler T, Herbst H et al: Eruption cyst formation associated with cyclosporin A: a case report, *J Clin Periodontol* 30:462-466, 2003.

Seward MH: Eruption cyst: an analysis of its clinical features, *J Oral Surg* 31:31-35, 1973.

Primordial Cyst

Brannon RB: The odontogenic keratocyst—a clinicopathologic study of 312 cases. Part I: Clinical features, *Oral Surg Oral Med Oral Pathol* 42:54-72, 1976.

Robinson HBG: Classification of cysts of the jaws, *Am J Orthod Oral Surg* 31:370-375, 1945.

Odontogenic Keratocyst

Ahlfors E, Larsson A, Sjögren S: The odontogenic keratocyst: a benign cystic tumor? *J Oral Maxillofac Surg* 42:10-19, 1984.

Ali M, Baughman RA: Maxillary odontogenic keratocyst: a common and serious clinical misdiagnosis, *J Am Dent Assoc* 134:877-883, 2003.

Agaram NP, Collins BM, Barnes L et al: Molecular analysis to demonstrate that odontogenic keratocysts are neoplastic, *Arch Pathol Lab Med* 128:313-317, 2004.

Barnes L, Eveson JW, Reichart P et al, editors: *World Health Organization classification of tumours: pathology and genetics of head and neck tumours,* Lyon, France, 2005, IARC Press.

Bataineh AB, Al Qudah MA: Treatment of mandibular odontogenic keratocysts, *Oral Surg Oral Med Oral Pathol Oral Radiol Endod* 86:42-47, 1988.

Blanas N, Freund B, Schwartz M et al: Systematic review of the treatment and prognosis of the odontogenic keratocyst, *Oral Surg Oral Med Oral Pathol Oral Radiol Endod* 90:553-558, 1988.

Brannon RB: The odontogenic keratocyst—a clinicopathologic study of 312 cases. Part I: Clinical features, *Oral Surg Oral Med Oral Pathol* 42:54-72, 1976.

Brannon RB: The odontogenic keratocyst—a clinicopathologic study of 312 cases. Part II: Histologic features, *Oral Surg Oral Med Oral Pathol* 43:233-255, 1977.

Brøndum N, Jensen VJ: Recurrence of keratocysts and decompression treatment: a long-term follow-up of forty-four cases, *Oral Surg Oral Med Oral Pathol* 72:265-269, 1991.

Chehade A, Daley TD, Wysocki GP et al: Peripheral odontogenic keratocyst, *Oral Surg Oral Med Oral Pathol* 77:494-497, 1994.

Chi AC, Owings JR, Muller S: Peripheral odontogenic keratocyst: report of two cases and review of the literature, *Oral Surg Oral Med Oral Pathol Oral Radiol Endod* 99:71-78, 2005.

Fornatora ML, Reich RF, Chotkowski G et al: Odontogenic keratocyst with mural cartilaginous metaplasia: a case report and a review of the literature, *Oral Surg Oral Med Oral Pathol Oral Radiol Endod* 92:430-434, 2001.

Forssell K, Forssell H, Kahnberg K-E: Recurrence of keratocysts: a long-term follow-up study, *Int J Oral Maxillofac Surg* 17:25-28, 1988.

Garlock JA, Pringle GA, Hicks ML: The odontogenic keratocyst: a potential endodontic misdiagnosis, *Oral Surg Oral Med Oral Pathol Oral Radiol Endod* 85:452-456, 1988.

Henley J, Summerlin D-J, Tomich C et al: Molecular evidence supporting the neoplastic nature of odontogenic keratocyst: a laser capture microdissection study of 15 cases, *Histopathology* 47:582-586, 2005.

Ide F, Shimoyama T, Horie N: Peripheral odontogenic keratocyst: a report of 2 cases, *J Periodontol* 73:1079-1081, 2002.

Jackson IT, Potparic Z, Fasching M et al: Penetration of the skull base by dissecting keratocyst, *J Craniomaxillofac Surg* 21:319-325, 1993.

Kakarantza-Angelopoulou E, Nicolatou O: Odontogenic keratocysts: clinicopathologic study of 87 cases, *J Oral Maxillofac Surg* 48:593-599, 1990.

Kolokythas A, Fernandes RP, Pazoki A et al: Odontogenic keratocyst: to decompress or not to decompress? A comparative study of decompression and enucleation versus resection/peripheral ostectomy, *J Oral Maxillofac Surg* 65:640-644, 2007.

Kratochvil FJ, Brannon RB: Cartilage in the walls of odontogenic keratocysts, *J Oral Pathol Med* 22:282-285, 1993.

Levanat S, Kappler R, Hemmerlein B et al: Analysis of the PTCH1 signaling pathway in ovarian dermoids, *Int J Mol Med* 14:793-799, 2004.

Makowski GJ, McGuff S, van Sickels JE: Squamous cell carcinoma in a maxillary odontogenic keratocyst, *J Oral Maxillofac Surg* 59:76-80, 2001.

Meiselman F: Surgical management of the odontogenic keratocyst: conservative approach, *J Oral Maxillofac Surg* 52:960-963, 1994.

Morgan TA, Burton CC, Qian F: A retrospective review of treatment of the odontogenic keratocyst, *J Oral Maxillofac Surg* 63:635-639, 2005.

Myoung H, Hong S-P, Hong S-D et al: Odontogenic keratocyst: review of 256 cases for recurrence and clinicopathologic parameters, *Oral Surg Oral Med Oral Pathol Oral Radiol Endod* 91:328-333, 2001.

Neville BW, Damm DD, Brock TR: Odontogenic keratocysts of the midline maxillary region, *J Oral Maxillofac Surg* 55:340-344, 1997.

Pogrel MA, Jordan RCK: Marsupialization as a definitive treatment for the odontogenic keratocyst, *J Oral Maxillofac Surg* 62:651-655, 2004.

Preston RD, Narayana N: Peripheral odontogenic keratocyst, *J Periodontol* 76:2312-2315, 2005.

Rodu B, Tate AL, Martinez MG: The implications of inflammation in odontogenic keratocysts, *J Oral Pathol* 16:518-521, 1987.

Shear M: The aggressive nature of the odontogenic keratocyst: is it a benign cystic neoplasm? Part 1. Clinical and early experimental evidence of aggressive behavior, *Oral Oncol* 38:219-226, 2002.

Shear M: The aggressive nature of the odontogenic keratocyst: is it a benign cystic neoplasm? Part 2. Proliferation and genetic studies, *Oral Oncol* 38:323-331, 2002.

Shear M: The aggressive nature of the odontogenic keratocyst: is it a benign cystic neoplasm? Part 3. Immunocytochemistry of cytokeratin and other epithelial cell markers, *Oral Oncol* 38:407-415, 2002.

Voorsmit RACA: The incredible keratocyst: a new approach to treatment, *Dtsch Zahnarztl Z* 40:641-644, 1985.

Williams TP, Connor Jr FA: Surgical management of the odontogenic keratocyst: aggressive approach, *J Oral Maxillofac Surg* 52:964-966, 1994.

Yamazaki M, Cheng J, Nomura T et al: Maxillary odontogenic keratocyst with respiratory epithelium: a case report, *J Oral Pathol Med* 32:496-498, 2003.

Yoon JH, Kim SG, Lee SH et al: Simultaneous occurrence of an odontogenic keratocyst and giant cell granuloma-like lesion in the mandible, *Int J Oral Maxillofac Surg* 33:615-617, 2004.

Orthokeratinized Odontogenic Cysts

Crowley TE, Kaugars GE, Gunsolley JC: Odontogenic keratocysts: a clinical and histologic comparison of the parakeratin and orthokeratin variants, *J Oral Maxillofac Surg* 50:22-26, 1992.

Li T-J, Kitano M, Chen X-M et al: Orthokeratinized odontogenic cyst: a clinicopathological and immunocytochemical study of 15 cases, *Histopathology* 32:242-251, 1998.

Siar CH, Ng KH: Orthokeratinised odontogenic keratocysts in Malaysians, *Br J Oral Maxillofac Surg* 26:215-220, 1988.

Vuhahula E, Nikai H, Ijuhin N et al: Jaw cysts with orthokeratinization: analysis of 12 cases, *J Oral Pathol Med* 22:35-40, 1993.

Wright JM: The odontogenic keratocyst: orthokeratinized variant, *Oral Surg Oral Med Oral Pathol* 51:609-618, 1981.

Nevoid Basal Cell Carcinoma Syndrome

Cohen MM Jr: Nevoid basal cell carcinoma syndrome: molecular biology and new hypotheses, *Int J Oral Maxillofac Surg* 28:216-223, 1999.

Evans DGR, Ladusans EJ, Rimmer S et al: Complications of the naevoid basal cell carcinoma syndrome: results of a population based study, *J Med Genet* 30:460-464, 1993.

Goldstein AM, Pastakia B, DeGiovanna JJ et al: Clinical findings in two African-American families with the nevoid basal cell carcinoma syndrome (NBCC), *Am J Med Genet* 50:272-281, 1994.

Gorlin RJ: Nevoid basal cell carcinoma (Gorlin) syndrome, *Genet Med* 6:530-539, 2004.

Gorlin RJ, Goltz R: Multiple nevoid basal cell epithelioma, jaw cysts and bifid rib syndrome, *N Engl J Med* 262:908-914, 1960.

Kimonis VE, Goldstein AM, Pastakia B et al: Clinical manifestations in 105 persons with nevoid basal cell carcinoma syndrome, *Am J Med Genet* 69:299-308, 1997.

Lo Muzio L, Nocini P, Bucci P et al: Early diagnosis of nevoid basal cell carcinoma syndrome, *J Am Dent Assoc* 130:669-674, 1999.

Lo Muzio L, Staibano S, Pannone G et al: Expression of cell cycle and apoptosis-related proteins in sporadic odontogenic keratocysts and odontogenic keratocysts associated with the nevoid basal cell carcinoma syndrome, *J Dent Res* 78:1345-1353, 1999.

Manfredi M, Vescovi P, Bonanini M et al: Nevoid basal cell carcinoma syndrome: a review of the literature, *Int J Oral Maxillofac Surg* 33:117-124, 2004.

Shanley S, Ratcliffe J, Hockey A et al: Nevoid basal cell carcinoma syndrome: review of 118 affected individuals, *Am J Med Genet* 50:282-290, 1994.

Woolgar JA, Rippin JW, Browne RM: A comparative histologic study of odontogenic keratocysts in basal cell nevus syndrome and non-syndrome patients, *J Oral Pathol* 16:75-80, 1987.

Woolgar JA, Rippin JW, Browne RM: The odontogenic keratocyst and its occurrence in the nevoid basal cell carcinoma syndrome, *Oral Surg Oral Med Oral Pathol* 64:727-730, 1987.

Gingival Cyst of the Newborn

Cataldo E, Berkman M: Cysts of the oral mucosa in newborns, *Am J Dis Child* 116:44-48, 1968.

Donley CL, Nelson LP: Comparison of palatal and alveolar cysts of the newborn in premature and full term infants, *Pediatr Dent* 22:321-324, 2000.

Fromm A: Epstein's pearls, Bohn's nodules and inclusion cysts of the oral cavity, *J Dent Child* 34:275-287, 1967.

Jorgenson RJ, Shapiro SD, Salinas CF et al: Intraoral findings and anomalies in neonates, *Pediatrics* 69:577-582, 1982.

Paula JDR, Dezan CC, Frossard WTG et al: Oral and facial inclusion cysts in newborns, *J Clin Pediatr Dent* 31:127-129, 2006.

Gingival Cyst of the Adult

Bell RC, Chauvin PJ, Tyler MT: Gingival cyst of the adult: a review and report of eight cases, *J Can Dent Assoc* 63:533-535, 1997.

Breault LG, Billman MA, Lewis DM: Report of a gingival "surgical cyst" developing secondarily to a subepithelial connective tissue graft, *J Periodontol* 68:392-395, 1997.

Buchner A, Hansen LS: The histomorphologic spectrum of the gingival cyst in the adult, *Oral Surg Oral Med Oral Pathol* 48:532-539, 1979.

Cairo F, Rotundo R, Ficarra G: A rare lesion of the periodontium: the gingival cyst of the adult—a report of three cases, *Int J Periodontics Restorative Dent* 22:79-83, 2002.

Cunha KG, Carvalho Neto LG, Saraiva FM et al: Gingival cyst of the adult: a case report, *Gen Dent* 53:215-216, 2005.

Nxumalo TN, Shear M: Gingival cyst in adults, *J Oral Pathol Med* 21:309-313, 1992.

Lateral Periodontal Cyst

Altini M, Shear M: The lateral periodontal cyst: an update, *J Oral Pathol Med* 21:245-250, 1992.

Baker RD, D'Onofrio ED, Corio RL: Squamous-cell carcinoma arising in a lateral periodontal cyst, *Oral Surg Oral Med Oral Pathol* 47:495-499, 1979.

Carter LC, Carney YL, Perez-Pudlewski D: Lateral periodontal cyst: multifactorial analysis of a previously unreported series, *Oral Surg Oral Med Oral Pathol Oral Radiol Endod* 81:210-216, 1996.

Cohen D, Neville B, Damm D et al: The lateral periodontal cyst: a report of 37 cases, *J Periodontol* 55:230-234, 1984.

Fantasia JE: Lateral periodontal cyst: an analysis of forty-six cases, *Oral Surg Oral Med Oral Pathol* 48:237-243, 1979.

Greer RO, Johnson M: Botryoid odontogenic cyst: clinicopathologic analysis of ten cases with three recurrences, *J Oral Maxillofac Surg* 46:574-579, 1988.

Gurol M, Burkes EJ Jr, Jacoway J: Botryoid odontogenic cyst: analysis of 33 cases, *J Periodontol* 66:1069-1073, 1995.

Kerezoudis NP, Donta-Bakoyianni C, Siskos G: The lateral periodontal cyst: aetiology, clinical significance and diagnosis, *Endod Dent Traumatol* 16:144-150, 2000.

Ramer M, Valauri D: Multicystic lateral periodontal cyst and botryoid odontogenic cyst: multifactorial analysis of previously unreported series and review of literature, *N Y State Dent J* 71:47-51, 2005.

Rasmusson LG, Magnusson BC, Borrman H: The lateral periodontal cyst: a histopathological and radiographic study of 32 cases, *Br J Oral Maxillofac Surg* 29:54-57, 1991.

Wysocki GP, Brannon RB, Gardner DG et al: Histogenesis of the lateral periodontal cyst and the gingival cyst of the adult, *Oral Surg Oral Med Oral Pathol* 50:327-334, 1980.

Calcifying Odontogenic Cyst

Barnes L, Eveson JW, Reichart P et al, editors: *World Health Organization classification of tumours: pathology and genetics of head and neck tumours*, Lyon, France, 2005, IARC Press.

Buchner A: The central (intraosseous) calcifying odontogenic cyst: an analysis of 215 cases, *J Oral Maxillofac Surg* 49:330-339, 1991.

Buchner A, Merrell PW, Hansen LS et al: Peripheral (extraosseous) calcifying odontogenic cyst, *Oral Surg Oral Med Oral Pathol* 72:65-70, 1991.

Daniels JSM: Recurrent calcifying odontogenic cyst involving the maxillary sinus, *Oral Surg Oral Med Oral Pathol Oral Radiol Endod* 98:660-664, 2004.

Ellis GL: Odontogenic ghost cell tumor, *Semin Diagn Pathol* 16:288-292, 1999.

Ellis GL, Shmookler BM: Aggressive (malignant?) epithelial odontogenic ghost cell tumor, *Oral Surg Oral Med Oral Pathol* 61:471-478, 1986.

Fregnani ER, Pires FR, Quezada RD et al: Calcifying odontogenic cyst: clinicopathological features and immunohistochemical profile of 10 cases, *J Oral Pathol Med* 32:163-170, 2003.

Goldenberg D, Sciubba J, Tufano RP: Odontogenic ghost cell carcinoma, *Head Neck* 26:378-381, 2004.

Gorlin RJ, Pindborg JJ, Clausen FP et al: The calcifying odontogenic cyst—a possible analogue to the cutaneous calcifying epithelioma of Malherbe: an analysis of fifteen cases, *Oral Surg* 15:1235-1243, 1962.

Hong SP, Ellis GL, Hartman KS: Calcifying odontogenic cyst: a review of ninety-two cases with reevaluation of their nature as cysts or neoplasms, the nature of the ghost cells and subclassification, *Oral Surg Oral Med Oral Pathol* 72:56-64, 1991.

Iida S, Fukuda Y, Ueda T et al: Calcifying odontogenic cyst: radiologic findings in 11 cases, *Oral Surg Oral Med Oral Pathol Oral Radiol Endod* 101:356-362, 2006.

Johnson A III, Fletcher M, Gold L et al: Calcifying odontogenic cyst: a clinicopathologic study of 57 cases with immunohistochemical evaluation for cytokeratin, *J Oral Maxillofac Surg* 55:679-683, 1997.

Li T-J, Yu S-F: Clinicopathologic spectrum of the so-called calcifying odontogenic cysts: a study of 21 intraosseous cases with reconsideration of the terminology and classification, *Am J Surg Pathol* 27:372-384, 2003.

Lu Y, Mock D, Takata T et al: Odontogenic ghost cell carcinoma: report of four new cases and review of the literature, *J Oral Pathol Med* 28:323-329, 1999.

Praetorius F, Hjørting-Hansen E, Gorlin RJ et al: Calcifying odontogenic cyst: range, variations and neoplastic potential, *Acta Odontol Scand* 39:227-240, 1981.

Tajima Y, Yokose S, Sakamoto E et al: Ameloblastoma arising in calcifying odontogenic cyst, *Oral Surg Oral Med Oral Pathol* 74:776-779, 1992.

Toida M: So-called calcifying odontogenic cyst: review and discussion on the terminology and classification, *J Oral Pathol Med* 27:49-52, 1998.

Yoshida M, Kumamoto H, Ooya K et al: Histopathological and immunohistochemical analysis of calcifying odontogenic cysts, *J Oral Pathol Med* 30:582-588, 2001.

Glandular Odontogenic Cyst

Gardner DG, Kessler HP, Morency R et al: The glandular odontogenic cyst: an apparent entity, *J Oral Pathol* 17:359-366, 1988.

High AS, Main DMG, Khoo SP et al: The polymorphous odontogenic cyst, *J Oral Pathol Med* 25:25-31, 1996.

Hussain K, Edmondson HD, Browne RM: Glandular odontogenic cysts: diagnosis and treatment, *Oral Surg Oral Med Oral Pathol Oral Radiol Endod* 79:593-602, 1995.

Kaplan I, Gal G, Anavi Y et al: Glandular odontogenic cyst: treatment and recurrence, *J Oral Maxillofac Surg* 63:435-441, 2005.

Koppang HS, Johannessen S, Haugen LK et al: Glandular odontogenic cyst (sialo-odontogenic cyst): report of two cases and literature review of 45 previously reported cases, *J Oral Pathol Med* 27:455-462, 1998.

Magnusson B, Göransson L, Ödesjö B et al: Glandular odontogenic cyst: report of seven cases, *Dentomaxillofac Radiol* 26:26-31, 1997.

Manor R, Anavi Y, Kaplan I et al: Radiological features of glandular odontogenic cyst, *Dentomaxillofac Radiol* 32:73-79, 2003.

Noffke C, Raubenheimer EJ: The glandular odontogenic cyst: clinical and radiological features; review of the literature and report of nine cases, *Dentomaxillofac Radiol* 31:333-338, 2002.

Qin X-N, Li J-R, Chen X-M et al: The glandular odontogenic cyst: clinicopathologic features and treatment of 14 cases, *J Oral Maxillofac Surg* 63:694-699, 2005.

Shen J, Fan M, Chen X et al: Glandular odontogenic cyst in China: report of 12 cases and immunohistochemical study, *J Oral Pathol Med* 35:175-182, 2006.

Tran P-T, Cunningham CJ, Baughman RA: Glandular odontogenic cyst, *J Endod* 30:182-184, 2004.

Buccal Bifurcation Cyst

Colgan CM, Henry J, Napier SS et al: Paradental cysts: a role for food impaction in the pathogenesis? A review of cases from Northern Ireland, *Br J Oral Maxillofac Surg* 40:163-168, 2002.

Craig GT: The paradental cyst: a specific inflammatory odontogenic cyst, *Br Dent J* 141:9-14, 1976.

David LA, Sàndor GKB, Stoneman DW: The buccal bifurcation cyst: is non-surgical treatment an option? *J Can Dent Assoc* 64:712-716, 1998.

Fowler CB, Brannon RB: The paradental cyst: a clinicopathologic study of six new cases and review of the literature, *J Oral Maxillofac Surg* 47:243-248, 1989.

Pompura JR, Sàndor GKB, Stoneman DW: The buccal bifurcation cyst: a prospective study of treatment outcomes in 44 sites, *Oral Surg Oral Med Oral Pathol Oral Radiol Endod* 83:215-221, 1997.

Shohat I, Buchner A, Taicher S: Mandibular buccal bifurcation cyst: enucleation without extraction, *Int J Oral Maxillofac Surg* 32:610-613, 2003.

Stoneman DW, Worth HM: The mandibular infected buccal cyst-molar area, *Dent Radiogr Photogr* 56:1-14, 1983.

Carcinoma Arising in Odontogenic Cysts

Cavalcanti MGP, Veltrini VC, Ruprecht A et al: Squamous-cell carcinoma arising from an odontogenic cyst—the importance of computed tomography in the diagnosis of malignancy, *Oral Surg Oral Med Oral Pathol Oral Radiol Endod* 100:365-368, 2005.

Chaisuparat R, Coletti D, Kolokythas A et al: Primary intraosseous odontogenic carcinoma arising in an odontogenic cyst or de novo: a clinicopathologic study of six new cases, *Oral Surg Oral Med Oral Pathol Oral Radiol Endod* 101:196-202, 2006.

Gardner AF: The odontogenic cyst as a potential carcinoma: a clinicopathologic appraisal, *J Am Dent Assoc* 78:746-755, 1969.

Hennis HL, Stewart WC, Neville B et al: Carcinoma arising in an odontogenic keratocyst with orbital invasion, *Doc Ophthalmol* 77:73-79, 1991.

Makowski GJ, McGuff S, van Sickels JE: Squamous cell carcinoma in a maxillary odontogenic keratocyst, *J Oral Maxillofac Surg* 59:76-80, 2001.

Scheer M, Koch AM, Drebber U et al: Primary intraosseous carcinoma of the jaws arising from an odontogenic cyst—a case report, *J Craniomaxillofac Surg* 32:166-169, 2004.

Stoelinga PJ, Bronkhorst FB: The incidence, multiple presentation and recurrence of aggressive cysts of the jaws, *J Craniomaxillofac Surg* 16:184-195, 1988.

Swinson BD, Jerjes W, Thomas GJ: Squamous cell carcinoma arising in a residual odontogenic cyst: case report, *J Oral Maxillofac Surg* 63:1231-1233, 2005.

van der Waal I, Rauhamaa R, van der Kwast WAM et al: Squamous cell carcinoma arising in the lining of odontogenic cysts: report of 5 cases, *Int J Oral Surg* 14:146-152, 1985.

Waldron CA, Mustoe TA: Primary intraosseous carcinoma of the mandible with probable origin in an odontogenic cyst, *Oral Surg Oral Med Oral Pathol* 67:716-724, 1989.

Yasuoka T, Yonemoto K, Kato Y et al: Squamous cell carcinoma arising in a dentigerous cyst, *J Oral Maxillofac Surg* 58:900-905, 2000.

Yoshida H, Onizawa K, Yusa H: Squamous cell carcinoma arising in association with an orthokeratinized odontogenic keratocyst. Report of a case, *J Oral Maxillofac Surg* 54:647-651, 1996.

Ameloblastoma

Buchner A, Merrell PW, Carpenter WM: Relative frequency of central odontogenic tumors: a study of 1,088 cases from northern California and comparison to studies from other parts of the world, *J Oral Maxillofac Surg* 64:1343-1352, 2006.

Carlson ER, Marx RE: The ameloblastoma: primary, curative surgical management, *J Oral Maxillofac Surg* 64:484-494, 2006.

Eversole LR, Leider AS, Hansen LS: Ameloblastomas with pronounced desmoplasia, *J Oral Maxillofac Surg* 42:735-740, 1984.

Gardner DG: Some current concepts on the pathology of ameloblastomas, *Oral Surg Oral Med Oral Pathol Oral Radiol Endod* 82:660-669, 1996.

Gardner DG: Critique of the 1995 review by Reichart et al of the biologic profile of 3677 ameloblastomas, *Oral Oncol* 35:443-449, 1999.

Gardner DG, Pecak AMJ: The treatment of ameloblastoma based on pathologic and anatomic principles, *Cancer* 46:2514-2519, 1980.

Ghandhi D, Ayoub AF, Pogrel MA et al: Ameloblastoma: a surgeon's dilemma, *J Oral Maxillofac Surg* 64:1010-1014, 2006.

Gortzak RA, Latief BS, Lekkas C et al: Growth characteristics of large mandibular ameloblastomas: report of 5 cases with implications for the approach to surgery, *Int J Oral Maxillofac Surg* 35:691-695, 2006.

Hirota M, Aoki S, Kawabe R et al: Desmoplastic ameloblastoma featuring basal cell ameloblastoma: a case report, *Oral Surg Oral Med Oral Pathol Oral Radiol Endod* 99:160-164, 2005.

Hong J, Yun P-Y, Chung I-H et al: Long-term follow up on recurrence of 305 ameloblastoma cases, *Int J Oral Maxillofac Surg* 36:283-288, 2007.

Keszler A, Paparella ML, Dominguez FV: Desmoplastic and non-desmoplastic ameloblastoma: a comparative clinicopathological analysis, *Oral Dis* 2:228-231, 1996.

Kishino M, Murakami S, Fukuda Y et al: Pathology of the desmoplastic ameloblastoma, *J Oral Pathol Med* 30:35-40, 2001.

Leibovitch I, Schwarcz RM, Modjtahedi S et al: Orbital invasion by recurrent maxillary ameloblastoma, *Ophthalmology* 113:1227-1230, 2006.

Leider AS, Eversole LR, Barkin ME: Cystic ameloblastoma: a clinicopathologic analysis, *Oral Surg Oral Med Oral Pathol* 60:624-630, 1985.

Martins WD, Fávaro DM: Recurrence of an ameloblastoma in an autogenous iliac bone graft, *Oral Surg Oral Med Oral Pathol Oral Radiol Endod* 98:657-659, 2004.

Melrose RJ: Benign epithelial odontogenic tumors, *Semin Diagn Pathol* 16:271-287, 1999.

Miller RS, Biddinger PW, Marciani RD et al: Simultaneously occurring ameloblastoma of the maxilla and mandible: case report, *Otolaryngol Head Neck Surg* 131:324-326, 2004.

Philipsen HP, Ormiston IW, Reichart PA: The desmo- and osteoplastic ameloblastoma: histologic variant or clinicopathologic entity? *Int J Oral Maxillofac Surg* 21:352-357, 1992.

Philipsen HP, Reichart PA, Takata T: Desmoplastic ameloblastoma (including "hybrid" lesion of ameloblastoma): biological profile based on 100 cases from the literature and own files, *Oral Oncol* 37:455-460, 2001.

Philipsen HP, Reichart PA: Classification of odontogenic tumours: a historical review, *J Oral Pathol Med* 35:525-529, 2006.

Raubenheimer EJ, van Heerden WFP, Noffke CEE: Infrequent clinicopathological findings in 108 ameloblastomas, *J Oral Pathol Med* 24:227-232, 1995.

Reichart PA, Philipsen HP, Sonner S: Ameloblastoma: biological profile of 3677 cases, *Oral Oncol* 31B:86-99, 1995.

Richard BM, Thyveetil M, Sharif H et al: Ameloblastoma with stromal multinucleated giant cells, *Histopathology* 25:497-499, 1994.

Sachs SA: Surgical excision with peripheral ostectomy: a definitive, yet conservative, approach to the surgical management of ameloblastoma, *J Oral Maxillofac Surg* 64:476-483, 2006.

Said-Al-Naief NAH, Lumerman H, Ramer M et al: Keratoameloblastoma of the maxilla: a case report and review of the literature, *Oral Surg Oral Med Oral Pathol Oral Radiol Endod* 84:535-539, 1997.

Sampson DE, Pogrel MA: Management of mandibular ameloblastoma: the clinical basis for a treatment algorithm, *J Oral Maxillofac Surg* 57:1074-1077, 1999.

Schafer DR, Thompson LDR, Smith BC et al: Primary ameloblastoma of the sinonasal tract, *Cancer* 82:667-674, 1998.

Small IA, Waldron CA: Ameloblastoma of the jaws, *Oral Surg Oral Med Oral Pathol* 8:281-297, 1955.

Takata T, Miyauchi M, Ito H et al: Clinical and histopathological analyses of desmoplastic ameloblastoma, *Pathol Res Pract* 195:669-675, 1999.

Takata T, Miyauchi M, Ogawa I et al: Immunoexpression of transforming growth factor β in desmoplastic ameloblastoma, *Virchows Arch* 436:319-323, 2000.

Waldron CA, El-Mofty S: A histopathologic study of 116 ameloblastomas with special reference to the desmoplastic variant, *Oral Surg Oral Med Oral Pathol* 63:441-451, 1987.

Unicystic Ameloblastoma

Ackerman GL, Altini M, Shear M: The unicystic ameloblastoma: a clinicopathologic study of 57 cases, *J Oral Pathol* 17:541-546, 1988.

Cunha EM, Fernandes AV, Versiani MA et al: Unicystic ameloblastoma: a possible pitfall in periapical diagnosis, *Int Endod J* 38:334-340, 2005.

Gardner DG, Corio RL: The relationship of plexiform unicystic ameloblastoma to conventional ameloblastoma, *Oral Surg Oral Med Oral Pathol* 56:54-60, 1983.

Lau SL, Samman N: Recurrence related to treatment modalities of unicystic ameloblastoma: a systematic review, *Int J Oral Maxillofac Surg* 35:681-690, 2006.

Li T-J, Browne RM, Matthews JB: Expression of proliferating cell nuclear antigen (PCNA) and Ki-67 unicystic ameloblastoma, *Histopathology* 26:219-228, 1995.

Philipsen HP, Reichart PA: Unicystic ameloblastoma: a review of 193 cases from the literature, *Oral Oncol* 34:317-325, 1998.

Robinson L, Martinez MG: Unicystic ameloblastoma: a prognostically distinct entity, *Cancer* 40:2278-2285, 1977.

Vickers RA, Gorlin RJ: Ameloblastoma: delineation of early histopathologic features of neoplasia, *Cancer* 26:699-710, 1970.

Peripheral (Extraosseous) Ameloblastoma

Baden E, Doyle JL, Petriella V: Malignant transformation of peripheral ameloblastoma, *Oral Surg Oral Med Oral Pathol* 75:214-219, 1993.

Buchner A, Merrell PW, Carpenter WM: Relative frequency of peripheral odontogenic tumors: a study of 45 new cases and comparison with studies from the literature, *J Oral Pathol Med* 35:385-391, 2006.

Gardner DG: Peripheral ameloblastoma: a study of 21 cases including 5 reported as basal cell carcinoma of the gingiva, *Cancer* 39:1625-1633, 1977.

Ide F, Kusama K: Difficulty in predicting biological behavior of peripheral ameloblastoma, *Oral Oncol* 40:651-652, 2004.

Ide F, Kusama K, Tanaka A et al: Peripheral ameloblastoma is not a hamartoma but rather more of a neoplasm, *Oral Oncol* 38:318-320, 2002.

LeCorn DW, Bhattacharyya I, Vertucci FJ: Peripheral ameloblastoma: a case report and review of the literature, *J Endod* 32:152-154, 2006.

Martelli-Júnior H, Souza LN, Santos LA et al: Peripheral ameloblastoma: a case report, *Oral Surg Oral Med Oral Pathol Oral Radiol Endod* 99:e31-e33, 2005.

Philipsen HP, Reichart PA, Nikai H et al: Peripheral ameloblastoma: biological profile based on 160 cases from the literature, *Oral Oncol* 37:17-27, 2001.

Woo SB, Smith-Williams JE, Sciubba JJ et al: Peripheral ameloblastoma of the buccal mucosa: case report and review of the English language literature, *Oral Surg Oral Med Oral Pathol* 63:78-84, 1987.

Yamanishi T, Ando S, Aikawa T et al: A case of extragingival peripheral ameloblastoma in the buccal mucosa, *J Oral Pathol Med* 36:184-186, 2007.

Malignant Ameloblastoma and Ameloblastic Carcinoma

Akrish S, Buchner JA, Shoshani Y et al: Ameloblastic carcinoma: report of a new case, literature review, and comparison to ameloblastoma, *J Oral Maxillofac Surg* 65:777-783, 2007.

Corio RL, Goldblatt LI, Edwards PA et al: Ameloblastic carcinoma: a clinicopathologic assessment of eight cases, *Oral Surg Oral Med Oral Pathol* 64:570-576, 1987.

Eliasson A, Moser RJ III, Tenholder MF: Diagnosis and treatment of metastatic ameloblastoma, *South Med J* 82:1165-1168, 1989.

Eversole LR: Malignant epithelial odontogenic tumors, *Semin Diagn Pathol* 16:317-324, 1999.

Goldenberg D, Sciubba J, Koch W et al: Malignant odontogenic tumors: a 22-year experience, *Laryngoscope* 114:1770-1774, 2004.

Hall JM, Weathers DR, Unni KK: Ameloblastic carcinoma: an analysis of 14 cases, *Oral Surg Oral Med Oral Pathol Oral Radiol Endod*103:799-807, 2007.

Lau SK, Tideman H, Wu PC: Ameloblastic carcinoma of the jaws: a report of two cases, *Oral Surg Oral Med Oral Pathol Oral Radiol Endod* 85:78-81, 1998.

Okada H, Davies JE, Yamamoto H: Malignant ameloblastoma: a case study and review, *J Oral Maxillofac Surg* 57:725-730, 1999.

Simko EJ, Brannon RB, Eibling DE: Ameloblastic carcinoma of the mandible, *Head Neck* 20:654-659, 1998.

Slootweg PJ, Müller H: Malignant ameloblastoma or ameloblastic carcinoma, *Oral Surg Oral Med Oral Pathol* 57:168-176, 1984.

Suomalainen A, Hietanen J, Robinson S et al: Ameloblastic carcinoma of the mandible resembling odontogenic cyst in a panoramic radiograph, *Oral Surg Oral Med Oral Pathol Oral Radiol Endod* 101:638-642, 2006.

Üzüm N, Akyol G, Asal K et al: Ameloblastic carcinoma containing melanocyte and melanin pigment in the mandible: a case report and review of the literature, *J Oral Pathol Med* 34:618-620, 2005.

Clear Cell Odontogenic Tumor

August M, Faquin W, Troulis M et al: Clear cell odontogenic carcinoma: evaluation of reported cases, *J Oral Maxillofac Surg* 61:580-586, 2003.

Bang G, Koppang HS, Hansen LS et al: Clear cell odontogenic carcinoma: report of three cases and lymph node metastasis, *J Oral Pathol Med* 18:113-118, 1989.

Brandwein M, Said-Al-Naief N, Gordon R et al: Clear cell odontogenic carcinoma: report of a case and analysis of the literature, *Arch Otolaryngol Head Neck Surg* 128:1089-1095, 2002.

Ebert CS, Dubin MG, Hart CF et al: Clear cell odontogenic carcinoma: a comprehensive analysis of treatment strategies, *Head Neck* 27:536-542, 2005.

Eversole LR: On the differential diagnosis of clear cell tumours of the head and neck, *Eur J Cancer B Oral Oncol* 29B:173-179, 1993.

Fan J, Kubota E, Imamura H et al: Clear cell odontogenic carcinoma: a case report with massive invasion of neighboring organs and lymph node metastasis, *Oral Surg Oral Med Oral Pathol* 74:768-775, 1992.

Hansen LS, Eversole LR, Green TL et al: Clear cell odontogenic tumor—a new histologic variant with aggressive potential, *Head Neck Surg* 8:115-123, 1985.

Kumamoto H, Kawamura H, Ooya K: Clear cell odontogenic tumor in the mandible: report of a case with an immunohistochemical study of epithelial cell markers, *Pathol Int* 48:618-622, 1998.

Kumamoto H, Yamazaki S, Sato A et al: Clear cell odontogenic tumor in the mandible: report of a case with duct-like appearances and dentinoid induction, *J Oral Pathol Med* 29:43-47, 2000.

Waldron CA, Small IA, Silverman H: Clear cell ameloblastoma—an odontogenic carcinoma, *J Oral Maxillofac Surg* 43:709-717, 1985.

Yamamoto H, Inui M, Mori A et al: Clear cell odontogenic carcinoma. A case report and literature review of odontogenic tumors with clear cells, *Oral Surg Oral Med Oral Pathol Oral Radiol Endod* 86:86-89, 1998.

Adenomatoid Odontogenic Tumor

Courtney RM, Kerr DA: The odontogenic adenomatoid tumor: a comprehensive review of 21 cases, *Oral Surg Oral Med Oral Pathol* 39:424-435, 1975.

Damm DD, White DK, Drummond JF et al: Combined epithelial odontogenic tumor: adenomatoid odontogenic tumor and calcifying epithelial odontogenic tumor, *Oral Surg Oral Med Oral Pathol* 55:487-496, 1983.

Giansanti JS, Someren A, Waldron CA: Odontogenic adenomatoid tumor (adenoameloblastoma), *Oral Surg Oral Med Oral Pathol* 30:69-86, 1970.

Leon JE, Mata GM, Fregnani ER et al: Clinicopathological and immunohistochemical study of 39 cases of adenomatoid odontogenic tumour: a multicentric study, *Oral Oncol* 41:835-842, 2005.

Miyake M, Nagahata S, Nishihara J et al: Combined adenomatoid odontogenic tumor and calcifying epithelial odontogenic tumor: report of a case and ultrastructural study, *J Oral Maxillofac Surg* 54:788-793, 1996.

Philipsen HP, Reichart PA: Adenomatoid odontogenic tumour: facts and figures, *Oral Oncol* 35:125-131, 1999.

Philipsen HP, Srisuwan T, Reichart PA: Adenomatoid odontogenic tumor mimicking a periapical (radicular) cyst: a case report, *Oral Surg Oral Med Oral Pathol Oral Radiol Endod* 94:246-248, 2002.

Poulson TC, Greer RO: Adenomatoid odontogenic tumor: clinicopathologic and ultrastructural concepts, *J Oral Maxillofac Surg* 41:818-824, 1983.

Calcifying Epithelial Odontogenic Tumor

Anavi Y, Kaplan I, Citir M et al: Clear-cell variant of calcifying epithelial odontogenic tumor: clinical and radiographic characteristics, *Oral Surg Oral Med Oral Pathol Oral Radiol Endod* 95:332-339, 2003.

Aviel-Ronen S, Liokumovich P, Rahima D et al: The amyloid deposit in calcifying epithelial odontogenic tumor is immunoreactive for cytokeratins, *Arch Pathol Lab Med* 124:872-876, 2000.

Basu MK, Matthews JB, Sear AJ et al: Calcifying epithelial odontogenic tumour: a case showing features of malignancy, *J Oral Pathol* 13:310-319, 1984.

Bridle C, Visram K, Piper K et al: Maxillary calcifying epithelial odontogenic (Pindborg) tumor presenting with abnormal eye signs: case report and literature review, *Oral Surg Oral Med Oral Pathol Oral Radiol Endod* 102:e12-e15, 2006.

Cheng Y-SL, Wright JM, Walstad WR et al: Calcifying epithelial odontogenic tumor showing microscopic features of potential malignant behavior, *Oral Surg Oral Med Oral Pathol Oral Radiol Endod* 93:287-295, 2002.

Dantas da Silveira EJ, Gordón-Núñez MA, Guerra Seabra FR et al: Peripheral calcifying epithelial odontogenic tumor associated with generalized drug-induced gingival growth: a case report, *J Oral Maxillofac Surg* 65:341-345, 2007.

Franklin CD, Pindborg JJ: The calcifying epithelial odontogenic tumor: a review and analysis of 113 cases, *Oral Surg Oral Med Oral Pathol* 42:753-765, 1976.

Germanier Y, Bornstein MM, Stauffer E et al: Calcifying epithelial odontogenic (Pindborg) tumor of the mandible with clear cell component treated by conservative surgery: report of a case, *J Oral Maxillofac Surg* 63:1377-1382, 2005.

Gopalakrishnan R, Simonton S, Rohrer MD et al: Cystic variant of calcifying epithelial odontogenic tumor, *Oral Surg Oral Med Oral Pathol Oral Radiol Endod* 102:773-777, 2006.

Houston GD, Fowler CB: Extraosseous calcifying epithelial odontogenic tumor: report of two cases and review of the literature, *Oral Surg Oral Med Oral Pathol Oral Radiol Endod* 83:577-583, 1997.

Kaplan I, Buchner A, Calderon S et al: Radiological and clinical features of calcifying epithelial odontogenic tumour, *Dentomaxillofac Radiol* 30:22-28, 2001.

Kawano K, Ono K, Yada N et al: Malignant calcifying epithelial odontogenic tumor of the mandible: report of a case with pulmonary metastasis showing remarkable response to platinum derivatives, *Oral Surg Oral Med Oral Pathol Oral Radiol Endod* 104:76-81, 2007.

Kumamoto H, Sato I, Tateno H et al: Clear cell variant of calcifying epithelial odontogenic tumor (CEOT) in the maxilla: report of a case with immunohistochemical and ultrastructural investigations, *J Oral Pathol Med* 28:187-191, 1999.

Philipsen HP, Reichart PA: Calcifying epithelial odontogenic tumour: biological profile based on 181 cases from the literature, *Oral Oncol* 36:17-26, 2000.

Pindborg JJ: A calcifying epithelial odontogenic tumor, *Cancer* 11:838-843, 1958.

Seim P, Regezi JA, O'Ryan F: Hybrid ameloblastoma and calcifying epithelial odontogenic tumor: case report, *J Oral Maxillofac Surg* 63:852-855, 2005.

Solomon A, Murphy CL, Weaver K et al: Calcifying epithelial odontogenic (Pindborg) tumor-associated amyloid consists of a novel human protein, *J Lab Clin Med* 142:348-355, 2003.

Veness MJ, Morgan G, Collins AP et al: Calcifying epithelial odontogenic (Pindborg) tumor with malignant transformation and metastatic spread, *Head Neck* 23:692-696, 2001.

Squamous Odontogenic Tumor

Baden E, Doyle J, Mesa M et al: Squamous odontogenic tumor: report of three cases including the first extraosseous case, *Oral Surg Oral Med Oral Pathol* 75:733-738, 1993.

Goldblatt LI, Brannon RB, Ellis GL: Squamous odontogenic tumor: report of five cases and review of the literature, *Oral Surg Oral Med Oral Pathol* 54:187-196, 1982.

Haghighat K, Kalmar JR, Mariotti AJ: Squamous odontogenic tumor: diagnosis and management, *J Periodontol* 73:653-656, 2002.

Ide F, Shimoyama T, Horie N et al: Intraosseous squamous cell carcinoma arising in association with a squamous odontogenic tumour of the mandible, *Oral Oncol* 35:431-434, 1999.

Kim K, Mintz SM, Stevens J: Squamous odontogenic tumor causing erosion of the lingual cortical plate in the mandible: a report of 2 cases, *J Oral Maxillofac Surg* 65:1227-1231, 2007.

Krithika C, Vardhan BG, Saraswathy K et al: Radiolucency in the anterior maxilla associated with an impacted tooth, *Oral Surg Oral Med Oral Pathol Oral Radiol Endod* 103:164-168, 2007.

Kusama K, Kawashima A, Nagai H et al: Squamous odontogenic tumor of the maxilla: report of a case, *J Oral Sci* 40:119-122, 1998.

Leider AS, Jonker A, Cook HE: Multicentric familial squamous odontogenic tumor, *Oral Surg Oral Med Oral Pathol* 68:175-181, 1989.

Mills WP, Davilla MA, Beattenmuller EA et al: Squamous odontogenic tumor: report of a case with lesions in three quadrants, *Oral Surg Oral Med Oral Pathol* 61:557-563, 1986.

Philipsen HP, Reichart PA: Squamous odontogenic tumor (SOT): a benign neoplasm of the periodontium. A review of 36 reported cases, *J Clin Periodontol* 23:922-926, 1996.

Pullon PA, Shafer WG, Elzay RP et al: Squamous odontogenic tumor: report of six cases of a previously undescribed lesion, *Oral Surg Oral Med Oral Pathol* 40:616-630, 1975.

Wright JM: Squamous odontogenic tumor-like proliferations in odontogenic cysts, *Oral Surg Oral Med Oral Pathol* 47:354-358, 1979.

Mixed Odontogenic Tumors

Gardner DG: The mixed odontogenic tumors, *Oral Surg Oral Med Oral Pathol* 58:166-168, 1984.

Hansen LS, Ficarra G: Mixed odontogenic tumors: an analysis of 23 new cases, *Head Neck Surg* 10:330-343, 1988.

Philipsen HP, Reichart PA: Classification of odontogenic tumors: a historical review, *J Oral Pathol Med* 35:525-529, 2006.

Philipsen HP, Reichart PA, Praetorius F: Mixed odontogenic tumours and odontomas. Considerations on interrelationship. Review of the literature and presentation of 134 new cases of odontomas, *Oral Oncol* 33:86-99, 1997.

Slootweg PJ: An analysis of the interrelationship of the mixed odontogenic tumors—ameloblastic fibroma, ameloblastic fibro-odontoma and the odontomas, *Oral Surg Oral Med Oral Pathol* 51:266-276, 1981.

Tomich CE: Benign mixed odontogenic tumors, *Semin Diagn Pathol* 16:308-316, 1999.

Ameloblastic Fibroma

Chen Y, Li T-J, Gao Y et al: Ameloblastic fibroma and related lesions: a clinicopathologic study with reference to their nature and interrelationship, *J Oral Pathol Med* 34:588-595, 2005.

Cohen DM, Bhattacharyya I: Ameloblastic fibroma, ameloblastic fibro-odontoma, and odontoma, *Oral Maxillofac Surg Clin North Am* 16:375-384, 2004.

Dallera P, Bertoni F, Marchetti C et al: Ameloblastic fibroma: a follow-up of six cases, *Int J Oral Maxillofac Surg* 25:199-202, 1996.

Darling MR, Daley TD: Peripheral ameloblastic fibroma, *J Oral Pathol Med* 35:190-192, 2006.

Lin C-C, Chen C-H, Lin L-M et al: Calcifying odontogenic cyst with ameloblastic fibroma: report of three cases, *Oral Surg Oral Med Oral Pathol Oral Radiol Endod* 98:451-460, 2004.

Mosby EL, Russell D, Noren S et al: Ameloblastic fibroma in a 7-week-old infant: a case report and review of the literature, *J Oral Maxillofac Surg* 56:368-372, 1998.

Sawyer DR, Nwoku AL, Mosadomi A: Recurrent ameloblastic fibroma: report of 2 cases, *Oral Surg Oral Med Oral Pathol* 53:19-24, 1982.

Takeda Y: Ameloblastic fibroma and related lesions: current pathologic concept, *Oral Oncol* 35:535-540, 1999.

Trodahl JN: Ameloblastic fibroma: a survey of cases from the Armed Forces Institute of Pathology, *Oral Surg Oral Med Oral Pathol* 33:547-558, 1972.

Yoon JH, Kim HJ, Yook JI et al: Hybrid odontogenic tumor of calcifying odontogenic cyst and ameloblastic fibroma, *Oral Surg Oral Med Oral Pathol Oral Radiol Endod* 98:80-84, 2004.

Zallen RD, Preskar MH, McClary SA: Ameloblastic fibroma, *J Oral Maxillofac Surg* 40:513-517, 1982.

Ameloblastic Fibro-Odontoma

Chang H, Shimizu MS, Precious DS: Ameloblastic fibro-odontoma: a case report, *J Can Dent Assoc* 68:243-246, 2002.

Cohen DM, Bhattacharyya I: Ameloblastic fibroma, ameloblastic fibro-odontoma, and odontoma, *Oral Maxillofac Surg Clin North Am* 16:375-384, 2004.

Dhanuthai K, Kongin K: Ameloblastic fibro-odontoma: a case report, *J Clin Pediatr Dent* 29:75-78, 2004.

Favia GF, Di Alberti L, Scarano A et al: Ameloblastic fibro-odontoma: report of two cases, *Oral Oncol* 33:444-446, 1997.

Furst I, Pharoah M, Phillips J: Recurrence of an ameloblastic fibro-odontoma in a 9-year-old boy, *J Oral Maxillofac Surg* 57:620-623, 1999.

Howell RM, Burkes EJ: Malignant transformation of ameloblastic fibro-odontoma to ameloblastic fibrosarcoma, *Oral Surg Oral Med Oral Pathol* 43:391-401, 1977.

Miller AS, Lopez CF, Pullon PA et al: Ameloblastic fibro-odontoma, *Oral Surg Oral Med Oral Pathol* 41:354-365, 1976.

Sekine J, Kitamura A, Ueno K et al: Cell kinetics in mandibular ameloblastic fibro-odontoma evaluated by bromodeoxyuridine and proliferating cell nuclear antigen immunohistochemistry: case report, *Br J Oral Maxillofac Surg* 34:450-453, 1996.

Slootweg PJ: Epithelio-mesenchymal morphology in ameloblastic fibro-odontoma: a light and electron microscopic study, *J Oral Pathol* 9:29-40, 1980.

Van Wyk CW, Van der Vyver PC: Ameloblastic fibroma with dentinoid formation/immature dentinoma: a microscopic and ultrastructural study of the epithelial-connective tissue interface, *J Oral Pathol* 12:37-46, 1983.

Ameloblastic Fibrosarcoma

Altini M, Thompson SH, Lownie JF et al: Ameloblastic sarcoma of the mandible, *J Oral Maxillofac Surg* 43:789-794, 1985.

Carlos-Bregni R, Mosqueda-Taylor A, Meneses-Garcia A: Ameloblastic fibrosarcoma of the mandible: report of two cases and review of the literature, *J Oral Pathol Med* 30:316-320, 2001.

Chomette G, Auriol M, Guilbert F et al: Ameloblastic fibrosarcoma of the jaws—report of three cases, *Pathol Res Pract* 178:40-47, 1983.

DeLair D, Bejarano PA, Peleg M et al: Ameloblastic carcinosarcoma of the mandible arising in ameloblastic fibroma: a case report and review of the literature, *Oral Surg Oral Med Oral Pathol Oral Radiol Endod* 103:516-520, 2007.

Kobayashi K, Murakami R, Fujii T et al: Malignant transformation of ameloblastic fibroma to ameloblastic fibrosarcoma: case report and review of the literature, *J Craniomaxillofac Surg* 33:352-355, 2005.

Kunkel M, Ghalibafian M, Radner H et al: Ameloblastic fibrosarcoma or odontogenic carcinosarcoma: a matter of classification? *Oral Oncol* 40:444-449, 2004.

Leider AS, Nelson JF, Trodahl JN: Ameloblastic fibrosarcoma of the jaws, *Oral Surg Oral Med Oral Pathol* 33:559-569, 1972.

Muller S, Parker DC, Kapadia SB et al: Ameloblastic fibrosarcoma of the jaws: a clinicopathologic and DNA analysis of five cases and review of the literature with discussion of its relationship to ameloblastic fibroma, *Oral Surg Oral Med Oral Pathol Oral Radiol Endod* 79:469-477, 1995.

Slater LJ: Odontogenic sarcoma and carcinosarcoma, *Semin Diagn Pathol* 16:325-332, 1999.

Williams MD, Hanna EY, El-Naggar AK: Anaplastic ameloblastic fibrosarcoma arising from recurrent ameloblastic fibroma: restricted molecular abnormalities of certain genes to the malignant transformation, *Oral Surg Oral Med Oral Pathol Oral Radiol Endod* 104:72-75, 2007.

Wood RM, Markle TL, Barker BF et al: Ameloblastic fibrosarcoma, *Oral Surg Oral Med Oral Pathol* 66:74-77, 1988.

Odontoameloblastoma

Mosqueda-Taylor A, Carlos-Bregni R, Ramírez-Amador V et al: Odontoameloblastoma. Clinico-pathologic study of three cases and critical review of the literature, *Oral Oncol* 38:800-805, 2002.

Gupta DS, Gupta MK: Odontoameloblastoma, *J Oral Maxillofac Surg* 44:146-148, 1986.

Kaugars GE: Ameloblastic odontoma (odonto-ameloblastoma), *Oral Surg Oral Med Oral Pathol* 71:371-373, 1991.

LaBriola JD, Steiner M, Bernstein ML et al: Odontoameloblastoma, *J Oral Surg* 38:139-143, 1980.

Odontoma

Ashkenazi M, Greenberg BP, Chodik G et al: Postoperative prognosis of unerupted teeth after removal of supernumerary teeth or odontomas, *Am J Orthod Dentofacial Orthop* 131:614-619, 2007.

Budnick SD: Compound and complex odontomas, *Oral Surg Oral Med Oral Pathol* 42:501-506, 1976.

Cohen DM, Bhattacharyya I: Ameloblastic fibroma, ameloblastic fibro-odontoma, and odontoma, *Oral Maxillofac Surg Clin North Am* 16:375-384, 2004.

Ide F, Shimoyama T, Horie N: Gingival peripheral odontoma in an adult: case report, *J Periodontol* 71:830-832, 2000.

Kaugars GE, Miller ME, Abbey LM: Odontomas, *Oral Surg Oral Med Oral Pathol* 67:172-176, 1989.

Miki Y, Oda Y, Iwaya N et al: Clinicopathological studies of odontoma in 47 patients, *J Oral Sci* 41:173-176, 1999.

Owens BM, Schuman NJ, Mincer HH et al: Dental odontomas: a retrospective study of 104 cases, *J Clin Pediatr Dent* 21:261-264, 1997.

Sapp JP, Gardner DG: An ultrastructural study of the calcifications in calcifying odontogenic cysts and odontomas, *Oral Surg Oral Med Oral Pathol* 44:754-766, 1977.

Sedano HO, Pindborg JJ: Ghost cell epithelium in odontomas, *J Oral Pathol* 4:27-30, 1975.

Tomizawa M, Otsuka Y, Noda T: Clinical observations of odontomas in Japanese children: 39 cases including one recurrent case, *Int J Paediatr Dent* 15:37-43, 2005.

Central Odontogenic Fibroma

Allen CM, Hammond HL, Stimson PG: Central odontogenic fibroma WHO type: a report of 3 cases with an unusual associated giant cell reaction, *Oral Surg Oral Med Oral Pathol* 73:62-66, 1992.

Daniels JSM: Central odontogenic fibroma of the mandible: a case report and review of the literature, *Oral Surg Oral Med Oral Pathol Oral Radiol Endod* 98:295-300, 2004.

Dunlap CL: Odontogenic fibroma, *Semin Diagn Pathol* 16:293-296, 1999.

Gardner DG: The central odontogenic fibroma: an attempt at clarification, *Oral Surg Oral Med Oral Pathol* 50:425-432, 1980.

Gardner DG: Central odontogenic fibroma current concepts, *J Oral Pathol Med* 25:556-561, 1996.

Handlers JP, Abrams AM, Melrose RJ et al: Central odontogenic fibroma: clinicopathologic features of 19 cases and review of the literature, *J Oral Maxillofac Surg* 49:46-54, 1991.

Ide F, Sakashita H, Kusama K: Ameloblastomatoid, central odontogenic fibroma: an epithelium-rich variant, *J Oral Pathol Med* 31:612-614, 2002.

Kaffe I, Buchner A: Radiologic features of central odontogenic fibroma, *Oral Surg Oral Med Oral Pathol* 78:811-818, 1994.

Mosqueda Taylor A, Bermudez Flores V, Diaz Franco MA: Combined central odontogenic fibroma and giant cell granuloma-like lesion of the mandible: report of a case and review of the literature, *J Oral Maxillofac Surg* 57:1258-1262, 1999.

Odell EW, Lombardi T, Barrett AW et al: Hybrid central giant cell granuloma and central odontogenic fibroma-like lesions of the jaws, *Histopathology* 30:165-171, 1997.

Ramer M, Buonocore P, Krost B: Central odontogenic fibroma—report of a case and review of the literature, *Periodontal Clin Investig* 24:27-30, 2002.

Slootweg PJ, Müller H: Central fibroma of the jaw: odontogenic or desmoplastic, *Oral Surg Oral Med Oral Pathol* 56:61-70, 1983.

Peripheral Odontogenic Fibroma

Baden E, Moskow BS, Moskow R: Odontogenic epithelial hamartoma, *J Oral Surg* 26:702-714, 1968.

Buchner A: Peripheral odontogenic fibroma, *J Craniomaxillofac Surg* 17:134-138, 1989.

Buchner A, Ficarra G, Hansen LS: Peripheral odontogenic fibroma, *Oral Surg Oral Med Oral Pathol* 64:432-438, 1987.

Buchner A, Merrell PW, Carpenter WM: Relative frequency of peripheral odontogenic tumors: a study of 45 new cases and comparison with studies from the literature, *J Oral Pathol Med* 35:385-391, 2006.

Daley TD, Wysocki GP: Peripheral odontogenic fibroma, *Oral Surg Oral Med Oral Pathol* 78:329-336, 1994.

Ficarra G, Sapp JP, Eversole LR: Multiple peripheral odontogenic fibroma, World Health Organization type, and central giant cell granuloma: a case report of an unusual association, *J Oral Maxillofac Surg* 51:325-328, 1993.

Ide F, Obara K, Mishima K et al: Peripheral odontogenic tumor: a clinicopathologic study of 30 cases. General features and hamartomatous lesions, *J Oral Pathol Med* 34:552-557, 2005.

Martelli-Junior H, Mesquita RA, de Paula AM et al: Peripheral odontogenic fibroma (WHO type) of the newborn: a case report, *Int J Paediatr Dent* 16:376-379, 2006.

Siar CH, Ng KH: Clinicopathological study of peripheral odontogenic fibromas (WHO-type) in Malaysians (1967-95), *Br J Oral Maxillofac Surg* 38:19-22, 2000.

Slabben H, Altini M: Peripheral odontogenic fibroma: a clinicopathologic study, *Oral Surg Oral Med Oral Pathol* 72:86-90, 1991.

Weber A, van Heerden WF, Ligthelm AJ et al: Diffuse peripheral odontogenic fibroma: report of 3 cases, *J Oral Pathol Med* 21:82-84, 1992.

Granular Cell Odontogenic Tumor

Brannon RB, Goode RK, Eversole LR et al: The central granular cell odontogenic tumor: report of 5 new cases, *Oral Surg Oral Med Oral Pathol Oral Radiol Endod* 94:614-621, 2002.

Gesek DJ, Adrian JC, Reid EN: Central granular cell odontogenic tumor: a case report including light microscopy, immunohistochemistry, and literature review, *J Oral Maxillofac Surg* 53:945-949, 1995.

Meer S, Altini M, Coleman H et al: Central granular cell odontogenic tumor: immunohistochemistry and ultrastructure, *Am J Otolaryngol* 25:73-78, 2004.

Orsini Machado de Sousa S, Soares de Araújo N, Maia Melhado R et al: Central odontogenic granular cell tumor: immunohistochemical study of two cases, *J Oral Maxillofac Surg* 56:787-791, 1998.

Piattelli A, Rubini C, Goteri G et al: Central granular cell odontogenic tumour: report of the first malignant case and review of the literature, *Oral Oncol* 39:78-82, 2003.

Rinaggio J, Cleveland D, Koshy R et al: Peripheral granular cell odontogenic fibroma, *Oral Surg Oral Med Oral Pathol Oral Radiol Endod* 104:676-679, 2007.

Vincent SD, Hammond HL, Ellis GL et al: Central granular cell odontogenic fibroma, *Oral Surg Oral Med Oral Pathol* 63:715-721, 1987.

Waldron CA, Thompson CW, Conner WA: Granular cell ameloblastic fibroma, *Oral Surg Oral Med Oral Pathol* 16:1202-1213, 1963.

White DK, Chen S-Y, Hartman KS et al: Central granular cell tumor of the jaws (the so-called granular cell ameloblastic fibroma), *Oral Surg Oral Med Oral Pathol* 45:396-405, 1978.

Yih W-Y, Thompson C, Meshul CK et al: Central odontogenic granular cell tumor of the jaw: report of case and immunohistochemical and electron microscopic study, *J Oral Maxillofac Surg* 53:453-459, 1995.

Myxoma

Barker BF: Odontogenic myxoma, *Semin Diagn Pathol* 16:297-301, 1999.

Barros RE, Domingnez PV, Cabrini RL: Myxoma of the jaws, *Oral Surg Oral Med Oral Pathol* 27:225-236, 1969.

Chiodo AA, Strumas N, Gilbert RW et al: Management of odontogenic myxoma of the maxilla, *Otolaryngol Head Neck Surg* 117:S73-76, 1997.

Goldblatt LI: Ultrastructural study of an odontogenic myxoma, *Oral Surg Oral Med Oral Pathol* 42:206-220, 1976.

Gosh BC, Huvos AG, Gerald FP et al: Myxoma of the jaw bones, *Cancer* 31:237-240, 1973.

Kaffe I, Naor H, Buchner A: Clinical and radiological features of odontogenic myxoma of the jaws, *Dentomaxillofac Radiol* 26:299-303, 1997.

Lamberg MA, Calonius BP, Makinen JE et al: A case of malignant myxoma (myxosarcoma) of the maxilla, *Scan J Dent Res* 92:352-357, 1984.

Li T-J, Sun L-S, Luo H-Y: Odontogenic myxomas: a clinicopathologic study of 25 cases, *Arch Pathol Lab Med* 130:1799-1806, 2006.

Lo Muzio L, Nocini PF, Favia G et al: Odontogenic myxoma of the jaws: a clinical, radiologic, immunohistochemical, and ultrastructural study, *Oral Surg Oral Med Oral Pathol Oral Radiol Endod* 82:426-433, 1996.

Noffke CEE, Raubenheimer EJ, Chabikuli NJ et al: Odontogenic myxoma: review of the literature and report of 30 cases from South Africa, *Oral Surg Oral Med Oral Pathol Oral Radiol Endod* 104:101-109, 2007.

Pahl S, Henn W, Binger T et al: Malignant odontogenic myxoma of the maxilla: case with cytogenetic confirmation, *J Laryngol Otol* 114:533-535, 2000.

Peltola J, Magnusson B, Happonen R-P et al: Odontogenic myxoma—a radiographic study of 21 tumours, *Br J Oral Maxillofac Surg* 32:298-302, 1994.

Schmidt-Westhausen A, Becker J, Schuppan D et al: Odontogenic myxoma—characterisation of the extracellular matrix (ECM) of the tumour stroma, *Eur J Cancer B Oral Oncol* 30B:377-380, 1994.

Simon ENM, Merkx MAW, Vuhahula E et al: Odontogenic myxomas: a clinicopathologic study of 33 cases, *Int J Oral Maxillofac Surg* 33:333-337, 2004.

White DK, Chen SY, Mohnae AM et al: Odontogenic myxoma: a clinical and ultrastructural study, *Oral Surg Oral Med Oral Pathol* 39:901-917, 1975.

Zhao M, Lu Y, Takata T et al: Immunohistochemical and histochemical characterisation of the mucosubstances of odontogenic myxoma: histogenesis and differential diagnosis, *Pathol Res Pract* 195:391-397, 1999.

Zimmerman DC, Dahlin DC: Myxomatous tumors of the jaws, *Oral Surg Oral Med Oral Pathol* 11:1069-1080, 1958.

16

Dermatologic Diseases

CHAPTER OUTLINE

ECTODERMAL DYSPLASIA

Ectodermal dysplasia represents a group of inherited conditions in which two or more ectodermally derived anatomic structures fail to develop. Thus depending on the type of ectodermal dysplasia, hypoplasia or aplasia of tissues (e.g., skin, hair, nails, teeth, sweat glands) may be seen. The various types of this disorder may be inherited in any one of several genetic patterns, including autosomal dominant, autosomal recessive, and X-linked patterns. Even though by some accounts more than 170 different subtypes of ectodermal dysplasia can be defined, these disorders are considered to be relatively rare, with an estimated frequency of seven cases occurring in every 10,000 births. For fewer than 20% of these conditions, the specific genetic mutations and their chromosomal locations have been identified. Systematically classifying these conditions can be challenging because of their wide-ranging clinical features; however, some investigators have suggested that a classification scheme based on the molecular genetic alteration associated with each type might be appropriate. Thus groups of ectodermal dysplasia syndromes could be categorized as being caused by mutations in genes encoding cell-cell signals, genes encoding adhesion molecules, or genes regulating transcription.

CLINICAL FEATURES

Perhaps the best known of the ectodermal dysplasia syndromes is **hypohidrotic ectodermal dysplasia**. In most instances, this disorder seems to show an

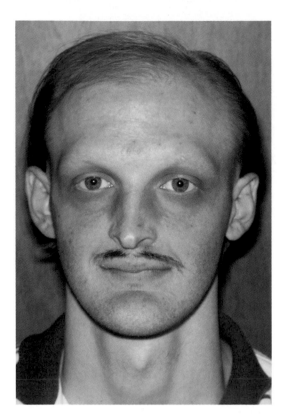

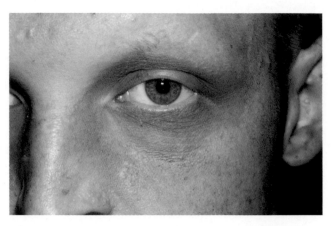

Fig. 16-2 Ectodermal dysplasia. Closer view of the same patient depicted in Fig. 16-1. Fine periocular wrinkling, as well as sparse eyelash and eyebrow hair, can be observed.

Fig. 16-1 Ectodermal dysplasia. The sparse hair, periocular hyperpigmentation, and mild midfacial hypoplasia are characteristic features evident in this affected patient.

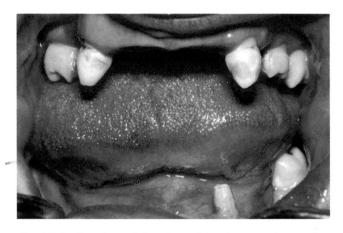

Fig. 16-3 Ectodermal dysplasia. Oligodontia and conical crown forms are typical oral manifestations. *(Courtesy of Dr. Charles Hook and Dr. Bob Gellin.)*

X-linked inheritance pattern, with the gene mapping to Xq12-q13.1; therefore, a male predominance is usually seen. However, a few families have been identified that show autosomal recessive or autosomal dominant patterns of inheritance.

Affected individuals typically display heat intolerance because of a reduced number of eccrine sweat glands. Sometimes the diagnosis is made during infancy because the baby appears to have a fever of undetermined origin; however, the infant simply cannot regulate body temperature appropriately because of the decreased number of sweat glands. Uncommonly, death results from the markedly elevated body temperature, although this generally happens only when the condition is not identified. Sometimes, as a diagnostic aid, a special impression can be made of the patient's fingertips and then examined microscopically to count the density of the sweat glands. Such findings should be interpreted in conjunction with appropriate age-matched controls.

Other signs of this disorder include fine, sparse hair, including a reduced density of eyebrow and eyelash hair (Fig. 16-1). The periocular skin may show a fine wrinkling with hyperpigmentation (Fig. 16-2), and midface hypoplasia is frequently observed, often result-

ing in protuberant lips. Because the salivary glands are ectodermally derived, these glands may be hypoplastic or absent, and patients may exhibit varying degrees of xerostomia. The nails may also appear dystrophic and brittle.

The teeth are usually markedly reduced in number (**oligodontia** or **hypodontia**), and their crown shapes are characteristically abnormal (Fig. 16-3). The incisor crowns usually appear tapered, conical, or pointed, and the molar crowns are reduced in diameter. Complete lack of tooth development (**anodontia**) has also been reported, but this appears to be uncommon.

Female patients may show partial expression of the abnormal gene; that is, their teeth may be reduced in number or may have mild structural changes. This incomplete presentation can be explained by the **Lyon hypothesis**, with half of the female patient's X chromosomes expressing the normal gene, and the other half expressing the defective gene.

HISTOPATHOLOGIC FEATURES

Histopathologic examination of the skin from a patient with hypohidrotic ectodermal dysplasia shows a decreased number of sweat glands and hair follicles. The adnexal structures that are present are hypoplastic and malformed.

TREATMENT AND PROGNOSIS

Management of hypohidrotic ectodermal dysplasia warrants genetic counseling for the parents and the patient. The dental problems are best managed by prosthetic replacement of the dentition with complete dentures, overdentures, or fixed appliances, depending on the number and location of the remaining teeth. With careful site selection, endosseous dental implants may be considered for facilitating prosthetic management of patients older than 5 years of age.

WHITE SPONGE NEVUS (CANNON'S DISEASE; FAMILIAL WHITE FOLDED DYSPLASIA)

White sponge nevus is a relatively rare genodermatosis (a genetically determined skin disorder) that is inherited as an autosomal dominant trait displaying a high degree of penetrance and variable expressivity. This condition is due to a defect in the normal keratinization of the oral mucosa. In the 30-member family of keratin filaments, the pair of keratins known as *keratin 4* and *keratin 13* is specifically expressed in the spinous cell layer of mucosal epithelium. Mutations in either of these keratin genes have been shown to be responsible for the clinical manifestations of white sponge nevus.

CLINICAL FEATURES

The lesions of white sponge nevus usually appear at birth or in early childhood, but sometimes the condition develops during adolescence. Symmetrical, thickened, white, corrugated or velvety, diffuse plaques affect the buccal mucosa bilaterally in most instances (Fig. 16-4). Other common intraoral sites of involvement include the ventral tongue, labial mucosa, soft palate, alveolar mucosa, and floor of the mouth, although the extent of involvement can vary from patient to patient. Extraoral mucosal sites, such as the nasal, esophageal, laryngeal, and anogenital mucosa, appear to be less commonly affected. Patients are usually asymptomatic.

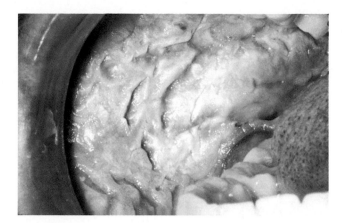

Fig. 16-4   White sponge nevus. Diffuse, thickened white plaques of the buccal mucosa.

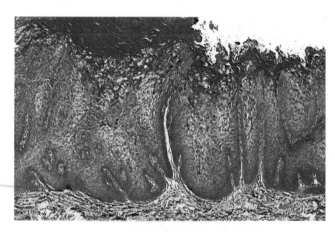

Fig. 16-5   White sponge nevus. This low-power photomicrograph shows prominent hyperparakeratosis, marked thickening (acanthosis), and vacuolation of the spinous cell layer.

HISTOPATHOLOGIC FEATURES

The microscopic features of white sponge nevus are characteristic but not necessarily pathognomonic. Prominent hyperparakeratosis and marked acanthosis with clearing of the cytoplasm of the cells in the spinous layer are common features (Figs. 16-5 and 16-6); however, similar microscopic findings may be associated with leukoedema and hereditary benign intraepithelial dyskeratosis (HBID). In some instances, an eosinophilic condensation is noted in the perinuclear region of the cells in the superficial layers of the epithelium, a feature that is unique to white sponge nevus. Ultrastructurally, this condensed material can be identified as tangled masses of keratin tonofilaments.

Exfoliative cytologic studies may provide more definitive diagnostic information. A cytologic preparation stained with the Papanicolaou method often shows

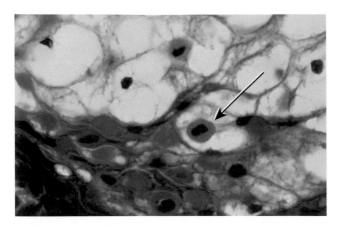

Fig. 16-6   White sponge nevus. This high-power photomicrograph shows vacuolation of the cytoplasm of the cells of the spinous layer, with no evidence of epithelial atypia. Perinuclear condensation of keratin tonofilaments can also be observed in some cells.

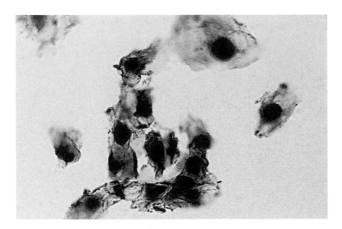

Fig. 16-7   White sponge nevus. This high-power photomicrograph of a Papanicolaou-stained cytologic preparation shows the pathognomonic perinuclear condensation of keratin tonofilaments.

the eosinophilic perinuclear condensation of the epithelial cell cytoplasm to a greater extent than does the histopathologic section (Fig. 16-7).

TREATMENT AND PROGNOSIS

Because this is a benign condition, no treatment is necessary. The prognosis is good.

HEREDITARY BENIGN INTRAEPITHELIAL DYSKERATOSIS (WITKOP-VON SALLMANN SYNDROME)

Hereditary benign intraepithelial dyskeratosis (HBID) is a rare autosomal dominant genodermatosis primarily affecting descendants of a triracial isolate

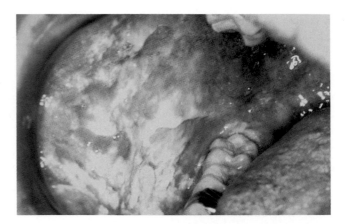

Fig. 16-8   Hereditary benign intraepithelial dyskeratosis (HBID). Oral lesions appear as corrugated white plaques of the buccal mucosa. *(Courtesy of Dr. John McDonald.)*

(Native American, black, and white) of people who originally lived in North Carolina. Examples of HBID have sporadically been reported from other areas of the United States because of migration of affected individuals, and descriptions of affected patients with no apparent connection to North Carolina have also appeared in the literature.

CLINICAL FEATURES

The lesions of HBID usually develop during childhood, in most instances affecting the oral and conjunctival mucosa. The oral lesions are similar to those of white sponge nevus, with both conditions showing thick, corrugated white plaques involving the buccal and labial mucosa (Fig. 16-8). Milder cases may exhibit the opalescent appearance of leukoedema. Other oral mucosal sites, such as the floor of the mouth and lateral tongue, may also be affected. These oral lesions may exhibit a superimposed candidal infection as well.

The most interesting feature of HBID is the ocular lesions, which begin to develop very early in life. These appear as thick, opaque, gelatinous plaques affecting the bulbar conjunctiva adjacent to the cornea (Fig. 16-9) and sometimes involving the cornea itself. When the lesions are active, patients may experience tearing, photophobia, and itching of the eyes. In many patients, the plaques are most prominent in the spring and tend to regress during the summer or autumn. Sometimes blindness may result from the induction of vascularity of the cornea secondary to the shedding process.

HISTOPATHOLOGIC FEATURES

The histopathologic features of HBID include prominent parakeratin production in addition to marked acanthosis. A peculiar dyskeratotic process, similar to

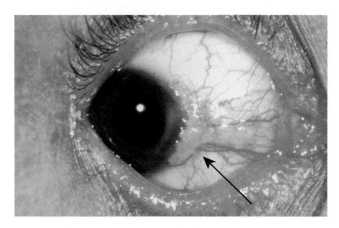

Fig. 16-9 **Hereditary benign intraepithelial dyskeratosis (HBID).** Ocular lesions appear as gelatinous plaques *(arrow)* of the bulbar conjunctivae. *(Courtesy of Dr. Carl Witkop.)*

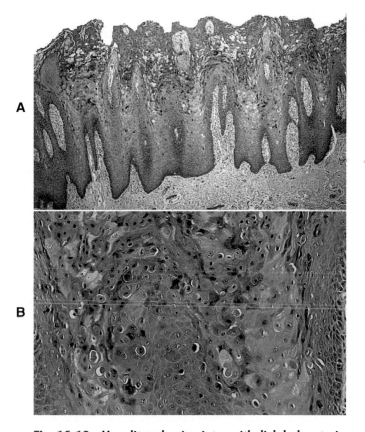

A

B

Fig. 16-10 **Hereditary benign intraepithelial dyskeratosis (HBID). A,** Medium-power photomicrograph exhibiting hyperparakeratosis, acanthosis, and dyskeratosis. **B,** Higher magnification showing dyskeratotic cells.

that of Darier's disease, is scattered throughout the upper spinous layer of the surface oral epithelium (Fig. 16-10). With this dyskeratotic process, an epithelial cell appears to be surrounded or engulfed by an adjacent epithelial cell, resulting in the so-called *cell-within-a-cell* phenomenon.

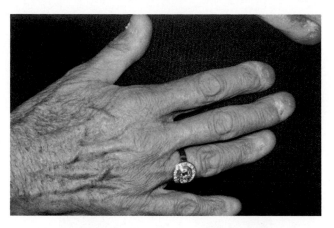

Fig. 16-11 **Pachyonychia congenita.** Loss of fingernails. *(Courtesy of Dr. John Lenox.)*

TREATMENT AND PROGNOSIS

Because HBID is a benign condition, no treatment is generally required or indicated for the oral lesions. If superimposed candidiasis develops, then an antifungal medication can be used. Patients with symptomatic ocular lesions should be referred to an ophthalmologist. Typically, the plaques that obscure vision must be surgically excised. This procedure, however, is recognized as a temporary measure because the lesions often recur.

PACHYONYCHIA CONGENITA (JADASSOHN-LEWANDOWSKY TYPE; JACKSON-LAWLER TYPE)

Pachyonychia congenita is a group of rare genodermatoses that are usually inherited as an autosomal dominant trait. The nails are dramatically affected in most patients, but oral lesions are seen only in patients affected by the Jadassohn-Lewandowsky form of the disease (pachyonychia congenita type 1). Fewer than 500 cases have been reported. Specific mutations in either the keratin 6a or keratin 16 gene have been detected for the Jadassohn-Lewandowsky type of pachyonychia congenita, whereas mutations of either the keratin 6b or keratin 17 gene are associated with the Jackson-Lawler form (pachyonychia congenita type 2).

CLINICAL FEATURES

Virtually all patients with pachyonychia congenita exhibit characteristic nail changes, either at birth or in the early neonatal period. The free margins of the nails are lifted up because of an accumulation of keratinaceous material in the nail beds. This results in a pinched, tubular configuration. Ultimately, nail loss may occur (Fig. 16-11).

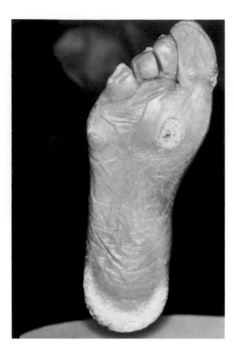

Fig. 16-12   Pachyonychia congenita. The soles of the feet of affected patients typically show marked calluslike thickenings. *(Courtesy of Dr. Lou Young.)*

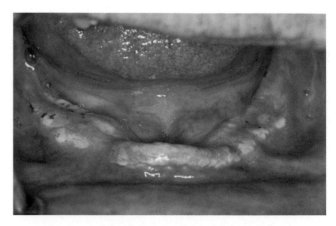

Fig. 16-13   Pachyonychia congenita. Although tongue lesions are more common in patients with pachyonychia congenita, other oral mucosal sites exposed to minor trauma, such as the alveolar mucosa, may develop thickened white patches. *(Courtesy of Dr. John Lenox.)*

Other skin changes that may occur include marked hyperkeratosis of the palmar and plantar surfaces, producing thick, calluslike lesions (Fig. 16-12). Hyperhidrosis of the palms and soles is also commonly present. The rest of the skin shows punctate papules, representing an abnormal accumulation of keratin in the hair follicles. One disabling feature of the syndrome is the formation of painful blisters on the soles of the feet after a few minutes of walking during warm weather.

The oral lesions seen in the Jadassohn-Lewandowsky form consist of thickened white plaques that involve the lateral margins and dorsal surface of the tongue. Other oral mucosal regions that are frequently exposed to mild trauma, such as the palate, buccal mucosa, and alveolar mucosa, may also be affected (Fig. 16-13). Neonatal teeth have been reported in patients affected by the Jackson-Lawler form, but these individuals do not have oral white lesions. Hoarseness and dyspnea have been described in some patients as a result of laryngeal mucosal involvement.

HISTOPATHOLOGIC FEATURES

Microscopic examination of lesional oral mucosa shows marked hyperparakeratosis and acanthosis with perinuclear clearing of the epithelial cells.

TREATMENT AND PROGNOSIS

Because the oral lesions of pachyonychia congenita show no apparent tendency for malignant transformation, no treatment is required. The nails are often lost or may need to be surgically removed because of the deformity. In addition, the keratin accumulation on the palms and soles can be quite uncomfortable and distressing to many of the affected individuals. Most patients have to pay continuous attention to removal of the excess keratin, and issues related to quality of life often arise. Patients should receive genetic counseling, as an aid in family planning. Identification of the various keratin mutations associated with these disorders is now possible, using molecular techniques to evaluate material obtained from chorionic villus sampling, thereby allowing prenatal diagnosis.

DYSKERATOSIS CONGENITA (COLE-ENGMAN SYNDROME; ZINSSER-COLE-ENGMAN SYNDROME)

Dyskeratosis congenita is a rare genodermatosis that is usually inherited as an X-linked recessive trait, resulting in a striking male predilection. Autosomal dominant and autosomal recessive forms, although less common, have been reported. Mutations in the *DKC1* gene have been determined to cause the X-linked form of dyskeratosis congenita. The mutated gene appears to disrupt the normal maintenance of telomerase, an enzyme that is critical in determining normal cellular longevity. The clinician should be aware of the condition because the oral lesions may undergo malignant transformation, and patients are susceptible to aplastic anemia.

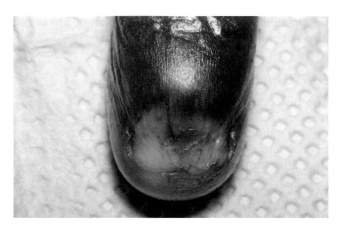

Fig. 16-14   Dyskeratosis congenita. Dysplastic nail changes.

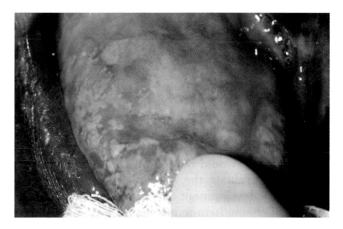

Fig. 16-15   Dyskeratosis congenita. Atrophy and hyperkeratosis of the dorsal tongue mucosa are visible.

CLINICAL FEATURES

Dyskeratosis congenita usually becomes evident during the first 10 years of life. A reticular pattern of skin hyperpigmentation develops, affecting the face, neck, and upper chest. In addition, abnormal, dysplastic changes of the nails are evident at this time (Fig. 16-14).

Intraorally, the tongue and buccal mucosa develop bullae; these are followed by erosions and, eventually, leukoplakic lesions (Fig. 16-15). The leukoplakic lesions are considered to be premalignant, and approximately one third of them become malignant in a 10- to 30-year period. The actual rate of transformation may be higher, but this may not be appreciated because of the shortened life span of these patients. Rapidly progressive periodontal disease has been reported sporadically.

Thrombocytopenia is usually the first hematologic problem that develops, typically during the second decade of life, followed by anemia. Ultimately, aplastic anemia develops in approximately 70% of these patients (see page 580). Mild to moderate mental retardation may also be present. Generally, the autosomal recessive and X-linked recessive forms show a more severe pattern of disease expression.

HISTOPATHOLOGIC FEATURES

Biopsy specimens of the early oral mucosal lesions show hyperorthokeratosis with epithelial atrophy. As the lesions progress, epithelial dysplasia develops until frank squamous cell carcinoma evolves.

TREATMENT AND PROGNOSIS

The discomfort of the oral lesions is managed symptomatically, and careful periodic oral mucosal examinations are performed to check for evidence of malignant transformation. Routine medical evaluation is warranted to monitor the patient for the development of aplastic anemia. Selected patients may be considered for allogeneic bone marrow transplantation once the aplastic anemia is identified.

As a result of these potentially life-threatening complications, the prognosis is guarded. The average life span for the more severely affected patients is 32 years of age. The parents and the patient should receive genetic counseling, but identification of the *DKC1* gene should allow for accurate confirmation of carriers of the gene and for prenatal diagnosis.

XERODERMA PIGMENTOSUM

Xeroderma pigmentosum is a rare genodermatosis in which numerous cutaneous malignancies develop at a very early age. The prevalence of the condition in the United States is estimated to be 1 in 250,000 to 500,000. The condition is inherited as an autosomal recessive trait and is caused by one of several defects in the excision repair and/or postreplication repair mechanism of DNA. As a result of the inability of the epithelial cells to repair ultraviolet (UV) light-induced damage, mutations in the epithelial cells occur, leading to the development of skin cancer at a rate 1000 to 4000 times what would normally be expected in people younger than 20 years of age.

CLINICAL FEATURES

During the first few years of life, patients affected by xeroderma pigmentosum show a markedly increased tendency to sunburn. Skin changes, such as atrophy, freckled pigmentation, and patchy depigmentation, soon follow (Fig. 16-16). In early childhood, **actinic keratoses** begin developing, a process that normally

HISTOPATHOLOGIC FEATURES

The gastrointestinal polyps of Peutz-Jeghers syndrome histopathologically represent benign overgrowths of intestinal glandular epithelium supported by a core of smooth muscle. Epithelial atypia is not usually a prominent feature, unlike the polyps of Gardner syndrome (see page 651).

Microscopic evaluation of the pigmented cutaneous lesions shows slight acanthosis of the epithelium with elongation of the rete ridges. No apparent increase in melanocyte number is detected by electron microscopy, but the dendritic processes of the melanocytes are elongated. Furthermore, the melanin pigment appears to be retained in the melanocytes rather than being transferred to adjacent keratinocytes.

TREATMENT AND PROGNOSIS

Patients with Peutz-Jeghers syndrome should be monitored for development of intussusception or tumor formation. Genetic counseling is also appropriate.

HEREDITARY HEMORRHAGIC TELANGIECTASIA (OSLER-WEBER-RENDU SYNDROME)

Hereditary hemorrhagic telangiectasia (HHT) is an uncommon mucocutaneous disorder that is inherited as an autosomal dominant trait, and recent epidemiologic studies suggest a prevalence of at least 1 in 10,000 people. Mutation of either one of two different genes at two separate loci is responsible for the condition. HHT1 is caused by a mutation of the *ENG* (endoglin) gene on chromosome 9, whereas mutation of *ALK1* (activin receptor-like kinase-1; *ACVRL1*), a gene located on chromosome 12, produces HHT2. The proteins produced by these genes may play a role in blood vessel wall integrity. With both types of HHT, numerous vascular hamartomas develop, affecting the skin and mucosa; however, other vascular problems, such as arteriovenous fistulas, may also be seen. Patients affected with HHT1 tend to have more pulmonary involvement, whereas those with HHT2 generally have a later onset of their telangiectasias and a greater degree of hepatic involvement. The clinician should be familiar with HHT because the oral lesions are often the most dramatic and most easily identified component of this syndrome.

CLINICAL FEATURES

Patients with HHT are often diagnosed initially because of frequent episodes of epistaxis. On further examination, the nasal and oropharyngeal mucosae exhibit

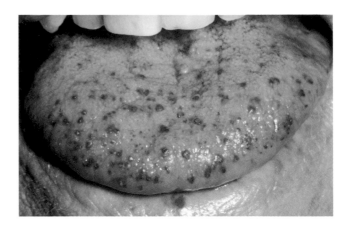

Fig. 16-29 Hereditary hemorrhagic telangiectasia (HHT). The tongue of this patient shows multiple red papules, which represent superficial collections of dilated capillary spaces.

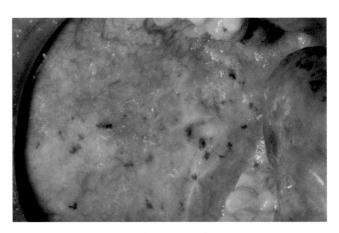

Fig. 16-30 Hereditary hemorrhagic telangiectasia (HHT). Red macules similar to the tongue lesions are observed on the buccal mucosa.

numerous scattered red papules, 1 to 2 mm in size, which blanch when diascopy is used. This blanching indicates that the red color is due to blood contained within blood vessels (in this case, small collections of dilated capillaries [**telangiectasias**] that are close to the surface of the mucosa). These telangiectatic vessels are most frequently found on the vermilion zone of the lips, tongue, and buccal mucosa, although any oral mucosal site may be affected (Figs. 16-29 and 16-30). With aging, the telangiectasias tend to become more numerous and slightly larger.

In many patients, telangiectasias are seen on the hands and feet. The lesions are often distributed throughout the gastrointestinal mucosa, the genitourinary mucosa, and the conjunctival mucosa. The gastrointestinal telangiectasias have a tendency to rupture, which may cause significant blood loss. Chronic iron-deficiency anemia is often a problem for such individu-

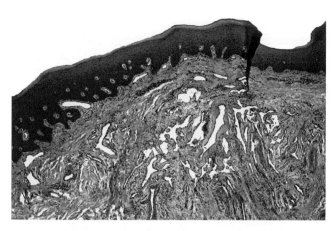

Fig. 16-31 Hereditary hemorrhagic telangiectasia (HHT). This low-power photomicrograph shows multiple dilated vascular spaces located immediately subjacent to the epithelium.

als. Significantly, arteriovenous fistulas may develop in the lungs (30% of HHT patients), liver (30%), or brain (10% to 20%). The brain lesions seem to predispose these patients to the development of brain abscesses. In at least one instance, periodontal vascular malformations were felt to be the cause of septic pulmonary emboli that resolved only after several teeth with periodontal abscesses were extracted.

A diagnosis of HHT can be made if a patient has three of the following four criteria:

1. Recurrent spontaneous epistaxis
2. Telangiectasias of the mucosa and skin
3. Arteriovenous malformation involving the lungs, liver, or CNS
4. Family history of HHT

In some instances, CREST syndrome (**C**alcinosis cutis, **R**aynaud's phenomenon, **E**sophageal dysfunction, **S**clerodactyly, and **T**elangiectasia) (see page 801) must be considered in the differential diagnosis. In these cases, serologic studies for anticentromere autoantibodies often help to distinguish between the two conditions because these antibodies typically would be present only in CREST syndrome.

HISTOPATHOLOGIC FEATURES

If one of the telangiectasias is submitted for biopsy, the microscopic features essentially show a superficially located collection of thin-walled vascular spaces that contain erythrocytes (Fig. 16-31).

TREATMENT AND PROGNOSIS

For mild cases of HHT, no treatment may be required. Moderate cases may be managed by selective cryosurgery or electrocautery of the most bothersome of the telangiectatic vessels. Laser ablation of the telangiectatic lesions has also been used, although this approach appears to be most successful for patients with mild to moderate disease. More severely affected patients, particularly those troubled by repeated episodes of epistaxis, may require a surgical procedure of the nasal septum (septal dermoplasty). The involved nasal mucosa is removed and replaced by a skin graft; however, some long-term follow-up studies suggest that the grafts eventually become revascularized, resulting in recurrence of the problem. Nasal closure is another surgical technique that has been performed for patients with severe epistaxis in whom other methods have failed.

Combined progesterone and estrogen therapy may benefit some patients, but because of the potentially serious side effects, this should be limited to the most severely affected individuals. Iron replacement therapy is indicated for the iron-deficient patient, and occasionally blood transfusions may be necessary to compensate for blood loss.

From a dental standpoint, some authors recommend the use of prophylactic antibiotics before dental procedures that might cause bacteremia in patients with HHT and evidence of a pulmonary arteriovenous malformation. For patients with a history of HHT, such antibiotics are advocated until a pulmonary arteriovenous malformation is ruled out because of the 1% prevalence of brain abscesses in affected individuals. Researchers believe that antibiotic coverage, similar to that for endocarditis prophylaxis, may prevent this serious complication. Patients with a history of HHT should be screened for arteriovenous malformations, which can be eliminated by embolization or other vasodestructive techniques using interventional radiologic methods.

The prognosis is generally good, although a 1% to 2% mortality rate is reported from complications related to blood loss. For patients with brain abscesses, the mortality rate is 10%, even with early diagnosis and appropriate therapy.

EHLERS-DANLOS SYNDROMES

The **Ehlers-Danlos syndromes**, a group of inherited connective tissue disorders, are relatively heterogeneous. At least 10 types have been described over the years, but recent clinical and molecular evidence suggests that seven categories of this disease may be more appropriate. The patient exhibits problems that are usually attributed to the production of abnormal collagen, the protein that is the main structural component of the connective tissue. Because the production of collagen necessitates many biochemical steps that are controlled by several genes, the potential exists for any

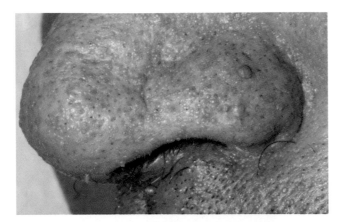

Fig. 16-39 Multiple hamartoma syndrome. These tiny cutaneous facial papules represent hair follicle hamartomas (trichilemmomas).

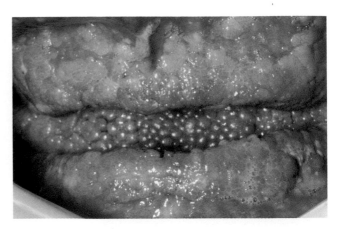

Fig. 16-40 Multiple hamartoma syndrome. Multiple, irregular fibroepithelial papules involve the tongue (*center*) and alveolar ridge mucosa.

MULTIPLE HAMARTOMA SYNDROME (COWDEN SYNDROME; *PTEN* HAMARTOMA-TUMOR SYNDROME)

Multiple hamartoma syndrome is a rare condition that has important implications for the affected patient, because malignancies, in addition to the benign hamartomatous growths, develop in a high percentage of these individuals. Usually, the syndrome is inherited as an autosomal dominant trait showing a high degree of penetrance and a range of expressivity. The gene responsible for this disorder has been mapped to chromosome 10, and a mutation of the *PTEN* (phosphatase and tensin homolog deleted on chromosome 10) gene has been implicated in its pathogenesis. The estimated prevalence of this condition is approximately 1 in 200,000, and more than 300 affected patients have been described in the literature. In recent years, overlapping clinical features of multiple hamartoma syndrome with **Lhermitte-Duclos disease**, **Bannayan-Riley-Ruvalcaba syndrome**, and **Proteus-like syndrome** have been noted, and all of these disorders have demonstrated mutations of the *PTEN* gene.

CLINICAL FEATURES

Cutaneous manifestations are present in almost all patients with multiple hamartoma syndrome, usually developing during the second decade of life. The majority of the skin lesions appear as multiple, small (less than 1 mm) papules, primarily on the facial skin, especially around the mouth, nose, and ears (Fig. 16-39). Microscopically, most of these papules represent hair follicle hamartomas called **trichilemmomas**. Other commonly noted skin lesions are **acral keratosis**, a warty-appearing growth that develops on the dorsal surface of the hand, and **palmoplantar keratosis**, a prominent calluslike lesion on the palms or soles. Cutaneous **hemangiomas, neuromas, xanthomas,** and **lipomas** have also been described.

Other problems can appear in these patients as well. Thyroid disease usually appears as either a goiter or a thyroid adenoma, but follicular adenocarcinoma may develop. In women, fibrocystic disease of the breast is frequently observed. Unfortunately, breast cancer occurs with a relatively high frequency (25% to 50%) in these patients. The mean age at diagnosis of breast malignancy is 40 years, which is much younger than usual. In the gastrointestinal tract, multiple benign hamartomatous polyps may be present. In addition, several types of benign and malignant tumors of the female genitourinary tract occur more often than in the normal population.

The oral lesions vary in severity from patient to patient and usually consist of multiple papules affecting the gingivae, dorsal tongue, and buccal mucosa (Figs. 16-40 and 16-41). These lesions have been reported in more than 80% of affected patients and generally produce no symptoms. Other possible oral findings include a high-arched palate, periodontitis, and extensive dental caries, although it is unclear whether the latter two conditions are significantly related to the syndrome.

HISTOPATHOLOGIC FEATURES

The histopathologic features of the oral lesions are rather nonspecific, essentially representing fibroepithelial hyperplasia. Other lesions associated with this syndrome have their own characteristic histopathologic findings, depending on the hamartomatous or neoplastic tissue origin.

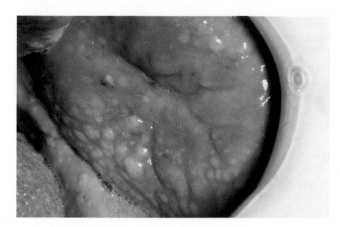

Fig. 16-41   Multiple hamartoma syndrome. Multiple papules on the left buccal mucosa.

DIAGNOSIS

The diagnosis can be based on the finding of two of the following three pathognomonic signs:

1. Multiple facial trichilemmomas
2. Multiple oral papules
3. Acral keratoses

A variety of other major and minor diagnostic criteria, as well as a positive family history, are also helpful in confirming the diagnosis. Genetic testing for mutations of the *PTEN* gene are clinically available, but 20% of patients who otherwise have characteristic multiple hamartoma syndrome will not demonstrate a genetic abnormality; therefore, a negative test does not necessarily preclude the diagnosis of multiple hamartoma syndrome.

TREATMENT AND PROGNOSIS

Treatment of multiple hamartoma syndrome is controversial. Although most of the tumors that develop are benign, the prevalence of malignancy is higher than in the general population; therefore, annual physical examinations that focus specifically on anatomic sites of increased tumor prevalence are appropriate. Some investigators recommend bilateral prophylactic mastectomies as early as the third decade of life for female patients because of the associated increased risk of breast cancer.

EPIDERMOLYSIS BULLOSA

The term **epidermolysis bullosa** describes a heterogeneous group of inherited blistering mucocutaneous disorders. Each has a specific defect in the attachment mechanisms of the epithelial cells, either to each other or to the underlying connective tissue. Recent advances

in the understanding of the clinical, epidemiologic, and molecular genetic abnormalities of these conditions have led to the identification of approximately 25 different forms. Depending on the defective mechanism of cellular cohesion, there are four broad categories:

1. Simplex
2. Junctional
3. Dystrophic
4. Hemidesmosomal

Each category consists of several forms of the disorder. A variety of inheritance patterns may be seen, depending on the particular form. The degree of severity can range from relatively mild, annoying forms, such as the **simplex** types, through a spectrum that includes severe, fatal disease. For example, many cases of **junctional** epidermolysis bullosa result in death at birth because of the significant sloughing of the skin during passage through the birth canal. Specific mutations in the genes encoding keratin 5 and keratin 14 have been identified as being responsible for most of the **simplex** types, whereas mutations in the genetic codes for the $\alpha3$, $\beta3$, and $\gamma2$ subunits of laminin have been documented for the **junctional** types. Most of the **dystrophic** types appear to be caused by mutations in the genes responsible for type VII collagen production, with nearly 200 distinctly different mutations identified to date. The **hemidesmosomal** type is the most recently characterized pattern of this group of disorders, and mutations of genes associated with various hemidesmosomal attachment proteins, such as plectin, type XVII collagen (BP180), and $\alpha6\beta4$ integrin, have been established.

A few representative examples of the types of epidermolysis bullosa are summarized in Table 16-2. Because oral lesions are most commonly observed in the dystrophic forms, this discussion centers on these forms. Dental abnormalities, such as anodontia, enamel hypoplasia, pitting of the enamel, neonatal teeth, and severe dental caries, have been variably associated with several of the different types of epidermolysis bullosa, although studies have suggested that the prevalence of dental abnormalities is significantly increased only with the **junctional** type. A disorder termed **epidermolysis bullosa acquisita** is mentioned because of the similarity of its name; however, this appears to be an unrelated condition, having an autoimmune (rather than a genetic) origin (see page 744).

CLINICAL FEATURES

DOMINANT DYSTROPHIC TYPES

The **dystrophic** forms of epidermolysis bullosa that are inherited in an autosomal dominant fashion are not usually life threatening, although they may certainly be disfiguring and pose many problems. The initial lesions

Table **16-2**   **Examples of Epidermolysis Bullosa**

Form	Inheritance	Clinical Features	Defect
EB simplex	AD	Blistering of the hands and feet; mucosal involvement uncommon; blisters heal without scarring; prognosis usually good	Keratin gene defects
Junctional EB, generalized gravis variant	AR	Severe blistering at birth; granulation tissue around the mouth; oral erosions common; pitted enamel hypoplasia; often fatal (previously called *EB letalis*)	Defects of hemidesmosomes
Dominant, dystrophic EB, Pasini type	AD	Generalized blistering, white papules	Defect in type VII collagen
Dominant, dystrophic EB, Cockayne-Touraine type	AD	Extremities primarily affected	Defect in type VII collagen
Recessive, dystrophic EB, generalized gravis type	AR	Severe mucosal involvement; mittenlike scarring; deformities of hands and feet; patients usually do not survive past early adulthood	Defect in type VII collagen
Recessive, dystrophic EB, inverse type	AR	Involvement of groin and axilla; severe oral and esophageal lesions	Defect in type VII collagen

EB, Epidermolysis bullosa; *AD*, autosomal dominant; *AR*, autosomal recessive.

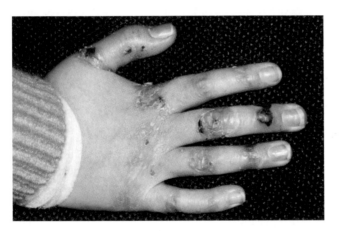

Fig. 16-42   Epidermolysis bullosa. A young girl, affected by the dominant dystrophic form of epidermolysis bullosa, shows the characteristic hemorrhagic bullae, scarring, and erosion associated with minimal trauma to the hands.

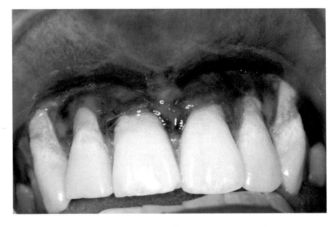

Fig. 16-43   Epidermolysis bullosa. A teenaged boy, affected by dominant dystrophic epidermolysis bullosa, shows a reduced depth of the labial vestibule caused by repeated mucosal tearing and healing with scarring.

are vesicles or bullae, which are seen early in life and develop on areas exposed to low-grade, chronic trauma, such as the knuckles or knees (Fig. 16-42). The bullae rupture, resulting in erosions or ulcerations that ultimately heal with scarring. In the process, appendages such as fingernails may be lost.

The oral manifestations are typically mild, with some gingival erythema and tenderness. Gingival recession and reduction in the depth of the buccal vestibule may be observed (Fig. 16-43).

RECESSIVE DYSTROPHIC TYPES

Generalized recessive dystrophic epidermolysis bullosa represents one of the more debilitating forms of the disease. Vesicles and bullae form with even minor trauma. Secondary infections are often a problem because of the large surface areas that may be involved. If the patient manages to survive into the second decade, then hand function is often greatly diminished because of the repeated episodes of cutaneous break-

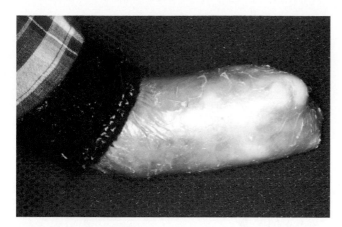

Fig. 16-44   Epidermolysis bullosa. A 19-year-old man, affected by recessive dystrophic epidermolysis bullosa, shows the typical mittenlike deformity of the hand caused by scarring of the tissue after damage associated with normal activity.

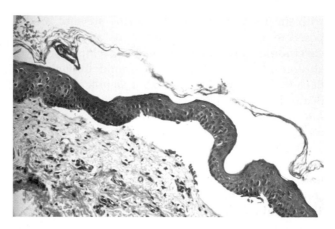

Fig. 16-46   Epidermolysis bullosa. Complete separation of the epithelium from the connective tissue is seen in this photomicrograph of a tissue section obtained from a patient affected by a junctional form of epidermolysis bullosa.

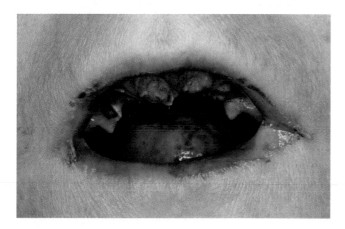

Fig. 16-45   Epidermolysis bullosa. Same patient as depicted in Fig. 16-44. Microstomia has been caused by repeated trauma and healing with scarring. Note the severe dental caries activity associated with a soft cariogenic diet.

Junctional, **dystrophic**, and **hemidesmosomal** forms show subepithelial clefting (Fig. 16-46). Electron microscopic examination, which is still considered the diagnostic "gold standard," reveals clefting at the level of the lamina lucida of the basement membrane in the **junctional** forms and below the lamina densa of the basement membrane in the **dystrophic** forms. In contrast, the **hemidesmosomal** form shows clefting just below the basal cell layer, at its interface with the lamina lucida. Immunohistochemical evaluation of perilesional tissue may help to identify specific defects to classify and subtype the condition further. Molecular genetic analysis is now being used to confirm the diagnosis in some instances.

TREATMENT AND PROGNOSIS

Treatment of epidermolysis bullosa varies with the type. For milder cases, no treatment other than local wound care may be needed. Sterile drainage of larger blisters and the use of topical antibiotics are often indicated in these situations. For the more severe cases, intensive management with oral antibiotics may be necessary if cellulitis develops; despite intensive medical care, some patients die as a result of infectious complications.

The "mitten" deformity of the hands, seen in recessive dystrophic epidermolysis bullosa, can be corrected with plastic surgery, but the problem usually recurs after a period of time, and surgical intervention is required every 2 years on average. With esophageal involvement, dysphagia may be a significant problem, resulting in malnutrition and weight loss. Placement of a gastrostomy tube may be necessary at times. Patients

down and healing with scarring, resulting in fusion of the fingers into a mittenlike deformity (Fig. 16-44).

The oral problems are no less severe. Bulla and vesicle formation is induced by virtually any food having some degree of texture. Even with a soft diet, the repeated cycles of scarring often result in microstomia (Fig. 16-45) and ankyloglossia. Similar mucosal injury and scarring may cause severe stricture of the esophagus. Because a soft diet is usually highly cariogenic, carious destruction of the dentition at an early age is common.

HISTOPATHOLOGIC FEATURES

The histopathologic features of epidermolysis bullosa vary with the type being examined. The **simplex** form shows intraepithelial clefting by light microscopy.

with the recessive dystrophic forms are also predisposed to development of **cutaneous squamous cell carcinoma.** This malignancy often develops in areas of chronic ulceration during the second through third decades of life and represents a significant cause of death for these patients. Infrequently, the lingual mucosa of affected patients has been reported to undergo malignant transformation as well.

Management of the oral manifestations also depends on the type of the disease. For patients who are susceptible to mucosal bulla formation, dental manipulation should be kept to a minimum. To achieve this, topical 1% neutral sodium fluoride solution should be administered daily to prevent dental caries. A soft diet that is as noncariogenic as possible, as well as atraumatic oral hygiene procedures, should be encouraged. Maintaining adequate nutrition for affected patients is critical to ensure optimal wound healing.

If dental restorative care is required, the lips should be lubricated to minimize trauma. Injections for local anesthesia can usually be accomplished by depositing the anesthetic slowly and deeply within the tissues. For extensive dental care, endotracheal anesthesia may be performed without significant problems in most cases.

Unfortunately, because of the genetic nature of these diseases, no cure exists. Genetic counseling of affected families is indicated. Both prenatal diagnosis and pre-implantation diagnosis are available as adjuncts to family planning.

Immune-Mediated Diseases and Their Evaluation

Several conditions discussed in this chapter are the result of inappropriate production of antibodies by the patient (autoantibodies). These autoantibodies are directed against various constituents of the molecular apparatus that hold epithelial cells together or that bind the surface epithelium to the underlying connective tissue. The ensuing damage produced by the interaction of these autoantibodies with the host tissue is seen clinically as a disease process, often termed an **immunobullous** disease. Because each disease is characterized by production of specific types of autoantibodies, identification of the antibodies and the tissues against which they are targeted is important diagnostically. The two techniques that are widely used to investigate the immunobullous diseases are (1) direct immunofluorescence and (2) indirect immunofluorescence studies. Following is a brief overview of how they work.

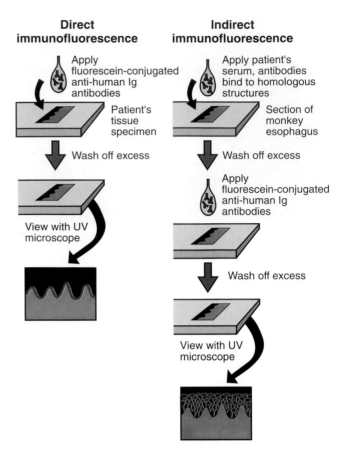

Fig. 16-47   Immunofluorescence techniques. Comparison of the techniques for direct and indirect immunofluorescence. The left side depicts the direct immunofluorescent findings in cicatricial pemphigoid, a disease that has autoantibodies directed toward the basement zone. The right side shows the indirect immunofluorescent findings for pemphigus vulgaris, a disease that has autoantibodies directed toward the intercellular areas between the spinous cells of the epithelium. *Ig,* Immunoglobulin; *UV,* ultraviolet.

Direct immunofluorescence is used to detect autoantibodies that are bound to the patient's tissue. Before testing can take place, several procedures must occur. Inoculating human immunoglobulins into a goat creates antibodies directed against these human immunoglobulins. The antibodies raised in response to the human immunoglobulins are harvested from the animal and tagged with fluorescein, a dye that glows when viewed with ultraviolet (UV) light. As illustrated on the left side of Fig. 16-47, a frozen section of the patient's tissue is placed on a slide, and this is incubated with fluorescein-conjugated goat antihuman antibodies. These antibodies bind to the tissue at any site where human immunoglobulin is present. The excess antibody suspension is washed off, and the section is then viewed with a microscope having a UV light source.

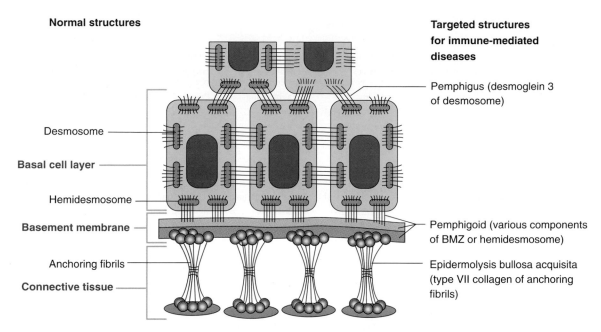

Normal structures

**Targeted structures
for immune-mediated
diseases**

Pemphigus (desmoglein 3
of desmosome)

Desmosome

Basal cell layer

Hemidesmosome

Basement membrane

Pemphigoid (various components
of BMZ or hemidesmosome)

Anchoring fibrils

Connective tissue

Epidermolysis bullosa acquisita
(type VII collagen of anchoring
fibrils)

Fig. 16-48   Epithelial attachment apparatus. Schematic diagram demonstrating targeted structures in several immune-mediated diseases. *BMZ,* Basement membrane zone.

With indirect immunofluorescence studies, the patient is being evaluated for presence of antibodies that are circulating in the blood. As shown on the right side of Fig. 16-47, a frozen section of tissue that is similar to human oral mucosa (e.g., Old World monkey esophagus) is placed on a slide and incubated with the patient's serum. If there are autoantibodies directed against epithelial attachment structures in the patient's serum, then they will attach to the homologous structures on the monkey esophagus. The excess serum is washed off, and fluorescein-conjugated goat antihuman antibody is incubated with the section. The excess is washed off, and the section is examined with UV light to detect the presence of autoantibodies that might have been in the serum.

Examples of the molecular sites of attack of the autoantibodies are seen diagrammatically in Fig. 16-48. Each site is distinctive for a particular disease; however, the complexities of the epithelial attachment mechanisms are still being elucidated, and more precise mapping may be possible in the future. A summary of the clinical, microscopic, and immunopathologic features of the more important immune-mediated mucocutaneous diseases is found in Table 16-3.

PEMPHIGUS

The condition known as **pemphigus** represents four related diseases of an autoimmune origin:

1. Pemphigus vulgaris
2. Pemphigus vegetans

3. Pemphigus erythematosus
4. Pemphigus foliaceus

Only the first two of these affect the oral mucosa, and the discussion is limited to **pemphigus vulgaris. Pemphigus vegetans** is rare; most authorities now feel it represents simply a variant of pemphigus vulgaris.

Pemphigus vulgaris is the most common of these disorders (*vulgaris* is Latin for *common*). Even so, it is not seen very often. The estimated incidence is one to five cases per million people diagnosed each year in the general population. Nevertheless, pemphigus vulgaris is an important condition because, if untreated, it often results in the patient's death. Furthermore, the oral lesions are often the first sign of the disease, and they are the most difficult to resolve with therapy. This has prompted the description of the oral lesions as "the first to show, and the last to go."

The blistering that typifies this disease is due to an abnormal production, for unknown reasons, of autoantibodies that are directed against the epidermal cell surface glycoproteins, desmoglein 3 and desmoglein 1. These desmogleins are components of **desmosomes** (structures that bond epithelial cells to each other), and the autoantibodies attach to these desmosomal components, effectively inhibiting the molecular interaction that is responsible for adherence. As a result of this immunologic attack on the desmosomes, a split develops within the epithelium, causing a blister to form. Desmoglein 3 is preferentially expressed in the parabasal region of the epidermis and oral epithelium,

Table **16-3**　**Chronic Vesiculoulcerative Diseases**

Condition	Mean Age	Sex Predilection	Clinical Features	Histopathologic Features	Direct Immunofluorescence	Indirect Immunofluorescence
Pemphigus vulgaris	Fourth to sixth decade	Equal	Vesicles, erosions, and ulcerations on any oral mucosal or skin surface	Intraepithelial clefting	Positive intercellular	Positive
Paraneoplastic pemphigus	Sixth to seventh decade	Equal	Vesicles, erosions, and ulcerations on any mucosal or skin surface	Subepithelial and intraepithelial clefting	Positive, intercellular and basement membrane zone	Positive (rat bladder)
Mucous membrane pemphigoid	Sixth to seventh decade	Female	Primarily mucosal lesions	Subepithelial clefting	Positive, basement membrane zone	Negative
Bullous pemphigoid	Seventh to eighth decade	Equal	Primarily skin lesions	Subepithelial clefting	Positive, basement membrane zone	Positive
Erythema multiforme	Third to fourth decade	Male	Skin and mucosa involved; target lesions on skin	Subepithelial edema and perivascular inflammations	Nondiagnostic	Negative
Lichen planus	Fifth to sixth decade	Female	Oral and/or skin lesions; may or may not be erosive	Hyperkeratosis, saw-toothed rete ridges, bandlike infiltrate of lymphocytes	Fibrinogen, basement membrane zone	Negative

whereas desmoglein 1 is found primarily in the superficial portion of the epidermis, with minimal expression in oral epithelium. Patients who have developed autoantibodies directed against desmoglein 3, with or without desmoglein 1, will histopathologically show intraepithelial clefting just above the basal layer, and clinically oral mucosal blisters of pemphigus vulgaris will form. Patients who develop autoantibodies directed against only desmoglein 1 will histopathologically show superficial intraepithelial clefting of the epidermis, but oral mucosa will not be affected. Clinically, the fine scaly red lesions of pemphigus foliaceous or pemphigus erythematosus will be evident.

Occasionally, a pemphigus-like oral and cutaneous eruption may occur in patients taking certain medications (e.g., penicillamine, angiotensin-converting enzyme [ACE] inhibitors, nonsteroidal antiinflammatory drugs [NSAIDs]) or in patients with malignancy, especially lymphoreticular malignancies (so-called **paraneoplastic pemphigus**) (see page 769). Similarly, a variety of other conditions may produce chronic vesiculoulcerative or erosive lesions of the oral mucosa, and these often need to be considered in the differential diagnosis (see Table 16-3). In addition, a rare genetic condition termed **chronic benign familial pemphigus** or **Hailey-Hailey disease** may have erosive cutaneous lesions, but oral involvement in that process appears to be uncommon.

CLINICAL FEATURES

The initial manifestations of pemphigus vulgaris often involve the oral mucosa, typically in adults. The average age at diagnosis is 50 years, although rare cases may be seen in childhood. No sex predilection is observed, and the condition seems to be more common in persons of Mediterranean, South Asian, or Jewish heritage.

Patients usually complain of oral soreness, and examination shows superficial, ragged erosions and ulcerations distributed haphazardly on the oral mucosa (Figs. 16-49 to 16-52). Such lesions may affect virtually any oral mucosal location, although the palate, labial

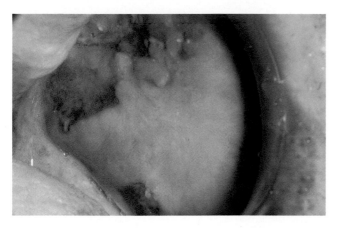

Fig. 16-49   Pemphigus vulgaris. Multiple erosions of the left buccal mucosa.

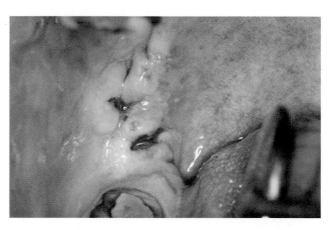

Fig. 16-52   Pemphigus vulgaris. The patient, with a known diagnosis of pemphigus vulgaris, had been treated with immunosuppressive therapy. The oral erosions shown here were the only persistent manifestation of her disease.

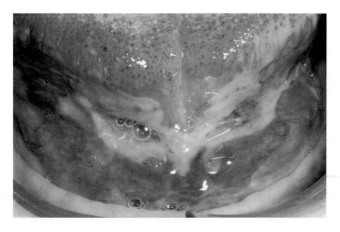

Fig. 16-50   Pemphigus vulgaris. Large, irregularly shaped ulcerations involving the floor of the mouth and ventral tongue.

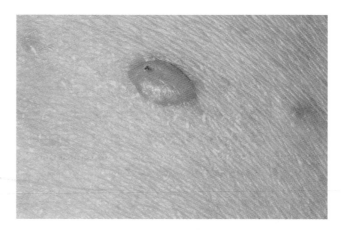

Fig. 16-53   Pemphigus vulgaris. This flaccid cutaneous bulla is characteristic of skin involvement.

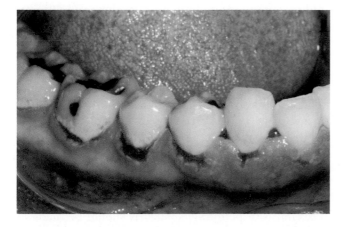

Fig. 16-51   Pemphigus vulgaris. Multiple erosions affecting the marginal gingiva.

mucosa, buccal mucosa, ventral tongue, and gingivae are often involved. Patients rarely report vesicle or bulla formation intraorally, and such lesions can seldom be identified by the examining clinician, probably because of early rupture of the thin, friable roof of the blisters. More than 50% of the patients have oral mucosal lesions before the onset of cutaneous lesions, sometimes by as much as 1 year or more. Eventually, however, nearly all patients have intraoral involvement. The skin lesions appear as flaccid vesicles and bullae (Fig. 16-53) that rupture quickly, usually within hours to a few days, leaving an erythematous, denuded surface. Infrequently ocular involvement may be seen, usually appearing as bilateral conjunctivitis. Unlike cicatricial pemphigoid, the ocular lesions of pemphigus do not tend to produce scarring and symblepharon formation (see page 772).

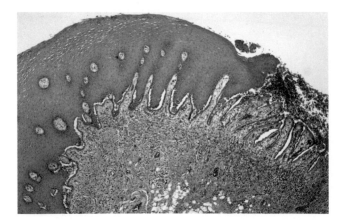

Fig. 16-54 Pemphigus vulgaris. Low-power photomicrograph of perilesional mucosa affected by pemphigus vulgaris. An intraepithelial cleft is located just above the basal cell layer.

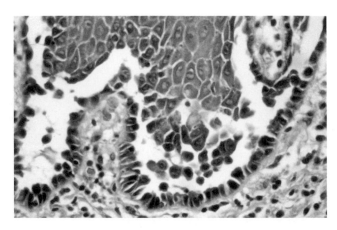

Fig. 16-55 Pemphigus vulgaris. High-power photomicrograph showing rounded, acantholytic epithelial cells sitting within the intraepithelial cleft.

Without proper treatment, the oral and cutaneous lesions tend to persist and progressively involve more surface area. A characteristic feature of pemphigus vulgaris is that a bulla can be induced on normal-appearing skin if firm lateral pressure is exerted. This is called a **positive Nikolsky sign**.

HISTOPATHOLOGIC FEATURES

Biopsy specimens of perilesional tissue show characteristic intraepithelial separation, which occurs just above the basal cell layer of the epithelium (Fig. 16-54). Sometimes the entire superficial layers of the epithelium are stripped away, leaving only the basal cells, which have been described as resembling a "row of tombstones." The cells of the spinous layer of the surface epithelium typically appear to fall apart, a feature that has been termed **acantholysis**, and the loose cells tend to assume a rounded shape (Fig. 16-55). This feature of pemphigus vulgaris can be used in making a diagnosis based on the identification of these rounded cells **(Tzanck cells)** in an exfoliative cytologic preparation. A mild-to-moderate chronic inflammatory cell infiltrate is usually seen in the underlying connective tissue.

The diagnosis of pemphigus vulgaris should be confirmed by direct immunofluorescence examination of fresh perilesional tissue or tissue submitted in Michel's solution. With this procedure, antibodies (usually IgG or IgM) and complement components (usually C3) can be demonstrated in the intercellular spaces between the epithelial cells (Fig. 16-56) in almost all patients with this disease. Indirect immunofluorescence is also typically positive in 80% to 90% of cases, demonstrating the presence of circulating autoantibodies in the

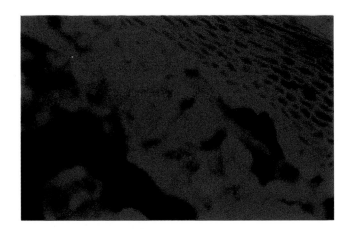

Fig. 16-56 Pemphigus vulgaris. Photomicrograph depicting the direct immunofluorescence pattern of pemphigus vulgaris. Immunoreactants are deposited in the intercellular areas between the surface epithelial cells.

patient's serum. Enzyme-linked immunosorbent assays (ELISAs) have been developed to detect circulating autoantibodies as well.

It is critical that perilesional tissue be obtained for both light microscopy and direct immunofluorescence to maximize the probability of a diagnostic sample. If ulcerated mucosa is submitted for testing, then the results are often inconclusive because of either a lack of an intact interface between the epithelium and connective tissue or a great deal of nonspecific inflammation.

TREATMENT AND PROGNOSIS

A diagnosis of pemphigus vulgaris should be made as early in its course as possible because control is generally easier to achieve. Pemphigus is a systemic disease;

therefore, treatment consists primarily of systemic corticosteroids (usually prednisone), often in combination with other immunosuppressive drugs (so-called steroid-sparing agents), such as azathioprine. Although some clinicians have advocated the use of topical corticosteroids in the management of oral lesions, the observed improvement is undoubtedly because of the absorption of the topical agents, resulting in a greater systemic dose. The potential side effects associated with the long-term use of systemic corticosteroids are significant and include the following:

- Diabetes mellitus
- Adrenal suppression
- Weight gain
- Osteoporosis
- Peptic ulcers
- Severe mood swings
- Increased susceptibility to a wide range of infections

Ideally, a physician with expertise in immunosuppressive therapy should manage the patient. The most common approach is to use relatively high doses of systemic corticosteroids initially to clear the lesions, then attempt to maintain the patient on as low a dose of corticosteroids as is necessary to control the condition. Often the clinician can monitor the success of therapy by measuring the titers of circulating autoantibodies using indirect immunofluorescence, because disease activity frequently correlates with the abnormal antibody levels. Pemphigus may undergo complete resolution, although remissions and exacerbations are common. One study suggested that up to 75% of patients will have disease resolution after 10 years of treatment.

Before the development of corticosteroid therapy, as many as 60% to 90% of these patients died, primarily as a result of infections and electrolyte imbalances. Even today, the mortality rate associated with pemphigus vulgaris is in the range of 5% to 10%, usually because of the complications of long-term systemic corticosteroid use.

PARANEOPLASTIC PEMPHIGUS (NEOPLASIA-INDUCED PEMPHIGUS; PARANEOPLASTIC AUTOIMMUNE MULTIORGAN SYNDROME)

Paraneoplastic pemphigus is a rare vesiculobullous disorder that affects patients who have a neoplasm, usually **lymphoma** or **chronic lymphocytic leukemia**. Approximately 150 cases have been documented. Although the precise pathogenetic mechanisms are unknown, some evidence suggests abnormal levels of the cytokine, interleukin 6 (IL-6), could be produced by host lymphocytes in response to the patient's tumor.

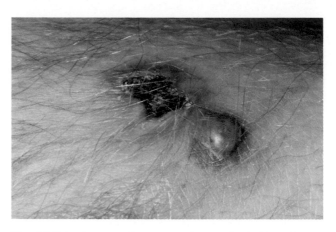

Fig. 16-57   Paraneoplastic pemphigus. The bulla and crusted ulcerations on this patient's arm are representative of the polymorphous cutaneous lesions.

IL-6 may then be responsible for stimulating the abnormal production of antibodies directed against antigens associated with the desmosomal complex and the basement membrane zone of the epithelium. In addition to a variety of different antibodies that attack these epithelial adherence structures, recent reports have described cutaneous and mucosal damage that appears to be mediated by cytotoxic T lymphocytes in some cases of paraneoplastic pemphigus. As a result of this multifaceted immunologic attack, the disease manifests in an array of clinical features, histopathologic findings, and immunopathologic findings that may be perplexing if the clinician is unfamiliar with this condition.

CLINICAL FEATURES

Patients typically have a history of a malignant lymphoreticular neoplasm, or less commonly, a benign lymphoproliferative disorder such as angiofollicular lymph node hyperplasia (Castleman's disease) or thymoma. In approximately one third of reported cases, paraneoplastic pemphigus developed before a malignancy was identified, thus signaling the presence of a tumor. The neoplastic disease may or may not be under control at the time of onset of the paraneoplastic condition. Signs and symptoms of paraneoplastic pemphigus usually begin suddenly and may appear polymorphous. In some instances, multiple vesiculobullous lesions affect the skin (Fig. 16-57) and oral mucosa. Palmar or plantar bullae may be evident, a feature that is uncommon in pemphigus vulgaris. For other patients, skin lesions can appear more papular and pruritic, similar to cutaneous lichen planus. The lips often show hemorrhagic crusting similar to that of erythema multiforme (Fig. 16-58). The oral mucosa shows multiple areas of erythema and

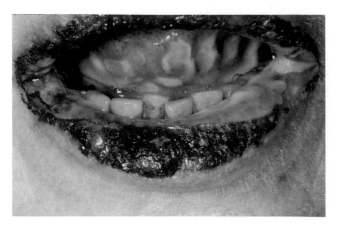

Fig. 16-58   Paraneoplastic pemphigus. Crusted, hemorrhagic lip lesions may be mistaken for erythema multiforme or herpes simplex infection.

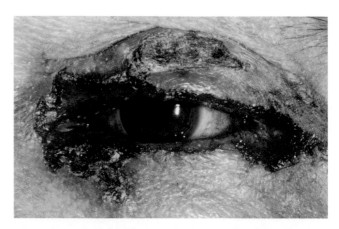

Fig. 16-60   Paraneoplastic pemphigus. Ocular involvement.

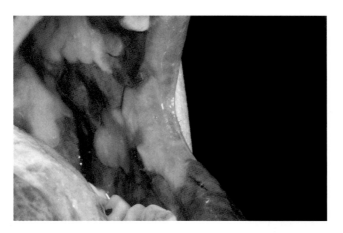

Fig. 16-59   Paraneoplastic pemphigus. These diffuse oral ulcerations are quite painful.

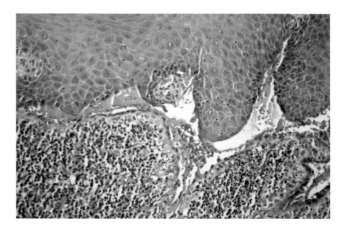

Fig. 16-61   Paraneoplastic pemphigus. This medium-power photomicrograph shows both intraepithelial and subepithelial clefting.

diffuse, irregular ulceration (Fig. 16-59), affecting virtually any oral mucosal surface. If the lesions remain untreated, then they persist and worsen. Some patients may develop only oropharyngeal lesions, without cutaneous involvement.

Other mucosal surfaces are also commonly affected, with 70% of patients having involvement of the conjunctival mucosa. In this area, a cicatrizing (scarring) conjunctivitis develops, similar to that seen with cicatricial pemphigoid (Fig. 16-60). The vaginal mucosa and mucosa of the respiratory tract may be involved.

HISTOPATHOLOGIC FEATURES

The features of paraneoplastic pemphigus on light microscopic examination may be as diverse as the clinical features. In most cases, a lichenoid mucositis is seen, usually with subepithelial clefting (like pemphigoid) or intraepithelial clefting (like pemphigus) (Fig. 16-61).

Direct immunofluorescence studies may show a weakly positive deposition of immunoreactants (IgG and complement) in the intercellular zones of the epithelium and/or a linear deposition of immunoreactants at the basement membrane zone. Indirect immunofluorescence should be conducted using a transitional type of epithelium (e.g., rat urinary bladder mucosa) as the substrate. This shows a fairly specific pattern of antibody localization to the intercellular areas of the epithelium. Immunoprecipitation studies remain the gold standard for the diagnosis of paraneoplastic pemphigus, however, because the various antibodies that characterize this condition can be identified with a considerable degree of specificity. Antibodies directed against desmoplakin I and II, major bullous pemphigoid antigen, envoplakin, and periplakin, in addition to desmoglein 1 and 3, are typically detected. Examples of paraneoplastic pemphigus that show only a lichenoid reaction with no demonstrable autoantibody production have infrequently been described.

TREATMENT AND PROGNOSIS

Paraneoplastic pemphigus is often a very serious condition with a high morbidity and mortality rate. For the infrequent cases associated with a benign lymphoproliferative condition, surgical removal of the tumor may result in regression of the paraneoplastic pemphigus. For those cases associated with malignancy, treatment essentially consists of systemic prednisone, typically combined with another immunosuppressive agent, such as azathioprine, methotrexate, or cyclophosphamide. As with pemphigus vulgaris, the skin lesions usually respond more quickly to treatment than the oral lesions. Unfortunately, although the immunosuppressive therapy often manages to control the autoimmune disease, this immunosuppression often seems to trigger a reactivation of the malignant neoplasm. Thus a high mortality rate is seen, with patients succumbing to complications of the vesiculobullous lesions, complications of immune suppressive therapy, or progression of malignant disease. Occasionally, long-term survivors are reported, but these seem to be in the minority. As more of these patients are identified, therapeutic strategies can be better evaluated and modified for optimal care in the future.

MUCOUS MEMBRANE PEMPHIGOID (CICATRICIAL PEMPHIGOID; BENIGN MUCOUS MEMBRANE PEMPHIGOID)

Evidence has accumulated to suggest that **mucous membrane pemphigoid** represents a group of chronic, blistering, mucocutaneous autoimmune diseases in which tissue-bound autoantibodies are directed against one or more components of the basement membrane. As such, this condition has a heterogeneous origin, with autoantibodies being produced against any one of a variety of basement membrane components, all of which produce similar clinical manifestations. The precise incidence is unknown, but most authors believe that it is at least twice as common as pemphigus vulgaris.

The term **pemphigoid** is used because clinically it often appears similar (the meaning of the *-oid* suffix) to **pemphigus**. The prognosis and microscopic features of pemphigoid, however, are very different.

Although a variety of terms have been used over the decades to designate this condition, a group of experts from both medicine and dentistry met in 1999 and came to an agreement that **mucous membrane pemphigoid** would be the most appropriate name for the disease. **Cicatricial pemphigoid**, another commonly

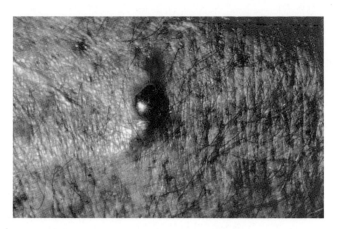

Fig. 16-62   Mucous membrane pemphigoid. Although cutaneous lesions are not common, tense bullae such as these may develop on the skin of 20% of affected patients. *(Courtesy of Dr. Charles Camisa.)*

used name for this process, is derived from the word **cicatrix**, meaning *scar*. When the conjunctival mucosa is affected, the scarring that results is the most significant aspect of this disorder because it invariably results in blindness unless the condition is recognized and treated. Interestingly, the oral lesions seldom exhibit this tendency for scar formation.

CLINICAL FEATURES

Mucous membrane pemphigoid usually affects older adults, with an average age of 50 to 60 years at the onset of disease. Females are affected more frequently than males by a 2:1 ratio. Oral lesions are seen in most patients, but other sites, such as conjunctival, nasal, esophageal, laryngeal, and vaginal mucosa, as well as the skin (Fig. 16-62), may be involved.

The oral lesions of pemphigoid begin as either vesicles or bullae that may occasionally be identified clinically (Fig. 16-63). In contrast, patients with pemphigus rarely display such blisters. The most likely explanation for this difference is that the pemphigoid blister forms in a subepithelial location, producing a thicker, stronger roof than the intraepithelial, acantholytic pemphigus blister. Eventually, the oral blisters rupture, leaving large, superficial, ulcerated, and denuded areas of mucosa (Fig. 16-64). The ulcerated lesions are usually painful and persist for weeks to months if untreated.

Often this process is seen diffusely throughout the mouth, but it may be limited to certain areas, especially the gingiva (Fig. 16-65). Gingival involvement produces a clinical reaction pattern termed **desquamative gingivitis** (see page 162). This pattern may also be seen in other conditions, such as **erosive lichen planus** or, much less frequently, **pemphigus vulgaris**.

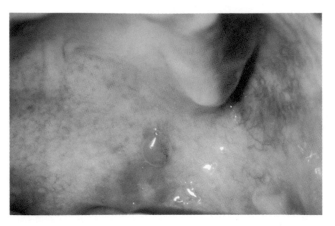

Fig. 16-63   Mucous membrane pemphigoid. One or more intraoral vesicles, as seen on the soft palate, may be detected in patients with cicatricial pemphigoid. Usually, ulcerations of the oral mucosa are also present.

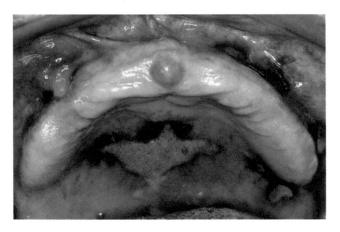

Fig. 16-64   Mucous membrane pemphigoid. Large, irregular oral ulcerations characterize the lesions after the initial bullae rupture.

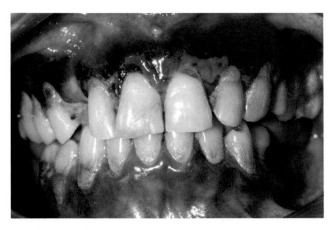

Fig. 16-65   Mucous membrane pemphigoid. Often the gingival tissues are the only affected site, resulting in a clinical pattern known as *desquamative gingivitis*. Such a pattern may also be seen with lichen planus and pemphigus vulgaris.

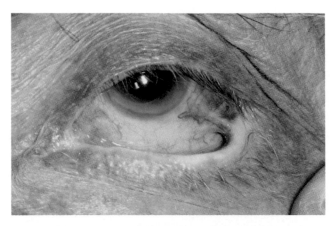

Fig. 16-66   Mucous membrane pemphigoid. Although the earliest ocular changes are difficult to identify, patients with ocular involvement may show adhesions (symblepharons) between the bulbar and palpebral conjunctivae before severe ocular damage occurs.

The most significant complication of mucous membrane pemphigoid, however, is ocular involvement. Although exact figures are not available, up to 25% of patients with oral lesions may eventually develop ocular disease. One eye may be affected before the other. The earliest change is subconjunctival fibrosis, which usually can be detected by an ophthalmologist using slit-lamp examination. As the disease progresses, the conjunctiva becomes inflamed and eroded. Attempts at healing lead to scarring between the bulbar (lining the globe of the eye) and palpebral (lining the inner surface of the eyelid) conjunctivae. Adhesions called **symblepharons** result (Fig. 16-66). Without treatment the inflammatory changes become more severe, although conjunctival vesicle formation is rarely seen (Fig. 16-67). Scarring can ultimately cause the eyelids to turn inward **(entropion)**. This causes the eyelashes to rub against the cornea and globe **(trichiasis)** (Fig. 16-68). The scarring closes off the openings of the lacrimal glands as well, and with the loss of tears, the eye becomes extremely dry. The cornea then produces keratin as a protective mechanism; however, keratin is an opaque material, and blindness ensues. End-stage ocular involvement may also be characterized by adhesions between the upper and lower eyelids themselves (Fig. 16-69).

Other mucosal sites may also be involved and cause considerable difficulty for the patient. In females, the vaginal mucosal lesions may cause considerable pain during attempts at intercourse **(dyspareunia)**.

Laryngeal lesions, which are fairly uncommon, may be especially significant because of the possibility of airway obstruction by the bullae that are formed. Patients who experience a sudden change in vocaliza-

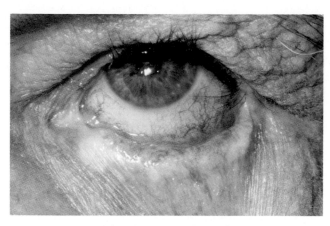

Fig. 16-67 **Mucous membrane pemphigoid.** The disease has caused the upper eyelid of this patient to turn inward (entropion), resulting in the eyelashes rubbing against the eye itself (trichiasis). Also note the obliteration of the lower fornix of the eye.

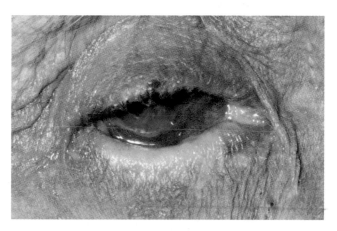

Fig. 16-68 **Mucous membrane pemphigoid.** A patient with ocular involvement shows severe conjunctival inflammation. An ophthalmologist removed the lower eyelashes because of trichiasis associated with entropion.

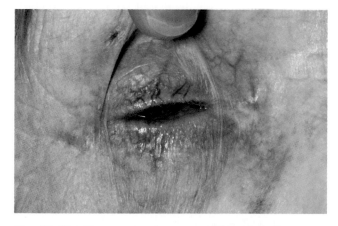

Fig. 16-69 **Mucous membrane pemphigoid.** In this patient, the ocular involvement has resulted in nearly complete scarring between the conjunctival mucosa and the eyelids themselves, producing blindness.

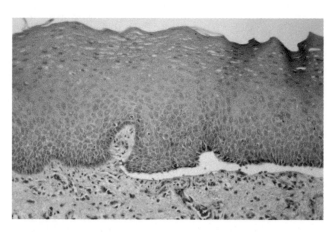

Fig. 16-70 **Mucous membrane pemphigoid.** Medium-power photomicrograph of perilesional tissue shows characteristic subepithelial clefting.

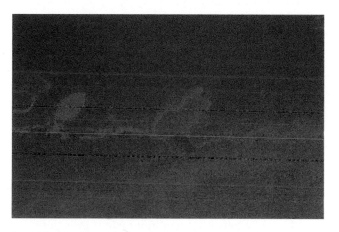

Fig. 16-71 **Mucous membrane pemphigoid.** Direct immunofluorescence studies show a deposition of immunoreactants at the basement membrane zone of the epithelium. *(Courtesy of Dr. Ronald Grimwood.)*

tion or who have difficulty breathing should undergo examination with laryngoscopy.

HISTOPATHOLOGIC FEATURES

Biopsy of perilesional mucosa shows a split between the surface epithelium and the underlying connective tissue in the region of the basement membrane (Fig. 16-70). A mild chronic inflammatory cell infiltrate is present in the superficial submucosa.

Direct immunofluorescence studies of perilesional mucosa show a continuous linear band of immunoreactants at the basement membrane zone in nearly 90% of affected patients (Fig. 16-71). The immune deposits consist primarily of IgG and C3, although IgA and IgM may also be identified. One study has suggested that, when IgG and IgA deposits are found in the same patient, the disease may be more severe. All of these immunoreactants may play a role in the pathogenesis of the subepithelial vesicle formation by weakening the attachment of the basement membrane through a variety of mechanisms, including complement activation with recruitment of inflammatory cells, particularly neutrophils.

Indirect immunofluorescence is positive in only 5% to 25% of these patients, indicating a relatively consistent lack of readily detectable circulating autoantibodies. One type of mucous membrane pemphigoid produces low levels of circulating autoantibodies to epiligrin (laminin-5), a component of the basement membrane. Antiepiligrin mucous membrane pemphigoid seems to have more widespread involvement, affecting oral, nasal, ocular, and laryngeal mucosa, compared with other forms of mucous membrane pemphigoid. In contrast, another group of investigators has shown that pemphigoid patients with only oral mucosal involvement have circulating autoantibodies to α6 integrin, a component of the hemidesmosome.

For an accurate diagnosis, perilesional tissue—rather than the ulcerated lesion itself—should be obtained. Often the epithelium in the area of the lesion is so loose that it strips off as the clinician attempts to perform the biopsy. Such tissue is not usually adequate for diagnostic purposes because the interface between the epithelium and connective tissue is no longer intact (although some investigators have shown positive immunofluorescence with this tissue).

Other relatively rare conditions can mimic pemphigoid histopathologically. These include **linear IgA bullous dermatosis**, **angina bullosa hemorrhagica**, and **epidermolysis bullosa acquisita**.

LINEAR IgA BULLOUS DERMATOSIS

Linear IgA bullous dermatosis, as the name indicates, is characterized by the linear deposition of only IgA along the basement membrane zone. Even though some cases of mucous membrane pemphigoid may have IgA antibodies, linear IgA bullous dermatosis predominantly affects the skin and, therefore, can usually be distinguished from mucous membrane pemphigoid on a clinical basis.

ANGINA BULLOSA HEMORRHAGICA

Angina bullosa hemorrhagica is a rare, poorly characterized oral mucosal disorder that exhibits variably painful, blood-filled vesicles or bullae, usually affecting the soft palate of middle-aged or older adults. The blisters typically rupture spontaneously and heal without scarring. A subepithelial cleft is noted microscopically. No hematologic or immunopathologic abnormalities

have been detected, and although the cause is unknown, many patients have a history of trauma or corticosteroid inhaler use.

EPIDERMOLYSIS BULLOSA ACQUISITA

Epidermolysis bullosa acquisita is an immunologically mediated condition characterized by autoantibodies directed against type VII collagen, the principal component of the anchoring fibrils. The anchoring fibrils play an important role in bonding the epithelium to the underlying connective tissue. As a result, their immunologic destruction leads to the formation of bullous lesions of the skin and mucosa with minimal trauma.

Oral lesions are present in nearly 50% of the cases, although such lesions are uncommon in the absence of cutaneous lesions. To distinguish epidermolysis bullosa acquisita from other immunobullous diseases with subepithelial clefting, a special technique is performed. A sample of the patient's perilesional skin is incubated in a concentrated salt solution; this causes the epithelium to separate from the connective tissue, forming an artificially induced bulla. Immunohistochemical evaluation shows deposition of IgG autoantibodies on the floor (connective tissue side) of the bulla where type VII collagen resides. This finding is in contrast to that of most forms of mucous membrane pemphigoid, in which the autoantibodies are usually localized to the roof of the induced blister.

TREATMENT AND PROGNOSIS

Once the diagnosis of mucous membrane pemphigoid has been established by light microscopy and direct immunofluorescence, the patient should be referred to an ophthalmologist who is familiar with the ocular lesions of this condition for a baseline examination of the conjunctivae. This should be done whether or not the patient is experiencing ocular complaints. In addition, if the patient is experiencing symptoms at other anatomic sites, then the appropriate specialist should be consulted.

Because this condition is characterized by heterogeneous pathogenetic mechanisms, it is not surprising that treatments advocated over the years have been varied. In fact, there is no single good therapy for every patient; treatment must be individualized, depending on lesional distribution, disease activity, and therapeutic response. Perhaps as the various forms of pemphigoid are better defined immunopathologically, more specific, directed therapy can be devised.

TOPICAL AGENTS

If only oral lesions are present, sometimes the disease can be controlled with application of one of the more potent topical corticosteroids to the lesions several times each day. Once control is achieved, the applications can be discontinued, although the lesions are certain to flare up again. Sometimes alternate-day application prevents such exacerbations of disease activity.

Patients with only gingival lesions often benefit from good oral hygiene measures, which can help to decrease the severity of the lesions and reduce the amount of topical corticosteroids required. As an additional aid in treating gingival lesions, a flexible mouth guard may be fabricated to use as a carrier for the corticosteroid medication.

SYSTEMIC AGENTS

If topical corticosteroids are unsuccessful, systemic corticosteroids plus other immunosuppressive agents (particularly cyclophosphamide) may be used if the patient has no medical contraindications. This type of aggressive treatment is absolutely indicated in the presence of advancing ocular disease. Recent studies have suggested that treatment with intravenous (IV) human immunoglobulin may be more effective in managing ocular lesions of pemphigoid than systemic corticosteroid therapy. Attempts at surgical correction of any symblepharons that might have formed must be done when the disease is under control or quiescent; otherwise, the manipulation often induces an acute flare of the ocular lesions.

For patients with mild-to-moderate involvement by mucous membrane pemphigoid, an alternative systemic therapy that may produce fewer serious side effects is the use of dapsone, a sulfa drug derivative. Some centers report good results with dapsone, but others observe that a minority of patients respond adequately. Contraindications to its use include glucose-6-phosphate dehydrogenase deficiency or allergy to sulfa drugs.

Another alternative systemic therapy that may be used for patients with less severe disease is tetracycline or minocycline and niacinamide (nicotinamide). Systemic daily divided doses of 0.5 to 2.0 g of each drug have been reported (in open-label trials) to be effective in controlling mucous membrane pemphigoid. Double-blind, placebo-controlled studies on larger groups of patients should be done to confirm this form of therapy, however.

BULLOUS PEMPHIGOID

Bullous pemphigoid is the most common of the autoimmune blistering conditions, occurring at an estimated rate of 10 cases per million population per year. The disease is characterized by the production of autoantibodies directed against components of the basement membrane. In many respects, bullous pemphigoid

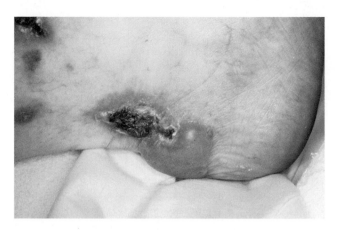

Fig. 16-72 Bullous pemphigoid. Cutaneous vesiculobullous lesions of the heel. The bullae eventually rupture, leaving hemorrhagic crusted areas.

resembles **mucous membrane pemphigoid**, but most investigators note that there are enough differences to consider these diseases as distinct but related entities. One significant difference is that the clinical course in patients with bullous pemphigoid is usually limited, whereas the course in patients with cicatricial pemphigoid is usually protracted and progressive.

CLINICAL FEATURES

Bullous pemphigoid typically develops in older people; most patients are between 60 and 80 years of age. No sex or racial predilection is generally reported, although one group of investigators noted that men are overrepresented in this disease by a 2:1 margin when one corrects for the skewing of the aging population toward the female gender. Pruritus may be an early symptom. This is followed by the development of multiple, tense bullae on either normal or erythematous skin (Fig. 16-72). These lesions eventually rupture after several days, causing a superficial crust to form. Eventually, healing takes place without scarring.

Oral mucosal involvement is uncommon, although the reported prevalence in several series of cases has ranged from 8% to 39%. Referral bias may explain the discrepancy in prevalence rates. The oral lesions, like the skin lesions, begin as bullae, but they tend to rupture sooner, probably as a result of the constant low-grade trauma to which the oral mucosa is subjected. Large, shallow ulcerations with smooth, distinct margins are present after the bullae rupture (Fig. 16-73).

HISTOPATHOLOGIC FEATURES

Microscopic examination of tissue obtained from the perilesional margin of a bulla shows separation of the epithelium from the connective tissue at the basement

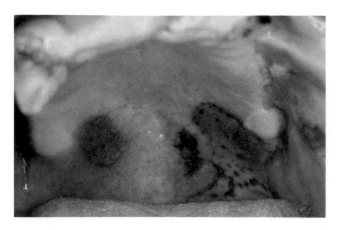

Fig. 16-73   Bullous pemphigoid. These oral lesions appear as large, shallow ulcerations involving the soft palate.

membrane zone, resulting in a subepithelial separation. Modest numbers of both acute and chronic inflammatory cells are typically seen in the lesional area, and the presence of eosinophils within the bulla itself is characteristic.

Direct immunofluorescence studies show a continuous linear band of immunoreactants, usually IgG and C3, localized to the basement membrane zone in 90% to 100% of affected patients. These antibodies may bind to proteins associated with **hemidesmosomes**, structures that bind the basal cell layer of the epithelium to the basement membrane and the underlying connective tissue. These proteins have been designated as **bullous pemphigoid antigens (BP180 and BP230)**, and immunoelectron microscopy has demonstrated the localization of BP180 to the upper portion of the lamina lucida of the basement membrane.

In addition to the tissue-bound autoantibodies, 50% to 90% of the patients also have circulating autoantibodies in the serum, producing an indirect immunofluorescent pattern that is identical to that of the direct immunofluorescence. Unlike pemphigus vulgaris, the antibody titers seen in bullous pemphigoid do not appear to correlate with disease activity. The antibodies alone do not appear to be capable of inducing bullae in this disease. Instead, binding of the antibodies to the basement membrane initiates the complement cascade, which in turn results in degranulation of mast cells, with recruitment of neutrophils and eosinophils to the area. The damage to the basement membrane is thought to be mediated by elastases and matrix metalloproteinases released by these inflammatory cells.

TREATMENT AND PROGNOSIS

Management of the patient with bullous pemphigoid consists of systemic immunosuppressive therapy. Moderate daily doses of systemic prednisone usually control the condition, after which alternate-day therapy may be given to reduce the risk of corticosteroid complications. If the lesions do not respond to prednisone alone, then another immunosuppressive agent, such as azathioprine, may be added to the regimen. Dapsone, a sulfa derivative, may be used as an alternative therapeutic agent, and tetracycline and niacinamide therapy is reported to be effective for some patients. The more severe, resistant cases require prednisone combined with cyclophosphamide; however, this regimen has the potential for significant side effects.

The prognosis is generally good, with many patients experiencing spontaneous remission after 2 to 5 years. Problems may develop with immunosuppressive therapy in this older adult population, however, and mortality rates of up to 27% have been reported in some series.

ERYTHEMA MULTIFORME

Erythema multiforme is a blistering, ulcerative mucocutaneous condition of uncertain etiopathogenesis. This is probably an immunologically mediated process, although the cause is poorly understood. In about 50% of the cases, the clinician can identify either a preceding infection, such as **herpes simplex** or *Mycoplasma pneumoniae*, or exposure to any one of a variety of drugs and medications, particularly antibiotics or analgesics. These agents may trigger the immunologic derangement that produces the disease. Sophisticated techniques in molecular biology have demonstrated the presence of herpes simplex DNA in patients with recurrent erythema multiforme, thus supporting the concept of an immunologic precipitating event. Interestingly, direct and indirect immunofluorescence studies are nonspecific and are not really very useful diagnostically except to rule out other vesiculobullous diseases.

A spectrum of severity of this disease has been recognized for many years, ranging from **erythema multiforme minor** through **erythema multiforme major** (traditionally thought to be synonymous with **Stevens-Johnson syndrome**) and **toxic epidermal necrolysis (Lyell's disease).** Recent publications have suggested that erythema multiforme minor and major may represent a distinctly different process from the latter two conditions. However, considerable overlap in the clinical features of erythema multiforme major and Stevens-Johnson syndrome is seen, and this classification scheme remains controversial.

CLINICAL FEATURES

Erythema multiforme usually has an acute onset and may display a wide spectrum of clinical disease. On the mild end of the spectrum, ulcerations develop, affect-

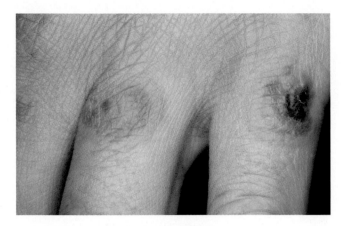

Fig. 16-74 **Erythema multiforme.** The concentric erythematous pattern of the cutaneous lesions on the fingers resembles a target or bull's-eye.

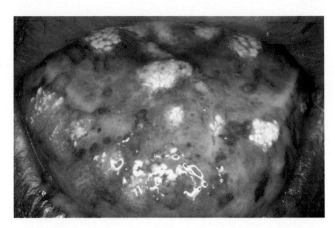

Fig. 16-75 **Erythema multiforme.** Diffuse ulcerations and erosions involving the dorsal surface of this patient's tongue.

ing the oral mucosa primarily. In its most severe form, diffuse sloughing and ulceration of the entire skin and mucosal surfaces may be seen (toxic epidermal necrolysis or Lyell's disease).

Patients affected by erythema multiforme are usually young adults in their 20s or 30s. Men are affected more frequently than women.

Prodromal symptoms include fever, malaise, headache, cough, and sore throat, occurring approximately 1 week before onset. Although the disease is self-limiting, usually lasting 2 to 6 weeks, about 20% of patients experience recurrent episodes, usually in the spring and autumn.

Erythematous skin lesions develop in about 50% of cases. A variety of appearances (*multiforme* means *many forms*) may be present. Typically, early lesions appear on the extremities and are flat, round, and dusky-red in hue. These become slightly elevated and may evolve into bullae with necrotic centers. Sometimes particular skin lesions develop that are highly characteristic for the disease. These lesions appear as concentric circular erythematous rings resembling a target or bull's-eye **(target lesions)** (Fig. 16-74).

The oral lesions begin as erythematous patches that undergo epithelial necrosis and evolve into large, shallow erosions and ulcerations with irregular borders (Fig. 16-75). Hemorrhagic crusting of the vermilion zone of the lips is common (Fig. 16-76). These oral lesions, like the skin lesions, emerge quickly and are uncomfortable. Sometimes patients are dehydrated because they are unable to ingest liquids as a result of mouth pain. The ulcerations often have a diffuse distribution. The lips, labial mucosa, buccal mucosa, tongue, floor of the mouth, and soft palate are the most common

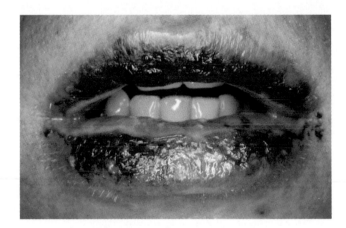

Fig. 16-76 **Erythema multiforme.** Ulceration of the labial mucosa, with hemorrhagic crusting of the vermilion zone of the lips.

sites of involvement. Usually, the gingivae and hard palate are relatively spared.

ERYTHEMA MULTIFORME MAJOR

A more severe form of the disease, known as *erythema multiforme major* or *Stevens-Johnson syndrome*, is usually triggered by a drug rather than infection. For such a diagnosis to be made, either the ocular (Fig. 16-77) or genital (Fig. 16-78) mucosae should be affected in conjunction with the oral and skin lesions. With severe ocular involvement, scarring (symblepharon formation) may occur, similar to that in cicatricial pemphigoid (see page 772).

TOXIC EPIDERMAL NECROLYSIS

Many dermatologists consider toxic epidermal necrolysis to represent the most severe form of erythema

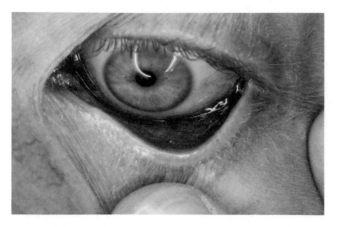

Fig. 16-77   Stevens-Johnson syndrome. With erythema multiforme major (Stevens-Johnson syndrome), other mucosal surfaces may show involvement, such as the severe conjunctivitis depicted in this photograph.

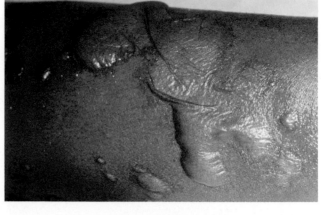

Fig. 16-79   Toxic epidermal necrolysis. This severe form of erythema multiforme exhibits diffuse bullous skin lesions. *(Courtesy of Dr. Peter Larsen.)*

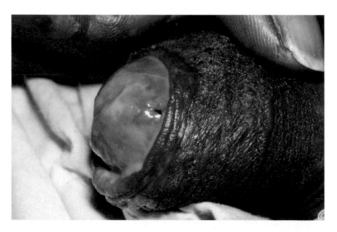

Fig. 16-78   Stevens-Johnson syndrome. Genital ulcerations, demonstrated in this patient by the involvement of the glans penis, may also be a component.

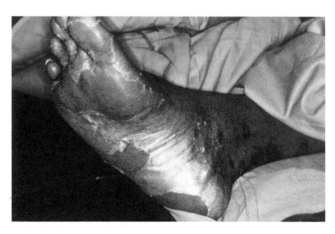

Fig. 16-80   Toxic epidermal necrolysis. The desquamation of the skin of the foot is characteristic of the diffuse sloughing cutaneous lesions. *(Courtesy of Dr. Peter Larsen.)*

multiforme. It is almost always triggered by drug exposure, with more than 200 different medications having been implicated. Recent studies have shown that the damage to the epithelium is due to increased apoptosis of the epithelial cells. Diffuse sloughing of a significant proportion of the skin and mucosal surfaces makes it appear as if the patient had been badly scalded (Figs. 16-79 and 16-80). In contrast to erythema multiforme major, toxic epidermal necrolysis tends to occur in older people. A female predilection is observed. If the patient survives, then the cutaneous process resolves in 2 to 4 weeks; however, oral lesions may take longer to heal, and significant residual ocular damage is evident in half the patients. These more severe presentations of erythema multiforme are rare. Erythema multiforme major occurs at an average rate of five cases per million population per year, and toxic epider-

mal necrolysis occurs at a rate of about one case per million per year.

HISTOPATHOLOGIC FEATURES

Histopathologic examination of the perilesional mucosa in erythema multiforme reveals a pattern that is characteristic but not pathognomonic. Subepithelial or intraepithelial vesiculation may be seen in association with necrotic basal keratinocytes (Fig. 16-81). A mixed inflammatory infiltrate is present, consisting of lymphocytes, neutrophils, and often eosinophils. Sometimes these cells are arranged in a perivascular orientation (Fig. 16-82). Because the immunopathologic features are also nonspecific, the diagnosis is often based on the clinical presentation and the exclusion of other vesiculobullous disorders.

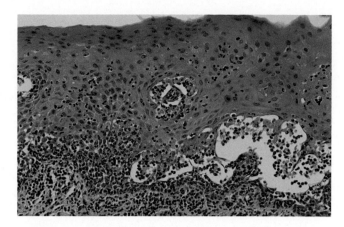

Fig. 16-81   Erythema multiforme. This medium-power photomicrograph shows inflammation and intraepithelial vesicle formation in the basilar portion of the epithelium. Numerous necrotic eosinophilic keratinocytes are present in the blister area.

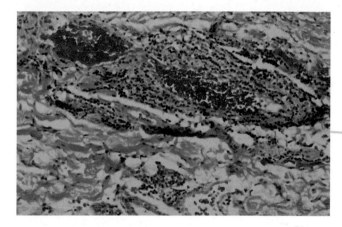

Fig. 16-82   Erythema multiforme. This medium-power photomicrograph shows the perivascular inflammatory infiltrate, typically seen in erythema multiforme.

TREATMENT AND PROGNOSIS

Management of erythema multiforme, in many respects, remains controversial. In the past, the use of systemic or topical corticosteroids was often advocated, especially in the early stages of the disease. There is little good clinical evidence that such treatment alters the course of this disease, however. If a causative drug is identified or suspected, then it should be discontinued immediately.

If the patient is dehydrated as a result of an inability to eat because of oral pain, then intravenous rehydration may be necessary along with topical anesthetic agents to decrease discomfort.

If recurrent episodes of erythema multiforme are a problem, then an initiating factor, such as recurrent herpesvirus infection or drug exposure, should be sought. If disease is triggered by herpes simplex, then continuous oral acyclovir or valacyclovir therapy can prevent recurrences.

Generally, erythema multiforme is not life threatening except in its most severe forms. The mortality rate in patients with toxic epidermal necrolysis historically has been approximately 34%; the rate in those with Stevens-Johnson syndrome is 2% to 10%. Corticosteroids should be avoided in the management of toxic epidermal necrolysis because some investigators have found that such drugs may be detrimental. Intravenous administration of pooled human immunoglobulins has been shown in several open-label trials to produce remarkable resolution of toxic epidermal necrolysis, presumably because of blockade of Fas ligand, which is believed to be responsible for inducing epithelial cell apoptosis. Because the lesions of toxic epidermal necrolysis are analogous to those suffered by burn patients, management of these patients in the burn unit of the hospital is recommended.

ERYTHEMA MIGRANS (GEOGRAPHIC TONGUE; BENIGN MIGRATORY GLOSSITIS; WANDERING RASH OF THE TONGUE; ERYTHEMA AREATA MIGRANS; STOMATITIS AREATA MIGRANS)

Erythema migrans is a common benign condition that primarily affects the tongue. It is often detected on routine examination of the oral mucosa. The lesion occurs in 1% to 3% of the population. Females are affected more frequently than males by a 2:1 ratio. Patients may occasionally consult a health care professional if they happen to notice the unusual appearance of their tongue or if the lingual mucosa becomes sensitive to hot or spicy foods as a result of the process.

Even though erythema migrans has been documented for many years, the etiopathogenesis is still unknown. Some investigators have suggested that erythema migrans occurs with increased frequency in atopic individuals; however, one recent large epidemiologic study in the United States found no statistically significant association between erythema migrans and a variety of conditions that had previously been postulated either to cause or influence this process. Erythema migrans was not seen as frequently in cigarette smokers, while there seemed to be no significant differences in frequency related to age, sex, oral contraceptive use, presence of allergies, diabetes mellitus, or psychological or dermatologic conditions.

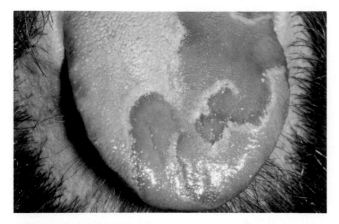

Fig. 16-83   Erythema migrans. The erythematous, well-demarcated areas of papillary atrophy are characteristic of erythema migrans affecting the tongue (benign migratory glossitis). Note the asymmetrical distribution and the tendency to involve the lateral aspects of the tongue.

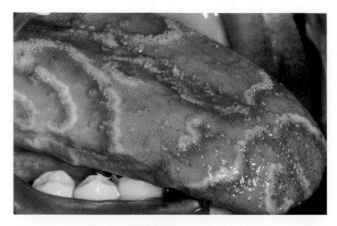

Fig. 16-85   Erythema migrans. Striking involvement of the dorsal and lateral surfaces of the tongue.

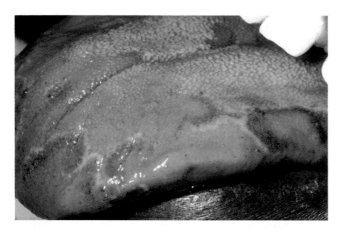

Fig. 16-84   Erythema migrans. Lingual mucosa of a different patient than the one in Fig. 16-83. The lateral distribution of the lesions is shown.

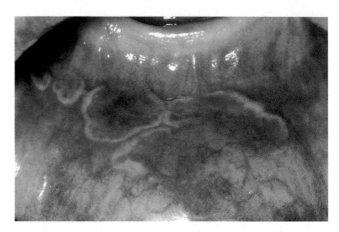

Fig. 16-86   Erythema migrans. Lesions of the lower labial mucosa.

CLINICAL FEATURES

The characteristic lesions of erythema migrans are seen on the anterior two thirds of the dorsal tongue mucosa. They appear as multiple, well-demarcated zones of erythema (Figs. 16-83 and 16-84), concentrated at the tip and lateral borders of the tongue. This erythema is due to atrophy of the filiform papillae, and these atrophic areas are typically surrounded at least partially by a slightly elevated, yellow-white, serpentine or scalloped border (Fig. 16-85). The patient who is aware of the process is often able to describe the lesions as appearing quickly in one area, healing within a few days or weeks, then developing in a very different area. Frequently, the lesion begins as a small white patch, which then develops a central erythematous atrophic zone and enlarges centrifugally. Often patients with **fissured tongue** (see page 13) are affected with erythema migrans as well. Some patients may have only a solitary lesion, but this is uncommon. The lesions are usually asymptomatic, although a burning sensation or sensitivity to hot or spicy foods may be noted when the lesions are active. Only rarely is the burning sensation more constant and severe.

Very infrequently, erythema migrans may occur on oral mucosal sites other than the tongue. In these instances, the tongue is almost always affected; however, other lesions develop on the buccal mucosa, on the labial mucosa, and (less frequently) on the soft palate (Figs. 16-86 and 16-87). These lesions typically produce no symptoms and can be identified by a yellow-white serpentine or scalloped border that surrounds an erythematous zone. These features should prevent confusion with such conditions as candidiasis or erythroplakia.

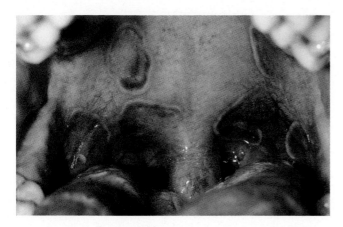

Fig. 16-87   Erythema migrans. These palatal lesions show well-demarcated erythematous areas surrounded by a white border, similar to the process involving the tongue.

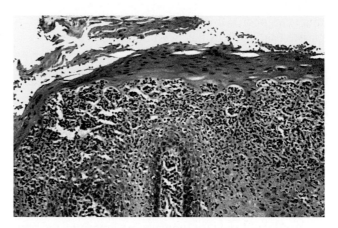

Fig. 16-89   Erythema migrans. This medium-power photomicrograph shows collections of neutrophils in the superficial spinous layer of the epithelium.

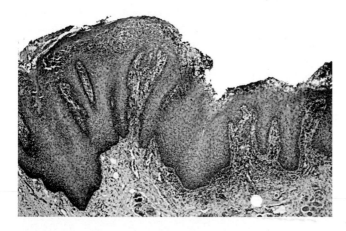

Fig. 16-88   Erythema migrans. This low-power photomicrograph shows the elongation of the rete ridges with parakeratosis and neutrophilic infiltration. Such features are also common in psoriasis, which explains why this is known as a *psoriasiform mucositis.*

HISTOPATHOLOGIC FEATURES

If a biopsy specimen of the peripheral region of erythema migrans is examined, a characteristic histopathologic pattern is observed. Hyperparakeratosis, spongiosis, acanthosis, and elongation of the epithelial rete ridges are seen (Fig. 16-88). In addition, collections of neutrophils (**Munro abscesses**) are observed within the epithelium (Fig. 16-89); lymphocytes and neutrophils involve the lamina propria. The intense neutrophilic infiltrate may be responsible for the destruction of the superficial portion of the epithelium, thus producing an atrophic, reddened mucosa as the lesion progresses. Because these histopathologic features are reminiscent of **psoriasis**, this is called a **psoriasiform mucositis**. Despite the apparent lack of

association between dermatologic conditions and erythema migrans in one recent report, another case-control study of psoriatic patients showed that erythema migrans occurred at a rate of about 10%; only 2.5% of an age-matched and sex-matched population were affected. A Brazilian study determined that both patients with psoriasis and those with benign migratory glossitis were more likely to have the same human leukocyte antigen (HLA) group, namely HLA-Cw6. Whether these findings mean that erythema migrans represents oral psoriasis or that patients with psoriasis are just more susceptible to erythema migrans is open to debate.

TREATMENT AND PROGNOSIS

Generally no treatment is indicated for patients with erythema migrans. Reassuring the patient that the condition is completely benign is often all that is necessary. Infrequently, patients may complain of tenderness or a burning sensation that is so severe that it disrupts their lifestyle. In such cases, topical corticosteroids, such as fluocinonide or betamethasone gel, may provide relief when applied as a thin film several times a day to the lesional areas.

REACTIVE ARTHRITIS (REITER'S SYNDROME)

Reactive arthritis represents a group of uncommon diseases that most likely have an immunologically mediated cause. Current evidence suggests that these disorders may be triggered by any one of several infectious agents in a genetically susceptible person. In some instances, the arthritis will be accompanied by mucocutaneous findings, including oral lesions. A classic triad of signs has been described:

1. Nongonococcal urethritis
2. Arthritis
3. Conjunctivitis

However, most patients do not exhibit all three of these signs. Although reactive arthritis with a mucocutaneous component is also known as **Reiter syndrome**, some authors have advocated removing the *Reiter* eponym because of Hans Reiter's Nazi criminal activities during World War II and he was not the first to describe this syndrome.

It is interesting that reactive arthritis has been reported with some frequency in patients infected with the human immunodeficiency virus (HIV).

CLINICAL FEATURES

Reactive arthritis is particularly prevalent in young adult men. According to most series, there is a male-to-female ratio of 9:1. The majority (60% to 90%) of these patients are positive for HLA-B27, a haplotype present in only 4% to 8% of the population. The syndrome usually develops 1 to 4 weeks after an episode of dysentery or venereal disease; in fact, two French physicians published a description of this entity affecting four postdysenteric soldiers 1 week before Reiter's paper appeared.

Urethritis is often the first sign and is seen in both affected males and females. Females may also have inflammation of the uterine cervix. Conjunctivitis usually appears concurrently with the urethritis, and after several days, arthritis ensues. The arthritis usually affects the joints of the lower extremities, although TMJ involvement has been identified in one third of these patients, typically as erosion of the condylar head. Skin lesions often take the form of a characteristic lesion of the glans penis **(balanitis circinata)**. These lesions develop in about 20% to 30% of patients with reactive arthritis, and they appear as well-circumscribed erythematous erosions with a scalloped, whitish linear boundary.

The oral lesions, which occur in slightly less than 20% of patients with this disorder, are described in various ways. Some reports mention painless erythematous papules distributed on the buccal mucosa and palate; other reports describe shallow, painless ulcers that affect the tongue, buccal mucosa, palate, and gingiva. Some authors have even implied that **geographic tongue** may be a component of reactive arthritis, probably because geographic tongue bears a superficial resemblance to the lesions of balanitis circinata.

The American Rheumatism Association has defined reactive arthritis based on the clinical findings of a peripheral arthritis that lasts longer than 1 month in conjunction with urethritis, cervicitis, or both.

HISTOPATHOLOGIC FEATURES

The histopathologic findings of the cutaneous lesions in patients with reactive arthritis are frequently similar to those found in patients with **psoriasis**, particularly with respect to the presence of microabscesses within the superficial layers of the surface epithelium. Other features in common with psoriasis include hyperparakeratosis with elongated, thin rete ridges.

TREATMENT AND PROGNOSIS

Some patients with reactive arthritis experience spontaneous resolution of their disease after 3 to 12 months, but many others have chronic symptoms that may wax and wane. Treatment may not be necessary for the milder cases. Nonsteroidal antiinflammatory drugs (NSAIDs) are initially used for managing arthritis, and sulfasalazine may be helpful in resolving cases that do not respond. Immunosuppressive agents, including corticosteroids, azathioprine, and methotrexate, are reserved for the most resistant cases if they are not associated with HIV infection.

Physical therapy probably helps to reduce joint fibrosis associated with arthritis. About 10% to 25% of patients with this disorder have severe disability, usually from arthritis.

LICHEN PLANUS

Lichen planus is a relatively common, chronic dermatologic disease that often affects the oral mucosa. The strange name of the condition was provided by the British physician Erasmus Wilson, who first described it in 1869. Lichens are primitive plants composed of symbiotic algae and fungi. The term *planus* is Latin for *flat*. Wilson probably thought that the skin lesions looked similar enough to the lichens growing on rocks to merit this designation. Even though the term *lichen planus* suggests a flat, fungal condition, current evidence indicates that this is an immunologically mediated mucocutaneous disorder.

A variety of medications may induce lesions that can appear clinically very similar to the idiopathic form of the condition; however, the term **lichenoid mucositis** (or **lichenoid dermatitis**, depending on the site involved) is probably a better name for the drug-related alterations (see page 347). Similarly, foreign material that becomes inadvertently embedded in the gingiva may elicit a host response that is termed **lichenoid foreign body gingivitis** (see page 160). Reports of hepatitis C infection associated with oral lichen planus occasionally have appeared in the literature, usually from the Mediterranean countries, but this does not appear to be a significant association in the United States or Great Britain. More recent, carefully controlled epidemiologic studies do not appear to support an association of oral lichen planus with hepatitis C. However, genetic influences presumably may have an effect on the expression of lichen planus in select populations.

The relationship of stress or anxiety to the development of lichen planus is controversial, and most cited cases appear to be anecdotal or lack appropriate controls. Those studies that have applied psychologic questionnaires often find increased levels of anxiety in these patients; however, many patients who have been told that they have lichen planus are aware that anxiety has been linked to the disorder. Whether this awareness may influence the manner in which they answer the psychologic questionnaires could be debated. In one study that used psychologic questionnaires to attempt to resolve this question, patients with oral lichen planus had no greater degree of stress in their lives than did age-matched and sex-matched control patients. It might be that stress has no bearing on the pathogenesis of lichen planus; however, an alternative explanation might be that those patients who have lichen planus simply respond in this fashion to levels of stress that do not induce lesions in other people.

CLINICAL FEATURES

Most patients with lichen planus are middle-aged adults. It is rare for children to be affected. Women predominate in most series of cases, usually by a 3:2 ratio over men. Approximately 1% of the population may have cutaneous lichen planus. The prevalence of oral lichen planus is between 0.1% and 2.2%.

The skin lesions of lichen planus have been classically described as purple, pruritic, polygonal papules (Fig. 16-90). These usually affect the flexor surfaces of the extremities. Excoriations may not be visible, despite the fact that the lesions itch, because it hurts the patient when he or she scratches them.

Careful examination of the surface of the skin papules reveals a fine, lacelike network of white lines **(Wickham's striae)**. Other sites of extraoral involvement include the glans penis, the vulvar mucosa, and the nails (Fig. 16-91). Essentially there are two forms of oral lesions: reticular and erosive.

RETICULAR LICHEN PLANUS

Reticular lichen planus is much more common than the erosive form, but the erosive form predominates in several studies. This is probably because of referral bias (because the erosive form is symptomatic and, there-

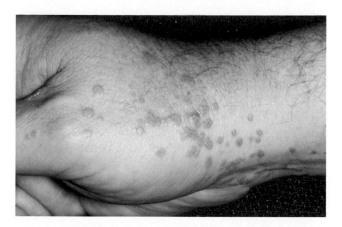

Fig. 16-90 Lichen planus. The cutaneous lesions on the wrist appear as purple, polygonal papules. Careful examination shows a network of fine white lines (Wickham's striae) on the surface of the papules.

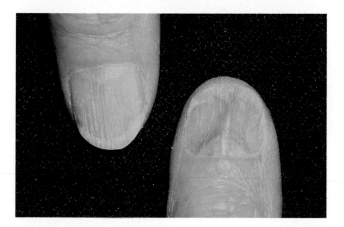

Fig. 16-91 Lichen planus. Dysplastic appearance of the fingernails.

fore, the patient is more likely to be referred to an academic center for evaluation). The reticular form usually causes no symptoms and involves the posterior buccal mucosa bilaterally (Figs. 16-92 and 16-93). Other oral mucosal surfaces may also be involved concurrently, such as the lateral and dorsal tongue, the gingivae, the palate, and vermilion border (Fig. 16-94).

Reticular lichen planus is thus named because of its characteristic pattern of interlacing white lines (also referred to as *Wickham's striae*); however, the white lesions may appear as papules in some instances. These lesions are typically not static but wax and wane over weeks or months (Fig. 16-95). The reticular pattern may not be as evident in some sites, such as the dorsal tongue, where the lesions appear more as keratotic plaques with atrophy of the papillae (Fig. 16-96). In

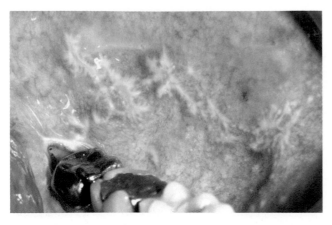

Fig. 16-92   Lichen planus. The interlacing white lines are typical of reticular lichen planus involving the posterior buccal mucosa, the most common site of oral involvement.

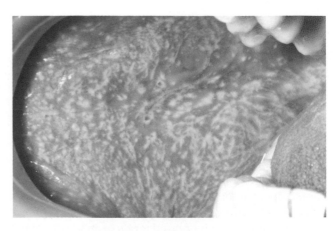

Fig. 16-93   Lichen planus. Diffuse papular and reticular lesions of the right buccal mucosa.

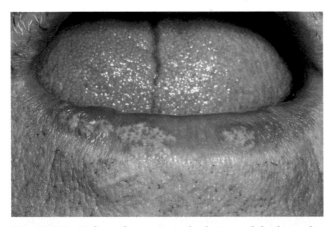

Fig. 16-94   Lichen planus. Reticular lesions of the lower lip vermilion.

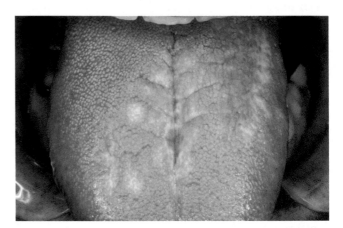

Fig. 16-96   Lichen planus. With involvement of the dorsal tongue by reticular lichen planus, the characteristic interlacing striae seen in the buccal mucosal lesions are usually not present. Instead, smooth white plaques are typically observed replacing the normal papillary surface of the tongue.

A

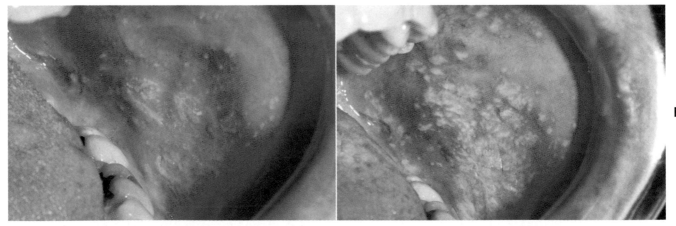

B

Fig. 16-95   Lichen planus. A, A middle-aged woman with mild reticular lichen planus of the left buccal mucosa. **B,** Same patient 2 weeks later, showing exacerbation of the lesions. Such waxing and waning is characteristic of lichen planus.

addition, superficial mucoceles may develop within, or adjacent to, mucosal areas that are involved by lichen planus.

EROSIVE LICHEN PLANUS

Erosive lichen planus, although not as common as the reticular form, is more significant for the patient because the lesions are usually symptomatic. Clinically, there are atrophic, erythematous areas with central ulceration of varying degrees. The periphery of the atrophic regions is usually bordered by fine, white radiating striae (Figs. 16-97 and 16-98). Sometimes the atrophy and ulceration are confined to the gingival mucosa, producing the reaction pattern called **desquamative gingivitis** (see page 162) (Fig. 16-99). In such cases, biopsy specimens should be obtained for light microscopic and immunofluorescent studies of perile-

sional tissue, because mucous membrane pemphigoid (see page 771) and pemphigus vulgaris (see page 765) may appear in a similar fashion.

If the erosive component is severe, epithelial separation from the underlying connective tissue may occur. This results in the relatively rare presentation of **bullous lichen planus**.

HISTOPATHOLOGIC FEATURES

The histopathologic features of lichen planus are characteristic but may not be specific, because other conditions, such as **lichenoid drug reaction**, **lichenoid amalgam reaction**, **oral graft-versus-host disease** (GVHD), **lupus erythematosus** (LE), **chronic ulcerative stomatitis**, and **oral mucosal cinnamon reaction** may also show a similar histopathologic pattern.

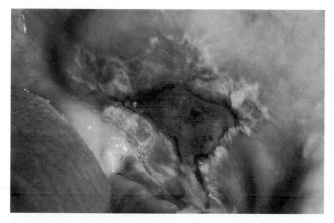

Fig. 16-97   Lichen planus. Ulceration of the buccal mucosa shows peripheral radiating keratotic striae, characteristic of oral erosive lichen planus.

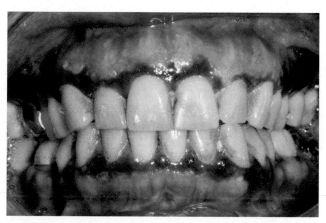

Fig. 16-99   Lichen planus. Erosive lichen planus often appears as a desquamative gingivitis, producing gingival erythema and tenderness.

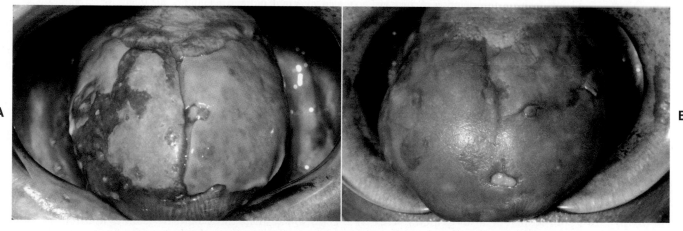

Fig. 16-98   Lichen planus. A, The dorsal surface of the tongue shows extensive ulceration caused by erosive lichen planus. Note the fine white streaks at the periphery of the ulcerations. **B,** Same patient after systemic corticosteroid therapy. Much of the mucosa has reepithelialized, with only focal ulcerations remaining.

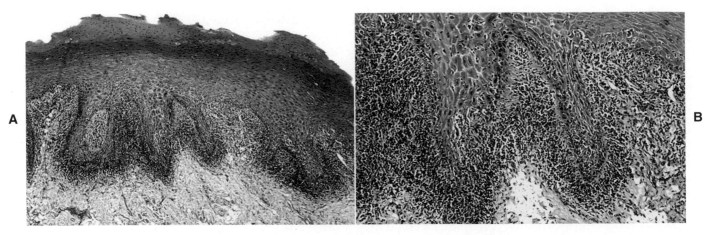

Fig. 16-100   Lichen planus. A, This low-power photomicrograph of an oral lesion shows hyperkeratosis, saw-toothed rete ridges, and a bandlike infiltrate of lymphocytes immediately subjacent to the epithelium. **B,** Higher-power view showing migration of lymphocytes into the lower epithelium with interface degeneration of the basal cell layer.

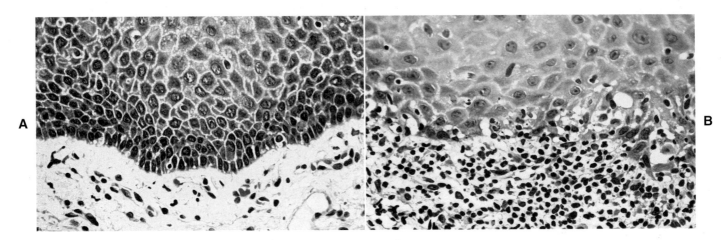

Fig. 16-101   Lichen planus. A, High-power photomicrograph of normal epithelium showing an intact basal cell layer and no inflammation. **B,** High-power photomicrograph of lichen planus showing degeneration of the basal epithelial layer and an intense lymphocytic infiltrate in the superficial lamina propria.

Varying degrees of orthokeratosis and parakeratosis may be present on the surface of the epithelium, depending on whether the biopsy specimen is taken from an erosive or reticular lesion.

The thickness of the spinous layer can also vary. The rete ridges may be absent or hyperplastic, but they classically have a pointed or "saw-toothed" shape (Fig. 16-100).

Destruction of the basal cell layer of the epithelium **(hydropic degeneration)** is also evident. This is accompanied by an intense, bandlike infiltrate of predominantly T lymphocytes immediately subjacent to the epithelium (Fig. 16-101). Degenerating keratinocytes may be seen in the area of the epithelium and

connective tissue interface and have been termed **colloid, cytoid, hyaline,** or **Civatte bodies.** No significant degree of epithelial atypia is expected in oral lichen planus, although lesions having a superimposed candidal infection may appear worrisome. These should be reevaluated histopathologically after the candidal infection is treated. On occasion, the chronic inflammatory host response to the atypical cells of **epithelial dysplasia** can appear virtually indistinguishable histopathologically from lichen planus, particularly in milder cases of epithelial dysplasia. Such ambiguity may contribute to the controversy related to the malignant transformation potential of lichen planus.

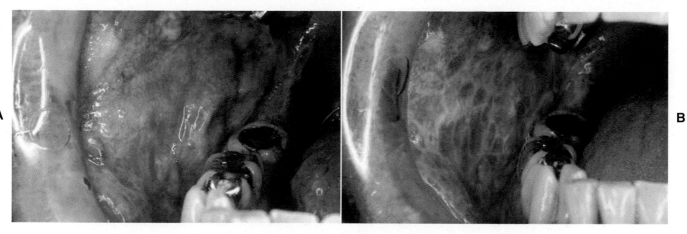

A

B

Fig. 16-102   Lichen planus. A, These relatively nondescript white lesions affected the buccal mucosa of a patient who had complained of a burning sensation. Histopathologic evaluation of the lesion showed a lichenoid mucositis with superimposed candidiasis. **B,** Same patient 2 weeks after antifungal therapy. Once the mucosal reaction to the candidal organism was eliminated, the characteristic white striae of reticular lichen planus were identified.

The immunopathologic features of lichen planus are nonspecific. Most lesions show the deposition of a shaggy band of fibrinogen at the basement membrane zone.

DIAGNOSIS

The diagnosis of **reticular lichen planus** can often be made based on the clinical findings alone. The interlacing white striae appearing bilaterally on the posterior buccal mucosa are virtually pathognomonic. Difficulties in diagnosis may arise if candidiasis is superimposed on the lesions because the organism may disturb the characteristic reticular pattern of the lichen planus (Fig. 16-102).

Erosive lichen planus is sometimes more challenging to diagnose (based on clinical features alone) than the reticular form. If the typical radiating white striae and erythematous, atrophic mucosa are present at the periphery of well-demarcated ulcerations on the posterior buccal mucosa bilaterally, then the diagnosis can sometimes be rendered without the support of histopathologic findings. However, a biopsy is often necessary to rule out other ulcerative or erosive diseases, such as lupus erythematosus or chronic ulcerative stomatitis.

Specimens of isolated erosive lichenoid lesions, particularly those of the soft palate, the lateral and ventral tongue, or the floor of the mouth, should be obtained for biopsy to rule out premalignant changes or malignancy. Another condition that may mimic an isolated lesion of lichen planus, both clinically and histopatho-

logically, is a **lichenoid reaction to dental amalgam** (see page 354).

TREATMENT AND PROGNOSIS

Reticular lichen planus typically produces no symptoms, and no treatment is needed. Occasionally, affected patients may have superimposed candidiasis, in which case they may complain of a burning sensation of the oral mucosa. Antifungal therapy is necessary in such a case. Some investigators recommend annual reevaluation of the reticular lesions of oral lichen planus.

Erosive lichen planus is often bothersome because of the open sores in the mouth. Because it is an immunologically mediated condition, corticosteroids are recommended. The lesions respond to systemic corticosteroids, but such drastic therapy is usually not necessary. One of the stronger topical corticosteroids (e.g., fluocinonide, betamethasone, clobetasol gel) applied several times per day to the most symptomatic areas is usually sufficient to induce healing within 1 or 2 weeks. Some investigators have recommended compounding corticosteroid ointments with an adhesive methylcellulose base, but patient compliance may be reduced because this material is difficult to apply. The patient should be warned that the condition will undoubtedly flare up again, in which case the corticosteroids should be reapplied. In addition, the possibility of iatrogenic candidiasis associated with corticosteroid use should be monitored (Fig. 16-103). Although the use of agents such as topical retinoids,

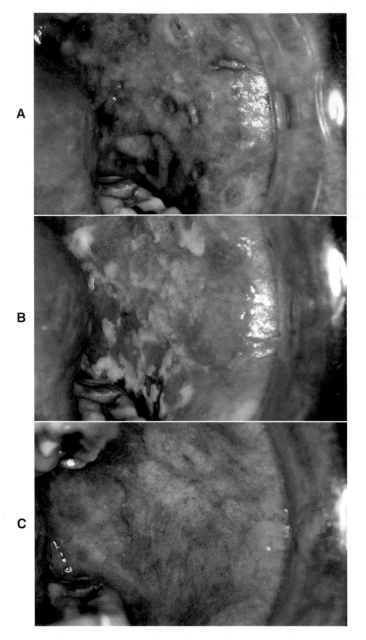

Fig. 16-103 **Lichen planus. A,** This patient was diagnosed with erosive lichen planus affecting the buccal mucosa and was treated with topical corticosteroids. **B,** Same patient 2 weeks later. The creamy-white plaques of pseudomembranous candidiasis have developed as a result of the corticosteroid therapy. **C,** Same patient after antifungal therapy. At this point, he was asymptomatic.

tacrolimus, or cyclosporine has occasionally been advocated for recalcitrant cases of erosive lichen planus, reports of their efficacy have been contradictory. Furthermore, their side effects can be significant, and in the case of cyclosporine, the cost of the drug may be prohibitive. Some investigators suggest that patients with oral erosive lichen planus be evaluated every 3 to 6 months, particularly if the lesions are not typical.

The question of the malignant potential of lichen planus, particularly the erosive form, is yet to be resolved. Most cases of reported malignant transformation are rather poorly documented. Some of these reported cases may not have been true lichen planus, but rather they may have actually been dysplastic leukoplakias with a secondary lichenoid inflammatory infiltrate that mimicked lichen planus ("lichenoid dysplasia"). In addition, the argument can be made that because both lichen planus and squamous cell carcinoma are not rare, some people may have both problems simultaneously, and the two processes may be unrelated to one another. Conversely, some investigators say that the atrophic epithelium of lichen planus may be more susceptible to the action of carcinogens, resulting in an increased risk of malignant transformation. One study examined the molecular characteristics of classic reticular lichen planus, comparing the loss of heterozygosity at purported tumor suppressor gene loci in these lesions with that of varying grades of oral epithelial dysplasia, squamous cell carcinoma, normal oral mucosa, and oral reactive lesions. The molecular profile of oral lichen planus more closely resembled that of normal or reactive oral mucosa, a finding that provides less support for the concept of lichen planus being precancerous. Another study evaluated the malignant transformation rate of typical oral lichen planus compared with oral "lichenoid" lesions. The lichenoid lesions had some features of lichen planus, but were not completely representative, either clinically or histopathologically, of that disease. These investigators found that there was no transformation of characteristic lichen planus, although several of the lichenoid lesions developed into squamous cell carcinoma. Additional prospective clinical studies with strict clinical and histopathologic criteria for the definition of oral lichen planus will need to be performed to resolve this question. If the potential for malignant transformation exists, then it appears to be small. Most of the reported cases have been confined to patients with either the erosive or so-called plaque-type form of lichen planus.

CHRONIC ULCERATIVE STOMATITIS

Chronic ulcerative stomatitis is another immune-mediated disorder that affects the oral mucosa. This condition was initially described in 1989, and slightly more than 40 cases have been reported. Although the precise pathogenetic mechanisms are unknown, these patients develop autoantibodies against a 70-kD nuclear protein that is very similar to p63 and may play a role in epithelial growth and differentiation.

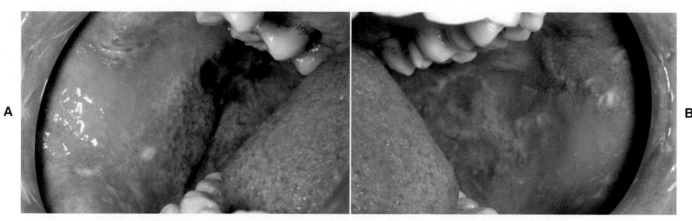

Fig. 16-104 Chronic ulcerative stomatitis. A, White lesions with central erosion on the buccal mucosa. **B,** Opposite buccal mucosa in the same patient. The lesions appear somewhat lichenoid, although classic Wickham's striae are not evident.

The prevalence of this disease may be more common than is realized. Because of its clinical similarity to erosive lichen planus, it is possible that only a clinical diagnosis is made when an affected patient is encountered, and a biopsy is not performed. Even if a biopsy is done, the tissue is often submitted for routine light microscopy alone, and the direct immunofluorescence studies that are required for its diagnosis are not ordered. Distinction from lichen planus should be made because chronic ulcerative stomatitis typically does not respond as well to corticosteroid therapy, and just as is the case with lupus erythematosus, chronic ulcerative stomatitis often can be effectively treated using antimalarial drugs.

CLINICAL FEATURES

Chronic ulcerative stomatitis usually affects adult women, and the mean age at diagnosis is late in the sixth decade of life. The condition may appear as desquamative gingivitis, although ulcerations or erosions of the tongue or buccal mucosa are also quite common (Fig. 16-104). The ulcers are generally surrounded by patchy zones of erythema and streaky keratosis that somewhat resemble lichen planus, although classic striae formation is not evident. The ulcers heal without scarring and often migrate around the oral mucosa. As is typical with most immune-mediated conditions, the severity of the oral lesions tends to wax and wane. Fewer than 20% of affected patients will develop concurrent lichenoid skin lesions.

HISTOPATHOLOGIC FEATURES

Although the histopathologic features of chronic ulcerative stomatitis are similar to those of lichen planus, the epithelium is generally more atrophic and the inflammatory infiltrate usually contains significant numbers of plasma cells in addition to lymphocytes (Fig. 16-105). Artifactual epithelial separation from the underlying connective tissue is not unusual.

DIAGNOSIS

The diagnosis of chronic ulcerative stomatitis is essentially based on its characteristic immunopathologic pattern. Although it may not be economically feasible to do immunologic testing on every case of lichen planus, this procedure should be considered for erosive lichenoid lesions that do not have a characteristic appearance or distribution, as well as for erosive lesions that do not respond to topical corticosteroid therapy. With direct immunofluorescence studies, autoantibodies (usually IgG) that are directed against the nuclei of stratified squamous epithelial cells in the basal and parabasal regions of the epithelium are detected (Fig. 16-106). Indirect immunofluorescence studies are also positive for these stratified epithelium-specific antinuclear antibodies (ANAs), and some investigators believe that confirmation of the diagnosis is necessary using serum for indirect immunofluorescence evaluation. Other immune-mediated conditions (e.g., systemic sclerosis and lupus erythematosus) may show ANA deposition with direct immunofluorescence; however, nuclei throughout the entire thickness of the epithelium are positive with those diseases.

TREATMENT AND PROGNOSIS

Unlike the lesions of erosive lichen planus, the lesions associated with chronic ulcerative stomatitis may not respond as well to topical or systemic corticosteroid therapy. If the lesions are not adequately controlled with corticosteroids, then management with hydroxy-

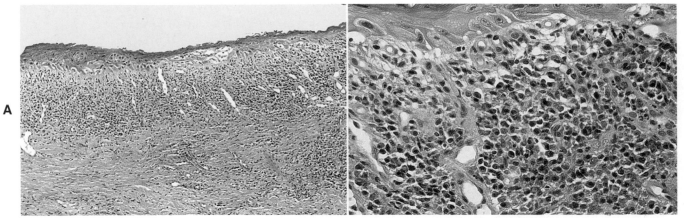

Fig. 16-105   Chronic ulcerative stomatitis. A, Low-power photomicrograph showing epithelial atrophy with a heavy chronic inflammatory cell infiltrate in the superficial lamina propria. **B,** High-power photomicrograph showing interface degeneration of the basilar epithelium in association with the inflammation. Unlike lichen planus, this infiltrate includes numerous plasma cells, as well as lymphocytes.

Fig. 16-106   Chronic ulcerative stomatitis. Direct immunofluorescence studies show presence of IgG in the basal and parabasal epithelial nuclei.

chloroquine, an antimalarial drug, should be considered. Hydroxychloroquine therapy, however, requires both periodic ophthalmologic evaluation to monitor for drug-related retinopathy and periodic hematologic evaluation.

GRAFT-VERSUS-HOST DISEASE

Graft-versus-host disease (GVHD) occurs mainly in recipients of allogeneic bone marrow transplantation, a procedure performed on approximately 4000 patients in the United States each year. Such transplants are performed at major medical centers to treat life-threatening diseases of the blood or bone marrow, such as leukemia, lymphoma, multiple myeloma, aplastic anemia, thalassemia, sickle cell anemia, or disseminated metastatic disease. Cytotoxic drugs, radiation, or both may be used to destroy the malignant cells, but in the process the normal hematopoietic cells of the patient are destroyed. To provide the patient with an immune system, an HLA-matched donor must be found. The donor supplies hematopoietic stem cells obtained from bone marrow, peripheral blood, or umbilical cord blood. These stem cells are transfused into the patient, whose own hematopoietic and immune cells have been destroyed. The transfused hematopoietic cells make their way to the recipient's bone marrow and begin to reestablish normal function.

Unfortunately, the HLA match is not always exact, and despite the use of immunomodulating and immunosuppressive drugs, such as cyclosporine, methotrexate, and prednisone, the engrafted cells often recognize that they are not in their own environment. When this happens, these cells start attacking what they perceive as a foreign body. The result of this attack is GVHD, and it can be quite devastating to the patient.

In recent years, oncologists have taken advantage of this type of immunologic attack when treating leukemia patients, and often a beneficial "graft-versus-leukemia" effect is seen when the donor cells interpret the leukemic cells as being foreign. For older patients, who tend to have more significant side effects with traditional bone marrow transplantation, the concept of a "miniallograft" has been developed. Not all of the patient's white blood cells (WBCs) are destroyed in this procedure, which is also known as *nonmyeloablative allogenic hematopoietic cell transplantation,* to allow the donor cells to mount a more aggressive assault on the patient's leukemic cells.

Autologous stem cell transplantation has also become an increasingly popular method of treatment for some of these life-threatening diseases. Because these cells are derived from the patient, there is no risk of GVHD in this setting.

CLINICAL FEATURES

The systemic signs of GVHD are varied, depending on the organ system involved and whether the problem is acute or chronic. The severity of GVHD depends on several factors, with milder disease seen in patients who have a better histocompatibility match, are younger, have received cord blood, and are female.

Acute GVHD is typically observed within the first few weeks after bone marrow transplantation. Although acute GVHD has arbitrarily been defined as occurring within 100 days after the procedure, most investigators make this diagnosis based on the clinical features rather than a specific time point. The disease affects about 50% of bone marrow transplant patients. The skin lesions that develop may range from a mild rash to a diffuse severe sloughing that resembles toxic epidermal necrolysis (see page 777). These signs may be accompanied by diarrhea, nausea, vomiting, abdominal pain, and liver dysfunction.

Chronic GVHD may represent a continuation of a previously diagnosed case of acute GVHD, or it may develop later than 100 days after bone marrow transplantation, sometimes not appearing for several years after the procedure. Chronic GVHD can be expected to develop in 30% to 70% of bone marrow transplant recipients, and it often mimics any one of a variety of autoimmune conditions, such as systemic lupus erythematosus (SLE), Sjögren syndrome, or primary biliary cirrhosis. Skin involvement, which is the most common manifestation, may resemble lichen planus or even systemic sclerosis.

The oral mucosal manifestations of GVHD can also vary, depending on the duration and severity of the attack and the targeted oral tissues. Of patients with acute GVHD, 33% to 75% will have oral involvement; of patients with chronic GVHD, 80% or more will have oral lesions. Sometimes the oral lesions of GVHD are the only sign of the disorder. In most patients with oral GVHD, there is a fine, reticular network of white striae that resembles oral lichen planus, although a more diffuse pattern of pinpoint white papules has also been described (Figs. 16-107 to 16-109). The tongue, the labial mucosa, and the buccal mucosa are the oral mucosal sites most frequently involved. Patients often complain of a burning sensation of the oral mucosa, and care must be taken not to overlook possible candidiasis. Atrophy of the oral mucosa may be present, and this can contribute to the mucosal discomfort. Ulcerations that are related to the chemotherapeutic conditioning and neutropenic state of the patient often develop during the first 2 weeks after bone marrow transplantation. Ulcers that persist longer than 2 weeks

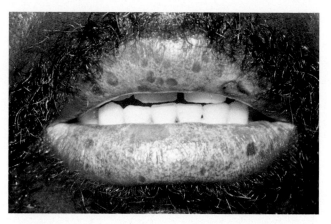

Fig. 16-107   Graft-versus-host disease (GVHD). Confluent, interlacing white linear lesions of the vermilion zone superficially resemble oral lichen planus.

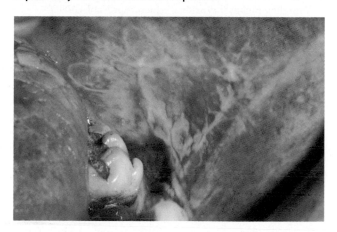

Fig. 16-108   Graft-versus-host disease (GVHD). Lichenoid lesions of the left buccal mucosa.

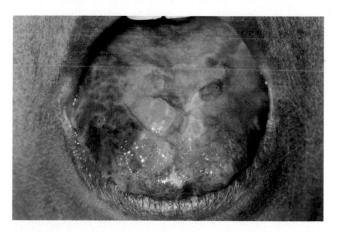

Fig. 16-109   Graft-versus-host disease (GVHD). Involvement of the tongue showing erosions and ulcerations that resemble erosive lichen planus.

may represent acute GVHD, and these should be differentiated from intraoral herpesvirus infection or bacterial infection. Bone marrow transplant patients have a small but increased risk for the development of both oral and cutaneous epithelial dysplasia and squamous

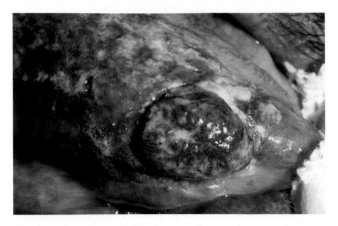

Fig. 16-110   Squamous cell carcinoma arising in graft-versus-host disease (GVHD). Erythematous, ulcerated mass arising on the lateral border of the tongue. Note the surrounding mucosal erosions, which represent GVHD.

cell carcinoma. Demarcated white or red plaques of the oral mucosa that do not have the characteristic lichenoid features should be biopsied to rule out preneoplastic or neoplastic changes (Fig. 16-110).

Xerostomia is also a common complaint. If the patient is not taking drugs that dry the mouth, it is likely that the immunologic response is destroying the salivary gland tissue. Other evidence of salivary gland involvement includes the development of small superficial mucoceles, particularly on the soft palate.

HISTOPATHOLOGIC FEATURES

The histopathologic features of GVHD resemble those of oral lichen planus to a certain degree. Both lesions display hyperorthokeratosis, short and pointed rete ridges, and degeneration of the basal cell layer. The inflammatory response in GVHD is usually not as intense as in lichen planus. With advanced cases, an abnormal deposition of collagen is present, similar to the pattern in systemic sclerosis. Minor salivary gland tissue usually shows periductal inflammation in the early stages, with gradual acinar destruction and extensive periductal fibrosis appearing later.

DIAGNOSIS

The diagnosis of GVHD may be difficult because of the varied clinical manifestations. Such a diagnosis is of great clinical significance to the patient because complications of the condition and its treatment may be lethal. Although the diagnosis of GVHD is based on the clinical and histopathologic findings, each patient may have a different constellation of signs and symptoms. Oral lesions appear to have value as a highly predictive index of the presence of GVHD.

TREATMENT AND PROGNOSIS

The primary strategy for dealing with GVHD is to reduce or prevent its occurrence. Careful tissue histocompatibility matching is performed, and the patient is given prophylactic therapy with immunomodulatory and immunosuppressive agents, such as prednisone in combination with either cyclosporine or tacrolimus. If GVHD develops, then the doses of these drugs may be increased or similar pharmacologic agents, such as mycophenolate mofetil, or azathioprine, may be added. The drug thalidomide has shown some promise for cases of chronic GVHD that have been resistant to standard therapy.

Topical corticosteroids may facilitate the healing of focal oral ulcerations associated with GVHD. Topical anesthetic agents are administered to provide patient comfort while the lesions are present, although narcotic analgesics may be required in some cases. Several case reports have described the efficacy of topical tacrolimus for management of oral ulceration caused by GVHD. The use of **p**soralen and **u**ltraviolet **A** (PUVA) therapy also has been shown to improve the cutaneous and oral lesions of patients with the lichenoid form of GVHD. If significant xerostomia is present in a dentulous patient, then topical fluorides should be used daily to prevent xerostomia-related caries. If significant amounts of salivary acinar tissue remain, then treatment with pilocarpine hydrochloride or cevimeline hydrochloride may improve the salivary flow. Current recommendations are to evaluate the oral status of patients before bone marrow transplantation and eliminate any potential sources of infection. Interestingly, one recent study showed no differences in posttransplant infections or survival between a group of patients who received dental treatment before their transplant and a group who did not.

In general, some degree of GVHD is expected in most allogeneic bone marrow transplant recipients. The prognosis depends on the extent to which the condition progresses and whether or not it can be controlled. The significance of this complication is reflected in the survival of more than 70% of patients with relatively mild GVHD at 6 years posttransplant, compared with approximately 15% of patients with severe GVHD.

PSORIASIS

Psoriasis is a common chronic skin disease affecting approximately 2% of people in the United States. According to some estimates, roughly 6 million people in this country have psoriasis, and up to 250,000 new cases are diagnosed each year.

Psoriasis is characterized by an increased proliferative activity of the cutaneous keratinocytes. Recent advances in cell kinetics, immunology, and molecular biology have increased the understanding of the etiopathogenesis of the keratinocyte proliferation in this disorder. Although the triggering agent has yet to be identified, activated T lymphocytes appear to orchestrate a complex scenario that includes abnormal production of cytokines, adhesion molecules, chemotactic polypeptides, and growth factors. Genetic factors also seem to play a role, because as many as one third of these patients have affected relatives. Currently nine different genetic loci have been identified that may be related to the development of psoriasis. Yet, if one twin in a set of identical twins has psoriasis, there is only a 35% chance that the other twin will have it. This suggests that genetic factors are not entirely responsible for the condition, and that one or more unidentified environmental agents must influence its pathogenesis.

CLINICAL FEATURES

Psoriasis often has its onset during the second or third decade of life and tends to persist for years, with periods of exacerbation and quiescence. Patients often report that the lesions improve during the summer and worsen during the winter, an observation that may be related to lesional exposure to ultraviolet (UV) light. The lesions are often symmetrically distributed in certain favored locations, such as the scalp, elbows, and knees. The classic description is a well-demarcated, erythematous plaque with a silvery scale on its surface (Fig. 16-111). The lesions are often asymptomatic, but it is not unusual for a patient to complain of itching—in fact, the term *psoriasis* is derived from the Greek word for itching. An unfortunate complication affecting approximately 11% of these patients is **psoriatic arthritis**, which may involve the TMJ.

Oral lesions may occur in patients with psoriasis, but they are distinctly uncommon. Because descriptions of these lesions have ranged from white plaques to red plaques to ulcerations, it is difficult to determine the true nature of intraoral psoriasis (Fig. 16-112). To render a diagnosis of intraoral psoriasis, some investigators say that the activity of the oral lesions should parallel that of the cutaneous lesions. Some authors refer to **erythema migrans** (see page 779) as *intraoral psoriasis*, and the prevalence of erythema migrans in psoriatic patients appears to be slightly greater than that seen in the rest of the population. It is difficult, however, to prove a direct correlation of that common mucosal alteration with psoriasis.

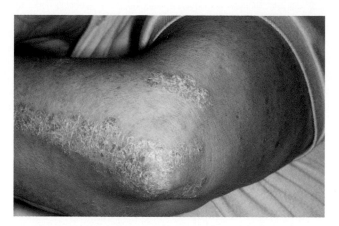

Fig. 16-111   Psoriasis. Characteristic cutaneous lesions on the skin of the elbow. Note the erythematous plaques surmounted by silvery keratotic scales.

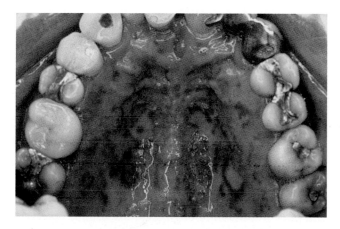

Fig. 16-112   Psoriasis. This is an example of relatively rare involvement of the oral mucosa by psoriasis. The erythematous linear patches tended to flare with the patient's cutaneous lesions. *(Courtesy of Dr. George Blozis.)*

HISTOPATHOLOGIC FEATURES

Microscopically, psoriasis has a characteristic pattern. The surface epithelium shows marked parakeratin production, and the epithelial rete ridges are elongated (Fig. 16-113). The connective tissue papillae, which contain dilated capillaries, approach close to the epithelial surface, and a perivascular chronic inflammatory cell infiltrate is present. In addition, collections of neutrophils (**Munro abscesses**), are seen within the parakeratin layer.

With respect to oral lesions, good correlation with skin disease activity should be seen in addition to the characteristic histopathologic features, because other intraoral lesions, such as erythema migrans and oral mucosal cinnamon reaction (see page 352), exhibit a psoriasiform microscopic appearance.

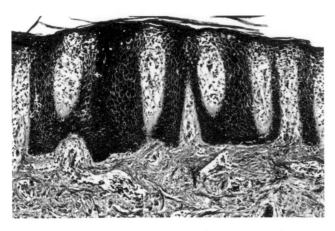

Fig. 16-113   Psoriasis. Low-power photomicrograph showing elongation of the rete ridges, hyperkeratosis, and inflammation of the papillary dermis.

TREATMENT AND PROGNOSIS

The treatment of psoriasis depends on the severity of the disease activity. For mild lesions, no treatment may be necessary.

For moderate involvement, topical corticosteroids are commonly prescribed in the United States. Coal tar derivatives and keratolytic agents also may be used. Other topical drugs that have proven effective include calcipotriene, a vitamin D_3 analog, and tazarotene, a retinoid (vitamin A) compound. Newer topical biologic agents include the calcineurin inhibitors, tacrolimus and pimecrolimus, although these are usually reserved for recalcitrant lesions. Exposure to UV radiation may also be helpful for mild to moderate disease.

For severe cases, **p**soralen and **u**ltraviolet **A** (PUVA) therapy or ultraviolet B (UVB) therapy may be needed. Methotrexate or cyclosporine may also be used as systemic treatments for severe disease; however, these drugs have significant side effects. Newer systemic biologic agents that target specific disease-related components include infliximab and etanercept (directed against tumor necrosis factor-α [TNF-α]) or alefacept and efalizumab (directed against T-cell receptors).

Although the mortality rate is not increased in patients with psoriasis, the condition often persists for years despite therapy. Some studies have shown a modest increase in the risk for cutaneous squamous cell carcinoma in psoriasis patients, possibly related to their PUVA or methotrexate therapy.

LUPUS ERYTHEMATOSUS

Lupus erythematosus (LE) is a classic example of an immunologically mediated condition, and is the most common of the so-called collagen vascular or connective tissue diseases in the United States, with more than 1.5 million people affected. It may exhibit any one of several clinicopathologic forms.

Systemic lupus erythematosus (SLE) is a serious multisystem disease with a variety of cutaneous and oral manifestations. There is an increase in the activity of the humoral limb (B lymphocytes) of the immune system in conjunction with abnormal function of the T lymphocytes. Although genetic factors probably play a role in the pathogenesis of SLE, the precise cause is unknown. Undoubtedly, interplay between genetic and environmental factors occurs, for if SLE develops in one monozygotic (identical) twin, then the other twin has a 24% chance of having SLE as well. In contrast, if one dizygotic (fraternal) twin has SLE, then the other twin has only a 2% chance of being affected.

Chronic cutaneous lupus erythematosus (CCLE) may represent a different, but related, process. It primarily affects the skin and oral mucosa, and the prognosis is good.

Subacute cutaneous lupus erythematosus (SCLE) is a third form of the disease, which has clinical features intermediate between those of SLE and CCLE.

CLINICAL FEATURES
SYSTEMIC LUPUS ERYTHEMATOSUS

SLE can be a very difficult disease to diagnose in its early stages because it often appears in a nonspecific, vague fashion, frequently with periods of remission or disease inactivity. Women are affected nearly 8 to 10 times more frequently than men. The average age at diagnosis is 31 years. Common findings include fever, weight loss, arthritis, fatigue, and general malaise. In 40% to 50% of affected patients, a characteristic rash, having the pattern of a butterfly, develops over the malar area and nose (Fig. 16-114), typically sparing the nasolabial folds. Sunlight often makes the lesions worse.

The kidneys are affected in approximately 40% to 50% of SLE patients. This complication may ultimately lead to kidney failure; thus it is typically the most significant aspect of the disease.

Cardiac involvement is also common, with pericarditis being the most frequent complication. At autopsy nearly 50% of SLE patients display warty vegetations affecting the heart valves **(Libman-Sacks endocarditis)**. Its significance is debatable, although some patients may develop superimposed subacute bacterial endocarditis on these otherwise sterile outgrowths of fibrinoid material and connective tissue cells.

Oral lesions of SLE develop in 5% to 25% of these patients, although some studies indicate prevalence as high as 40%. The lesions usually affect the palate, buccal mucosa, and gingivae. Sometimes they appear as lichenoid areas, but they may also look nonspecific or even somewhat granulomatous (Fig. 16-115). Involve-

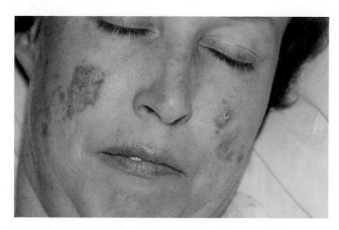

Fig. 16-114   Systemic lupus erythematosus (SLE). The erythematous patches seen in the malar regions are a characteristic sign.

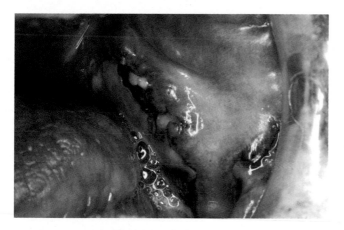

Fig. 16-115   Systemic lupus erythematosus (SLE). Irregularly shaped ulcerations of the buccal mucosa.

ment of the vermilion zone of the lower lip **(lupus cheilitis)** is sometimes seen. Varying degrees of ulceration, pain, erythema, and hyperkeratosis may be present. Other oral complaints such as xerostomia, stomatodynia, candidiasis, periodontal disease, and dysgeusia have been described, but the direct association of these problems with SLE remains to be proven.

Confirming the diagnosis of SLE can often be difficult, particularly in the early stages. Criteria for making the diagnosis of SLE have been established by the American Rheumatism Association, and these include both clinical and laboratory findings (Table 16-4).

CHRONIC CUTANEOUS LUPUS ERYTHEMATOSUS

Patients with CCLE usually have few or no systemic signs or symptoms, with lesions being limited to skin or mucosal surfaces. The skin lesions of CCLE most commonly present as **discoid lupus erythematosus**. They begin as scaly, erythematous patches that are frequently distributed on sun-exposed skin, especially in the head and neck area (Fig. 16-116). Patients may

Table 16-4   Prevalence of Clinical and Laboratory Manifestations of Systemic Lupus Erythematosus

Findings	Affected Patients (%)
SYSTEMIC SIGNS AND SYMPTOMS: FATIGUE, MALAISE, FEVER, ANOREXIA, WEIGHT LOSS	95%
MUSCULOSKELETAL SYMPTOMS	95%
Arthralgia/myalgia	95%
Nonerosive polyarthritis	60%
CUTANEOUS SIGNS	80%
Photosensitivity	70%
Malar rash	50%
Oral ulcers	40%
Discoid rash	20%
HEMATOLOGIC SIGNS	85%
Anemia (chronic disease)	70%
Leukopenia (<4000/μL)	65%
Lymphopenia (<1500/μL)	50%
Thrombocytopenia (<100,000/μL)	15%
Hemolytic anemia	10%
NEUROLOGIC SIGNS AND SYMPTOMS	60%
Cognitive disorder	50%
Headache	25%
Seizures	20%
CARDIOPULMONARY SIGNS	60%
Pleurisy, pericarditis, effusions	30%-50%
Myocarditis, endocarditis	10%
RENAL SIGNS	30%-50%
Proteinuria >500 mg/24 hours, cellular casts	30%-50%
Nephrotic syndrome	25%
End-stage renal disease	5%-10%

Adapted from Hahn BH: Systemic lupus erythematosus. In Kasper DL, Braunwald E, Fanci AS et al, editors: *Harrison's principles of internal medicine,* ed 16, pp 1960-1967, New York, 2005, McGraw-Hill. Reproduced with permission of The McGraw-Hill Companies.

indicate that the lesions are exacerbated by sun exposure. With time, the lesions may heal spontaneously in one area, only to appear in another area. The healing process usually results in cutaneous atrophy with scarring and hypopigmentation or hyperpigmentation of the resolving lesion. Conjunctival involvement by CCLE has rarely been reported to cause cicatrizing conjunctivitis, clinically similar to mucous membrane pemphigoid.

In most cases the oral manifestations of CCLE essentially appear clinically identical to the lesions

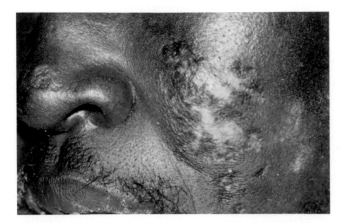

Fig. 16-116   Chronic cutaneous lupus erythematosus (CCLE). The skin lesions are characterized by scaling, atrophy, and pigmentary disturbances, which are most evident on sun-exposed skin.

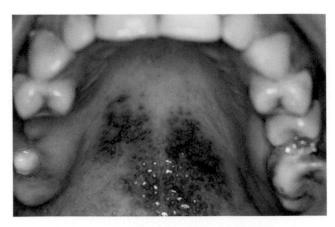

Fig. 16-118   Chronic cutaneous lupus erythematosus (CCLE). Oral involvement may also include relatively nondescript erythematous patches, such as this one in the palate.

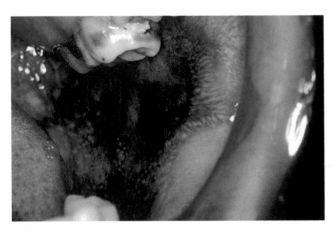

Fig. 16-117   Chronic cutaneous lupus erythematosus (CCLE). Radiating keratotic striae surround erythematous zones of the buccal mucosa. These features are similar to those of erosive lichen planus.

of erosive lichen planus. Unlike the oral lesions of lichen planus, however, the oral lesions of CCLE seldom occur in the absence of skin lesions. An ulcerated or atrophic, erythematous central zone, surrounded by white, fine, radiating striae, characterizes the oral lesion of CCLE (Figs. 16-117 and 16-118). Sometimes the erythematous, atrophic central region of a lesion may show a fine stippling of white dots. As with erosive lichen planus, the ulcerative and atrophic oral lesions of CCLE may be painful, especially when exposed to acidic or salty foods.

SUBACUTE CUTANEOUS LUPUS ERYTHEMATOSUS

Patients with SCLE have clinical manifestations intermediate between those of SLE and CCLE. The skin lesions are the most prominent feature of this varia-

tion. They are characterized by photosensitivity and are, therefore, generally present in sun-exposed areas. These lesions do not show the induration and scarring seen with the skin lesions of CCLE. Usually, the renal or neurologic abnormalities associated with SLE are not present either, with most patients having arthritis or musculoskeletal problems. SCLE may be triggered by any one of a variety of medications (see page 347).

HISTOPATHOLOGIC FEATURES

The histopathologic features of the skin and oral lesions of the various forms of LE show some features in common but are different enough to warrant separate discussions.

The skin lesions of CCLE are characterized by hyperkeratosis, often displaying keratin packed into the openings of hair follicles ("follicular plugging"). In all forms of LE, degeneration of the basal cell layer is frequently observed, and the underlying connective tissue supports patchy to dense aggregates of chronic inflammatory cells (Figs. 16-119 and 16-120). In the deeper connective tissue, the inflammatory infiltrate often surrounds the small blood vessels.

The oral lesions demonstrate hyperkeratosis, alternating atrophy and thickening of the spinous cell layer, degeneration of the basal cell layer, and subepithelial lymphocytic infiltration. These features may also be seen in oral lichen planus; however, the two conditions can usually be distinguished by the presence in LE of patchy deposits of a periodic acid-Schiff (PAS)-positive material in the basement membrane zone, subepithelial edema (sometimes to the point of vesicle formation), and a more diffuse, deep inflammatory infiltrate,

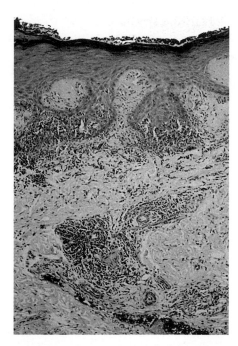

Fig. 16-119   Lupus erythematosus (LE). Low-power photomicrograph showing hyperparakeratosis with interface mucositis and perivascular inflammation.

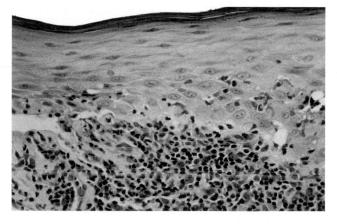

Fig. 16-120   Lupus erythematosus (LE). High-power photomicrograph of the interface mucositis.

often in a perivascular orientation. Some authorities, however, feel that differentiating lichen planus from LE is best done by direct immunofluorescence studies or histopathologic examination of the cutaneous lesions.

DIAGNOSIS

In addition to the clinical and microscopic features, a number of additional immunologic studies may be helpful in making the diagnosis of LE.

Direct immunofluorescence testing of lesional tissue shows deposition of one or more immunoreactants (usually IgM, IgG, or C3) in a shaggy or granular band at the basement membrane zone. In addition, direct immunofluorescence testing of clinically normal skin of SLE patients often shows a similar deposition of IgG, IgM, or complement components. This finding is known as a **positive lupus band test**. Although a positive lupus band test is consistent with the diagnosis of LE, it is now known that other conditions, such as rheumatoid arthritis, Sjögren syndrome, and systemic sclerosis, may also have similar positive findings. Furthermore, some patients with LE may not have a positive lupus band test; therefore, this study must always be interpreted in the context of other clinical signs.

Evaluation of serum obtained from a patient with SLE shows various immunologic abnormalities. Approximately 95% of these patients have antibodies directed against multiple nuclear antigens (i.e., antinuclear antibodies [ANAs]). Although this is a nonspecific finding that may be seen in other autoimmune diseases, as well as in otherwise healthy older individuals, it is nevertheless useful as a screening study. Furthermore, if results are negative on multiple occasions, then the diagnosis of SLE should probably be doubted. Antibodies directed against double-stranded DNA are noted in 70% of patients with SLE, and these are more specific for the disease. Another 30% of patients show antibodies directed against Sm, a protein that is complexed with small nuclear RNA. This finding is very specific for SLE.

A summary of selected immunologic findings in LE is shown in Table 16-5.

TREATMENT AND PROGNOSIS

Patients with SLE should avoid excessive exposure to sunlight because ultraviolet light may precipitate disease activity. Mild active disease may be effectively managed using nonsteroidal antiinflammatory drugs (NSAIDs) combined with antimalarial drugs, such as hydroxychloroquine. For more severe, acute episodes that involve arthritis, pericarditis, thrombocytopenia, or nephritis, systemic corticosteroids are generally indicated; these may be combined with other immunosuppressive agents. If oral lesions are present, they typically respond to the systemic therapy.

As with SLE patients, patients with CCLE should avoid excessive sunlight exposure. Because most of the manifestations of CCLE are cutaneous, topical corticosteroids are often reasonably effective. For cases that are resistant to topical therapy, systemic antimalarial drugs or low-dose thalidomide may produce a response. Topical corticosteroids are also helpful in treating the oral lesions of CCLE.

Table **16-5**   **Selected Abnormal Immunologic Findings in Lupus Erythematosus**

Findings	Frequency	Significance
Direct immunofluorescence, lesional skin	CCLE: 90% SLE: 95%	May help distinguish among the various types of LE
Direct immunofluorescence, normal skin	CCLE: 0% SLE: 25%-60%	Lupus band test
Antinuclear antibodies	CCLE: 0%-10% SLE: 95%	Very sensitive for SLE, but not very specific; not useful for CCLE diagnosis
Antidouble-stranded DNA antibodies	CCLE: 0% SLE: 70%-80%	Specific for SLE; may indicate disease activity or kidney involvement
Anti-Sm antibodies	CCLE: 0% SLE: 10%-30%	Specific for SLE

CCLE, Chronic cutaneous lupus erythematosus; *SLE,* systemic lupus erythematosus; *LE,* lupus erythematosus.

The prognosis for the patient with SLE is variable. For patients undergoing treatment today, the 5-year survival rate is approximately 82% to 90%; however, by 20 years, the survival rate falls to 63% to 75%. Ultimately, the prognosis depends on which organs are affected and how frequently the disease is reactivated. The most common cause of death is renal failure; however, chronic immunosuppression also predisposes these patients to increased mortality because of infection and development of malignancy. For reasons that are poorly understood, the prognosis is worse for men than for women. In addition, blacks tend to fare more poorly than whites.

The prognosis for patients with CCLE is considerably better than that for patients with SLE, although transformation to SLE may be seen in approximately 5% of CCLE patients. Usually, CCLE remains confined to the skin, but it may persist and be quite a nuisance. For about 50% of CCLE patients, the problem eventually resolves after several years.

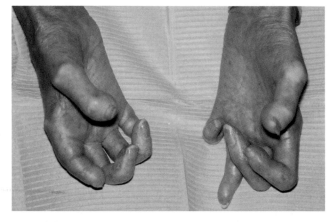

Fig. 16-121   Systemic sclerosis. The tense, shiny appearance of the skin is evident. Note that the fingers are fixed in a clawlike position, with some showing shortening as a result of acro-osteolysis.

SYSTEMIC SCLEROSIS (PROGRESSIVE SYSTEMIC SCLEROSIS; SCLERODERMA; HIDE-BOUND DISEASE)

Systemic sclerosis is a relatively rare condition that probably has an immunologically mediated pathogenesis. For reasons that are not understood, dense collagen is deposited in the tissues of the body in extraordinary amounts. Although its most dramatic effects are seen in association with the skin, the disease is often quite serious, with most organs of the body affected.

CLINICAL AND RADIOGRAPHIC FEATURES

Systemic sclerosis affects approximately 19 persons per million population each year. Women have the condition three to five times more frequently than do men. Most patients are adults. The onset of the disease is generally insidious, with the cutaneous changes often responsible for bringing the problem to the patient's attention.

Often one of the first signs of the disease is **Raynaud's phenomenon**, a vasoconstrictive event triggered by emotional distress or exposure to cold. Raynaud's phenomenon (see CREST syndrome, on page 801) is not specific for systemic sclerosis, however, because it may be present in other immunologically mediated diseases and in otherwise healthy people. Resorption of the terminal phalanges (**acro-osteolysis**) and flexion contractures produce shortened, clawlike fingers (Fig. 16-121). The vascular events and the abnormal collagen deposition contribute to the production of ulcerations on the fingertips (Fig. 16-122).

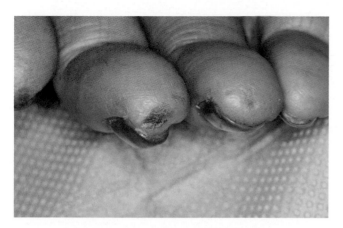

Fig. 16-122 **Systemic sclerosis.** Ulcerations of the fingertips.

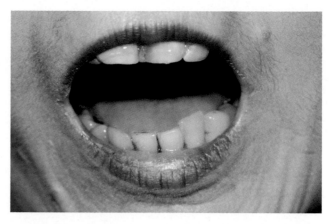

Fig. 16-124 **Systemic sclerosis.** Same patient as depicted in Fig. 16-123. Because of the associated microstomia, this is the patient's maximal opening.

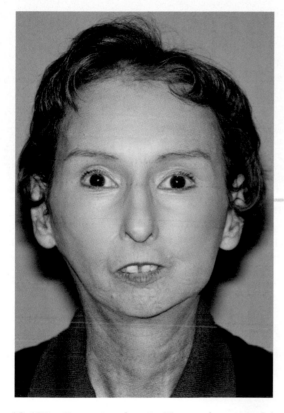

Fig. 16-123 **Systemic sclerosis.** The involvement of the facial skin with abnormal collagen deposition produces a masklike facies. Note the loss of the alae of the nose.

The skin develops a diffuse, hard texture (*sclero* = hard; *derma* = skin), and its surface is usually smooth. Involvement of the facial skin by subcutaneous collagen deposition results in the characteristic smooth, taut, masklike facies (Fig. 16-123). Similarly, the nasal alae become atrophied, resulting in a pinched appearance to the nose, called a *mouse facies*.

Involvement of other organs may be subtle at first, but the results are more serious. Fibrosis of the lungs, heart, kidneys, and gastrointestinal tract leads to organ failure, typically within the first 3 years after the diagnosis is made. Pulmonary fibrosis is particularly significant, leading to pulmonary hypertension and heart failure, a primary cause of death for these patients.

The oral manifestations occur in varying degrees. **Microstomia** often develops as a result of collagen deposition in the perioral tissues. This causes a limitation of opening the mouth in nearly 70% of these patients (Fig. 16-124). Characteristic furrows radiating from the mouth produce a "purse string" appearance. Loss of attached gingival mucosa and multiple areas of gingival recession may occur in some patients. Dysphagia often develops as a result of deposition of collagen in the lingual and esophageal submucosa, producing a firm, hypomobile (boardlike) tongue and an inelastic esophagus, thus hindering swallowing. Xerostomia is frequently identified in these patients, and the possibility of concurrent secondary Sjögren syndrome may require consideration.

On dental radiographs, diffuse widening of the periodontal ligament space is often present throughout the dentition. The extent of the widening may vary, with some examples being subtle and others quite dramatic (Fig. 16-125). Varying degrees of resorption of the posterior ramus of the mandible, the coronoid process, the chin, and the condyle may be detected on panoramic radiographs, affecting approximately 10% to 20% of patients (Fig. 16-126). In theory, these areas are resorbed because of the increased pressure associated with the abnormal collagen production. Individual tooth resorption has also been reported to occur at a higher frequency in these patients.

A mild variant of this condition, called **localized scleroderma**, usually affects only a solitary patch of skin. Because these lesions often look like scars, the name *en coup de sabre* ("strike of the sword") is used to describe them (Fig. 16-127). This problem is primarily cosmetic and, unlike systemic sclerosis, it is rarely life threatening.

HISTOPATHOLOGIC FEATURES

Microscopic examination of tissue involved by systemic sclerosis shows diffuse deposition of dense collagen within and around the normal structures (Fig. 16-128). This abnormal collagen replaces and destroys the normal tissue, causing the loss of normal tissue function.

DIAGNOSIS

During the early phases, it may be difficult to make a diagnosis of systemic sclerosis. Generally, the clinical signs of stiffened skin texture along with the development of Raynaud's phenomenon are suggestive of the diagnosis. A skin biopsy may be supportive of the diagnoses if abundant collagen deposition is observed microscopically.

Laboratory studies may be helpful to the diagnostic process if anticentromere antibodies or anti-Scl 70 (topoisomerase I) is detected. Antitopoisomerase I antibodies are seen more often with systemic sclerosis;

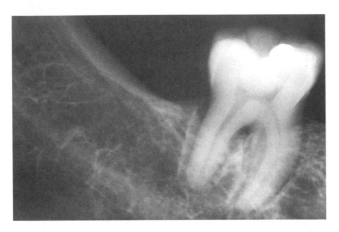

Fig. 16-125   Systemic sclerosis. Diffuse widening of the periodontal ligament space is often identified on evaluation of periapical radiographs.

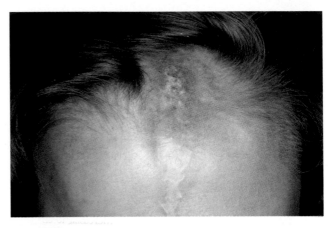

Fig. 16-127   Localized scleroderma. The cutaneous alteration on the patient's forehead represents a limited form of scleroderma called *en coup de sabre*, because the lesion resembles a scar that might result from a cut with a sword.

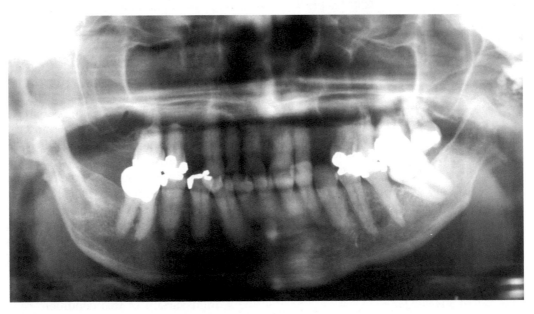

Fig. 16-126   Systemic sclerosis. Panoramic radiographic evaluation may show a characteristic resorption of the ramus, coronoid process, or condyle.

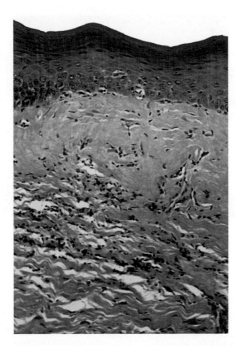

Fig. 16-128   Systemic sclerosis. Medium-power photomicrograph of an oral biopsy specimen. Diffuse deposition of collagen is apparent throughout the lamina propria.

anticentromere antibodies are usually associated with more limited forms of scleroderma or **CREST syndrome** (see next topic). In addition, increasing levels of endothelial cell autoantibodies appear to correlate with disease severity.

TREATMENT AND PROGNOSIS

The management of systemic sclerosis is difficult. Unfortunately, many of the recommended treatments have not been examined in controlled trials, and the natural waxing and waning course of the disease makes it difficult to assess the effectiveness of a given treatment in an open-label trial. Systemic medications, such as penicillamine, are prescribed in an attempt to inhibit collagen production. A recent double-blind study, however, showed no difference in measured patient outcomes with high-dose versus low-dose penicillamine, suggesting that perhaps this medication has limited efficacy. Surprisingly, corticosteroids are of little benefit. Extracorporeal photochemotherapy has shown some beneficial effect on the skin lesions; however, no improvement of the pulmonary function tests is observed.

Other management strategies are directed at controlling symptoms. Such techniques as esophageal dilation are used, for example, to temporarily correct the esophageal dysfunction and dysphagia. Calcium channel blocking agents help to increase peripheral blood flow and lessen the symptoms of Raynaud's phenomenon, but many patients can reduce episodes by keeping warm (especially their hands and feet) or by stopping cigarette smoking. Angiotensin-converting enzyme (ACE) inhibitors often effectively control hypertension if kidney involvement is prominent.

From a dental standpoint, problems may develop for patients who wear prostheses because of the microstomia and inelasticity of the mouth. Collapsible dental appliances with special hinges have been made to facilitate the insertion and removal of dentures. Microstomia and inelastic soft tissue also hamper the maintenance of good oral hygiene, and affected patients have a decreased ability to manipulate a toothbrush as a result of sclerotic changes in the fingers and hands. Surgical correction of open bite associated with condylar resorption has been described. Infrequently, the resorption of the mandible may become so great as to cause a pathologic fracture.

The prognosis is poor, although the outlook is better for patients with limited cutaneous involvement than for those with diffuse involvement. If the heart is affected, then the prognosis is particularly poor, but most patients die because of pulmonary involvement. Overall survival figures are difficult to calculate because of a variety of factors, including the rarity of the disease, the inherent variability of its natural course, and the variation in treatments provided at medical centers around the world. With current treatment regimens, it is estimated that 10-year survival rates for patients with limited cutaneous scleroderma approach 80% to 90%, whereas survival drops to 60% to 75% for patients with diffuse systemic sclerosis.

CREST SYNDROME (ACROSCLEROSIS; LIMITED SCLERODERMA)

CREST syndrome is an uncommon condition that may be a relatively mild variant of systemic sclerosis. The term *CREST* is an acronym for **C**alcinosis cutis, **R**aynaud's phenomenon, **E**sophageal dysfunction, **S**clerodactyly, and **T**elangiectasia.

CLINICAL FEATURES

As with systemic sclerosis, most patients with CREST syndrome are women in the sixth or seventh decade of life. The characteristic signs may not appear synchronously but instead may develop sequentially over a period of months to years.

Calcinosis cutis occurs in the form of movable, nontender, subcutaneous nodules, 0.5 to 2.0 cm in size, which are usually multiple (Fig. 16-129). Larger, more numerous or superficial calcifications may occasionally become bothersome and require removal.

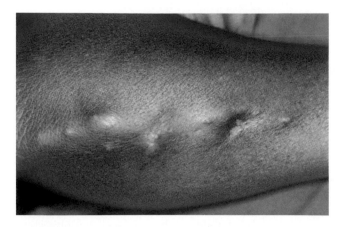

Fig. 16-129   CREST syndrome. The subcutaneous nodules on this patient's arm represent deposition of calcium salts (calcinosis cutis). *(Courtesy of Dr. Román Carlos.)*

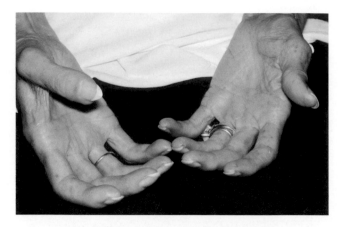

Fig. 16-130   CREST syndrome. Clawlike deformity affecting the hands (sclerodactyly).

Raynaud's phenomenon may be observed when a person's hands or feet are exposed to cold temperatures. The initial clinical sign is a dramatic blanching of the digits, which appear dead-white in color as a result of severe vasospasm. A few minutes later, the affected extremity takes on a bluish color because of venous stasis. After warming, increased blood flow results in a dusky-red hue with the return of hyperemic blood flow. This may be accompanied by varying degrees of throbbing pain.

Esophageal dysfunction, caused by abnormal collagen deposition in the esophageal submucosa, may not be noticeable in the early phases of CREST syndrome. Often the subtle initial signs of this problem must be demonstrated by barium swallow radiologic studies.

The **sclerodactyly** of CREST syndrome is rather remarkable. The fingers become stiff, and the skin takes on a smooth, shiny appearance. Often the fingers undergo permanent flexure, resulting in a characteristic "claw" deformity (Fig. 16-130). As with **systemic sclerosis**, this change is due to abnormal deposition of collagen within the dermis in these areas.

The **telangiectasias** in this syndrome are similar to those seen in hereditary hemorrhagic telangiectasia (HHT) (see page 754). As with that condition, significant bleeding from the superficial dilated capillaries may occur. The facial skin and the vermilion zone of the lips are commonly affected (Fig. 16-131).

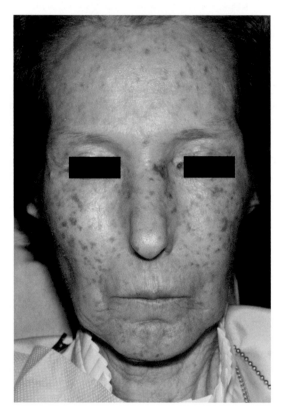

Fig. 16-131   CREST syndrome. The patient shows numerous red facial macules representing telangiectatic blood vessels.

if a telangiectatic vessel is included in the biopsy specimen.

HISTOPATHOLOGIC FEATURES

The histopathologic findings in CREST syndrome are similar, although milder, to those seen in systemic sclerosis. Superficial dilated capillaries are observed

DIAGNOSIS

Sometimes, HHT may be considered in the differential diagnosis if the history is unclear and the other signs of CREST syndrome are not yet evident. In these cases, laboratory studies directed at identifying anticentromere antibodies may be useful, because this test is relatively specific for CREST syndrome.

TREATMENT AND PROGNOSIS

The treatment of patients with CREST syndrome is essentially the same as that of those with systemic sclerosis. Because CREST syndrome usually is not as severe, the treatment does not have to be as aggressive. Although the prognosis for this condition is much better than that for systemic sclerosis, patients should be monitored for an increased risk of developing pulmonary hypertension or primary biliary cirrhosis, generally more than 10 years after the initial diagnosis.

ACANTHOSIS NIGRICANS

Acanthosis nigricans is an acquired dermatologic problem characterized by the development of a velvety, brownish alteration of the skin. In some instances, this unusual condition develops in conjunction with gastrointestinal cancer and is termed **malignant acanthosis nigricans**. The cutaneous lesion itself is benign, yet it is significant because it represents a cutaneous marker for internal malignancy. The cause of malignant acanthosis nigricans is unknown, although a cytokine-like peptide capable of affecting the epidermal cells may be produced by the malignancy.

Most cases, estimated to affect as many as 5% of adults, are not associated with a malignancy and are termed **benign acanthosis nigricans**. A clinically similar form, **pseudoacanthosis nigricans**, may occur in some obese people. Some benign forms of acanthosis nigricans may be inherited or may occur in association with various endocrinopathies, such as diabetes mellitus, Addison's disease, hypothyroidism, and acromegaly. Furthermore, benign acanthosis nigricans may occur with certain syndromes (e.g., Crouzon syndrome) or drug ingestion (e.g., oral contraceptives, corticosteroids). These forms of the condition are typically associated with resistance of the tissues to the effects of insulin, similar to the insulin resistance seen in non-insulin-dependent diabetes mellitus (NIDDM). Even though the affected individuals may not have overt diabetes mellitus, they often show increased levels of insulin or an abnormal response to exogenously administered insulin.

CLINICAL FEATURES

The malignant form of acanthosis nigricans develops in association with an internal malignancy, particularly adenocarcinoma of the gastrointestinal tract. Approximately 20% of the cases of malignant acanthosis nigri-

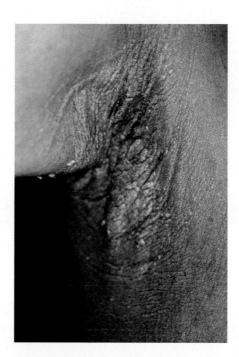

Fig. 16-132   Acanthosis nigricans. The lesions are characterized by numerous fine, almost velvety, confluent papules. The lesions most often affect the flexural areas, such as the axilla depicted in this photograph. *(From Hall JM, Moreland A, Cox GJ et al: Oral acanthosis nigricans: report of a case and comparison of oral and cutaneous pathology, Am J Dermatopathol 10:68-73, 1988.)*

cans are identified before the malignancy is found, but most appear at about the same time as discovery of the gastrointestinal tumor or thereafter.

Both forms of acanthosis nigricans affect the flexural areas of the skin predominantly, appearing as finely papillary, hyperkeratotic, brownish patches that are usually asymptomatic (Fig. 16-132). The texture of the lesions has been variably described as either velvety or leathery.

Oral lesions of acanthosis nigricans have also been reported and may occur in 25% to 50% of affected patients, especially those with the malignant form. These lesions appear as diffuse, finely papillary areas of mucosal alteration that most often involve the tongue or lips, particularly the upper lip (Figs. 16-133 and 16-134). The buccal mucosa may also be affected. The brownish pigmentation associated with the cutaneous lesions is usually not seen in oral acanthosis nigricans.

HISTOPATHOLOGIC FEATURES

The histopathologic features of the various forms of acanthosis nigricans are essentially identical. The epidermis exhibits hyperorthokeratosis and papillomatosis. Usually, some degree of increased melanin depo-

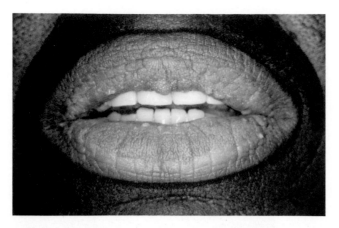

Fig. 16-133 Acanthosis nigricans. The vermilion zone of the lips is affected. *(Courtesy of Dr. George Blozis.)*

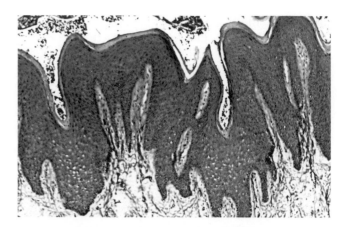

Fig. 16-135 Acanthosis nigricans. Medium-power photomicrograph of an oral lesion showing papillomatosis, mild hyperkeratosis, and acanthosis of the epithelium.

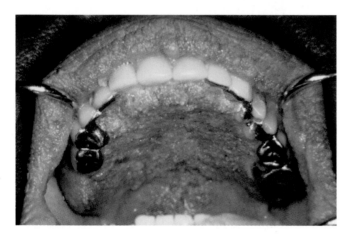

Fig. 16-134 Acanthosis nigricans. Same patient as depicted in Fig. 16-133. Note involvement of the palatal mucosa. *(Courtesy of Dr. George Blozis.)*

sition is noted, but the extent of acanthosis (thickening of the spinous layer) is really rather mild. The oral lesions have much more acanthosis, but show minimal increased melanin pigmentation (Fig. 16-135).

TREATMENT AND PROGNOSIS

Although acanthosis nigricans itself is a harmless process, the patient should be evaluated to ascertain which form of the disease is present. Identification and treatment of the underlying malignancy obviously are important for patients with the malignant type; unfortunately, the prognosis for these individuals is very poor. Interestingly, malignant acanthosis nigricans may resolve when the cancer is treated. Keratolytic agents may improve the appearance of the benign forms.

BIBLIOGRAPHY

Ectodermal Dysplasia

Aswegan AL, Josephson KD, Mowbray R et al: Autosomal dominant hypohidrotic ectodermal dysplasia in a large family, *Am J Med Genet* 72:462-467, 1997.

Berg D, Weingold DH, Abson KG et al: Sweating in ectodermal dysplasia syndromes, *Arch Dermatol* 126:1075-1079, 1990.

Bonilla ED, Guerra L, Luna O: Overdenture prosthesis for oral rehabilitation of hypohidrotic ectodermal dysplasia: a case report, *Quintessence Int* 28:657-665, 1997.

Cambiaghi S, Restano L, Paakkonen K et al: Clinical findings in mosaic carriers of hypohidrotic ectodermal dysplasia, *Arch Dermatol* 136:217-224, 2000.

Ho L, Williams MS, Spritz RA: A gene for autosomal dominant hypohidrotic ectodermal dysplasia (EDA3) maps to chromosome 2q11-q13, *Am J Hum Genet* 62:1102-1106, 1998.

Itin PH, Fistarol SK: Ectodermal dysplasias, *Am J Med Genet* 131C:45-51, 2004.

Jorgenson RJ, Salinas CF, Dowben JS et al: A population study on the density of palmar sweat pores, *Birth Defects Orig Artic Ser* 24:51-63, 1988.

Kantaputra PN, Hamada T, Kumchai T et al: Heterozygous mutation in the SAM domain of p63 underlies Rapp-Hodgkin ectodermal dysplasia, *J Dent Res* 82:433-437, 2003.

Kearns G, Sharma A, Perrott D et al: Placement of endosseous implants in children and adolescents with hereditary ectodermal dysplasia, *Oral Surg Oral Med Oral Pathol Oral Radiol Endod* 88:5-10, 1999.

Lamartine J: Towards a new classification of ectodermal dysplasias, *Clin Exp Dermatol* 28:351-355, 2003.

Levin LS: Dental and oral abnormalities in selected ectodermal dysplasia syndromes, *Birth Defects Orig Artic Ser* 24:205-227, 1988.

Lo Muzio L, Bucci P, Carile F et al: Prosthetic rehabilitation of a child affected from anhydrotic ectodermal dysplasia: a case report, *J Contemp Dent Pract* 6:1-7, 2005.

Mills R, Montague M-L, Naysmith L: Ear, nose and throat manifestations of ectodermal dysplasia, *J Laryngol Otol* 118:406-408, 2004.

Munoz F, Lestringant G, Sybert V et al: Definitive evidence for an autosomal recessive form of hypohidrotic ectodermal dysplasia clinically indistinguishable from the more common X-linked disorder, *Am J Hum Genet* 61:94-100, 1997.

Nordgarden H, Johannessen S, Storhaug K et al: Salivary gland involvement in hypohidrotic ectodermal dysplasia, *Oral Dis* 4:152-154, 1998.

Shankly PE, Mackie IC, McCord FJ: The use of tricalcium phosphate to preserve alveolar bone in a patient with ectodermal dysplasia: a case report, *Spec Care Dentist* 19:35-39, 1999.

Singh P, Warnakulasuriya S: Aplasia of submandibular salivary glands associated with ectodermal dysplasia, *J Oral Pathol Med* 33:634-636, 2004.

White Sponge Nevus

Jorgenson RJ, Levin LS: White sponge nevus, *Arch Dermatol* 117:73-76, 1981.

Krajewska IA, Moore L, Brown JH: White sponge nevus presenting in the esophagus—case report and literature review, *Pathology* 24:112-115, 1992.

Marcushamer M, King DL, McGuff S: White sponge nevus: case report, *Pediatr Dent* 17:458-459, 1995.

Martelli H, Mourão-Pereira S, Martins-Rocha T et al: White sponge nevus: report of a three-generation family, *Oral Surg Oral Med Oral Pathol Oral Radiol Endod* 103:43-47, 2007.

Morris R, Gansler TS, Rudisill MT et al: White sponge nevus: diagnosis by light microscopic and ultrastructural cytology, *Acta Cytol* 32:357-361, 1988.

Richard G, De Laurenzi V, Didona B et al: Keratin 13 point mutation underlies the hereditary mucosal disorder white sponge nevus, *Nat Genet* 11:453-455, 1995.

Rugg EL, Magee GJ, Wilson NJ et al: Identification of two novel mutations in keratin 13 as the cause of white sponge naevus, *Oral Dis* 5:321-324, 1999.

Rugg EL, McLean WHI, Allison WE et al: A mutation in the mucosal keratin K4 is associated with oral white sponge nevus, *Nat Genet* 11:450-452, 1995.

Terrinoni A, Candi E, Oddi S et al: A glutamine insertion in the 1A alpha helical domain of the keratin 4 gene in a familial case of white sponge nevus, *J Invest Dermatol* 114:388-391, 2000.

Terrinoni A, Rugg EL, Lane EB et al: A novel mutation in the keratin 13 gene causing oral white sponge nevus, *J Dent Res* 80:919-923, 2001.

Hereditary Benign Intraepithelial Dyskeratosis

McLean IW, Riddle PJ, Scruggs JH et al: Hereditary benign intraepithelial dyskeratosis. A report of two cases from Texas, *J Ophthalmol* 88:164-168, 1981.

Reed JW, Cashwell LF, Klintworth GK: Corneal manifestations of hereditary benign intraepithelial dyskeratosis, *Arch Ophthalmol* 97:297-300, 1979.

Sadeghi EM, Witkop CJ: The presence of *Candida albicans* in hereditary benign intraepithelial dyskeratosis: an ultrastructural observation, *Oral Surg Oral Med Oral Pathol* 48:342-346, 1979.

Shields CL, Shields JA, Eagle RC: Hereditary benign intraepithelial dyskeratosis, *Arch Ophthalmol* 105:422-423, 1987.

Pachyonychia Congenita

Feinstein A, Friedman J, Schewach-Millet M: Pachyonychia congenita, *J Am Acad Dermatol* 19:705-711, 1988.

García-Rio I, Peñas PF, García-Díez A et al: A severe case of pachyonychia congenital type I due to a novel praline mutation in keratin 6a, *Br J Dermatol* 152:800-802, 2005.

Leachman SA, Kaspar RL, Fleckman P et al: Clinical and pathological features of pachyonychia congenita, *J Investig Dermatol Symp Proc* 10:3-17, 2005.

McLean WHI, Rugg EL, Lunny DP et al: Keratin 16 and keratin 17 mutations cause pachyonychia congenita, *Nat Genet* 9:273-278, 1995.

Milstone LM, Fleckman P, Leachman SA et al: Treatment of pachyonychia congenita, *J Investig Dermatol Symp Proc* 10:18-20, 2005.

Pradeep AR, Nagaraja C: Pachyonychia congenita with unusual dental findings: a case report, *Oral Surg Oral Med Oral Pathol Oral Radiol Endod* 104:89-93, 2007.

Smith FJD, Liao H, Cassidy AJ et al: The genetic basis of pachyonychia congenita, *J Investig Dermatol Symp Proc* 10:21-30, 2005.

Smith FJD, McKusick VA, Nielsen K et al: Cloning of multiple keratin 16 genes facilitates prenatal diagnosis of pachyonychia congenita type 1, *Prenat Diag* 19:941-946, 1999.

Stieglitz JB, Centerwall WR: Pachyonychia congenita (Jadassohn-Lewandowsky syndrome): a seventeen member, four-generation pedigree with unusual respiratory and dental involvement, *Am J Med Genet* 14:21-28, 1983.

Dyskeratosis Congenita

Baykal C, Kavak A, Gülcan P et al: Dyskeratosis congenita associated with three malignancies, *J Eur Acad Dermatol Venereol* 17:216-218, 2003.

Davidovitch E, Eimerl D, Aker M et al: Dyskeratosis congenita: dental management of a medically complex child, *Pediatr Dent* 27:244-248, 2005.

Dokal I, Vulliamy T: Dyskeratosis congenita: its link to telomerase and aplastic anemia, *Blood Rev* 17:217-225, 2003.

Elliot AM, Graham GE, Bernstein M et al: Dyskeratosis congenita: an autosomal recessive variant, *Am J Med Genet* 83:178-182, 1999.

Fernandes-Gomes M, Pinheiro de Abreu P, de Freitas-Banzi ÉC et al: Interdisciplinary approach to treat dyskeratosis congenita associated with severe aplastic anemia: a case report, *Spec Care Dentist* 26:81-85, 2006.

Ghavamzadeh A, Alimoghadam K, Nasseri P et al: Correction of bone marrow failure in dyskeratosis congenita by bone marrow transplantation, *Bone Marrow Transplant* 23:299-301, 1999.

Handley TPB, McCaul JA, Ogden GR: Dyskeratosis congenita, *Oral Oncol* 42:331-336, 2006.

Handley TPB, Ogden GR: Dyskeratosis congenita: oral hyperkeratosis in association with lichenoid reaction, *J Oral Pathol Med* 35:508-512, 2006.

Hyodo M, Sadamoto A, Hinohira Y et al: Tongue cancer as a complication of dyskeratosis congenita in a woman, *Am J Otolaryngol* 20:405-407, 1999.

Kanegane H, Kasahara Y, Okamura J et al: Identification of DKC1 gene mutations in Japanese patients with X-linked dyskeratosis congenita, *Br J Haematol* 129:432-434, 2005.

Knight SW, Heiss NS, Vulliamy TJ et al: X-linked dyskeratosis congenita is predominantly caused by missense mutations in the DKC1 gene, *Am J Hum Genet* 65:50-58, 1999.

Marrone A, Mason PJ: Human genome and diseases: review. Dyskeratosis congenita, *Cell Mol Life Sci* 60:507-517, 2003.

Mason PJ, Wilson DB, Bessler M: Dyskeratosis congenita—a disease of dysfunctional telomere maintenance, *Curr Mol Med* 5:159-170, 2005.

Mitchell JR, Wood E, Collins K: A telomerase component is defective in the human disease dyskeratosis congenita, *Nature* 402:551-555, 1999.

Tanaka A, Kumagai S, Nakagawa K et al: Cole-Engman syndrome associated with leukoplakia of the tongue: a case report, *J Oral Maxillofac Surg* 57:1138-1141, 1999.

Vulliamy TJ, Marrone A, Knight SW et al: Mutations in dyskeratosis congenita: their impact on telomere length and the diversity of clinical presentation, *Blood* 107:2680-2685, 2006.

Vulliamy T, Dokal I: Dyskeratosis congenita, *Semin Hematol* 43:157-166, 2006.

Xeroderma Pigmentosum

Benhamou S, Sarasin A: Variability in nucleotide excision repair and cancer risk: a review, *Mutat Res* 462:149-158, 2000.

Cleaver JE: Common pathways for ultraviolet skin carcinogenesis in the repair and replication defective groups of xeroderma pigmentosum, *J Dermatol Sci* 23:1-11, 2000.

Cleaver JE: Cancer in xeroderma pigmentosum and related disorders of DNA repair, *Nature Rev* 5:564-573, 2005.

Goyal JL, Rao, VA, Srinivasan R et al: Oculocutaneous manifestations in xeroderma pigmentosa, *Br J Ophthalmol* 78:295-297, 1994.

Kraemer KH, Lee MM, Scotto J: Xeroderma pigmentosum: cutaneous, ocular, and neurologic abnormalities in 830 published cases, *Arch Dermatol* 123:241-250, 1987.

Magnaldo T, Sarasin A: Xeroderma pigmentosum: from symptoms and genetics to gene-based skin therapy, *Cells Tissues Organs* 177:189-198, 2004.

Park S, Dock M: Xeroderma pigmentosum: a case report, *Pediatr Dent* 25:397-400, 2003.

Patton LL, Valdez IH: Xeroderma pigmentosum: review and report of a case, *Oral Surg Oral Med Oral Pathol* 71:297-300, 1991.

van Steeg H, Kraemer KH: Xeroderma pigmentosum and the role of UV-induced DNA damage in skin cancer, *Mol Med Today* 5:86-94, 1999.

Hereditary Mucoepithelial Dysplasia

Boralevi F, Haftek M, Vabres P et al: Hereditary mucoepithelial dysplasia: clinical, ultrastructural and genetic study of eight patients and literature review, *Br J Dermatol* 153:310-318, 2005.

Rogers M, Kourt G, Cameron A: Hereditary mucoepithelial dysplasia, *Pediatr Dermatol* 11:133-138, 1994.

Scheman AJ, Ray DJ, Witkop CJ et al: Hereditary mucoepithelial dysplasia: case report and review of the literature, *J Am Acad Dermatol* 21:351-357, 1989.

Urban MD, Schosser R, Spohn W et al: New clinical aspects of hereditary mucoepithelial dysplasia, *Am J Med Genet* 39:338-341, 1991.

Witkop CJ, White JG, Sauk JJ et al: Clinical, histologic, cytologic and ultrastructural characteristics of the oral lesions from hereditary mucoepithelial dysplasia, *Oral Surg Oral Med Oral Pathol* 46:645-657, 1978.

Incontinentia Pigmenti

Bentolila R, Rivera H, Sanchez-Quevedo MC: Incontinentia pigmenti: a case report, *Pediatr Dent* 28:54-57, 2006.

Berlin AL, Paller AS, Chan LS: Incontinentia pigmenti: a review and update on the molecular basis of pathophysiology, *J Am Acad Dermatol* 47:169-187, 2002.

Bruckner AL: Incontinentia pigmenti: a window to the role of NF-κB function, *Semin Cutan Med Surg* 23:116-124, 2004.

Emery MM, Siegfried EC, Stone MS et al: Incontinentia pigmenti: transmission from father to daughter, *J Am Acad Dermatol* 29:368-372, 1993.

Faloyin M, Levitt J, Bercowitz E et al: All that is vesicular is not herpes: incontinentia pigmenti masquerading as herpes simplex virus in a newborn, *Pediatrics* 114:270-272, 2004.

Fusco F, Fimiani G, Tadini G et al: Clinical diagnosis of incontinentia pigmenti in a cohort of male patients, *J Am Acad Dermatol* 56:264-267, 2007.

Landy SJ, Donnai D: Incontinentia pigmenti (Bloch-Sulzberger syndrome), *J Med Genet* 30:53-59, 1993.

Pacheco TR, Levy M, Collyer JC et al: Incontinentia pigmenti in male patients, *J Am Acad Dermatol* 55:251-255, 2006.

Phan TA, Wargon O, Turner AM: Incontinentia pigmenti case series: clinical spectrum of incontinentia pigmenti in 53 female patients and their relatives, *Clin Exp Dermatol* 30:474-480, 2005.

Welbury TA, Welbury RR: Incontinentia pigmenti (Bloch-Sulzberger syndrome): report of a case, *ASDC J Dent Child* 66:213-215, 1999.

Darier's Disease

Adams AM, Macleod RI, Munro CS: Symptomatic and asymptomatic salivary duct abnormalities in Darier's disease: a sialographic study, *Dentomaxillofac Radiol* 23:25-28, 1994.

Burge SM, Wilkinson JD: Darier-White disease: a review of the clinical features in 163 patients, *J Am Acad Dermatol* 27:40-50, 1992.

Cooper SM, Burge SM: Darier's disease: epidemiology, pathophysiology, and management, *Am J Clin Dermatol* 4:97-105, 2003.

Dhitavat J, Dode L, Leslie N et al: Mutations in the sarcoplasmic/endoplasmic reticulum Ca²⁺ ATPase isoform cause Darier's disease, *J Invest Dermatol* 121:486-489, 2003.

Foggia L, Hovnanian A: Calcium pump disorders of the skin, *Am J Med Genet* 131C:20-31, 2004.

Frezzini C, Cedro M, Leao JC et al: Darier disease affecting the gingival and oral mucosal surfaces, *Oral Surg Oral Med Oral Pathol Oral Radiol Endod* 102:e29-e33, 2006.

Jalil AA, Zain RB, van der Waal I: Darier disease: a case report, *Br J Oral Maxillofac Surg* 43:336-338, 2005.

Macleod RI, Munro CS: The incidence and distribution of oral lesions in patients with Darier's disease, *Br Dent J* 171:133-136, 1991.

Munro CS: The phenotype of Darier's disease: penetrance and expressivity in adults and children, *Br J Dermatol* 127:126-130, 1992.

Sakuntabhai A, Ruiz-Perez V, Carter S et al: Mutations in ATP2A2, encoding a Ca²⁺ pump, cause Darier's disease, *Nat Genet* 21:271-277, 1999.

Sehgal VN, Srivastava G: Darier's (Darier-White) disease/keratosis follicularis, *Int J Dermatol* 44:184-192, 2005.

Zeglaoui F, Zaraa I, Fazaa B et al: Dyskeratosis follicularis disease: case reports and review of the literature, *J Eur Acad Dermatol Venereol* 19:114-117, 2005.

Warty Dyskeratoma

Chau MNY, Radden BG: Oral warty dyskeratoma, *J Oral Pathol* 13:546-556, 1984.

Kaddu S, Dong H, Mayer G et al: Warty dyskeratoma—"follicular dyskeratoma": analysis of clinicopathologic features of a distinctive follicular adnexal neoplasm, *J Am Acad Dermatol* 47:423-428, 2002.

Kaugars GE, Lieb RJ, Abbey LM: Focal oral warty dyskeratoma, *Int J Dermatol* 23:123-130, 1984.

Laskaris G, Sklavounou A: Warty dyskeratoma of the oral mucosa, *Br J Oral Maxillofac Surg* 23:371-375, 1985.

Mesa ML, Lambert WC, Schneider LC et al: Oral warty dyskeratoma, *Cutis* 33:293-296, 1984.

Peutz-Jeghers Syndrome

Giardiello FM, Trimbath JD: Peutz-Jeghers syndrome and management recommendations, *Clin Gastroenterol Hepatol* 4:408-415, 2006.

Hearle N, Schumacher V, Menko FH et al: Frequency and spectrum of cancers in the Peutz-Jeghers syndrome, *Clin Cancer Res* 12:3209-3215, 2006.

Hemminki A: The molecular basis and clinical aspects of Peutz-Jeghers syndrome, *Cell Mol Life Sci* 55:735-750, 1999.

Jenne DE, Reimann H, Nezu J-I et al: Peutz-Jeghers syndrome is caused by mutations in a novel serine threonine kinase, *Nat Genet* 18:38-43, 1998.

Le Meur N, Martin C, Saugier-Veber P et al: Complete germline deletion of the STK11 gene in a family with Peutz-Jeghers syndrome, *Eur J Human Genet* 12:415-418, 2004.

McGarrity TJ, Amos C: Peutz-Jeghers syndrome: clinicopathology and molecular alterations, *Cell Mol Life Sci* 63:2135-2144, 2006.

McGarrity TJ, Kulin HE, Zaino RJ: Peutz-Jeghers syndrome, *Am J Gastroenterol* 95:596-604, 2000.

Uno A, Hori Y: Disturbance of melanosome transfer in pigmented macules of Peutz-Jeghers syndrome. In Fitzpatrick TB et al: *Brown melanoderma*, pp 173-178, Tokyo, 1986, University of Tokyo Press.

Westerman AM, Entius MM, de Baar E et al: Peutz-Jeghers syndrome: 78-year follow-up of the original family, *Lancet* 353:1211-1215, 1999.

Hereditary Hemorrhagic Telangiectasia

Abdalla SA, Letarte M: Hereditary haemorrhagic telangiectasia: current views on genetics and mechanisms of disease, *J Med Genet* 43:97-110, 2006.

Abdalla SA, Pece-Barbara N, Vera S et al: Analysis of ALK-1 and endoglin in newborns from families with hereditary hemorrhagic telangiectasia type 2, *Hum Mol Genet* 9:1227-1237, 2000.

Bayrak-Toydemir P, McDonald J, Markewitz B et al: Genotype-phenotype correlation in hereditary hemorrhagic telangiectasia: mutations and manifestations, *Am J Med Genet* 140A:463-470, 2006.

Begbie ME, Wallace GMF, Shovlin CL: Hereditary haemorrhagic telangiectasia (Osler-Weber-Rendu syndrome): a view from the 21st century, *Postgrad Med J* 79:18-24, 2003.

Bergler W, Götte K: Hereditary hemorrhagic telangiectasias: a challenge for the clinician, *Eur Arch Otorhinolaryngol* 256:10-15, 1999.

Braveman IM, Keh A, Jacobson BS: Ultrastructure and three-dimensional organization of the telangiectases of hereditary hemorrhagic telangiectasia, *J Invest Dermatol* 95:422-427, 1990.

Cymerman U, Vera S, Pece-Barbara N et al: Identification of hereditary hemorrhagic telangiectasia type 1 in newborns by protein expression and mutation analysis of endoglin, *Pediatr Res* 47:24-35, 2000.

Fiorella ML, Ross D, Henderson KJ et al: Outcome of septal dermoplasty in patients with hereditary hemorrhagic telangiectasia, *Laryngoscope* 115:301-305, 2005.

Guttmacher AE, Marchuk DA, White RI: Hereditary hemorrhagic telangiectasia, *N Engl J Med* 333:918-924, 1995.

Hitchings AE, Lennox PA, Lund VJ et al: The effect of treatment for epistaxis secondary to hereditary hemorrhagic telangiectasia, *Am J Rhinol* 19:75-78, 2005.

Kjeldsen AD, Vase P, Green A: Hereditary haemorrhagic telangiectasia: a population-based study of prevalence and mortality in Danish patients, *J Intern Med* 245:31-39, 1999.

McAllister KA, Grogg KM, Johnson DW et al: Endoglin, a TGF-β binding protein of endothelial cells, is the gene for hereditary haemorrhagic telangiectasia type 1, *Nat Genet* 8:345-351, 1994.

Russi EW, Dazzi H, Gäumann N: Septic pulmonary embolism due to periodontal disease in a patient with hereditary hemorrhagic telangiectasia, *Respiration* 63:117-119, 1996.

Swanson DL, Dahl MV: Embolic abscesses in hereditary hemorrhagic telangiectasia, *J Am Acad Dermatol* 24:580-583, 1991.

Ehlers-Danlos Syndromes

Abel MD, Carrasco LR: Ehlers-Danlos syndrome: classifications, oral manifestations, and dental considerations, *Oral Surg Oral Med Oral Pathol Oral Radiol Endod* 102:582-590, 2006.

Beighton P, De Paepe A, Steinmann B et al: Ehlers-Danlos syndromes: revised nosology, Villefranche, 1997, *Am J Med Genet* 77:31-37, 1998.

Burrows NP: The molecular genetics of the Ehlers-Danlos syndrome, *Clin Exp Dermatol* 24:99-106, 1999.

De Coster PJ, Malfait F, Martens LC et al: Unusual oral findings in dermatosparaxis (Ehlers-Danlos syndrome type VIIC), *J Oral Pathol Med* 32:568-570, 2003.

De Coster PJ, Martens LC, De Paepe A: Oral health in prevalent types of Ehlers-Danlos syndromes, *J Oral Pathol Med* 34:298-307, 2005.

Dyne KM, Vitellaro-Zuccarello L, Bacchella L et al: Ehlers-Danlos syndrome type VIII: biochemical, stereological and immunocytochemical studies on dermis from a child with clinical signs of Ehlers-Danlos syndrome and a family history of premature loss of permanent teeth, *Br J Dermatol* 128:458-463, 1993.

Fridrich KL, Fridrich HH, Kempf KK et al: Dental implications in Ehlers-Danlos syndrome: a case report, *Oral Surg Oral Med Oral Pathol* 69:431-435, 1990.

Hartsfield JK, Kousseff BG: Phenotypic overlap of Ehlers-Danlos syndrome types IV and VIII, *Am J Med Genet* 37:465-470, 1990.

Malfait F, De Coster P, Hausser I et al: The natural history, including orofacial features of three patients with Ehlers-Danlos syndrome, dermatosparaxis type (EDS type VIIC), *Am J Med Genet* 131A:18-28, 2004.

Norton LA, Assael LA: Orthodontic and temporomandibular joint considerations in treatment of patients with Ehlers-Danlos syndrome, *Am J Orthod Dentofac Orthop* 111:75-84, 1997.

Nuytinck L, Freund M, Lagae L et al: Classical Ehlers-Danlos syndrome caused by a mutation in type I collagen, *Am J Hum Genet* 66:1398-1402, 2000.

Pepin M, Schwarze U, Superti-Furga A et al: Clinical and genetic features of Ehlers-Danlos syndrome type IV, the vascular type, *N Engl J Med* 342:673-680, 2000.

Pope FM, Komorowska A, Lee KW et al: Ehlers Danlos syndrome type I with novel dental features, *J Oral Pathol Med* 21:418-421, 1992.

Rahman N, Dunstan M, Teare MD et al: Ehlers-Danlos syndrome with severe early-onset periodontal disease (EDS-VIII) is a distinct, heterogeneous disorder with one predisposition gene at chromosome 12p13, *Am J Hum Genet* 73:198-204, 2003.

Sacks H, Zelig D, Schabes G: Recurrent temporomandibular joint subluxation and facial ecchymosis leading to diagnosis of Ehlers-Danlos syndrome: report of surgical management and review of the literature, *J Oral Maxillofac Surg* 48:641-647, 1990.

Yassin OM, Rihani FB: Multiple developmental dental anomalies and hypermobility type Ehlers-Danlos syndrome, *J Clin Pediatr Dent* 30:337-341, 2006.

Tuberous Sclerosis

Barron RP, Kainulainen VT, Forrest CR et al: Tuberous sclerosis: clinicopathologic features and review of the literature, *J Craniomaxillofac Surg* 30:361-366, 2002.

Çelenk P, Alkan A, Canger EM et al: Fibrolipomatous hamartoma in a patient with tuberous sclerosis: report of a case, *Oral Surg Oral Med Oral Pathol Oral Radiol Endod* 99:202-206, 2005.

Crino PB, Nathanson KL, Henske EP: The tuberous sclerosis complex, *N Engl J Med* 355:1345-1356, 2006.

Damm DD, Tomich CE, White DK et al: Intraosseous fibrous lesions of the jaws. A manifestation of tuberous sclerosis, *Oral Surg Oral Med Oral Pathol Oral Radiol Endod* 87:334-340, 1999.

Franz DN: Diagnosis and management of tuberous sclerosis complex, *Semin Pediatr Neurol* 5:253-268, 1998.

Franz DN: Non-neurologic manifestations of tuberous sclerosis complex, *J Child Neurol* 19:690-698, 2004.

Houser OW, Shepherd CW, Gomez MR: Imaging of intracranial tuberous sclerosis, *Ann N Y Acad Sci* 615:81-93, 1991.

Hurst JS, Wilcoski S: Recognizing an index case of tuberous sclerosis, *Am Fam Physician* 61:703-708, 710, 2000.

Hyman MH, Whittemore VH: National Institutes of Health consensus conference: tuberous sclerosis complex, *Arch Neurol* 57:662-665, 2000.

Jones AC, Shyamsundar MM, Thomas MW et al: Comprehensive mutation analysis of TSC1 and TSC2—and phenotypic correlations in 150 families with tuberous sclerosis, *Am J Hum Genet* 64:1305-1315, 1999.

Lendvay TS, Marshall FF: The tuberous sclerosis complex and its highly variable manifestations, *J Urol* 169:1635-1642, 2003.

Lygidakis NA, Lindenhum RH: Oral fibromatosis in tuberous sclerosis, *Oral Surg Oral Med Oral Pathol* 68:725-728, 1989.

O'Callaghan FJ, Osborne JP: Advances in the understanding of tuberous sclerosis, *Arch Dis Child* 83:140-142, 2000.

Roach ES, Sparagana SP: Diagnosis of tuberous sclerosis complex, *J Child Neurol* 19:643-649, 2004.

Rosser T, Panigrahy A, McClintock W: The diverse clinical manifestations of tuberous sclerosis complex: a review, *Semin Pediatr Neurol* 13:27-36, 2006.

Sampson JR, Attwood D, Al Mughery AS et al: Pitted enamel hypoplasia in tuberous sclerosis, *Clin Genet* 42:50-52, 1992.

Shepherd CW, Gomez MR: Mortality in the Mayo Clinic tuberous sclerosis complex study, *Ann N Y Acad Sci* 615:375-377, 1991.

Thomas D, Rapley J, Strathman R et al: Tuberous sclerosis with gingival overgrowth, *J Periodontol* 63:713-717, 1992.

Multiple Hamartoma Syndrome

Albrecht S, Haber RM, Goodman JC et al: Cowden syndrome and Lhermitte-Duclos disease, *Cancer* 70:869-876, 1992.

Bagan JV, Penarrocha M, Vera-Sempere F: Cowden syndrome: clinical and pathological considerations in two new cases, *J Oral Maxillofac Surg* 47:291-294, 1989.

Bonneau D, Longy M: Mutations of the human PTEN gene, *Hum Mutat* 16:109-122, 2000.

Devlin MF, Barrie R, Ward-Booth RP: Cowden's disease: a rare but important manifestation of oral papillomatosis, *Br J Oral Maxillofac Surg* 30:335-336, 1992.

Eng C: Genetics of Cowden syndrome: through the looking glass of oncology (Review), *Int J Oncol* 12:701-710, 1998.

Hand JL, Rogers RS: Oral manifestations of genodermatoses, *Dermatol Clin* 21:183-194, 2003.

Leão JC, Batista V, Guimarães PB et al: Cowden's syndrome affecting the mouth, gastrointestinal, and central nervous system: a case report and review of the literature, *Oral Surg Oral Med Oral Pathol Oral Radiol Endod* 99:569-572, 2005.

Mallory SB: Cowden syndrome (multiple hamartoma syndrome), *Dermatol Clin* 13:27-31, 1995.

Merks JHM, de Vries LS, Zhou X-P et al: PTEN hamartoma tumor syndrome: variability of an entity, *J Med Genet* 40:e111, 2003.

Mignogna MD, Lo Muzio L, Ruocco V et al: Early diagnosis of multiple hamartoma and neoplasia syndrome (Cowden disease). The role of the dentist, *Oral Surg Oral Med Oral Pathol Oral Radiol Endod* 79:295-299, 1995.

Nelen MR, Padberg GW, Peeters EAJ et al: Localization of the gene for Cowden disease to chromosome 10q22-23, *Nat Genet* 13:114-116, 1996.

Pilarski R, Eng C: Will the real Cowden syndrome please stand up (again)? Expanding mutational and clinical spectra of the PTEN hamartoma tumour syndrome, *J Med Genet* 41:323-326, 2004.

Porter S, Cawson R, Scully C et al: Multiple hamartoma syndrome presenting with oral lesions, *Oral Surg Oral Med Oral Pathol Oral Radiol Endod* 82:295-301, 1996.

Schaffer JV, Kamino H, Witkiewicz A et al: Mucocutaneous neuromas: an underrecognized manifestation of PTEN hamartoma-tumor syndrome, *Arch Dermatol* 142:625-632, 2006.

Scheper MA, Nikitakis NG, Sarlani E et al: Cowden syndrome: report of a case with immunohistochemical analysis and review of the literature, *Oral Surg Oral Med Oral Pathol Oral Radiol Endod* 101:625-631, 2006.

Takenoshita Y, Kubo S, Takeuchi T et al: Oral and facial lesions in Cowden's disease: report of two cases and a review of the literature, *J Oral Maxillofac Surg* 51:682-687, 1993.

Wright DD, Whitney J: Multiple hamartoma syndrome (Cowden's syndrome): case report and literature review, *Gen Dent* 54:417-419, 2006.

Epidermolysis Bullosa

Azrak B, Kaevel K, Hofmann L et al: Dystrophic epidermolysis bullosa: oral findings and problems, *Spec Care Dentist* 26:111-115, 2006.

Bello YM, Falabella AF, Schachner LA: Management of epidermolysis bullosa in infants and children, *Clin Dermatol* 21:278-282, 2003.

Brain JH, Paul BF, Assad DA: Periodontal plastic surgery in a dystrophic epidermolysis bullosa patient: review and case report, *J Periodontol* 70:1392-1396, 1999.

Bruckner-Tuderman L: Hereditary skin diseases of anchoring fibrils, *J Dermatol Sci* 20:122-133, 1999.

Çagirankaya LB, Hatipoglu MG, Hatipoglu H: Localized epidermolysis bullosa simplex with generalized enamel hypoplasia in a child, *Pediatr Dermatol* 23:167-168, 2006.

Das BB, Sahoo S: Dystrophic epidermolysis bullosa, *J Perinatol* 24:41-47, 2004.

De Benedittis M, Petruzzi M, Favia G et al: Oro-dental manifestations in Hallopeau-Siemens type recessive dystrophic epidermolysis bullosa, *Clin Exp Dermatol* 29:128-132, 2004.

Dunnill MGS, Eady RAJ: The management of dystrophic epidermolysis bullosa, *Clin Exp Dermatol* 20:179-188, 1995.

Fine J-D, Eady RAJ, Bauer EA et al: Revised classification system for inherited epidermolysis bullosa: report of the Second International Consensus Meeting on diagnosis and classification of epidermolysis bullosa, *J Am Acad Dermatol* 42:1051-1066, 2000.

Jonkman MF: Hereditary skin diseases of hemidesmosomes, *J Dermatol Sci* 20:103-121, 1999.

Lin AN: Management of patients with epidermolysis bullosa, *Dermatol Clin* 14:381-387, 1996.

Marinkovich MP: Update on inherited bullous dermatoses, *Dermatol Clin* 17:473-485, 1999.

McAllister JC, Marinkovich MP: Advances in inherited epidermolysis bullosa, *Adv Dermatol* 21:303-334, 2005.

McGrath JA, O'Grady A, Mayou BJ et al: Mitten deformity in severe generalized recessive dystrophic epidermolysis bullosa: histological, immunofluorescence, and ultrastructural study, *J Cutan Pathol* 19:385-389, 1992.

Momeni A, Pieper K: Junctional epidermolysis bullosa: a case report, *Int J Paediatr Dent* 15:146-150, 2005.

Mullett F: A review of the management of the hand in dystrophic epidermolysis bullosa, *J Hand Ther* 11:261-265, 1998.

Pai S, Marinkovich MP: Epidermolysis bullosa: new and emerging trends, *Am J Clin Dermatol* 3:371-380, 2002.

Pekiner FN, Yücelten D, Özbayrak S et al: Oral-clinical findings and management of epidermolysis bullosa, *J Clin Pediatr Dent* 30:59-66, 2005.

Pulkkinen L, Uitto J: Mutation analysis and molecular genetics of epidermolysis bullosa, *Matrix Biol* 18:29-42, 1999.

Serrano-Martínez MC, Bagán JV, Silvestre FJ et al: Oral lesions in recessive dystrophic epidermolysis bullosa, *Oral Dis* 9:264-268, 2003.

Silva LC, Cruz RA, Abou-Id LR et al: Clinical evaluation of patients with epidermolysis bullosa: review of the literature and case reports, *Spec Care Dentist* 24:22-27, 2004.

Uitto J: Molecular diagnostics of epidermolysis bullosa: novel pathomechanisms and surprising genetics, *Exp Dermatol* 8:92-95, 1999.

Uitto J, Richard G: Progress in epidermolysis bullosa: genetic classification and clinical implications, *Am J Med Genet* 131C:61-74, 2004.

Uitto J, Richard G: Progress in epidermolysis bullosa: from eponyms to molecular genetic classification, *Clin Dermatol* 23:33-40, 2005.

Wright JT: Oral manifestations of epidermolysis bullosa. In Fine J-D, Bauer EA, McGuire J et al, editors: *Epidermolysis bullosa. Clinical, epidemiologic, and laboratory advances and the findings of the National Epidermolysis Bullosa Registry*, pp 236-256, Baltimore and London, 1999, The Johns Hopkins University Press.

Pemphigus

Black M, Mignogna MD, Scully C: Pemphigus vulgaris, *Oral Dis* 11:119-130, 2005.

Brenner S, Bialy-Golan A, Ruocco V: Drug-induced pemphigus, *Clin Dermatol* 16:393-397, 1998.

Bystryn J-C, Rudolph JL: Pemphigus, *Lancet* 366:61-73, 2005.

Bystryn J-C, Rudolph JL: IVIg treatment of pemphigus: how it works and how to use it, *J Invest Dermatol* 125:1093-1098, 2005.

Calebotta A, Sáenz AM, González F et al: Pemphigus vulgaris: benefits of tetracycline as adjuvant therapy in a series of thirteen patients, *Int J Dermatol* 38:217-221, 1999.

Carson PJ, Hameed A, Ahmed AR: Influence of treatment on the clinical course of pemphigus vulgaris, *J Am Acad Dermatol* 34:645-652, 1996.

Dabelsteen E: Molecular biological aspects of acquired bullous diseases, *Crit Rev Oral Biol Med* 9:162-178, 1998.

Darling MR, Daley T: Blistering mucocutaneous diseases of the oral mucosa—a review: Part 2. Pemphigus vulgaris, *J Can Dent Assoc* 72:63-66, 2006.

Eisenberg E, Ballow M, Wolfe SH et al: Pemphigus-like mucosal lesions: a side effect of penicillamine therapy, *Oral Surg Oral Med Oral Pathol* 51:409-414, 1981.

El Tal AK, Posner MR, Spigelman Z et al: Rituximab: a monoclonal antibody to CD20 used in the treatment of pemphigus vulgaris, *J Am Acad Dermatol* 55:449-459, 2006.

Enk AH, Knop J: Mycophenolate is effective in the treatment of pemphigus vulgaris, *Arch Dermatol* 135:54-56, 1999.

Harman KE, Seed PT, Gratian MJ et al: The severity of cutaneous and oral pemphigus is related to desmoglein 1 and 3 antibody levels, *Br J Dermatol* 144:775-780, 2001.

Herbst A, Bystryn JC: Patterns of remission in pemphigus vulgaris, *J Am Acad Dermatol* 42:422-427, 2000.

Ioannides D, Chrysomallis F, Bystryn J-C: Ineffectiveness of cyclosporine as an adjuvant to corticosteroids in the treatment of pemphigus, *Arch Dermatol* 136:868-872, 2000.

Laforest C, Huilgol SC, Casson R et al: Autoimmune bullous diseases: ocular manifestations and management, *Drugs* 65:1767-1779, 2005.

Laskaris G, Stoufi E: Oral pemphigus vulgaris in a 6-year-old girl, *Oral Surg Oral Med Oral Pathol* 69:609-613, 1990.

Martel P, Joly P: Pemphigus: autoimmune diseases of keratinocyte's adhesion molecules, *Clin Dermatol* 19:662-674, 2001.

Mignogna MD, Lo Muzio L, Mignogna RE et al: Oral pemphigus: long term behaviour and clinical response to treatment with deflazacort in sixteen cases, *J Oral Pathol Med* 29:145-152, 2000.

Mignogna MD, Lo Muzio L, Bucci E: Clinical features of gingival pemphigus vulgaris, *J Clin Periodontol* 28:489-493, 2001.

Nousari HC, Anhalt GJ: Pemphigus and bullous pemphigoid, *Lancet* 354:667-672, 1999.

Scully C, Challacombe SJ: Pemphigus vulgaris: update on etiopathogenesis, oral manifestations, and management, *Crit Rev Oral Biol Med* 13:397-408, 2002.

Tóth GG, Jonkman MF: Therapy of pemphigus, *Clin Dermatol* 19:761-767, 2001.

Yeh SW, Sami N, Ahmed RA: Treatment of pemphigus vulgaris: current and emerging options, *Am J Clin Dermatol* 6:327-342, 2005.

Paraneoplastic Pemphigus

Ahmed AR, Avram MM, Duncan LM: Case 23-2003: a 79-year-old woman with gastric lymphoma and erosive mucosal and cutaneous lesions, *N Engl J Med* 349:382-391, 2003.

Allen CM, Camisa C: Paraneoplastic pemphigus: a review of the literature, *Oral Dis* 6:208-214, 2000.

Anhalt GJ: Paraneoplastic pemphigus, *J Investig Dermatol Symp Proc* 9:29-33, 2004.

Anhalt GJ, Kim SC, Stanley JR et al: Paraneoplastic pemphigus: an autoimmune mucocutaneous disease associated with neoplasia, *N Engl J Med* 323:1729-1735, 1990.

Billet SE, Grando SA, Pittelkow MR: Paraneoplastic autoimmune multiorgan syndrome: review of the literature and support for a cytotoxic role in pathogenesis, *Autoimmunity* 36:617-630, 2006.

Cummins DL, Mimouni D, Tzu J et al: Lichenoid paraneoplastic pemphigus in the absence of detectable antibodies, *J Am Acad Dermatol* 56:153-159, 2007.

Hashimoto T: Immunopathology of paraneoplastic pemphigus, *Clin Dermatol* 19:675-682, 2001.

Helm TN, Camisa C, Valenzuela R et al: Paraneoplastic pemphigus: a distinct autoimmune vesiculobullous disorder associated with neoplasia, *Oral Surg Oral Med Oral Pathol* 75:209-213, 1993.

Hoque SR, Black MM, Cliff S: Paraneoplastic pemphigus associated with CD20-positive follicular non-Hodgkin's lymphoma treated with rituximab: a third case resistant to rituximab therapy, *Clin Exp Dermatol* 32:172-175, 2007.

Kaplan I, Hodak E, Ackerman L et al: Neoplasms associated with paraneoplastic pemphigus: a review with emphasis on non-hematologic malignancy and oral mucosal manifestations, *Oral Oncol* 40:553-562, 2004.

Laforest C, Huilgol SC, Casson R et al: Autoimmune bullous diseases: ocular manifestations and management, *Drugs* 65:1767-1779, 2005.

Meyers SJ, Varley GA, Meisler DM et al: Conjunctival involvement in paraneoplastic pemphigus, *Am J Ophthalmol* 114:621-624, 1992.

Mimouni D, Anhalt GJ, Lazarova Z et al: Paraneoplastic pemphigus in children and adolescents, *Br J Dermatol* 147:725-732, 2002.

Nousari HC, Deterding R, Wojtczack H et al: The mechanism of respiratory failure in paraneoplastic pemphigus, *N Engl J Med* 340:1406-1410, 1999.

Nguyen VT, Ndoye A, Bassler KD et al: Classification, clinical manifestations, and immunopathological mechanisms of the epithelial variant of paraneoplastic autoimmune multiorgan syndrome: a reappraisal of paraneoplastic pemphigus, *Arch Dermatol* 137:193-206, 2001.

Schmidt E, Hunzelmann N, Zillikens D et al: Rituximab in refractory autoimmune bullous diseases, *Clin Exp Dermatol* 31:503-508, 2006.

Sklavounou A, Laskaris G: Paraneoplastic pemphigus: a review, *Oral Oncol* 35:437-440, 1998.

Van Rossum MM, Verhaegen NTM, Jonkman MF et al: Follicular non-Hodgkin's lymphoma with refractory paraneoplastic pemphigus: case report with review of novel treatment modalities, *Leuk Lymphoma* 45:2327-2332, 2004.

Yokokura H, Demitsu T, Kakurai M et al: Paraneoplastic pemphigus mimicking erosive mucosal lichen planus associated with primary hepatocellular carcinoma, *J Dermatol* 33:842-845, 2006.

Cicatricial Pemphigoid

Ahmed AR, Colón JE: Comparison between intravenous immunoglobulin and conventional immunosuppressive therapy regimens in patients with severe oral pemphigoid: effects on disease progression in patients nonresponsive to dapsone therapy, *Arch Dermatol* 137:1181-1189, 2001.

Ahmed M, Zein G, Khawaja F et al: Ocular cicatricial pemphigoid: pathogenesis, diagnosis and treatment, *Prog Retin Eye Res* 23:579-592, 2004.

Bagan J, Muzio LL, Scully C: Mucous membrane pemphigoid, *Oral Dis* 11:197-218, 2005.

Bhol KC, Goss L, Kumari S et al: Autoantibodies to human α6 integrin in patients with oral pemphigoid, *J Dent Res* 80:1711-1715, 2001.

Calabresi V, Carrozzo M, Cozzani E et al: Oral pemphigoid autoantibodies preferentially target BP180 ectodomain, *Clin Immunol* 122:207-213, 2007.

Casiglia J, Woo S-B, Ahmed AR: Oral involvement in autoimmune blistering diseases, *Clin Dermatol* 19:737-741, 2001.

Chaidemenos G: Tetracycline and niacinamide in the treatment of blistering skin diseases, *Clin Dermatol* 19:781-785, 2001.

Chan LS: Mucous membrane pemphigoid, *Clin Dermatol* 19:703-711, 2001.

Chan LS, Ahmed AR, Anhalt GJ et al: The first international consensus on mucous membrane pemphigoid: definition, diagnostic criteria, pathogenic factors, medical treatment, and prognostic indicators, *Arch Dermatol* 138:370-379, 2002.

Darling MR, Daley T: Blistering mucocutaneous diseases of the oral mucosa—a review: Part 1. Mucous membrane pemphigoid, *J Can Dent Assoc* 71:851-854, 2005.

Egan CA, Lazarova Z, Darling TN et al: Anti-epiligrin cicatricial pemphigoid: clinical findings, immunopathogenesis and significant associations, *Medicine* 82:177-186, 2003.

Egan CA, Taylor TB, Meyer LJ et al: The immunoglobulin A antibody response in clinical subsets of mucous membrane pemphigoid, *Dermatology* 198:330-335, 1999.

Ekong AS, Foster CS, Roque MR: Eye involvement in autoimmune blistering diseases, *Clin Dermatol* 19:742-749, 2001.

Fatahzadeh M, Radfar L, Sirois DA: Dental care of patients with autoimmune vesiculobullous diseases: case reports and literature review, *Quintessence Int* 37:777-787, 2006.

González-Moles MA, Scully C: Vesiculo-erosive oral mucosal disease—management with topical corticosteroids: (1) fundamental principles and specific agents available, *J Dent Res* 84:294-301, 2005.

Grinspan D, Abulafia J, Lanfranchi H: Angina bullosa hemorrhagica, *Int J Dermatol* 38:525-528, 1999.

Guiliani M, Favia GF, Lajolo C et al: Angina bullosa haemorrhagica: presentation of eight new cases and review of the literature, *Oral Dis* 8:54-58, 2002.

Letko E, Bhol K, Anzaar F et al: Chronic cicatrizing conjunctivitis in a patient with epidermolysis bullosa acquisita, *Arch Ophthalmol* 124:1615-1618, 2006.

Letko E, Miserocchi E, Daoud YJ et al: A nonrandomized comparison of the clinical outcome of ocular involvement in patients with mucous membrane (cicatricial) pemphigoid between conventional immunosuppressive and intravenous immunoglobulin therapies, *Clin Immunol* 111:303-310, 2004.

Leverkus M, Schmidt E, Lazarova Z et al: Antiepiligrin cicatricial pemphigoid. An underdiagnosed entity within the spectrum of scarring autoimmune subepidermal bullous diseases? *Arch Dermatol* 135:1091-1098, 1999.

Luke MC, Darling TN, Hsu R et al: Mucosal morbidity in patients with epidermolysis bullosa acquisita, *Arch Dermatol* 135:954-959, 1999.

O'Regan E, Bane A, Flint S et al: Linear IgA disease presenting as desquamative gingivitis, *Arch Otolaryngol Head Neck Surg* 130:469-472, 2004.

Oyama N, Setterfield JF, Powell AM et al: Bullous pemphigoid antigen II (BP180) and its soluble extracellular domains are major autoantigens in mucous membrane pemphigoid: the pathogenic relevance to HLA class II alleles and disease severity, *Br J Dermatol* 154:90-98, 2006.

Rashid KA, Gürcan HM, Ahmed AR: Antigen specificity in subsets of mucous membrane pemphigoid, *J Invest Dermatol* 126:2631-2636, 2006.

Sacher C, Hunzelmann N: Cicatricial pemphigoid (mucous membrane pemphigoid): current and emerging therapeutic approaches, *Am J Clin Dermatol* 6:93-103, 2005.

Sami N, Bhol KC, Ahmed AR: Intravenous immunoglobulin therapy in patients with multiple mucosal involvement in mucous membrane pemphigoid, *Clin Immunol* 102:59-67, 2002.

Sánchez AR, Rogers III RS, Kupp LI et al: Desquamative gingivitis associated with IgG/IgA pemphigoid presents a challenging diagnosis and treatment: a case report, *J Periodontol* 75:1714-1719, 2004.

Sapadin AN, Fleischmajer R: Tetracyclines: nonantibiotic properties and their clinical implications, *J Am Acad Dermatol* 54:258-265, 2006.

Scully C, Porter SR: The clinical spectrum of desquamative gingivitis, *Sem Cutan Med Surg* 16:308-313, 1997.

Setterfield J, Shirlaw PJ, Kerr-Muir M et al: Mucous membrane pemphigoid: a dual circulating antibody response with IgG and IgA signifies a more severe and persistent disease, *Br J Dermatol* 138:602-610, 1998.

Siegel MA, Anhalt GJ: Direct immunofluorescence of detached gingival epithelium for diagnosis of cicatricial pemphigoid: report of five cases, *Oral Surg Oral Med Oral Pathol* 75:296-302, 1993.

Sollecito TP, Parisi E: Mucous membrane pemphigoid, *Dent Clin North Am* 49:91-106, 2005.

Stephenson P, Lamey P-J, Scully C et al: Angina bullosa haemorrhagica: clinical and laboratory features in 30 patients, *Oral Surg Oral Med Oral Pathol* 63:560-565, 1987.

Thorne JE, Anhalt GJ, Jabs DA: Mucous membrane pemphigoid and pseudopemphigoid, *Ophthalmology* 111:45-52, 2004.

Vincent SD, Lilly GE, Baker KA: Clinical, historic, and therapeutic features of cicatricial pemphigoid: a literature review and open therapeutic trial with corticosteroids, *Oral Surg Oral Med Oral Pathol* 76:453-459, 1993.

Wojnarowska F, Kirtschig G, Khumalo N: Treatment of subepidermal immunobullous diseases, *Clin Dermatol* 19:768-777, 2001.

Woodley DT, Chang C, Saadat P et al: Evidence that anti-type VII collagen antibodies are pathogenic and responsible for the clinical, histological, and immunological features of epidermolysis bullosa acquisita, *J Invest Dermatol* 124:958-964, 2005.

Yamamoto K, Fujimoto M, Inoue M et al: Angina bullosa hemorrhagica of the soft palate: report of 11 cases and literature review, *J Oral Maxillofac Surg* 64:1433-1436, 2006.

Bullous Pemphigoid

Anhalt GJ, Monison LH: Bullous and cicatricial pemphigoid, *J Autoimmun* 4:17-35, 1991.

Korman NJ: Bullous pemphigoid. The latest in diagnosis, prognosis, and therapy, *Arch Dermatol* 134:1137-1141, 1998.

Walsh SRA, Hogg D, Mydlarski PR: Bullous pemphigoid: from bench to bedside, *Drugs* 65:905-926, 2005.

Williams DM: Vesiculo-bullous mucocutaneous disease: benign mucous membrane and bullous pemphigoid, *J Oral Pathol Med* 19:16-23, 1990.

Erythema Multiforme

Aslanzadeh J, Helm K, Espy MJ et al: Detection of HSV-specific DNA in biopsy tissue of patients with erythema multiforme by polymerase chain reaction, *Br J Dermatol* 126:19-23, 1992.

Auqier-Dunant A, Mockenhaupt M, Naldi L et al: Correlations between clinical patterns and causes of erythema multiforme majus, Stevens-Johnson syndrome, and toxic epidermal necrolysis, *Arch Dermatol* 138:1019-1024, 2002.

Ayangco L, Rogers RS: Oral manifestations of erythema multiforme, *Dermatol Clin* 21:195-205, 2003.

Bastuji-Garin S, Rzany B, Stern RS et al: Clinical classification of cases of toxic epidermal necrolysis, Stevens-Johnson syndrome, and erythema multiforme, *Arch Dermatol* 129:92-96, 1993.

Chang Y-S, Huang F-C, Tseng S-H et al: Erythema multiforme, Stevens-Johnson syndrome, and toxic epidermal necrolysis: acute ocular manifestations, causes, and management, *Cornea* 26:1123-129, 2007.

Farthing P, Bagan J-V, Scully C: Erythema multiforme, *Oral Dis* 11:261-267, 2005.

French LE: Toxic epidermal necrolysis and Stevens Johnson syndrome: our current understanding, *Allergol Int* 55:9-16, 2006.

Garcia-Doval I, LeCleach L, Bocquet H et al: Toxic epidermal necrolysis and Stevens-Johnson syndrome. Does early withdrawal of causative drugs decrease the risk of death? *Arch Dermatol* 136:323-327, 2000.

Kakourou T, Klontza D, Soteropoulou F et al: Corticosteroid treatment of erythema multiforme major (Stevens-Johnson syndrome) in children, *Eur J Pediatr* 156:90-93, 1997.

Lamoreux MR, Sternbach MR, Hsu WT: Erythema multiforme, *Am Fam Physician* 74:1883-1888, 2006.

Lozada-Nur F, Cram D, Gorsky M: Clinical response to levamisole in thirty-nine patients with erythema multiforme: an open prospective study, *Oral Surg Oral Med Oral Pathol* 74:294-298, 1992.

Lyell A: Toxic epidermal necrolysis: an eruption resembling scalding of the skin, *Br J Dermatol* 68:355-361, 1956.

Mittmann N, Chan B, Knowles S et al: Intravenous immunoglobulin use in patients with toxic epidermal necrolysis and Stevens-Johnson syndrome, *Am J Clin Dermatol* 7:359-368, 2006.

Paquet P, Piérard GE: Erythema multiforme and toxic epidermal necrolysis: a comparative study, *Am J Dermatopathol* 19:127-132, 1997.

Pereira FA, Mudgil AV, Rosmarin DM: Toxic epidermal necrolysis, *J Am Acad Dermatol* 56:181-200, 2007.

Schofield JK, Tatnail FM, Leigh IM: Recurrent erythema multiforme: clinical features and treatment in a large series of patients, *Br J Dermatol* 128:542-545, 1993.

Shortt R, Gomez M, Mittman N et al: Intravenous immunoglobulin does not improve outcome in toxic epidermal necrolysis, *J Burn Care Rehabil* 25:246-255, 2004.

Singla R, Brodell RT: Erythema multiforme due to herpes simplex virus: recurring target lesions are the clue to diagnosis, *Postgrad Med* 106:151-154, 1999.

Stern RS: Improving the outcome of patients with toxic epidermal necrolysis and Stevens-Johnson syndrome, *Arch Dermatol* 136:410-411, 2000.

Trent J, Halem M, French L et al: Toxic epidermal necrolysis and intravenous immunoglobulin: a review, *Semin Cutan Med Surg* 25:91-93, 2006.

Tripathi A, Ditto AM, Grammer LC et al: Corticosteroid therapy in an additional 13 cases of Stevens-Johnson syndrome: a total series of 67 cases, *Allergy Asthma Proc* 21:101-105, 2000.

Vanfleteren I, Van Gysel D, De Brandt C: Stevens-Johnson syndrome: a diagnostic challenge in the absence of skin lesions, *Pediatr Dermatol* 20:52-56, 2003.

Viard I, Wehrli P, Bullani R et al: Inhibition of toxic epidermal necrolysis by blockade of CD95 with human intravenous immunoglobulin, *Science* 282:490-493, 1998.

Wilkins J, Morrison L, White CR: Oculocutaneous manifestations of the erythema multiforme/Stevens-Johnson syndrome/toxic epidermal necrolysis spectrum, *Dermatol Clin* 10:571-582, 1992.

Williams PM, Conklin RJ: Erythema multiforme: a review and contrast from Stevens-Johnson syndrome/toxic epidermal necrolysis, *Dent Clin North Am* 49:67-76, 2005.

Erythema Migrans

Espelid M, Bang G, Johannessen AC et al: Geographic stomatitis: report of 6 cases, *J Oral Pathol Med* 20:425-428, 1991.

Gonzaga HFS, Torres EA, Alchorne MMA et al: Both psoriasis and benign migratory glossitis are associated with HLA-Cw6, *Br J Dermatol* 135:368-370, 1996.

Jainkittivong A, Langlais RP: Geographic tongue: clinical characteristics of 188 cases, *J Contemp Dent Pract* 6:123-135, 2005.

Marks R, Radden BG: Geographic tongue: a clinico-pathological review, *Australas J Dermatol* 22:75-79, 1981.

Morris LF, Phillips CM, Binnie WH et al: Oral lesions in patients with psoriasis: a controlled study, *Cutis* 49:339-344, 1992.

Shulman JD, Carpenter WM: Prevalence and risk factors associated with geographic tongue among US adults, *Oral Dis* 12:381-386, 2006.

Sigal MJ, Mock D: Symptomatic benign migratory glossitis: report of two cases and literature review, *Pediatr Dent* 14:392-396, 1992.

Waltimo J: Geographic tongue during a year of oral contraceptive cycles, *Br Dent J* 171:94-96, 1991.

Zagari O: The prevalence and significance of fissured tongue and geographical tongue in psoriatic patients, *Clin Exp Dermatol* 31:192-195, 2006.

Reactive Arthritis

Edwards L, Hartsen RC: Reiter's syndrome of the vulva, *Arch Dermatol* 128:811-814, 1992.

Kataria RK, Brent LH: Spondyloarthropathies, *Am Fam Physician* 69:2853-2860, 2004.

Keat A, Rowe I: Reiter's syndrome and associated arthritides, *Rheum Dis Clin North Am* 17:25-42, 1991.

Könönen M, Kovero O, Wenneberg B et al: Radiographic signs in the temporomandibular joint in Reiter's disease, *J Orofac Pain* 16:143-147, 2002.

Lu DW, Katz KA: Declining use of the eponym "Reiter's syndrome" in the medical literature, 1998-2003, *J Am Acad Dermatol* 53:720-723, 2005.

Panush RS, Wallace DJ, Dorff EN et al: Retraction of the suggestion to use the term "Reiter's syndrome" sixty-five years later: the legacy of Reiter, a war criminal, should not be eponymic honor but rather condemnation (letter), *Arthritis Rheum* 56:693-694, 2007.

Rothe MJ, Kerdel FA: Reiter syndrome, *Int J Dermatol* 30:173-180, 1991.

Schneider JM, Matthews JH, Graham BS: Reiter's syndrome, *Cutis* 71:198-200, 2003.

Lichen Planus

Al-Hashimi I, Schifter M, Lockhart PB et al: Oral lichen planus and oral lichenoid lesions: diagnostic and therapeutic considerations, *Oral Surg Oral Med Oral Pathol Oral Radiol Endod* 103(suppl):S25e1-S25e12, January 2007 (Epub).

Belfiore P, Di Fede O, Cabibi D et al: Prevalence of vulval lichen planus in a cohort of women with oral lichen planus: an interdisciplinary study, *Br J Dermatol* 155:994-998, 2006.

Borghelli RF, Pettinari IL, Chuchurru JA et al: Oral lichen planus in patients with diabetes: an epidemiologic study, *Oral Surg Oral Med Oral Pathol* 75:498-500, 1993.

Bornstein MM, Kalas L, Lemp S et al: Oral lichen planus and malignant transformation: a retrospective follow-up study of clinical and histopathologic data, *Quintessence Int* 37:261-271, 2006.

Campana F, Sibaud V, Chauvel A et al: Recurrent superficial mucoceles associated with lichenoid disorders, *J Oral Maxillofac Surg* 64:1830-1833, 2006.

Campisi G, Di Fede O, Craxì A et al: Oral lichen planus, hepatitis C virus, and HIV: no association in a cohort study from an area of high hepatitis C virus endemicity, *J Am Acad Dermatol* 51:364-370, 2004.

Carrozzo M, Francia di Celle P, Gandolfo S et al: Increased frequency of HLA-DR6 allele in Italian patients with hepatitis C virus-associated oral lichen planus, *Br J Dermatol* 144:803-808, 2001.

DeRossi SS, Ciarrocca KN: Lichen planus, lichenoid drug reactions, and lichenoid mucositis, *Dent Clin North Am* 49:77-89, 2005.

Eisen D: The clinical features, malignant potential, and systemic associations of oral lichen planus: a study of 723 patients, *J Am Acad Dermatol* 46:207-214, 2002.

Eisen D, Carrozzo M, Bagan-Sebastian J-V et al: Oral lichen planus: clinical features and management, *Oral Dis* 11:338-349, 2005.

Eisenberg E: Oral lichen planus: a benign lesion, *J Oral Maxillofac Surg* 58:1278-1285, 2000.

Epstein JB, Wan LS, Gorsky M et al: Oral lichen planus: progress in understanding its malignant potential and the implications for clinical management, *Oral Surg Oral Med Oral Pathol Oral Radiol Endod* 96:32-37, 2003.

Fatahzadeh M, Rinaggio J, Chiodo T: Squamous cell carcinoma arising in an oral lichenoid lesion, *J Am Dent Assoc* 135:754-759, 2004.

Firth NA, Rich AM, Radden BG et al: Assessment of the value of immunofluorescence microscopy in the diagnosis of oral mucosal lichen planus, *J Oral Pathol Med* 19:295-297, 1990.

González-García A, Diniz-Freitas M, Gándara-Vila P et al: Triamcinolone acetonide mouth rinses for treatment of erosive oral lichen planus: efficacy and risk of fungal over-infection, *Oral Dis* 12:559-565, 2006.

Gordon SC, Daley TD: Foreign body gingivitis. Clinical and microscopic features of 61 cases, *Oral Surg Oral Med Oral Pathol Oral Radiol Endod* 83:562-570,1997.

Harden D, Skelton H, Smith KJ: Lichen planus associated with hepatitis C virus: no viral transcripts are found in the lichen planus, and effective therapy for hepatitis C virus does not clear lichen planus, *J Am Acad Dermatol* 49:847-852, 2003.

Hietanen J, Paasonen M-R, Kuhlefelt M et al: A retrospective study of oral lichen planus patients with concurrent or subsequent development of malignancy, *Oral Oncol* 35:278-282, 1999.

Holzberg M: Common nail disorders, *Dermatol Clin* 24:349-354, 2006.

Ingafou M, Leao JC, Porter SR et al: Oral lichen planus: a retrospective study of 690 British patients, *Oral Dis* 12:463-468, 2006.

Jainkittivong A, Kuvatanasuchati J, Pipattanagovit P et al: *Candida* in oral lichen planus patients undergoing topical steroid therapy, *Oral Surg Oral Med Oral Pathol Oral Radiol Endod* 104:61-66, 2007.

Jungell P, Malmström M: Cyclosporin A mouthwash in the treatment of oral lichen planus, *Int J Oral Maxillofac Surg* 25:60-62, 1996.

Kalmar JR: Diagnosis and management of oral lichen planus, *J Calif Dent Assoc* 35:405-412, 2007.

Laeijendecker R, Tank B, Dekker SK et al: A comparison of treatment of oral lichen planus with topical tacrolimus and triamcinolone acetonide ointment, *Acta Derm Venereol* 86:227-229, 2006.

Lodi G, Scully C, Carrozzo M et al: Current controversies in oral lichen planus: report of an international consensus meeting. Part 1. Viral infections and etiopathogenesis, *Oral Surg Oral Med Oral Pathol Oral Radiol Endod* 100:40-51, 2005.

Lodi G, Scully C, Carrozzo M et al: Current controversies in oral lichen planus: report of an international consensus meeting. Part 2. Clinical management and malignant transformation, *Oral Surg Oral Med Oral Pathol Oral Radiol Endod* 100:164-178, 2005.

Lozada-Nur FI, Sroussi HY: Tacrolimus powder in Orabase 0.1% for the treatment of oral lichen planus and oral lichenoid lesions: an open clinical trial, *Oral Surg Oral Med Oral Pathol Oral Radiol Endod* 102:744-749, 2006.

Mattsson U, Jontell M, Holmstrup P: Oral lichen planus and malignant transformation: is a recall of patients justified? *Crit Rev Oral Biol Med* 13:390-396, 2002.

McCartan BE, McCreary CE: Oral lichenoid drug eruptions, *Oral Dis* 3:58-63, 1997.

Patel S, Yeoman CM, Murphy R: Oral lichen planus in childhood: a report of three cases, *Int J Paediatr Dent* 15:118-122, 2005.

Petruzzi M, De Benedittis M, Pastore L et al: Peno-gingival lichen planus, *J Periodontol* 76:2293-2298, 2005.

Piboonniyom S, Treister N, Pitiphat W et al: Scoring system for monitoring oral lichenoid lesions: a preliminary study, *Oral Surg Oral Med Oral Pathol Oral Radiol Endod* 99:696-703, 2005.

Ramer MA, Altchek A, Deligdisch L et al: Lichen planus and the vulvovaginal-gingival syndrome, *J Periodontol* 74:1385-1393, 2003.

Roosaar A, Yin L, Sandborgh-Englund G et al: On the natural course of oral lichen lesions in a Swedish population-based sample, *J Oral Pathol Med* 35:257-261, 2006.

Roy KM, Bagg J: Hepatitis C virus and oral disease: a critical review, *Oral Dis* 5:270-277, 1999.

Setterfield JF, Neill S, Shirlaw PJ et al: The vulvovaginal gingival syndrome: a severe subgroup of lichen planus with characteristic clinical features and a novel association with the class II HLA DQB1*0201 allele, *J Am Acad Dermatol* 55:98-113, 2006.

Silverman S, Gorsky M, Lozada-Nur F et al: A prospective study of findings and management in 214 patients with oral lichen planus, *Oral Surg Oral Med Oral Pathol* 72:665-670, 1991.

Sugerman PB, Savage NW, Walsh LJ et al: The pathogenesis of oral lichen planus, *Crit Rev Oral Biol Med* 13:350-365, 2002.

Thorne JE, Jabs DA, Nikolskaia OV et al: Lichen planus and cicatrizing conjunctivitis: characterization of five cases, *Am J Ophthalmol* 136:239-243, 2003.

Thornhill MH, Sankar V, Xu X-J et al: The role of histopathological characteristics in distinguishing amalgam-associated oral lichenoid reactions and oral lichen planus, *J Oral Pathol Med* 35:233-240, 2006.

Tucker SC, Coulson IH: Lichen planus is not associated with hepatitis C infection in patients from North West England, *Acta Derm Venereol* 79:378-379, 1999.

Van der Meij EH, Mast H, van der Waal I: The possible premalignant character of oral lichen planus and oral lichenoid lesions: a prospective follow-up study of 192 patients, *Oral Oncol* 43:742-748, 2007.

Van der Meij EH, Slootweg PJ, van der Wal JE et al: Interobserver and intraobserver variability in the histologic assessment of oral lichen planus, *J Oral Pathol Med* 28:274-277, 1999.

Van der Meij EH, van der Waal I: Lack of clinicopathologic correlation in the diagnosis of oral lichen planus based on the presently available diagnostic criteria and suggestions for modifications, *J Oral Pathol Med* 32:507-512, 2003.

Voûte ABE, Schulten EAJM, Langendijk PNJ et al: Fluocinonide in an adhesive base for treatment of oral lichen planus: a double-blind, placebo-controlled clinical study, *Oral Surg Oral Med Oral Pathol* 75:181-185, 1993.

Zakrzewska JM, Chan ES-Y, Thornhill MH: A systematic review of placebo-controlled randomized clinical trials of treatments used in oral lichen planus, *Br J Dermatol* 153:336-341, 2005.

Zhang LW, Michelsen C, Cheng X et al: Molecular analysis of oral lichen planus. A premalignant lesion? *Am J Pathol* 151:323-327, 1997.

Chronic Ulcerative Stomatitis

Church LF, Schosser RH: Chronic ulcerative stomatitis associated with stratified epithelial specific antinuclear antibodies: a case report of a newly described entity, *Oral Surg Oral Med Oral Pathol* 73:579-582, 1992.

Jaremko WM, Beutner EH, Kumar V et al: Chronic ulcerative stomatitis associated with a specific immunologic marker, *J Am Acad Dermatol* 22:2115-2120, 1990.

Lee LA, Walsh P, Prater CA et al: Characterization of an autoantigen associated with chronic ulcerative stomatitis: the CUSP autoantigen is a member of the p53 family, *J Invest Dermatol* 113:146-151, 1999.

Lewis JE, Beutner EH: Chronic ulcerative stomatitis with stratified epithelium-specific antinuclear antibodies, *Int J Dermatol* 35:272-275, 1996.

Lorenzana ER, Rees TD, Glass M et al: Chronic ulcerative stomatitis: a case report, *J Periodontol* 71:104-111, 2000.

Solomon LW, Aguirre A, Neiders M et al: Chronic ulcerative stomatitis: clinical, histopathologic, and immunopathologic findings, *Oral Surg Oral Med Oral Pathol Oral Radiol Endod* 96:718-726, 2003.

Wörle B, Wollenberg A, Schaller M et al: Chronic ulcerative stomatitis, *Br J Dermatol* 137:262-265, 1997.

Graft-Versus-Host Disease

Abdelsayed RA, Sumner T, Allen CM et al: Oral precancerous and malignant lesions associated with graft-versus-host disease: report of 2 cases, *Oral Surg Oral Med Oral Pathol Oral Radiol Endod* 93:75-80, 2002.

Alborghetti MR, Corrêa MEP, Adam RL et al: Late effect of chronic graft-versus-host disease in minor salivary glands, *J Oral Pathol Med* 34:486-493, 2005.

Bridge AT, Nelson RP, Schwartz JE et al: Histological evaluation of acute mucocutaneous graft-versus-host disease in non-myeloablative hematologic stem cell transplants with an observation predicting an increased risk of progression to chronic graft-versus-host disease, *Am J Dermatopathol* 29:1-6, 2007.

Centers for Disease Control: Guidelines for preventing opportunistic infections among hematopoietic stem cell transplant recipients, *MMWR Morb Mortal Wkly Rep* 49(RR-10):1-128, 2000.

Chao NJ, Schmidt GM, Niland JC et al: Cyclosporine, methotrexate, and prednisone compared with cyclosporine and prednisone for prophylaxis of acute graft-versus-host disease, *N Engl J Med* 329:1225-1230, 1993.

Couriel D, Caldera H, Champlin R et al: Acute graft-versus-host disease: pathophysiology, clinical manifestations, and management, *Cancer* 101:1936-1946, 2004.

Deeg HJ, Antin JH: The clinical spectrum of acute graft-versus-host disease, *Semin Hematol* 43:24-31, 2006.

Demarosi F, Soligo D, Lodi G et al: Squamous cell carcinoma of the oral cavity associated with graft versus host disease: report of a case and review of the literature, *Oral Surg Oral Med Oral Pathol Oral Radiol Endod* 100:63-69, 2005.

Easaw SJ, Lake DE, Beer M et al: Graft-versus-host disease. Possible higher risk for African American patients, *Cancer* 78:1492-1497, 1996.

Eckardt A, Starke O, Stadler M et al: Severe oral chronic graft-versus-host disease following allogeneic bone marrow transplantation: highly effective treatment with topical tacrolimus, *Oral Oncol* 40:811-814, 2004.

Euvrard S, Kanitakis J, Claudy A: Medical progress: skin cancers after organ transplantation, *N Engl J Med* 348:1681-1691, 2003.

García-F-Villalta MJ, Pascual-López M, Elices M et al: Superficial mucoceles and lichenoid graft versus host disease: report of three cases, *Acta Derm Venereol* 82:453-455, 2002.

Gilman AL, Serody J: Diagnosis and treatment of chronic graft-versus-host disease, *Semin Hematol* 43:70-80, 2006.

Goldman KE: Dental management of patients with bone marrow and solid organ transplantation, *Dent Clin North Am* 50:659-676, 2006.

Horwitz ME, Sullivan KM: Chronic graft-versus-host disease, *Blood Rev* 20:15-27, 2006.

Johnson ML, Farmer ER: Graft-versus-host reactions in dermatology, *J Am Acad Dermatol* 38:369-392, 1998.

Lee SJ, Klein JP, Barrett AJ et al: Severity of chronic graft-versus-host disease: association with treatment-related mortality and relapse, *Blood* 100:406-414, 2002.

Melkos AB, Massenkeil G, Arnold R et al: Dental treatment prior to stem cell transplantation and its influence on the posttransplantation outcome, *Clin Oral Invest* 7:113-115, 2003.

Nagler RM, Nagler A: Pilocarpine hydrochloride relieves xerostomia in chronic graft-versus-host disease: a sialometrical study, *Bone Marrow Transplant* 23:1007-1011, 1999.

Nagler RM, Nagler A: Salivary gland involvement in graft-versus-host disease: the underlying mechanism and implicated treatment, *Isr Med Assoc J* 6:167-172, 2004.

Pérez-Simón JA, Sánchez-Abarca I, Díez-Campelo M et al: Chronic graft-versus-host disease: pathogenesis and clinical management, *Drugs* 66:1041-1057, 2006.

Rocha V, Wagner JE, Sobocinski KA et al: Graft-versus-host disease in children who have received a cord-blood or bone marrow transplant from an HLA-identical sibling, *N Engl J Med* 342:1846-1854, 2000.

Rodu B, Gockerman JP: Oral manifestations of the chronic graft-v-host reaction, *JAMA* 249:504-507, 1983.

Sánchez AR, Sheridan PJ, Rogers RS: Successful treatment of oral lichen planus-like chronic graft-versus-host disease with topical tacrolimus: a case report, *J Periodontol* 75:613-619, 2004.

Sato M, Tokuda N, Fukumoto T et al: Immunohistopathological study of the oral lichenoid lesions of chronic GVHD, *J Oral Pathol Med* 35:33-36, 2006.

Schubert MM, Williams BE, Lloid ME et al: Clinical assessment scale for the rating of oral mucosal changes associated with bone marrow transplantation: development of an oral mucositis index, *Cancer* 69:2469-2477, 1992.

Sedghizadeh PP, Allen CM, Anderson KE et al: Oral graft-versus-host disease and programmed cell death: pathogenetic and clinical correlates, *Oral Surg Oral Med Oral Pathol Oral Radiol Endod* 97:491-498, 2004.

Shulman HM, Kleiner D, Lee SJ et al: Histopathologic diagnosis of chronic graft-versus-host disease: National Institutes of Health consensus development project on criteria for clinical trials in chronic graft-versus-host disease: II. Pathology working group report, *Biol Blood Marrow Transplant* 12:31-47, 2006.

Soares AB, Faria PR, Magna LA et al: Chronic GVHD in minor salivary glands and oral mucosa: histopathological and immunohistochemical evaluation of 25 patients, *J Oral Pathol Med* 34:368-373, 2005.

Szeto CH, Shek TWH, Lie AKW et al: Squamous cell carcinoma of the tongue complicating chronic oral mucosal graft-versus-host disease after allogeneic hematopoietic stem cell transplantation, *Am J Hematol* 77:200-202, 2004.

Thomas ED: Bone marrow transplantation: a review, *Semin Hematol* 36 (suppl7):95-103, 1999.

Treister NS, Woo S-B, O'Holleran EW et al: Oral chronic graft-versus-host disease in pediatric patients after hematopoietic stem cell transplantation, *Biol Blood Marrow Transplant* 11:721-731, 2005.

Vogelsang GB: Acute and chronic graft-versus-host disease, *Curr Opin Oncol* 5:276-281, 1993.

Woo S-B, Lee SJ, Schubert MM: Graft-vs-host disease, *Crit Rev Oral Biol Med* 8:201-216, 1997.

Woo S-B, Sonis ST, Monopoli MM et al: A longitudinal study of oral ulcerative mucositis in bone marrow transplant recipients, *Cancer* 72:1612-1617, 1993.

Psoriasis

Bruce AJ, Rogers RS: Oral psoriasis, *Dermatol Clin* 21:99-104, 2003.

Camisa C: Psoriasis: a clinical update on diagnosis and new therapies, *Cleve Clin J Med* 67:105-106, 109-113, 117-119, 2000.

Doffy DL, Spelman LS, Martin NG: Psoriasis in Australian twins, *J Am Acad Dermatol* 29:428-434, 1993.

Eastman JR, Goldblatt LI: Psoriasis: palatal manifestations and physiologic considerations, *J Periodontol* 54:736-739, 1983.

Gelfand JM, Gladman DD, Mease PJ et al: Epidemiology of psoriatic arthritis in the population of the United States, *J Am Acad Dermatol* 53:573, 2005.

Lowes MA, Bowcock AM, Krueger JG: Pathogenesis and therapy of psoriasis, *Nature* 445:866-873, 2007.

Myers WA, Gottlieb AB, Mease P: Psoriasis and psoriatic arthritis: clinical features and disease mechanisms, *Clin Dermatol* 24:438-447, 2006.

Richardson LJ, Kratochvil FJ, Zieper MB: Unusual palatal presentation of oral psoriasis, *J Can Dent Assoc* 66:80-82, 2000.

Smith CH, Barker JNWN: Psoriasis and its management, *Br Med J* 333:380-384, 2006.

Stern RS, Laird N: The carcinogenic risk of treatments for severe psoriasis, *Cancer* 73:2759-2764, 1994.

Younai FS, Phelan JA: Oral mucositis with features of psoriasis: report of a case and review of the literature, *Oral Surg Oral Med Oral Pathol Oral Radiol Endod* 84:61-67, 1997.

Lupus Erythematosus

Brennan MT, Valerin MA, Napeñas JJ et al: Oral manifestations of patients with lupus erythematosus, *Dent Clin North Am* 49:127-141, 2005.

Burge SM, Frith PA, Millard PR et al: Mucosal involvement in systemic and chronic cutaneous lupus erythematosus, *Br J Dermatol* 121:727-741, 1989.

Callen JP: Oral manifestations of collagen vascular disease, *Semin Cutan Med Surg* 16:323-327, 1997.

Cervera R, Khamashta MA, Font J et al: Morbidity and mortality in systemic lupus erythematosus during a 5-year period, *Medicine (Baltimore)* 78:167-175, 1999.

Deapen D, Escalante A, Weinrib L et al: A revised estimate of twin concordance in systemic lupus erythematosus, *Arthritis Rheum* 35:311-318, 1992.

D'Cruz DP: Systemic lupus erythematosus, *Br Med J* 332:890-894, 2006.

D'Cruz DP, Khamashta MA, Hughes GRV: Systemic lupus erythematosus, *Lancet* 369:587-596, 2007

De Rossi SS, Glick M: Lupus erythematosus: considerations for dentistry, *J Am Dent Assoc* 129:330-339, 1998.

Doria A, Iaccarino L, Ghirardello A et al: Long-term prognosis and causes of death in systemic lupus erythematosus, *Am J Med* 119:700-706, 2006.

Duong DJ, Spigel GT, Moxley RT et al: American experience with low-dose thalidomide therapy for severe cutaneous lupus erythematosus, *Arch Dermatol* 135:1079-1087, 1999.

Fabbri P, Cardinali C, Giomi B et al: Cutaneous lupus erythematosus: diagnosis and management, *Am J Clin Dermatol* 4:449-465, 2003.

Ginzler EM, Dooley MA, Aranow C et al: Mycophenolate mofetil or intravenous cyclophosphamide for lupus nephritis, *N Engl J Med* 353:2219-2228, 2005.

Hahn BH: Systemic lupus erythematosus. In Kasper DL, Braunwald E, Fauci AS et al: *Harrison's principles of internal medicine,* ed 16, pp 1960-1967, New York, 2005, McGraw-Hill.

Rhodus NL, Johnson DK: The prevalence of oral manifestations of systemic lupus erythematosus, *Quintessence Int* 21:461-465, 1990.

Rothfield N, Sontheimer RD, Bernstein M: Lupus erythematosus: systemic and cutaneous manifestations, *Clin Dermatol* 24:348-362, 2006.

Tebbe B: Clinical course and prognosis of cutaneous lupus erythematosus, *Clin Dermatol* 22:121-124, 2004.

Thorne JE, Jabs DA, Nikolskaia O et al: Discoid lupus erythematosus and cicatrizing conjunctivitis: clinicopathologic study of two cases, *Ocul Immunol Inflamm* 10:287-292, 2002.

Velthuis PJ, Kater L, Baart de la Faille H: Direct immunofluorescence patterns in clinically healthy skin of patients with collagen diseases, *Clin Dermatol* 10:423-430, 1993.

Werth VP: Clinical manifestations of cutaneous lupus erythematosus, *Autoimmun Rev* 4:296-302, 2005.

Systemic Sclerosis

Chung L, Lin J, Furst DE et al: Systemic and localized scleroderma, *Clin Dermatol* 24:374-392, 2006.

Demir Y, Karaaslan T, Aktepe F et al: Linear scleroderma "en coup de sabre" of the cheek, *J Oral Maxillofac Surg* 61:1091-1094, 2003.

Eversole LR, Jacobsen PL, Stone CE: Oral and gingival changes in systemic sclerosis (scleroderma), *J Periodontol* 55:175-178, 1984.

Generini S, Fiori G, Moggi-Pignone A et al: Systemic sclerosis: a clinical overview, *Adv Exp Med Biol* 455:73-83, 1999.

Gonzales TS, Coleman GC: Periodontal manifestations of collagen vascular disorders, *Periodontol 2000* 21:94-105, 1999.

Haers PE, Sailer HF: Mandibular resorption due to systemic sclerosis: case report of surgical correction of a secondary open bite deformity, *Int J Oral Maxillofac Surg* 24:261-267, 1995.

Ioannidis JPA, Vlachoyiannopoulos PG, Haidich A-B et al: Mortality in systemic sclerosis: an international meta-analysis of individual patient data, *Am J Med* 118:2-10, 2005.

Knobler RM, French LE, Kim Y et al: A randomized, double-blind, placebo-controlled trial of photopheresis in systemic sclerosis, *J Am Acad Dermatol* 54:793-799, 2006.

Marmary Y, Glaiss R, Pisanty S: Scleroderma: oral manifestations, *Oral Surg Oral Med Oral Pathol* 52:32-37, 1981.

Medsger TA: Natural history of systemic sclerosis and the assessment of disease activity, severity, functional status, and psychologic well-being, *Rheum Dis Clin North Am* 29:255-273, 2003.

Naylor WP: Oral management of the scleroderma patient, *J Am Dent Assoc* 105:814-817, 1982.

Ong VH, Brough G, Denton CP: Management of systemic sclerosis, *Clin Med* 5:214-219, 2005.

Rook AH, Freundlich B, Jegasothy BV et al: Treatment of systemic sclerosis with extracorporeal photochemotherapy: results of a multicenter trial, *Arch Dermatol* 128:337-346, 1992.

Rout PGJ, Hamburger J, Potts AJC: Orofacial radiological manifestations of systemic sclerosis, *Dentomaxillofac Radiol* 25:193-196, 1996.

Salojin KV, Tonquèze ML, Saraux A et al: Antiendothelial cell antibodies: useful markers of systemic sclerosis, *Am J Med* 102:178-185, 1997.

Spackman GK: Scleroderma: what the general dentist should know, *Gen Dent* 47:576-579, 1999.

Wollheim FA: Classification of systemic sclerosis. Visions and reality, *Rheumatol* 44:1212-1216, 2005.

Yenisey M, Külünk T, Kurt Ş et al: A prosthodontics management alternative for scleroderma patients, *J Oral Rehabil* 32:696-700, 2005.

CREST Syndrome

Chamberlain AJ, Walker NPJ: Successful palliation and significant remission of cutaneous calcinosis in CREST syndrome with carbon dioxide laser, *Dermatol Surg* 968-970, 2003.

Paley M, McLoughlin P: Oral problems associated with CREST syndrome: a case report, *Br Dent J* 175:295-296, 1993.

Sparsa A, Lesaux N, Kessler E et al: Treatment of cutaneous calcinosis in CREST syndrome by extracorporeal shock wave lithotripsy, *J Am Acad Dermatol* 53:S263-S265, 2005.

Stanford TW, Peterson J, Machen RL: CREST syndrome and periodontal surgery: a case report, *J Periodontol* 70:536-541, 1999.

Ueda M, Abe Y, Fujiwara H et al: Prominent telangiectasia associated with marked bleeding in CREST syndrome, *J Dermatol* 20:180-184, 1993.

Acanthosis Nigricans

Cairo F, Rubino I, Rotundo R et al: Oral acanthosis nigricans as a marker of internal malignancy. A case report, *J Periodontol* 72:1271-1275, 2001.

Hall JM, Moreland A, Cox GJ et al: Oral acanthosis nigricans: report of a case and comparison of oral and cutaneous pathology, *Am J Dermatopathol* 10:68-73, 1988.

McGuinness J, Greer K: Malignant acanthosis nigricans and tripe palms associated with pancreatic adenocarcinoma, *Cutis* 78:37-40, 2006.

Mostofi RS, Hayden NP, Soltani K: Oral malignant acanthosis nigricans, *Oral Surg Oral Med Oral Pathol* 56:372-374, 1983.

Pentenero M, Carrozzo M, Pagano M et al: Oral acanthosis nigricans, tripe palms and sign of Leser-Trélat in a patient with gastric adenocarcinoma, *Int J Dermatol* 43:530-532, 2004.

Ramírez-Amador V, Esquivel-Pedraza L, Caballero-Mendoza E et al: Oral manifestations as a hallmark of malignant acanthosis nigricans, *J Oral Pathol Med* 28:278-281, 1999.

Schwartz RA: Acanthosis nigricans, *J Am Acad Dermatol* 31:1-19, 1994.

Scully C, Barrett WA, Gilkes J et al: Oral acanthosis nigricans, the sign of Leser-Trélat and cholangiocarcinoma, *Br J Dermatol* 145:505-526, 2001.

Stuart CA, Driscoll MS, Lundquist KF et al: Acanthosis nigricans, *J Basic Clin Physiol Pharmacol* 9:407-418, 1998.

17

Oral Manifestations of Systemic Diseases

CHAPTER OUTLINE

MUCOPOLYSACCHARIDOSIS

The **mucopolysaccharidoses** are a heterogeneous group of metabolic disorders that are usually inherited in an autosomal recessive fashion. These disorders are all characterized by the lack of any one of several normal enzymes needed to process the important intercellular substances known as *glycosaminoglycans*. These substances used to be known as *mucopolysaccharides*, thus the term *mucopolysaccharidosis*. Examples of glycosaminoglycans include the following:

- Heparan sulfate
- Dermatan sulfate
- Keratan sulfate
- Chondroitin sulfate

The type of mucopolysaccharidosis that is seen clinically depends on which of these substrates lacks its particular enzyme. The mucopolysaccharidoses as a group occur with a frequency of approximately 1 in 15,000 to 29,000 live births, although some types are much less common.

Table **17-1**   **Features of Selected Mucopolysaccharidosis Syndromes**

Type	Eponym	Inheritance	Enzyme Deficiency	Stored Substrate	Clinical Features
I-H	Hurler	AR	α-L-Iduronidase	HS and DS	Appears in infancy; cloudy corneas, growth retardation, reduced intelligence, coronary artery disease; rarely live 10 years
I-S	Scheie	AR	α-L-Iduronidase	HS and DS	Onset in late childhood; cloudy corneas, normal intelligence, aortic regurgitation; survive to adulthood
II	Hunter	X-Linked R	Iduronate-2-sulfatase	HS and DS	Appears at 1 to 2 years of age; clear corneas, reduced intelligence, growth retardation, stiff joints
III-A	Sanfilippo-A	AR	Sulfamidase	HS	Appears at 4 to 6 years of age; clear corneas, reduced intelligence, mild skeletal changes; death in adolescence
III-B	Sanfilippo-B	AR	α-N-acetylglucosaminidase	HS	Generally same as Sanfilippo-A
IV-A	Morquio-A	AR	Galactosamine-6-sulfatase	KS, CS, GalNAc6S	Appears at 1 to 2 years of age; cloudy corneas, normal intelligence, lax joints; may survive to middle age
IV-B	Morquio-B	AR	β-galactosidase	KS	Generally similar to Morquio-A
VI	Maroteaux-Lamy	AR	N-acetylgalactosamine-4-sulfatase	DS, CS, GalNAc4S, GalNAc4, 6dis	Appears at 2 to 6 years of age; cloudy corneas, normal intelligence, growth retardation, stiff joints; may survive to adulthood

AR, Autosomal recessive; *CS*, chondroitin sulfate; *dis*, disulfate; *DS*, dermatan sulfate; *GalNAc*, N-acetylgalactosamine; *HS*, heparan sulfate; *KS*, keratan sulfate; *R*, recessive; *S*, sulfate.

CLINICAL AND RADIOGRAPHIC FEATURES

The clinical features of the mucopolysaccharidoses vary, depending on the particular syndrome that is examined (Table 17-1). Furthermore, affected patients with a particular type of this disorder often exhibit a wide range of severity of involvement. Most types of mucopolysaccharidosis display some degree of mental retardation. Often the facial features of affected patients

are somewhat coarse, with heavy browridges (Fig. 17-1), and there are other skeletal changes, such as stiff joints. Cloudy degeneration of the corneas, a problem that frequently leads to blindness, is seen in several forms of mucopolysaccharidosis.

The oral manifestations vary according to the particular type of mucopolysaccharidosis. Most types show some degree of macroglossia. Gingival hyperplasia may be present, particularly in the anterior regions, as a result of the drying and irritating effects of mouth

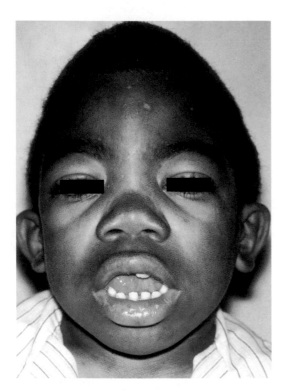

Fig. 17-1 Mucopolysaccharidosis. This patient affected by Hunter syndrome exhibits the characteristic facial features of this disorder.

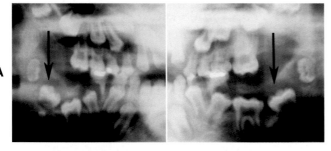

Fig. 17-2 Mucopolysaccharidosis. Radiographic examination of the dentition of a child affected by Hunter syndrome typically shows radiolucencies *(arrows)* associated with the crowns of unerupted teeth.

breathing. The dental changes include thin enamel with pointed cusps on the posterior teeth, although this seems to be a feature unique to mucopolysaccharidosis type IVA. Other dental manifestations include numerous impacted teeth with prominent follicular spaces (Fig. 17-2), possibly caused by the accumulation of glycosaminoglycans in the follicular connective tissue. Some investigators have reported the occurrence of multiple impacted teeth that are congregated in a single large follicle, forming a rosette pattern radiographically.

Although the clinical findings may suggest that a patient is affected by one of the mucopolysaccharidoses, the diagnosis is confirmed by finding elevated levels of glycosaminoglycans in the urine, as well as deficiencies of the specific enzymes in the patient's leukocytes and fibroblasts.

TREATMENT AND PROGNOSIS

No satisfactory systemic treatment of the mucopolysaccharidoses exists at this time. Several forms of mucopolysaccharidosis are associated with a markedly reduced life span and with mental retardation. Attempts to improve the survival and quality of life of these patients using allogeneic bone marrow transplantation have met with some success. Unfortunately, not all aspects of the disease are corrected, and the complications associated with transplantation must be addressed. Such complications are associated with a 15% to 20% mortality rate. Enzyme replacement therapy currently is available for mucopolysaccharidosis I. Initiation of the enzyme, laronidase, early in the patient's life appears to improve significantly many of the aspects of the disease, although complete resolution does not occur. Enzyme replacement strategies are also being developed for several of the other forms of this condition. Because of the rarity of these conditions and the expense of developing the treatments, the annual cost for such therapy typically exceeds $340,000. Genetic counseling is indicated for the parents and siblings of a patient affected by one of the mucopolysaccharidosis syndromes. Prenatal diagnosis is available for family planning as well.

Management of the dental problems of these patients is essentially no different from that of other patients. However, several factors may have to be taken into account:

- Degree of mental retardation (if any)
- Presence or absence of a seizure disorder
- Degree of joint stiffening
- Extent of other related medical problems

Depending on which of these factors is present and the extent of involvement, dental care may warrant sedation, hospitalization, or general anesthesia of the patient for optimal results. General anesthesia and sedation may be challenging, however, because of excess amounts of pharyngeal tissues that often produce a smaller than normal airway. In severely affected patients, general anesthesia probably should be considered only in life-threatening situations.

LIPID RETICULOENDOTHELIOSES

The **lipid reticuloendothelioses** are a relatively rare group of inherited disorders. These include the following conditions:

- Gaucher disease
- Niemann-Pick disease
- Tay-Sachs disease

These conditions are seen with increased frequency in patients with Ashkenazi Jewish heritage. Affected patients lack certain enzymes necessary for processing specific lipids, and this results in an accumulation of the lipids within a variety of cells. Because of this accumulation, it appeared that cells were attempting to store these substances; therefore, the term *storage disease* was commonly used for these disorders.

In **Gaucher disease** (the most common of the reticuloendothelioses), a lack of glucocerebrosidase results in the accumulation of glucosylceramide, particularly within the lysosomes of cells of the macrophage and monocyte lineage. Three types of Gaucher disease are now recognized: type 1 (nonneuronopathic) is seen primarily in the Ashkenazi Jewish population, and types 2 and 3 (neuronopathic) have a panethnic distribution.

Niemann-Pick disease is characterized by a deficiency of acid sphingomyelinase, resulting in the accumulation of sphingomyelin, also within the lysosomes of macrophages.

Tay-Sachs disease is caused by a lack of β-hexosaminidase A, which results in the accumulation of a ganglioside, principally within the lysosomes of neurons.

All these disorders are inherited as autosomal recessive traits. When the genetic mutation known to cause Gaucher disease was evaluated for the Ashkenazi Jewish population, researchers found that approximately 1 in 10 persons carried the defective gene. Most of the persons identified as having the gene, however, were heterozygous and, therefore, asymptomatic.

CLINICAL AND RADIOGRAPHIC FEATURES

GAUCHER DISEASE

The clinical features of Gaucher disease are generally the result of the effects of the abnormal storage of glucosylceramide. Macrophages laden with this glucocerebroside are typically rendered relatively nonfunctional, and they tend to accumulate within the bone marrow of the affected patient. This accumulation displaces the normal hematopoietic cells and produces anemia and thrombocytopenia. In addition, these patients are susceptible to bone infarctions. The resulting bone pain is often the presenting complaint. Characteristic *Erlenmeyer flask* deformities of the long bones, particularly of the femur, are often identified. Accumulations of the macrophages in the spleen and liver result in visceral enlargement. Many affected patients show a significant degree of growth retardation. Neurologic deterioration occurs in patients with the less common types 2 and 3 Gaucher disease. Jaw lesions

typically appear as ill-defined radiolucencies that usually affect the mandible without causing devitalization of the teeth or resorption of the lamina dura. Decreased salivary flow has been documented for patients with Gaucher disease compared with an age- and sex-matched population, although this decrease may not be clinically significant.

NIEMANN-PICK DISEASE

Niemann-Pick disease occurs as three different types, each associated with a different clinical expression and prognosis. Types A and B are caused by a deficiency of acid sphingomyelinase, whereas type C is primarily the result of mutation of *NPC-1*, a gene involved with cholesterol processing. Types A and C have **neuronopathic** features, characterized by psychomotor retardation, dementia, spasticity, and hepatosplenomegaly, with death occurring during the first or second decade of life. Type B patients normally survive into adulthood and exhibit **visceral signs**, primarily hepatosplenomegaly, and sometimes pulmonary involvement.

TAY-SACHS DISEASE

Tay-Sachs disease may have a wide clinical range because the condition is genetically heterogeneous. Some forms are mild, with patients surviving into adulthood. In the severe infantile form, however, rapidly progressive neuronal degeneration develops shortly after birth. Signs and symptoms include blindness, developmental retardation, and intractable seizures. Death usually occurs by 3 to 5 years of age.

HISTOPATHOLOGIC FEATURES

Histopathologic examination of an osseous lesion of Gaucher disease shows sheets of lipid-engorged macrophages (Gaucher cells) exhibiting abundant bluish cytoplasm, which has a fine texture resembling wrinkled silk. In Niemann-Pick disease, the characteristic cell seen on examination of a bone marrow aspirate is the "sea blue" histiocyte.

TREATMENT AND PROGNOSIS

GAUCHER DISEASE

For patients with a mild expression of Gaucher disease, no treatment may be necessary. For more severe forms of Gaucher disease, enzyme replacement therapy with macrophage-targeted glucocerebrosidase (imiglucerase for injection) is used; however, this is quite expensive, often costing more than $200,000 per year for treatment. After 9 to 12 months of therapy, patients exhibit improvement in the status of their anemia, a decrease in plasma glucocerebroside levels, and a decrease in hepatosplenomegaly. Resolution of the radiographic bone changes takes place over a longer period. Children treated with this regimen may show significant gain in height. Unfortunately enzyme replacement therapy has shown minimal effect on the neuronopathic Gaucher disease types 2 and 3. Bone marrow transplantation has also been attempted; however, the problems inherent in graft-versus-host disease (GVHD) are still present with that form of therapy, and thus it is not recommended. A case-control study showed that adults with Gaucher disease have an increased risk for hematologic malignancies, particularly lymphoma and multiple myeloma. Genetic counseling should be provided to all affected patients.

NIEMANN-PICK AND TAY-SACHS DISEASE

The neuronopathic forms of Niemann-Pick disease and the infantile form of Tay-Sachs disease are associated with a poor prognosis. Genetic counseling should be provided for affected families. Molecular markers of these disorders have been developed to identify carriers. Such identification allows earlier intervention in terms of counseling, and targeted population screening for the gene that causes Tay-Sachs disease has resulted in a marked decrease in affected patients during the past 3 decades.

LIPOID PROTEINOSIS (HYALINOSIS CUTIS ET MUCOSAE; URBACH-WIETHE SYNDROME)

A rare condition, **lipoid proteinosis** is inherited as an autosomal recessive trait. It is characterized by the deposition of a waxy material in the dermis and submucosal connective tissue of affected patients. The earliest thorough description of lipoid proteinosis was by Urbach and Wiethe in 1929, and more than 300 patients, most of whom are of European background, have been reported to date. Mutations of the *ECM1* gene, which encodes a glycoprotein known as *extracellular matrix protein 1*, have recently been identified as the cause for this condition.

CLINICAL FEATURES

The laryngeal mucosa and vocal cords are usually the sites that are initially affected by lipoid proteinosis. Therefore, the first sign of the disease may be one of the following:
- An inability of the infant to make a crying sound
- A hoarse cry in infancy
- The development of a hoarse voice during early childhood

The vocal cords become thickened as the accumulation of an amorphous material begins to affect the laryngeal mucosa. This infiltrative mucosal process may also involve the pharynx, esophagus, tonsils, vulva,

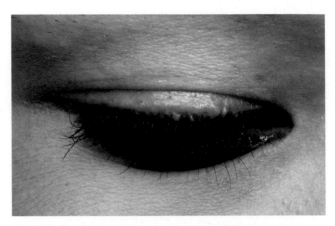

Fig. 17-3 Lipoid proteinosis. Thickened papules are present along the margin of the eyelid. *(Courtesy of Dr. Maria Copete.)*

and rectum. Skin lesions also develop early in life, appearing as thickened, yellowish, waxy papules; plaques; or nodules that often affect the face, particularly the lips and the margins of the eyelids (Fig. 17-3). Some lesions may begin as dark-crusted vesicles that heal as atrophic hyperpigmented patches.

Eventually, most patients exhibit a thickened, furrowed appearance of the skin. Other areas of the skin that may be involved include the neck, palms, axillae, elbows, scrotum, knees, and digits. In those areas subjected to chronic trauma, a hyperkeratotic, verrucous surface often develops. In addition to the cutaneous manifestations, symmetrical intracranial calcifications of the medial temporal lobes have been identified in approximately 70% of affected patients. These lesions are usually asymptomatic, although a few patients with such calcifications have been reported to have a seizure disorder.

The oral mucosal abnormalities typically become evident in the second decade of life. The tongue, labial mucosa, and buccal mucosa become nodular, diffusely enlarged, and thickened because of infiltration with waxy, yellow-white plaques and nodules (Fig. 17-4). The dorsal tongue papillae are eventually destroyed, and the tongue develops a smooth surface. The accumulation of the amorphous material within the tongue may result in its being bound to the floor of the mouth. Therefore, the patient may not be able to protrude the tongue. Gingival enlargement appears to be an infrequent finding.

HISTOPATHOLOGIC FEATURES

A biopsy specimen of an early lesion of lipoid proteinosis typically reveals the deposition of a lamellar material around the blood vessels, nerves, hair follicles, and sweat glands. This material stains positively with the periodic acid-Schiff (PAS) method and is not digested by diastase. The location of this material, its staining properties, and the presence of increased laminin, type IV collagen, and type V collagen suggest a basement membrane origin.

A biopsy specimen of a lesion in its later stages usually shows not only the lamellar material but also deposition of an amorphous substance within the dermal connective tissue (Fig. 17-5).

TREATMENT AND PROGNOSIS

Generally, no specific treatment is available for lipoid proteinosis other than genetic counseling. In rare instances, the infiltration of the laryngeal mucosa may produce difficult breathing for some infants, in which case debulking of the mucosal lesions may be neces-

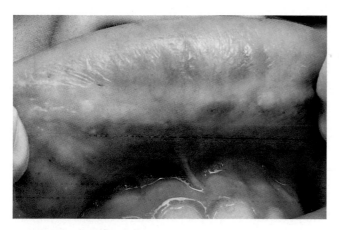

Fig. 17-4 Lipoid proteinosis. The upper labial mucosa exhibits yellow-white, nodular thickening. *(Courtesy of Dr. Maria Copete.)*

sary. Most patients with lipoid proteinosis have a normal life span. Certainly, however, the vocal hoarseness and the appearance of the skin may influence the quality of life for affected patients.

JAUNDICE (ICTERUS)

Jaundice is a condition characterized by excess bilirubin in the bloodstream. The bilirubin accumulates in the tissues, which results in a yellowish discoloration of the skin and mucosa. To understand jaundice, it is important to know something about the metabolism of bilirubin. Most bilirubin is derived from the breakdown of hemoglobin, the oxygen-carrying pigment of erythrocytes. The average life span of an erythrocyte in the circulation is 120 days. After this time, it undergoes physiologic breakdown. The hemoglobin is degraded and processed by the cells of the reticuloendothelial system, and bilirubin is liberated into the bloodstream in an unconjugated state. In the liver, bilirubin is taken up by the hepatocytes and conjugated with glucuronic acid, which produces conjugated bilirubin, a soluble product that can be excreted in the bile.

There are numerous causes for increased serum levels of bilirubin; some are physiologic, and many are pathologic. Therefore, the presence of jaundice is not a specific sign and generally necessitates physical examination and laboratory studies to determine the precise cause. The basic disturbances associated with increased bilirubin levels include an increased production of bilirubin. This occurs when the red blood cells (RBCs) are being broken down at such a rapid rate that the liver cannot keep pace with processing. This breakdown is seen in such conditions as **autoimmune hemolytic anemia** or **sickle cell anemia**.

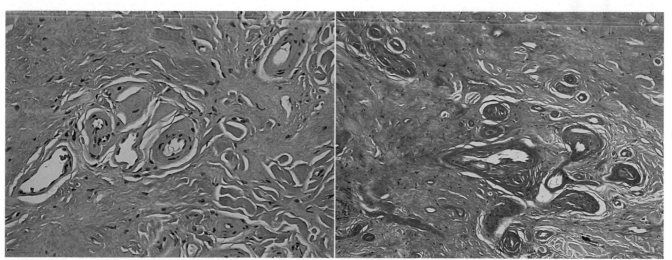

Fig. 17-5 Lipoid proteinosis. A, This medium-power photomicrograph shows perivascular deposition of a lamellar, acellular material. **B,** The periodic acid-Schiff (PAS) method is used to stain and highlight the perivascular deposits. *(Courtesy of Dr. Maria Copete.)*

In addition, the liver may not be functioning correctly, resulting in decreased uptake of the bilirubin from the circulation or decreased conjugation of bilirubin in the liver cells. Jaundice is frequently present at birth as a result of the low level of activity of the enzyme system that conjugates bilirubin. Defects in this enzyme system may also be seen with certain inherited problems, one of the more common of which is **Gilbert syndrome**. This innocuous condition is often detected on routine examination, and it is estimated to affect up to 5% of people in the United States. Because most of these examples of jaundice occur with impaired processing of bilirubin, laboratory studies usually show unconjugated bilirubin in the serum.

The presence of conjugated bilirubinemia in jaundice can usually be explained by the reduced excretion of bilirubin into the bile ducts. This can be the result of swelling of the hepatocytes (resulting in an occlusion of the bile canaliculi) or hepatocyte necrosis, with disruption of the bile canaliculi and liberation of conjugated bilirubin. Thus liver function may be disturbed because of any one of a variety of infections (e.g., viruses) or toxins (e.g., alcohol). Occlusion of the bile duct from gallstones, stricture, or cancer can also force conjugated bilirubin into the bloodstream.

CLINICAL FEATURES

The patient affected by jaundice exhibits a diffuse, uniform, yellowish discoloration of the skin and mucosa. The color varies in intensity, depending on the serum level of bilirubin and the anatomic site. Because elastin fibers have an affinity for bilirubin, tissues that have a high content of elastin, including the sclera, lingual frenum, and soft palate, are prominently affected. The sclera of the eye is often the first site at which the yellow color is noted (Fig. 17-6). The yellow discoloration caused by **hypercarotenemia** (resulting from excess ingestion of carotene, a vitamin-A precursor found in yellow vegetables and fruits) may be confused with jaundice, but the sclera is not involved in that condition.

Other signs and symptoms associated with jaundice vary with the underlying cause of the hyperbilirubinemia. For example, patients with viral hepatitis usually have a fever, abdominal pain, anorexia, and fatigue. The patient with jaundice typically requires a complete medical evaluation to determine the precise cause of the condition so that proper therapy can be instituted.

TREATMENT AND PROGNOSIS

The treatment and prognosis of the patient with jaundice vary with the cause. The jaundice that is commonly noted at birth often resolves spontaneously;

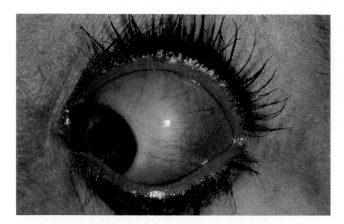

Fig. 17-6   Jaundice. The yellow color of the sclera represents a common finding.

however, if the infant is placed under special lights, then the clearing will occur more quickly because conjugation of the bilirubin molecule is triggered by exposure to blue light. If the episode of jaundice is due to significant liver damage, as may be seen with viral hepatitis B or hepatotoxic chemical injury, then the prognosis will vary, depending on the extent of liver damage. The prognosis for patients with jaundice secondary to liver damage associated with metastatic malignancy is poor.

AMYLOIDOSIS

Amyloidosis represents a heterogeneous group of conditions characterized by the deposition of an extracellular proteinaceous substance called **amyloid**. Virchow coined the term *amyloid* in the middle of the nineteenth century because he believed it to be a starchlike material (*amyl* = starch; *oid* = resembling). We now understand that amyloid can be formed in a variety of settings, each with its own specific type of amyloid protein. Many of these amyloid proteins have been identified precisely with respect to their biochemical composition, and ideally an attempt should be made to categorize the type of amyloid specifically when this diagnosis is made. The various amyloid proteins are designated with an A, to indicate amyloid, followed by an abbreviation for the specific amyloid protein. For example, *AL* would identify amyloid composed of immunoglobulin light (L) chain molecules. Although amyloid may have several sources, all types of amyloid have the common feature of a β-pleated sheet molecular configuration, which can be seen with x-ray diffraction crystallographic analysis. Because of this similarity of molecular structure, the different types of amyloid have similar staining patterns with special stains.

Amyloidosis can produce a variety of effects, depending on the organ of involvement and the extent to which the amyloid is deposited. With limited cutaneous forms of amyloidosis, virtually no effect on survival is seen. With some forms of systemic amyloidosis, however, death may occur within a few years of the diagnosis as a result of cardiac or renal failure. Furthermore, the presence of amyloid may be associated with other problems, such as multiple myeloma or chronic infections.

CLINICAL FEATURES

Several classifications of amyloidosis have been proposed in the past decade, each evolving as the knowledge of this unusual condition increases. None of the classifications is completely satisfactory, although in recent years, the biochemical makeup of these proteins has figured more prominently in most classifications. This discussion attempts to be as concise and direct as possible. Essentially, amyloidosis may be divided into **organ-limited** and **systemic** forms from a clinical standpoint.

ORGAN-LIMITED AMYLOIDOSIS

Although organ-limited amyloidosis may occur in a variety of organs, it has rarely been reported in the oral soft tissues. An example of a limited form of amyloidosis is the amyloid nodule, which appears as a solitary, otherwise asymptomatic, submucosal deposit. Most of the organ-limited forms of amyloidosis consist of aggregates of immunoglobulin light chains, which in some cases are produced by a focal collection of monoclonal plasma cells. By definition, such amyloid deposits are not associated with any systemic alteration.

SYSTEMIC AMYLOIDOSIS

Systemic amyloidosis may occur in several forms:
- Primary
- Myeloma associated
- Secondary
- Hemodialysis associated
- Heredofamilial

PRIMARY AND MYELOMA-ASSOCIATED AMYLOIDOSIS

The primary and myeloma-associated forms of amyloidosis usually affect older adults (average age, 65 years), and a slight male predilection is present. These types of amyloidosis are caused by deposition of light chain molecules (thus the designation *AL*), with most cases being idiopathic, although approximately 15% to 20% are associated with multiple myeloma. The initial signs and symptoms may be nonspecific, often resulting in a delayed diagnosis. Fatigue, weight loss, paresthesia, hoarseness, edema, and orthostatic hypotension are

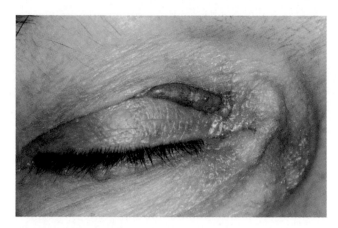

Fig. 17-7   Amyloidosis. This patient exhibits a firm, waxy nodular lesion in the periocular region, a finding that is characteristic of this condition.

among the first indications of this disease process. Eventually, carpal tunnel syndrome, mucocutaneous lesions, hepatomegaly, and macroglossia develop as a result of the deposition of the amyloid protein. The skin lesions appear as smooth-surfaced, firm, waxy papules and plaques. These most commonly affect the eyelid region (Fig. 17-7), the retroauricular region, the neck, and the lips. The lesions are often associated with petechiae and ecchymoses. Macroglossia has been reported in 10% to 40% of these patients and may appear as diffuse or nodular enlargement of the tongue (Fig. 17-8). Sometimes oral amyloid nodules show ulceration and submucosal hemorrhage overlying the lesions. Infrequently, patients may complain of dry eyes or dry mouth, which is secondary to amyloid infiltration and destruction of the lacrimal and salivary glands. When significant blood vessel infiltration has occurred, claudication of the jaw musculature may be noticed.

SECONDARY AMYLOIDOSIS

Secondary amyloidosis is so named because it characteristically develops as a result of a chronic inflammatory process, such as long-standing osteomyelitis, tuberculosis, or sarcoidosis. Cleavage fragments of a circulating acute-phase reactant protein appear to comprise this type of amyloidosis, which is thus designated AA. The heart is usually not affected as in other forms of amyloidosis. Liver, kidney, spleen, and adrenal involvement are typical, however. With the advent of modern antibiotic therapy, this form of amyloidosis has become much less common in the United States.

HEMODIALYSIS-ASSOCIATED AMYLOIDOSIS

Patients who have undergone long-term renal dialysis also are susceptible to amyloidosis, although in this case the amyloid protein has been identified as β_2-microglobulin, and this type of amyloidosis is

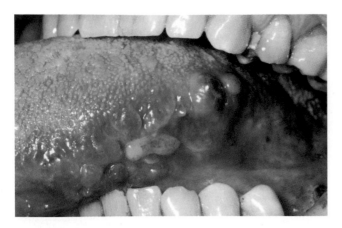

Fig. 17-8 Amyloidosis. Same patient as depicted in Fig. 17-7. Note amyloid nodules of lateral tongue, some of which are ulcerated. The patient's amyloidosis was the result of previously undiagnosed multiple myeloma.

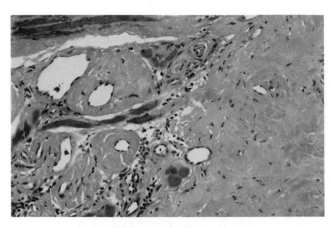

Fig. 17-9 Amyloidosis. This medium-power photomicrograph shows the eosinophilic, acellular deposits that are characteristic of amyloid deposition.

designated as $A\beta_2M$. β_2-Microglobulin is a normally occurring protein that is not removed by the dialysis procedure, and it accumulates in the plasma. Eventually, it forms deposits, particularly in the bones and joints. Often, carpal tunnel syndrome occurs, as well as cervical spine pain and dysfunction. Tongue involvement has been reported.

HEREDOFAMILIAL AMYLOIDOSIS

Heredofamilial amyloidosis is an uncommon but significant form of the disease. Several kindred have been identified in Swedish, Portuguese, and Japanese populations, and most types are inherited as autosomal dominant traits. An autosomal recessive form, known as *familial Mediterranean fever*, has also been described. Several of these conditions appear as polyneuropathies, although other manifestations, such as cardiomyopathy, cardiac arrhythmias, congestive heart failure, and renal failure, eventually develop as the amyloid deposition continues.

HISTOPATHOLOGIC FEATURES

Biopsy of rectal mucosa has classically been used to confirm a diagnosis of primary or myeloma-associated amyloidosis, with up to 80% of such biopsy specimens being positive. Aspiration biopsy of abdominal subcutaneous fat is a simpler procedure, however, and the sensitivity of this technique has been reported to range from 55% to 75%. Alternative tissue sources, however, are the gingiva and labial salivary glands. Histopathologic examination of gingival tissue that has been affected by amyloidosis shows extracellular deposition in the submucosal connective tissue of an amorphous,

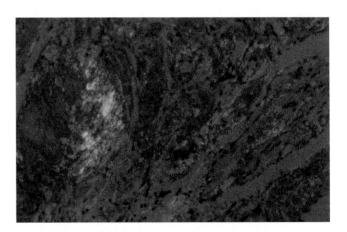

Fig. 17-10 Amyloidosis. High-power photomicrograph of a Congo red-stained section, demonstrating characteristic apple-green birefringence when viewed with polarized light. *(Courtesy of Dr. John Kalmar.)*

eosinophilic material, which may be arranged in a perivascular orientation or may be diffusely present throughout the tissue (Fig. 17-9). Relatively low sensitivity has been reported for gingival biopsies, whereas labial salivary gland tissue shows deposition of amyloid in a periductal or perivascular location in more than 80% of the cases.

A standard means of identifying amyloid uses the dye, Congo red, which has an affinity for the abnormal protein. In tissue sections stained with Congo red, the amyloid appears red. When the tissue is viewed with polarized light, it exhibits an apple-green birefringence (Fig. 17-10). Microscopic sections stained with crystal violet reveal a characteristic metachromasia; this normally purple dye appears more reddish when it reacts with amyloid. Staining with thioflavine T, a fluorescent dye, also gives positive results if amyloid is present. Ultrastructurally, amyloid is seen as a collection of 7.5- to 10-nm diameter, nonbranching, linear fibrils.

DIAGNOSIS

Once the histopathologic diagnosis of amyloidosis has been made, the patient must be evaluated medically to determine the type of amyloidosis that is present. This often entails a workup that includes serum immunoelectrophoresis to determine whether a monoclonal gammopathy exists so that multiple myeloma can be ruled out. Immunohistochemical studies are proving to be very useful in distinguishing the specific type of amyloid protein. Family history and physical examination findings are also important.

TREATMENT AND PROGNOSIS

In most instances, no effective therapy is available for amyloidosis. Surgical debulking of amyloid deposition in the tongue has met with limited success. Selected forms of amyloidosis may respond to treatment, or at least their progression may be slowed, depending on the underlying cause. In cases of secondary amyloidosis associated with an infectious agent, treatment of the infection and reduction of the inflammation often result in clinical improvement. Renal transplantation may arrest the progression of the bone lesions in hemodialysis-associated amyloidosis, but this procedure apparently does not reverse the process. Liver transplantation can improve the prognosis of several forms of inherited amyloidosis, particularly the transthyretin variant. Familial Mediterranean fever may respond to systemic colchicine therapy. Genetic counseling is also appropriate for patients affected by the inherited forms of amyloidosis. Treatment of primary amyloidosis (AL) with colchicine, prednisone, and melphalan appears to improve the prognosis of patients who do not have cardiac or renal involvement, although the outlook is guarded to poor in most instances. Most patients die of cardiac failure, arrhythmia, or renal disease within months to a few years after the diagnosis.

VITAMIN DEFICIENCY

In the United States today, significant vitamin deficiencies are not common. Patients with malabsorption syndromes or eating disorders, persons who follow "fad diets," and alcoholics are the groups most commonly affected.

Vitamin A (retinol) is essential for the maintenance of vision, and it also plays a role in growth and tissue differentiation. Vitamin A can be obtained directly from dietary sources, such as organ meats (particularly liver), or the body can synthesize it from β-carotene, which is abundant in red and yellow vegetables.

Vitamin B_1 (thiamin) acts as a coenzyme for several metabolic reactions and is thought to maintain the proper functioning of neurons. Thiamin is found in many animal and vegetable food sources.

Vitamin B_2 (riboflavin) is necessary for cellular oxidation-reduction reactions. Foods that contain significant amounts of riboflavin include milk, green vegetables, lean meat, fish, legumes, and eggs.

Vitamin B_3 (niacin) acts as a coenzyme for oxidation-reduction reactions. Rich sources include food from animal sources, especially lean meat and liver, milk, eggs, whole grains, peanuts, yeast, and cereal bran or germ.

Vitamin B_6 (pyridoxine) serves as a cofactor associated with enzymes that participate in amino acid synthesis. It is found in many animal and vegetable food sources.

Vitamin C (ascorbic acid) is necessary for the proper synthesis of collagen. This vitamin is present in a wide variety of vegetables and fruits, although it is particularly abundant in citrus fruits.

Vitamin D, which is now considered to be a hormone, can be synthesized in adequate amounts within the epidermis if the skin is exposed to a moderate degree of sunlight. Most milk and processed cereal is fortified with vitamin D in the United States today, however. Appropriate levels of vitamin D and its active metabolites are necessary for calcium absorption from the gut.

Vitamin E (α-tocopherol) is a fat-soluble vitamin that is widely stored throughout the body. It probably functions as an antioxidant. Vegetable oils, meats, nuts, cereal grains, and fresh greens and vegetables are good sources of vitamin E.

Vitamin K is a fat-soluble vitamin found in a wide variety of green vegetables, as well as milk, butter, and liver; intestinal bacteria also produce it. This vitamin is necessary for the proper synthesis of various proteins, including the clotting factors II, VII, IX, and X.

CLINICAL FEATURES

VITAMIN A

A severe deficiency of vitamin A during infancy may result in blindness. The early changes associated with a lack of this vitamin later in life include an inability of the eye to adapt to reduced light conditions (i.e., night blindness). With more severe, prolonged deficiency, dryness of the skin and conjunctiva develop, and the ocular changes may progress to ulceration of the cornea, leading to blindness.

THIAMIN

A deficiency of thiamin results in a condition called **beriberi,** a problem that is relatively uncommon in the Western world except in alcoholics or other individuals who do not receive a balanced diet. Thiamin deficiency has also been documented in patients who have had gastric bypass surgery for weight control, presumably because an adequate amount of the vitamin is not obtained in the diet. The condition became prevalent in southeast Asia when the practice of removing the outer husks of the rice grain by machine was introduced. Because these outer husks contained nearly all of the thiamin, people who subsisted on the "polished" rice became deficient in this vitamin. The disorder is manifested by cardiovascular problems (e.g., peripheral vasodilation, heart failure, edema) and neurologic problems (including peripheral neuropathy and Wernicke's encephalopathy). Patients with Wernicke's encephalopathy experience vomiting, nystagmus, and progressive mental deterioration, which may lead to coma and death.

RIBOFLAVIN

A diet that is chronically deficient in riboflavin causes a number of oral alterations, including glossitis, angular cheilitis, sore throat, and swelling and erythema of the oral mucosa. A normocytic, normochromic anemia may be present, and seborrheic dermatitis may affect the skin.

NIACIN

A deficiency of niacin causes a condition known as **pellagra**, a term derived from the Italian words *pelle agra,* meaning *rough skin.* This condition may occur in populations that use maize as a principal component of their diets, because corn is a poor source of niacin. Pellagra was once common in the southeastern United States and may still be seen in some parts of the world. The classic systemic signs and symptoms include the triad of dermatitis, dementia, and diarrhea. The dermatitis is distributed symmetrically; sun-exposed areas, such as the face, neck, and forearms, are affected most severely (Fig. 17-11). The oral manifestations have been described as stomatitis and glossitis, with the tongue appearing red, smooth, and raw. Without correction of the niacin deficiency, the disease may evolve and persist over a period of years, eventually leading to death.

PYRIDOXINE

A deficiency of pyridoxine is unusual because of its widespread occurrence in a variety of foods. A number of drugs, such as the antituberculosis drug isoniazid, act as pyridoxine antagonists; therefore, patients who

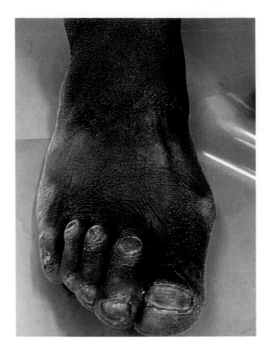

Fig. 17-11   Pellagra. The skin on the foot is rough and hyperpigmented, except for a central band that was protected from sunlight by a sandal strap. (*Courtesy of Dr. Sylvie Brener.*)

receive these medications may have a deficiency state. Because the vitamin plays a role in neuronal function, patients may show weakness, dizziness, or seizure disorders. Cheilitis and glossitis, reported in people with pellagra, are also reported in patients with pyridoxine deficiency.

VITAMIN C

A deficiency of vitamin C is known as **scurvy,** and its occurrence in the United States is usually limited to people whose diets lack fresh fruits and vegetables. Commonly affected groups include inner-city infants (whose diets often consist entirely of milk) and older edentulous men, particularly those who live alone.

The clinical signs of scurvy are typically related to inadequate collagen synthesis. For example, weakened vascular walls may result in widespread petechial hemorrhage and ecchymosis. Similarly, wound healing is delayed, and recently healed wounds may break down. In childhood, painful subperiosteal hemorrhages may occur.

The oral manifestations are well documented and include generalized gingival swelling with spontaneous hemorrhage, ulceration, tooth mobility, and increased severity of periodontal infection and periodontal bone loss. The gingival lesions have been termed **scorbutic gingivitis** (Fig. 17-12). If untreated, scurvy may ultimately lead to death, often as a result of intracranial hemorrhage.

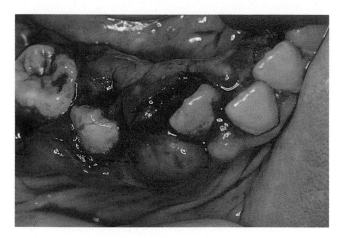

Fig. 17-12   Scurvy. Hemorrhagic gingival enlargement (scorbutic gingivitis) because of capillary fragility. (*Courtesy of Dr. James Hargan.*)

VITAMIN D

A deficiency of vitamin D during infancy results in a condition called **rickets**; adults who are deficient in this vitamin develop **osteomalacia**. With the vitamin-D supplementation of milk and cereal, rickets is a relatively uncommon disease today in the United States. In past centuries, however, rickets was often seen, particularly in the temperate zones of the world, which often do not receive adequate sunlight to ensure physiologic levels of vitamin D. Even today in the United States, children who are dark skinned and do not receive adequate sun exposure, as well as solely breast-fed infants, remain at risk for developing rickets. Nutritional rickets remains a problem in many developing countries, although the condition is thought to be associated more with calcium deficiency than vitamin-D deficiency.

Clinical manifestations of rickets include irritability, growth retardation, and prominence of the costochondral junctions (*rachitic rosary*). As the child ages and begins to put weight on the long bones of the legs, significant bowing results because of the poor mineralization of the skeleton.

A similar pattern of poorly mineralized bone is seen in osteomalacia in adults. Bone normally undergoes continuous remodeling and turnover, and the osteoid that is produced during this process does not have sufficient calcium to mineralize completely. Thus a weak, fragile bone structure results. Patients affected by osteomalacia frequently complain of diffuse skeletal pain, and their bones are susceptible to fracture with relatively minor injury.

VITAMIN E

A deficiency of vitamin E is rare and occurs primarily in children who suffer from chronic cholestatic liver disease. These patients have severe malabsorption of all fat-soluble vitamins, but particularly vitamin E. Multiple neurologic signs develop as a result of abnormalities in the central nervous system (CNS) and peripheral nervous system.

VITAMIN K

A deficiency of vitamin K may be seen in patients with malabsorption syndromes or in those whose intestinal microflora has been eliminated by long-term, broad-spectrum antibiotic use. Oral anticoagulants in the dicumarol family also inhibit the normal enzymatic activity of vitamin K. A deficiency or inhibition of synthesis of vitamin K leads to a coagulopathy because of the inadequate synthesis of prothrombin and other clotting factors. Intraorally, this coagulopathy is most often manifested by gingival bleeding. If the coagulopathy is not corrected, death may result from uncontrolled systemic hemorrhage.

TREATMENT AND PROGNOSIS

Replacement therapy is indicated for vitamin deficiencies. However, such deficiencies are uncommon, except for the situations described earlier. In fact, vitamin excess is perhaps more likely to be encountered in the United States today because so many people self-medicate with unnecessary and potentially harmful vitamin supplements. For example, excess vitamin A may cause abdominal pain, vomiting, headache, joint pain, and exostoses, whereas excess vitamin C may induce the formation of additional kidney stones in individuals with a history of nephrolithiasis.

IRON-DEFICIENCY ANEMIA

Iron-deficiency anemia is the most common cause of anemia in the United States and throughout the world. This form of anemia develops when the amount of iron available to the body cannot keep pace with the need for iron in the production of red blood cells (RBCs). This type of anemia develops under four conditions:

1. Excessive blood loss
2. Increased demand for RBCs
3. Decreased intake of iron
4. Decreased absorption of iron

It is estimated that 20% of women of childbearing age in the United States are iron deficient as a result of the chronic blood loss associated with excessive menstrual flow (**menorrhagia**). Similarly, 2% of adult men are iron deficient because of chronic blood loss, usually associated with gastrointestinal disease, such as peptic ulcer disease, diverticulosis, hiatal hernia, or malignancy.

An increased demand for erythrocyte production occurs during childhood growth spurts and during pregnancy. A decreased intake of iron may be seen during infancy when the diet consists of relatively iron-poor foods, such as cereals and milk. Likewise, the diets of older people may be deficient if their dental condition prohibits them from eating the proper foods or if they cannot afford iron-rich foods, such as meats and vegetables. In the developing world, intestinal parasites (especially hookworms) are a common cause of iron deficiency in children and pregnant women.

Decreased absorption is a much less common problem; however, it can be seen in patients who have had a complete gastrectomy or who have **celiac sprue**, a condition that results in severe chronic diarrhea because of sensitivity to the plant protein, gluten.

CLINICAL FEATURES

Patients with iron-deficiency anemia that is severe enough to cause symptoms may complain of fatigue, easy tiring, palpitations, lightheadedness, and lack of energy. Oral manifestations include angular cheilitis and atrophic glossitis or generalized oral mucosal atrophy. The glossitis has been described as a diffuse or patchy atrophy of the dorsal tongue papillae, often accompanied by tenderness or a burning sensation. Such findings are also evident in oral candidiasis, and some investigators have suggested that iron deficiency predisposes the patient to candidal infection, which results in the changes seen at the corners of the mouth and on the tongue. Such lesions are rarely seen in the United States, perhaps because the anemia is usually detected relatively early before the oral mucosal changes have had a chance to develop.

LABORATORY FINDINGS

The diagnosis should be established by means of a complete blood count with RBC indices because many other conditions, such as hypothyroidism, other anemias, or chronic depression, may elicit similar systemic clinical complaints. The laboratory evaluation characteristically shows hypochromic microcytic RBCs in addition to reduced numbers of erythrocytes. Additional supporting evidence for iron deficiency includes the findings of low serum iron levels and ferritin concentration together with elevated total iron-binding capacity.

TREATMENT AND PROGNOSIS

Therapy for most cases of iron-deficiency anemia consists of dietary iron supplementation by means of oral ferrous sulfate. For patients with malabsorption prob-

lems, parenteral iron may be given periodically. The response to therapy is usually prompt, with red cell parameters returning to normal within 1 to 2 months. The underlying cause of the anemia should be identified so that it may be addressed, if feasible.

PLUMMER-VINSON SYNDROME (PATERSON-KELLY SYNDROME; SIDEROPENIC DYSPHAGIA)

Plummer-Vinson syndrome is a rare condition characterized by iron-deficiency anemia, seen in conjunction with glossitis and dysphagia. Its incidence in developed countries has been declining, probably as a result of the improved nutritional status of the populations. The condition is significant in that it has been associated with a high frequency of both oral and esophageal squamous cell carcinoma; therefore, it is considered a premalignant process.

CLINICAL AND RADIOGRAPHIC FEATURES

Most reported patients with Plummer-Vinson syndrome have been women of Scandinavian or Northern European background, between 30 and 50 years of age. Patients typically complain of a burning sensation associated with the tongue and oral mucosa. Sometimes this discomfort is so severe that dentures cannot be worn. Angular cheilitis is often present and may be severe (Fig. 17-13). Marked atrophy of the lingual papillae, which produces a smooth, red appearance of the dorsal tongue, is seen clinically (Fig. 17-14).

Patients also frequently complain of difficulty in swallowing (**dysphagia**) or pain on swallowing. An evaluation with endoscopy or esophageal barium contrast radiographic studies usually shows the presence

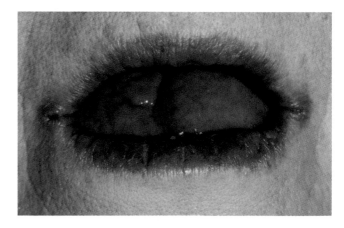

Fig. 17-13   Plummer-Vinson syndrome. Patients often show angular cheilitis.

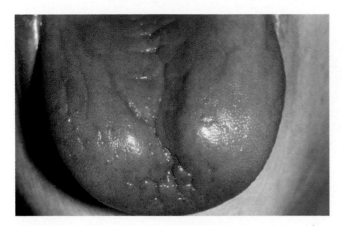

Fig. 17-14   Plummer-Vinson syndrome. The diffuse papillary atrophy of the dorsal tongue is characteristic of the oral changes. *(From Neville BW, Damm DD, White DK: Color atlas of clinical oral pathology, ed 2, Philadelphia, 1999, Lippincott Williams & Wilkins.)*

of abnormal bands of tissue in the esophagus, called **esophageal webs**. Another sign is an alteration of the growth pattern of the nails, which results in a spoon-shaped configuration **(koilonychia)**. The nails may also be brittle.

Symptoms of anemia may prompt patients with Plummer-Vinson syndrome to seek medical care. Fatigue, shortness of breath, and weakness are characteristic symptoms.

LABORATORY FINDINGS

Hematologic studies show a hypochromic microcytic anemia that is consistent with an iron-deficiency anemia.

HISTOPATHOLOGIC FEATURES

A biopsy specimen of involved mucosa from a patient with Plummer-Vinson syndrome typically shows epithelial atrophy with varying degrees of submucosal chronic inflammation. In advanced cases, evidence of epithelial atypia or dysplasia may be seen.

TREATMENT AND PROGNOSIS

Treatment of Plummer-Vinson syndrome is primarily directed at correcting the iron-deficiency anemia by means of dietary iron supplementation. This therapy usually resolves the anemia, relieves the glossodynia, and may reduce the severity of the esophageal symptoms. Occasionally, esophageal dilation is necessary to help improve the symptoms of dysphagia. Patients with Plummer-Vinson syndrome should be evaluated

periodically for oral, hypopharyngeal, and esophageal cancer because a 5% to 50% prevalence of upper aerodigestive tract malignancy has been reported in affected persons.

PERNICIOUS ANEMIA

Pernicious anemia is an uncommon condition that occurs with greatest frequency among older patients of Northern European heritage, although recent studies have identified the disease in black and Hispanic populations as well. The disease is a megaloblastic anemia caused by poor absorption of cobalamin (vitamin B_{12}, extrinsic factor). Intrinsic factor, which is produced by the parietal cells of the stomach lining, is needed for vitamin-B_{12} absorption. Normally, when cobalamin is ingested, it binds to intrinsic factor in the duodenum. Because the lining cells of the intestine preferentially take up the cobalamin-intrinsic factor complex, significant amounts of the vitamin cannot be absorbed unless both components are present.

In the case of pernicious anemia, most patients lack intrinsic factor because of an autoimmune destruction of the parietal cells of the stomach, and this results in decreased absorption of cobalamin. Antibodies directed against intrinsic factor are also found in the serum of these patients. Vitamin B_{12} deficiency may occur for other reasons, and although the resulting signs and symptoms may be identical to those of pernicious anemia, these should be considered as distinctly different deficiency disorders. For example, a decreased ability to absorb cobalamin may also occur after gastrointestinal bypass operations. In addition, because cobalamin is primarily derived from animal sources, some strict vegetarians (vegans) may develop vitamin B_{12} deficiency. In older patients, gastritis associated with *Helicobacter pylori* infection can result in decreased vitamin B_{12} absorption.

Because cobalamin is necessary for normal nucleic acid synthesis, anything that disrupts the absorption of the vitamin causes problems, especially for cells that are multiplying rapidly and, therefore, synthesizing large amounts of nucleic acids. The cells that are the most mitotically active are affected to the greatest degree, especially the hematopoietic cells and the gastrointestinal lining epithelial cells.

CLINICAL FEATURES

With respect to systemic complaints, patients with pernicious anemia often report fatigue, weakness, shortness of breath, headache, and feeling faint. Such symptoms are associated with most anemias and probably reflect the reduced oxygen-carrying capacity of the blood. In addition, many patients report

Fig. 17-15 Pernicious anemia. A, The dorsal tongue shows erythema and atrophy. **B,** After therapy with vitamin B₁₂, the mucosal alteration resolved.

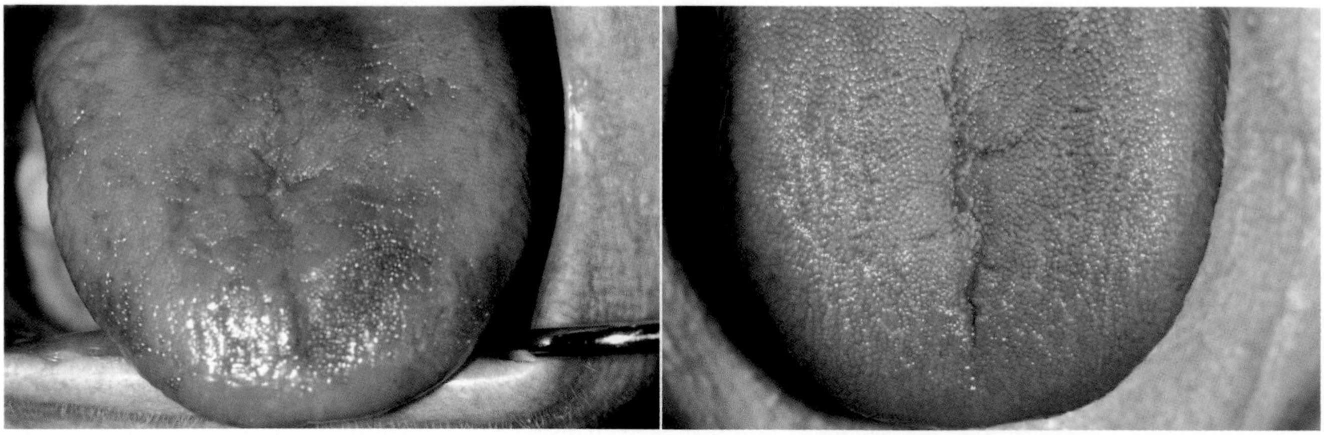

paresthesia, tingling, or numbness of the extremities. Difficulty in walking and diminished vibratory and positional sense may be present. Psychiatric symptoms of memory loss, irritability, depression, and dementia have also been described.

Oral symptoms often consist of a burning sensation of the tongue, lips, buccal mucosa, or other mucosal sites. Clinical examination may show focal patchy areas of oral mucosal erythema and atrophy (Fig. 17-15), or the process may be more diffuse, depending on the severity and duration of the condition. The tongue may be affected in as many as 50% to 60% of patients with pernicious anemia, but it may not show as much involvement as other areas of the oral mucosa in some instances. The atrophy and erythema may be easier to appreciate on the dorsal tongue than at other sites, however.

HISTOPATHOLOGIC FEATURES

Histopathologic examination of an erythematous portion of the oral mucosa shows marked epithelial atrophy with loss of rete ridges, an increased nuclear-to-cytoplasmic ratio, and prominent nucleoli (Fig. 17-16). This pattern can be misinterpreted as epithelial dysplasia at times, although the nuclei in pernicious anemia typically are pale staining and show peripheral chromatin clumping. A patchy diffuse chronic inflammatory cell infiltrate is usually noted in the underlying connective tissue.

LABORATORY FINDINGS

Hematologic evaluation of vitamin B₁₂ deficiency shows a macrocytic anemia and reduced serum cobalamin levels. The Schilling test for pernicious anemia

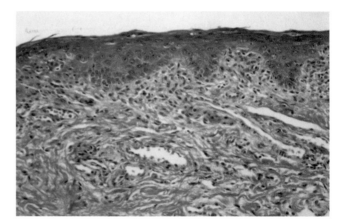

Fig. 17-16 Pernicious anemia. This medium-power photomicrograph shows epithelial atrophy and atypia with chronic inflammation of the underlying connective tissue. These features are characteristic of a megaloblastic anemia, such as pernicious anemia.

has been used to determine the pathogenesis of the cobalamin deficiency by comparing absorption and excretion rates of radiolabeled cobalamin. However, this study is rather complicated to perform, and it appears to be falling out of favor. The presence of serum antibodies directed against intrinsic factor is quite specific for pernicious anemia.

TREATMENT AND PROGNOSIS

Once the diagnosis of pernicious anemia is established, treatment traditionally has consisted of monthly intramuscular injections of cyanocobalamin. The condition responds rapidly once therapy is initiated, with reports of clearing of oral lesions within 5 days. High-dose oral cobalamin therapy has also been shown to be an equally effective treatment, however, with advantages being its cost-effectiveness and the elimination of painful injections. One study has confirmed an increased risk of malignancy, particularly gastric carcinoma, a complication that affects between 1% and 2% of pernicious anemia patients.

PITUITARY DWARFISM

Pituitary dwarfism is a relatively rare condition that results from either the diminished production of growth hormone by the anterior pituitary gland or a reduced capacity of the tissues to respond to growth hormone. Affected patients are typically much shorter than normal, although their body proportions are generally appropriate.

Several conditions may cause short stature, and a careful evaluation of the patient must be performed to rule out other possible causes, such as the following:

1. Intrinsic defects in the patient's tissues (e.g., certain skeletal dysplasias, chromosomal abnormalities, idiopathic short stature)
2. Alterations in the environment of the growing tissues (e.g., malnutrition, hypothyroidism, diabetes mellitus)

If a lack of growth hormone is detected, the cause should be determined. Sometimes the fault lies with the pituitary gland itself (e.g., aplasia, hypoplasia). In other instances, the problem may be related to destruction of the pituitary or hypothalamus by tumors, therapeutic radiation, or infection.

If the hypothalamus is affected, a deficiency in growth hormone-releasing hormone, which is produced by the hypothalamus, results in a deficiency of growth hormone. Often deficiencies in other hormones, such as thyroid hormone and cortisol, are also detected in patients with primary pituitary or hypothalamic disorders.

Some patients exhibit normal or even elevated levels of growth hormone, yet still show little evidence of growth. These individuals usually have inherited an autosomal recessive trait, resulting in abnormal and reduced growth hormone receptors on the patients' cells. Thus normal growth cannot proceed.

CLINICAL FEATURES

Perhaps the most striking feature of pituitary dwarfism is the remarkably short stature of the affected patient. Sometimes this is not noticed until the early years of childhood, but a review of the patient's growth history should show a consistent pattern of failure to achieve the minimal height on the standard growth chart. Often the patient's height may be as much as three standard deviations below normal for a given age. Unlike the body proportions in many of the dysmorphic syndromes and skeletal dysplasias, the body proportions of patients affected by a lack of growth hormone are usually normal. One possible exception is the size of the skull, which is usually within normal limits. Because the facial skeleton does not keep pace with the skull, however, the face of an affected patient may appear smaller than it should be. Mental status is generally within normal limits.

The maxilla and mandible of affected patients are smaller than normal, and the teeth show a delayed pattern of eruption. The delay ranges from 1 to 3 years for teeth that normally erupt during the first decade of life and from 3 to 10 years for teeth that normally erupt in the second decade of life. Often the shedding of deciduous teeth is delayed by several years, and the development of the roots of the permanent teeth also appears to be delayed. A lack of development of the third molars seems to be a common finding. The size of the teeth is usually reduced in proportion to the other anatomic structures.

LABORATORY FINDINGS

Radioimmunoassay for human growth hormone shows levels that are markedly below normal.

TREATMENT AND PROGNOSIS

Replacement therapy with human growth hormone is the treatment of choice for patients with pituitary dwarfism if the disorder is detected before closure of the epiphyseal growth plates. In the past, growth hormone was extracted from cadaveric pituitary glands; today, genetically engineered human growth hormone is produced with recombinant DNA technology. For patients with a growth hormone deficiency caused by a hypothalamic defect, treatment with growth hormone-releasing hormone is appropriate. If patients are identified and treated at an early age, they can be expected to achieve a relatively normal height. The craniofacial bone structure also assumes a less childlike pattern. Evaluation of a series of patients who had been treated for long periods with growth hormone determined that up to half developed acromegalic features, including larger feet and a larger mandible. For patients who lack growth hormone receptors, no treatment is available.

GIGANTISM

Gigantism is a rare condition caused by an increased production of growth hormone, usually related to a functional pituitary adenoma. The increased production of growth hormone takes place before closure of the epiphyseal plates, and the affected person grows at a much more rapid pace, becoming abnormally tall. Although the average height of the population of the United States has been gradually increasing during the past several decades, individuals who exceed the mean height by more than three standard deviations may be considered candidates for endocrinologic evaluation. Familial examples of gigantism have also been described.

CLINICAL AND RADIOGRAPHIC FEATURES

Patients with gigantism usually show markedly accelerated growth during childhood, irrespective of normal growth spurts. Radiographic evaluation of the skull often shows an enlarged sella as a result of the presence of a pituitary adenoma. The adenoma may result in hormonal deficiencies, such as hypothyroidism and hypoadrenocorticism, if the remaining normal pituitary gland tissue is compressed and destroyed. **McCune-Albright syndrome** (polyostotic fibrous dysplasia and *café au lait* pigmentation with associated endocrinologic disturbances) (see page 636) may account for as many as 20% of the cases of gigantism.

If the condition remains uncorrected for a prolonged period, extreme height (more than 7 feet tall) will be achieved, and enlargement of the facial soft tissues, the mandible, and the hands and feet will become apparent. These changes often resemble those seen in **acromegaly** (discussed later). Another oral finding is true generalized macrodontia.

TREATMENT AND PROGNOSIS

Appropriate management of gigantism involves the surgical removal of the functioning pituitary adenoma, usually by a transsphenoidal approach. Radiation therapy may also be used.

The life span of patients with gigantism is usually markedly reduced. Complications associated with hypertension, peripheral neuropathy, osteoporosis, and pulmonary disease contribute to increased morbidity and mortality.

ACROMEGALY

Acromegaly is an uncommon condition characterized by the excess production of growth hormone after closure of the epiphyseal plates in the affected patient. Usually, this increase in growth hormone is due to a functional pituitary adenoma. The incidence is estimated to be approximately three to five new cases diagnosed per million population per year. The prevalence is believed to be 66 affected patients per million.

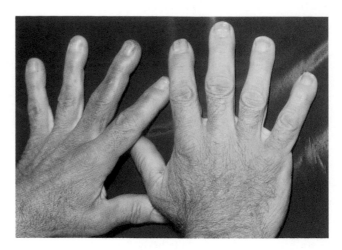

Fig. 17-17   Acromegaly. Enlargement of the bones of the hands. *(Courtesy of Dr. William Bruce.)*

CLINICAL AND RADIOGRAPHIC FEATURES

Because most patients with acromegaly have a pituitary adenoma, symptoms related directly to the space-occupying mass of the tumor may be present. These symptoms include headaches, visual disturbances, and other signs of a brain tumor. Sometimes pressure atrophy of the residual normal pituitary by the adenoma results in diminished production of other pituitary hormones and causes other indirect endocrine problems. The direct effects of increased levels of growth hormone include a variety of problems, such as hypertension, heart disease, hyperhidrosis, arthritis, and peripheral neuropathy.

Renewed growth in the small bones of the hands and feet (Fig. 17-17) and in the membranous bones of the skull and jaws is typically observed. Patients may complain of gloves or hats becoming "too small." The soft tissue is also often affected, producing a coarse facial appearance (Fig. 17-18). Hypertrophy of the soft palatal tissues may cause or accentuate sleep apnea. Because these signs and symptoms are slow to develop and are vague at the onset, an average time of nearly 9 years elapses from the onset of symptoms to the diagnosis of disease. The average age at diagnosis is 42 years, and no sex predilection is seen.

From a dental perspective, these patients have mandibular prognathism as a result of the increased growth of the mandible (Fig. 17-19), which may cause apertognathia (anterior open bite). Growth of the jaws also may cause spacing of the teeth, resulting in diastema formation. Soft tissue growth often produces uniform macroglossia in affected patients.

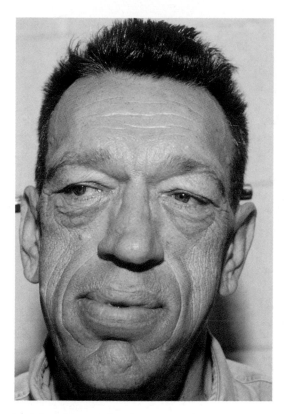

Fig. 17-18   Acromegaly. This patient shows the typical coarse facial features. *(Courtesy of Dr. William Bruce.)*

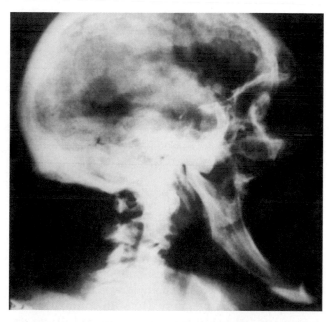

Fig. 17-19   Acromegaly. This lateral skull film shows the dramatic degree of mandibular enlargement that may occur.

LABORATORY FINDINGS AND DIAGNOSIS

If acromegaly is suspected, measurement of serum growth hormone levels is done after giving the patient a measured quantity of glucose orally. Normally, this glucose challenge will reduce the production of growth hormone, but if the patient has acromegaly, growth hormone will not be suppressed. Usually magnetic resonance imaging (MRI) will identify the pituitary adenoma that is responsible for inappropriate growth hormone secretion.

TREATMENT AND PROGNOSIS

The treatment of a patient with acromegaly is typically directed at the removal of the pituitary tumor mass and the return of the growth hormone levels to normal. The most effective treatment with the least associated morbidity is surgical excision by a transsphenoidal approach. The prognosis for such a procedure is good, although a mortality rate of approximately 1% is still expected. The condition is usually controlled with this procedure, but patients with larger tumors and markedly elevated growth hormone levels are less likely to be controlled.

Radiation therapy may be used in some instances, but the return of the growth hormone levels to normal is not as rapid or as predictable as with surgery. Because some patients also experience hypopituitarism caused by radiation effects on the rest of the gland, some centers may offer radiation therapy as treatment only when surgery fails or is too risky. Pharmacotherapy with one of the somatostatin analogues (e.g., octreotide, lanreotide, vapreotide) helps to control acromegaly if surgical treatment is unsuccessful or if surgery is contraindicated. A growth hormone receptor-blocking agent, pegvisomant, has also been developed and may be used in conjunction with one of the somatostatin analogues or by itself if the patient cannot tolerate the somatostatin analogue. Pegvisomant is injected daily and acts in the peripheral tissues to inhibit the action of growth hormone. These drugs are also used as an adjunct to radiation therapy during the prolonged period that is sometimes necessary for that treatment to take effect.

The prognosis for untreated patients is guarded, with an increased mortality rate compared with that of the general population. Hypertension, diabetes mellitus, coronary artery disease, congestive heart failure, respiratory disease, and colon cancer are seen with increased frequency in acromegalic patients, and each of these contributes to the increased mortality rate. Although treatment of the patient with acromegaly helps to control many of the other complicating problems and improves the prognosis, the life span of these patients still is shortened.

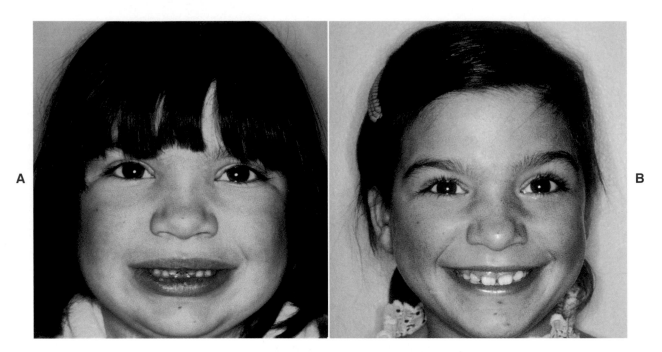

Fig. 17-20 **Hypothyroidism. A,** The facial appearance of this 9-year-old child is due to the accumulation of tissue edema secondary to severe hypothyroidism. **B,** Same patient after 1 year of thyroid hormone replacement therapy. Note the eruption of the maxillary permanent teeth.

HYPOTHYROIDISM (CRETINISM; MYXEDEMA)

Hypothyroidism is a condition that is characterized by decreased levels of thyroid hormone. When this decrease occurs during infancy, the resulting clinical problem is known as **cretinism**. If an adult has markedly decreased thyroid hormone levels for a prolonged period, then deposition of a glycosaminoglycan ground substance is seen in the subcutaneous tissues, producing a nonpitting edema. Some call this severe form of hypothyroidism **myxedema**; others use the terms *myxedema* and *hypothyroidism* interchangeably.

Hypothyroidism may be classified as either **primary** or **secondary**. In primary hypothyroidism, the thyroid gland itself is in some way abnormal; in secondary hypothyroidism, the pituitary gland does not produce an adequate amount of thyroid-stimulating hormone (TSH), which is necessary for the appropriate release of thyroid hormone. Secondary hypothyroidism, for example, often develops after radiation therapy for brain tumors, resulting in unavoidable radiation damage to the pituitary gland. Most cases, however, represent the primary form of the disease.

Screening for this disorder is routinely carried out at birth, and the prevalence of congenital hypothyroidism in North America is approximately 1 in 4000 births. Usually, this is due to hypoplasia or agenesis of the thyroid gland. In other areas of the world, hypothyroidism in infancy is usually due to a lack of dietary iodine. In adults, hypothyroidism is often caused by autoimmune destruction of the thyroid gland (known as **Hashimoto's thyroiditis**) or iatrogenic factors, such as radioactive iodine therapy or surgery for the treatment of hyperthyroidism. Because thyroid hormone is necessary for normal cellular metabolism, many of the clinical signs and symptoms of hypothyroidism can be related to the decreased metabolic rate in these patients.

CLINICAL FEATURES

The most common features of hypothyroidism include such signs and symptoms as lethargy, dry and coarse skin, swelling of the face (Fig. 17-20) and extremities, huskiness of the voice, constipation, weakness, and fatigue. The heart rate is usually slowed **(bradycardia)**. Reduced body temperature **(hypothermia)** may be present, and the skin often feels cool and dry to the touch. In the infant, these signs may not be readily apparent, and the failure to grow normally may be the first indication of the disease.

With respect to the oral findings, the lips may appear thickened because of the accumulation of glycosaminoglycans. Diffuse enlargement of the tongue occurs

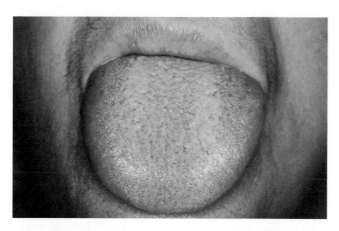

Fig. 17-21   Hypothyroidism. The enlarged tongue (macroglossia) is secondary to edema associated with adult hypothyroidism (myxedema). *(Courtesy of Dr. George Blozis.)*

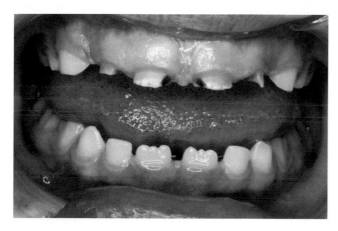

Fig. 17-22   Hypothyroidism. Photograph of the same patient depicted in Fig. 17-20 before hormone replacement therapy. Note the retained deciduous teeth, for which the patient was initially referred.

for the same reason (Fig. 17-21). If the condition develops during childhood, the teeth may fail to erupt, although tooth formation may not be impaired (Figs. 17-22 and 17-23).

LABORATORY FINDINGS

The diagnosis is made by assaying the free thyroxine (T_4) levels. If these levels are low, then TSH levels are measured to determine whether primary or secondary hypothyroidism is present. With primary thyroid disease, TSH levels are elevated. With secondary disease caused by pituitary dysfunction, TSH levels are normal or borderline.

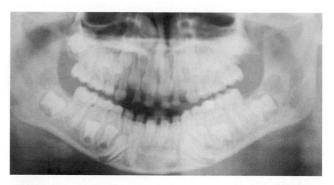

Fig. 17-23   Hypothyroidism. Panoramic radiograph of the same patient in Figs. 17-20 and 17-22. Note the unerupted, yet fully developed permanent dentition.

TREATMENT AND PROGNOSIS

Thyroid replacement therapy, usually with levothyroxine, is indicated for confirmed cases of hypothyroidism. The prognosis is generally good for adult patients. If the condition is recognized within a reasonable time, the prognosis is also good for children. If the condition is not identified in a timely manner, however, permanent damage to the central nervous system may occur, resulting in mental retardation. For affected children, thyroid hormone replacement therapy often results in a dramatic resolution of the condition (see Fig. 17-20).

HYPERTHYROIDISM (THYROTOXICOSIS; GRAVES' DISEASE)

Hyperthyroidism is a condition caused by excess production of thyroid hormone. This excess production results in a state of markedly increased metabolism in the affected patient. Most cases (60% to 90%) are due to **Graves' disease**, a condition that was initially described in the early nineteenth century. It is thought to be triggered by autoantibodies that are directed against receptors for thyroid-stimulating hormone (TSH) on the surface of the thyroid cells. When the autoantibodies bind to these receptors, they seem to stimulate the thyroid cells to release inappropriate thyroid hormone.

Other causes of hyperthyroidism include hyperplastic thyroid tissue and thyroid tumors, both benign and malignant, which secrete inappropriate thyroid hormone. Similarly, a pituitary adenoma may produce TSH, which can then stimulate the thyroid to secrete excess thyroid hormone.

CLINICAL FEATURES

Graves' disease is five to 10 times more common in women than in men and is seen with some frequency. It affects almost 2% of the adult female population.

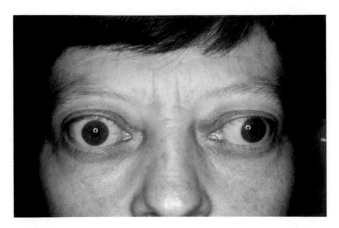

Fig. 17-24 Hyperthyroidism. The prominent eyes are characteristic of the exophthalmos associated with Graves' disease.

Graves' disease is most commonly diagnosed in patients during the third and fourth decades of life.

Most patients with Graves' disease exhibit diffuse thyroid enlargement. Many of the signs and symptoms of hyperthyroidism can be attributed to an increased metabolic rate caused by the excess thyroid hormone. Patients usually complain about nervousness, heart palpitations, heat intolerance, emotional lability, and muscle weakness. The following are often noted during the clinical evaluation:

- Weight loss despite increased appetite
- Tachycardia
- Excessive perspiration
- Widened pulse pressure (increased systolic and decreased diastolic pressures)
- Warm, smooth skin
- Tremor

Ocular involvement, which develops in 20% to 40% of affected patients, is perhaps the most striking feature of this disease. In the early stages of hyperthyroidism, patients have a characteristic stare with eyelid retraction and lid lag. With some forms of Graves' disease, protrusion of the eyes (**exophthalmos** or **proptosis**) develops (Fig. 17-24). This bulging of the eyes is due to an accumulation of glycosaminoglycans in the retro-orbital connective tissues.

LABORATORY FINDINGS

The diagnosis of hyperthyroidism is made by assaying free T_4 (thyroxine) and TSH levels in the serum. In affected patients, the T_4 levels should be elevated and the TSH concentration is typically depressed.

HISTOPATHOLOGIC FEATURES

Diffuse enlargement and hypercellularity of the thyroid gland are seen in patients with Graves' disease, typically with hyperplastic thyroid epithelium and little apparent colloid production. Lymphocytic infiltration of the glandular parenchyma is also often noted.

TREATMENT AND PROGNOSIS

In the United States, radioactive iodine (^{131}I) is the most commonly used form of therapy for adult patients with Graves' disease. The thyroid gland normally takes up iodine from the bloodstream because this element is a critical component of thyroid hormone. When radioactive iodine is given to a patient with Graves' disease, the thyroid gland quickly removes it from the bloodstream and sequesters the radioactive material within the glandular tissue. The radioactivity then destroys the hyperactive thyroid tissue, bringing the thyroid hormone levels back to normal. Most of the radiation is received during the first few weeks because the half-life of ^{131}I is short.

Other techniques include drug therapy with agents that block the normal use of iodine by the thyroid gland, and this form of therapy is initially favored in most European centers. The two widely used drugs are propylthiouracil and methimazole. At times, they are used before the radioactive iodine therapy. Sometimes they may be administered chronically in the hope that a remission may be induced. In addition, a portion of the thyroid gland may be removed surgically, thereby reducing thyroid hormone production.

Drug therapy alone is often unsuccessful in controlling hyperthyroidism. Unfortunately, with radioactive iodine and surgery, the risk of hypothyroidism is relatively great, although thyroid hormone replacement therapy can be instituted, if needed.

In a patient with uncontrolled hyperthyroidism, a definite risk exists with respect to an inappropriate release of large amounts of thyroid hormone at one time, resulting in a condition called a **thyroid storm**. A thyroid storm may be precipitated by infection, psychologic trauma, or stress. Clinically, patients may have delirium, convulsions, an elevated temperature (up to 106° F), and tachycardia (sometimes more than 140 beats/minute). Such individuals should be hospitalized immediately because the mortality rate associated with thyroid storm is 20% to 50%. The clinician should be aware of the potential for this problem, and patients with hyperthyroidism should ideally have the condition under control before dental treatment.

HYPOPARATHYROIDISM

Calcium levels in extracellular tissues are normally regulated by parathyroid hormone (PTH) (parathormone) in conjunction with vitamin D. If calcium levels drop below a certain point, then the release of PTH is stimulated. The hormone then acts directly on the kidney and the osteoclasts of the bone to restore the calcium to normal levels. In the kidney, calcium reabsorption is promoted, phosphate excretion is enhanced, and the production of vitamin D is stimulated, which increases the absorption of calcium from the gut. Osteoclasts are activated to resorb bone and thus liberate calcium.

If a reduced amount of PTH is produced, the relatively rare condition known as **hypoparathyroidism** results. Usually, hypoparathyroidism is due to inadvertent surgical removal of the parathyroid glands when the thyroid gland is excised for other reasons, but sometimes it is the result of autoimmune destruction of the parathyroid tissue. Rare syndromes, such as **DiGeorge syndrome** and the **autoimmune polyendocrinopathy-candidiasis-ectodermal dystrophy syndrome (endocrine-candidiasis syndrome)**, may be associated with hypoparathyroidism.

CLINICAL FEATURES

With the loss of parathyroid function, the serum levels of calcium drop, resulting in hypocalcemia. Often the patient with chronic hypoparathyroidism adapts to the presence of hypocalcemia and is asymptomatic unless situations that further reduce the calcium levels are encountered. Such situations include metabolic alkalosis, as seen during hyperventilation, when a state of tetany may become evident.

Chvostek's sign is an oral finding of significance, characterized by a twitching of the upper lip when the facial nerve is tapped just below the zygomatic process. A positive response suggests a latent degree of tetany. If the hypoparathyroidism develops early in life during odontogenesis, then a pitting enamel hypoplasia and failure of tooth eruption may occur (Fig. 17-25). The presence of persistent oral candidiasis in a young patient may signal the onset of autoimmune polyendocrinopathy-candidiasis-ectodermal dystrophy syndrome (see page 219). Hypoparathyroidism may be only one of several endocrine deficiencies associated with this condition.

LABORATORY FINDINGS

PTH can be measured by means of a radioimmunoassay. If serum PTH levels are decreased in conjunction with a decreased serum calcium concentration, ele-

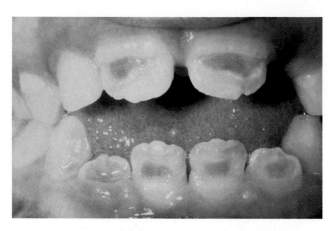

Fig. 17-25   Hypoparathyroidism. Enamel hypoplasia has affected the dentition of this patient, who had hypoparathyroidism while the teeth were forming.

vated serum phosphate level, and normal renal function, then a diagnosis of hypoparathyroidism can be made.

TREATMENT AND PROGNOSIS

Patients with hypoparathyroidism are usually treated with oral doses of a vitamin-D precursor (ergocalciferol, vitamin D_2). Additional supplements of dietary calcium may also be necessary to maintain the proper serum calcium levels. With this regimen, patients can often live a fairly normal life. Teriparatide, a recombinant form of the active component of human parathormone, has been developed recently. When given twice daily as subcutaneous injections, this drug has also shown promise as an alternative management strategy for hypoparathyroidism, although it is relatively expensive.

PSEUDOHYPOPARATHYROIDISM (ALBRIGHT HEREDITARY OSTEODYSTROPHY; ACRODYSOSTOSIS)

The rare condition known as **pseudohypoparathyroidism** represents at least two broad disorders in which normal parathyroid hormone (PTH) is present in adequate amounts but the biochemical pathways responsible for activating the target cells are not functioning properly. The clinical result is a patient who appears to have hypoparathyroidism.

In the case of pseudohypoparathyroidism type I, three subcategories have been defined. For type Ia, a molecular defect of a specific intracellular binding protein known as $G_s\alpha$ seems to prevent the formation of cyclic adenosine monophosphate (cAMP), a critical component in the activation of cell metabolism.

Because other hormones also require binding with $G_s\alpha$ to carry out their functions, patients have multiple problems with other endocrine organs and functions. This condition is usually inherited as an autosomal dominant trait.

With respect to pseudohypoparathyroidism type Ib, the problem is thought to be caused by defective receptors for the PTH on the surface of the target cells (the proximal renal tubules). For this reason, no other endocrine tissues or functions are affected. An autosomal dominant mode of inheritance has been suggested for a few families affected by type Ib pseudohypoparathyroidism, but most cases are apparently sporadic. The mechanism of action for pseudohypoparathyroidism type Ic is less clear, but it may involve a defect in adenylate cyclase or a subtle $G_s\alpha$ alteration.

Pseudohypoparathyroidism type II is characterized by the induction of cAMP by PTH in the target cells; however, a functional response by the cells is not invoked. All of the reported cases of this form of the disease appear to be sporadic.

CLINICAL FEATURES

Pseudohypoparathyroidism most commonly appears as type Ia disease. Patients affected by pseudohypoparathyroidism, either type Ia or Ic, have a characteristic array of features that includes mild mental retardation, obesity, round face, short neck, and markedly short stature. Midfacial hypoplasia is also commonly observed. The metacarpals and metatarsals are usually shortened, and the fingers appear short and thick. Subcutaneous calcifications (osteoma cutis) may be identified in some patients. Other endocrine abnormalities that are typically encountered include hypogonadism and hypothyroidism.

Patients with type Ib and II disease clinically appear normal, aside from their symptoms of hypocalcemia.

Dental manifestations of pseudohypoparathyroidism include generalized enamel hypoplasia, widened pulp chambers with intrapulpal calcifications, oligodontia, delayed eruption, and blunting of the apices of the teeth. The pulpal calcifications are often described as "dagger" shaped.

The diagnosis of pseudohypoparathyroidism is made based on elevated serum levels of PTH seen concurrently with hypocalcemia, hyperphosphatemia, and otherwise normal renal function. More sophisticated studies are necessary to delineate the various subtypes.

TREATMENT AND PROGNOSIS

Pseudohypoparathyroidism is managed by the administration of vitamin D and calcium. The serum calcium levels and urinary calcium excretion are carefully monitored. Because of individual patient differences, the medication may need to be carefully adjusted; however, the prognosis is considered to be good.

HYPERPARATHYROIDISM

Excess production of parathyroid hormone (PTH) results in the condition known as **hyperparathyroidism**. PTH normally is produced by the parathyroid glands in response to a decrease in serum calcium levels.

Primary hyperparathyroidism is the uncontrolled production of PTH, usually as a result of a parathyroid adenoma (80% to 90% of cases) or parathyroid hyperplasia (10% to 15% of cases). Rarely (approximately 1% of cases), a parathyroid carcinoma may be the cause of primary hyperparathyroidism. Infrequently this endocrine disturbance is caused by any one of several inherited syndromes, including **multiple endocrine neoplasia type 1** or **type 2a**, or **hyperparathyroidism-jaw tumor syndrome.** In the latter condition, affected patients develop multiple jaw lesions that histopathologically are consistent with central cemento-ossifying fibroma. There also appears to be an increased risk for these patients to develop parathyroid carcinoma.

Secondary hyperparathyroidism develops when PTH is continuously produced in response to chronic low levels of serum calcium, a situation usually associated with chronic renal disease. The kidney processes vitamin D, which is necessary for calcium absorption from the gut. Therefore, in a patient with chronic renal disease, active vitamin D is not produced and less calcium is absorbed from the gut, resulting in lowered serum calcium levels.

CLINICAL AND RADIOGRAPHIC FEATURES

Most patients with primary hyperparathyroidism are older than 60 years of age. Women have this condition two to four times more often than men do. Typically the condition is identified on routine serologic testing, and the majority of patients are relatively asymptomatic.

Patients with the classic triad of signs and symptoms of hyperparathyroidism are described as having "stones, bones, and abdominal groans."

Stones refers to the fact that these patients, particularly those with primary hyperparathyroidism, have a marked tendency to develop renal calculi (kidney stones, nephrolithiasis) because of the elevated serum calcium levels. Metastatic calcifications are also seen, frequently involving other soft tissues, such as blood

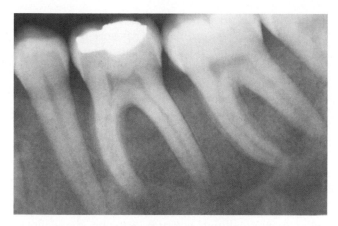

Fig. 17-26 Hyperparathyroidism. This periapical radiograph reveals the "ground glass" appearance of the trabeculae and loss of lamina dura in a patient with secondary hyperparathyroidism. *(Courtesy of Dr. Randy Anderson.)*

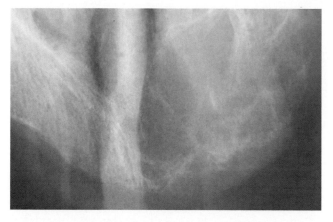

Fig. 17-27 Hyperparathyroidism. This occlusal radiograph of the edentulous maxillary anterior region shows a multilocular radiolucency characteristic of a brown tumor of primary hyperparathyroidism. *(Courtesy of Dr. Brian Blocher.)*

vessel walls, subcutaneous soft tissues, the sclera, the dura, and the regions around the joints.

Bones refers to a variety of osseous changes that may occur in conjunction with hyperparathyroidism. One of the first clinical signs of this disease is seen radiographically as subperiosteal resorption of the phalanges of the index and middle fingers. Generalized loss of the lamina dura surrounding the roots of the teeth is also seen as an early manifestation of the condition (Fig. 17-26). Alterations in trabecular pattern characteristically develop next. A decrease in trabecular density and blurring of the normal trabecular pattern occur; often a "ground glass" appearance results.

With persistent disease, other osseous lesions develop, such as the so-called **brown tumor** of hyperparathyroidism. This lesion derives its name from the color of the tissue specimen, which is usually a dark red-brown because of the abundant hemorrhage and hemosiderin deposition within the tumor. These lesions appear radiographically as well-demarcated unilocular or multilocular radiolucencies (Fig. 17-27). They commonly affect the mandible, clavicles, ribs, and pelvis. They may be solitary but are often multiple, and long-standing lesions may produce significant cortical expansion. Typically, the other osseous changes are observable if brown tumors are present. The most severe skeletal manifestation of chronic hyperparathyroidism has been called **osteitis fibrosa cystica**, a condition that develops from the central degeneration and fibrosis of long-standing brown tumors. In patients with secondary hyperparathyroidism caused by end-stage renal disease (**renal osteodystrophy**), striking enlargement of the jaws has been known to occur (Fig. 17-28) and produce a "ground-glass" radiographic pattern (see Fig. 17-26).

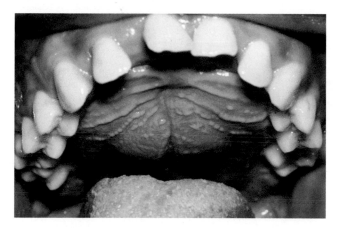

Fig. 17-28 Hyperparathyroidism. Palatal enlargement is characteristic of the renal osteodystrophy associated with secondary hyperparathyroidism.

Abdominal groans refers to the tendency for the development of duodenal ulcers. In addition, changes in mental status are often seen, ranging from lethargy and weakness to confusion or dementia.

HISTOPATHOLOGIC FEATURES

The brown tumor of hyperparathyroidism is histopathologically identical to the **central giant cell granuloma** of the jaws, a benign tumorlike lesion that usually affects teenagers and young adults (see page 626). Both lesions are characterized by a proliferation of exceedingly vascular granulation tissue, which serves as a background for numerous multinucleated osteoclast-type giant cells (Fig. 17-29). Some lesions may also show a proliferative response characterized by a parallel arrangement of spicules of woven bone set in a cellular fibroblastic background with variable

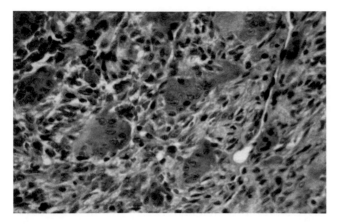

Fig. 17-29 Hyperparathyroidism. This high-power photomicrograph of a brown tumor of hyperparathyroidism shows scattered multinucleated giant cells within a vascular and proliferative fibroblastic background.

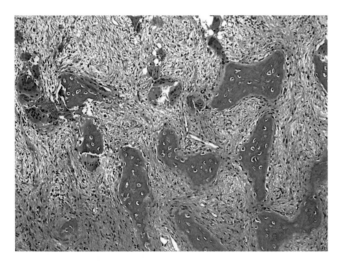

Fig. 17-30 Hyperparathyroidism. This medium-power photomicrograph shows trabeculae of cellular woven bone and clusters of multinucleated giant cells within a background of cellular fibrous connective tissue. These features are characteristic of tissue changes seen in renal osteodystrophy.

numbers of multinucleated giant cells (Fig. 17-30). This pattern is often associated with secondary hyperparathyroidism related to chronic renal disease (renal osteodystrophy).

TREATMENT AND PROGNOSIS

In **primary hyperparathyroidism**, the hyperplastic parathyroid tissue or the functional tumor must be removed surgically to reduce PTH levels to normal.

Secondary hyperparathyroidism may evolve to produce signs and symptoms related to renal calculi or renal osteodystrophy. Restriction of dietary phosphate, use of phosphate-binding agents, and pharmacologic treatment with an active vitamin D metabolite (e.g., calcitriol) may avert problems. Exposure to aluminum salts, which inhibit bone mineralization, should be eliminated also. Patients who do not respond to medical therapy may require parathyroidectomy. Renal transplantation may restore the normal physiologic processing of vitamin D, as well as phosphorus and calcium reabsorption and excretion; however, this does not occur in every case. Cinacalcet is a recently approved medical treatment for managing the overproduction of parathormone associated with secondary hyperparathyroidism. This medication is a calcimimetic agent that sensitizes the calcium receptors of the parathyroid cells to extracellular calcium, causing the cells to reduce their output of parathormone.

HYPERCORTISOLISM (CUSHING'S SYNDROME)

Hypercortisolism is a clinical condition that results from a sustained increase in glucocorticoid levels. In most cases this increase is due to corticosteroid therapy that is prescribed for other medical purposes. If the increase is caused by an endogenous source, such as an adrenal or pituitary (adrenocorticotropic hormone [ACTH]-secreting) tumor, then the condition is known as **Cushing's disease**. This latter condition is rather rare and usually affects young adult women.

CLINICAL FEATURES

The signs of Cushing's syndrome usually develop slowly. The most consistent clinical observation is weight gain, particularly in the central areas of the body. The accumulation of fat in the dorsocervical spine region results in a "buffalo hump" appearance; fatty tissue deposition in the facial area results in the characteristic rounded facial appearance known as *moon facies* (Fig. 17-31). Other common findings include the following:
- Red-purple abdominal striae
- Hirsutism
- Poor healing
- Osteoporosis
- Hypertension
- Mood changes (particularly depression)
- Hyperglycemia with thirst and polyuria
- Muscle wasting with weakness

DIAGNOSIS

If the patient has been receiving large amounts of corticosteroids (greater than the equivalent of 20 mg of prednisone) on a daily basis for several months, then the diagnosis is rather obvious, given the classic signs

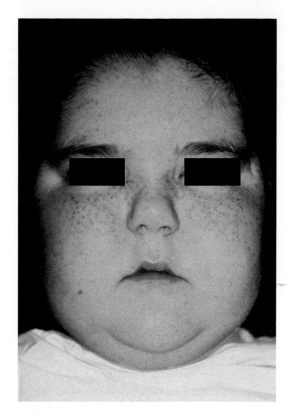

Fig. 17-31   Cushing's syndrome. The rounded facial features ("moon facies") of this patient are due to the abnormal deposition of fat, which is induced by excess corticosteroid hormone. *(Courtesy of Dr. George Blozis.)*

and symptoms described earlier. The diagnosis may be more difficult to establish in patients with a functioning adrenal cortical tumor or an ACTH-secreting pituitary adenoma. Evaluation of these patients should include the measurement of free cortisol in the urine and an assay of the effect of dexamethasone (a potent artificial corticosteroid) on the serum ACTH and cortisol levels. In an unaffected patient, the levels of free cortisol should be within normal limits, and the administration of an exogenous corticosteroid, such as dexamethasone, should suppress the normal level of ACTH, with a concomitant decrease in the cortisol levels. Because functioning tumors do not respond to normal feedback mechanisms, the anticipated decreases in ACTH and cortisol would not be seen in a patient with such a tumor.

TREATMENT AND PROGNOSIS

The clinician should be aware of the signs and symptoms of hypercortisolism to refer affected patients for appropriate endocrinologic evaluation and diagnosis. Once the diagnosis is established and the cause is determined to be an adrenal or pituitary tumor, surgi-

cal removal of the lesion is the treatment of choice. Radiation therapy also may be effective, particularly in younger patients. For patients with unresectable tumors, drugs that inhibit cortisol synthesis, such as ketoconazole, metyrapone, or aminoglutethimide, may be used to help control the excess production of cortisol.

Most cases of hypercortisolism, however, are caused by systemic corticosteroid therapy that is given for a variety of immunologic reasons, including treatment of autoimmune diseases and allogeneic transplant recipients. Certain strategies, such as the use of corticosteroid-sparing agents or alternate-day therapy, may minimize the corticosteroid dose needed. The goal should be for patients to use the lowest dose possible to manage immunologic disease.

In normal situations, cortisol is critical to the function of the body, particularly in dealing with stress. As the hormone is metabolized and serum levels drop, feedback to the pituitary gland signals it to produce ACTH, which stimulates the adrenal gland to produce additional cortisol. Unfortunately, therapeutic corticosteroids suppress the production of ACTH by the pituitary gland to the extent that the pituitary gland may not be able to produce ACTH in response to stress, and an acute episode of hypoadrenocorticism (*addisonian crisis*) may be precipitated. Therefore, the clinician must be aware of the potential side effects of chronic high-dose corticosteroid use and must be able to adapt the treatment of the patient accordingly. For stressful dental and surgical procedures especially, it is often necessary to increase the corticosteroid dose because of the greater need of the body for cortisol. Consultation with the physician who is managing the corticosteroid therapy is advised to determine to what extent the dose should be adjusted.

ADDISON'S DISEASE (HYPOADRENOCORTICISM)

Insufficient production of adrenal corticosteroid hormones caused by the destruction of the adrenal cortex results in the condition known as **Addison's disease**, or **primary hypoadrenocorticism**. The incidence of new cases diagnosed in the Western hemisphere is 110 to 140 per million population per year. The causes are diverse and include the following:
- Autoimmune destruction
- Infections (e.g., tuberculosis and deep fungal diseases, particularly in patients with acquired immunodeficiency syndrome [AIDS])
- Rarely, metastatic tumors, sarcoidosis, hemochromatosis, or amyloidosis

If the pituitary gland is not functioning properly, **secondary hypoadrenocorticism** may develop

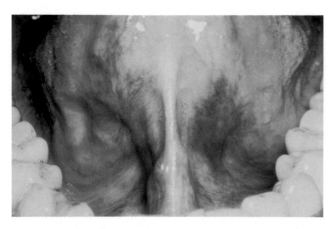

Fig. 17-32　Addison's disease. Diffuse pigmentation of the floor of the mouth and ventral tongue in a patient with Addison's disease. *(Courtesy of Dr. George Blozis.)*

because of decreased production of ACTH, the hormone responsible for maintaining normal levels of serum cortisol.

CLINICAL FEATURES

The clinical features of hypoadrenocorticism do not actually begin to appear until at least 90% of the glandular tissue has been destroyed. With gradual destruction of the adrenal cortex, an insidious onset of fatigue, irritability, depression, weakness, and hypotension is noted over a period of months. A generalized hyperpigmentation of the skin occurs, classically described as *bronzing*. The hyperpigmentation is generally more prominent on sun-exposed skin and over pressure points, such as the elbows and knees; it is caused by increased levels of beta-lipotropin or ACTH, each of which can stimulate melanocytes. The patient usually complains of gastrointestinal upset with anorexia, nausea, vomiting, diarrhea, weight loss, and a peculiar craving for salt. When hypoadrenocorticism is accompanied by hypoparathyroidism and mucocutaneous candidiasis, the possibility of autoimmune polyendocrinopathy-candidiasis-ectodermal dystrophy syndrome should be considered (see page 219).

The oral manifestations include diffuse or patchy, brown, macular pigmentation of the oral mucosa caused by excess melanin production (Fig. 17-32). Often the oral mucosal changes are the first manifestation of the disease, with the skin hyperpigmentation occurring afterward. Sometimes the oral hypermelanosis may be difficult to distinguish from physiologic racial pigmentation, but a history of a recent onset of oral pigmentation should suggest the possibility of Addison's disease.

LABORATORY FINDINGS

The diagnosis of hypoadrenocorticism is confirmed by a rapid ACTH stimulation test and measurement of serum cortisol levels and plasma ACTH levels. If serum cortisol levels are below 20 µg/dL, then the patient has adrenal insufficiency. In primary hypoadrenocorticism, the plasma ACTH levels are high (>100 ng/L). In secondary hypoadrenocorticism, the levels are normal (9 to 52 ng/L) or low, as would be expected because the condition results from decreased ACTH production by the pituitary gland.

TREATMENT AND PROGNOSIS

Addison's disease is managed with corticosteroid replacement therapy. The physiologic dose of corticosteroid is considered to be approximately 5.0 to 7.5 mg of prednisone or its equivalent per day, usually given in divided doses. Because the body's need for corticosteroid hormones increases during stressful events, the patient must take this into account and increase the dose accordingly. This adjustment is generally not required for dental procedures performed using local anesthesia and lasting less than 1 hour, but an increased dose may be necessary for certain dental and oral surgical procedures that are more lengthy or are done under general anesthesia.

Before the availability of corticosteroids, the prognosis for patients with hypoadrenocorticism was poor, with most patients surviving less than 2 years. Even today, if the condition is not recognized promptly, death may result in a relatively short period of time. With proper diagnosis and management, most affected patients can expect to have a normal life span.

DIABETES MELLITUS

Diabetes mellitus is a common disorder of carbohydrate metabolism that is thought to have several causes, although the basic problem is one of either decreased production of insulin or tissue resistance to the effects of insulin. The net result of this abnormal state is an increase in the blood glucose level (**hyperglycemia**).

Diabetes mellitus is usually divided into two presentations:

1. Type I—insulin-dependent diabetes mellitus (IDDM) or juvenile-onset diabetes
2. Type II—non–insulin-dependent diabetes mellitus (NIDDM) or adult-onset diabetes

Type I diabetes mellitus is characterized by a lack of insulin production. Patients usually exhibit severe hyperglycemia and ketoacidosis. The disease is typically diagnosed during childhood, and patients require exogenous insulin injections to survive.

Type II diabetes mellitus is sometimes more difficult to diagnose. It usually occurs in older, obese adults. Although hyperglycemia is present, ketoacidosis rarely develops. Furthermore, patients can produce some endogenous insulin. A few patients may take insulin to help control their disease; the insulin injections, however, are usually not necessary for the patient's survival.

With respect to epidemiology, in the United States diabetes mellitus affects approximately 7% of the population, or 21 million people, although nearly 6 million of these cases remain undiagnosed. More than 1 million new cases are identified each year in the United States. Of these affected patients, most have type II diabetes; only 5% to 10% have type I.

Diabetes is an important disease when we consider the many complications associated with it and the economic effect it has on society. One of the main complications of diabetes is **peripheral vascular disease**, a problem that results in kidney failure, as well as ischemia and gangrenous involvement of the limbs. By some estimates, 25% of all new cases of kidney failure occur in diabetic patients. Thus diabetes is the leading cause of kidney failure in the United States. Each year more than 50,000 amputations are performed for the gangrenous complications of diabetes. This disease is the leading cause of lower limb amputations in the United States. Retinal involvement often results in blindness; thus the leading cause of new cases of blindness in working-age adults in the United States is diabetes, with more than 12,000 people affected annually. Complications because of diabetes are estimated to contribute to the deaths of more than 200,000 Americans each year.

The cause of diabetes mellitus is essentially unknown, although most cases of type I diabetes appear to be caused by autoimmune destruction of the pancreatic islet cells, and this immunologic attack may be precipitated by a viral infection in a genetically susceptible individual. Type II diabetes does not appear to have an autoimmune cause, however, because no destruction of the islet cells is seen microscopically. Instead, genetic abnormalities have been detected in patients with certain types of type II diabetes, which may explain why the condition occurs so often in families. If one parent is affected by type II diabetes, then the chances of a child having the disorder is about 40%. Similarly, if one identical twin has type II diabetes, then the chances are 90% that the disease will also develop in the other twin.

CLINICAL FEATURES

Although a complete review of the pathophysiology of diabetes mellitus is beyond the scope of this text, the clinical signs and symptoms of a patient with this disease are easier to understand with some basic knowledge of the process. The hormone insulin, produced by the beta cells of the pancreatic islets of Langerhans, is necessary for the uptake of glucose by the cells of the body. When insulin binds to its specific cell surface receptor, a resulting cascade of intracellular molecular events causes the recruitment of intracellular glucose-binding proteins, which facilitate the uptake of glucose by each cell.

TYPE I DIABETES MELLITUS

Because patients with type I diabetes have a deficiency in the amount of insulin, the body's cells cannot absorb glucose and it remains in the blood. Normal blood glucose levels are between 70 and 120 mg/dL; in diabetic patients, these levels are often between 200 and 400 mg/dL. Above 300 mg/dL, the kidneys can no longer reabsorb the glucose; therefore, it spills over into the urine. Because glucose is the main source of energy for the body, and because none of this energy can be used because glucose cannot be absorbed, the patient feels tired and lethargic. The body begins to use other energy sources, such as fat and protein, resulting in the production of ketones as a by-product of those energy consumption pathways. The patient often loses weight, despite increased food intake (**polyphagia**). With the hyperglycemia, the osmolarity of the blood and urine increases. The increased osmolarity results in frequent urination (**polyuria**) and thirst, which leads to increased water intake (**polydipsia**). Clinically, most patients with type I diabetes are younger (average age at diagnosis being 14 years), and they have a thin body habitus.

TYPE II DIABETES MELLITUS

By contrast, patients with type II diabetes are usually older than 40 years of age at diagnosis, and 80% to 90% of them are obese. In this situation, it is thought that a decrease in the number of insulin receptors or abnormal postbinding molecular events related to glucose uptake results in glucose not being absorbed by the body's cells. Thus patients are said to show "insulin resistance" because serum insulin levels are usually within normal limits or even elevated. If the hyperglycemia is taken into account, however, the amount of circulating insulin is typically not as much as would be present in a normal person with a similar level of blood glucose. Therefore, many of these patients are described as having a relative lack of insulin.

The symptoms associated with type II diabetes are much more subtle in comparison to those seen with type I. The first sign of type II diabetes is often detected with routine hematologic examination rather than any specific patient complaint. Ketoacidosis is almost never seen in patients with type II diabetes. Nevertheless, many of the other complications of diabetes are still associated with this form of the disease.

COMPLICATIONS

Many complications of diabetes mellitus are directly related to the **microangiopathy** caused by the disease. The microangiopathy results in occlusion of the small blood vessels, producing peripheral vascular disease. The resultant decrease in tissue perfusion results in ischemia. The ischemia predisposes the patient to infection, particularly severe infections such as gangrene. Another contributing factor is the impairment of neutrophil function, particularly neutrophil chemotaxis.

Amputation of the lower extremity often is necessary because of the lack of tissue perfusion and the patient's inability to cope with infection. Similar vascular occlusion may affect the coronary arteries (which places the patient at risk for myocardial infarction) or the carotid arteries and their branches (predisposing the patient to cerebrovascular accident, or stroke). When microvascular occlusion affects the retinal vessels, blindness typically results. Kidney failure is the outcome of renal blood vessel involvement. If the ketoacidosis is not corrected in type I diabetes, the patient may lapse into a diabetic coma.

The oral manifestations of diabetes mellitus are generally limited to patients with type I diabetes. Problems include periodontal disease, which occurs more frequently and progresses more rapidly than in normal patients. Healing after surgery may be delayed, and the likelihood of infection is probably increased. Diffuse, nontender, bilateral enlargement of the parotid glands, called **diabetic sialadenosis** (see page 470), may be seen in patients with either form of diabetes. In uncontrolled or poorly controlled diabetic patients, a striking enlargement and erythema of the attached gingiva has been described (Fig. 17-33). In addition, these patients appear to be more susceptible to **oral candidiasis** in its various clinical forms (see page 213). Erythematous candidiasis, which appears as central papillary atrophy of the dorsal tongue papillae, is reported in up to 30% of these patients. **Zygomycosis** (see page 232) may occur in patients with poorly controlled type I diabetes. Some investigators have identified an increased prevalence of **benign migratory glossitis** (see page 779) in patients with type I diabetes; however, others have not been able to confirm this finding. **Xerostomia**, a subjective feeling of dryness of the oral mucosa, has been reported as a complaint in one third of diabetic patients. Unfortunately, studies that attempt to confirm an actual decrease in salivary flow rate in diabetic patients have produced conflicting results. Some studies show a decrease in salivary flow; some, no difference from normal; and some, an increased salivary flow rate.

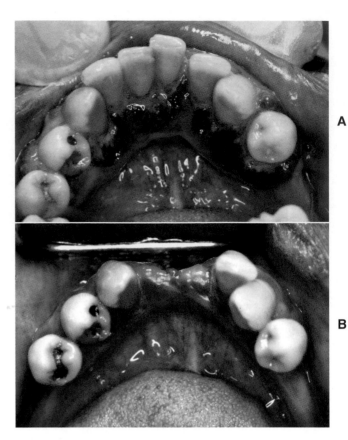

Fig. 17-33 Diabetes mellitus. **A,** This diffuse, erythematous enlargement of the gingival tissues developed in a diabetic patient who discontinued taking her insulin. **B,** The gingival tissues have greatly improved after reinstitution of regular insulin injections. Several incisors were extracted because of severe periodontal bone loss.

TREATMENT AND PROGNOSIS

For patients with type II diabetes, dietary modification coupled with exercise may be the only treatment necessary, with the goal being weight loss. The dietary and lifestyle changes may need to be coupled with one or more oral hypoglycemic agents. These drugs are designed to affect different pathophysiologic aspects of the disease. For example, secretagogues increase the insulin supply. These include the second-generation sulfonylurea medications such as glipizide or glyburide. Metformin is a biguanide that increases glucose utilization and decreases insulin resistance and hepatic glucose production. Thiazolidinediones, such as rosiglitazone and pioglitazone, also reduce insulin resistance. Acarbose and miglitol are α-glucosidase inhibitors that reduce the absorption of glucose from the gastrointestinal tract by inhibiting enzymatic degradation of more complex sugars. If these modalities do not control the blood glucose levels, then treatment with insulin is necessary.

For patients with type I diabetes, injections of insulin are required to control blood glucose levels. Different types of insulin are marketed, each type having different degrees of duration and times of peak activity. Insulin was previously extracted primarily from beef and pork pancreata. In some patients, however, antibodies developed to this foreign protein and rendered the insulin useless. To overcome this problem, pharmaceutical companies have developed brands of insulin that have the molecular structure of human insulin. Laboratories produce this human insulin with genetically engineered bacteria using recombinant DNA technology.

The patient's schedule of insulin injections must be carefully structured and monitored to provide optimal control of blood glucose levels. This schedule is carefully formulated by the patient's physician and takes into account such factors as the patient's activity level and the severity of the insulin deficiency. It is imperative that adequate dietary carbohydrates be ingested after the administration of the insulin; otherwise, a condition known as **insulin shock** may occur. If carbohydrates are not consumed after an insulin injection, then the blood glucose levels may fall to dangerously low levels. The brain is virtually dependent on blood glucose as its energy source. If the blood glucose level drops below 40 mg/dL, the patient may go into shock. This condition can be treated by administration of sublingual dextrose paste, intravenous (IV) infusion of a dextrose solution, or injection of glucagon.

In summary, diabetes mellitus is a common, complex medical problem with many complications. The prognosis is guarded. Studies suggest that strict control of blood glucose levels results in a slowing of the development of the late complications of type I diabetes (e.g., blindness, kidney damage, neuropathy) and reduces the frequency of these complications. Health care practitioners should be aware of the problems these patients may have and should be prepared to deal with them. Consultation with the patient's physician may be necessary, particularly for patients with type I diabetes who show poor blood glucose control, have active infections, or require extensive oral surgical procedures.

HYPOPHOSPHATASIA

Hypophosphatasia is a rare metabolic bone disease that is characterized by a deficiency of tissue-nonspecific alkaline phosphatase. Approximately 150 distinct mutations of the gene responsible for alkaline phosphatase production have been described. One of the first presenting signs of hypophosphatasia may be the premature loss of the primary teeth, presumably caused by a lack of cementum on the root surfaces. In the homozygous autosomal recessive form, there are rather severe manifestations, and many of these patients are identified in infancy. The milder forms of the disease are inherited in an autosomal dominant or recessive fashion, appearing in childhood or even adulthood, with variable degrees of expression. Generally, the younger the age of onset, the more severe the expression of the disease. The common factors in all types include the following:

- Reduced levels of the bone, liver, and kidney isozyme of alkaline phosphatase
- Increased levels of blood and urinary phosphoethanolamine
- Bone abnormalities that resemble rickets

Most authorities believe that the decreased alkaline phosphatase levels probably are responsible for the clinically observed abnormalities. Alkaline phosphatase is thought to play a role in the production of bone, but its precise mechanism of action is unknown.

CLINICAL AND RADIOGRAPHIC FEATURES

Four types of hypophosphatasia are generally recognized, depending on the severity and the age of onset of the symptoms:

1. Perinatal
2. Infantile
3. Childhood
4. Adult

PERINATAL HYPOPHOSPHATASIA

The **perinatal** form has the most severe manifestations. It is usually diagnosed at birth, and the infant rarely survives for more than a few hours. Death is due to respiratory failure. Marked hypocalcification of the skeletal structures is observed.

INFANTILE HYPOPHOSPHATASIA

Babies affected by **infantile** hypophosphatasia may appear normal up to 6 months of age; after this time, they begin to show a failure to grow. Vomiting and hypotonia may develop as well. Skeletal malformations that suggest rickets are typically observed; these malformations include shortened, bowed limbs. Deformities of the ribs predispose these patients to pneumonia, and skull deformities cause increased intracranial pressure. Nephrocalcinosis and nephrolithiasis also produce problems for these infants. Radiographs show a markedly reduced degree of ossification with a preponderance of hypomineralized osteoid. If these infants survive, premature shedding of the deciduous teeth is often seen.

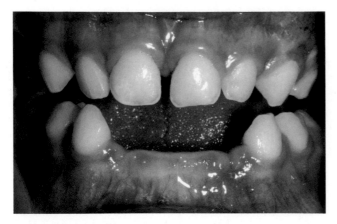

Fig. 17-34   Hypophosphatasia. Premature loss of the mandibular anterior teeth. *(Courtesy of Dr. Jackie Banahan.)*

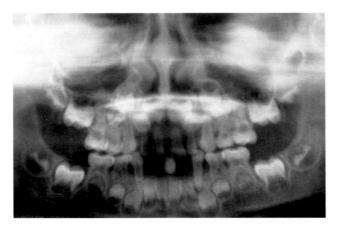

Fig. 17-35   Hypophosphatasia. This panoramic radiograph shows the loss of the mandibular anterior teeth. *(Courtesy of Dr. Jackie Banahan.)*

CHILDHOOD HYPOPHOSPHATASIA

The **childhood** form is usually detected at a later age and has a wide range of clinical expression. One of the more consistent features is the premature loss of the primary teeth without evidence of a significant inflammatory response (Figs. 17-34 and 17-35). The deciduous incisor teeth are usually affected first and may be the only teeth involved. In some patients, this may be the only expression of the disease. The teeth may show enlarged pulp chambers in some instances, and a significant degree of alveolar bone loss may be seen. More severely affected patients may have open fontanelles with premature fusion of cranial sutures. This early fusion occasionally leads to increased intracranial pressure and subsequent brain damage. Affected patients typically have a short stature, bowed legs, and a waddling gait. The development of motor skills is often delayed.

Radiographically, the skull has the appearance of "beaten copper," and it shows uniformly spaced, poorly defined, small radiolucencies. This pattern may be the result of areas of thinning of the inner cortical plate produced by the cerebral gyri.

ADULT HYPOPHOSPHATASIA

The **adult** form is typically mild. Patients often have a history of premature loss of their primary or permanent dentition, and many of these patients are edentulous. Stress fractures that involve the metatarsal bones of the feet may be a presenting sign of the condition, or an increased number of fractures associated with relatively minor trauma may alert the clinician to this disorder.

DIAGNOSIS

The diagnosis of hypophosphatasia is based on the clinical manifestations and the finding of decreased levels of serum alkaline phosphatase and increased amounts of phosphoethanolamine in both the urine and the blood. Interestingly, as some patients grow older, serum alkaline phosphatase levels may approach normal.

HISTOPATHOLOGIC FEATURES

The histopathologic evaluation of bone sampled from a patient affected with the **infantile** form of hypophosphatasia shows abundant production of poorly mineralized osteoid. In the **childhood** or **adult** form, the bone may appear relatively normal or it may show an increased amount of woven bone, which is a less mature form of osseous tissue.

The histopathologic examination of either a primary or permanent tooth that has been exfoliated from an affected patient often shows an absence or a marked reduction of cementum that covers the root's surface (Fig. 17-36). This reduced amount of cementum is thought to predispose to tooth loss because of the inability of periodontal ligament fibers to attach to the tooth and to maintain it in its normal position.

TREATMENT AND PROGNOSIS

The treatment of hypophosphatasia is essentially symptomatic because the lack of alkaline phosphatase cannot be corrected. Attempts to treat this condition by infusing alkaline phosphatase have been unsuccessful, presumably because the enzyme functions within the cell rather than in the extracellular environment. Basically, fractures are treated with orthopedic surgery, followed by rehabilitation. Prosthetic appliances are indicated to replace missing teeth, but satisfactory

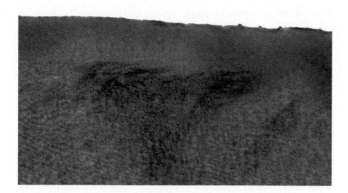

Fig. 17-36   Hypophosphatasia. This medium-power photomicrograph of an exfoliated tooth shows no cementum associated with the root surface.

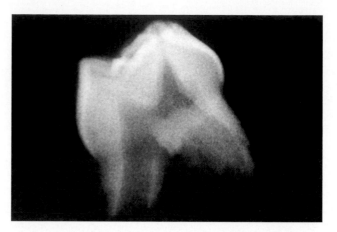

Fig. 17-37   Vitamin D-resistant rickets. This radiograph of an extracted tooth shows a prominent pulp chamber with pulp horns extending out toward the dentinoenamel junction.

results are not always possible because the alveolar bone is hypoplastic. Because mutational analysis of DNA can identify carriers of the defective gene, patients and their parents should be provided with genetic counseling. As stated earlier, the prognosis varies with the onset of symptoms; the perinatal and infantile types are associated with a rather poor outcome. The childhood and adult forms are usually compatible with a normal life span.

VITAMIN D-RESISTANT RICKETS (HEREDITARY HYPOPHOSPHATEMIA; FAMILIAL HYPOPHOSPHATEMIC RICKETS)

After the use of vitamin D to treat rickets became widespread, it was recognized that some individuals with clinical features characteristic of rickets did not seem to respond to therapeutic doses of the vitamin. For this reason, this condition in these patients was called **vitamin D-resistant rickets**. Most cases of this rare condition appear to be inherited as an X-linked dominant trait; therefore, males are usually affected more severely than females, who presumably have attenuated features because of lyonization. In the United States, this condition occurs at a frequency of 1 in 20,000 births. In addition to the rachitic changes, these patients are also hypophosphatemic and show a decreased capacity for reabsorption of phosphate from the renal tubules. The disorder is caused by mutations in a zinc metalloproteinase gene known as *PHEX* (phosphate-regulating gene with endopeptidase activity on the X chromosome). Although the precise mechanisms of action of this gene are unclear, it appears to play a role in vitamin D metabolism.

In contrast, patients affected by the rare autosomal recessive condition known as **vitamin D-dependent rickets** exhibit hypocalcification of the teeth, unlike those with vitamin D-resistant rickets. Otherwise, the two disorders have similar clinical features. Vitamin D-dependent rickets is caused by a lack of 1α-hydroxylase, the enzyme responsible for converting the relatively inactive vitamin D precursor, 25-hydroxycholecalciferol (calcifediol) to the active metabolite 1,25-dihydroxycholecalciferol (calcitriol) in the kidney. Therefore, these patients respond to replacement therapy with active vitamin D (calcitriol).

CLINICAL FEATURES

Patients with vitamin D-resistant rickets have a short stature. The upper body segment appears more normal, but the lower body segment is shortened. The lower limbs are generally shortened and bowed.

Laboratory investigation reveals hypophosphatemia with diminished renal reabsorption of phosphate and decreased intestinal absorption of calcium. This typically results in rachitic changes that are unresponsive to vitamin D (calciferol). With aging, ankylosis of the spine frequently develops.

From a dental standpoint, the teeth have large pulp chambers, with pulp horns extending almost to the dentinoenamel junction (Figs. 17-37 and 17-38). In some cases the cuspal enamel may be worn down by attrition to the level of the pulp horn, causing pulpal exposure and pulp death. The exposure may be so small that the resulting periapical abscesses and gingival sinus tracts seem to affect what appear to be otherwise normal teeth (Fig. 17-39). Studies have also shown that microclefts may develop in the enamel, giving the

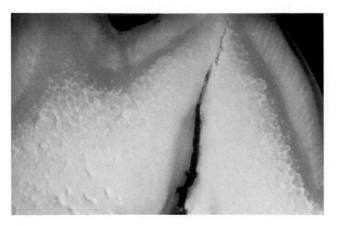

Fig. 17-38 **Vitamin D-resistant rickets.** Ground section of the same tooth depicted in Fig. 17-37. A pulp horn extends to the dentinoenamel junction. *(Courtesy of Dr. Carl Witkop.)*

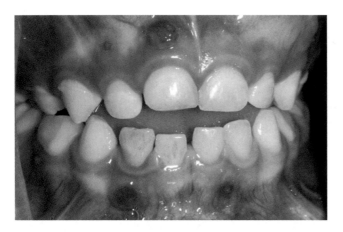

Fig. 17-39 **Vitamin D-resistant rickets.** This patient exhibits multiple nonvital teeth with associated parulides. This arose in the absence of caries or trauma.

oral microflora access to the dentinal tubules and subsequently to the pulp. One study examined a series of affected children and found that 25% of these patients had multiple abscesses involving the primary dentition.

HISTOPATHOLOGIC FEATURES

Microscopic examination of an erupted tooth from a patient with vitamin D-resistant rickets usually shows markedly enlarged pulp horns. The dentin appears abnormal and is characterized by the deposition of globular dentin, which often exhibits clefting. The clefts may extend from the pulp chamber to the dentino-enamel junction. Microclefts are also seen within the enamel. The pulp frequently is nonvital, presumably because of the bacterial contamination associated with both the enamel and the dentinal clefts.

TREATMENT AND PROGNOSIS

For a normal stature to develop, patients with vitamin D-resistant rickets usually need early treatment with calcitriol and multiple daily doses of phosphate. Endodontic therapy is necessary for the pulpally involved teeth. Initiating therapy in early childhood with a synthetic vitamin D compound (1α-hydroxycholecalciferol) appears to reduce dental problems in affected patients when compared with untreated historic controls. Interestingly, the radiographic dental abnormalities do not seem to be improved. Although serum and urine calcium levels must be monitored carefully to prevent nephrocalcinosis with its potential for kidney damage, patients generally have a normal life span.

CROHN'S DISEASE (REGIONAL ILEITIS; REGIONAL ENTERITIS)

Crohn's disease is an inflammatory and probably an immunologically mediated condition of unknown cause that primarily affects the distal portion of the small bowel and the proximal colon. It is now well established that the manifestations of Crohn's disease may be seen anywhere in the gastrointestinal tract, from the mouth to the anus. In addition, other extraintestinal sites of disease involvement, such as the skin, eyes, and joints, have also been identified. The oral lesions are significant because they may precede the gastrointestinal lesions in as many as 30% of the cases that have both oral and gastrointestinal involvement. It is interesting that the prevalence of Crohn's disease appears to be increasing, but the reasons for this increase have not been determined.

CLINICAL FEATURES

Most patients with Crohn's disease are teenagers when the disease first becomes evident, although another diagnostic peak of disease activity occurs in patients more than 60 years of age. Gastrointestinal signs and symptoms usually include abdominal cramping and pain, nausea, and diarrhea, occasionally accompanied by fever. Weight loss and malnutrition may develop, which can lead to anemia, decreased growth, and short stature.

A wide range of oral lesions has been clinically reported in Crohn's disease; however, many of the abnormalities described are relatively nonspecific and may be associated with other conditions that cause **orofacial granulomatosis** (see page 341). The more prominent findings include diffuse or nodular swelling of the oral and perioral tissues, a cobblestone appearance of the mucosa, and deep, granulomatous-appear-

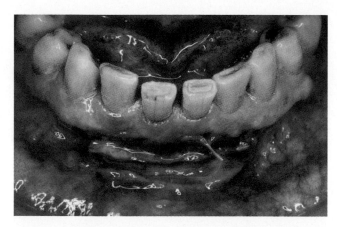

Fig. 17-40   Crohn's disease. This patient has a linear ulceration of the mandibular vestibule. An adhesion between the alveolar and labial mucosae was caused by repeated ulceration and healing of the mucosa at this site.

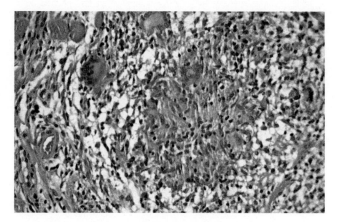

Fig. 17-41   Crohn's disease. This medium-power photomicrograph of an oral lesion shows a nonnecrotizing granuloma in the submucosal connective tissue.

ing ulcers. The ulcers are often linear and develop in the buccal vestibule (Fig. 17-40). Patchy erythematous macules and plaques involving the attached and un-attached gingivae have been termed *mucogingivitis* and may represent one of the more common lesions related to Crohn's disease. Soft tissue swellings that resemble denture-related fibrous hyperplasia may be seen, as well as smaller mucosal tags. Another manifestation that has been reported is aphthouslike oral ulcerations, although the significance of this finding is uncertain because aphthous ulcerations are found rather frequently in the general population, including the same age group that is affected by Crohn's disease. One large study showed no difference in the prevalence of aphthous ulcers in patients with Crohn's disease compared with a control population. Fewer than 1% of patients with Crohn's disease may develop diffuse stomatitis, with some cases apparently caused by *Staphylococcus aureus*, and others being nonspecific. In at least one instance, recurrent severe buccal space infections resulted in cutaneous salivary fistula formation. Infrequently, pyostomatitis vegetans (see next topic) has been associated with Crohn's disease.

HISTOPATHOLOGIC FEATURES

Microscopic examination of lesional tissue obtained from the intestine or from the oral mucosa should show nonnecrotizing granulomatous inflammation within the submucosal connective tissue (Fig. 17-41). The severity of the granulomatous inflammation may vary tremendously from patient to patient and from various sites in the same patient. Therefore, a negative biopsy result at any one site and time may not necessarily rule out a diagnosis of Crohn's disease. As with the clinical lesions, the histopathologic pattern is rela-

tively nonspecific, resembling orofacial granulomatosis. Special stains should be performed to rule out the possibility of deep fungal infection, tertiary syphilis, or mycobacterial infection.

TREATMENT AND PROGNOSIS

Most patients with Crohn's disease are initially treated medically with a sulfa type of drug (sulfasalazine), and some patients respond well to this medication. Metronidazole may be used if no response is seen with sulfasalazine therapy. With moderate to severe involvement, systemic prednisone may be used and is often effective, particularly when combined with the immunosuppressive drug, azathioprine. Infliximab, a monoclonal antibody directed against tumor necrosis factor-α (TNF-α), has shown promise in refractory cases of Crohn's disease. Sometimes the disease cannot be maintained in remission by medical therapy, and complications develop that require surgical intervention. Complications may include bowel obstruction or fistula or abscess formation. If a significant segment of the terminal ileum has been removed surgically or is involved with the disease, then periodic injections of vitamin B_{12} may be necessary to prevent megaloblastic anemia secondary to the lack of ability to absorb the vitamin. Similar supplementation of magnesium, iron, the fat-soluble vitamins, and folate may also be required because of malabsorption.

Oral lesions have been reported to clear with treatment of the gastrointestinal process in many cases. Occasionally persistent oral ulcerations will develop, and these may have to be treated with topical or intralesional corticosteroids. Systemic thalidomide and infliximab have been used successfully to manage refractory oral ulcers of Crohn's disease.

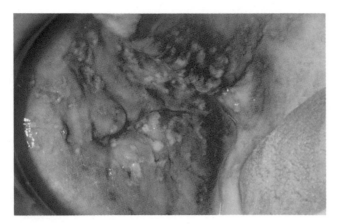

Fig. 17-42 Pyostomatitis vegetans. The characteristic lesions are seen on the buccal mucosa, appearing as yellow-white pustules.

PYOSTOMATITIS VEGETANS

Pyostomatitis vegetans is a relatively rare condition that has a controversial history. It has been associated in the past with diseases such as pemphigus or pyodermatitis vegetans. Most investigators today, however, believe that pyostomatitis vegetans is an unusual oral expression of inflammatory bowel disease, particularly **ulcerative colitis** or **Crohn's disease**. The pathogenesis of the condition, like that of inflammatory bowel disease, is poorly understood. A few patients with pyostomatitis vegetans have also been noted to have one of several concurrent liver abnormalities.

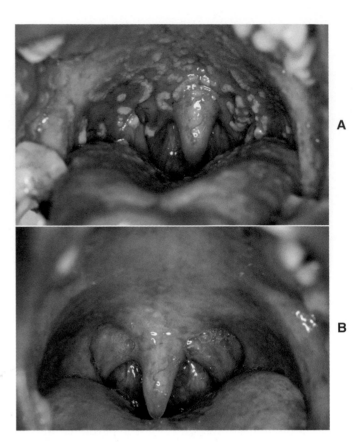

Fig. 17-43 Pyostomatitis vegetans. A, Characteristic "snail track" lesions involve the soft palate. **B,** Same patient after 5 days of prednisone therapy. *(From Neville BW, Laden SA, Smith SE et al: Pyostomatitis vegetans, Am J Dermatopathol 7:69-77, 1985.)*

CLINICAL FEATURES

Patients with pyostomatitis vegetans exhibit characteristic yellowish, slightly elevated, linear, serpentine pustules set on an erythematous oral mucosa. The lesions primarily affect the buccal and labial mucosa, soft palate, and ventral tongue (Figs. 17-42 and 17-43). These lesions have been called "snail track" ulcerations, although in most instances the lesions are probably not truly ulcerated. Oral discomfort is variable but can be surprisingly minimal in some patients. This variation in symptoms may be related to the number of pustules that have ruptured to form ulcerations. The oral lesions may appear concurrently with the bowel symptoms, or they may precede the intestinal involvement.

HISTOPATHOLOGIC FEATURES

A biopsy specimen of an oral lesion of pyostomatitis vegetans usually shows marked edema, causing an acantholytic appearance of the involved epithelium. This may be the result of the accumulation of numerous eosinophils within the spinous layer, often forming intraepithelial abscesses (Fig. 17-44). Subepithelial eosinophilic abscesses have been reported in some instances. The underlying connective tissue usually supports a dense mixed infiltrate of inflammatory cells that consists of eosinophils, neutrophils, and lymphocytes. Perivascular inflammation may also be present.

TREATMENT AND PROGNOSIS

Usually, the intestinal signs and symptoms of inflammatory bowel disease are of most concern for patients with pyostomatitis vegetans. Medical management of the bowel disease with sulfasalazine or systemic corticosteroids also produces clearing of the oral lesions (see Fig. 17-40). Often the oral lesions clear within days after systemic corticosteroid therapy is begun, and they may recur if the medication is withdrawn. If the bowel symptoms are relatively mild, then the oral lesions have been reported to respond to topical therapy with some of the more potent corticosteroid preparations.

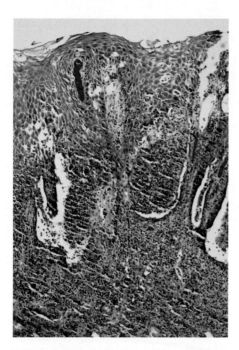

Fig. 17-44 Pyostomatitis vegetans. Medium-power photomicrograph showing intraepithelial abscesses composed of eosinophils.

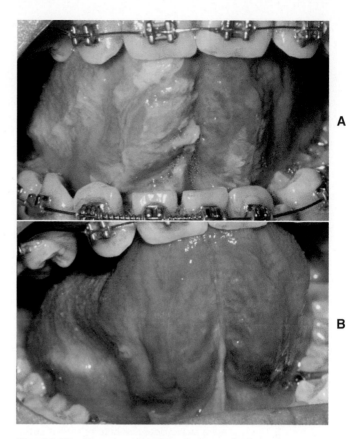

Fig. 17-45 Uremic stomatitis. A, Ragged white plaques affect the ventral tongue and floor of the mouth. **B,** Same patient after renal dialysis. *(From Ross WF, Salisbury PL: Uremic stomatitis associated with undiagnosed renal failure, Gen Dent 42:410-412, 1994.)*

UREMIC STOMATITIS

Patients who have either acute or chronic renal failure typically show markedly elevated levels of urea and other nitrogenous wastes in the bloodstream. **Uremic stomatitis** represents a relatively uncommon complication of renal failure. In two series that included 562 patients with renal failure, only eight examples of this oral mucosal condition were documented. Nevertheless, for the patients in whom uremic stomatitis develops, this can be a painful disorder. The cause of the oral lesions is unclear, but some investigators suggest that urease, an enzyme produced by the oral microflora, may degrade urea secreted in the saliva. This degradation results in the liberation of free ammonia, which presumably damages the oral mucosa.

CLINICAL FEATURES

Most cases of uremic stomatitis have been reported in patients with acute renal failure. The onset may be abrupt, with white plaques distributed predominantly on the buccal mucosa, tongue, and floor of the mouth (Fig. 17-45). Patients may complain of unpleasant taste, oral pain, or a burning sensation with the lesions, and the clinician may detect an odor of ammonia or urine on the patient's breath. The clinical appearance occasionally has been known to mimic oral hairy leukoplakia.

TREATMENT AND PROGNOSIS

In some instances, uremic stomatitis may clear within a few days after renal dialysis, although such resolution may take place over 2 to 3 weeks. In other instances, treatment with a mildly acidic mouth rinse, such as diluted hydrogen peroxide, seems to clear the oral lesions. For control of pain while the lesions heal, patients may be given palliative therapy with ice chips or a topical anesthetic, such as viscous lidocaine or dyclonine hydrochloride. Although renal failure itself is life threatening, at least one example of a uremic plaque that presumably caused a patient's death has been recorded. This event was thought to have been caused by the dislodging of the plaque with subsequent obstruction of the patient's airway.

BIBLIOGRAPHY

Mucopolysaccharidosis

Alpöz AR, Çoker M, Çelen E et al: The oral manifestations of Maroteaux-Lamy syndrome (mucopolysaccharidosis VI): a case report, *Oral Surg Oral Med Oral Pathol Oral Radiol Endod* 101:632-637, 2006.

Brady RO: Enzyme replacement for lysosomal diseases, *Annu Rev Med* 57:283-296, 2006.

Danos O, Heard J-M: Mucopolysaccharidosis, *Mol Cell Biol Hum Dis Ser* 5:350-367, 1995.

Downs AT, Crisp T, Ferretti G: Hunter's syndrome and oral manifestations: a review, *Pediatr Dent* 17:98-100, 1995.

Fahnehjelm KT, Törnquist A-L, Malm G et al: Ocular findings in four children with mucopolysaccharidosis I-Hurler (MPS I-H) treated early with haematopoietic stem cell transplantation, *Acta Ophthalmol Scand* 84:781-785, 2006.

Harmatz P, Giugliani R, Schwartz I et al: Enzyme replacement therapy for mucopolysaccharidosis VI: a phase 3, randomized, double-blind, placebo-controlled, multinational study of recombinant human N-acetylgalactosamine 4-sulfatase (recombinant human arylsulfatase B or RHASB) and follow-on, open-label extension study, *J Pediatr* 148:533-539, 2006.

Kinirons MJ, Nelson J: Dental findings in mucopolysaccharidosis type IV A (Morquio's disease type A), *Oral Surg Oral Med Oral Pathol* 70:176-179, 1990.

Meikle PJ, Hopwood JJ, Clague AE et al: Prevalence of lysosomal storage disorders, *JAMA* 281:249-254, 1999.

Mikles M, Stanton RP: A review of Morquio syndrome, *Am J Orthop* 26:533-540, 1997.

Muenzer J: The mucopolysaccharidoses: a heterogeneous group of disorders with variable pediatric presentations, *J Pediatr* 144:S27-S34, 2004.

Nakamura T, Miwa K, Kanda S et al: Rosette formation of impacted molar teeth in mucopolysaccharidoses and related disorders, *Dentomaxillofac Radiol* 21:45-49, 1992.

Nelson J, Crowhurst J, Carey B et al: Incidence of the mucopolysaccharidoses in Western Australia, *Am J Med Genet* 123A:310-313, 2003.

Northover H, Cowie RA, Wraith JE: Mucopolysaccharidosis type IVA (Morquio syndrome): a clinical review, *J Inherit Metab Dis* 19:357-365, 1996.

Nussbaum BL: Dentistry for the at-risk patient—mucopolysaccharidosis III (Sanfilippo syndrome): a nine-year case study, *ASDC J Dent Child* 57:466-469, 1990.

Pastores GM, Arn P, Beck M et al: The MPS I registry: design, methodology, and early findings of a global disease registry for monitoring patients with mucopolysaccharidosis type I, *Mol Genet Metab* 91:37-47, 2007.

Peters C, Shapiro EG, Anderson J et al: Hurler syndrome: II. Outcome of HLA-genotypically identical sibling and HLSA-haploidentical related donor bone marrow transplantation in fifty-four children, *Blood* 91:2601-2608, 1998.

Scott HS, Bunge S, Gal A et al: Molecular genetics of mucopolysaccharidosis type I: diagnostic, clinical, and biological implications, *Hum Mutat* 6:288-302, 1995.

Sifuentes M, Doroshow R, Hoft R et al: A follow-up study of MPS I patients treated with laronidase enzyme replacement therapy for 6 years, *Mol Genet Metab* 90:171-180, 2007.

Simmons MA, Bruce IA, Penney S et al: Otorhinolaryogological manifestations of the mucopolysaccharidoses, *Int J Pediatr Otorhinolaryngol* 69:589-595, 2005.

Smith KS, Hallett KB, Hall RK et al: Mucopolysaccharidosis: MPS VI and associated delayed tooth eruption, *Int J Oral Maxillofac Surg* 24:176-180, 1995.

Staba SL, Escolar ML, Poe M et al: Cord-blood transplants from unrelated donors in patients with Hurler's syndrome, *N Engl J Med* 350:1960-1969, 2004.

Vellodi A, Young EP, Cooper A et al: Bone marrow transplantation for mucopolysaccharidosis type I: experience of two British centres, *Arch Dis Child* 76:92-99, 1997.

Vijay S, Wraith JE: Clinical presentation and follow-up of patients with the attenuated phenotype of mucopolysaccharidosis type I, *Acta Paediatrica* 94:872-877, 2005.

Wraith JE: The mucopolysaccharidoses: a clinical review and guide to management, *Arch Dis Child* 72:263-267, 1995.

Wraith JE, Hopwood JJ, Fuller M et al: Laronidase treatment of mucopolysaccharidosis I, *BioDrugs* 19:1-7, 2005.

Lipid Reticuloendothelioses

Barranger JA, Rice E, Sakallah SA et al: Enzymatic and molecular diagnosis of Gaucher disease, *Clin Lab Med* 15:899-913, 1995.

Beutler E: Lysosomal storage diseases: natural history and ethical and economic aspects, *Mol Genet Metab* 88:208-215, 2006.

Beutler E, Nguyen NJ, Henneberger MW et al: Gaucher disease: gene frequencies in the Ashkenazi Jewish population, *Am J Hum Genet* 52:85-88, 1993.

Blitzer MG, McDowell CA: Tay-Sachs disease as a model for screening inborn errors, *Clin Lab Med* 12:463-479, 1992.

Dayan B, Elstein D, Zimran A et al: Decreased salivary output in patients with Gaucher disease, *Q J Med* 96:53-56, 2003.

Fernandes-Filho JA, Shapiro BE: Tay-Sachs disease, *Arch Neurol* 61:1466-1468, 2004.

Gieselmann V: Lysosomal storage diseases, *Biochim Biophys Acta* 1270:103-136, 1995.

Grabowski GA: Recent clinical progress in Gaucher disease, *Curr Opin Pediatr* 17:519-524, 2005.

Gravel RA, Triggs-Raine BL, Mahuran DJ: Biochemistry and genetics of Tay-Sachs disease, *Can J Neurol Sci* 18:419-423, 1991.

Imrie J, Dasgupta S, Besley GTN et al: The natural history of Niemann-Pick disease type C in the UK, *J Inherit Metab Dis* 30:51-59, 2007.

Kolodny EH: Niemann-Pick disease, *Curr Opin Hematol* 7:48-52, 2000.

Levran O, Desnick RJ, Schuchman EH: Niemann-Pick disease: a frequent missense mutation in the acid sphingomyelinase gene of Ashkenazi Jewish type A and B patients, *Proc Natl Acad Sci U S A* 88:3748-3752, 1991.

Lustmann J, Ben-Yehuda D, Somer M et al: Gaucher's disease affecting the mandible and maxilla: report of a case, *Int J Oral Maxillofac Surg* 20:7-8, 1991.

McGovern MM, Aron A, Brodie SE et al: Natural history of type A Niemann-Pick disease. Possible endpoints for therapeutic trials, *Neurology* 66:228-232, 2006.

Morales LE: Gaucher's disease: a review, *Ann Pharmacother* 30:381-388, 1996.

Morris JA, Carstea ED: Niemann-Pick disease: cholesterol handling gone awry, *Mol Med Today* 4:525-531, 1998.

Rosenthal DI, Doppelt SH, Mankin HJ et al: Enzyme replacement therapy for Gaucher disease: skeletal responses to macrophage-targeted glucocerebrosidase, *Pediatrics* 96:629-637, 1995.

Sévin M, Lesca G, Baumann N et al: The adult form of Niemann-Pick disease type C, *Brain* 130:120-133, 2007.

Shiran A, Brenner B, Laor A et al: Increased risk of cancer in patients with Gaucher disease, *Cancer* 72:219-224, 1993.

Sidransky E, Tayebi N, Ginns EI: Diagnosing Gaucher disease. Early recognition, implications for treatment, and genetic counseling, *Clin Pediatr (Phila)* 34:365-371, 1995.

Starzyk K, Richards S, Yee J et al: The long-term international safety experience of imiglucerase therapy for Gaucher disease, *Mol Genet Metab* 90:157-163, 2007.

Tamura H, Takahashi T, Ban N et al: Niemann-Pick type C disease: Novel NPC1 mutations and characterization of the concomitant acid sphingomyelinase deficiency, *Mol Genet Metab* 87:113-121, 2006.

Vanier MT: Prenatal diagnosis of Niemann-Pick diseases types A, B and C, *Prenat Diagn* 22:630-632, 2002.

Weinstein LB: Selected genetic disorders affecting Ashkenazi Jewish families, *Fam Community Health* 30:50-62, 2007.

Lipoid Proteinosis

Aroni K, Lazaris AC, Papadimitriou K et al: Lipoid proteinosis of the oral mucosa: case report and review of the literature, *Pathol Res Pract* 194:855-859, 1998.

Bahadir S, Çobanoğlu Ü, Kapicioğlu Z et al: Lipoid proteinosis: a case with ophthalmological and psychiatric findings, *J Dermatol* 3:215-218, 2006.

Bazopoulou-Kyrkanidou E, Tosios KI, Zabelis G et al: Hyalinosis cutis et mucosae: gingival involvement, *J Oral Pathol Med* 27:233-237, 1998.

Botha P: Oral lipoid proteinosis, *SADJ* 54:371-373, 1999.

Chaudhary SJ, Dayal PK: Hyalinosis cutis et mucosae. Review with a case report, *Oral Surg Oral Med Oral Pathol Oral Radiol Endod* 80:168-171, 1995.

Hamada T: Lipoid proteinosis, *Clin Exp Dermatol* 27:624-629, 2002.

Hamada T, Wessagowit V, South AP et al: Extracellular matrix protein 1 gene (ECM1) mutations in lipoid proteinosis and genotype-phenotype correlation, *J Invest Dermatol* 120:345-350, 2003.

Horev L, Potikha T, Ayalon S et al: A novel splice-site mutation in ECM-1 gene in a consanguineous family with lipoid proteinosis, *Exp Dermatol* 14:891-897, 2005.

Lupo I, Cefalu AB, Bongiorno MR et al: A novel mutation of the extracellular matrix protein 1 gene (ECM1) in a patient with lipoid proteinosis (Urbach-Wiethe disease) from Sicily, *Br J Dermatol* 153:1019-1022, 2005.

Muda AO, Paradisi M, Angelo C et al: Lipoid proteinosis: clinical, histologic, and ultrastructural investigations, *Cutis* 56, 220-224, 1995.

Staut CCV, Naidich TP: Urbach-Wiethe disease (lipoid proteinosis), *Pediatr Neurosurg* 28:212-214, 1998.

Jaundice

Bansal V, Schuchert VD: Jaundice in the intensive care unit, *Surg Clin North Am* 86:1495-1502, 2006.

Cohen SM: Jaundice in the full-term newborn, *Pediatr Nurs* 32:202-208, 2006.

Gordon SC: Jaundice and cholestasis, *Postgrad Med* 90:65-71, 1991.

Hass PL: Differentiation and diagnosis of jaundice, *AACN Clin Issues* 10:433-441, 1999.

Pratt DS, Kaplan MM: Jaundice. In Kasper DL, Braunwald E, Fauci AS et al: *Harrison's principles of internal medicine*, pp 238-243, ed 16, New York, 2005, McGraw-Hill.

Murtagh J: Jaundice, *Aust Fam Physician* 20:457-466, 1991.

Roche SP, Kobos R: Jaundice in the adult patient, *Am Fam Physician* 69:299-304, 2004.

Amyloidosis

Fahrner KS, Black CC, Gosselin BJ: Localized amyloidosis of the tongue: a review, *Am J Otolaryngol* 25:186-189, 2004.

Falk RH, Comenzo RL, Skinner M: The systemic amyloidoses, *N Engl J Med* 337:898-909, 1997.

Gertz MA, Lacy MQ, Dispenzieri A: Amyloidosis: recognition, confirmation, prognosis, and therapy, *Mayo Clin Proc* 74:490-494, 1999.

Hachulla E, Grateau G: Diagnostic tools for amyloidosis, *Joint Bone Spine* 69:538-545, 2002.

Hachulla E, Janin A, Flipo RM et al: Labial salivary gland biopsy as a reliable test for the diagnosis of primary and secondary amyloidosis: a prospective clinical and immunohistologic study in 59 patients, *Arthritis Rheum* 36:691-697, 1993.

Hirschfield GM: Amyloidosis: a clinico-pathophysiological synopsis, *Semin Cell Dev Biol* 15:39-44, 2004.

Johansson I, Ryberg M, Steen L et al: Salivary hypofunction in patients with familial amyloidotic polyneuropathy, *Oral Surg Oral Med Oral Pathol* 74:742-748, 1992.

Kaplan B, Martin BM, Livneh A et al: Biochemical subtyping of amyloid in formalin-fixed tissue samples confirms and supplements immunohistologic data, *Am J Clin Pathol* 121:794-800, 2004.

Lachmann HJ, Hawkins PN: Systemic amyloidosis, *Curr Opin Pharmacol* 6:214-220, 2006.

Mardinger O, Rotenberg L, Chaushu G et al: Surgical management of macroglossia due to primary amyloidosis, *Int J Oral Maxillofac Surg* 28:129-131, 1999.

Merlini G, Westermark P: The systemic amyloidoses: clearer understanding of the molecular mechanisms offers hope for more effective therapies, *J Intern Med* 255:159-178, 2004.

Nandapalan V, Jones TM, Morar P et al: Localized amyloidosis of the parotid gland: a case report and review of the localized amyloidosis of the head and neck, *Head Neck* 20:73-78, 1998.

Penner CR, Müller S: Head and neck amyloidosis: a clinicopathologic study of 15 cases, *Oral Oncol* 42:421-429, 2006.

Raymond AK, Sneige N, Batsakis JG: Amyloidosis in the upper aerodigestive tract, *Ann Otol Rhinol Laryngol* 101:794-796, 1992.

Skinner M, Anderson JJ, Simms R et al: Treatment of 100 patients with primary amyloidosis: a randomized trial of melphalan, prednisone, and colchicine versus colchicine only, *Am J Med* 100:290-298, 1996.

Stoopler ET, Alawi F, Laudenbach JM et al: Bullous amyloidosis of the oral cavity: a rare clinical presentation and review, *Oral Surg Oral Med Oral Pathol Oral Radiol Endod* 101:734-740, 2006.

Stoopler ET, Sollecito TP, Chen S-Y: Amyloid deposition in the oral cavity: a retrospective study and review of the literature, *Oral Surg Oral Med Oral Pathol Oral Radiol Endod* 95:674-680, 2003.

Westermark P, Benson MD, Buxbaum JN et al: Amyloid: toward terminology clarification. Report from the Nomenclature Committee of the International Society of Amyloidosis, *Amyloid* 12:1-4, 2005.

Xavier SD, Filho IB, Müller H: Macroglossia secondary to systemic amyloidosis: case report and literature review, *Ear Nose Throat J* 84:358-361, 2005.

Vitamin Deficiency

Blanck HM, Bowman BA, Serdula MK et al: Angular stomatitis and riboflavin status among adolescent Bhutanese refugees living in southeastern Nepal, *Am J Clin Nutr* 76:430-435, 2002.

Fairfield KM, Fletcher RH: Vitamins for chronic disease prevention in adults, *JAMA* 287:3116-3126, 2002.

Halligan TJ, Russell NG, Dunn WJ et al: Identification and treatment of scurvy: a case report, *Oral Surg Oral Med Oral Pathol Oral Radiol Endod* 100:688-692, 2005.

Harper C: Thiamine (vitamin B₁) deficiency and associated brain damage is still common throughout the world and prevention is simple and safe! *Eur J Neurol* 13:1078-1082, 2006.

Heath ML, Sidbury R: Cutaneous manifestations of nutritional deficiency, *Curr Opin Pediatr* 18:417-422, 2006.

Hirschmann JV, Raugi GJ: Adult scurvy, *J Am Acad Dermatol* 41:895-906, 1999.

Mason ME, Jalagani H, Vinik AI: Metabolic complications of bariatric surgery: diagnosis and management issues, *Gastroenterol Clin North Am* 34:25-33, 2005.

Nield LS, Mahajan P, Joshi A et al: Rickets: not a disease of the past, *Am Fam Physician* 74:619-626, 629-630, 2006.

Olmedo JM, Yiannias JA, Windgassen EB et al: Scurvy: a disease almost forgotten, *Int J Dermatol* 45:909-913, 2006.

Powers HJ: Riboflavin (vitamin B₂) and health, *Am J Clin Nutr* 77:1352-1360, 2003.

Sethuraman U: Vitamins, *Pediatr Rev* 27:44-55, 2006.

Thacher TD, Fischer PR, Pettifor JM et al: A comparison of calcium, vitamin D, or both for nutritional rickets in Nigerian children, *N Engl J Med* 341:563-568, 1999.

Touyz LZG: Oral scurvy and periodontal disease, *J Can Dent Assoc* 63:837-845, 1997.

Russell RM: Vitamin and trace mineral deficiency and excess. In Kasper DL, Braunwald E, Fauci AS et al: *Harrison's principles of internal medicine*, pp 403-411, ed 16, New York, 2005, McGraw-Hill.

Wolpowitz D, Gilchrest BA: The vitamin D questions: how much do you need and how should you get it? *J Am Acad Dermatol* 54:301-317, 2006.

Iron-Deficiency Anemia

Brigden ML: Iron deficiency anemia: every case is instructive, *Postgrad Med* 93:181-192, 1993.

Brown RG: Normocytic and macrocytic anemias, *Postgrad Med* 89:125-136, 1991.

Cook JD: Diagnosis and management of iron-deficiency anaemia, *Best Pract Res Clin Haematol* 18:319-332, 2005.

Killip S, Bennett JM, Chambers MD: Iron deficiency anemia, *Am Fam Physician* 75:671-678, 2007.

Massey AC: Microcytic anemia: differential diagnosis and management of iron deficiency anemia, *Med Clin North Am* 76:549-566, 1992.

Osaki T, Ueta E, Arisawa K et al: The pathophysiology of glossal pain in patients with iron deficiency anemia, *Am J Med Sci* 318:324-329, 1999.

Provan D: Mechanisms and management of iron deficiency anaemia, *Br J Haematol* 105(suppl 1):19-26, 1999.

Umbreit J: Iron deficiency: a concise review, *Am J Hematol* 78:225-231, 2005.

Plummer-Vinson Syndrome

Atmatzidis K, Papaziogas B, Pavlidis T et al: Plummer-Vinson syndrome, *Dis Esophagus* 16:154-157, 2003.

Bredenkamp JK, Castro D J, Mickel RA: Importance of iron repletion in the management of Plummer-Vinson syndrome, *Ann Otol Rhinol Laryngol* 99:51-54, 1990.

Chen TSN, Chen PSY: Rise and fall of the Plummer-Vinson syndrome, *J Gastroenterol Hepatol* 9:654-658, 1994.

Dantas RO, Villanova MG: Esophageal motility impairment in Plummer-Vinson syndrome: correction by iron treatment, *Dig Dis Sci* 38:968-971, 1993.

Geerlings SE, Statius van Eps LW: Pathogenesis and consequences of Plummer-Vinson syndrome, *Clin Invest* 70:629-630, 1992.

Hoffman RM, Jaffe PE: Plummer-Vinson syndrome: a case report and literature review, *Arch Intern Med* 155:2008-2011, 1995.

Nagai T, Susami E, Ebiham T: Plummer-Vinson syndrome complicated by gastric cancer: a case report, *Keio J Med* 39:106-111, 1990.

Seitz ML, Sabatino D: Plummer-Vinson syndrome in an adolescent, *J Adolesc Health* 12:279-281, 1991.

Wahlberg PCG, Andersson KEH, Biörklund AT et al: Carcinoma of the hypopharynx: analysis of incidence and survival in Sweden in over a 30-year period, *Head Neck* 20:714-719, 1998.

Yukselen V, Karaoglu AO, Yasa MH: Plummer-Vinson syndrome: a report of three cases, *Int J Clin Pract* 57:646-648, 2003.

Pernicious Anemia

Colon-Otero G, Menke D, Hook CC: A practical approach to the differential diagnosis and evaluation of the adult patient with macrocytic anemia, *Med Clin North Am* 76:581-596, 1992.

Dharmarajan TS, Adiga GU, Norkus EP: Vitamin B₁₂ deficiency: recognizing subtle symptoms in older adults, *Geriatrics* 58:30-38, 2003.

Drummond JF, White DK, Damm DD: Megaloblastic anemia with oral lesions: a consequence of gastric bypass surgery, *Oral Surg Oral Med Oral Pathol* 59:149-153, 1985.

Field EA, Speechley JA, Rugman FR et al: Oral signs and symptoms in patients with undiagnosed vitamin B₁₂ deficiency, *J Oral Pathol Med* 24:468-470, 1995.

Greenberg M: Clinical and histologic changes of the oral mucosa in pernicious anemia, *Oral Surg Oral Med Oral Pathol* 52:38-42, 1981.

Hsing AW, Hansson L-E, McLaughlin JK et al: Pernicious anemia and subsequent cancer: a population-based cohort study, *Cancer* 71:745-750, 1993.

Kleinegger CL, Krolls SO: Severe pernicious anemia presenting with burning mouth symptoms, *Miss Dent Assoc J* 52:12-14, 1996.

Lehman JS, Bruce AJ, Rogers RS: Atrophic glossitis from vitamin B₁₂ deficiency: a case misdiagnosed as burning mouth disorder, *J Periodontol* 77:2090-2092, 2006.

Loffeld BCAJ, van Spreeuwel JP: The gastrointestinal tract in pernicious anemia, *Dig Dis* 9:70-77, 1991.

Oh RC, Brown DL: Vitamin B₁₂ deficiency, *Am Fam Physician* 67:979-986, 993-994, 2003.

Toh B-H, Alderuccio F: Pernicious anemia, *Autoimmunity* 37:357-361, 2004.

Toh B-H, van Driel IR, Gleeson PA: Pernicious anemia, *N Engl J Med* 337:1441-1448, 1997.

Pituitary Dwarfism

Ayuk J, Sheppard MC: Growth hormone and its disorders, *Postgrad Med J* 82:24-30, 2006.

Buduneli N, Alpoz AR, Candan U et al: Dental management of isolated growth hormone deficiency: a case report, *J Clin Pediatr Dent* 29:263-266, 2005.

Carvalho LR, Justamante de Faria ME, Farah-Osorio MG et al: Acromegalic features in growth hormone (GH)-deficient patients after long-term GH therapy, *Clin Endocrinol* 59:788-792, 2003.

Funatsu M, Sato K, Mitani H: Effects of growth hormone on craniofacial growth, *Angle Orthod* 76:970-977, 2006.

Grumbach MM, Bin-Abbas BS, Kaplan SL: The growth hormone cascade: progress and long-term results of growth hormone treatment in growth hormone deficiency, *Horm Res* 49(suppl 2):41-57, 1998.

Kosowicz J, Rzymski K: Abnormalities of tooth development in pituitary dwarfism, *Oral Surg Oral Med Oral Pathol* 44:853-863, 1977.

Lamberts SWJ, de Herder WW, van der Lely AJ: Pituitary insufficiency, *Lancet* 352:127-134, 1998.

Laron Z: Short stature due to genetic defects affecting growth hormone activity, *N Engl J Med* 334:463-465, 1996.

Gigantism

Daughaday WH: Pituitary gigantism, *Endocrinol Metab Clin North Am* 21:633-647, 1992.

Eugster EA, Pescovitz OH: Gigantism, *J Clin Endocrinol Metab* 84:4379-4384, 1999.

Kant SG, Wit JM, Breuning MH: Genetic analysis of tall stature, *Horm Res* 64:149-156, 2005.

Van Haelst MM, Hoogeboom JJM, Baujat G et al: Familial gigantism caused by an NSD1 mutation, *Am J Med Genet* 139A:40-44, 2005.

Acromegaly

Ayuk J, Sheppard MC: Growth hormone and its disorders, *Postgrad Med J* 82:24-30, 2006.

Ben-Shlomo A, Melmed S: Skin manifestations in acromegaly, *Clin Dermatol* 24:256-259, 2006.

Burt MG, Ho KKY: Newer options in the management of acromegaly, *Intern Med J* 36:437-444, 2006.

Cohen RB, Wilcox CW: A case of acromegaly identified after patient complaint of apertognathia, *Oral Surg Oral Med Oral Pathol* 75:583-586, 1993.

Farinazzo-Vitral RW, Motohiro-Tanaka O, Reis-Fraga M et al: Acromegaly in an orthodontic patient, *Am J Orthod Dentofacial Orthop* 130:388-390, 2006.

Gayle C, Sonksen P: The presentation of acromegaly in general practice, *Practitioner* 243:110-117, 1999.

Guistina A, Barkan A, Casanueva FF et al: Criteria for cure of acromegaly: a consensus statement, *J Clin Endocrinol Metab* 85:526-529, 2000.

Laws ER, Vance ML, Thapar K: Pituitary surgery for the management of acromegaly, *Horm Res* 53(suppl 3):71-75, 2000.

Melmed S: Acromegaly, *N Engl J Med* 355:2558-2573, 2006.

Newman CB: Medical therapy for acromegaly, *Endocrinol Metab Clin North Am* 28:171-190, 1999.

Ron E, Gridley G, Hrubec Z et al: Acromegaly and gastrointestinal cancer, *Cancer* 68:1673-1677, 1991.

Hypothyroidism

Burman KD, McKinley-Grant L: Dermatologic aspects of thyroid disease, *Clin Dermatol* 24:247-255, 2006.

LaFranchi S: Congenital hypothyroidism: etiologies, diagnosis, and management, *Thyroid* 9:735-740, 1999.

Lazarus JH, Obuobie K: Thyroid disorders—an update, *Postgrad Med J* 76:529-536, 2000.

Martinez M, Derksen D, Kapsner P: Making sense of hypothyroidism, *Postgrad Med* 93:135-145, 1993.

Mg'ang'a PM, Chindia ML: Dental and skeletal changes in juvenile hypothyroidism following treatment: case report, *Odontostomatol Trop* 13:25-27, 1990.

Roberts CGP, Ladenson PW: Hypothyroidism, *Lancet* 363:793-803, 2004.

Topliss DJ, Eastman CJ: Diagnosis and management of hyperthyroidism and hypothyroidism, *Med J Aust* 180:186-193, 2004.

Woeber KA: Update on the management of hyperthyroidism and hypothyroidism, *Arch Fam Med* 9:743-747, 2000.

Hyperthyroidism

Caruso DR, Mazzaferri EL: Intervention in Graves' disease, *Postgrad Med* 92:117-134, 1992.

Cooper DS: Hyperthyroidism, *Lancet* 362:459-468, 2003.

McKeown NJ, Tews MC, Gossain VV et al: Hyperthyroidism, *Emerg Med Clin North Am* 23:669-685, 2005.

Pearce EN: Diagnosis and management of thyrotoxicosis, *Br Med J* 332:1369-1373, 2006.

Pérusse R, Goulet J-P, Turcotte J-Y: Contraindications to vasoconstrictors in dentistry. Part II: hyperthyroidism, diabetes, sulfite sensitivity, cortico-dependent asthma, and pheochromocytoma, *Oral Surg Oral Med Oral Pathol* 74:687-691, 1992.

Reid JR, Wheeler SF: Hyperthyroidism: diagnosis and treatment, *Am Fam Physician* 72:623-30, 635-636, 2005.

Singer PA, Cooper DS, Levy EG et al: Treatment guidelines for patients with hyperthyroidism and hypothyroidism, *JAMA* 273:808-812, 1995.

Tietgens ST, Leinung MC: Thyroid storm, *Med Clin North Am* 79:169-184, 1995.

Topliss DJ, Eastman CJ: Diagnosis and management of hyperthyroidism and hypothyroidism, *Med J Aust* 180:186-193, 2004.

Yeatts RP: Graves' ophthalmopathy, *Med Clin North Am* 79:195-209, 1995.

Hypoparathyroidism

Ahonen P, Myllärniemi S, Sipilä I et al: Clinical variation of autoimmune polyendocrinopathy-candidiasis-ectodermal dystrophy (APECED) in a series of 68 patients, *N Engl J Med* 322:1829-1836, 1990.

Angelopoulos NG, Goula A, Tolis G: Sporadic hypoparathyroidism treated with teriparatide: a case report and literature review, *Exp Clin Endocrinol Diabetes* 115:50-54, 2007.

Greenberg MS, Brightman VJ, Lynch MA et al: Idiopathic hypoparathyroidism, chronic candidiasis, and dental hypoplasia, *Oral Surg Oral Med Oral Pathol* 28:42-53, 1969.

Perheentupa J: Autoimmune polyendocrinopathy-candidiasis-ectodermal dystrophy, *J Clin Endocrinol Metab* 91:2843-2850, 2006.

Walls AWG, Soames JV: Dental manifestations of autoimmune hypoparathyroidism, *Oral Surg Oral Med Oral Pathol* 75:452-454, 1993.

Winer KK, Ko CW, Reynolds JC et al: Long-term treatment of hypoparathyroidism: a randomized controlled study comparing parathyroid hormone-(1-34) versus calcitriol and calcium, *J Clin Endocrinol Metab* 88:4214-4220, 2003.

Yasuda T, Niimi H: Hypoparathyroidism and pseudohypoparathyroidism, *Acta Paediatr Jpn* 39:485-490, 1997.

Pseudohypoparathyroidism

Brown MD, Aaron G: Pseudohypoparathyroidism: case report, *Pediatr Dent* 13:106-109, 1991.

Faull CM, Welbury RR, Paul B et al: Pseudohypoparathyroidism: its phenotypic variability and associated disorders in a large family, *Q J Med* 78:251-264, 1991.

Gelfand IM, Eugster EA, DiMeglio LA: Presentation and clinical progression of pseudohypoparathyroidism with multi-hormone resistance and Albright hereditary osteodystrophy: a case series, *J Pediatr* 149:877-880, 2006.

Goeteyn V, De Potter CR, Naeyaert JM: Osteoma cutis in pseudohypoparathyroidism, *Dermatology* 198:209-211, 1999.

Jüppner H, Linglart A, Fröhlich LF et al: Autosomal-dominant pseudohypoparathyroidism type Ib is caused by different microdeletions within or upstream of the GNAS locus, *Ann N Y Acad Sci* 1068:250-255, 2006.

Levine MA: Pseudohypoparathyroidism: from bedside to bench and back, *J Bone Miner Res* 14:1255-1260, 1999.

Mallette LE: Pseudohypoparathyroidism, *Curr Ther Endocrinol Metab* 6:577-581, 1997.

Potts JT: Diseases of the parathyroid gland and other hyper- and hypocalcemic disorders. In Kasper DL, Braunwald E, Fauci AS et al: *Harrison's principles of internal medicine*, pp 2249-2268, ed 16, New York, 2005, McGraw-Hill.

Simon A, Koppeschaar HP, Roijers JF et al: Pseudohypoparathyroidism type Ia, Albright hereditary osteodystrophy: a model for research on G protein-coupled receptors and genomic imprinting, Neth J Med 56:100-109, 2000.

Hyperparathyroidism

Aggunlu L, Akpek S, Coskun B: Leontiasis ossea in a patient with hyperparathyroidism secondary to chronic renal failure, Pediatr Radiol 34:630-632, 2004.

Antonelli JR, Hottel TL: Oral manifestations of renal osteodystrophy: case report and review of the literature, Spec Care Dentist 23:28-34, 2003.

Daniels JSM: Primary hyperparathyroidism presenting as a palatal brown tumor, Oral Surg Oral Med Oral Pathol Oral Radiol Endod 98:409-413, 2004.

Farford B, Presutti J, Moraghan TJ: Nonsurgical management of primary hyperparathyroidism, Mayo Clin Proc 82:351-355, 2007.

Gavaldá C, Bagán JV, Scully C et al: Renal hemodialysis patients: oral, salivary, dental and periodontal findings in 105 adult cases, Oral Dis 5:299-302, 1999.

Hata T, Irei I, Tanaka K et al: Macrognathia secondary to dialysis-related renal osteodystrophy treated successfully by parathyroidectomy, Int J Oral Maxillofac Surg 35:378-382, 2006.

Kalyvas D, Tosios KI, Leventis MD et al: Localized jaw enlargement in renal osteodystrophy: report of a case and review of the literature, Oral Surg Oral Med Oral Pathol Oral Radiol Endod 97:68-74, 2004.

Khan A, Bilezikian J: Primary hyperparathyroidism: pathophysiology and impact on bone, CMAJ 163:173-175, 2000.

Ogata H, Koiwa F, Ito H et al: Therapeutic strategies for secondary hyperparathyroidism in dialysis patients, Ther Apher Dial 10:355-363, 2006.

Prado FO, Rosales AC, Rodrigues CI et al: Brown tumor of the mandible associated with secondary hyperparathyroidism: a case report and review of the literature, Gen Dent 54:341-343, 2006.

Sakhaee K, Gonzalez GB: Update on renal osteodystrophy: pathogenesis and clinical management, Am J Med Sci 317:251-260, 1999.

Silverman S Jr, Gordon G, Grant T et al: The dental structures in primary hyperparathyroidism. Studies in forty-two consecutive patients, Oral Surg Oral Med Oral Pathol 15:426-436, 1962.

Silverman S Jr, Ware WH, Gillooly C: Dental aspects of hyperparathyroidism, Oral Surg Oral Med Oral Pathol 26:184-189, 1968.

Slatopolsky E, Brown A, Dusso A: Pathogenesis of secondary hyperparathyroidism, Kidney Int Suppl 73:S14-19, 1999.

Solt DB: The pathogenesis, oral manifestations, and implications for dentistry of metabolic bone disease, Curr Opin Dent 1:783-791, 1991.

Tejwani NC, Schachter AK, Immerman I et al: Renal osteodystrophy, J Am Acad Orthop Surg 14:303-311, 2006.

Triantafillidou K, Zouloumis L, Karakinaris G et al: Brown tumors of the jaws associated with primary or secondary hyperparathyroidism. A clinical study and review of the literature, Am J Otolaryngol 27:281-286, 2006.

Cushing's Disease

Findling JW, Raff H: Cushing's syndrome: important issues in diagnosis and management, J Clin Endocrinol Metab 91:3746-3753, 2006.

Gabrilove JL: Cushing's syndrome, Compr Ther 18:13-16, 1992.

Katz J, Bouloux P-MG: Cushing's: how to make the diagnosis, Practitioner 243:118-124, 1999.

Newell-Price J, Bertagna X, Grossman AB et al: Cushing's syndrome, Lancet 367:1605-1617, 2006.

Shibli-Rahhal A, Van Beek M, Schlechte JA: Cushing's syndrome, Clin Dermatol 24:260-265, 2006.

Tsigos C: Differential diagnosis and management of Cushing's syndrome, Annu Rev Med 47:443-461, 1996.

Addison's Disease

Coursin DB, Wood KE: Corticosteroid supplementation for adrenal insufficiency, JAMA 287:236-240, 2002.

Jabbour SA: Cutaneous manifestations of endocrine disorders: a guide for dermatologists, Am J Clin Dermatol 4:315-331, 2003.

Marzotti S, Falorni A: Addison's disease, Autoimmunity 37:333-336, 2004.

Neiman LK, Chanco-Turner ML: Addison's disease, Clin Dermatol 24:276-280, 2006.

Porter SR, Haria S, Scully C et al: Chronic candidiasis, enamel hypoplasia, and pigmentary anomalies, Oral Surg Oral Med Oral Pathol 74:312-314, 1992.

Shah SS, Oh CH, Coffin SE et al: Addisonian pigmentation of the oral mucosa, Cutis 76:97-99, 2005.

Werbel SS, Ober KP: Acute adrenal insufficiency, Endocrinol Metab Clin North Am 22:303-328, 1993.

Ziccardi VB, Abubaker AO, Sotereanos GC et al: Precipitation of an addisonian crisis during dental surgery: recognition and management, Compend Contin Educ Dent 13:518-523, 1992.

Diabetes Mellitus

Belazi M, Velegraki A, Fleva A et al: Candidal overgrowth in diabetic patients: potential predisposing factors, Mycoses 48:192-196, 2005.

Bergman SA: Perioperative management of the diabetic patient, Oral Surg Oral Med Oral Pathol Oral Radiol Endod 103:731-737, 2007.

Cianciola LJ, Park BH, Bruck E et al: Prevalence of periodontal disease in insulin-dependent diabetes mellitus (juvenile diabetes), J Am Dent Assoc 104:653-660, 1982.

Emancipator K: Laboratory diagnosis and monitoring of diabetes mellitus, Am J Clin Pathol 112:665-674, 1999.

Franco OH, Steyerberg EW, Hu FB et al: Associations of diabetes mellitus with total life expectancy and life expectancy with and without cardiovascular disease, Arch Intern Med 167:1145-1151, 2007.

Guggenheimer J, Moore PA, Rossie K et al: Insulin-dependent diabetes mellitus and oral soft tissue pathologies: II. Prevalence and characteristics of non-candidal lesions, Oral Surg Oral Med Oral Pathol Oral Radiol Endod 89:563-569, 2000.

Guggenheimer J, Moore PA, Rossie K et al: Insulin-dependent diabetes mellitus and oral soft tissue pathologies: II. Prevalence and characteristics of Candida and candidal lesions, Oral Surg Oral Med Oral Pathol Oral Radiol Endod 89:570-576, 2000.

Manfredi M, Al-Karaawi Z, McCullough MJ et al: The isolation, identification and molecular analysis of Candida spp. isolated from the oral cavities of patients with diabetes mellitus, Oral Microbiol Immunol 17:181-185, 2002.

Manfredi M, McCollough MJ, Vescovi P et al: Update on diabetes mellitus and related oral diseases, Oral Dis 10:187-200, 2004.

McKenna SJ: Dental management of patients with diabetes, Dent Clin North Am 50:591-606, 2006.

Mealey BL, Oates TW: Diabetes mellitus and periodontal diseases, J Periodontol 77:1289-1303, 2006.

Miley DD, Terezhalmy GT: The patient with diabetes mellitus: etiology, epidemiology, principles of medical management, oral disease burden, and principles of dental management, *Quintessence Int* 36:779-795, 2005.

Moore PA, Weyant RJ, Mongelluzzo MB et al: Type 1 diabetes mellitus and oral health: assessment of tooth loss and edentulism, *J Public Health Dent* 58:135-142, 1998.

Murrah VA: Diabetes mellitus and associated oral manifestations: a review, *J Oral Pathol* 14:271-281, 1985.

Newton CA, Raskin P: Diabetic ketoacidosis in type 1 and type 2 diabetes mellitus: clinical and biochemical differences, *Arch Intern Med* 164:1925-1931, 2004.

Seppälä B, Seppälä M, Ainamo J: A longitudinal study on insulin-dependent diabetes mellitus and periodontal disease, *J Clin Periodontol* 20:161-165, 1993.

Tsai C, Hayes C, Taylor GW: Glycemic control of type 2 diabetes and severe periodontal disease in the US adult population, *Community Dent Oral Epidemiol* 30:182-192, 2002.

Wang PH, Lau J, Chalmers TC: Meta-analysis of effects of intensive blood-glucose control on late complications of type I diabetes, *Lancet* 341:1306-1309, 1993.

Winer N, Sowers JR: Epidemiology of diabetes, *J Clin Pharmacol* 44:397-405, 2004.

Wysocki GP, Daley T: Benign migratory glossitis in patients with juvenile diabetes, *Oral Surg Oral Med Oral Pathol* 63:68-70, 1987.

Zachariasen RD: Diabetes mellitus and xerostomia, *Compend Contin Educ Dent* 13:314-322, 1992.

Hypophosphatasia

Brun-Heath I, Taillandier A, Serre J-L et al: Characterization of 11 novel mutations in the tissue non-specific alkaline phosphatase gene responsible for hypophosphatasia and genotype-phenotype correlations, *Mol Genet Metab* 84:273-277, 2005.

Caswell AM, Whyte MP, Russell RGG: Hypophosphatasia and the extracellular metabolism of inorganic pyrophosphate: clinical and laboratory aspects, *Crit Rev Clin Lab Sci* 28:175-232, 1991.

Fallon MD, Teitelbaum SL, Weinstein RS et al: Hypophosphatasia: clinicopathologic comparison of the infantile, childhood, and adult forms, *Medicine* 63:12-24, 1984.

Hu C-C, King DL, Thomas HF et al: A clinical and research protocol for characterizing patients with hypophosphatasia, *Pediatr Dent* 18:17-23, 1996.

Mornet E: Hypophosphatasia: the mutations in the tissue-non-specific alkaline phosphatase gene, *Hum Mutat* 15:309-315, 2000.

Olsson A, Matsson L, Blomquist HK et al: Hypophosphatasia affecting the permanent dentition, *J Oral Pathol Med* 25:343-347, 1996.

Plagmann H-H, Kocher T, Kuhrau N et al: Periodontal manifestation of hypophosphatasia. A family case report, *J Clin Periodontol* 21:710-716, 1994.

Spentchian M, Merrien Y, Herasse M et al: Severe hypophosphatasia: characterization of fifteen novel mutations in the ALPL gene, *Hum Mutat* 22:105-106, 2003.

Van den Bos T, Handoko G, Niehof A et al: Cementum and dentin in hypophosphatasia, *J Dent Res* 84:1021-1025, 2005.

Vitamin D-Resistant Rickets

Archard HO, Witkop CJ: Hereditary hypophosphatemia (vitamin D-resistant rickets) presenting primary dental manifestations, *Oral Surg Oral Med Oral Pathol* 22:184-193, 1966.

Batra P, Tejani Z, Mars M: X-linked hypophosphatemia: dental and histologic findings, *J Can Dent Assoc* 72:69-72, 2006.

Berndt M, Ehrich JHH, Lazovic D et al: Clinical course of hypophosphatemic rickets in 23 adults, *Clin Nephrol* 45:33-41, 1996.

Carpenter TO: New perspectives on the biology and treatment of X-linked hypophosphatemic rickets, *Pediatr Clin North Am* 44:443-466, 1997.

Chaussin-Miller C, Sinding C, Wolikow M et al: Dental abnormalities in patients with familial hypophosphatemic vitamin D-resistant rickets: prevention by early treatment with 1-hydroxyvitamin D, *J Pediatr* 142:324-331, 2003.

Fadavi S, Rowold E: Familial hypophosphatemic vitamin D-resistant rickets: review of the literature and report of case, *ASDC J Dent Child* 57:212-215, 1990.

Hanna JD, Niimi K, Chart JCM: X-linked hypophosphatemia: genetic and clinical correlates, *Am J Dis Child* 145:865-870, 1991.

Hillman G, Geurtsen W: Pathohistology of undecalcified primary teeth in vitamin D-resistant rickets. Review and report of two cases, *Oral Surg Oral Med Oral Pathol Oral Radiol Endod* 82:218-224, 1996.

McWhorter AG, Seale NS: Prevalence of dental abscess in a population of children with vitamin D-resistant rickets, *Pediatr Dent* 13:91-96, 1991.

Miller WL, Portale AA: Genetic causes of rickets, *Curr Opin Pediatr* 11:333-339, 1999.

Murayama T, Iwatsubo R, Akiyama S et al: Familial hypophosphatemic vitamin D-resistant rickets: dental findings and histologic study of teeth, *Oral Surg Oral Med Oral Pathol Oral Radiol Endod* 90:310-316, 2000.

Pereira CM, de Andrade CR, Vargas PA et al: Dental alterations associated with X-linked hypophosphatemic rickets, *J Endod* 30:241-245, 2004.

Scriver CR, Tenenhouse HS, Glorieux HI: X-linked hypophosphatemia: an appreciation of a classic paper and a survey of progress since 1958, *Medicine (Baltimore)* 70:218-228, 1991.

Seow WK, Needleman HL, Holm IA: Effect of familial hypophosphatemic rickets on dental development: a controlled, longitudinal study, *Pediatr Dent* 17:346-350, 1995.

Shroff DV, McWhorter AG, Seale NS: Evaluation of aggressive pulp therapy in a population of vitamin D-resistant rickets patients: a follow-up of 4 cases, *Pediatr Dent* 24:347-349, 2002.

Wang JT, Lin C-J, Burridge SM et al: Genetics of vitamin D 1α-hydroxylase deficiency in 17 families, *Am J Hum Genet* 63:1694-1702, 1998.

Zambrano M, Nikitakis NG, Sanchez-Quevedo MC et al: Oral and dental manifestations of vitamin D-dependent rickets type I: report of a pediatric case, *Oral Surg Oral Med Oral Pathol Oral Radiol Endod* 95:705-709, 2003.

Crohn's Disease

Brunner B, Hirschi C, Weimann R et al: Treatment-resistant lingual Crohn's disease disappears after infliximab, *Scand J Gastroenterol* 40:1255-1259, 2005.

Challacombe SJ: Oro-facial granulomatosis and oral Crohn's disease: are they specific diseases and do they predict systemic Crohn's disease? *Oral Dis* 3:127-129, 1997.

Dunlap CL, Friesen CA, Shultz R: Chronic stomatitis: an early sign of Crohn's disease, *J Am Dent Assoc* 128:347-348, 1997.

Dupuy A, Cosnes J, Revuz J et al: Oral Crohn disease: clinical characteristics and long-term follow-up of 9 cases, *Arch Dermatol* 135:439-442, 1999.

Galbraith SS, Drolet BA, Kugathasan S et al: Asymptomatic inflammatory bowel disease presenting with mucocutaneous findings, *Pediatrics* 116:e439-e444, 2005.

Girlich C, Bogenrieder T, Palitzsch K-D et al: Orofacial granulomatosis as initial manifestation of Crohn's disease: a report of two cases, *Eur J Gastroenterol Hepatol* 14:873-876, 2002.

Friedman S, Blumberg RS: Inflammatory bowel disease. In Kasper DL, Braunwald E, Fauci AS et al: *Harrison's principles of internal medicine*, pp 1776-1789, ed 16, New York, 2005, McGraw-Hill.

Harty S, Fleming P, Rowland M et al: A prospective study of the oral manifestations of Crohn's disease, *Clin Gastroenterol Hepatol* 3:886-891, 2005.

Hegarty A, Hodgson T, Porter S: Thalidomide for the treatment of recalcitrant oral Crohn's disease and orofacial granulomatosis, *Oral Surg Oral Med Oral Pathol Oral Radiol Endod* 95:576-585, 2003.

Hoffmann JC, Zeitz M: Treatment of Crohn's disease, *Hepatogastroenterology* 47:90-100, 2000.

Kalmar JR: Crohn's disease: orofacial considerations and disease pathogenesis, *Periodontol 2000* 6:101-115, 1994.

Lisciandrano D, Ranzi T, Carrassi A et al: Prevalence of oral lesions in inflammatory bowel disease, *Am J Gastroenterol* 91:7-10, 1996.

Mills CC, Amin M, Manisali M: Salivary duct fistula and recurrent buccal space infection: a complication of Crohn's disease, *J Oral Maxillofac Surg* 61:1485-1487, 2003.

Ottaviani F, Schindler A, Capaccio P et al: New therapy for orolaryngeal manifestations of Crohn's disease, *Ann Otol Rhinol Laryngol* 112:37-39, 2003.

Plauth M, Jenss H, Meyle J: Oral manifestations of Crohn's disease: an analysis of 79 cases, *J Clin Gastroenterol* 13:29-37, 1991.

Podolsky DK: Inflammatory bowel disease, *N Engl J Med* 347:417-429, 2002.

Rehberger A, Püspök A, Stallmeister T et al: Crohn's disease masquerading as aphthous ulcers, *Eur J Dermatol* 8:274-276, 1998.

Sánchez AR, Rogers RS, Sheridan PJ: Oral ulcerations are associated with the loss of response to infliximab in Crohn's disease, *J Oral Pathol Med* 34:53-55, 2005.

Scheper HJ, Brand HS: Oral aspects of Crohn's disease, *Int Dent J* 52:163-172, 2002.

Scully C, Cochran KM, Russell RI et al: Crohn's disease of the mouth: an indicator of intestinal involvement, *Gut* 23:198-201, 1982.

Van de Scheur MR, van der Waal RIF, Völker-Dieben HJ et al: Orofacial granulomatosis in a patient with Crohn's disease, *J Am Acad Dermatol* 49:952-954, 2003.

Weinstein TA, Sciubba JJ, Levine J: Thalidomide for the treatment of oral aphthous ulcers in Crohn's disease, *J Pediatr Gastroenterol Nutr* 28:214-216, 1999.

Pyostomatitis Vegetans

Ayangco L, Rogers RS, Sheridan PJ: Pyostomatitis vegetans as an early sign of reactivation of Crohn's disease: a case report, *J Periodontol* 73:1512-1516, 2002.

Ballo FS, Camisa C, Allen CM: Pyostomatitis vegetans: report of a case and review of the literature, *J Am Acad Dermatol* 21:381-387, 1989.

Calobrisi SD, Mutasim DF, McDonald JS: Pyostomatitis vegetans associated with ulcerative colitis. Temporary clearance with fluocinonide gel and complete remission after colectomy, *Oral Surg Oral Med Oral Pathol Oral Radiol Endod* 79:452-454, 1995.

Chan SWY, Scully C, Prime SS et al: Pyostomatitis vegetans: oral manifestation of ulcerative colitis, *Oral Surg Oral Med Oral Pathol* 72:689-692, 1991.

Chaudhry SI, Philpot NS, Odell EW et al: Pyostomatitis vegetans associated with asymptomatic ulcerative colitis: a case report, *Oral Surg Oral Med Oral Pathol Oral Radiol Endod* 87:327-330, 1999.

Ficarra G, Cicchi P, Amorosi A et al: Oral Crohn's disease and pyostomatitis vegetans: an unusual association, *Oral Surg Oral Med Oral Pathol* 75:220-224, 1993.

Healy CM, Farthing PM, Williams DM et al: Pyostomatitis vegetans and associated systemic disease. A review and two case reports, *Oral Surg Oral Med Oral Pathol* 78:323-328, 1994.

Hegarty AM, Barrett AW, Scully C: Pyostomatitis vegetans, *Clin Exp Dermatol* 29:1-7, 2004.

Markiewicz M, Suresh L, Margarone J et al: Pyostomatitis vegetans: a clinical marker of silent ulcerative colitis, *J Oral Maxillofac Surg* 65:346-348, 2007.

Neville BW, Laden SA, Smith SE et al: Pyostomatitis vegetans, *Am J Dermatopathol* 7:69-77, 1985.

Philpot HC, Elewski BE, Banwell JG et al: Pyostomatitis vegetans and primary sclerosing cholangitis: markers of inflammatory bowel disease, *Gastroenterology* 103:668-674, 1992.

Thornhill MH, Zakrzewska JM, Gilkes JJH: Pyostomatitis vegetans: report of three cases and review of the literature, *J Oral Pathol Med* 21:128-133, 1992.

Uremic Stomatitis

Halazonetis J, Harley A: Uremic stomatitis: report of a case, *Oral Surg Oral Med Oral Pathol* 23:573-577, 1967.

Hovinga J, Roodvoets AP, Gailliard J: Some findings in patients with uraemic stomatitis, *J Maxillofac Surg* 3:124-127, 1975.

Larato DC: Uremic stomatitis: report of a case, *J Periodontol* 46:731-733, 1975.

Leão JC, Gueiros LAM, Segundo AVL et al: Uremic stomatitis in chronic renal failure, *Clinics* 60:259-262, 2005.

McCreary CE, Flint SR, McCartan BE et al: Uremic stomatitis mimicking oral hairy leukoplakia. Report of a case, *Oral Surg Oral Med Oral Pathol Oral Radiol Endod* 83:350-353, 1997.

Proctor R, Kumar N, Stein A et al: Oral and dental aspects of chronic renal failure, *J Dent Res* 84:199-208, 2005.

Ross WF, Salisbury PL: Uremic stomatitis associated with undiagnosed renal failure, *Gen Dent* 42:410-412, 1994.

18

Facial Pain and Neuromuscular Diseases

Revised by THERESA S. GONZALES

CHAPTER OUTLINE

BELL'S PALSY (IDIOPATHIC SEVENTH NERVE PARALYSIS; IDIOPATHIC FACIAL PARALYSIS)

Bell's palsy is a dramatic but self-limiting, unilateral facial paralysis. It represents the most common form of facial paralysis. A variety of potential triggering events are known (Box 18-1), although a trigger cannot be identified in at least one fourth of all cases. The precise cause remains unclear; however, familial occurrences have been reported, and suspected causes include reactivation of herpes simplex or zoster in the geniculate ganglion, nerve demyelination, nerve edema or ischemia, autoimmune damage to nerves, and vasospasm of vessels associated with nerves.

A similar presentation can be seen with obvious damage to the facial nerve (e.g., from facial and salivary gland tumors or from severance of the nerve caused by trauma or surgery). When the cause is known, the term *Bell's palsy* is not usually used.

Bell's palsy is diagnosed in 24 of every 100,000 persons each year, with increased frequency in the fall and winter seasons. In demyelinating diseases, such as multiple sclerosis (MS), it occurs much more frequently (one in five cases), usually appearing late in the disease but occasionally being the first symptom. Rarely, other anatomic sites also will become paralyzed, usually in persons with Melkersson-Rosenthal syndrome (see page 342), Lyme disease (*Borrelia burgdorferi* infection, Lyme peripheral facial palsy, transient facial nerve palsy), or sarcoidosis.

CLINICAL FEATURES

People of all ages are susceptible to Bell's palsy, but middle-aged people are affected most frequently. Women are affected more often (71%) than men. Childhood involvement is usually associated with a viral infection, Lyme disease, or earache.

Considerable variation exists in the severity of signs and symptoms. The palsy is characterized by an abrupt loss of muscular control on one side of the face, imparting a rigid masklike appearance and resulting in the inability to smile, to close the eye, to wink, or to raise the eyebrow (Fig. 18-1). A few patients, especially those with MS, experience prodromal pain on the affected side before the onset of paralysis. Infrequently, bilateral involvement is seen. The paralysis may take several

hours to become complete, but patients frequently awaken in the morning with a full-fledged case. Rapid onset of bilateral facial weakness should alert the clinician to the possibility of such diseases as **Guillain-Barre syndrome,** a form of sarcoidosis known as *uveoparotid fever* (see Heerfordt's syndrome, page 339), or other types of vasculitis causing multiple cranial neuropathies. If multiple cranial nerve deficits accompany the observed facial weakness, then central nervous system (CNS) infectious diseases and basilar skull tumors must be considered in the differential diagnosis. When vertigo or tinnitus is a major symptom, an occult herpes zoster ear infection should be suspected, and the diagnosis may be changed to Ramsay Hunt syndrome (see page 252).

The corner of the mouth usually droops, causing saliva to drool onto the skin. Speech becomes slurred and taste may be abnormal. Because the eyelid cannot close, conjunctival dryness or ulceration may occur.

TREATMENT AND PROGNOSIS

No universally preferred treatment exists for Bell's palsy. Histamine and other vasodilators may shorten

Box 18-1

Triggering Events or Phenomena Related to Bell's Palsy

- Acute otitis media
- Atmospheric pressure change (diving, flying)
- Exposure to cold
- Ischemia of the nerve near the stylomastoid foramen
- Local and systemic infections (viral, bacterial, fungal)
- Melkersson-Rosenthal syndrome
- Multiple sclerosis (MS)
- Pregnancy (third trimester, early eclampsia)

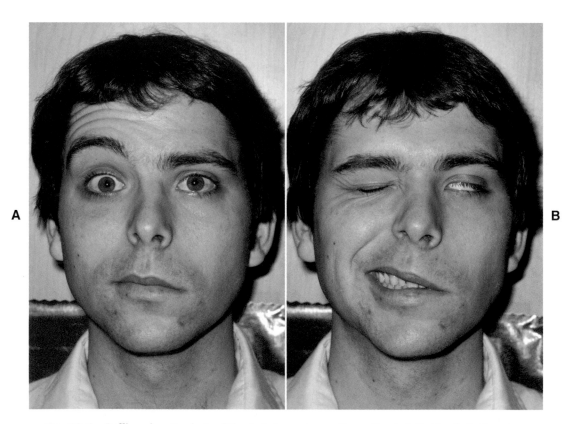

Fig. 18-1   Bell's palsy. Paralysis of the facial muscles on the patient's left side. **A,** Patient is trying to raise the eyebrows. **B,** Patient is attempting to close the eyes and smile. *(Courtesy of Dr. Bruce B. Brehm.)*

the duration, as will systemic corticosteroids and hyperbaric oxygen therapy. Surgical decompression of the intratemporal facial nerve is used in select cases. Topical ocular antibiotics and artificial tears may be required to prevent corneal ulceration, and the eyelid may have to be taped shut.

Symptoms usually begin to regress slowly and spontaneously within 1 to 2 months of onset; more severe cases take longer, as do those in older patients. Overall, more than 82% of patients recover completely within 6 months. Residual symptoms that remain after 1 year will probably remain indefinitely. Recurrence is rare, except in Melkersson-Rosenthal syndrome.

TRIGEMINAL NEURALGIA (TIC DOULOUREUX; TIC)

The head and neck region is a common site for neuralgias (pain extending along the course of a nerve) (Box 18-2). Because facial neuralgias produce pain that often mimics pain of dental origin, the dental profession is frequently called on to rule out odontogenic or inflammatory causes. **Trigeminal neuralgia**, the most serious and the most common of the facial neuralgias, is characterized by an extremely severe electric shock-like or lancinating (i.e., sharp, jabbing) pain limited to one or more branches of the trigeminal nerve. In the majority of cases the pain is located in the maxillary (V2) or the mandibular (V3) distribution of the nerve. It is often idiopathic but is usually associated with pathosis somewhere along the course of the nerve. Occasionally, trigeminal neuralgia results from a brainstem tumor or infarction and is referred to as *secondary trigeminal neuralgia.*

Trigeminal neuralgia is diagnosed in 6 of every 100,000 persons each year, but it develops in 4% of persons with multiple sclerosis (MS). Moreover, patients with **neuralgia-inducing cavitational osteonecrosis**

(NICO) of the jaws (see page 866), Gradenigo syndrome (suppurative otitis media, trigeminal nerve pain, abducens nerve palsy), and chronic paroxysmal hemicrania-tic syndrome may have pain so similar as to be virtually indistinguishable from trigeminal neuralgia.

Because so many of its features are consistent with a CNS disease, trigeminal neuralgia has been called "a pain syndrome with a peripheral cause but a central pathogenesis." The seriousness of the disorder is underscored by the fact that it has one of the highest suicide rates of any disease and is regarded as one of the most painful afflictions known.

CLINICAL FEATURES

Trigeminal neuralgia characteristically affects individuals older than 40 years of age (the average age at onset is 50 years), although it may affect persons as early as puberty. Women are affected slightly more often than men, and the right side is involved more often than the left. Any branch of the trigeminal nerve may be involved, but the ophthalmic division is affected in only 5% of cases. More than one branch may be involved, and the pain is occasionally bilateral.

Specific and strict criteria must be met for an accurate diagnosis (Box 18-3). If the pain pattern does not meet these criteria, then a different diagnosis should be considered. When these criteria are partially fulfilled, alternative terms such as *atypical trigeminal neuralgia, atypical facial pain,* and *atypical facial neuralgia* are applied.

Box 18-2

Types of Facial and Cervical Neuralgias

- Atypical pain/neuralgia
- Geniculate neuralgia
- Glossopharyngeal neuralgia
- Migrainous neuralgia
- Occipital neuralgia
- Raeder's paratrigeminal neuralgia
- Postherpetic facial neuralgia
- Sphenopalatine ganglion neuralgia
- Superior laryngeal neuralgia
- Trigeminal neuralgia
- Tympanic plexus neuralgia

Box 18-3

Necessary Criteria for a Diagnosis of Trigeminal Neuralgia

- The onset of a pain "attack" is abrupt, often initiated by a light touch to a specific and constant trigger point.
- The pain is extreme, paroxysmal, and lancinating.
- The duration of a single pain "spasm" is less than 2 minutes, although the overall attack may consist of numerous repeating spasms of short duration.
- For several minutes after an attack (the "refractory period"), touching the trigger point usually cannot induce additional attacks.
- The pain must be limited to the known distribution of one or more branches of the trigeminal nerve with no motor deficit in the affected area.
- The pain is dramatically diminished, at least initially, with the use of carbamazepine.
- Spontaneous remissions occur, often lasting more than 6 months, especially during the early phase of the disease.

In the early stages, the pain of trigeminal neuralgia may be rather mild and is often described by the patient as a twinge, dull ache, or burning sensation. This clinical presentation may be erroneously attributed to disorders of the teeth, jaws, and paranasal sinuses and lead to escalation of treatment and a variety of therapeutic misadventures. Many documented cases of idiopathic trigeminal neuralgia are preceded by this dull, continuous, aching type of jaw pain that may persist for days to years without obvious dental pathology before the onset of the characteristic paroxysmal pain in the same region of the face. This has come to be regarded in the literature as *pretrigeminal neuralgia*. Pretrigeminal neuralgia has been reported in approximately 18% of documented trigeminal neuralgia cases. Moreover, pretrigeminal neuralgia has shown a dramatic response to carbamazepine in controlled clinical drug trials.

There are long, asymptomatic refractory periods between painful attacks. With time, the attacks occur at more frequent intervals and the pain becomes increasingly intense. At this point, patients often state that the pain is like "a lightning bolt" or a "hot ice pick jabbed into the face." A distinguishing feature of trigeminal neuralgia is that objective signs of sensory loss cannot be demonstrated on physical examination. The presence of objective facial sensory loss, facial weakness, or ataxia should raise the distinct possibility of a CNS tumor.

Although individual pains or pain spasms last only a few seconds, several attacks may follow each other for up to 30 minutes of rapidly repeating volleys. Patients often clutch at the face and experience spasmodic contractions of the facial muscles during attacks, a feature that long ago led to the use of the term *tic douloureux* (i.e., painful jerking) for this disease. Similar to other neuralgic disorders, a refractory period follows a paroxysm of pain during which time the pain cannot be elicited. This refractory period can be useful, clinically, in distinguishing neuralgic pain from a stimulus-provoked odontogenic pain source. The paroxysmal facial pain is occasionally accompanied by excess lacrimation, conjunctival injection, and intense headache. This presentation may represent the SUNCT (**s**hort-lasting, **u**nilateral, **n**euralgiform headache with **c**onjunctival injection and **t**earing) syndrome rather than trigeminal neuralgia. Other differential considerations include but are not limited to glossopharyngeal neuralgia, Raeder's syndrome, atypical facial pain, and cluster headache. Raeder's syndrome is applied to pain of trigeminal distribution usually in the ophthalmic distribution in association with an ocular sympathetic deficit comprising ptosis, miosis, and an impairment of sweating limited to the medial aspect of the forehead. Because this constellation of clinical findings may have a variety of causes, the recognition of Raeder's syndrome serves only to draw attention to the region of the disturbance and does not imply causation.

When an obvious trigger point is present in trigeminal neuralgia, a pain attack may be brought on by a stimulus to the area as mild as a breeze, a gentle movement, or a feather-light touch. Trigger points are found most frequently on the nasolabial fold, the vermilion border of the lip, or the midfacial and periorbital skin. Intraoral trigger points are uncommon but do occur, especially on the alveolus.

HISTOPATHOLOGIC FEATURES

No unique histopathologic characteristic to the nerves in trigeminal neuralgia exists, although the trigger points may show fibrosis and infiltration by small numbers of chronic inflammatory cells. Focal areas of myelin degeneration have been reported within the gasserian ganglion and along the course of the cranial nerve itself, but these also have been occasionally seen in persons without trigeminal neuralgia. MS patients with trigeminal neuralgia show unique amorphous plaques in the ganglion.

TREATMENT AND PROGNOSIS

There have been rare reports of spontaneous permanent remissions of trigeminal neuralgia. However, more often than not, this disease is characterized by a protean and protracted clinical course with regard to the frequency and severity of exacerbations. The initial treatment for trigeminal neuralgia is medical. Topical capsaicin cream (a nociceptive substance-P suppressor) over the affected skin may be effective. Almost all patients with trigeminal neuralgia respond favorably to the anticonvulsant, carbamazepine, and an unequivocal response to this medication can be used as a diagnostic test for this disease. Anticonvulsant medications (phenytoin, carbamazepine, gabapentin) often are effective in pain control, probably because they decrease conductance in Na+ channels and inhibit ectopic (i.e., arising from abnormal sites) discharges. These drugs, unfortunately, often have severe side effects and may not be tolerated for long by the patient. Moreover, the pain usually returns on discontinuance of the medication. If drug treatment fails, then surgical therapy may be considered.

Various neurosurgical procedures such as microvascular decompression and radiofrequency rhizotomy also are effective in severe or refractory cases, especially in younger patients (Box 18-4). Recent reports have shown some success with gamma knife radiosurgery of the gasserian ganglion and its associated nerves.

Box 18-4

Intracranial Neurosurgical Therapies for Trigeminal Neuralgia

- Injection of caustic material near nerves leaving or entering the gasserian ganglion (glycerol rhizotomy)
- Removal of skull base bony irregularities impinging on trigeminal nerve (decompression)
- Repositioning of blood vessels impinging on trigeminal nerve (microvascular decompression)
- Selective destruction of the sensory fibers of the nerve by crushing or by the application of heat (percutaneous radiofrequency rhizotomy)
- Severing the trigeminal sensory roots (neurectomy)

Neurosurgical methods provide relief for years in the majority of trigeminal neuralgia patients. Repeated surgical procedures often are necessary, however, and techniques that deliberately damage neural tissues leave the patient with a sensory deficit. After surgery, up to 8% of patients develop distorted sensations of the facial skin (**facial dysesthesia**) or a combination of anesthesia and spontaneous pain (**anesthesia dolorosa**). Anesthesia dolorosa is a dreaded form of central pain that can occur after any neurosurgical procedure that causes a variable amount of sensory loss, but this complication occurs more commonly with procedures that totally denervate a region. Overall, long-term success from surgical procedures is 70% to 85%.

GLOSSOPHARYNGEAL NEURALGIA (VAGOGLOSSOPHARYNGEAL NEURALGIA)

Neuralgia of the ninth cranial nerve, **glossopharyngeal neuralgia**, is similar in every way to trigeminal neuralgia (see previous topic) except in the anatomic location of the pain. In glossopharyngeal neuralgia, the pain is centered on the tonsil and the ear. The pain often radiates from the throat to the ear because of the involvement of the tympanic branch of the glossopharyngeal nerve. Some unfortunate individuals have a combination of glossopharyngeal neuralgia and trigeminal neuralgia.

Glossopharyngeal neuralgia is rare, occurring only once for every 100 cases of trigeminal neuralgia. The pain also may affect sensory areas supplied by the pharyngeal and auricular branches of the vagus nerve. As with trigeminal neuralgia, the cause is unknown.

CLINICAL FEATURES

The age of onset for glossopharyngeal neuralgia varies from 15 to 85 years, but the average age is 50 years. There is no sex predilection, and only rarely is there bilateral involvement. The paroxysmal pain may be felt in the ear (**tympanic plexus neuralgia**), infra-auricular area, tonsil, base of the tongue, posterior mandible, or lateral wall of the pharynx; however, the patient often has difficulty localizing the pain in the oropharynx.

The episodic pain in this unilateral neuralgia is sharp, lancinating (jabbing), and extremely intense. Attacks have an abrupt onset and a short duration (30- to 60-second bursts that may repeat for 5 to 30 minutes). The pain typically radiates upward from the oropharynx to the ipsilateral ear. Talking, chewing, swallowing, yawning, or touching a blunt instrument to the tonsil on the affected side may precipitate the pain, but a definite trigger zone is not easily identified. Because the pain is related to jaw movement, it may be difficult to differentiate it from the severe pain of **temporomandibular joint dysfunction** (TMD).

Patients frequently point to the neck immediately below the angle of the mandible as the site of greatest pain, but trigger points are not found on the external skin, except within the ear canal. Rarely, syncope, hypotension, seizures, arrhythmia, or cardiac arrest may accompany the paroxysmal pain, as may coughing or excessive salivation. As with trigeminal neuralgia, idiopathic and secondary forms of glossopharyngeal neuralgia exist. The clinician should be careful to rule out Eagle syndrome (see page 23) and other conditions before applying the glossopharyngeal neuralgia diagnosis. The literature suggests that approximately 25% of cases of glossopharyngeal neuralgia are the result of secondary causes such as neoplasms involving the skull base or aneurysms in the posterior cranial fossa.

TREATMENT AND PROGNOSIS

As in trigeminal neuralgia, glossopharyngeal neuralgia is subject to unpredictable remissions and recurrences. It is not unusual during the early stages for remissions to last 6 months or more. Painful episodes are of varying severity but generally become more severe and more frequent with time.

Approximately 80% of patients experience immediate pain relief when a topical anesthetic agent is applied to the tonsil and pharynx on the side of the pain. Because this relief lasts only 60 to 90 minutes, it is used more as a diagnostic tool and emergency measure than a long-term treatment. Repeated applications to a trigger point for 2 or 3 days may extend the pain-free episode enough to allow the patient to obtain much needed rest and nutrition. Carbamazepine, oxcarbazepine, baclofen, phenytoin, and lamotrigine may relieve the neuralgic pain for a long period, but no therapy is considered to be uniformly effective or even adequate.

Moreover, glossopharyngeal neuralgia is considerably less responsive than trigeminal neuralgia to treatment with anticonvulsant medications. If the patient fails drug therapy, then surgical options should be considered. The preferred neurosurgical treatments are microvascular decompression or surgical sectioning of the glossopharyngeal nerve and the upper two rootlets of the vagus nerve.

POSTHERPETIC NEURALGIA

An acute painful disorder (herpes zoster) (see page 250) and a chronic pain syndrome (postherpetic neuralgia [PHN]) are associated with the varicella-zoster virus (VZV). Herpes zoster, commonly referred to as *shingles,* is characterized by a unilateral vesicular eruption within a dermatome. More often than not, this eruption is accompanied by severe pain. Herpes zoster usually involves the thoracic dermatomes; in 23% of cases, the rash and its associated pain follow a trigeminal distribution. The ophthalmic division of the trigeminal nerve (V1) is affected most frequently. Herpes zoster is caused by the reactivation of the latent VZV that is thought to lie dormant in the gasserian, geniculate, and dorsal root ganglia after chickenpox infection in early life. The onset of acute herpes zoster is frequently preceded by exquisite pain in the affected dermatome. Approximately 48 to 72 hours later, an erythematous maculopapular rash evolves rapidly into vesicular lesions (see discussion of herpes zoster, page 250).

When the trigeminal nerve is involved, the lesions may appear on the face, the eye, and the tongue. **Herpes zoster ophthalmicus** is a debilitating condition that can result in blindness if aggressive antiviral therapy is not promptly instituted. The combination of a herpetic rash in the external auditory canal and a facial palsy secondary to viral invasion of the geniculate ganglion of the sensory branch of the facial nerve is known as **Ramsay Hunt syndrome** (see page 252). Often these patients lose their taste discrimination in the anterior two thirds of the tongue before the development of the ipsilateral facial palsy.

CLINICAL FEATURES

The most significant complication of herpes zoster is the pain that is associated with acute neuritis and PHN. PHN is defined as pain persisting for anywhere from 1 to 6 months or more after the onset of the rash. Postherpetic pain is described as a burning sensation with episodic "stabbing" pains. Light touch over the previously involved area may elicit a painful response (**tac-tile allodynia**) from the patient. Changes in sensation within the affected area may result in hypoesthesia or hyperesthesia.

The pain of PHN should not be confused with "shocklike" pain of trigeminal neuralgia that can be triggered by similar stimuli. The pain is constant and described as "burning and aching." The burning character of the pain is thought to be the result of spontaneous activity in nociceptor C fibers. The VZV damages the peripheral nerve by a combination of demyelination, wallerian degeneration, fibrosis, and sclerosis. The pain associated with PHN is thought to arise from a disturbed pattern of afferent impulses combined with the loss of some central inhibitory influence in the pain modulatory systems. The mechanism of the pain in PHN is characteristic of deafferentation pain. Pathologically, degenerative lesions are observed in the axons, the dorsal root ganglion, and the dorsal horn of the spinal cord.

Age appears to be the major risk factor associated with the development of PHN. Approximately 50% of patients over the age of 50 with herpes zoster report some pain in the affected dermatome after the resolution of the cutaneous presentation, and 75% of patients older than 70 years of age are afflicted. Severe pain in the acute phase of the disease (acute neuritis) combined with advanced age appears to make the patient more prone to the development of PHN. Another susceptible group consists of those patients with diseases that compromise immunity.

Clinically, scarring and pigmentary changes are observed within the affected dermatome. The pain is usually accompanied by a sensory deficit. Researchers have found lowered sensory thresholds for cold, warmth, vibration, and two-point discrimination in patients whose rash was followed by neuralgia pain. In one recent study, allodynia (i.e., pain in response to a nonnoxious stimulus) was present in 85% of patients with PHN.

TREATMENT AND PROGNOSIS

As with most diseases, the best treatment option is prevention. Many argue that the administration of antiviral medication (most notably famciclovir) or corticosteroids, either alone or in combination, early in the course of herpes zoster possibly could prevent the development of PHN. Patients with acute herpes zoster benefit from the administration of oral antivirals. Accelerated healing of the lesions and an attenuation of zoster-associated pain have both been reported in placebo-controlled clinical drug trials. Further research is necessary to determine the most predictable way of preventing PHN.

Once PHN has established itself, a variety of treatment options are available for pain management. In addition to the judicious use of analgesics, including both nonnarcotic and narcotic preparations, a wide variety of drugs ranging from gabapentin, pregabalin, and amitriptyline hydrochloride to topical agents, such as lidocaine patches, EMLA (eutectic mixture of lidocaine and prilocaine), and capsaicin (0.025%), have been reported to be beneficial in pain relief. The topical application of capsaicin, an extract of hot chili peppers, has been reported to deplete the neurotransmitter substance P from nerve terminals, thereby desensitizing them.

Tricyclic antidepressants such as amitriptyline, nortriptyline, and desiprimine have proven to be quite useful in the management of the persistent pain that characterizes PHN; however, the anticholinergic and cardiovascular side effects may limit their utility, especially in older patients. Amitriptyline has consistently proven to be the single most effective drug, with approximately 60% of patients reporting relief with this agent. Patients are started at a low dose (10 mg) and titrated to effect, with the majority of patients obtaining significant relief with a median dose of 75 mg daily. These medications are usually given at bedtime to prevent daytime somnolence and to improve tolerance. Patients who report a stabbing pain in addition to the burning sensation may derive additional benefit from the use of anticonvulsant medications such as carbamazepine or phenytoin. In recent studies, gabapentin and pregabalin have been shown to reduce pain associated with PHN by more than 30%, and these drugs are typically well tolerated in all patient cohorts.

Patients who fail medical therapy have a limited range of surgical treatments available to them. However, the outcome of procedures (e.g., blockade of peripheral nerves, roots, or sympathetic nervous system; surgery at the level of the affected nerve [neurectomy] or dorsal root) is far from certain with regard to pain management.

ATYPICAL FACIAL PAIN (ATYPICAL FACIAL NEURALGIA; IDIOPATHIC FACIAL PAIN; ATYPICAL TRIGEMINAL NEURALGIA; TRIGEMINAL NEUROPATHIC PAIN)

The International Headache Society (IHS) defines **atypical facial pain** as "persistent facial pain that does not have the characteristics of the cranial neuralgias classified above and is not associated with physical signs or a demonstrable organic cause." In short, atypical facial pain is defined less in terms of *what it is* but rather in terms of *what it is not*. In other words, it is

---

> **Box 18-5**
>
> ### Diseases That Must Be Ruled Out Before Making a Diagnosis of Atypical Facial Pain
>
> - Allergy of sinuses
> - Cracked tooth syndrome
> - Headache with referred pain to face
> - Impingement of bone or blood vessel on nerve
> - Infection: dental, periodontal, sinuses, ear
> - Ischemic and inflammatory marrow disease
> - Myofascial pain
> - Neuralgias, other
> - Temporomandibular joint disorder (TMD)
> - Trauma to nerve (including traumatic neuroma)
> - Tumors

---

a diagnosis of exclusion, and its use by the clinician implies that all potential causes of pain have been ruled out (Box 18-5). Although not the most common facial pain, this condition is the facial disease that most often brings a patient to a pain clinic. No acceptable population studies are available.

Atypical facial pain is such a difficult diagnostic and therapeutic condition that patients travel from one health professional to another and receive many different diagnoses and treatments in a frustrated attempt to find relief. Patients are often described as being neurotic ("hysterical") and suffering from hypochondriasis, obsessive-compulsive disorder, anxiety disorder, depression, somatization disorder, or a "lack of insight." Whether this is true or not, the strong emotional overtones of this condition make it difficult to distinguish functional (psychogenic) from organic (physiologic) pain.

CLINICAL FEATURES

Atypical facial pain affects women far more frequently than men. It usually develops during the fourth through sixth decades of life, but can occur as early as the teenage years. The pain may be localized to a small area of the face or alveolus (e.g., atypical odontalgia, "phantom" toothache) but more frequently affects most of a quadrant and may extend to the temple, neck, or occipital area. Patients have great difficulty describing the pain, but most often portray it as a continuous, deep, diffuse, gnawing ache; an intense burning sensation; a pressure; or a sharp pain. The patient may nominally describe the pain using such terms as "drawing, aching, or pulling." It is important to differentiate the pain from that of trigeminal neuralgia (see page 861).

Bilateral involvement occasionally occurs, and patients frequently attribute the onset of the pain to trauma or a dental procedure. The mucosa of the affected quadrant appears normal but typically contains a zone of increased temperature, tenderness, or bone marrow activity ("hot spot" on technetium-99m methylene diphosphonate [MDP] bone scan). Radiographic changes are not present. In some cases initially diagnosed as atypical facial pain, significant underlying disease has ultimately been identified (e.g., nasopharyngeal carcinoma, occult lung tumors).

TREATMENT AND PROGNOSIS

Occasional cases of spontaneous remission are noted, but the great majority of atypical facial pain patients will obtain little relief without therapy. Symptoms tend to become more intense gradually, and patients become irritable, fatigued, and depressed. Most patients are not benefited substantially from the drugs used for trigeminal neuralgia, although the new anticonvulsant, gabapentin, dramatically reduces the pain in one third of affected patients. Opioid analgesics (codeine, fentanyl, hydrocodone, morphine, and oxycodone) may be of considerable benefit, but their effectiveness characteristically diminishes over time and, of course, they are associated with the risk of abuse and addiction.

The tricyclic antidepressants (amitriptyline, nortriptyline) are popular therapies for neuropathic pain. They appear to block reuptake of norepinephrine and serotonin, transmitters released by pain-modulating systems in the spinal cord and brain stem, thereby allowing long periods of diminished neural activity. Other antidepressants (e.g., the selective serotonin reuptake inhibitors, paroxetine and citalopram) are generally not as effective as the tricyclic antidepressants for managing atypical facial pain, although some patients may respond to this therapy. It is important to remember, however, that antidepressant medications may be quite hazardous to frail older adults or to patients with coronary disease. When a localized area (usually alveolar) of tenderness can be found in the quadrant of pain, the application of topical capsaicin or injection with local anesthetics may be temporarily beneficial. Psychotherapy, behavior modification, transcutaneous electric nerve stimulation, and sympathetic nerve blocks are helpful in a subset of patients with atypical facial pain.

The frequent failure of medical treatment for atypical facial pain may lead to surgical intervention, usually the removal of a portion of the affected trigeminal nerve branch or the injection of a caustic solution

(phenol, glycerol, alcohol) into the nerve, designed to destroy a portion of the nerve. These therapies often provide relief for several weeks or months, but there is seldom a permanent cure.

NEURALGIA-INDUCING CAVITATIONAL OSTEONECROSIS (NICO; ALVEOLAR CAVITATIONAL OSTEOPATHOSIS; ISCHEMIC OSTEONECROSIS; BONE MARROW EDEMA)

One of the most controversial topics in the diagnosis and management of orofacial pain is the entity referred to as **neuralgia-inducing cavitational osteonecrosis** (NICO). Since this concept first appeared in the scientific literature in the late 1970s, there have been numerous attempts by science-based investigators to define the clinical and radiographic features, as well as the histopathology and neuropathology of these lesions. However, to date, there is no consensus among pain practitioners regarding this entity. The following information is presented in the context of completeness with regard to orofacial pain and to facial neuralgias in particular.

Ischemic osteonecrosis is a bone disease characterized by degeneration and death of marrow and bone from a slow or abrupt decrease in marrow blood flow. Along with its lesser variants, bone marrow edema and regional ischemic osteoporosis, it is one of the most common bone diseases in humans, but only recently has it been appreciated as a disorder of the head and neck region. Numerous local and systemic factors are associated with ischemic damage to marrow (Box 18-6), the most common being a hereditary (autosomal dominant) tendency toward blood clot formation within blood vessels. Bone is particularly susceptible to this problem, which in the jaws may be accentuated by dental infections and the vasoconstrictors in local anesthetics.

The ischemia and infarctions of osteonecrosis are typically associated with pain, often with an ill-defined neuralgic or neuropathic character. Because of this, presumed examples of this process in the jaws have been referred to as NICO. NICO is included in this chapter because of its strong association with pain, but it should be remembered that osteonecrosis is not necessarily a painful condition and our understanding of this disease is still incomplete.

Ischemic osteonecrosis most often affects the hips, maxillofacial bones, and knees. NICO has been found in 1 of every 11,000 adults, a prevalence rate similar to that of hip cases. The NICO prevalence rate for women (1 per 2000) is much higher than the rate for men (1 per 20,000).

BOX 18-6

Diseases and Phenomena Associated with Ischemic Osteonecrosis

COMMONLY ASSOCIATED

- Coagulation disorders (thrombophilia, hypofibrinolysis)
- Alcohol abuse
- Trauma
- Prednisone, prednisolone
- Estrogen, pregnancy
- Sickle cell disease
- Lupus erythematosus
- Cancer chemotherapy (including prednisone)

LESS COMMONLY ASSOCIATED

- Tobacco use
- Arteriosclerosis
- Deep-sea diving ("bends")
- Shwartzman reaction (serum sickness)

RARELY ASSOCIATED

- Osteomyelitis
- Starvation (anorexia nervosa)

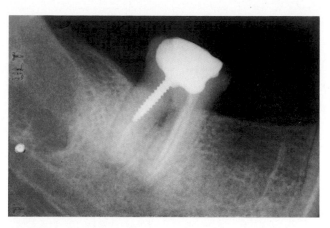

Fig. 18-2 Neuralgia-inducing cavitational osteonecrosis (NICO). Periapical radiograph demonstrates an oval radiolucency in the third molar region and thin lamina dura remnants (residual socket) more anteriorly.

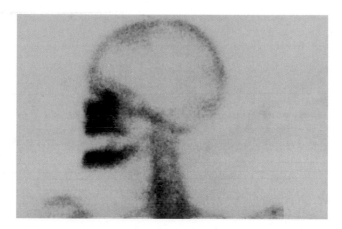

Fig. 18-3 Neuralgia-inducing cavitational osteonecrosis (NICO). Technetium-99m bone scan reveals multifocal and extensive NICO involvement (hot spots) years after extraction of the entire dentition for "atypical facial pain." None of the sites were visualized by radiographs, magnetic resonance imaging (MRI), computed tomography (CT) scans, or other forms of radioisotope bone scans.

CLINICAL AND RADIOGRAPHIC FEATURES

NICO characteristically affects women 35 to 60 years of age but has been diagnosed in men and in teenagers. Third molar regions are affected in half of all cases, but any alveolar site may become involved, as may the walls of the sinuses and the mandibular condyle. At least one third of patients have more than one maxillofacial site of involvement, and 10% have lesions in all four alveolar quadrants.

Patients often have trouble describing and localizing their pain, which can be intermittent or constant, deep or superficial, aching or sharp, mild or extremely intense. Most often the pain is described as a deep ache or sharp bone pain. It typically begins as quite mild and vague, increasing slowly in frequency and intensity over months and years, but may also have a sudden onset, especially after a dental procedure using vasoconstrictors in the anesthetic. The pain may roam in the general anatomic area or be referred some distance from the affected bone (neck, shoulder). Many describe pressure and deep burning sensations, and local anesthesia typically relieves the pain.

Osteonecrosis is not visualized readily on radiographs, but when visible it usually appears as an area of regional osteoporosis or ill-defined radiolucency, often with irregular vertical remnants of lamina dura representing old extraction sites (Fig. 18-2). Occasional lesions show an admixture of irregular sclerotic and radiolucent areas (ischemic osteosclerosis), or there may be a faint central sclerotic oval surrounded by a thick radiolucent circle that is, in turn, surrounded by a thick but faint sclerotic ring **(bull's-eye lesion)**. More than 60% of the lesions will exhibit a hot spot of increased isotope uptake with the technetium-99m MDP bone scan (Fig. 18-3).

HISTOPATHOLOGIC FEATURES

The microscopic appearance of ischemic osteonecrosis depends on the duration and intensity of the diminished marrow blood flow. The features of bone

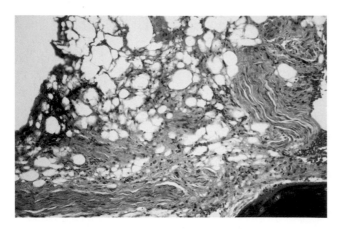

Fig. 18-4 Neuralgia-inducing cavitational osteonecrosis (NICO). Photomicrograph showing ischemic myelofibrosis with a sprinkling of chronic inflammatory cells and serous ooze.

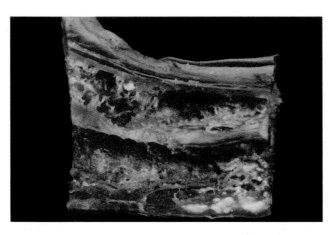

Fig. 18-5 Neuralgia-inducing cavitational osteonecrosis (NICO). Gross photo of section of posterior mandible showing extensive cavitation that has hollowed out most of the bone. *(From Bouquot JE, McMahon RE: Neuropathic pain in maxillofacial osteonecrosis, J Oral Maxillofacial Surg 58:1003-1020, 2000.)*

marrow edema include dilated marrow capillaries and sinusoids, serous ooze **(plasmostasis)** around blood vessels and adipocytes, wispy fibrous streaming **(ischemic myelofibrosis)** between fat cells, areas of dense fibrosis **(intramedullary fibrous scar)**, and a light sprinkling of chronic inflammatory cells in regions of myelofibrosis (Fig. 18-4). Bony trabeculae usually remain viable at this stage but are inactive, thin, and often widely spaced.

Degenerative extracellular cystic spaces **(cavitations)** are commonly seen and may dominate the picture, eventually coalescing to form spaces large enough to extend from cortex to cortex (Fig. 18-5). Focal areas of marrow hemorrhage **(microinfarction)** are frequently present and considered by some to be pathognomonic for osteonecrosis.

Bubbles of coalesced, liquefied fat (oil cysts) may be seen. However, because high-speed rotary instruments can produce similar bubbles as an artifact, it is important that only hand-curetted marrow samples be submitted for histopathologic evaluation.

Bone death, when present, is represented by focal loss of osteocytes. However, this feature can be evaluated properly only if formic acid or another very weak acid is used for slow, gentle laboratory decalcification. In addition, smudged, globular, often dark masses of **calcific necrotic detritus** may be seen. These represent destroyed trabeculae that have literally dissolved over time and contributed their calcium to other salts precipitated within necrotic fat. The heat of high-speed rotary instrumentation can create similar calcific debris, but this debris remains at the edges of tissue fragments.

TREATMENT AND PROGNOSIS

Antibiotics may temporarily diminish the associated pain of NICO in those cases with a superimposed low-grade infection (chronic nonsuppurative osteomyelitis), but the pain typically returns when antibiotics are stopped. Usually the diseased marrow must be removed surgically by decortication and curettage. Once removed, the defect frequently heals and the intense facial pain subsides dramatically or disappears completely, although pain abatement may take several months to occur. Unfortunately, one third of patients thus treated experience no pain relief. In addition, the disease has a strong tendency to recur or to develop in additional jawbone sites. A repetition of the surgical procedure is, therefore, often necessary. Overall, the cure rate (free of pain for at least 5 years) for curettage is better than 70%.

CLUSTER HEADACHE (MIGRAINOUS NEURALGIA; SPHENOPALATINE NEURALGIA; HISTAMINIC CEPHALGIA; HORTON'S SYNDROME)

Cluster headache is an exquisitely painful affliction of the midface and upper face, particularly in and around the eye. The name is derived from the fact that the headache attacks occur in temporal groups or clusters, with extended periods of remission between attacks. Cluster headache is an uncommon disease of unknown origin and has been called "the most severe pain syndrome known to humans." A vascular (vasodilation) cause has been suggested, possibly related to abnormal hypothalamic function, head trauma, or abnormal release of histamine from mast cells. The majority of patients suffer from sleep apnea and diminished oxygen saturation, but it is not known whether this is a cause or effect of the disease. Headache can be initiated by alcohol, cocaine, and nitroglycerin; 80% of affected persons are cigarette smokers.

This disorder is diagnosed in 10 of every 100,000 persons each year, and there is a predilection for blacks. There is also a strong familial influence: when a first-degree relative has the headache, there is a fiftyfold increase in the chance that another family member also will be affected.

CLINICAL FEATURES

Cluster headache may occur at any age, although it usually affects persons in the third and fourth decades of life and is rare before puberty. There is a strong male predilection (a 6:1 male-to-female ratio). The pain is almost always unilateral and follows the distribution of the ophthalmic division of the trigeminal nerve.

It is usually felt deep within or behind the orbit, radiating to the temporal and upper cheek regions. However, it may simulate a toothache or neuralgic jaw pain in the anterior maxillary region. Because of this, patients may be treated inappropriately for dental pain with endodontic therapy or tooth extraction, which is thought to be successful when the pain subsequently resolves. When each successive cluster returns, the next tooth is treated, sometimes resulting in multiple, repeated episodes of unnecessary dental therapy.

The pain is described as paroxysmal (i.e., abrupt onset) and intense, with a burning or lancinating quality and without a trigger zone. The attacks may last from 15 minutes to 3 hours and occur up to eight times daily (or on alternate days). The cluster periods typically last for weeks, with the intervening periods of remission usually lasting for months (sometimes years). The pain often begins at the same time in a given 24-hour period **(alarm clock headache)**, with most attacks occurring in the middle of the night.

A chronic form occurs occasionally, with no remissions for years at a time, and episodic forms may convert to the constant, chronic form. In addition, cluster headache is rarely accompanied by the aura so common to migraine headache. An important behavioral difference between migraine and cluster headache is that the patient is usually hyperactive during the latter and retreats to a dark, quiet room during the former.

In addition to the pain, the patient may experience autonomic alterations such as nasal stuffiness, tearing, facial flush, or congestion of conjunctival blood vessels. The latter sign, especially when associated with increased intraocular pressure, may indicate chronic paroxysmal hemicrania (Sjaastad syndrome), a rare syndrome with short-duration, highly recurring, non-clustered pain (see following topic).

TREATMENT AND PROGNOSIS

The proper diagnosis is important to avoid sequential, unnecessary endodontic or extraction procedures. Systemic prednisone, ergotamine, lithium carbonate, indomethacin, methysergide maleate, and verapamil all provide relief in some cases. Sumatriptan (agonistic to 5-HTID receptors) and other drugs of this class shorten the symptoms in 74% of cases. However, no single drug is universally effective. Inhaling oxygen may abort impending attacks, and various neurosurgical interventions to the affected nerve have provided relief in some patients, as has the recently reported use of gamma knife radiosurgery. Overall, only 50% of patients with cluster headache benefit significantly and permanently from the available therapeutic modalities.

It is important to distinguish cluster headache from chronic paroxysmal hemicrania because the latter disease responds almost universally to indomethacin.

PAROXYSMAL HEMICRANIA

Paroxysmal hemicrania has a clinical presentation similar to cluster headache. The headaches are strictly unilateral, brief, and excruciating and have associated autonomic features. Paroxysmal hemicrania can be differentiated from cluster headache primarily by the high frequency but shorter duration of the attacks. Although the differentiation can be subtle, it is worth pursuing because paroxysmal hemicrania responds dramatically and predictably to indomethacin. Therefore, an "indomethacin challenge" can be used to rule out other trigeminal autonomic cephalgias. A predictable response to indomethacin is also observed in **hemicrania continua**, a type of chronic daily headache that is unilateral, moderately severe, and associated with autonomic signs similar to those of cluster headache.

CLINICAL FEATURES

In contradistinction to cluster headache, paroxysmal hemicrania is more common in women by a ratio of 2:1. The headache is for the most part strictly unilateral, and the pain is centered on the ocular, maxillary, temporal, and frontal regions. The symptoms typically last from 2 to 30 minutes, and the pain is described as a "boring" sensation that can be excruciating in terms of severity. The headache has an abrupt onset and an equally abrupt cessation. Ipsilateral cranial autonomic features such as lacrimation, conjunctival injection, and rhinorrhea also invariably occur. The patient may experience anywhere from 2 to 40 attacks daily, and the mean attack frequency is 14 per day. The headaches occur regularly throughout the 24-hour day and do not demonstrate a preponderance of nocturnal attacks as is commonly observed in cluster headache. About half of these patients desire reductions in stimuli similar to the preference demonstrated by those with migraines; the remaining 50% prefer hyperactivity during the attack similar to the response preference of individuals with cluster headache.

TREATMENT AND PROGNOSIS

Indomethacin is the treatment of choice for paroxysmal hemicrania. Effective resolution of the headache is prompt, typically occurring within 1 to 2 days of initiating the effective dose. The therapeutic trial of oral indomethacin should be initiated at 25 mg three times daily for 10 days. If the response is suboptimal, then the dosage should be increased to 50 mg three times daily for an additional 10 days. If there is a suspicion that the optimal dose has not been achieved, the dosage can be increased further to 75 mg three times daily for an additional 14 days. The typical maintenance dose is between 25 mg and 100 mg daily, but higher doses can be tolerated relatively well. A "drug holiday" should be attempted at least once every 6 months because long-lasting remissions have been reported in some patients after cessation of indomethacin. Long-term treatment with indomethacin may result in the gastrointestinal side effects common to this class of drugs. These side effects can be effectively managed with antacids, histamine H_2-receptor antagonists, or proton pump inhibitors. In patients who fail to demonstrate a predictable response to indomethacin, the diagnosis of paroxysmal hemicrania should be reconsidered.

MIGRAINE (MIGRAINE SYNDROME; MIGRAINE HEADACHE)

Migraine is a common, disabling, paroxysmal, unilateral headache that is experienced at least once by more than 14% of teenagers and young adults (lifetime risk: 21%). More than 400 new cases are diagnosed each year for every 100,000 persons. At least 14 different types of migraine exist; they are broadly classified into two groups: (1) **migraine with aura** and (2) **migraine without aura**.

The cause of migraine is still unclear, but it appears to be related to vasoconstriction or vasospasm of portions of the cerebral arteries, possibly in response to a chronically reduced activity of serotonin (5-hydroxytryptamine, 5-HT$_1$). The vasoconstriction apparently leads to cerebral ischemia, which is followed by a compensating vasodilation (mediated by nitric oxide), with subsequent pain and cerebral edema. Many affected persons (migraineurs) have a family history of migraine,

Table **18-1** **Common Triggers for Migraine Headache**

Type of Trigger	Subtypes
Hormonal	Menstruation
	Ovulation
	Oral contraceptives
	Hormonal replacement therapy
Dietary	Alcohol
	Nitrite-laden meat
	Monosodium glutamate
	Aspartame
	Chocolate
	Aged cheese
	Missing a meal
Psychologic	Stress/poststress
	Anxiety/worry
	Depression
Physical/environmental	Glare
	Flashing lights
	Fluorescent lights
	Odors
	Weather changes
	High altitude
Sleep related	Lack of sleep
	Excessive sleep
Drugs	Nitroglycerine
	Histamine
	Reserpine
	Hydralazine
	Ranitidine
	Estrogen
Miscellaneous	Head trauma
	Physical exertion
	Fatigue

From Campbell JK, Sakai F: Diagnosis and differential diagnosis. In Olesen J, Tfelt-Hansen P, Welch KMA: *The headaches*, ed 2, Philadelphia, 2000, Lippincott, Williams & Wilkins.

sometimes with a clear autosomal dominant inheritance pattern. Migraine headaches are often associated with endogenous or environmental triggers. Common triggering events are listed in Table 18-1.

CLINICAL FEATURES

Migraine affects women three times more frequently than men, and women tend to experience more severe attacks than men. The disease is most prevalent in the third through fifth decades of life, but the first symptoms often begin at puberty or shortly thereafter.

The unilateral headache lasts for 4 to 72 hours and is usually felt in the temporal, frontal, and orbital regions, as well as occasionally in the parietal, postauricular, or occipital areas. It begins as a poorly localized discomfort in the head that soon becomes a mild ache and then increases in severity over the next 30 minutes to 2 hours. At its peak, the pain has a throbbing quality, is quite severe, and is typically associated with nausea, vomiting, diarrhea, photophobia, and phonophobia. Usually, the pain is so severe as to be incapacitating, and the patient must lie down in a dark, quiet room. The headache recurs frequently, although the time between attacks varies widely. Rarely, bilateral examples occur.

It is important for the dentist to remember that referred migraine pain may initially mimic a toothache, especially of the anterior maxilla. Symptoms may also mimic sinusitis or allergic rhinitis.

Many migraineurs experience an "aura" before the actual headache pain. The aura may appear as visual hallucination, "seeing sparks" (**scintillation**), temporary and partial blindness, partial or complete loss of light perception (**scotoma**), nausea, vertigo, lethargy, mental confusion, loss of the ability to express thoughts (**aphasia**), or unilateral facial paresthesia or weakness.

TREATMENT AND PROGNOSIS

Nonpharmacologic approaches to the management of migraine involve the recognition and avoidance of known environmental triggers, as well as volitional modulation of the stress response (cognitive behavioral therapy). The pharmacologic treatment of migraine includes a wide variety of medications, and the two basic forms, with and without aura, respond in a similar fashion. The drugs that have shown the greatest efficacy in the treatment of migraine are members of the following three pharmacologic classes: (1) antiinflammatory agents, (2) 5-HT$_1$ agonists, and (3) dopamine antagonists. The optimal treatment regimen for a migraine attack depends primarily on the severity of the attack and must be individualized for each patient. Severe attacks frequently are diminished by ergotamine tartrate, perhaps combined with caffeine, aspirin, acetaminophen, phenobarbital, or belladonna. The drugs known as *triptans* are selective 5-HT$_1$ receptor agonists, and a variety of these medications are now available for the treatment of acute migraine attacks. Less severe but more frequent attacks are best treated prophylactically using other ergot compounds (e.g., methergine), β-adrenergic agents (e.g., propranolol, metoprolol), calcium channel blockers (e.g., nifedipine, diltiazem), or serotonin receptor agonists (e.g., methysergide, cyproheptadine). Some patients are aided by simple pressure on the ipsilateral carotid artery. The headaches tend to become less severe and less frequent over time, with or without effective therapy.

TEMPORAL ARTERITIS (GIANT CELL ARTERITIS; CRANIAL ARTERITIS)

Temporal arteritis is a multifocal vasculitis of cranial arteries, especially the superficial temporal artery. Its cause remains unknown, but autoimmunity to the elastic lamina of the artery has been proposed. The disease most often affects head and neck vessels, but it is considered to be a systemic problem. There may be a genetic predisposition.

The annual incidence rate of temporal arteritis in the United States is approximately 6 per 100,000 population. Incidence rises with age and has been increasing over time, perhaps because the population is aging. There is a strong predilection for whites.

CLINICAL FEATURES

Women are affected by temporal arteritis somewhat more often than men, and patients are usually older than 50 years of age at the time of diagnosis (average age, 70 years). The disease is most frequently a unilateral, throbbing headache that is gradually replaced by an intense, aching, burning temporal and facial pain. The throbbing frequently coincides with the patient's heartbeat (systole), and the pain may be lancinating. The superficial temporal artery is exquisitely sensitive to palpation and eventually appears erythematous, swollen, tortuous, or rarely ulcerated.

Most patients complain of pain during mastication (jaw claudication) or with the wearing of hats (pressure over the artery). The pain occasionally mimics toothache or a neuralgic jaw or tongue pain. Significantly, ocular symptoms, such as loss of vision or retro-orbital pain, may be the first complaint. Prompt recognition of signs and symptoms of temporal arteritis is important because it is a preventable cause of blindness. The blindness is caused by involvement of the posterior ciliary artery supplying the optic disc, which results in ischemic papillopathy. The visual loss may be transient or permanent, unilateral or bilateral.

Fever, malaise, fatigue, nausea, anorexia, vomiting, sore throat, and earache often occur, perhaps as prodromal symptoms, and the erythrocyte sedimentation rate is usually elevated. A generalized muscle aching and stiffness (**polymyalgia rheumatica**) frequently follow an acute attack. Because muscle and joint aches are quite common in older adults, the potential exists for missed opportunities in the diagnosis and management of temporal arteritis.

HISTOPATHOLOGIC FEATURES

Biopsy confirms the diagnosis of temporal arteritis. Microscopic changes tend to be segmental and can be missed if the specimen is too small. At least 1 cm of the affected vessel must, therefore, be examined for proper evaluation.

The disease is characterized by chronic inflammation of the tunica intima and tunica media of the involved artery, with narrowing of the lumen from edema and proliferation of the tunica intima. Necrosis of the smooth muscle and elastic lamina is frequent. A variable number of foreign body–type multinucleated giant cells are mixed with macrophages, plasma cells, and lymphocytes. Thrombosis or complete occlusion of the lumen is not unusual.

TREATMENT AND PROGNOSIS

Temporal arteritis responds well to systemic and local corticosteroids; the symptoms subside within a few days. However, many cases are chronic and need treatment for years. In addition, permanent loss of vision occurs in more than 50% of untreated patients (and even in the occasional patient refractory to treatment). With some individuals, vascular involvement is so widespread throughout the body that the disease is fatal, even with aggressive corticosteroid therapy.

MYASTHENIA GRAVIS

Myasthenia gravis is an autoimmune disease that affects the acetylcholine receptors (AChR) of muscle fibers and results in an abnormal and progressive fatigability of skeletal muscle. Defective neuromuscular transmission occurs, probably secondary to the coating of the AChRs by circulating antibodies to those receptors. Such antibodies are not normally found in humans; hence, the measurement of serum AChR antibody levels is an important diagnostic tool for this disease. The motor end plate itself is normal, and smooth and cardiac muscles are not affected.

Many patients demonstrate either thymus hyperplasia or an actual neoplasm (thymoma) of the thymus gland. Conversely, 75% of patients with thymoma have myasthenia gravis, and 90% have circulating AChR antibodies. The infant of an affected mother may be affected for several weeks or months by maternal antibodies that traverse the placenta. Almost half of the patients with myasthenia gravis have at least one additional autoimmune disorder, especially of the thyroid gland. Each year 1 person in every 100,000 is diagnosed with myasthenia gravis.

CLINICAL FEATURES

Myasthenia gravis is more common in females (1:2 male-to-female ratio). It can begin at any age, and congenital cases have been reported. The disease appears

Box 18-7

Head and Neck Manifestations of Myasthenia Gravis

- Inability to focus the eyes (extraocular muscular paresis)
- Drooping eyelids (ptosis)
- Double vision (diplopia)
- Difficulty in chewing
- Difficulty in swallowing (dysphagia)
- Slurring of words (dysarthria)

as a subtle but progressive muscle weakness that is most frequently noticed first in the small muscles of the head and neck (Box 18-7).

Repeated muscle contractions, in particular, lead to progressively less power in the contracting muscle; hence, affected patients usually become weaker as the day progresses. The muscles of mastication may become so weak from eating a single meal that the jaws literally "hang open." Bite force is especially weak when circulating AChR antibody titers are high. Lateral tongue forces exerted during swallowing, speech, and mastication, are reduced significantly in a number of patients.

DIAGNOSIS

The diagnosis of myasthenia gravis is based on the clinical symptoms, an elevated serum AChR antibody level, and improved strength after intravenous (IV) injection of edrophonium, a cholinesterase inhibitor. Degenerated muscle fibers are the only characteristic histopathologic feature, with fibers appearing much smaller than normal (hypotrophy, atrophy), having fewer nuclei, and showing a loss of the normal rounded cross-sectional appearance.

TREATMENT AND PROGNOSIS

The prognosis for myasthenia gravis is usually good. Spontaneous remission sometimes occurs, and approximately 10% of patients never have more than weak eye muscles. Unfortunately, more severe cases often progress, after months or years, to permanent muscular weakness and wasting of the neck, limbs, and trunk. Respiratory paralysis is sometimes a fatal complication.

The defective neuromuscular transmission can be reversed partially by cholinesterase inhibitors (e.g., edrophonium, neostigmine), often in combination with intermittent corticosteroid therapy. For patients with evidence of thymoma or with elevated AChR antibody titers, thymectomy is recommended. Complete, permanent recovery often results from thymectomy and, to a lesser extent, from medical therapy.

MOTOR NEURON DISEASE (PROGRESSIVE MUSCULAR ATROPHY; PROGRESSIVE BULBAR PALSY; AMYOTROPHIC LATERAL SCLEROSIS)

First described by Charcot in the 1870s, **motor neuron disease** is a fatal neurodegenerative disorder that is characterized by progressive weakness and wasting of muscles. The basic defect is progressive degeneration and death of the motor neurons of the cranial nerves, the anterior horn of the spinal cord, and the pyramidal tract.

There are three distinct clinical syndromes with considerable overlapping of signs and symptoms:

1. Progressive muscular atrophy
2. Progressive bulbar palsy
3. Amyotrophic lateral sclerosis (ALS)

Confusion exists over the appropriate terminology, because some authors have used ALS to include all three disease syndromes. Including all subtypes, new cases of motor neuron disease are diagnosed in 15 of every 100,000 persons each year.

Many cases appear to be genetic defects associated with mRNA processing. Progressive muscular atrophy is, for example, the most common autosomal recessive disorder (mutated *SMN* gene on chromosome 5q) lethal to infants; it now can be identified with a prenatal test for the involved gene. Likewise, up to 10% of cases of ALS are inherited as an autosomal dominant trait (mutated superoxide dismutase-1 gene on chromosome 21). Proposed causes for the nonhereditary cases include toxic accumulation of the neurotransmitter glutamate, trauma, and slow viruses, especially the poliovirus.

CLINICAL FEATURES

Progressive muscular atrophy occurs in childhood. Most cases occur at birth or within the first few months of life, although adult onset is rarely seen. Males and females are affected equally. There is progressive limb weakness and sensory disturbances, which result in difficulty in walking, leg pain, paresthesia, and atrophy of the feet and hands. Facial muscles are spared.

Progressive bulbar palsy typically affects children and young adults and has no gender predilection. It usually begins with a subtle but progressive difficulty in speaking or swallowing (**dysphagia**). Attempts to swallow food produce bouts of choking and regurgitation, with liquids frequently thrown into the naso-

pharynx and nasal sinuses because of palatal paralysis. Chronic hoarseness may develop. Atrophy of the facial muscles, tongue, and soft palate eventually occurs, as do weakness and spasticity of the limbs. There are no altered sensory perceptions.

ALS (commonly called *Lou Gehrig disease*, named after the professional baseball player who died of the disease) affects males more frequently than females and begins to manifest itself in middle age (the average age of onset is 59 years). The disease begins with difficulty in walking because of bilateral, generalized leg stiffness. Occasionally, one leg is affected more than the other, forcing the patient to drag it behind the other. Swallowing difficulty develops early in 29% of cases.

The physical examination in ALS reveals spastic quadriparesis, often with a remarkable increase in the tendon reflexes of all four limbs and with extensor plantar responses. Small, synchronous, subcutaneous muscle contractions (**fasciculation**) of the shoulders and thighs are an early symptom, with muscle atrophy eventually developing at affected sites. Central reflexes, such as those of the abdomen, are not altered until late in the disease, and there are no changes in sense perception. Dysfunction of the muscles controlled by the medulla oblongata (**bulbar paralysis**) appears late in the disease, predominantly as spasticity and weakness. Patients become completely disabled, often requiring respiratory support and gastrostomy.

TREATMENT AND PROGNOSIS

Although each of these conditions may have temporary remissions, the course of motor neuron disease is invariably fatal. Progressive muscular atrophy and progressive bulbar palsy almost always result in death within 2 years, usually from respiratory distress caused by weak intercostal muscles.

ALS usually results in death within 5 years of diagnosis, most often from respiratory failure or cachexia, although 20% of patients survive more than 10 years without ventilator use. The antiglutamate agent, riluzole, has shown some promise in slowing the progression of ALS and improving the morbidity in patients with disease of bulbar onset, but in general there is no cure at this time. Palliative and rehabilitative strategies are used to ease suffering.

BURNING MOUTH SYNDROME (STOMATOPYROSIS; STOMATODYNIA; GLOSSOPYROSIS; GLOSSODYNIA; BURNING TONGUE SYNDROME)

Burning mouth syndrome is a common dysesthesia (i.e., distortion of a sense) typically described by the patient as a burning sensation of the oral mucosa in the

Box 18-8

Local and Systemic Factors Reportedly Associated with Burning Tongue Syndrome (Glossopyrosis)

Local Factors	Systemic Factors
Xerostomia	Vitamin B deficiency
Chronic mouth breathing	Vitamin B_1 or B_2
Chronic tongue thrust habit	deficiency
Chronic mechanical trauma	Pernicious anemia (B_{12})
Referred pain from teeth or	Pellagra (niacin
tonsils	deficiency)
Trigeminal neuralgia	Folic acid deficiency
Atypical facial pain or	Diabetes mellitus
neuralgia	Chronic gastritis or
Angioedema (angioneurotic	regurgitation
edema)	Chronic gastric hypoacidity
Oral candidiasis	Hypothyroidism
Temporomandibular	Mercurialism
dysfunction	Estrogen deficiency
Oral submucous fibrosis	Anxiety, stress, depression
Fusospirochetal infection	Parkinson's disease
Contact stomatitis (allergy)	Acquired immunodeficiency
Trauma to lingual nerve	syndrome (AIDS)

absence of clinically apparent mucosal alterations. Although the tongue is most commonly affected (**glossopyrosis**), other mucosal surfaces may be symptomatic (**stomatopyrosis**). In addition to the burning sensation, some patients also experience mucosal pain that is often described as "rawness" (**stomatodynia, glossodynia**). Idiopathic burning and painful sensations (the "dynias") also can affect the urogenital (**vulvodynia**) and intestinal mucosa. The so-called scalded mouth syndrome is an apparently unrelated immune response to certain medications, especially angiotensin-converting enzyme (ACE) inhibitors.

Various local and systemic factors have been postulated to cause this condition (Box 18-8), but none have been proven. The fact that most patients are postmenopausal women has led to the common belief that estrogen or progesterone deficit is responsible, but a strong correlation between such deficits and burning tongue syndrome has not been established. Some evidence exists for an autoimmune origin. Abnormal levels of antinuclear antibodies (ANAs) and rheumatoid factor (RF), for example, are found in the serum of more than 50% of patients, although these may also be found in older persons without burning mouth syndrome. The disorder has been reported to be strongly associated with depression and anxiety states, leading some authorities to consider it a psychosomatic disease.

Well-controlled comparison studies, however, are lacking.

Burning tongue syndrome affects 2% to 3% of adults to some degree (14% of postmenopausal women). Asians and Native Americans have a considerably higher risk than whites or blacks, and there is increasing prevalence with advancing age, especially after 55 years of age. This disorder is one of the most common problems encountered in the clinical practice of oral and maxillofacial pathology.

CLINICAL FEATURES

Women are four to seven times more likely to have burning tongue syndrome than men. The syndrome is rare before the age of 30 years (40 years for men), and the onset in women usually occurs within 3 to 12 years after menopause.

This disorder also has a typically abrupt onset, although it may be quite gradual. The dorsum of the tongue develops a burning sensation, usually strongest in the anterior third. Occasionally, patients will describe an irritated or raw feeling. Mucosal changes are seldom visible, although some patients will show diminished numbers and size of filiform papillae, and individuals who rub the tongue against the teeth often have erythematous and edematous papillae on the tip of the tongue. If the dorsum is significantly erythematous and smooth, an underlying systemic or local infectious process, such as anemia or erythematous candidiasis, should be suspected.

Close questioning often determines that additional oral sites are affected similarly, especially the anterior hard palate and the lips. There is seldom a significant decrease in stimulated salivary output in tests, despite the frequent patient complaint of xerostomia. Salivary levels of various proteins, immunoglobulins, and phosphates may be elevated, and there may be a decreased salivary pH or buffering capacity.

One frequently described pattern is that of mild discomfort on awakening, with increasing intensity throughout the day. Other affected patients describe a waxing and waning pattern that occurs over several days or weeks. Usually the condition does not interfere with sleep. A persistently altered (salty, bitter) or diminished taste may accompany the burning sensation. Contact with hot food or liquid often intensifies the symptoms. A minority describe a constant degree of discomfort.

As with other chronic discomforts, affected patients frequently demonstrate psychologic dysfunction, usually depression, anxiety, or irritability. The dysfunction often disappears, however, with resolution of the burning or painful tongue condition, and there is no correlation between duration and intensity of the burning sensation and the amount of psychologic dysfunction.

TREATMENT AND PROGNOSIS

If an underlying systemic or local cause can be identified and corrected, the lingual symptoms should disappear. Almost two thirds of patients with idiopathic disease show at least some improvement of their symptoms when they take one of the mood-altering drugs (e.g., chlordiazepoxide). Additional therapies that have been used include clonazepam, α-lipoic acid (thioctic acid, a neuroprotective drug), amitriptyline, transcutaneous electrical nerve stimulation, analgesics, antibiotics, antifungals, vitamin B complex, and psychologic counseling. However, none of these treatments has been proven to be effective in a double-blind, placebo-controlled trial.

The long-term prognosis for idiopathic burning tongue or mouth syndrome is variable. It is reported that one third to one half of patients experience a spontaneous or gradual remission months or years after the onset of symptoms. However, other patients may continue to experience symptoms throughout the rest of their lives. Even though the condition is chronic and may not always respond to therapy, patients should be reassured that it is benign and not a symptom of oral cancer.

DYSGEUSIA AND HYPOGEUSIA (PHANTOM TASTE; DISTORTED TASTE)

Dysgeusia is defined as a persistent abnormal taste. It is much less common than simple deficiencies in smell (**hyposmia, anosmia**) and taste (**hypogeusia, ageusia**) perception, which are found in approximately 2 million adult Americans. Dysgeusia is less tolerated than hypogeusia or hyposmia, explaining why it accounts for more than a third of patients in chemosensory centers.

Most cases of dysgeusia are produced by or associated with an underlying systemic disorder or by radiation therapy to the head and neck region (Box 18-9). Trauma, tumors, or inflammation of the peripheral nerves of the gustatory system usually produce transient hypogeusia rather than dysgeusia. In contrast, relatively common upper respiratory tract infections produce a temporary and mild dysgeusia in almost one third of cases, although they seldom produce hypogeusia. CNS neoplasms predominantly produce dysgeusia, not hypogeusia or ageusia, and taste hallucinations are fairly common during migraine headaches, Bell's palsy, or herpes zoster of the geniculate ganglion. Ischemia and infarction of the brainstem can lead to

---

Box 18-9

Local and Systemic Factors Associated with Altered Taste Sensations (Dysgeusia) or Diminished Taste Sensations (Hypogeusia)

Local Factors	Systemic Factors
Oral candidiasis	Vitamin A deficiency
Oral trichomoniasis	Vitamin B_{12} deficiency
Desquamative gingivitis	Zinc deficiency
Oral galvanism	Iron deficiency
Periodontitis or gingivitis	Nutritional overdose (zinc, vitamin A, pyridoxine)
Chlorhexidine rinse	Food sensitivity or allergy
Oral lichen planus	Sjögren syndrome
Xerostomia	Chorda tympani nerve damage
	Anorexia, cachexia, bulimia
	Severe vomiting during pregnancy
	Liver dysfunction
	Crohn's disease
	Cystic fibrosis
	Familial dysautonomia
	Addison's disease
	Turner syndrome
	Alcoholism
	Medications (200 types)
	Psychosis or depression
	Pesticide ingestion
	Lead, copper, or mercury poisoning
	Temporal arteritis
	Brainstem ischemia or infarction
	Migraine headaches
	Temporal lobe central nervous system (CNS) tumor
	Nerve trauma, gustatory nerves
	Herpes zoster, geniculate ganglion
	Upper respiratory tract infection
	Chronic gastritis or regurgitation
	Bell's palsy
	Radiation therapy to head and neck

---

ageusia of only half of the tongue (**hemiageusia**) on the same side as the brainstem lesion.

The perception of a particular taste depends on its concentration in a liquid environment; hence, persons with severe dry mouth may suffer from both hypogeusia and dysgeusia. In addition, more than 200 drugs are known to produce taste disturbances (Table 18-2). Even without medication-induced alterations, 40% of persons with clinical depression complain of dysgeusia. The clinician should be especially diligent in assessing local, intraoral causes of dysgeusia, such as periodontal or dental abscess, oral candidiasis, and routine gingivitis or periodontitis. The latter may

Table **18-2** **Examples of Pharmaceutical Agents That May Be Associated with Altered Taste**

Pharmaceutical Action	Examples
Anticoagulant	Phenindione
Antihistamine	Chlorpheniramine maleate
Antihypertensive or diuretic	Captopril, diazoxide, ethacrynic acid
Antimicrobial	Amphotericin B, ampicillin, griseofulvin, idoxuridine, lincomycin, metronidazole, streptomycin, tetracycline, tyrothricin
Antineoplastic or immunosuppressant	Doxorubicin, methotrexate, vincristine, azathioprine, carmustine
Antiparkinsonian agent	Baclofen, chlormezanone, levodopa
Antipsychotic or anticonvulsant	Carbamazepine, lithium, phenytoin
Antirheumatic	Allopurinol, colchicine, gold, levamisole, penicillamine, phenylbutazone
Antiseptic	Hexetidine, chlorhexidine
Antithyroid agent	Carbimazole, methimazole, thiouracil
Hypoglycemic	Glipizide, phenformin
Opiate	Codeine, morphine
Sympathomimetic	Amphetamines, phenmetrazine
Vasodilator	Oxyfedrine, bamifylline

produce a salty taste because of the high sodium chloride content of oozing crevicular fluids.

CLINICAL FEATURES

In contrast to hypogeusia, dysgeusia is discerned promptly and distressingly by affected individuals. The clinician must be certain that the patient's alteration is, in fact, a taste disorder rather than an olfactory one, because 75% of "flavor" information (e.g., taste, aroma, texture, temperature, irritating properties) is derived from smell. Abnormal taste function should be verified through formal taste testing by using standard tastants that are representative of each of the four primary taste qualities (i.e., sweet, sour, salty, bitter) in a nonodorous solution. Additional electrical and chemical analysis of taste bud function is frequently required. Because this is outside the scope of most general practices, patients are typically referred to a *taste and smell center*.

Affected patients may describe their altered taste as one of the primary ones, but many describe the new taste as metallic, foul, or rancid. The latter two are more likely to be associated with aberrant odor perception **(parosmia)** than with dysgeusia. The altered taste may require a stimulus, such as certain foods or liquids, in which case the taste is said to be distorted. If no stimulus is required, then the dysgeusia is classified as a *phantom taste*.

TREATMENT AND PROGNOSIS

If an underlying disease or process is identified and treated successfully, the taste function should return to normal. For idiopathic cases there is no effective pharmacologic or surgical therapy. Dysgeusia in particular tends to affect lifestyles and interpersonal relationships significantly, perhaps leading to depression, anxiety, or nutritional deficiencies from altered eating habits. Fortunately, two thirds of dysgeusia patients experience spontaneous resolution (average duration, 10 months). Idiopathic hypogeusia is less of a problem for the patient, but tends to slowly become worse over time. Occasionally, even this will undergo spontaneous resolution.

FREY SYNDROME (AURICULOTEMPORAL SYNDROME; GUSTATORY SWEATING AND FLUSHING)

First described by Baillarger in 1853, **Frey syndrome** is characterized by facial flushing and sweating along the distribution of the auriculotemporal nerve. These signs occur in response to gustatory stimuli, and the syndrome results from injury to the nerve.

This nerve, in addition to supplying sensory fibers to the preauricular and temporal regions, carries parasympathetic fibers to the parotid gland and sympathetic vasomotor and sudomotor (sweat stimulating) fibers to the preauricular skin. After parotid abscess, trauma, mandibular surgery, or parotidectomy, the parasympathetic nerve fibers may be severed. In their attempt to reestablish innervation, these fibers occasionally become misdirected and regenerate along the sympathetic nerve pathways, establishing communication with the sympathetic nerve fibers of sweat glands and blood vessels of the facial skin. The most widely accepted mechanism of Frey's syndrome is aberrant neuronal regeneration. Subsequent to these aberrant neural connections, when salivation is stimulated, local sweat glands are activated inadvertently and the patient's cheek becomes flushed and moist.

More than 40% of patients with parotidectomies develop Frey syndrome as a complication of surgery. The condition is rare in infancy but has been seen after forceps delivery. Neonatal cases do not typically occur until the child begins to eat solid foods, at which time it is usually interpreted as an allergy. Additionally, more than one third of diabetics with neuropathy will experience gustatory sweating, especially those who also have severe kidney damage. The nerve damage in this case is presumably from chronic ischemia and immune attacks.

Related phenomena may accompany an operation or injury to the submandibular gland (**chorda tympani syndrome**) or the facial nerve proximal to the geniculate ganglion (**gustatory lacrimation syndrome, "crocodile tears"**). The chin and submental skin demonstrate sweating and flushing in the former. Chewing food in the latter syndrome produces abundant tear formation.

CLINICAL FEATURES

The presenting signs and symptoms of Frey syndrome include sweating, flushing, warmth, and occasionally pain in the preauricular and temporal regions during chewing. Within 2 months to 2 years (average, 9 months) after the nerve injury, the sweating and flushing reactions commence and become steadily more severe for several months, remaining constant thereafter. When flushing occurs, the local skin temperature may be raised as much as 2° C. This may occur without sweating, especially in females. Pain, when present, is usually mild, and hypesthesia (hypoesthesia) or hyperesthesia are common features.

To detect sweating, Minor's starch-iodine test may be used. A 1% iodine solution is painted on the affected area of the skin. This solution is allowed to dry, and the area is then coated with a layer of starch. When the patient is given something to eat, the moisture of the sweat that is produced will mix with the iodine on the skin. This allows the iodine to react with the starch and produce a blue color (Fig. 18-6). Iodine-sublimated paper, which changes color when wet, also can be used, and thermography or surface thermometers will document the temperature changes of the skin.

TREATMENT AND PROGNOSIS

Most cases are mild enough that treatment is not required. Moreover, approximately 5% of adult patients and almost all affected infants experience spontaneous resolution of the syndrome. About 5% of Frey syndrome patients with diabetically damaged kidneys will show

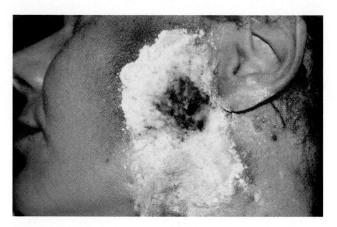

Fig. 18-6   Frey syndrome. This patient received an injury to her auriculotemporal nerve during orthognathic surgery 3 years earlier. Notice the region of sweating detected during mastication by a color change of the starch in the Minor's starch-iodine test.

considerable improvement or complete resolution of the facial problem after renal transplant.

Severing the auriculotemporal or glossopharyngeal nerve on the affected side inhibits or abolishes the sweating and flushing reaction of auriculotemporal syndrome, as may atropine injections, botulinum toxin injections, scopolamine creams, and the systemic use of oxybutynin chloride, an antimuscarinic agent. The risk of this syndrome is greatly diminished by positioning a temporoparietal fascia flap between the gland and the overlying skin of the cheek at the time of parotidectomy.

OSTEOARTHRITIS (DEGENERATIVE ARTHRITIS; DEGENERATIVE JOINT DISEASE)

Osteoarthritis is a common degenerative and destructive alteration of the joints that until recently was considered to be the inevitable result of simple wear and tear on aging anatomic structures. It is now known to have a strong inflammatory component as well, especially in small joints, such as the temporomandibular joint (TMJ), where there appears to be little association with the aging process. The disease represents approximately 10% of patients evaluated for TMJ pain.

Osteoarthritis is thought by some to be unavoidable; almost everyone older than 50 years of age is affected to some extent. The TMJ is less affected than the heavy weight–bearing joints, but even that joint is involved at the microscopic level in 40% of older adults and at the radiographic level in 14%. Although osteoarthritis is definitely an aging phenomenon, recent research also has identified osteoarthritis in a majority of young persons referred to a TMJ clinic for joint pain and dysfunction.

Presumably, with advancing age, there is slower and less complete replacement of chondroblasts and chondrocytes in joint cartilage. The cartilage matrix (fibrocartilage in the case of the TMJ) turns over less rapidly, forcing available fibers to work longer and become susceptible to fatigue. The matrix also holds less water, becoming desiccated and brittle, in part because underlying marrow blood flow diminishes, providing poor nutrition. With continued joint use, the surface fibers break down and portions of the hyaline or fibrocartilage are destroyed, often breaking away to expose underlying bone. The exposed bone then undergoes a dual process of degenerative destruction and proliferation.

CLINICAL AND RADIOGRAPHIC FEATURES

Osteoarthritis usually involves multiple joints, typically the large weight-bearing joints. The disease is characterized by a gradually intensifying deep ache and pain, usually worse in the evening than in the morning. Some degree of morning joint stiffness and stiffness after inactivity is present in 80% of cases. The affected joint may become swollen and warm to the touch, rarely with erythema of the overlying skin. Degenerative changes occur in areas of greatest impact, and the joint may become so deformed that it limits motion. Crepitation (i.e., crackling noise during motion) is a late sign of the disease and is, therefore, associated with more pronounced damage.

These changes are seen also when the TMJ is affected, except that patients seldom experience stiffness of the TMJ. In addition, the muscles of mastication frequently exhibit tenderness because of the constant strain of "muscle guarding" (i.e., attempting to keep the painful joint immobile).

On radiography, joints affected by osteoarthritis demonstrate a narrowing or obliteration of the joint space, surface irregularities and protuberances (**exostoses, osteophytes**), flattening of the articular surface, osteosclerosis and osteolysis of bone beneath the cartilage, radiolucent **subchondral cysts**, and ossification within the synovial membrane (**ossicles**). More sensitive diagnostic techniques, such as computed tomography (CT) scanning arthrography, magnetic resonance imaging (MRI), and arthroscopy, reveal the same features but in much more detail; hence, they are able to identify earlier changes. With arthroscopy, 90% of the joints will show evidence of synovitis, usually before cartilage surface changes are visible.

HISTOPATHOLOGIC FEATURES

The articulating surface of a joint affected by osteoarthritis has a diminished number of chondrocytes, is roughened, and contains variable numbers of vertical clefts; in older cases the clefts extend to the underlying bone. The surface is proliferative in some areas and degenerative in others. The bone beneath the cartilage shows a loss of osteocytes, minimal osteoblastic or osteoclastic activity, fatty degeneration or necrosis of the marrow, marrow fibrosis, infiltration by chronic inflammatory cells, and perhaps the formation of a large degenerative space beneath the articular cartilage (subchondral cyst). Inflammation and thickening of the synovial membrane is seen, sometimes with the formation of metaplastic bone (ossicles) or hyaline cartilage granules (chondral bodies), which may number in the hundreds within a single joint. The synovial joint fluid typically contains inflammatory and degradation molecules, the levels of which have prognostic significance.

The TMJ is unique because of its fibrocartilage covering and its meniscus. The disk may be centrally destroyed, and there is little vertical clefting of the articular surface. All other features of TMJ osteoarthritis, however, are similar to those noted in other joints.

TREATMENT AND PROGNOSIS

The treatment of osteoarthritis is usually palliative and consists of analgesics and nonsteroidal antiinflammatory drugs (NSAIDs) for the symptoms. Arthroplasty and joint replacement often are required for heavy weight-bearing joints and are used occasionally in the TMJ. Occlusal adjustment and occlusal splints may reduce symptoms by relieving the pressure on the joint surfaces, and orofacial physiotherapy and hot or cold packs may be helpful to relax involved muscles. Arthroscopic lavage provides short-term pain relief in many cases, and low-dose doxycycline (collagenase inhibitor, antimatrix metalloproteinase) recently has been shown to reduce symptoms. Glucosamine and chondroitin sulfate, common therapies for large joint arthritis, have shown some success in TMJ osteoarthritis patients.

Aggressive therapy might not be indicated for this disease except in its most severe form. A recent 30-year follow-up investigation found radiographic evidence of continued joint destruction, but the clinical signs and symptoms were no more severe than they had been initially.

RHEUMATOID ARTHRITIS

Rheumatoid arthritis is a chronic, presumably autoimmune disorder characterized by nonsuppurative inflammatory destruction of the joints. It may result from a cross-reaction of antibodies generated against hemolytic streptococci or other microorganisms, or it may represent an antibody attack against bacterial cell walls or viral capsule fragments deposited within the synovium. The cause is still unknown, although some examples show a familial pattern.

This disease affects 3% of people in the United States to at least some degree, and approximately 200,000 new cases are diagnosed yearly. The TMJ eventually becomes involved in 75% of patients, although the involvement is usually so mild as to be clinically insignificant.

In contrast to osteoarthritis (see previous topic), rheumatoid arthritis begins as an attack against the synovial membrane **(synovitis)**. A reactive macrophage-laden fibroblastic proliferation **(pannus)** from the synovium creeps onto the joint surface. This releases collagenases and other proteases, which destroy the cartilage and underlying bone. Attempted remodeling by the damaged bone results in a characteristic deformation of the joint.

CLINICAL AND RADIOGRAPHIC FEATURES

Rheumatoid arthritis affects women three times more frequently than men, although the condition in men is usually diagnosed at a somewhat younger age (25 to 35 years) than in women (35 to 45 years). The onset and course of the disease are extremely variable. For many patients, only one or two joints become involved and significant pain or limitation of motion never develops. In others, the disease rapidly progresses to debilitating **polyarthralgia**.

Typically, the signs and symptoms become more severe over time and include swelling, stiffness, pain, joint deformity, and disability, with possible fibrous or bony fusion of opposing articular surfaces **(ankylosis)**. Periods of remission often are interspersed with periods of exacerbation. Symmetrical involvement of the small joints of the hands and feet almost always is present, but it is not unusual for knees and elbows to be affected. The hip joint, the joint most often affected by osteoarthritis, is the joint least affected by rheumatoid arthritis. Twenty percent of patients have firm, partially movable, nontender **rheumatoid nodules** beneath the skin near the affected joint. These are pathognomonic for the disease.

Joints involved with rheumatoid arthritis have a characteristic "anvil" shape, with an irregular flattening of the central articular surface and a splaying of the lateral bone. Unlike the situation in osteoarthritis, narrowing of the joint space is seldom seen, except when ankylosis has occurred.

The TMJ is affected to some degree in more than 40% of persons with rheumatoid arthritis. When present, TMJ involvement is usually bilateral and occurs late in the disease. The signs and symptoms are seldom as severe as in other joints and include stiffness, crepitation, pain or ache, tenderness, or limitation of mouth opening. Swelling is less obvious than with other joints.

Frequently, the pain of TMJ rheumatoid arthritis is not related to motion but rather to pressure on the joint. Clenching the teeth on one side produces pain of the contralateral joint. Similarly, subluxation or ankylosis is less frequent in the TMJs than in other joints, but gross destruction of the condylar heads may be so severe that mandibular micrognathia causes a receding chin and malocclusion. Permanent TMJ subluxation has been reported.

Radiographically, involved TMJs demonstrate a flattened condylar head with irregular surface features, an irregular temporal fossa surface, perhaps with remodeling of the fossa itself, and anterior displacement of the condyle. Several diagnostic techniques are available besides routine TMJ radiographs. CT scans, scanning arthrography, and arthroscopy are excellent tools for assessing TMJ damage. Thermography is used commonly in Europe to detect early disease. Ultrasonography is valuable for larger joints but has been used little in TMJ disease. Nuclear medicine scans that use scintigraphy have, in recent years, been largely replaced by MRI scans. The latter are sensitive and have become the diagnostic tool of choice.

LABORATORY VALUES

Approximately 80% of patients with rheumatoid arthritis exhibit significant elevations of rheumatoid factor (RF), an autoantibody thought to be directed toward an altered host IgG antibody that is no longer recognized by the body as "self." In addition, antinuclear antibodies (ANAs) can be detected in about 50% of the patients with rheumatoid arthritis, although it is not diagnostically specific because it also may be associated with other autoimmune diseases. During active phases of the disease, almost all patients have an elevated erythrocyte sedimentation rate. In addition, some affected patients have mild anemia.

HISTOPATHOLOGIC FEATURES

Needle biopsy is the most popular technique for obtaining diagnostic synovial material, but aspiration and analysis of synovial fluid from the affected joint frequently are undertaken to rule out other forms of arthritis. These techniques are seldom used for TMJ involvement.

Microscopically, early cases of rheumatoid arthritis demonstrate hyperplasia of the synovial lining cells with deeper portions of the membrane showing hyperemia, edema, and infiltration by lymphocytes, macrophages, and occasional neutrophils. Neutrophils are the predominant inflammatory cell in the synovial fluid. Older lesions show continued, often pronounced synovial proliferation and edema, with cholesterol crystals and fewer inflammatory cells. Typically, the membrane protrudes into the joint space as villi or fingerlike projections. These projections occasionally undergo necrosis, producing **rice bodies**—small whitish villi fragments composed of cellular debris admixed with fibrin and collagen. When the TMJ is severely involved, the meniscus is typically perforated or replaced completely by fibrous scar.

The rheumatoid nodule is represented by a moderately well-demarcated area of amorphous, eosinophilic necrosis surrounded by a thick layer of mononuclear cells. The mononuclear cells closest to the amorphous center are typically large and palisaded. Neutrophils are frequently seen in the center.

TREATMENT AND PROGNOSIS

No cure exists for rheumatoid arthritis, and current treatments strive only to suppress the process as much as possible. The various therapies that are used are largely empirical and aimed at nonspecific suppression of the inflammatory or immunologic process in an effort to attenuate not only the symptoms but also the progressive damage to articular structures. Drug therapy in early and mild cases consists of nonsteroidal antiinflammatory drugs (NSAIDs), perhaps aided by occasional corticosteroid injections into the joint. The latter injections are used sparingly, however, because frequent use is associated with additional degenerative changes and fibrous ankylosis.

Second-line medications often are required, and the wide variability in responses to these drugs typically results in an extended course of constantly changing doses and agents in an effort to achieve optimal relief. Systemic glucocorticoid therapy has been shown to be effective in providing symptomatic relief for patients with rheumatoid arthritis. A number of agents appear to have the capacity to modify the course of rheumatoid arthritis, and these medications are referred to as *disease-modifying antirheumatic drugs*. Agents such as gold injections, D-penicillamine, sulfasalazine, the antimalarials, and methotrexate are included in this group. Patients report clinical improvement with the use of these medications; they also demonstrate an improvement in serologic evidence of disease activity with reductions in C-reactive protein, erythrocyte sedimentation rate, and RF. Emerging evidence indicates that the early and aggressive use of disease-modifying antirheumatic drugs may actually retard the development of bone erosions and potentially facilitate healing of existing lesions. However, toxicity is a problem with all of these agents, and at present, no one drug has demonstrated a consistent advantage over the others. Methotrexate, a folic acid antagonist, is the most frequently used first-line agent in the disease-modifying group. The literature suggests that patients who fail or who have shown a suboptimal response to disease-modulating therapy might benefit from tumor necrosis factor-α (TNF-α) neutralizing agents (e.g., etanercept and infliximab), used alone or in combination with standard disease-modulation algorithms.

Immunosuppressive drugs such as azathioprine, cyclosporine, and cyclophosphamide appear to be no more effective in the management of rheumatoid arthritis than the previously mentioned disease-modulating antirheumatic drugs, and the side effect profile of immunosuppressive therapy includes increased risk for serious infections and potential predisposition to the development of malignant neoplasms. Therefore, immunosuppressive therapy should be reserved for those patients who have failed all other efforts at disease modulation.

Severely damaged joints may require surgical replacement, with the goals of therapy being attenuation of pain and reduction of disability. Total joint replacement of the hips, knees, and shoulders are reported to have the highest satisfaction rates associated with surgical management of these patients.

TEMPOROMANDIBULAR JOINT DYSFUNCTION

Pain and dysfunction of the TMJ are common and have been proposed to result from a wide variety of etiologic factors, both traumatic and nontraumatic (Box 18-10). The syndrome of signs and symptoms (pain, altered function, joint noises) is termed **temporomandibular joint dysfunction** (TMD). TMD is a problem of the entire masticatory system: teeth, jaws, joints, and muscles. All facets must be evaluated to arrive at the most specific diagnosis and management protocol. Because of the extreme complexity of this disease, the present discussion is limited to a brief overview of those facets of the disorder that are appropriate to the production of pain.

Almost 15% of U.S. adults experience facial and cervical pain, facial tenderness, and headache from TMD, but fewer than 1% of those have symptoms severe enough to warrant professional evaluation or intervention.

CLINICAL AND RADIOGRAPHIC FEATURES

TMD is seen primarily in middle-aged women, but it may affect any age and either sex. Most patients have some degree of pain, which is the primary reason for

Box 18-10

Classification of Temporomandibular Disorders

MUSCULAR DISORDERS

- Hyperactivity, spasm, and trismus
- Inflammation (myositis)
- Trauma
- Myofascial pain and fibromyalgia
- Atrophy or hypertrophy

ARTHROGENIC DISORDERS

- Disc displacement (internal derangement)
- Hypomobility of the disc (adhesions or scars)
- Dislocation and subluxation
- Arthritis
- Infections
- Metabolic disease (gout, chondrocalcinosis)
- Capsulitis, synovitis
- Ankylosis (fibrous, bony)
- Fracture
- Condylar hyperplasia, hypoplasia, aplasia
- Neoplasia

Box 18-11

Medications Used to Treat the Symptoms of Temporomandibular Joint Dysfunction

- Aspirin
- Acetaminophen (with or without codeine)
- Other nonsteroidal antiinflammatory drugs (NSAIDs)
- Centrally acting muscle relaxants (methocarbamol, chlorzoxazone)
- Benzodiazepine derivatives (diazepam, chlordiazepoxide)
- Glucocorticoids (cortisone, prednisone)

seeking professional help. The pain is usually localized to the preauricular area but may radiate to the temporal, frontal, or occipital areas. The pain may be a headache, a ringing in the ears (**tinnitus**), an earache (**otalgia**), or a toothache.

Nonarthritic inflammatory disorders of the TMJ are characterized by continuous deep pain or ache. The pain is evoked by palpation of the affected joint or by mandibular movement, especially chewing and clenching. Both TMJs may be involved, at the same time or at differing times.

The pain may be associated more with the surrounding musculature and soft tissue than with the TMJ itself. Muscle splinting can lead to involuntary CNS-induced muscular contractions (**myospasm**), or the muscle fibers themselves may become inflamed (**myositis**).

Myofascial trigger point pain is common in TMD, but it is seldom noted in other TMJ disorders. It is characterized by circumscribed regions within the muscle ("trigger points") that elicit local or referred pain on palpation and may be a source of constant deep pain. In many instances, patients are aware only of the referred pain and not the trigger points themselves. The exact nature of the trigger points is not known, but they seem similar to small areas of myospasm and can, through their chronic nature, induce CNS excitatory effects.

Derangements of the condyle and meniscus complex are more often associated with dysfunction than with joint pain (**arthralgia**). When present, the pain associated with a deranged joint may be localized, nonspecific, or referred. It is not a reliable finding for diagnostic purposes. For TMD associated with internal joint damage or derangement, CT and MRI provide excellent diagnostic images of the TMJ. Transcranial and cephalometric radiographic images are much less detailed, but they are usually adequate and are used more commonly. The bone itself frequently appears normal, but a widened joint space, anteriorly displaced meniscus, or altered meniscus shape are common findings. Irregular joint surfaces with protuberances (**osteophytes**) are more likely to relate to arthritis than TMD (see previous two topics). Joint effusions seen with MRI are useful markers of arthritic degeneration.

TREATMENT AND PROGNOSIS

Therapies for TMD are numerous and should be recommended based on the exact pathogenesis of the pain. Conservative treatments include simple rest or immobilization of the joint, application of cold (usually reserved for acute injuries) or heat, occlusal splints and adjustment, and physical therapy. Various medications also have been used for TMD with some success (Box 18-11), although few TMD treatments have been examined in a blinded, controlled fashion. Long-term follow-up of large numbers of patients treated conservatively indicates that 75% to 88% experience significant or complete reduction of symptoms.

Surgical intervention may be required for severely affected joints, especially those with internal meniscal derangements, condylar dislocation or fracture, ankylosis, and degenerative or developmental deformities. Usually, TMD is treated conservatively for several years without improvement before surgery is attempted. For joints with pain from anterior disk displacement (with or without reduction), however, diskectomy is recommended within 6 months of TMD diagnosis; for those with ankylosis, surgery should occur even sooner. The indications for surgery are strict. Of all patients sent to a specialist for TMD surgery, fewer than 1% actually have the surgery.

TEMPOROMANDIBULAR JOINT ANKYLOSIS

Ankylosis refers literally to a "fusion" of body parts, in this case the opposing components of a joint. The fusion can be fibrous or bony in nature—usually fibrous when the TMJ is involved. Joint infection, usually after trauma, accounts for 50% of all TMJ ankylosis cases, but 30% result from aseptic trauma. The remaining cases are idiopathic or produced by rheumatoid arthritis.

The ankylosis may be intra-articular or extra-articular. **Intra-articular** ankylosis is characterized by the destruction of the meniscus and the temporal fossa, thickening and flattening of the condylar head, and a narrowing of the joint space. Opposing joint surfaces then develop fibrous adhesions that inhibit normal movements and may become ossified. Fibrotic intra-articular ankylosis is the most common type seen in the TMJ, especially after trauma-induced hemorrhage **(hemarthrosis)**. Osseous ankylosis is more likely with nonhemorrhagic infections of the joint.

Extra-articular involvement is less frequently seen and produces an external fibrous or osseous encapsulation with minimal destruction of the joint itself.

CLINICAL FEATURES

TMJ ankylosis occurs predominantly in the first decade of life, and males and females are equally affected. Almost all cases are unilateral. The condition results in a gradually worsening inability to open the jaws, with the mandible shifting toward the affected side on opening. Pain, tenderness, and malocclusion may be present, but this is not usually the case.

In severe examples, there is almost complete immobilization of the mandible, and the mandible may protrude forward as the excess tissues occupy the joint space. In very young children, unilateral micrognathia **(hemifacial microsomia)** may result from diminished growth on the affected side. Malocclusion may be severe in such cases.

HISTOPATHOLOGIC FEATURES

TMJ ankylosis is characterized by an excessive amount of dense, rather avascular fibrous connective tissue or new bone formation. Intra-articular ankylosis demonstrates irregular destruction of cartilage and bone with a sparse lymphocytic infiltration.

TREATMENT AND PROGNOSIS

Surgical osteoplasty of the joint with removal of excessive fibrous or calcific tissues is the treatment of choice for TMJ ankylosis. For severe cases, complete joint replacement may be necessary.

BIBLIOGRAPHY

Bell's Palsy

Cook SP, Macartney KK, Rose CD et al: Lyme disease and seventh nerve paralysis in children, *Am J Otolaryngol* 18:320-323, 1997.

Danielidis V, Skevas A, Van Cauwenberge P et al: A comparative study of age and degree of facial nerve recovery in patients with Bell's palsy, *Eur Arch Otorhinolaryngol* 256:520-522, 1999.

Friedman RA: The surgical management of Bell's palsy: a review, *Am J Otol* 21:139-144, 2000.

Furuta Y, Aizawa H, Ohtani F et al: Varicella-zoster virus DNA level and facial paralysis in Ramsay Hunt syndrome, *Ann Otol Rhinol Laryngol* 113(9):700-705, 2004

Jackson CG, von Doersten PG: The facial nerve: current trends in diagnosis, treatment, and rehabilitation, *Med Clin North Am* 83:179-195, 1999.

Morgan M, Moffat M, Ritchie L et al: Is Bell's palsy a reactivation of varicella zoster virus? *J Infect* 30(1): 29-36, 1995.

Peitersen E: Bell's palsy: the spontaneous course of 2,500 peripheral facial nerve palsies of different etiologies, *Acta Otolaryngol Suppl* 549:4-30, 2002.

Ramsey MJ, Der Simonian R, Holtel MR et al: Corticosteroid treatment for idiopathic facial nerve paralysis: a meta-analysis, *Laryngoscope* 110:335-341, 2000.

Sussman GL, Yang WH, Steinberg S: Melkersson-Rosenthal syndrome: clinical, pathologic, and therapeutic considerations, *Ann Allergy* 69:187-194, 1992.

Pretrigeminal and Trigeminal Neuralgia

Al-Din AS, Mirr, Davey R et al: Trigeminal cephalgias and facial pain syndromes associated with autonomic dysfunction, *Cephalalgia* 25(8):605-611, 2005.

Benoliel R, Sharav Y: SUNCT syndrome: case report and literature review, *Oral Surg Oral Med Oral Pathol Oral Radiol Endod* 85:158-161, 1998.

Brabant S, Van Zundert J, Van Buyten JP: *Pulsed radiofrequency treatment of the gasserian ganglion in patients with essential trigeminus neuralgia: a retrospective study*. Proceedings of the World Pain Congress, San Francisco, 2000.

Brisman R: Trigeminal neuralgia and multiple sclerosis, *Arch Neurol* 44:379-381, 1987.

Burchiel KJ, Slavin KV: On the natural history of trigeminal neuralgia, *Neurosurgery* 46:152-155, 2000.

Evans RW, Graff-Radford SB, Bassiur JP: Pretrigeminal neuralgia, *Headache* 45:242-244, 2005.

Fromm GH, Terrence CF, Maroon JCL: Trigeminal neuralgia-current concepts regarding etiology and pathogenesis, *Arch Neurol* 41:1204-1207, 1984.

Golby AJ, Norbash A, Silverberg GD: Trigeminal neuralgia resulting from infarction of the root entry zone of the trigeminal nerve: case report, *Neurosurgery* 43:620-623, 1998.

Headache Classification Subcommittee of the International Headache Society: The international classification of headache disorders, ed 2, *Cephalalgia* 24(suppl 1):9-160, 2004.

Khan OA: Gabapentin relieves trigeminal neuralgia in multiple sclerosis patients, *Neurology* 51:611-614, 1998.

Mathews ES, Scrivani SJ: Percutaneous stereotactic radiofrequency thermal rhizotomy for the treatment of trigeminal neuralgia, *Mt Sinai J Med* 67:288-299, 2000.

Merrill RL, Graff-Radford SB: Trigeminal neuralgia: how to rule out the wrong treatment, *J Am Dent Assoc* 123:63-68, 1992.

Perkins GD: Trigeminal neuralgia, *Curr Treat Options Neurol* 1:458-465, 1999.

Pollock BE, Foote RL, Stafford SL et al: Results of repeated gamma knife radiosurgery for medically unresponsive trigeminal neuralgia, *J Neurosurg* 93(suppl 3):162-164, 2000.

Sawaya RA: Trigeminal neuralgia associated with sinusitis, *ORL J Otorhinolaryngol Relat Spec* 62:160-163, 2000.

Schwartz AH: Trigeminal neuralgia in a patient with multiple sclerosis and chronic inflammatory demyelinating polyneuropathy, *J Am Dent Assoc* 136:469-476, 2005.

Tremont-Lukats IW, Megeff C, Backonja MM: Anticonvulsants for neuropathic pain syndromes: mechanisms of action and place in therapy, *Drugs* 60:1029-1052, 2000.

Truini A, Galeotti F, Cruccu G: New insight into trigeminal neuralgia, *J Headache Pain* 6(4):237-239, 2005.

Glossopharyngeal Neuralgia

Ceylan S, Karakus A, Duru S et al: Glossopharyngeal neuralgia: a study of 6 cases, *Neurosurg Rev* 20:196-200, 1997.

Olesen J, Tfelt-Hansen P, Welch KMA: *The headaches*, ed 2, pp 921-946, Philadelphia, 2000, Lippincott, Williams & Wilkins.

Rushton JG, Stevens C, Miller RH: Glossopharyngeal (vagoglossopharyngeal) neuralgia: a study of 217 cases, *Arch Neurol* 38:201-205, 1981.

Soh KB: The glossopharyngeal nerve, glossopharyngeal neuralgia and the Eagle's syndrome—current concepts and management, *Singapore Med J* 40:659-665, 1999.

Stevens JC: Cranial neuralgias, *J Craniomandib Disord* 1:51-53, 1987.

Postherpetic Neuralgia

Bennett GJ: Hypotheses on the pathogenesis of herpes-associated pain, *Ann Neurol* 35:538-541, 1994.

Donahue JG, Choo PW, Masson JE et al: The incidence of herpes zoster, *Arch Intern Med* 155:1605-1609, 1995.

Helgason S, Petursson G, Gudmundsson S et al: Prevalence of postherpetic neuralgia after first episode of herpes zoster: prospective study with long term follow up, *BMJ* 321(7264):794-796, 2000.

Higa K, Mori M, Hirata K et al: Severity of skin lesions of herpes zoster at the worst phase rather than age and involved region most influences the duration of acute herpetic pain, *Pain* 69:245-253, 1997.

Watson CPN, Gershon AA: Herpes zoster and postherpetic neuralgia, *Pain Res Clin Management* 11:90-93; 108-109, 2001.

Whitley RJ, Shukla S, Crooks RJ: The identification of risk factors associated with persistent pain following herpes zoster, *J Infect Dis* 178(suppl 1):S71-S75, 1998.

Atypical Facial Pain

DeNucci DJ, Chen CC, Sobiski C et al: The use of SPECT bone scans to evaluate patients with idiopathic jaw pain, *Oral Surg Oral Med Oral Pathol Oral Radiol Endod* 90:750-757, 2000.

Fricton JR: Atypical orofacial pain disorders: a study of diagnostic subtypes, *Curr Rev Pain* 4:142-147, 2000.

Gouda JJ, Brown JA: Atypical facial pain and other pain syndromes: differential diagnosis and treatment, *Neurosurg Clin North Am* 8:87-100, 1997.

Graff-Radford SB: Facial pain, *Curr Opin Neurol* 13:291-296, 2000.

Graff-Radford SB, Ketelaer MC, Gratt BM et al: Thermographic assessment of neuropathic facial pain, *J Orofac Pain* 9:138-146, 1995.

Headache Classification Committee of the International Headache Society: Classification and diagnostic criteria for headache disorders, cranial neuralgias and facial pain, *Cephalalgia* 8:1-96, 1988.

Hampf G, Aalberg V, Sunden B: Assessment of patients suffering from chronic orofacial pain of nonspecific origin, *J Craniomandib Disord* 4:30-34, 1990.

Lund JP, Lavigne GJ, Dubner R et al: *Orofacial pain: from basic science to clinical management*, Chicago, 2001, Quintessence.

Marbach JJ, Hulbrock J, Hohn C et al: Incidence of phantom tooth pain: an atypical facial neuralgia, *Oral Surg Oral Med Oral Pathol* 53:190-193, 1982.

Olesen J, Tfelt-Hansen P, Welch KMA: *The headaches*, ed 2, pp 593-598, Philadelphia, 2000, Lippincott, Williams & Wilkins.

Raskin NH: *Headache*, ed 2, pp 366-367, New York, 1998, Churchill Livingstone.

Scully C, Porter S: Orofacial disease: update for the clinical team: 9. Orofacial pain, *Dent Update* 26:410-417, 1999.

Sessle BJ: The neurobiology of facial and dental pain: present knowledge, future directions, *J Dent Res* 65:962-981, 1987.

Taha JM, Tew JM Jr: Honored guest presentation: therapeutic decisions in facial pain, *Clin Neurosurg* 46:410-431, 2000.

Turp JC, Gobetti JP: Trigeminal neuralgia versus atypical facial pain: a review of the literature and case report, *Oral Surg Oral Med Oral Pathol Oral Radiol Endod* 81:424-432, 1996.

Woda A, Pionchon P: A unified concept of idiopathic orofacial pain: clinical features, *J Orofac Pain* 13:172-195, 1999.

Neuralgia-Inducing Cavitational Osteonecrosis

Adams WR, Spolnick KJ, Bouquot JE: Maxillofacial osteonecrosis in a patient with multiple facial pains, *J Oral Pathol Med* 28:423-432, 1999.

Bouquot JE, LaMarche MG: Ischemic osteonecrosis under fixed partial denture pontics: radiographic and microscopic features in 38 patients with chronic pain, *J Prosthet Dent* 81:148-158, 1999.

Bouquot JE, McMahon RE: Neuropathic pain in maxillofacial osteonecrosis, *J Oral Maxillofac Surg* 58:1003-1020, 2000.

Bouquot J, Wrobleski G, Fenton S: The most common osteonecrosis? Prevalence of maxillofacial osteonecrosis (NICO), *J Oral Pathol Med* 29:345, 2000.

Glueck CJ, McMahon RE, Bouquot JE et al: Heterozygosity for the Leiden mutation V gene, a common pathoetiology for osteonecrosis of the jaw with thrombophilia augmented by exogenous estrogens, *J Lab Clin Med* 130:540-543, 1997.

Gruppo R, Glueck CJ, McMahon RE et al: The pathophysiology of osteonecrosis of the jaw: anticardiolipin antibodies, thrombophilia, and hypofibrinolysis, *J Lab Clin Med* 127:481-488, 1996.

Larheim TA, Westesson PL, Hicks DG et al: Osteonecrosis of the temporomandibular joint: correlation of magnetic resonance imaging and histology, *J Oral Maxillofac Surg* 57:888-898, 1999.

McMahon RE, Adams W, Spolnik KJ: Diagnostic anesthesia for referred trigeminal pain. Part 1, *Compendium* 13:870-876, 1992.

Cluster Headache

Benoliel R, Sharav Y: Paroxysmal hemicrania: case studies and review of the literature, *Oral Surg Oral Med Oral Pathol Oral Radiol Endod* 85:285-292, 1998.

Mathew NT: Cluster headache, *Semin Neurol* 17:313-323, 1997.

May A, Bahra A, Buchel C et al: PET and MRA findings in cluster headache and MRA in experimental pain, *Neurology* 55:1328-1335, 2000.

Olesen J, Tfelt-Hansen P, Welch KMA: *The headaches*, ed 2, pp 675-740, Philadelphia, 2000, Lippincott, Williams & Wilkins.

Penarrocha M, Bagan JV, Penarrocha MA et al: Cluster headache and cocaine use, *Oral Surg Oral Med Oral Pathol Oral Radiol Endod* 90:271-274, 2000.

Salvesen R: Cluster headache, *Curr Treat Options Neurol* 1:441-449, 1999.

Silberstein SD, Niknam R, Rozen TD et al: Cluster headache with aura, *Neurology* 54:219-221, 2000.

Chronic Paroxysmal Hemicrania

Boes CJ, Doddick DW: Redefining the clinical spectrum of chronic paroxysmal hemicrania: a review of 74 patients, *J Headache Pain* 42(8):699-708, 2002.

Goadsby PJ: Short-lasting primary headaches: focus on trigeminal autonomic cephalgias and indomethacin-sensitive headaches, *Curr Opin Neurol* 12(3):273-277, 1999.

Goadsby PJ, Lipton RB: A review of paroxysmal hemicranias, SUNCT syndrome and other short-lasting headaches with autonomic features, including new cases, *Brain* 120(pt 1):193-209, 1997.

Lance JW, Goadsby PJ: *Mechanism and management of headache*, London, 1998, Butterworth-Heinemann.

Russell D: Paroxysmal hemicrania. In Olessen J, Goadsby PJ, editors: *Cluster headache & related conditions*, pp 27-36, Oxford, UK, 1999, Oxford University Press.

Migraine

Ambrosini A, de Noordhout AM, Sandor PS et al: Electrophysiological studies in migraine: a comprehensive review of their interest and limitations, *Cephalalgia* 23(suppl 1):13-31, 2003.

Bolay H, Reuter U, Dunn AK et al: Intrinsic brain activity triggers trigeminal meningeal afferents in a migraine model, *Nat Med* 8:136-142, 2002.

Cady RK, Gutterman D, Saires JA et al: Responsiveness of non-HIS migraine and tension-type headache to sumatriptan, *Cephalalgia* 17:588-590, 1997.

Cologno D, Torelli P, Manzoni GC: Migraine with aura: a review of 81 patients with 10-20 years' follow-up, *Cephalalgia* 18:690-696, 1998.

Cutrer FM, O'Donnel A, del Rio MS: Functional neuroimaging: enhanced understanding of migraine, *Neurology* 55(suppl 2):S36-S45, 2000.

Olesen J: Some clinical features of acute migraine attack: an analysis of 750 patients, *Headache* 18:268-271, 1978.

Olesen J, Tfelt-Hansen P, Welch KMA: *The headaches*, ed 2, pp 223-542, Philadelphia, 2000, Lippincott, Williams & Wilkins.

Peatfield RC: Migraine, *Curr Treat Options Neurol* 1:450-457, 1999.

Silberstein SD, Lipton RB, Goadsby PJ: *Headache in clinical practice*, Oxford, UK, 1998, Isis Medical Media.

Ward TN: Providing relief from headache pain: current options for acute and prophylactic therapy, *Postgrad Med* 108:121-128, 2000.

Woods RP, Iacoboni M, Mazziotta JC: Bilateral spreading cerebral hypoperfusion during spontaneous migraine headache, *N Engl J Med* 331:1689-1692, 1994.

Temporal Arteritis

Blockmans D, Stroobants S, Maes A: Positron emission tomography in giant cell arteritis and polymyalgia rheumatica: evidence for inflammation of the aortic arch, *Am J Med* 108(3):246-249, 2000.

González-Gay MA, García-Porrúa C, Llorca J et al: Visual manifestations of giant cell arteritis. Trends and clinical spectrum in 161 patients, *Medicine (Balt)* 79:283-292, 2000.

Hunder GG: Giant cell arteritis, *Lupus* 7:266-269, 1998.

Kleinegger CL, Lilly GE: Cranial arteritis: a medical emergency with orofacial manifestations, *J Am Dent Assoc* 130:1203-1209, 1999.

Matteson EL, Gold KN, Bloch DA: Long-term survival of patients with giant cell arteritis in the American College of Rheumatology giant cell arteritis classification criteria cohort, *Am J Med* 100:193-196, 1996.

Neff AG, Greifenstein EM: Giant cell arteritis update, *Semin Ophthalmol* 14:109-112, 1999.

Nesher G, Sonnenblick M, Friedlander Y: Analysis of steroid related complications and mortality in temporal arteritis: a 15-year survey of 43 patients, *J Rheumatol* 21:1283-1286, 1994.

Turbin RE, Kupersmith MJ: Giant cell arteritis, *Curr Treat Options Neurol* 1:49-56, 1999.

van der Wal JE, van der Waal I: Oral manifestations of giant cell arteritis, *Mund Kiefer Gesichtschir* 1:65-67, 1997.

Myasthenia Gravis

Anlar B: Juvenile myasthenia: diagnosis and treatment, *Paediatr Drugs* 2:161-169, 2000.

Daskalakis GJ, Papageorgiou IS, Petrogiannis ND et al: Myasthenia gravis and pregnancy, *Eur J Obstet Gynecol Reprod Biol* 89:201-204, 2000.

Iani C, Caramia M, Morosetti M et al: The treatment of severe forms of myasthenia gravis, *Funct Neurol* 13:231-237, 1998.

Lisak RP: Myasthenia gravis, *Curr Treat Options Neurol* 1:239-250, 1999.

Mehta S: Neuromuscular disease causing acute respiratory failure, *Respir Care* 51:1016-1021; discussion 1021-1023, 2006.

Pascuzzi RM: Pearls and pitfalls in the diagnosis and management of neuromuscular junction disorders, *Semin Neurol* 21:425-440, 2001.

Robertson NP, Deans J, Compston DA: Myasthenia gravis: a population based epidemiological study in Cambridgeshire, UK, *J Neurol Neurosurg Psychiatry* 65:492-496, 1998.

Sasakura Y, Kumasaka S, Takahashi T et al: Myasthenia gravis associated with reduced masticatory function, *Int J Oral Maxillofac Surg* 29:381-383, 2000.

Scherer K, Bedlack RS, Simel DL: Does this patient have myasthenia gravis? *JAMA* 293:1906-1914, 2005.

Weijnen FG, Kuks JB, van der Bilt A et al: Tongue force in patients with myasthenia gravis, *Acta Neurol Scand* 102:303-308, 2000.

Motor Neuron Disease

Adams RD, Victor M, Ropper AH, editors: *Principles of neurology*, ed 6, pp 1089-1094, New York, 1997, McGraw-Hill.

Bromberg MB: Pathogenesis of amyotrophic lateral sclerosis: a critical review, *Curr Opin Neurol* 12:581-588, 1999.

Francis K, Bach JR, DeLisa JA: Evaluation and rehabilitation of patients with adult motor neuron disease, *Arch Phys Med Rehabil* 80:951-963, 1999.

Leighton SE, Burton MJ, Lund WS et al: Swallowing in motor neurone disease, *J R Soc Med* 87:801-805, 1994.

Rames CM, Newcombe RG, Harper PS et al: Risk estimates for developing motor neuron disease in first-degree relatives, *Clin Genet* 47:13-16, 1995.

Ross MA: Acquired motor neuron disorders, *Neurol Clin* 15:481-500, 1997.

Strober JB, Tennekoon GI: Progressive spinal muscular atrophies, *J Child Neurol* 14:691-695, 1999.

Williams DB, Windebank AJ: Motor neuron disease (amyotrophic lateral sclerosis), *Mayo Clin Proc* 66:54-82, 1991.

Wokke JH: Diseases that masquerade as motor neuron disease, *Lancet* 347:1347-1348, 1996.

Wong PC, Rothstein JD, Price DL: The genetic and molecular mechanisms of motor neuron disease, *Curr Opin Neurobiol* 8:791-799, 1998.

Yapijakis C, Kapaki E, Boussious M et al: Prenatal diagnosis of X-linked spinal and bulbar muscular atrophy in a Greek family, *Prenat Diagn* 16:262-265, 1996.

Burning Tongue Syndrome and Glossodynia

Bergdahl M, Bergdahl J: Burning mouth syndrome: prevalence and associated factors, *J Oral Pathol Med* 28:350-354, 1999.

Bessho K, Okubo Y, Hori S et al: Effectiveness of kampo medicine (sai-boku-to) in treatment of patients with glossodynia, *Oral Surg Oral Med Oral Pathol Oral Radiol Endod* 86:682-686, 1998.

Bogetto F, Maina G, Ferro G et al: Psychiatric comorbidity in patients with burning mouth syndrome, *Psychosom Med* 60:378-385, 1998.

Brown RS, Krakow AM, Douglas T et al: "Scalded mouth syndrome" caused by angiotensin converting enzyme inhibitors: two case reports, *Oral Surg Oral Med Oral Pathol Oral Radiol Endod* 83:665-667, 1997.

Formaker BK, Frank ME: Taste function in patients with oral burning, *Chem Senses* 25:575-581, 2000.

Grinspan D, Fernandez Blanco G, Allevato MA et al: Burning mouth syndrome, *Int J Dermatol* 34:483-487, 1995.

Grushka M, Bartoshuk LM: Burning mouth syndrome and oral dysesthesias, *Can J Diagnos* 99-109, June 2000.

Grushka M, Kawalec J, Epstein JB: Burning mouth syndrome: evolving concepts, *Oral Maxillofac Surg Clin North Am* 12:287-295, 2000.

Grushka M, Sessle BJ: Burning mouth syndrome, *Dent Clin North Am* 35:171-184, 1991.

Haberland CM, Allen CM, Beck FM: Referral patterns, lesion prevalence, and patient care parameters in a clinical oral pathology service, *Oral Surg Oral Med Oral Pathol Oral Radiol Endod* 87:583-588, 1999.

Lamey PJ: Burning mouth syndrome, *Dermatol Clin* 14:339-354, 1996.

Muzyka BC, De Rossi SS: A review of burning mouth syndrome, *Cutis* 64:29-35, 1999.

Yanagisawa L, Bartoshuk LM, Catalanotto FA et al: Anesthesia of the chorda tympani nerve and taste phantoms, *Physiol Behav* 63:329-335, 1998.

Wesselmann U, Reich SG: The dynias, *Semin Neurol* 16:63-74, 1996.

Dysgeusia and Hypogeusia

Ackerman BH, Kasbekar N: Disturbances of taste and smell induced by drugs, *Pharmacotherapy* 17:482-496, 1997.

Bromley SM: Smell and taste disorders: a primary care approach, *Am Fam Physician* 61:427-436, 438, 2000.

Deem DA, Yen DM, Kreshak A et al: Spontaneous resolution of dysgeusia, *Arch Otolaryngol Head Neck Surg* 122:961-963, 1996.

Nelson GM: Biology of taste buds and the clinical problem of taste loss, *Anat Rec* 253:70-78, 1998.

Osaki T, Ohshima M, Tomita Y et al: Clinical and physiological investigations in patients with taste abnormality, *J Oral Pathol Med* 25:38-43, 1996.

Schiffman SS, Graham BG, Suggs MS et al: Effect of psychotropic drugs on taste responses in young and elderly persons, *Ann N Y Acad Sci* 855:732-777, 1998.

Schiffman SS, Zervakis J, Suggs MS et al: Effect of tricyclic antidepressants on taste responses in humans and gerbils, *Pharmacol Biochem Behav* 65:599-609, 2000.

Frey Syndrome

Bonanno PC, Palaia D, Rosenberg M et al: Prophylaxis against Frey's syndrome in parotid surgery, *Ann Plast Surg* 44:498-501, 2000.

Dulguerov P, Quinodoz D, Cosendai G et al: Frey syndrome treatment with botulinum toxin, *Otolaryngol Head Neck Surg* 122:821-827, 2000.

Kaddu S, Smolle J, Komericki P et al: Auriculotemporal (Frey) syndrome in late childhood: an unusual variant presenting as gustatory flushing mimicking food allergy, *Pediatr Dermatol* 17:126-128, 2002.

Laskawi R, Drobik C, Schonebeck C: Up-to-date report of botulinum toxin type A treatment in patients with gustatory sweating (Frey's syndrome), *Laryngoscope* 108:381-384, 1998.

Laskawi R, Ellies M, Rodel R et al: Gustatory sweating: clinical implications and etiologic aspects, *J Oral Maxillofac Surg* 57:642-649, 1999.

Linder TE, Huber A, Schmid S: Frey's syndrome after parotidectomy: a retrospective and prospective analysis, *Laryngoscope* 107:1496-1501, 1997.

Mellor TK: Frey's syndrome following fracture of the mandibular condyle: case report and literature review, *Injury* 27:359-360, 1996.

Scrivani SJ, Keith DA et al: Posttraumatic gustatory neuralgia: a clinical model of trigeminal neuropathic pain, *J Orofac Pain* 12:287-292, 1998.

Shaw JE, Parker R, Hollis S et al: Gustatory sweating in diabetes mellitus, *Diabet Med* 13:1033-1037, 1996.

von Lindern JJ, Niederhagen B, Berge S et al: Frey syndrome, *Cancer* 89:1659-1663, 2000.

Osteoarthritis

Dahlstrom L: Diagnoses among referrals to a Swedish clinic specialized in temporomandibular disorders, *Acta Odontol Scand* 56:143-147, 1998.

de Bont LG, Boering G, Liem RS et al: Osteoarthritis and internal derangement of the temporomandibular joint: a light microscopic study, *J Oral Maxillofac Surg* 44:634-643, 1986.

de Leeuw R, Boering G, van der Kuijl B et al: Hard and soft tissue imaging of the temporomandibular joint 30 years after diagnosis of osteoarthrosis and internal derangement, *J Oral Maxillofac Surg* 54:1270-1280, 1996.

Dijkgraaf LC, Spijkervet FK, de Bont LG: Arthroscopic findings in osteoarthritic temporomandibular joints, *J Oral Maxillofac Surg* 57:255-268, 1999.

European Society of Osteoarthrology (ESOA): Joint destruction in arthritis and osteoarthritis: 19th symposium of the ESOA, *Agents Actions* 39(suppl):1-272, 1993.

Gynther GW, Holmlund AB, Reinholt FP et al: Temporomandibular joint involvement in generalized osteoarthritis and rheumatoid arthritis: a clinical, arthroscopic, histologic, and immunohistochemical study, *Int J Oral Maxillofac Surg* 26:10-16, 1997.

Ong TK, Franklin CD: A clinical and histopathological study of osteoarthrosis of the temporomandibular joint, *Br J Maxillofac Surg* 34:186-192, 1996.

Peyron JG, Altman RD: The epidemiology of osteoarthritis. In Moskowitz RW, Howell DS, Goldberg VM, editors: *Osteoarthritis, diagnosis and medical/surgical management*, ed 2, pp 15-37, Philadelphia, 1992, Saunders.

Rodrigo JJ, Gershwin ME: Management of the orthopedic joint. In Chapman MW, editor: *Chapman's orthopaedic surgery*, ed 3, pp 2551-2572, Philadelphia, 2001, Lippincott, Williams & Wilkins.

Rudisch A, Innerhofer K, Bertram S et al: Magnetic resonance imaging findings of internal derangement and effusion in patients with unilateral joint pain, *Oral Surg Oral Med Oral Pathol Oral Radiol Endod* 92:566-571, 2001.

Sano T, Westesson PL, Larheim TA et al: Osteoarthritis and abnormal bone marrow of the mandibular condyle, *Oral Surg Oral Med Oral Pathol Oral Radiol Endod* 87:243-252, 1999.

Takahashi T, Nagai H, Seki H et al: Relationship between joint effusion, joint pain, and protein levels in joint lavage fluid of patients with internal derangement and osteoarthritis of the temporomandibular joint, *J Oral Maxillofac Surg* 57:1187-1194, 1999.

Wiberg B, Wanman A: Signs of osteoarthrosis of the temporomandibular joints in young patients: a clinical and radiographic study, *Oral Surg Oral Med Oral Pathol Oral Radiol Endod* 86:158-164, 1998.

Rheumatoid Arthritis

Al-Mobireek AF, Darwazeh AM, Hassanin MB: Experimental induction of rheumatoid arthritis in temporomandibular joint of the guinea pig: a clinical and radiographic study, *Dentomaxillofac Radiol* 29:286-290, 2000.

Ericson S, Lundberg M: Alterations in the temporomandibular joint at various stages of rheumatoid arthritis, *Acta Rheum Scand* 13:257-274, 1967.

Gynther GW, Tronje G, Holmlund AB: Radiographic changes in the temporomandibular joint in patients with generalized osteoarthritis and rheumatoid arthritis, *Oral Surg Oral Med Oral Pathol Oral Radiol Endod* 81:613-618, 1996.

Hansson TL: Pathological aspects of arthritides and derangements. In Sarnat BG, Laskin DM, editors: *The temporomandibular joint: a biological basis for clinical practice,* ed 4, pp 165-182, Philadelphia, 1992, WB Saunders.

Harris ED: Pathogenesis of rheumatoid arthritis, *Am J Med* 80:4-10, 1986.

Larheim TA, Bjornland T: Arthrographic findings in the temporomandibular joint in patients with rheumatic disease, *J Oral Maxillofac Surg* 47:780-784, 1989.

Marbach JJ: Arthritis of the temporomandibular joints and facial pain, *Bull Rheum Dis* 27:918-921, 1976-1977.

Speculand B, Hensher R, Powell D: Total prosthetic replacement of the TMJ: experience with two systems 1988-1997, *Br J Oral Maxillofac Surg* 38:360-369, 2000.

Voog U, Alstergren P, Eliasson S et al: Progression of radiographic changes in the temporomandibular joints of patients with rheumatoid arthritis in relation to inflammatory markers and mediators in blood, *Acta Odontol Scand* 62:7-13, 2004.

Wenneberg B, Kononen M, Kallenberg A: Radiographic changes in the temporomandibular joint of patients with rheumatoid arthritis, psoriatic arthritis, and ankylosing spondylitis, *J Craniomandib Disord* 4:35-39, 1990.

Temporomandibular Joint Dysfunction

Adame CG, Monje F, Offnoz M et al: Effusion in magnetic resonance imaging of the temporomandibular joint: a study of 123 joints, *J Oral Maxillofac Surg* 56:314-318, 1998.

Burakoff RP, Kaplan AS: Temporomandibular disorders: current concepts of epidemiology, classification, and treatment, *J Pain Symptom Manage* 8:165-172, 1993.

Gaggl A, Schultes G, Santler G et al: Clinical and magnetic resonance findings in the temporomandibular joints of patients before and after orthognathic surgery, *Br J Oral Maxillofac Surg* 37:41-45, 1999.

Greene CS, Laskin DM: Long-term evaluation of treatment for myofascial pain-dysfunction syndrome: a comparative analysis, *J Am Dent Assoc* 107:235-238, 1983.

Kaplan AS, Assael LA: *Temporomandibular disorders: diagnosis and treatment,* Philadelphia, 1991, WB Saunders.

Laskin DM, Greene CS, Hylander WL: *Temporomandibular disorders: an evidence-based approach to diagnosis and treatment,* Chicago, 2006, Quintessence.

Lundh H, Westesson PL: Clinical signs of temporomandibular joint internal derangement in adults: an epidemiologic study, *Oral Surg Oral Med Oral Pathol* 72:637-641, 1991.

McQuary HJ, Tramer M, Nye BA et al: A systematic review of antidepressants in neuropathic pain, *Pain* 68:217-227, 1996.

Suvinen TI, Reade PC: Temporomandibular disorders: a critical review of the nature of pain and its assessment, *J Orofac Pain* 9:317-339, 1995.

Takahashi T, Nagai H, Seki H et al: Relationship between joint effusion, joint pain, and protein levels in joint lavage fluid of patients with internal derangement and osteoarthritis of the temporomandibular joint, *J Oral Maxillofac Surg* 57:1187-1194, 1999.

Vickers ER, Cousins MJ, Walker S et al: Analysis of 50 patients with atypical odontalgia: a preliminary report on pharmacological procedures for diagnosis and treatment, *Oral Surg Oral Med Oral Pathol Oral Radiol Endod* 85:24-32, 1998.

Vickers ER, Cousins MJ, Woodhouse A: Pain description and severity of chronic orofacial pain conditions, *Aust Dent J* 43:403-409, 1998.

Westesson P-L, Yamamoto M, Sano T et al: Temporomandibular joint. In Som PM, Curtin HD, editors: *Head and neck imaging,* ed 4, pp 995-1053, St Louis, 2003, Mosby.

Widmark G: On surgical intervention in the temporomandibular joint, *Swed Dent J* 123(suppl):1-87, 1997.

Wright WJ Jr: Temporomandibular disorders: occurrence of specific diagnoses and response to conservative management: clinical observations, *J Craniomandib Disord* 4:150-155, 1986.

Yatani H, Minakuchi H, Matsuka Y et al: The long-term effect of occlusal therapy on self-administered treatment outcomes of TMD, *J Orofacial Pain* 12:75-88, 1998.

Temporomandibular Joint Ankylosis

Chidzonga MM: Temporomandibular joint ankylosis: review of thirty-two cases, *Br J Oral Maxillofac Surg* 14:136-138, 1999.

Freedus MS, William DZ, Doyle PK: Principles of treatment of temporomandibular joint ankylosis, *J Oral Surg* 33:757-765, 1975.

Koorbusch GF, Zeitler DL, Fotos PG et al: Psoriatic arthritis of the temporomandibular joints with ankylosis, *Oral Surg Oral Med Oral Pathol* 71:267-274, 1991.

Manganello-Souza LC, Mariani PB: Temporomandibular joint ankylosis: report of 14 cases, *Int J Oral Maxillofac Surg* 32:24-29, 2002.

Rowe NL: Ankylosis of the temporomandibular joint. Part 1, *J R Coll Surg Edinb* 27:67-79, 1982.

Rowe NL: Ankylosis of the temporomandibular joint. Part 2, *J R Coll Surg Edinb* 27:167-173, 1982.

Rowe NL: Ankylosis of the temporomandibular joint. Part 3, *J R Coll Surg Edinb* 27:209-218, 1982.

Salins PC: New perspectives in the management of craniomandibular ankylosis, *Int J Oral Maxillofac Surg* 29:337-340, 2000.

Sarma UC, Dave PK: Temporomandibular joint ankylosis: an Indian experience, *Oral Surg Oral Med Oral Pathol* 72:660-664, 1991.

Su-Gwan K: Treatment of temporomandibular joint ankylosis with temporalis muscle and fascia flap, *Int J Oral Maxillofac Surg* 30:189-193, 2001.

19

Forensic Dentistry

EDWARD E. HERSCHAFT

CHAPTER OUTLINE

Forensic dentistry, which is also referred to as *forensic odontology*, is the area of dentistry concerned with the correct management, examination, evaluation, and presentation of dental evidence in criminal or civil legal proceedings in the interest of justice. Thus the forensic dentist must be knowledgeable in both dentistry and law.

Classically, forensic dentistry can be considered a subspecialty of oral and maxillofacial pathology. This is analogous to the relationship in medicine between forensic pathology and pathology. The requirements of forensic dental field work, however, often demand an interdisciplinary knowledge of dental science. This has resulted in other dental specialists and general dentists joining oral and maxillofacial pathologists in providing legal authorities with dental expertise.

Regardless of background, forensic dentists assist legal authorities by preparing dental evidence in the following situations:

- Management and maintenance of dental records that comply with legal requirements to document all unique dental information—these data are the foundation on which dental identification of the patient is accomplished and potential malpractice litigation is reduced.

- Identification of human remains, through the comparison of antemortem and postmortem dental information, in cases that involve the death of an individual or multiple deaths in mass fatality incident (MFI) situations.

- Collection and analysis of patterned marks (bite marks) in inanimate material or injured tissue—this evidence can be compared with, and potentially related to, a specific human or animal dentition.

- Recognition of the signs and symptoms of human abuse (including intimate-partner violence [IPV], elder abuse, and child abuse) and the dental health care practitioner's rights and responsibilities when reporting such abuse.

- Presentation of dental evidence as an expert witness in identification, bite mark, human abuse, malpractice, fraud, and personal injury cases.

RECORD MANAGEMENT

The dental record is a legal document, owned by the dentist or an incorporated dental practice, which contains all subjective and objective information about the patient. Initially, this information is secured when the patient's medical and dental history is obtained. Results

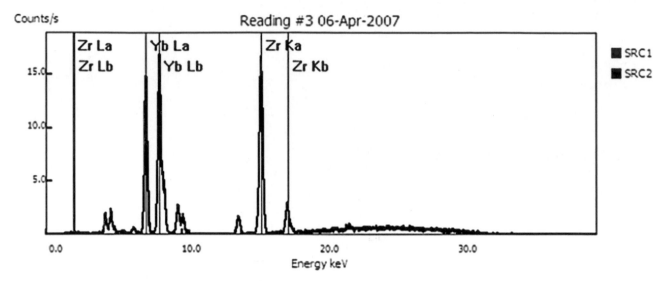

Fig. 19-1   The x-ray fluorescence (XRF) spectrum from a particle recovered from a cremation retort. The spectrum makes this a match for the restorative resin Four Seasons or Tetric Ceram (Ivoclar, Amherst, NY). *(Courtesy of Dr. Mary A. Bush and Peter J. Bush.)*

of the physical examination of the dentition and supporting oral and paraoral structures are recorded.

In addition, the results of clinical laboratory tests, study casts, photographs, and radiographs become components of the record. With this database, the dentist can develop a thorough assessment of all of the patient's medical and dental problems. Subsequent documentation of this "problem list" facilitates the development of a plan of treatment and prognosis for the patient.

The treatment plan addresses the management of both systemic and oral problems. It can then be periodically revised and updated as problems resolve or as new ones develop. Supplemental material, such as dental laboratory authorizations, referral letters from other practitioners, statements of informed consent, written prescriptions, and insurance and financial statements, also is included and stored in the record.

The progress notes (i.e., daily log of actual treatment rendered) should contain information about restorative and therapeutic procedures provided. This information should include documentation of the specific brand of dental material used in restorative procedures. This concept has forensic import because each dental restorative product contains inorganic materials, trace elements, and fillers that are unique to that product and can be detected by **x-ray fluorescence** (XRF) technology even after incineration. The XRF trace element and major element analysis of dental remains may be useful as an adjunct to traditional evaluation of dental information in some forensic settings, including cremation and dismemberment cases (Fig. 19-1).

Unusual physiologic and psychologic reactions and the patient's comments concerning therapy are entered in the record. Summaries of telephone conversations with patients, consultants, insurance company representatives, or legal authorities should be noted. All entries should be signed or initialed by recording personnel. Changes in the record should not be erased but corrected by a single line drawn through the incorrect material. This method permits the original entry to remain readable and removes any questions concerning fraudulent intent to alter recorded information.

It is becoming more common for dental records to be maintained electronically, and numerous commercial and individually designed computer software programs have been marketed to assist the dentist in collecting and preserving the patient's dental information. The obvious advantage of computer-generated dental records is that they can be easily networked and transferred for routine professional consultation or forensic cases requiring dental records for identification. Issues related to patient privacy in this regard are no different from those considered with paper documents.

In the United States, the Privacy Rule governing the use of protected health information (PHI) is regulated under the federal Health Insurance Portability and Accountability Act (HIPAA) of 1996. Despite the establishment of the Privacy Rule, the ability and necessity of forensic dentists, law enforcement personnel, medical examiners (MEs), and coroners to obtain released antemortem dental and medical records for forensic purposes was recognized and provided for in the HIPAA legislation.

The potential charge of insurance fraud associated with the enhancement of dental lesions or restorations on computer-generated or scanned **digital radiography** (DR) can be avoided if a clinician stores and maintains unaltered images. This is accomplished using programs with unchangeable, secure tagged block file extensions in their native file formats. When duplicates or copies are required, working images should be generated.

Computer-assisted management technology (e.g. WinID3 dental comparison software bridged with the Dexis digital radiography program) has been an asset in expediting the comparison of antemortem and postmortem dental record information in recent MFI events, including the World Trade Center terrorist attack, the Indian Ocean tsunami disaster, and the Hurricane Katrina recovery effort. Additionally, software such as Adobe Photoshop and Mideo Systems casePACS, facilitates the superimposition of digitally scanned radiographs and photographs for comparison.

Whether preserved in written form or by using a computer database, the principles of record management describe a mechanism that ensures that dental information, which may be required to resolve a forensic problem, is properly maintained and retrievable. Additionally, records preserved in this manner are reliable evidentiary material if subpoenaed in peer review or malpractice litigation proceedings.

Time limits concerning how long records must be retained vary among the states. As a rule, states mandate that records be kept for 7 to 10 years. Federal legislation related to the problem of missing persons in the United States requires that records of pediatric dental patients be retained until the patient reaches the age of majority.

IDENTIFICATION

Legal situations often revolve around the establishment of a person's proper identity. Any death not certified by an individual's own physician must be referred to the medical examiner (ME) or coroner for review. However, cases requiring an **autopsy** to determine the time, cause, and manner of death represent a small percentage of cases. When required, these tasks are the responsibility of a coroner or ME. These officials are charged with the role of establishing identification; determining the cause, mechanism, and mode or manner of death; and issuing a death certificate. Besides identification of the decedent, these key issues of death investigation for the coroner or ME are defined according to the following:

- **Cause of death.** The disease, injury, or chemical or physical agent responsible for initiating the lethal sequence of events (e.g., myocardial infarction, cancer, bullet, knife, poison, ligature, lightning, infectious agent)
- **Mechanism of death.** The pathologic process that results in death (e.g., congestive heart failure, cardiac

arrhythmias, asphyxia, sepsis, exsanguination, renal failure, and hepatic failure.)

- **Mode or manner of death.** According to the NASH classification, the mode or manner of death is considered to be **N**atural, **A**ccidental, **S**uicide, or **H**omicide. Natural deaths are caused exclusively by disease. Accidental deaths result from an environmental or human tragedy (e.g., lightning strike, vehicular incident).
- **Undetermined death.** Although the cause and mechanism of death may be resolved, the manner or mode may not be established because of decomposition, dismemberment, or postmortem destruction of the remains by insects or feral animals.

The coroner is an elected official and, depending on the laws of each state, does not necessarily have to be a physician or have advanced training in death investigation. An ME is an appointed official who is a pathologist specifically trained in forensic medicine. Many jurisdictions use forensic pathologists, and this trend has contributed to the professionalizing of a position increasingly involved with the interpretation of advanced scientific techniques requiring knowledge of toxicology, ballistics, pharmacology, and criminalistics, as well as pathology.

A death certificate, identifying the decedent, is required before probation of a will, release of life insurance claims, or resolution of other affairs associated with the settlement of an estate. Criminal cases involving homicide, suicide, and fraudulent misidentification may also require the expertise of forensic dentists and other forensic scientists trained in identification techniques. These professionals act as consultants to the coroner or ME and assist in this aspect of a death investigation.

Besides analysis of the dentition, the most common methods of identification include personal recognition, fingerprinting (friction ridge analysis), physical anthropologic examination of bones, and serologic and genetic (DNA) comparison techniques.

Additionally, the use of facial superimposition techniques (when the teeth are visible) and facial reconstruction techniques may also permit scientifically supported comparisons for identification. Each method has its advantages and disadvantages. However, all rely on the principle that identification is the positive correlation obtained by comparing known information about a suspect or victim with unique facts retrieved by physical examination of the suspect or victim.

Regardless of the method used to identify a decedent, the results of the antemortem and postmortem data comparison lead to one of the following four situations:

1. **Positive identification.** There is sufficient uniqueness among the comparable items in the antemor-

tem and postmortem databases, and no major differences are observed.

2. **Presumptive (possible) identification.** There are commonalities among the comparable items in the antemortem and postmortem databases; however, enough information may be missing from either source to prevent the establishment of a positive identification.

3. **Insufficient identification evidence.** There is insufficient supportive evidence available to compare and arrive at a conclusion based on scientific principles.

4. **Exclusion of identification evidence.** Either explainable or unexplainable discrepancies exist among comparable items in the antemortem and postmortem databases. This results in inconsistencies that prevent the establishment of any identification. Exclusion may be just as important as a determination of positive identification.

PERSONAL RECOGNITION

Personal recognition is the least reliable method used to identify an individual. It is often based on the visual identification of a decedent by a family member, friend, or acquaintance. This process assesses artifactual material, such as clothing, jewelry, keys, wallet contents, luggage, other personal effects, scars, and tattoos to determine identification. Evidence in this type of identification can be accidentally or purposely exchanged between bodies. This can occur in MFI situations or when there is criminal intent to create a misidentification in cases of identity theft or alias associated with criminal activity.

Even when a body is viewed shortly after death, distraught relatives can inadvertently misidentify the decedent. After the occurrence of postmortem changes associated with soft tissue decomposition, insect and burn artifact, or dismemberment, this method of identification may be precluded (Figs. 19-2 and 19-3).

FINGERPRINTING

Anthropometry was the first "scientific" system police used to identify criminals. The French law enforcement officer Alphonse Bertillon developed this system in the latter part of the nineteenth century. The method was unreliable and flawed because it relied on biometric physical measurements of the head and body, individual markings including scars and tattoos, and other personal characteristics. Bertillon's anthropometry identification process was eventually replaced by analysis of the epidermal friction ridges of the fingers, palms, and feet commonly referred to as **fingerprinting.**

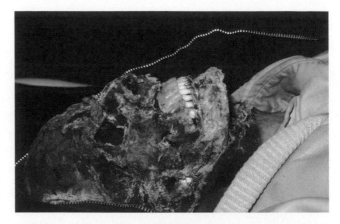

Fig. 19-2   Unrecognizable partially decomposed human remains with a maxillary removable partial denture in place. Notice that the skin tissue of the neck that has been protected by the windbreaker jacket has not reached the stage of decomposition of the tissues of the exposed face. *(Courtesy of Dr. Raymond D. Rawson.)*

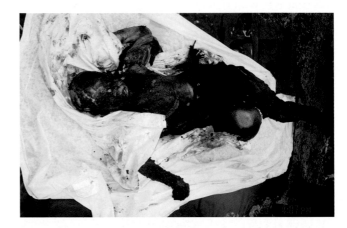

Fig. 19-3   A burn victim requiring identification by dental, DNA, or fingerprint methodology rather than personal recognition. *(Courtesy of Dr. Raymond D. Rawson.)*

By the beginning of the twentieth century, forensic science had recognized that the ridgelike patterns on the fingertips and palms are unique for each person. These friction ridges are genetically determined, and not even homozygous twins have the same patterns of loops, arches, and whorls. A principal variation in the fingerprints of twins is that they appear as mirror images of each other. The variation in combinations of the loops, arches, and whorls permits a scientific comparison of fingerprint records with the prints of an unidentified decedent.

Because the fingerprint pattern is inherited, it is a static characteristic and remains unchanged throughout life. This is an important advantage when one compares fingerprint identification with dental identification. The teeth and supporting structures have fluid characteristics. Dental patterns change as teeth erupt, exfoliate, decay, become restored, and, perhaps, are eventually extracted and replaced with implants or other prosthetic devices.

Unlike dental records, which are principally retained in private dental offices in the Americas and Western Europe, fingerprint information is maintained by governmental agencies. Several states retain records of noncriminals who work in sensitive occupations. In this regard, Nevada has a fingerprint database for employees in the gaming industry. The Criminal Justice Information Services (CJIS) Division of the Federal Bureau of Investigation (FBI) contains approximately 47 million fingerprint records in its Criminal Master File. This is the largest biometric database in the world, and it is retained within the Integrated Automated Fingerprint Identification System (IAFIS).

The establishment of the CJIS Division's IAFIS files permits automated computer data entry and search capabilities for matching and retrieval of fingerprint images. This information is available for electronic exchange among law enforcement agencies for identification purposes. Included in the IAFIS database are criminal and civil 10-print fingerprint records, latent fingerprint services, and subject and criminal history search capabilities. Information from this fingerprint repository is shared with international legal agencies such as Interpol and the Royal Canadian Mounted Police.

Fingerprint nomenclature is standardized in IAFIS, and all fingerprint experts use the same terminology worldwide. This advantage is not observed in dental identification, in which numerous charting and tooth-numbering systems are used. Because soft tissues decompose shortly after death, the friction ridge patterns within the epidermis may not be retrievable for fingerprint comparison. This is the principal disadvantage of fingerprint identification.

PHYSICAL ANTHROPOLOGIC EXAMINATION OF BONES AND TEETH

Forensic anthropologists and forensic dentists often work together to resolve problems associated with identification. Both disciplines are concerned with analysis of calcified structures of the body—bones and teeth. Historically, this anatomic material has assisted forensic anthropologists and dentists in determining the race, age, and sex of a person (Table 19-1). These characteristics have become less distinct in some populations as individuals from different cultures and races have intermarried and blended these genetically determined features in their offspring.

Determination of the age of an individual is helpful in cases involving limited population fatality incidents in which the ages of the victims vary. Immigration officials often deal with situations in which designation of juvenile or adult is important when considering the status of refugees or illegal aliens. In these settings the assessment of dental evidence may provide resolution.

In addition to the study of osseous material, the teeth can be evaluated clinically, radiographically, and biochemically to determine the age of the decedent. The basis for this analysis is related to progressive

Table **19-1**   **Skeletal Anthropologic Variations Associated with Racial and Sexual Characteristics of the Skull**

	RACIAL CHARACTERISTICS		
	White	**Black**	**Asian/Native American**
Width	Narrow	Narrow	Broad
Height	High	Low	Intermediate
Profile	Straight	Prognathic	Intermediate
Orbit	Triangular/teardrop	Square	Circular
Nasal opening	Tapered	Wide	Rounded
Palate	Narrow	Wide	Intermediate

	SEXUAL CHARACTERISTICS	
	Male	**Female**
Size	Large	Small
Glabellar (supraorbital) ridges	Pronounced	Not developed
Mastoid process	Large	Small
Occipital area	Pronounced muscle lines	Minimal muscle lines
Mandible	Larger, broader ramus	Smaller
Forehead	Steeper, slopes posteriorly	Rounded, more vertical

changes in forming and developing teeth, eruption patterns, and levels of metabolically stable tissue factors, including aspartic acid enantiomers. This information, combined with analysis of the calcification centers of the hand and wrist, can be used to estimate the precise age of a person who is younger than 20 years of age.

Depending on the type of case being studied, several techniques are available to estimate chronologic dental age. In individuals younger than 20 years old, this is most often accomplished through morphologic and histologic analysis of dental and skeletal material. Included in the methodology for this type of age evaluation is the radiographic assessment of the calcification stage of the third molars and analysis of ground sections of teeth for variations in the following patterns:

- Attrition
- Periodontal attachment
- Secondary dentin
- Cementum apposition
- Root resorption
- Transparency

There are variations in the calcification and eruption patterns among various ethnic and cultural groups, and studies have been undertaken to delineate these differences further. After the third molars, long bones, and bones of the wrist and hand are completely developed, evaluation of biochemical components of the calcified structures and collagen is the most accurate method for determining chronologic age.

Methods that rely on an analysis of the rate of racemization of the stereoisomers of aspartic acid in enamel and dentin can be used to determine an accurate chronologic age. This is related to the fact that the change from the L-form of this amino acid to its mirror image D-form occurs over time. Thus the ratio of the L- to D-forms of aspartic acid in the dentition is directly related to the age of the individual. Often, anthropologic and dental age analysis is helpful in arriving at a presumptive identification based on the criteria noted previously.

Positive identification may be achievable when the skull and facial bones are used as a foundation to reconstruct the facial soft tissues (Figs. 19-4 to 19-6). Three-dimensional (3D) computer images, computed tomography (CT) images, and radiographs have even been used in the replication of the face of Europe's oldest mummified human, a male dubbed Ötzi, whose 5300-year-old remains were removed from glacial ice in the Ötztal Alps on the Austrian-Italian border.

With knowledge of the anatomic relationships between the skull and face, antemortem facial photographs or radiographs can be superimposed for comparison with the skull of an unknown. Video superimposition with two television cameras and an electronic mixing device has been used successfully to

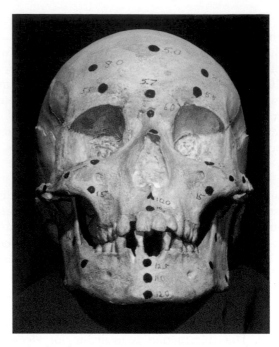

Fig. 19-4 Reconstruction of the facial soft tissue uses predetermined, standard anthropologic thickness measurements for specific points around the face. These measurements are based on variables that are related to racial and sexual characteristics. *(Courtesy of Dr. Cleve Smith.)*

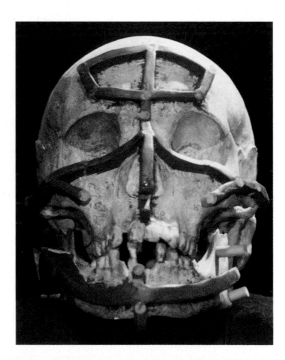

Fig. 19-5 The soft tissue thickness points can be connected with sculpting clay or digitized on a computer screen. The ultimate result of these techniques is a re-creation of the contour of the soft tissue features that permits a visual identification. *(Courtesy of Dr. Cleve Smith.)*

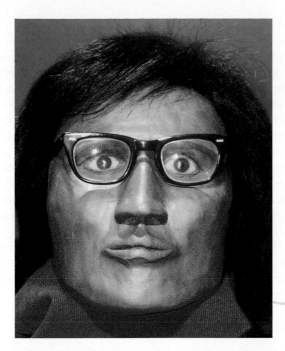

Fig. 19-6 The width of the mouth is related to the interpupillary distance. The length and shape of the nose are determined by the relationship between the inferior and superior nasal spines. If known, then the addition of a specific hairstyle, eyeglasses, and eye color can further individualize a facial reconstruction. *(Courtesy of Dr. Cleve Smith.)*

overlay a photograph of a human face on an image of a skull for identification. The development of computer software programs capable of superimposition has further facilitated the process.

The anterior dentition of the skull can be overlayed and compared with a smiling antemortem photograph. The shapes and positions of the individual teeth and their relationships to each other have been considered distinctive enough features on which to base identification, as have certain significant cranial and facial landmarks, including the orbits, nasal openings, malar eminence, and chin. Prosthetic joint replacements, intraosseous and dental implants, and radiographic signs of prior bone fracture are other anthropologic findings that can be used to facilitate identification.

Additionally, prosthetic devices, implanted defibrillators and pacemakers, and dental and osseous implants are designated with individual identification code numbers provided by their manufacturers. These codes can be visualized in the various devices and are useful in identifying individuals in cremation and dismemberment scenarios when the teeth and fingerprints are not available for evaluation.

SEROLOGIC AND GENETIC (DNA) COMPARISON

Every individual is unique by virtue of his or her chromosomal DNA—a polymer structured as a double helix and composed of four different nucleotides. The polymorphic sequencing of these nucleotides along the two strands of the DNA molecule accounts for the genetic diversity of all living things. This "ultimate identification material" was first used forensically to obtain a conviction in a criminal case in 1986, and DNA comparison has since become an accepted forensic method to resolve problems of identification.

Before 1986, comparison of antigenic markers found on red blood cells (RBCs) and in body fluids of secretors of these markers among the human population was traditionally used as a means of exculpatory (exclusionary) evidence. Because the ABH antigenic surface markers of RBCs are not discriminatory, this type of evidence was primarily used to exclude a suspect or victim when negative comparative results were achieved. Positive comparisons were justified only to place the suspect or victim in a population of individuals having similar serologic antigens.

Although DNA has become the principal biologic substance used to effect a positive identification, antigenic surface markers A, B, and H of the ABO blood group system, as well as various components of the rhesus (Rh) and Lewis systems, continue to be accepted for medicolegal comparison. The ability to secrete the ABH antigens in saliva and other body fluids is genetically determined, and more than 80% of individuals are secretors. With appropriate laboratory tests, even dried samples of fluid and blood can be analyzed for these markers.

DNA found in human cells is composed of chromosomal and mitochondrial DNA (mtDNA). Two copies of chromosomal DNA are incorporated into the nuclei of a person's cells by DNA provided from both parents. However, hundreds of copies of mtDNA are contained in the cytoplasm of these cells. This DNA is only maternally transferred and can be isolated from cells without nuclei such as RBCs. Unlike nuclear DNA, mtDNA is single stranded and circular. Because there is no mixing of sequence types from generation to generation in maternally transferred mtDNA, it can be compared with that of distant maternal relatives to effect identification when other reference sources are unavailable.

Restriction fragment length polymorphism (RFLP) and polymerase chain reaction (PCR) analyses are the principal laboratory techniques used to compare and evaluate fragments of DNA material from a suspect or victim's biologic forensic specimens (e.g., semen, vaginal fluid, teeth, soft tissues, saliva). Both are extremely accurate, precise, and reproducible; these methods are used when the conditions of the sample DNA presented dictate the need for their respective advantages.

RFLP methods result in splitting source DNA into thousands of fragments using "biologic scissors" known as *restriction enzymes*. Fragment size varies among individuals related to the variable number of tandem repeats (VNTR) of base pairs. These short segments of DNA contain a number of repeat units that differ among individuals. After gel separation of the fragments and transfer to a nylon mesh, specific DNA fragments are identified using oligonucleotides labeled with radioisotopes. Analysis of a series of different VNTR loci permits generation of an individual DNA profile.

A match of four or more VNTR loci is consistent with a positive match between DNA evidence gathered from suspect, victim, or crime scene evidence. The RFLP method requires large amounts of high molecular weight DNA, a major disadvantage. Small DNA samples (<100 ng) or degraded evidence in which the DNA has become denatured because of extreme heat or pH variation requires an analytic method other than RFLP.

The evaluation of minute quantities of DNA or DNA that has undergone degradation can be accomplished with the highly sensitive PCR test. Using this laboratory technique, smaller VNTR loci of a specific DNA sequence can be amplified into enough copies for sufficient analysis. Because of its high degree of sensitivity, PCR analysis has been used to evaluate small amounts of DNA from a suspect's clothing left at the scene of a crime, as well as from bone fragments from the Vietnam War. DNA amplification of microsatellite loci (referred to as *STRs*) and minisatellite loci (or *LTRs*) using PCR, is referred to as *AmpFLP analysis*.

The hard and soft tissues of the oral cavity and saliva are often good sources for DNA material. However, if the teeth or other hard structures of the mouth are to be used for the collection of DNA evidence, then the identification value of these structures should be considered (beyond their ability to yield a harvest DNA). A tooth or jaw fragment capriciously destroyed can result in the loss of valuable radiographic and anatomic sources for eventual dental identification. Besides the obvious source of DNA from human tissues, the forensic dentist often considers the evaluation of chewed gum, cigarette remains, licked envelopes, stamps, or similar inanimate objects as potential sources for DNA evidence using PCR analysis described previously.

Passage of the DNA Identification Act of 1994 and the establishment of the FBI's National DNA Index System (NDIS) in 1998 have facilitated the exchange and comparison of DNA profiles among federal, state, and local crime laboratories in the United States. This is accomplished electronically through the FBI Laboratory's Combined DNA Index System (CODIS). Through the CODIS computer program's forensic and offender indexes, biologic evidence from crime scenes can be linked to DNA profiles of individuals convicted of sex offenses and other felonies. As of March 2007, the total number of DNA profiles contained in the CODIS databases was more than 4.5 million. More than 47,000 successful comparisons ("hits") were made among cases in which the CODIS system was activated. This represents a 98% success rate linking DNA from a crime scene with similar material from the convicted offender profiles.

The U.S. Department of Defense has initiated a policy of obtaining DNA samples on all military personnel. This DNA "fingerprint" has significantly reduced the possibility of another unknown soldier among future military casualties. Despite the positive effects of DNA evidence in resolving questions of identity, the technique is not without controversy. Challenges have been made by population geneticists, concerned about random matching and variations among racial subgroups.

DENTAL EVALUATION
BASIC PRINCIPLES

In an identification case, the principal advantage of dental evidence is that, like other hard tissue, it is often preserved indefinitely after death. Although the status of a person's teeth changes throughout life, the combination of decayed, missing, and filled teeth is measurable, reproducible, and comparable at any fixed point in time. Therefore, like the comparison of unique patterns in a fingerprint, a scientific, objective analysis of antemortem and postmortem dental variables is achievable.

The presence and position of individual teeth and the respective anatomic, restorative, and pathologic components provide the database for the antemortem and postmortem comparison (Fig. 19-7). The pattern of the palatal ridge, ridges on the lip surface, and radiographic outline of the maxillary and frontal sinuses are also considered unique. In addition, the legal community accepts the fact that dentists can recognize procedures that they have performed.

Problems associated with dental identification information are often related to acquiring and interpreting antemortem records. Most antemortem dental records are retrieved from private-sector dental providers. However, dental records may be recovered from insurance carriers, dental schools, hospitals, clinics, state and federal prisons, military files, and the FBI National Crime Information Center (NCIC).

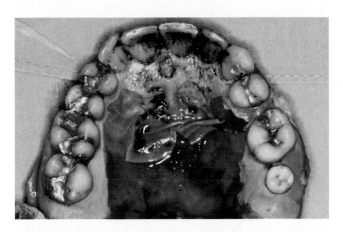

Fig. 19-7   The combination of decayed, missing, and filled teeth, along with unique anatomic and pathologic findings, provides the database for comparison in a dental identification. Note the microdont in the maxillary left quadrant.

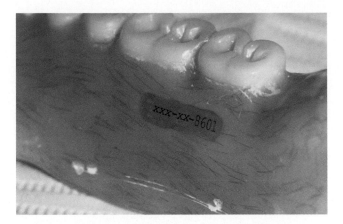

Fig. 19-8   Denture identification is accomplished by inserting a typed name or code number (i.e., Social Security number, hospital patient number) in an area of the denture that will not interfere with the aesthetics of the prosthesis. This procedure is performed in the laboratory during the final acrylic pack. Information can also be engraved in the framework of an all-metal appliance.

To initiate a request for antemortem records, a putative (suspected) identification is required. Reports of missing and unidentified persons, obtained from law enforcement agencies, are the principal source for this material. Thousands of victims who cannot be identified by fingerprint methods remain unidentified because a putative identification has not been established.

The FBI-NCIC computer registry of missing and unidentified persons was established to help rectify this problem. This computer system maintains demographic, dental, and medical information on missing persons. It attempts to match these data with similar facts obtained from unidentified bodies. The latter information is submitted by various investigative and legal agencies. Potentially, the otherwise unidentifiable victims of random violence, serial homicides, terrorist acts, and child abduction can now be identified without the need to determine a putative identification. A disadvantage of the NCIC computer identification system is that it does not have the capability to identify possible decedents based solely on dental information.

The National Dental Image Repository (NDIR) has been established to address this issue. Law enforcement agencies can voluntarily post supplemental dental images related to NCIC Missing, Unidentified, and Wanted Person records on the NDIR secure website. Thus access, retrieval, and review of dental information by qualified forensic odontologists who are members of the NDIR Review Panel can facilitate dental comparisons. The NDIR website is located at Law Enforcement Online (LEO) at http://cgate.leo.gov. This repository permits law enforcement, criminal justice, and public safety authorities to maintain a national and international method of electronic communication, education, and sharing of dental information.

The Armed Forces, Department of Veterans Affairs, and many states require that identifying markings be placed on removable dental prostheses (Fig. 19-8). The American Dental Association also supports this policy. It is an attempt to provide a basis for identification among the substantial population of completely or partially edentulous individuals in the United States.

Identifying markings in dental prostheses are important because even if dental records of an edentulous person can be obtained, they may not reflect the current status of the ridges and alveolar bone. Commonly used information for identifying marking in removable dental prostheses includes the person's name, driver's license number, and/or other identification number.

Even when a suspected identification is achieved, it may still be difficult to secure antemortem dental records. The family or acquaintances of the victim may not know where dental treatment was sought. Reviewing the victim's canceled bank checks or medical deductions on tax records may be helpful in locating antemortem dental records in such cases.

Although records obtained from institutional or governmental dental facilities routinely indicate all restored teeth, this is not true of charts forwarded from private dentists. In these instances, previously restored teeth often are not charted unless the current dentist intends to re-treat them. Therefore, in these records, the antemortem radiographs and progress notes become the principal sources for dental information.

Unfortunately, the nomenclature associated with dental charting systems is not standardized (Table 19-2). In 1984, the American Dental Association

Table **19-2** **Dental Numbering Systems**

PERMANENT TEETH		
Maxillary Right Mandibular Right		Maxillary Left Mandibular Left

UNIVERSAL NUMBERING SYSTEM

| 1 | 2 | 3 | 4 | 5 | 6 | 7 | 8 | 9 | 10 | 11 | 12 | 13 | 14 | 15 | 16 |
| 32 | 31 | 30 | 29 | 28 | 27 | 26 | 25 | 24 | 23 | 22 | 21 | 20 | 19 | 18 | 17 |

ZSIGMONDY/PALMER SYSTEM

| 8 | 7 | 6 | 5 | 4 | 3 | 2 | 1⏐1 | 2 | 3 | 4 | 5 | 6 | 7 | 8 |
| 8 | 7 | 6 | 5 | 4 | 3 | 2 | 1⏐1 | 2 | 3 | 4 | 5 | 6 | 7 | 8 |

FEDERATION DENTAIRE INTERNATIONALE TWO-DIGIT SYSTEM

| 18 | 17 | 16 | 15 | 14 | 13 | 12 | 11 | 21 | 22 | 23 | 24 | 25 | 26 | 27 | 28 |
| 48 | 47 | 46 | 45 | 44 | 43 | 42 | 41 | 31 | 32 | 33 | 34 | 35 | 36 | 37 | 38 |

DECIDUOUS TEETH		

UNIVERSAL NUMBERING SYSTEM

| A | B | C | D | E | F | G | H | I | J |
| T | S | R | Q | P | O | N | M | L | K |

ALTERNATE UNIVERSAL NUMBERING SYSTEM

| 4D | 5D | 6D | 7D | 8D | 9D | 10D | 11D | 12D | 13D |
| 29D | 28D | 27D | 26D | 25D | 24D | 23D | 22D | 21D | 20D |

ZSIGMONDY/PALMER SYSTEM

| E | D | C | B | A⏐A | B | C | D | E |
| E | D | C | B | A⏐A | B | C | D | E |

FEDERATION DENTAIRE INTERNATIONALE TWO-DIGIT SYSTEM

| 55 | 54 | 53 | 52 | 51 | 61 | 62 | 63 | 64 | 65 |
| 85 | 84 | 83 | 82 | 81 | 71 | 72 | 73 | 74 | 75 |

adopted the Universal Tooth Numbering System. All insurance companies, the Armed Forces, dental schools, and most dentists in the United States now use this system. It should be used in all forensic dental cases.

In the Universal Numbering System, a consecutive number from 1 to 32 is assigned to the adult dentition. It begins with the maxillary right third molar and ends with the mandibular right third molar. The deciduous dentition is identified by letters from A to T, beginning with the maxillary right deciduous second molar and ending with the mandibular right deciduous second molar. Thus the quadrants are identified in a clockwise direction, beginning with the maxillary right.

Other tooth numbering methods include the Zsigmondy/Palmer System and the Federation Dentaire Internationale (FDI) Two-Digit System. Each uses a different coding technique to identify dental quadrants and specific teeth.

The Zsigmondy/Palmer System stresses the anatomic likeness of the eight tooth types in each symbolically identified dental quadrant. Homologous permanent teeth are assigned the same number from 1 to 8. Deciduous teeth are assigned letters A through E.

The FDI Two-Digit System is endorsed by the World Health Organization (WHO) and is used in most developed countries, except the United States. The first digit represents the quadrant. Quadrants 1 to 4 are assigned for permanent teeth; 5 to 8 represent quadrants for the primary dentition. As in the Universal Numbering System, the quadrants are identified in a clockwise direction, beginning with the maxillary right. The second digit designates the permanent tooth type from 1 to 8, or deciduous tooth type from 1 to 5.

Thus in the Universal Numbering System, tooth 12 is the maxillary left first bicuspid. In the FDI Two-Digit System, tooth 12 (one-two) is the maxillary right lateral incisor. In the Zsigmondy/Palmer System, all lateral incisors are designated with a No. 2 code. The position of a specific No. 2 tooth is diagrammatically indicated by a symbolic quadrant.

Unless the forensic dentist knows which system has been used to encode the teeth in the antemortem record, all teeth should be referred to by their actual names. This method will prevent errors because all dentists use the same anatomic nomenclature when referring to individual teeth.

Dental identification problems may be further compounded because dental radiographs can be mounted and viewed from right to left or vice versa. Intraoral radiographic duplicating film does not contain a raised dot to assist the dentist in orienting the film for mounting. The lack of this orienting device can lead to transposition of dental evidence and potential misidentification based on an incorrect comparison. Panoramic radiographic duplicating film, however, does contain a series of notches on one side to indicate that the film is not an original.

With the advent of aesthetic materials for posterior restorations and the reduction in the incidence of caries, it may be difficult for the forensic dentist to determine whether restorations are present by simple visual assessment of the teeth. In addition, the postmortem dental evaluation is often performed in an autopsy room, temporary morgue, or funeral home. In these locations, proper lighting and access to dental instruments, which can facilitate analysis of the oral structures, are not readily available for detailed examination.

Often, there are additional demands for immediacy in providing a coroner, ME, or other legal agent with the results of a dental identification. These demands further compound the forensic dentist's technical and

Box 19-1

Suggested Instrument Kit for Forensic Identification

Dental explorers	Photographic mirrors
Dental mirrors	SLR film-based camera
Periodontal probes	Digital camera
Bite blocks	Photographic film, digital
Tissue scissors	memory card
Osteotome	Radiographic film and digital
Rubber air/water syringe	sensors
Cotton swabs	Rubber, latex, and nitrile gloves
Gauze	Tissue forceps
Flashlight or headlamp	Tissue clamp
Specimen containers	Tongue clamp
Scalpels and blades	Disclosing solution
Cheek retractors	Stryker saw
ABFO No. 2 ruler	Writing instruments
Bone mallet	Case labels
	Appropriate charts
	Masks and HEPA filters

ABFO, American Board of Forensic Odontology; *SLR*, single-lens reflex; *HEPA*, high-efficiency particulate air.

stress-related problems while performing the tasks related to this discipline. Because of the previous caveats, the forensic dentist should prepare an equipment kit (Box 19-1). The kit should be portable, containing instruments and supplies specifically required for the performance of dental procedures in an autopsy room environment.

GUIDELINES FOR DENTAL IDENTIFICATION

Although dental information can support the identification of a visually recognizable body, identification of dental remains is especially helpful when a decedent is skeletonized, decomposed, burned, or dismembered. Because each of these forensic situations presents different technical problems to the dentist, Body Identification Guidelines have been established by the American Board of Forensic Odontology (ABFO). The purpose of delineating these criteria is to assist dentists in comparing antemortem and postmortem dental information. Furthermore, the possibility of misidentification is reduced in both routine and mass-disaster cases.

Under the Body Identification Guidelines, provisions are made for the following:

- Examination of the postmortem dental remains in compliance with infection control and Occupational Safety and Health Administration (OSHA) requirements
- Examination of antemortem dental records
- Comparison of all dental and paradental information from the two databases

- Development of a written report listing conclusions and an opinion regarding the strength of the identification, for example positive, presumptive, insufficient, or exculpatory (Exculpatory evidence is favorable to the defendant in a criminal trial, clearing the defendant of guilt.)

POSTMORTEM EXAMINATION

The postmortem dental evidence is gathered by photographic, radiographic, and charting techniques. All records should include the case number, date, demographic and anthropologic information, the name of the authority that is requesting the dental examination, the location of the examination, and the name of the examining dentist.

Photographs should be taken of full head and face views. Images of the occlusal planes of both dental arches and individual views of unusual pathologic or restorative findings are also obtained. A single-lens reflex (SLR), 35-mm, film-based or digital camera and appropriate electronic flash and lens systems for close-up photography should be used. Routinely, both color and black-and-white exposures are recommended for use in each case.

Dental impressions and jaw resection may also be required after the initial full head photographs have been obtained. If requested by the coroner or ME, then the dental specimens from the autopsy may have to be retained and preserved in a 10% formalin solution.

The guidelines for body identification recognize that the dentist and dental auxiliary personnel involved in performing forensic dental procedures do so at the request and direction of a legal authority, such as a coroner or ME. Therefore, it is only with the permission of these individuals that techniques involving postmortem facial dissection or jaw resection are performed by the forensic dentist to achieve complete access to dental tissues.

These measures are used most often in decomposed, dismembered, or incinerated bodies to make postmortem dental charting and radiographic examination easier. Resection or soft tissue dissection may be necessary in visually recognizable bodies when the oral cavity is inaccessible because of rigor mortis.

When the jaws are removed with a reciprocating (Stryker) saw or osteotome and mallet, a Le Fort I fracture of the maxilla is created. The dissection instruments are placed above the inferior nasal spine and malar processes to ensure that the apices of the maxillary teeth are not transected. Similarly, if the mandible is not removed by disarticulation, then cuts into the mandibular rami should be high enough to prevent damage to impacted third molars.

While obtaining postmortem radiographic evidence, the forensic dentist may encounter technical obstacles that need to be addressed. It often is difficult to place intraoral radiographic film or digital radiographic sensors securely against the mandible or maxilla of a deceased individual. A modified Rinn XCP self-supporting film holder, which does not require active participation from the examinee, has been developed for postmortem identification. Because all dental evidence may eventually be required to be relinquished in court, the use of double-pack intraoral radiographs permits the forensic dentist to retain a set of films. Digital radiographic exposure and storage of images precludes this problem.

When the jaws cannot be resected, postmortem changes in rigor mortis cases and in bodies that are partially decomposed may prevent the positioning of intraoral periapical radiographic films or digital sensors. Occlusal films, 5 × 7 lateral plates, and panoramic radiographs are often used in these situations. Additionally, charting of dental evidence in fourth-degree burn cases, in which charring of soft tissues results in contraction of the muscles of mastication, may preclude the placement of these devices. With the coroner or ME's permission, the entire skull can be removed from the rest of the remains and placed in a panoramic radiographic machine.

Fifth-degree burn cases result in cremation (sometimes referred to as **cremains**). Dental evidence may be lost or compromised in these cases as temperatures range between 870° and 980° C (1600° and 1800° F). Most cremated skeletal and dental remains are structurally recognizable, and it is only the processing of these structures in commercial crematoria that creates the ash most associated with this process. Cremated bones and teeth are fragile, crumble easily, and require extreme care when handled.

Fragmentation of dental structures in dismemberment cases and total loss of soft tissues in skeletonized remains necessitate alterations in routine radiation exposure settings. Generally, when radiographs of this type of material are taken, 10-mA and 65-kVp exposure settings are used. Because there is little or no soft tissue, standard exposure times or impulse settings are halved to prevent overexposure of the radiograph.

The maxilla can be split along the midsagittal suture, and each half can be placed horizontally on an occlusal film. This projection can be used to simulate antemortem panoramic radiographs or bite-wing views. Similar exposures can be obtained from the mandible by mounting the jaw on the edge of a table or bracket tray and placing an occlusal film under the supporting half. Exposures of the opposite side of the arch are made by simply flipping the mandible and repeating the procedure.

The charting (odontogram) of the postmortem dentition should provide for situations in which teeth are

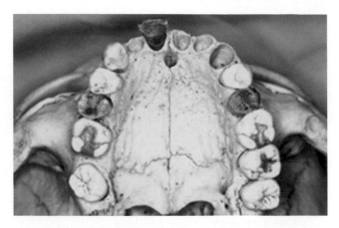

Fig. 19-9 Postmortem tooth loss results in an alveolar socket with unfractured margins and no reossification. In this example, teeth Nos. 7, 9, 10, and 11 represent postmortem tooth loss. Tooth No. 2 is a result of antemortem loss. Teeth Nos. 4, 8, and 13 were found near the body and reinserted into their respective sockets.

missing after death. If such a discrepancy remains unexplained, then it may preclude the positive identification of the body. Scavenging animals or poor investigation of a crime or disaster scene can cause postmortem loss of teeth. Environmental conditions at or around the time of death, such as tidal action in a saltwater drowning, can also contribute to perimortem loss of teeth. When teeth are lost in this manner, the crest of the alveolar bone remains intact. In addition, there is no reossification of the socket (Fig. 19-9). This pattern is inconsistent with what is observed after extraction of a tooth.

Postmortem tooth loss is associated with decomposition of the periodontal ligament. Thus the tooth simply falls out when the body is moved by animals or during crime scene recovery efforts. When this phenomenon occurs and is recognized, the charting abbreviation MPPA (missing postmortem, present antemortem) is used in that tooth's position in the dental odontogram.

ANTEMORTEM RECORD EXAMINATION

Antemortem records are usually obtained directly from the police, coroner, or ME. Before accepting this evidence, the forensic dentist should determine that the records indicate the name of the person to be identified and the name and address of the submitting dentist. In addition, most jurisdictions require an evidence transfer document to be signed. This form indicates that the continuity of evidence has been maintained and specifies who is currently in possession of the material.

Several antemortem records of the same person may be submitted from different dental practices for comparison with postmortem dental evidence. It is not uncommon for the general dental records of a decedent and those obtained from the oral and maxillofacial surgeon, endodontist, orthodontist, and other dental specialty practices to be forwarded for forensic analysis. Even if only one antemortem record is sent, then the forensic dentist should rechart all information obtained from the radiographs, progress notes, and odontograms on a standardized form. This record should be identical to the one on which the postmortem information was documented. All of this material should be appropriately labeled as the antemortem record.

The use of computer software, such as the WinID3 program, in mass-disaster situations accomplishes this same principle by entering all antemortem and postmortem dental information into the respective identification program. Besides making the comparison of records easier to manage, the creation of similar antemortem and postmortem analytic material is easier to present in court.

COMPARISON OF ANTEMORTEM AND POSTMORTEM RECORDS AND WRITTEN CONCLUSIONS

After all dental information has been collected from the antemortem and postmortem databases, it is compared for similarities and discrepancies. Comparison of dental evidence is unique among the techniques used to identify a decedent. A positive identification may still be established, even when some reconcilable discrepancies are observed.

Furthermore, the forensic dentist must routinely rely on the belief that antemortem records are truly those of the person they are purported to represent. The latter problem is best exemplified by the controversy associated with the antemortem dental records used to identify the bodies of Adolph Hitler and Eva Braun. Until recently, there was uncertainty concerning the reliability of those records. This uncertainty was based on the possibility that the records had been falsified to encourage the misidentification of Hitler and his wife.

The case demonstrated in Fig. 19-10 shows that all teeth, restorations, and anatomic structures are identical, except that deciduous tooth K is still present in the antemortem radiograph. Tooth No. 20 is erupted in the postmortem film. This difference could not support a positive identification if it were a component of fingerprint or DNA evidence. The facts that the deciduous tooth has exfoliated and the permanent tooth erupted before death are acceptable discrepancies in comparable dental evidence.

Comparison of dental evidence is often complicated by the quality of the evidence submitted. The physical status of the postmortem dental material can be

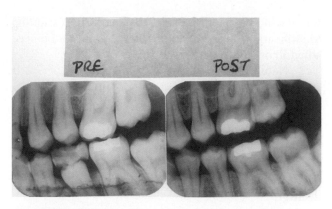

Fig. 19-10   Antemortem and postmortem radiographs demonstrating the fluid, changing nature of dental information.

compromised when teeth have fractured or are avulsed secondary to trauma. Often, only fragments of the jaws may be presented for comparison, and there may have been postmortem loss of teeth.

Dental restorations can be separated from the teeth or melted in a fire. Acrylic restorative material melts in temperatures less than 540° C (1000° F), gold and amalgam melt at 870° C (1600° F), and porcelain can withstand temperatures greater than 1100° C (2010° F). In addition, extreme temperature in a fire can cause the teeth to explode or appear shrunken. Although the principal role of the dentition of a fire victim is to provide data for identification, studies indicate that morphologic and microscopic tissue alterations of the teeth may assist forensic scientists, such as arson investigators, in determining temperature and duration of exposure to fire.

The problems associated with incomplete antemortem records are compounded when radiographs are of poor quality as a result of exposure and developing errors. Mischarted information in the antemortem record can also be considered a reconcilable discrepancy. This error often occurs when teeth have been extracted and adjoining teeth have moved into the position of the extraction site. Restorations may be inadvertently indicated on the wrong tooth when the clinician is charting or entering information into the progress record.

Regardless of the difficulties encountered when dental evidence is compared, the final conclusions must be based on an objective analysis of the data presented. The conclusions must be supportable and defensible when they are presented under oath in a court of law.

DENTISTRY'S ROLE IN MULTIPLE (MASS) FATALITY INCIDENT IDENTIFICATION

The term *multiple (mass) fatality incident* (MFI) evokes images of a chaotic event, initiated by a destructive force, which results in numerous deaths necessitating identification. These mass disaster events can be classified in one of three ways:

1. Natural
2. Accidental
3. Criminal (e.g., serial homicide, mass suicide, acts of terrorism)

Each type of MFI event results in the death of numerous victims. However, the problems faced by the forensic dental team responsible for identifying the decedents may vary, depending on the type of mass disaster.

NATURAL DISASTERS

Natural mass disasters include earthquakes, tornadoes, hurricanes, volcanic eruptions, fire storms, tsunamis, and floods. These may occur over relatively short periods or may be protracted over days or weeks. Victims may be scattered throughout broad areas, extending for miles. In addition, many victims in natural MFI situations may be unknowns who cannot be presumptively identified. Several countries or states can be affected, as in the 2004 Indian Ocean tsunami event.

Transients, homeless individuals, and tourists who are visiting an area involved in a natural MFI are often difficult to identify.

In a natural disaster, the principal problem for the dental identification team is that the environmental infrastructure is often compromised. For example, after Hurricane Katrina, medical and dental offices and hospital facilities containing antemortem records had been destroyed by tornado activity and flooding. In addition, communication lines and roads were damaged, preventing the retrieval of most available antemortem records. All of these factors delayed or precluded the prompt identification of many victims.

ACCIDENTS

Accidental MFI events are most often associated with transportation accidents, fires, industrial and mining accidents, and military accidents. These situations usually occur over short time periods and are associated with closed populations (e.g., airplane, bus, or train passengers; mine or factory workers).

Airlines maintain passenger logs of individuals who are registered on specific flights. However, it has been estimated that at any given time as many as 10% of air travelers may purchase their tickets using an alias for identification. The mining company, mill, or industrial plant can document those who have reported for work. In these examples, the victims of accidents should logically come from the closed population of employees on that shift. Therefore, antemortem records are first solicited from the families and health care providers of these individuals. Another source of medical and dental records in these cases is the occupational health files of workers, which are maintained by the employer.

Problems can be associated with the identification of victims of industrial and military accidents because these populations may be of similar age, sex, and ethnicity. Commonly, individuals working in industrial or military settings wear similar clothing. Thus military uniforms and protective industrial clothing decrease the potential use of personal recognition as an identification aid in these cases.

CRIMINAL DISASTERS

Unlike natural and accidental MFIs, criminal mass disasters involving death may occur over extremely long time periods and wide ranges of territory (e.g., different cities or states). This was the pattern of the rapes and murders committed by Ted Bundy, whose victims included young women residing in states from Washington to Florida from 1974 to 1978. The remains of the victims of serial killers can be hidden, as in the Green River homicides in the Pacific Northwest and the murders of young men committed by John Wayne Gacey in Chicago. Dismemberment and mutilation of victims is exemplified by the Jeffrey Dahmer case. Dental structures in these situations may not always be available for postmortem review.

Law enforcement agencies are often unaware of the victims of serial killers from other jurisdictions. Each agency may be investigating an individual homicide without recognizing a pattern of broader criminal involvement. Until the development of the FBI-NCIC computer registry, coordinated efforts at identification were hampered.

The rise in national and international terrorism in the twenty-first century has changed the paradigm associated with the traditional participation of the dental profession in an MFI setting. Until recently, forensic odontologists and other dental professionals were simply tasked as experts in the identification of the decedents. Currently, there are ongoing efforts within organized dentistry to develop effective responses to acts of bioterrorism. These efforts are exemplified by the profession's encouragement of legislation authorizing dental professionals, in federally declared emergencies, to perform various procedures that are routinely not within the practice of the profession. Under these provisions, dentists registered and trained in emerging medical diseases, bioterrorism, and emergency medical care would be indemnified for actions taken in the performance of these services.

Acts of terrorism may include exposure to biologic agents, chemical toxins, and the discharge of nuclear devices. Thus the dentist involved in MFI recovery and identification after an act of terrorism may additionally be required to assist medical workers in providing care for the injured. In these scenarios, dentists must consider their personal safety and that of their families. Civil defense and emergency preparedness organizational plans are beginning to include dentists among those charged with triaging the injured. Additional roles for the dental professional in future acts of bioterrorism and nuclear or chemical attack include providing first aid care and immunizations to injured and exposed survivors.

RESPONSIBILITIES

In the United States, the National Response Plan (NRP) provides a comprehensive, risk-based, emergency management plan to respond to any hazardous event. The NRP establishes guidelines to manage domestic response to radiological, technical, natural, or terrorist incidents by developing 12 emergency services functions and delineating the agencies charged with performing specific tasks in a response.

As part of the presidential directive that created the U.S. Department of Homeland Security after the September 11, 2001 terrorist attacks, the National Incident Management System (NIMS) was also developed. The overall objective of this system is coordination of governmental agencies, nongovernmental organizations, and the private sector in the resolution of nationally significant incidents.

Regardless of the type of MFI, the local coroner or ME is ultimately responsible for performing the autopsies and identifying the victims. In accidents that involve modes of public transportation, the National Transportation Safety Board (NTSB) is empowered to investigate and determine the cause of the crash. Other agencies with jurisdiction at a disaster scene may represent local police, public safety, and funeral home personnel. In addition, there may be representatives of the Federal Emergency Management Agency (FEMA), members of the FBI fingerprint team, members of the clergy, or personnel with the Disaster Mortuary Operational Response Team (DMORT) or Disaster Medical Assistance Team (DMAT).

Although DMORT and DMAT units include dental personnel, these teams may not be mobilized in all MFIs. In these situations, forensic dentists and support staff responsible for identification or care of the injured should also be organized into teams. Several state dental associations (including California, Washington, Michigan, New York, South Carolina, Nevada, and Iowa) have developed, supplied, and trained such groups in preparation for emergencies requiring their expertise. Training sessions include mock MFI exercises. These drills can prepare the dental team members for dealing with the technical problems of cases involving multiple fatalities.

In addition, training sessions can be used to counsel the dental team and to inform members of the post-traumatic stress often associated with this type of forensic work. This delayed stress is a result of the sensory and psychologic insults encountered by the dentist, hygienist, or dental assistant who is dealing with human death on a large scale.

During an MFI the National Disaster Medical System (NDMS), under its emergency support functions, is authorized and has responsibility to assist local authorities by establishing temporary morgue facilities; identifying victims using scientific techniques; and processing, preparing, and disposing of victims' remains to families, funeral homes, or proper legal representatives. This mission has been accomplished through the development of 10 regional DMORTs administered by the Department of Health and Human Services. Each DMORT is composed of funeral directors, MEs, coroners, pathologists, forensic anthropologists, medical records technicians and transcribers, fingerprint specialists, forensic dentists, dental hygienists, dental assistants, radiology technicians, mental health specialists, computer professionals, administrative support staff, and security and investigative personnel. These individuals are private citizens, each with a specific field of expertise, who are mobilized during a disaster. The licensure and certification of the DMORT members is recognized by all states because they are considered temporary federal employees during the emergency response.

Working with the authorization of the coroner or ME, a local dental disaster team or dental component of a DMORT is responsible for antemortem record assembly and interpretation, postmortem physical and dental radiographic examination, and final comparison of dental information. These are the same principles used to establish an individual identification. Yet, when numerous victims need to be identified in a short time, problems of identification are compounded exponentially.

Dividing the team into subsections responsible for each of the three identification domains permits a division of labor among the team members. This division reduces errors in identification, in that specific tasks in the identification process are assigned to separate subsections. A chain of command should be established, and the team leader of each shift should be directly responsible to the coroner or ME. This person is the only member of the team authorized to release the results of the dental identification process to appropriate investigative agencies.

TECHNOLOGIC AIDS IN MULTIPLE FATALITY INCIDENT ANALYSIS

Advances in photographic, radiographic, and computer technology have provided the forensic dental team with additional resources to enable recovery, documentation, storage, and comparison of forensic dental evidence in MFIs, as well as in other situations requiring forensic dental expertise (e.g., bite mark analysis, documentation of human abuse). Among these advances are developments in the following:

- **Digital photography.** The basic digital camera used for forensic evidence documentation should include a through-the-lens (TTL), light-metering, SLR, 35-mm digital camera body with interchangeable lenses or an adjustable lens capable of normal range (30 to 50 mm) to macro range (90 to 100 mm) focal length. A removable flash memory card with adequate storage capacity is also required. The Scientific Working Group on Imaging Technology (SWGIT) imaging guidelines provide the forensic odontologist with information regarding the limitations and parameters imposed by the judicial system regarding the manipulation and presentation of digital photographic evidence.
- **Digital radiography (DR) equipment.** Electronically generated and stored radiographic imaging can be accomplished by the following:
  - Scanning normally processed radiographic film into a computer
  - Using a phosphor substrate shaped and used like radiographic film to expose and scan radiographic information into the computer by a special proprietary device
  - Using a sensor sized and shaped like a radiographic film that is made of a scintillation screen and a charge-coupled device (CCD) or complementary metal oxide semiconductor (CMOS)
- **Direct digital radiography (DDR).** When energized by radiation, this device creates a direct image on the pixels of its CCD or CMOS. This radiographic image is then sent to a computer through wire or wireless technology. Thus because of its ability to save time, DDR technology is recommended for clinical and forensic casework. Additionally, DDR procedures reduce exposure times by requiring 90% less radiation than that required to expose a standard type D film radiograph and 50% less radiation than that required in exposure of type E film radiographs. The parameters by which the quality of a radiograph is evaluated include resolution and contrast sensitivity. Image resolution describes the detail an image holds. In film-based radiographs, this is expressed as a function of how close lines can be to each other and still be visibly distinguished. Digital imaging measures resolution as pixel counts. The contrast sensitivity is a measure of the smallest percentage change in an object's base thickness (density) that can be detected in a radiograph. The high resolution of the image produced by the DDR sensor is one of its most advantageous properties.

- **Cone-beam computed tomography (CBCT).** CBCT provides a 3D imaging modality to collect a complete maxillomandibular-facial anatomic volume of data. Computer software can be used to analyze the obtained image, and the diagnostic interpretation provided can be used for treatment planning, assessment of pathologic conditions, and evaluation of dental implants. Application of CBCT in forensic dental situations can overcome intraoral access problems with some specimens (e.g., fourth-degree burn cases).
- **Portable hand-held x-ray generation devices (e.g., Nomad manufactured by Aribex, and MinXray HF70DUL Type A).** The forensic dentist is able to expose film or digital radiographs quickly and effortlessly with a battery-powered unit that can be carried to the body on the gurney in the morgue. Additional applications for the use of these devices in the dental office include exposure of radiographs on pediatric or sedated patients or those having endodontic therapy.
- **X-ray fluorescence (XRF) methodology.** As discussed previously, analysis of dental materials in cremation and other difficult forensic identification cases may be facilitated by analysis of specimens with this technology.
- **Computer software technology.** The advent of computer software has assisted MFI dental identification teams in filing, storing, sorting, and matching bits of antemortem and postmortem information. Computer assistance has proved beneficial in disasters involving hundreds of victims. Commonly used programs include the following:
  - The FBI-NCIC program, based on the California Dental Identification System, developed by Dr. Norman Sperber and Dr. Robert Siegel (San Diego, Calif.)
  - CAPMI-4 (Computer-Assisted Postmortem identification–version 4.0), developed by Dr. Lewis Lorton of the U.S. Army Institute of Dental Research and maintained by the Armed Forces Institute of Pathology (It was first used in 1985 in support of the Arrow Air-U.S. military charter aviation runway accident in Gander, Newfoundland.)
  - WinID3 dental comparison software, developed by Dr. James McGivney (St. Louis, Mo.) (Bridged with the Dexis DR program, WinID3 facilitated comparison of antemortem and postmortem dental records in Hurricane Katrina recovery efforts and various transportation and industrial MFI events.)

Each of these computer software systems is user friendly, can be run on readily available and accessible hardware, is automated and capable of networking, and relies on objective data entry. The use of these computer software programs in MFI situations reduces the time and effort that had to be expended in past events. Before their use, an examiner in the dental identification team walked along tables with a postmortem record comparing the dental data and radiographs at each station containing an antemortem record.

Despite the fact that these technologic advances have facilitated forensic casework, the caveat for the forensic dentist remains that identification is the result of human thought processes and not the highly technical supportive procedures that provide the material being evaluated. To arrive at correct comparative conclusions based on the evidence, individual dental team members must evaluate the computer-generated matches for definitive identification.

BITE PATTERN EVIDENCE

BASIC PRINCIPLES

A bite mark is a patterned injury or surface disturbance produced by teeth on an individual's skin or inanimate object. Analysis of this type of evidence presumes that the dentition of the biter (animal or human) is unique and can be compared scientifically and related to the resultant pattern mark on the surface of a victim or object. Although studies indicate the uniqueness of the human dentition, the debate among forensic odontologists relates to the ability of these unique features to be transferred into skin, which is acknowledged as a poor impression material.

Despite the controversies related to this type of forensic evidence, 70% of respondents to a survey among specialists in the field indicated that trained forensic odontologists could positively identify a suspect from a bite mark on skin. Thus issues related to the validity, reliability, and admissibility of bite mark evidence continues to rest with the judicial system and its various rules pertaining to the introduction of scientific evidence in court.

Victims of mammalian animal bites account for most bite injuries reported annually. Bite-related injuries represent approximately 1% of all hospital emergency visits that require medical attention. Of these, nearly 370,000 were associated with dog bites in 2001. The second and third most likely mammalian biters are cats and humans, respectively. Each represents from 5% to 20% of cases reporting to urban emergency rooms.

As the habitats of wild animals in North America continue to recede, humans are more likely to come in contact with these dangerous carnivores. This is

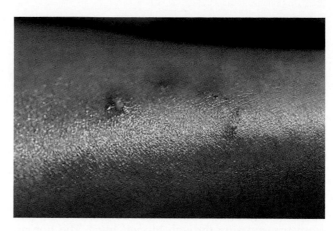

Fig. 19-11 Insect bites on the skin that mimic the pattern injury associated with bite mark trauma. In a decedent, this pattern may additionally be mistakenly interpreted as antemortem trauma. *(Courtesy of Dr. David K. Ord.)*

reflected in the increase in attacks on humans by mountain lions and brown, black, and grizzly bears, resulting in biting injuries or death from biting and clawing.

Animal bites may be observed postmortem when a body has not been buried or discovered quickly. Commonly, insect bites are made by ants and roaches, which leave pattern injuries that can be mistakenly interpreted as antemortem trauma (Fig. 19-11). Postmortem bites from rats and scavenging dogs and cats are often avulsive and of narrower or smaller diameter than human bites.

Injuries caused by human bites are routinely related to either aggressive or sexual behavior. Ironically, it is not uncommon for the perpetrator of an aggressive act to be bitten by the victim (as a means of self-defense). In children, biting is a form of expression that occurs when verbal communication fails. Biting injuries in children can result from playground altercations or sports competition. They are common among children who attend day care centers.

Self-inflicted bites are observed in **Lesch-Nyhan syndrome**. This syndrome is an X-linked, recessively transmitted disease manifesting insensitivity to pain and self-mutilation (among other signs) by chewing away the lips. This disease is rare, and self-inflicted bites are more commonly seen in adults and children who are victims of physical abuse or sexual assault. These individuals may bite their own forearms or hands in anguish or to prevent themselves from crying out while they are being traumatized.

Injuries resulting from animal or human bites may become septic or may progress to systemic infections. Secondary bacterial infections are more commonly associated with human bites than with animal bites, although 30% to 50% of cat bites become infected because bacteria are injected into the puncture wounds inflicted by their needlelike teeth. Infectious complications include tetanus, tuberculosis, syphilis, actinomycosis, cat-scratch disease (caused by *Bartonella henselae*), and those infectious complications related to streptococcal and staphylococcal organisms. Anaerobic organisms associated with bite injuries may eventually result in complications such as septic arthritis, tenosynovitis, meningitis, and infections of the lymphatic system.

Viral complications, including hepatitis B virus, herpes simplex, and cytomegalovirus, have resulted from transmission through human bites. The human immunodeficiency virus (HIV) can also potentially be transmitted through the exchange of blood and saliva in a bite injury. The risk of seroconversion from this mode of HIV transmission, however, is believed to be extremely low. An immunocompromised individual who is already infected with the HIV virus is at increased risk of secondary infection when bitten by a cat.

Rabies is the most serious infectious complication that results from mammalian animal bites. It is often necessary to identify the specific offending animal for rabies control or potential litigation. This identification is not routinely done by matching the animal's teeth to the pattern injury. When humans bite, however, the marks left in injured tissue or inanimate objects are often analyzed and compared with the alleged perpetrator's dentition.

HISTORICAL AND LEGAL ISSUES

References to biting during acts of passion or aggression can be found in the *Bible*, *Kama Sutra*, and Old English law. In colonial America, the Reverend George Burroughs was charged with the crime of biting one of the women accused of witchcraft during the Salem, Massachusetts, witch hunt incidents in 1692. He was hanged for this offense. Bite mark evidence was provided in expert dental testimony in the 1870 Ohio trial of Ansil L. Robinson, who was accused of murdering his mistress. Although the defendant was eventually acquitted, the expert dental presentation by Dr. Jonathan Taft became a benchmark for future experts in the discipline.

The concept of accepting evidence related to the analysis of patterns created by the dentition was first accepted by the appellate level courts of the United States justice system in 1954. At that time, *Doyle v. State of Texas* became the first modern case in which a criminal conviction was based on evidence relating a suspect's dentition to pattern marks in an inanimate object (a piece of cheese). Because of the *Doyle* case, more

than 260 decisions involving bite mark evidence have been entered into the case law records of the appellate courts of the United States.

The legal community has recognized tool mark and fingerprint pattern analysis as scientifically acceptable forensic disciplines for some time. The evidence presented by experts in these areas has been accepted in 20% of state courts under the *Frye* standard (*Frye v. United States*), and the remaining 80% of state courts and all federal courts under the Federal Rules of Evidence 702-705. These are special rules dealing with the admissibility of scientific evidence in the American judicial system. Thus they are also applicable to bite mark information.

The *Frye* test had been the standard for scientific admissibility in most state and federal courts since 1923. The three components of scientific evidence admissibility that are considered under the *Frye* test include the following:

1. The scientific principle must be recognizable.
2. The scientific principle must be sufficiently established.
3. The scientific principle must have gained general acceptance within the scientific discipline to which it belongs.

Among the three requirements, only the concept of "general acceptance" must be met to satisfy the *Frye* test of admissibility.

In 1993 the U.S. Supreme Court ruled on the admissibility of scientific evidence in *Daubert v. Merrell Dow Pharmaceuticals*. It was the Court's decision in this case that the general acceptance aspect of the *Frye* test should no longer be the sole, determining factor used in considering admissibility of scientific evidence. Essentially, the Court replaced this principle with one that stresses scientific validity. This decision removes the responsibility of determining sound scientific evidence from the scientific community in which it has gained general acceptance.

Instead, the *Daubert* ruling gives great latitude to the trial judge in considering the admissibility of scientific evidence. Trial judges often have limited knowledge of scientific methodology; however, under *Daubert* they are required to determine if the weight and admissibility of expert testimony is not only scientifically valid but also relevant and germane to the issues in individual cases. Thus the results of the Supreme Court's decision in *Daubert* are to make the judge a "gatekeeper" and the expert witness a provider of scientifically valid evidence.

The general acceptance concept is no longer the sole determinant of admissibility in *Daubert*. It becomes one of several factors that must be met for scientific evidence to be admissible. These factors include the following:

- Techniques used must be testable and tested.
- Peer review and publication of results are not required but may persuade the judge in admitting evidence.
- Standards should be established for evaluation of the scientific methods and error rates associated with the techniques used.
- Consideration is given to acceptance of scientific principles that have gained general acceptance within the scientific discipline to which they belong.

Because it is reasonable to consider the teeth as cutting or mashing tools, the basis for accepting bite pattern evidence can be supported on the same scientific principles used to evaluate tool marks. In addition, studies indicate that, like fingerprints, the human dentition is unique for each person. Variations in size, wear, and fractures; position in the dental arch; diastemata; and restored surfaces contribute to this principle.

Thus bite mark evidence is admissible under the *Frye* standard and Federal Rules of Evidence as determined by the *Daubert* decision. Although some legal experts believe the Federal Rules of Evidence provide better guidelines for admissibility decisions, no challenge to the scientific basis of bite mark evidence has been successful under either set of standards.

CHARACTERISTICS OF BITE MARKS

To evaluate a pattern mark, its characteristics must be recognizable and distinguishable. Reasonably, the mark should be consistent with the face of the instrument from which it was generated. Specific teeth can create representative patterns that are recognizable. These individual marks are described as internal characteristics of the entire bite mark. Human incisors make rectangular marks. Depending on the amount of attrition observed on the incisal edge of the cuspid, this surface may be associated with point or triangular patterns. Unlike mandibular bicuspid teeth, which have a diminutive lingual cusp, maxillary bicuspids often mark in a pattern that resembles a "figure eight."

Class characteristics of a human bite mark are related to the shapes that are created when groups of teeth from both dental arches are impressed into a bitten surface. Round, ovoid, or elliptical patterns are usually observed, but variations may be associated with tapered, square, and U-shaped arches. When only one arch contacts a surface, a crescent pattern may be formed. The greatest dimensions of an adult human bite mark do not usually exceed 4 cm (Fig. 19-12).

Internal and class characteristics of bite patterns are generated by groups of specific teeth. The dynamics of occlusion and muscle function must also be accounted

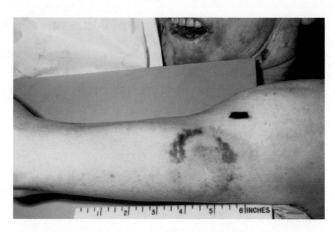

Fig. 19-12   A bite mark pattern demonstrating the internal and class characteristics associated with impressions made by the human dentition. An ecchymotic area in the center of the ovoid pattern is observed, which is not always related to the sucking action of a sexual bite. Therefore, this finding should not be overinterpreted to imply sexual intent on the part of the biter. The impressions made by the teeth of the mandibular arch are more delicate.

for when variations in internal and class characteristics of a bite mark are considered. Such variations can be caused by malocclusion, individual tooth mobility associated with periodontal disease, and movement of facial muscles during biting.

Class II malocclusion can cause the palatal surfaces of the maxillary anterior teeth, rather than their incisal edges, to contact the material being bitten. Shieldlike imprints of the palatal surfaces are generated in the bite mark rather than the rectangular patterns routinely associated with these teeth.

Aberrant muscle forces associated with tongue thrusting can alter the way the teeth contact a bitten surface. Temporomandibular joint dysfunction (TMD) can also contribute to variations in bite patterns. TMD can be associated with midline shifts or inability to achieve maximum opening while biting.

When bitten, many inanimate objects tend to act like dental-impression material, retaining the marks of the teeth. Such cases have involved bite marks in foods, chewing gum, paper toweling, and a roll of masking tape. Unlike inanimate material, the skin is a dynamic tissue that can change after it is injured. Swelling, caused by the acute inflammatory response of the tissue, can distort and affect the interpretation of the pattern. Bleeding into the area of a bite mark can mask the pattern.

The age of an injury is the time elapsed from its infliction to the analysis of the damaged tissue. Reliable determination of the age of antemortem skin injuries requires histopathologic and histochemical analysis to

Table **19-3** **Histopathologic and Clinical Changes Used to Monitor the Time Elapsed (Aging) in Skin Injuries Associated with Bite Marks**

Time	Predominant Cellular Infiltrate and Deposits	Healing	Variable Clinical Color
HOURS			
4-8	Polymorphonuclear leukocytes with a peripheral front		Red-blue-purple
12	Polymorphonuclear leukocytes		
16-24	Macrophages peak		Blue-black
24-36	Polymorphonuclear leukocytes peak	Peripheral fibroblasts	
DAYS			
1-3	Central necrosis		
3+	Hemosiderin		Green-blue
4		Collagen fibers	
4-5		Capillary growth	Brown-yellow-green
6		Lymphocytes peak at periphery	
10-14		Granulation tissue	Tan-yellow

relate the injury to the time of the alleged incident (Table 19-3). Color changes in the bitten tissue, associated with the degradation of hemoglobin from lysed RBCs, can be used only to broadly estimate the time of occurrence and qualify the age of a bruise as recent or old. Environmental factors, including seasonal temperature, location of the body, and presence or absence of clothing, may additionally act as important variables requiring consideration when attempting to determine the age of injury patterns.

Contusions and areas of ecchymosis are not unusual in bite marks made in living tissue. The absence of bleeding into the injury may imply that it was inflicted after death. Additional postmortem soft tissue changes that can affect the quality of a bite pattern injury and its eventual weight as evidence include artifacts created by lividity (caused by the settling of blood pigments in dependent body areas), decomposition, and embalming.

Bite marks from sexual attacks are commonly found on the neck, breasts, arms, buttocks, genitalia, and thighs. Axillary bites and bite patterns on the back, shoulder, penis, and scrotum are often associated with homosexual activity. Abused children may be bitten in areas of the face, particularly the cheek, ear, and nose. Assailants also can be bitten. The analysis of these bite pattern injuries is just as incriminating as those found on the victim of a violent act.

A review of 778 bite mark injuries concerning the anatomic locations most often bitten, victim and biter demographics, the type of crimes in which biting occurred, and legal disposition of cases revealed the following information:

- Females were bitten more often than males.
- Perpetrators were male more often than female.
- The most common sites bitten were the arms. Bites in these locations occurred more commonly among males.
- Females were bitten on the breast more often than males. This location accounted for the second most commonly bitten area of the body.
- The type of crime and the age of the victim were related to patterns in location, distribution, and number of bites.

GUIDELINES FOR BITE MARK ANALYSIS

In 1984 the American Board of Forensic Odontology (ABFO) established Guidelines for Bite Mark Analysis. Additional workshops held in 1993 and 1994 provided further insight into the techniques available to recover, store, analyze, and evaluate bite mark evidence based on the Guidelines. After the workshops, the ABFO Bite Mark Methodology Guidelines were revised in 1995. The development and revision of the Guidelines created a scientific approach to the description of the bite mark, collection of evidence from suspect and victim, and subsequent analysis of the evidence.

The guidelines do not mandate specific analytic methods for comparison. Through their careful use, however, the quality of the investigation and conclusions based on bite mark evidence follow customary procedures. Thus with these guidelines, it should be possible to determine the weight of bite mark evidence required to establish the validity of bite mark comparison.

DESCRIPTION OF THE BITE MARK

Demographic information (i.e., age, race, sex, and name of the victim; examination date; referring agency; case number) is obtained in cases involving both living and deceased victims. The names of the forensic dental examiner and referring agency contact person should also be included.

The location of the bite is then described. Attention is directed to the anatomic location, surface contour, and tissue characteristics of the bitten area. Underlying structures, such as bone or fat, may influence the analytic quality of the pattern injury. Relative skin mobility is also evaluated.

The shape, color, size, and type of injury are recorded. Metric measurements of the horizontal and vertical dimensions of the bite mark are determined. Irregularities and variations from the standard round, ovoid, and crescent shapes associated with human bite marks are noted. Injury types include abrasion, laceration, ecchymotic and petechial hemorrhage, incision, and avulsion. Artifactual injuries, such as proximate stab and bullet wounds, should be recorded because these may distort the pattern by separating anatomic cleavage lines of the skin (**Langer's lines**).

EVIDENCE COLLECTION
EXAMINATION OF THE VICTIM AND THE SUSPECT

Both the victim and the suspect are examined, and evidence from each is gathered for comparative study and evaluation. Collection of evidence must be performed in a manner that protects the rights of the person who is providing the evidence and that permits the eventual acceptance of the evidence in court.

A standard health history and informed consent are obtained before any evidence recovery procedure regarding the suspect is performed. An intraoral and extraoral examination of the suspect is completed, which includes dental charting, soft tissue and tongue evaluation, and probing of the periodontium. Therefore, knowledge of the medical history of the suspect relative to systemic problems associated with cardiovascular disease, allergy, seizure disorder, diabetes, or requirements for antibiotic prophylaxis has medicolegal importance in forensic casework, as well as in traditional patient evaluation.

A search warrant, court order, or legal consent may be required before evidence is collected from a suspect. A specific list of the dental-related evidence desired should be recorded in the legal document. This list usually includes facial and oral photographs, impressions of the teeth, occlusal registrations and bite exemplars, and saliva samples. These documents protect the rights of the suspect against unreasonable search and seizure and provide for due process, as guaranteed by the Fourth and Fourteenth Amendments, respectively, to the U.S. Constitution.

Bite marks are considered similar to such physical evidence as fingerprints, hair, blood, and semen samples, as well as to sobriety tests. Therefore, this material is not protected under provisions of the Fifth Amendment, which deals with self-incrimination.

PHOTOGRAPHY

Because evidence associated with bite marks, human abuse, and sexual and physical assault is transitory, there is an immediacy associated with the collection of physical evidence in these cases. Initial photographs of the pattern mark should be taken before any investigative procedures that may alter the pristine bite mark evidence (e.g., touching, removing, impressing, swabbing, cleansing).

Ideally, standard visible-light photographic techniques include the use of a 35-mm, SLR, film or digital camera with a flat-field macro lens and dedicated electronic flash. Numerous images using different camera and lighting positions, exposure settings, and color and black-and-white exposures should be obtained. If film is used, the submission of this evidence for development should strictly follow protocols for evidence preservation and maintenance of the chain of custody. Additional legal considerations and protocols related to the documentation of image enhancement, restoration, compression, and analysis have been established for digital bite mark images.

Orientation positions and close-up views with a reference scale are required. A reference scale permits the bite mark images to be measured and prepared as life-size (i.e., 1:1) representations of the pattern injury. Ultimately, these images can then be compared with casts and other exemplars obtained from the suspect. The scale should be stabilized and positioned next to, and in the same plane as, the bite mark to eliminate potential distortion artifacts in the resultant images. It should never be hand-held. Omitting the scale from at least one view documents that no marks or other injuries have been intentionally hidden by it.

The ABFO No. 2 reference scale (Lightning Powder Company, Inc; Salem, Ore.) was developed for use in bite mark photography (Fig. 19-13). This standardized, accurate scale has become the gold standard in bite mark photographic analysis. Variations of it have eventually come to be used in all varieties of forensic casework requiring accurate measurement of evidence at crime scenes or in the laboratory.

This instrument contains two metric scales, an 18% color gray scale, three circular symbols, and rectifying grids. Each of these components is used to account for photographic distortions, which can negate the value of the photographic evidence. Techniques using Adobe Photoshop and Mideo Systems casePACS computer software have been used to rectify distortions observed in the ABFO No. 2 reference scale and ultimately to eliminate these from a bite mark image being analyzed.

With living victims, serial pictures are taken over several days. This series provides documentation of the color changes associated with healing of the wound. In addition, special advanced photographic techniques, using nonvisible energy sources at the extremes of the electromagnetic spectrum and fluorescent alternative light sources, can be used to identify latent images of the teeth that may remain after the bite mark has clinically disappeared. These techniques require special films and illumination sources, bracketing of aperture (f-stop) openings, variations in shutter speeds, and/or lens filters to work within the desired wavelengths and include the following (Table 19-4):

- **Reflective ultraviolet (UV) photography.** This technique enhances the bite mark image by selectively identifying photoactive **chromophores** such as melanin and hemoglobin pigment in the superficial layers of the injured tissue. Variations in the amount of these natural light–absorbing organic pigments in the traumatized tissue are observable in images exposed with this energy source. This is based on the fluorescence created when the skin is exposed to UV light in the 200- to 400-nm wavelength range. Although there may be focusing problems associated with UV photography and exposures *must* be made with a tripod-mounted camera, the fact that this technique may permit recovery of latent evidence, even months after all clinical signs of a bite mark injury have disappeared, makes the effort worthwhile.
- **Infrared (IR) photography.** Tungsten lamps and quartz-halogen lamps are good sources of IR radiation when attempting to expose IR images from unfiltered light sources. To expose images specifically within the IR wavelengths of 750 to 1000 nm, a filter must be placed in front of the lens to absorb

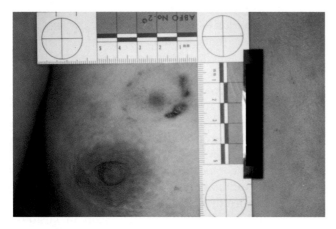

Fig. 19-13 The American Board of Forensic Odontology (ABFO) No. 2 Reference Scale.

Table **19-4**   **Comparison of Photographic Electromagnetic Energy Spectrum Sources and Their Forensic Imaging Capabilities**

	Visible Light	UV Light	IR Light	ALI Fluorescence
Light wavelength	400-700 nm	200-400 nm	700-1000 nm	450 nm
Filter	None	Kodak Wratten Filter No. 18A gel (visibly opaque glass filter)	Kodak gel 87	Kodak gel 15
TARGET PIGMENT OR MATERIAL				
Hemoglobin in pattern injuries and vessels	+	+	+	+
Melanin	+	+		+
Tattoos	+	+	+	+
Ink variations in document forgeries			+	+
Gunshot residues			+	+
Latent fingerprints				+
Serologic fluids (saliva, semen, blood)				+
Residual fibers				+

UV, Ultraviolet; *IR,* infrared; *ALI,* alternate light imaging.

visible light. The Kodak 87 gel filter accomplishes this task by limiting all transmittance of light except at the designated wavelengths. Additionally, IR photography requires that the camera lens be refocused (focus shift) after initial focusing under visible light and before exposure of the image. Like alternate light source photography, the focal plane for IR photography lies below the skin surface. The deeper focal depth permits visualization of faded tattoos and wound damage within a blood stain. This technique is not the best for identifying individual characteristics in bite mark injuries.

- **Alternate light source (alternate light imaging [ALI]) photography.** This technique is also referred to as *fluorescent photography*. It is advantageous in assisting investigators to locate and document evidence involving the presence of ink residues, fingerprint patterns, and the chromophores previously indicated. ALI enhances visualization of pigments derived from chromophores that may be found within evidence involving latent serologic fluids and subdermal bruises or pattern injuries of victims of violent or sexual crimes. ALI techniques illuminate deeper tissue targets by using a predominantly monochromatic band of light between the wavelengths of 430 and 460 nm. To accomplish the visualization of the weak fluorescent glow from the desired pigments, ALI photography must be performed by eliminating all other sources of light from striking the imaging surface (film or digital sensor). This requires that ALI techniques be performed in total darkness with yellow filters such as the Kodak gelatin No. 15. Because longer exposure times are also required, images exposed using ALI *must* be made with a tripod-mounted camera.

As previously stated, photographs of the suspect should involve the same attention to technical quality control. Extraoral, intraoral, and occlusal photographs are taken. Additional images of wax or acrylic test bites and measurements of maximum interincisal opening are also recorded.

SALIVA EVIDENCE

Although the forensic dentist is concerned principally with the analysis of the physical evidence associated with a bite mark, biologic evidence in the form of serologic and DNA material is also of probative importance. Collection of saliva trace evidence from the surface of the bite injury of the victim is performed before other evidence-gathering manipulation of the injury. There is an increase in the yield of recovered DNA for analysis when this procedure is carried out according to the two-swab protocol developed by Dr. David Sweet and others at the Bureau of Legal Dentistry, University of British Columbia.

Using this technique, a saliva sample is collected by first rubbing the bitten area with a cotton swab that has been moistened in sterile, distilled water. The swab should contain no preservatives. The bite mark is subsequently rolled with a second, dry, cotton swab. Both samples can be considered a single exhibit because they have been collected from the center of the pattern injury. They are placed in an evidence box and permitted to air-dry before submission to the laboratory. No control swabs are required from adjacent areas of the victim's skin.

DNA from the victim of a bite mark injury should be obtained from whole blood samples or buccal swabs. Additionally, autopsy tissue samples can be obtained from decedent victims. All samples can be used for DNA comparison with bodily fluid or tissue samples obtained from the suspect.

Because a victim may be bitten through the clothing, areas of garments that approximate a bite pattern injury should also be retained and evaluated for saliva. Many victims of sexual abuse wash the area of a bite mark before reporting for treatment. This is unfortunate because biologic evidence associated with DNA recovery can be lost. In this regard, emergency room personnel should be trained to recognize potential bite mark injuries and instructed not to wash or disinfect these areas until saliva evidence can be obtained.

IMPRESSIONS AND STUDY CASTS

When a bite injury exhibits indentations that can be related to the dentition of an alleged biter, accurate, 3D, life-sized exemplars (casts) can be obtained from molds of the area. Dental impression materials are used to create the molds that are then reinforced to prevent dimensional changes and distortions.

The Guidelines for Bite Mark Analysis deliberately do not dictate which impression materials should be used to create exemplars of a bite mark. Low- and medium-viscosity vinyl polysiloxane (VPS) impression materials are dimensionally stable, meet American Dental Association specifications, and are all acceptable. Hydrocolloid, polysulfide, polyether, and alginate materials are not recommended because of problems associated with long-term stability.

Orthopedic cast materials, heavy-body VPS materials, and nonexothermic resins have been used to create the rigid, stable trays for bite mark impressions. All impression trays and study casts should be appropriately labeled with demographic information for the specific case. Additionally, anatomic direction markers should be added to the impression tray before its removal from the skin surface. This will ensure that the impression is correctly oriented relative to the actual pattern injury.

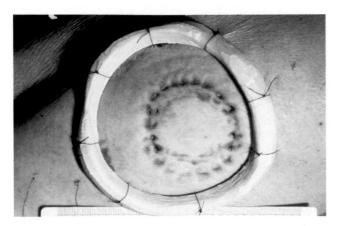

Fig. 19-14 An experimental bite pattern injury on a cadaver. This bite mark has had an acrylic stent glued and sutured around its circumference before dissection and fixation in 4% formalin. *(Courtesy of Dr. E. Steven Smith.)*

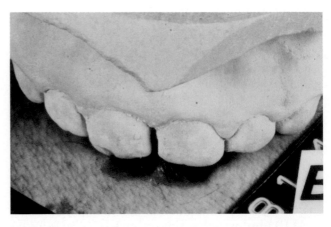

Fig. 19-15 An overlay of the maxillary cast of a suspect's dentition on a photograph of a bite pattern injury. Note the diastema between the central incisor teeth. The distal incisal surfaces of the lateral incisor teeth are not in the plane of occlusion.

Original impression trays and study casts are retained for eventual presentation in court. Working casts and models should be duplicated from the original impression or master casts. It is recommended that master casts be poured in type IV stone, according to the manufacturer's specifications, and that these casts remain pristine.

TISSUE SAMPLES

Tissue samples of a bite mark can be retained from decedents. With the permission of the ME or coroner, the epidermis, dermis, and underlying muscle and adipose tissue can be removed for transillumination analysis. Before excision, an acrylic ring or stent must be secured within 1 inch of the borders of the injured tissue sample. The ring or stent prevents shrinkage and distortion of the specimen when it is placed into a 4% formalin solution for fixation. The acrylic material is bound to the skin surface with cyanoacrylate and sutures (Fig. 19-14). These tissues samples can be transilluminated by backlighting. This process permits observation of the pattern injury in the bruised skin by a manner that is not possible when the tissue is *in situ*.

EVIDENCE ANALYSIS

The responsibility of comparing the photographs of the bite pattern injury with the dentition of the suspect rests with the forensic dentist. As an expert in the analysis of these patterns, this person objectively evaluates the evidence. The forensic dentist first determines whether the pattern is truly a result of biting or whether it is an artifact. Patterns of blood splatter around a wound, other tool marks, or insect artifacts unrelated to the teeth may be mistaken for bite marks in photographs provided for evaluation by crime scene investigators, police, and emergency room or autopsy personnel.

Once it is established that the pattern is related to the teeth, it can be matched to the suspect's dentition for inclusion or exclusionary purposes. An expert opinion is then made according to the results of the relationship of the bite pattern and suspect's teeth.

To accomplish these goals, the dentist uses numerous methods that have been accepted in the courts. Images of the bite mark and the teeth can be digitized in a computer. This information can then be enhanced and subsequently overlaid for matching purposes.

Clear overlays of the chewing surfaces of the teeth can be made by simply tracing these surfaces on a sheet of transparent acetate. Placing the incisal edges of the study casts on the glass of an office photocopier and duplicating on special paper achieves the same end. A similar effect is obtained by placing an opaque powder, such as barium sulfate, into wax or acrylic test bites and by obtaining radiographs of these exemplars. All of these overlays are then superimposed over the bite mark for comparison (Figs. 19-15 and 19-16). This process can also be accomplished using various computer programs to create a transparent computer-generated image of the dental casts of the alleged biter. These hollow outline images can then be superimposed over an equally standardized image of the bite pattern (Fig. 19-17).

A recent study indicates that there are limitations to the accuracy of the various overlay techniques. It has been suggested that subjective, hand-traced overlay methods be discontinued. Among the other techniques,

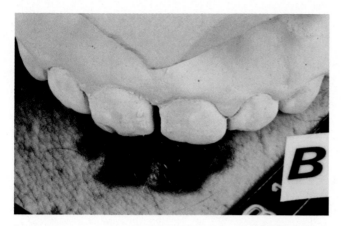

Fig. 19-16   A repositioned overlay of the maxillary cast of a suspect's dentition on a photograph of a bite pattern injury (same case as depicted in Fig. 19-15). The drag marks, diastema space, and mesial contact points of the lateral incisor teeth become apparent in the pattern. *(From Nuckles DB, Herschaft EE, Whatmough LN: Forensic odontology in solving crimes: dental techniques and bite mark evidence, Gen Dent 42:210-214, 1994.)*

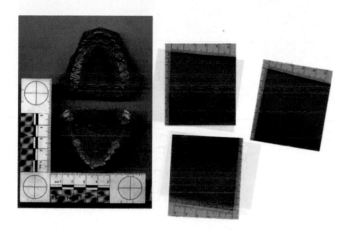

Fig. 19-17   On the left side, dental casts of an alleged suspect are being scanned and scaled to 1:1 before digitizing their image. The right half of the illustration shows three photographs of bite marks on the victim. Transparent overlays of the teeth of the alleged suspect have been digitally superimposed over 1:1 digital images of the victim's bite mark using a software program developed by Mideo Systems, Inc. *(Courtesy of Dr. David K. Ord.)*

computer-generated bite mark overlays are the most reproducible and accurate for analysis. The area of the biting edges of the teeth is best measured using overlays constructed from radiopaque material in wax dental impressions. Photocopiers, calibrated to create 100% images, are best used to record tooth rotation.

In court, bite mark evidence must be able to withstand legal challenges based on its scientific validity and the credibility of the expert witness who presents the evidence. This is true regardless of the techniques used to retrieve, compare, and determine a conclusion

based on the evidence. When the Guidelines for Bite Mark Analysis are used, such challenges can be minimized.

HUMAN ABUSE

EPIDEMIOLOGY AND CLASSIFICATION

Dental professionals are likely to encounter more victims of physical, neglective, sexual, and psychologic abuse as the scope of the problems associated with violent human behavior become more recognized and openly discussed. Currently in the United States, statistics reveal more than 3 million cases of child abuse, 2 million cases of elder abuse, and 4 million victims of intimate partner violence (IPV) annually.

Child abuse is the nonaccidental, physical, mental, emotional, or sexual trauma; exploitation; or neglect endured by a child younger than 18 years of age while under the care of a responsible person, such as a parent, sibling, babysitter, teacher, or other person acting *in loco parentis*. Elder abuse and abuse of the disabled are similar in all regards, except that they deal with geriatric victims or individuals who are physically and/or mentally impaired or disabled. These populations often require special care or have been institutionalized.

Victims of IPV are unique and differ from those of child, elder, or disabled abuse because they often have autonomy to choose their circumstances. Unlike the abused child, or geriatric or disabled resident in a nursing home, the abused intimate partner can make choices to leave the traumatic, violent environment.

Of the 3 million cases of alleged child abuse or neglect investigated by state and local child protective services (CPS) in the United States in 2004, 872,000 children were determined to be victims of child maltreatment and 1490 cases resulted in death. The National Child Abuse and Neglect Data System (NCANDS) is a federally sponsored program directed by the Department of Health and Human Services to collect and analyze annual data on child abuse and neglect.

Recognizing the global problem, in 2006 the United Nations released the first *UN Secretary-General's Study on Violence Against Children*. This document addresses violence against children in the home, school, workplace, community, and other settings. The project is the "first comprehensive, global study conducted by the United Nations on all forms of violence against children" (Box 19-2).

Victims and their abusers come from all racial, ethnic, religious, socioeconomic, and educational backgrounds. Reports concerning the distribution of cases among the different types of abuse vary widely. Up to 70% of child abuse cases may be the result of physical

Epidemiological, Statistical Overview of the *UN Secretary-General's Study on Violence Against Children*

- Almost 53,000 children died worldwide in 2002 as a result of homicide.
- Up to 80% to 98% of children suffer physical punishment in their homes, with one third or more experiencing severe physical punishment resulting from the use of implements.
- 150 million girls and 73 million boys younger than 18 years experienced forced sexual intercourse or other forms of sexual violence during 2002.
- Between 100 and 140 million girls and women in the world have undergone some form of female genital mutilation/cutting. In sub-Saharan Africa, Egypt, and the Sudan, 3 million girls and women are subjected to genital mutilation/cutting every year.
- In 2004, 218 million children were involved in child labor. Among these, 126 million did hazardous work.
- Estimates from 2000 suggest that 1.8 million children were forced into prostitution and pornography, and 1.2 million were victims of trafficking.

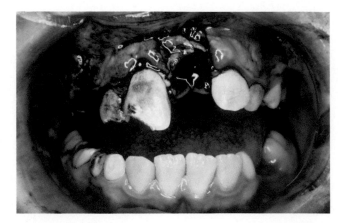

Fig. 19-18 An avulsed tooth, a fractured tooth, and a torn labial frenum associated with oral facial injuries in physical child abuse.

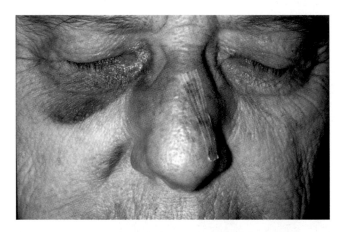

Fig. 19-19 Bilateral periorbital ecchymoses (raccoon mask) and fractured nasal bone in a 77-year-old white female victim of physical elder abuse. *(Courtesy of Dr. John D. McDowell.)*

trauma. Some studies relate 15% to 25% of the cases to sexual abuse and 50% to neglect. Neglective abuse is subclassified by the caretaker's neglect of the child's medical, dental, and safety needs; physical well-being; or education. Intentional drugging or poisoning and failure to thrive are additional types of maltreatment classified as abusive.

Many abusive individuals were themselves abused as children. Criminal charges are often lodged against an abusing caretaker. It is recognized, however, that counseling and psychologic and emotional support can also help to stabilize a violent, dysfunctional family unit.

SIGNS AND SYMPTOMS

Regardless of the overall statistical variations in subclassification of the problem of abuse, the dentist is most likely to encounter physical and sexual abuse, as well as health care and safety neglect among pediatric, older adult, and disabled dental patients. Of the children and older adults who are physically abused, 50% manifest orofacial and scalp injuries (Figs. 19-18 and 19-19). These unexplained injuries are inappropriately reported by the caretaker or are inconsistent with the history provided. Abusive trauma to the face and mouth includes the following:

- Laceration of the labial or lingual frenum, which results from a blow to the lip or forceful feeding
- Repeated fracture or the avulsion of teeth
- Zygomatic arch and nasal fractures
- Bilateral contusions of the lip commissures from the placement of a gag
- Bilateral periorbital ecchymoses (raccoon mask)
- Traumatic alopecia secondary to grabbing the head hair of the victim while throwing them

Pattern injuries can be associated with the semicircular or crescent shape of bite marks. Other instruments that contact the skin may leave parallel linear patterns; these include injuries made by a hanger, strap, belt, or ruler. Multiple parallel lines are associated with finger marks after an open-handed slap. Multiple circular, punched out, or ulcerated areas are caused by intentional burning with a cigarette or cigar. Loop patterns are created by electrical cord, rope, and wire (Figs. 19-20 and 19-21).

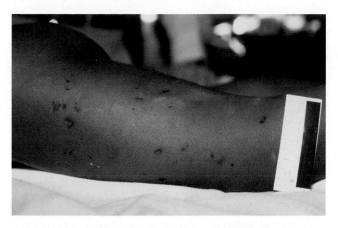

Fig. 19-20 Multiple circular ulcerated injuries are associated with intentional burns from a cigarette. When a child is accidentally burned by a cigarette, only one elliptic ulcer is observed.

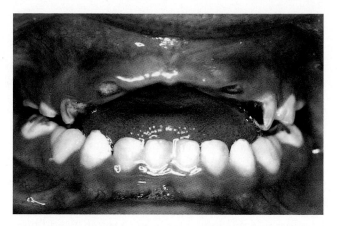

Fig. 19-22 Pseudoprognathism or pseudo-Class III malocclusion observed in a neglected child with nursing bottle (baby bottle) decay. *(Courtesy of Dr. Cynthia Hipp.)*

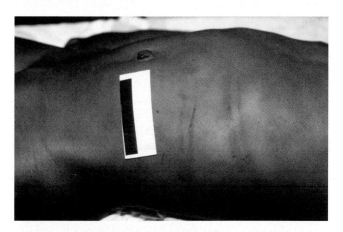

Fig. 19-21 Parallel linear ("railroad track") patterns are associated with blows to the skin with such straight-edged objects as a belt, a hanger, an electrical cord, and a ruler.

Other characteristics of child and elder abuse injuries are related to their multiplicity and repetitive nature. They often appear in various stages of resolution. Some injuries are acute; others are healing or even scarred. Therefore, the dentist should examine the skin of the pediatric, geriatric, or disabled dental patient. Suspicion of abuse is increased when the child or older patient appears overdressed for seasonal conditions; overdressing may be an attempt to mask or hide the physical signs of abuse.

By adulthood, 10% of men and 25% of women are the victims of sexual abuse. Oral infections associated with sexually transmitted diseases (STDs) are obviously signs of sexual abuse when they are observed in a minor. Erythematous or petechial lesions of the palate or ulceration of the sublingual area should be noted because these findings can result from the physical trauma associated with performing fellatio or cunnilingus (see page 307).

Among siblings, nursing or "baby bottle caries" is a sign of neglective abuse and indicates the caretaker's inattention to the dental needs of the children. When infants and toddlers are placed to bed with a nursing bottle filled with cariogenic solutions (e.g., milk, soft drinks, sweet juices), the maxillary incisors are bathed in the sugary solution and can manifest severe caries. The mandibular teeth, protected from the cariogenic material by the position of the tongue and nipple during sucking, are spared the destructive effects, and the child takes on the appearance of a pseudoprognathism or pseudo-Class III malocclusion (Fig., 19-22).

The dentist may become aware of other abusive behavior directed to a child or older patient by a responsible caretaker. Abusive behavior can involve refusal or delay in seeking treatment for serious medical or dental problems, abandonment, refusal to cooperate with planned treatment, and failure to return to the same physician or dentist for treatment.

ROLE OF DENTISTRY IN RECOGNIZING AND REPORTING HUMAN ABUSE

Awareness of the signs and symptoms of abuse among individuals of all ages should be a goal for every dentist. As a component of the dental relicensure process, New York state requires documentation of continuing education credits in the area of child abuse recognition and the dental professional's responsibility to report such cases.

By statute, all states require that dental personnel, other health care professionals, teachers, and day care and nursing home employees report suspected cases of child and elder abuse. Unfortunately, the reporting of IPV is limited in most jurisdictions to cases involving the use of a weapon while committing a violent act.

Although the dentist has no legal requirement to report IPV in these areas, the American Dental Association's Principles of Ethics and Code of Professional Conduct indicate a responsibility on behalf of dental professionals to intercede in cases involving family violence.

The agency to which the report is made varies among the different jurisdictions. Commonly, the police, social service, child welfare, senior services agencies, or family services departments are the governmental offices designated to accept reports. When a report is made in good faith, the dentist is immune from any counterprosecution or civil liability that might stem from a false report. Failure to report is considered a misdemeanor in most states. In addition, the dentist may be subject to license revocation or malpractice litigation by failing to make a report.

When a dentist determines that a report of child or elder abuse should be made, documentation of the physical evidence to support the charge is mandatory. All evidence is collected according to the principles described for identification and bite mark cases. Descriptions of the injuries and their locations, supporting photographs and radiographs, and information stating the basis for suspicion of abuse are included in the report. When abuse is considered, the dentist should examine the patient and assess the problem separately from the abusive caregiver. Parental consent is not required to obtain appropriate physical evidence from victims younger than the age of majority.

DENTISTS AS EXPERT WITNESSES

Observational, or lay, witnesses testify only to the facts known to them. They are referred to as *witnesses of fact*. Such witnesses are permitted to make inferences about physical facts based on ordinary experience. The witness of fact is not entitled to present hearsay evidence related by another person.

The judicial system recognizes that people with a scientific background or specialized field of study that is admissible under the *Frye* rule or Federal Rules of Evidence can provide the courts with analyses or explanations relative to that discipline. The facts and opinions offered by such a witness are beyond the scope of information that could be expected to be provided by a lay person or witness of fact. A witness who is qualified to testify under this standard is acknowledged as an "expert."

Members of the dental profession are experts. They are qualified to testify by the judge, who bases his or her opinion on educational background, dental and forensic expertise, publications, and other professional qualifications. Dentists who have additional training in one of the dental specialties may be called on to present specific information from that discipline.

Dental experts assist attorneys and, ultimately, the triers of fact (judges and juries) in understanding the scope and complexities of dental science and practice in relation to questions of law. The dentist should not become an advocate for either side in a case but should strive to be an educator and friend of the court.

As experts, dentists may be required to testify in civil litigation cases that involve the following situations:

- **Malpractice based on negligence.** This category includes battery (e.g., extraction of the wrong tooth); misdiagnosis; and failure to diagnose, refer, or inform. All of these actions fall outside the standard of care for the profession.
- **Personal injury.** Temporomandibular joint (TMJ) damage or dental trauma suffered in vehicular, home, sports, recreational, and work-related accidents fall under this category.
- **Dental fraud.** Charging for materials or procedures that were not used or performed are examples of fraud.
- **Identification of multiple fatality incident victims.**

In criminal court, dental expertise is requested in identification of homicide victims and in bite mark and human abuse cases.

Dentists are often unfamiliar with, and may be intimidated by, the adversarial nature of courtroom procedure and protocol. When presenting evidence, the dental expert should remember that his or her role in the legal process is to help the trier of fact understand the dental issues in the case. To this end, and as a scientist, the dental expert witness should present the evidence confidently, accurately, and objectively, relating information in nontechnical terms.

When cross-examined by the opposing attorney, the dental expert witness should remain composed and confident. As an expert, the dentist has the right to refer to records and exemplars prepared for the case. The dentist is entitled to read and review any books or articles proffered by the opposing attorney with the intent of discrediting the testimony.

Pretrial preparation is required if the dental expert and the attorney who has retained his or her services are to develop the evidence to be presented in court. Both must be aware of the strengths and weaknesses of the material and decide how best to provide the jury with this information. Adequate time must be allotted to prepare exhibits for court. It is also advantageous to attempt to determine the position that will be taken by dental experts called by the opposing side.

SUMMARY

Each practitioner has a responsibility to understand the forensic implications associated with the practice of his or her profession. This understanding should include more than ethics and jurisprudence, which were traditionally the only aspects of knowledge of the law acquired by dental professionals. Appreciation of forensic dental problems involving body identification permits clinicians to maintain legally acceptable records and assist legal authorities in the identification of victims of multiple fatality incidents and crimes.

The pursuit of justice in cases of rape, homicide, and human abuse often relies on dental testimony to interpret bite pattern injuries. The development of UV and IR wavelength photographic techniques and equipment has given forensic dentists the opportunity to provide objective scientific evidence in these types of cases. Evidence gathered using these resources can be analyzed and assessed with computer software, laboratory, and clinical procedures that also enhance the forensic odontologist's ability to interpret results.

The reliance of the legal community on the dental profession to continue to provide expertise in civil and criminal proceedings ensures that forensic dentistry will remain a viable component of the forensic sciences and the practice of dentistry.

BIBLIOGRAPHY

Arany S, Ohtani S, Yoshioka N et al: Age estimation from aspartic racemization of root dentin by internal standard method, *Forensic Sci Int* 141:127-130, 2004.

Austin-Smith D, Maples WR: The reliability of skull/photograph superimposition individual identification, *J Forensic Sci* 39:446-455, 1994.

Barsley RE: Forensic and legal issues in oral diagnosis, *Dent Clin North Am* 37:143-144, 1993.

Berger MA: Evidentiary framework. In Cecil JS et al: *Shepard's reference manual on scientific evidence*, pp 39-117, New York, 1994, McGraw-Hill.

Blankenship JA, Mincer HH, Anderson KM et al: Third molar development in the estimation of chronologic age in American blacks as compared with whites, *J Forensic Sci* 52:428-433, 2007.

Bowers CM, Johansen RJ: Photographic evidence protocol: the use of digital imaging methods to rectify angular distortion and create life size reproductions of bite mark evidence, *J Forensic Sci* 47:179-186, 2002.

Bush MA, Bush PJ, Miller RG: Detection and classification of composite resins in incinerated teeth for forensic purposes, *J Forensic Sci* 51:636-642, 2006.

Bush MA, Miller RG, Prutsman-Pfeiffer J et al: Identification through XRF analysis of dental restorative resin materials: a comprehensive study of non-cremated, and processed cremated individuals, *J Forensic Sci* 52:157-165, 2007.

Child Abuse Prevention and Treatment Act of 1974 (PL93-247), DHEW Pub No 78-30137, 42 USCS Section 5106 g (4), Washington, DC, 1988.

Chiodo GT, Tolle SW, Tilden VP: The dentist and family violence, *Gen Dent* 46:20-25, 1998.

CODIS, Combined DNA Index System. Available at http://www.fbi.gov/hq/lab/codis/clickmap.htm. Accessed January 15, 2008.

Cottone JA, Standish SM: *Outline of forensic dentistry*, Chicago, 1982, Year Book Medical Publishers.

Covell K: *The rights of children part three: child sexual exploitation and the age of consent*, 2006. Available at http://aboutkidshealth.ca/News/The-Rights-of-Children-Part-Three-Child-sexual-exploitation-and-the-age-of-consent.aspx?articleID=8226&categoryID=news-type. Accessed February 8, 2008.

da Fonseca MA, Feigal RJ, ten Bensel RW: Dental aspects of 1248 cases of child maltreatment on file at a major county hospital, *Pediatr Dent* 14:152-157, 1992.

Daubert v Merrell Dow Pharmaceuticals Inc, 113 S Ct 2786, 2798, 1993.

DiMaio DJ, DiMaio VJM: *Forensic pathology*, Boca Raton, 1993, CRC Press.

Dorion RBJ, editor: *Bitemark evidence*, New York, 2005, Marcel Dekker.

Doyle v State, 159 Tex C R 310, 263 S W 2d 779, January 20, 1954.

Epstein JB, Scully C: Mammalian bites: risk and management, *Am J Dent* 5:167-172, 1992.

Freeman AJ, Senn DR, Arendt DM: Seven hundred seventy eight bite marks: analysis by anatomical location, victim and biter demographics, type of crime, and legal disposition, *J Forensic Sci* 50:1436-1443, 2005.

Frair J, West MH: Ultraviolet forensic photography, *Kodak Tech Bits* 2:311, 1989.

Frye v United States, 293 F 1013 DC Cir, 1923.

Golden GS: Lessons learned from the WTC disaster: a first-person account, *J Can Dent Assoc* 32:675-680, 2004.

Golden GS: Use of alternative light source illumination in bite mark photography, *J Forensic Sci* 39:815-823, 1994.

Gorlin RJ, Cohen MM, Levin LS: *Syndromes of the head and neck*, ed 3, New York, 1990, Oxford University Press.

Gustafson G: Age determination on teeth, *J Am Dent Assoc* 41:445-454, 1950.

Herschaft EE, Alder ME, Ord DK et al, editors: *American Society of Forensic Odontology—manual of forensic odontology*, ed 4, Albany, NY, 2007, ImPress Printing.

Hopper J: *Child abuse, statistics, research, and resources*, 2007. Available at http://www.jimhopper.com/abstats/. Accessed on February 8, 2008.

Hyzer WG, Krauss TC: The bitemark standard reference scale ABFO no. 2, *J Forensic Sci* 33:498-506, 1988.

IAFIS: *Integrated automated fingerprint identification system*, 2005. Available at http://www.fbi.gov/hq/cjisd/iafis.htm#main. Accessed February 7, 2008.

Jakush J: Forensic dentistry, *J Am Dent Assoc* 119:355-368, 1989.

Kim YK, Kho HS, Lee KH: Age estimation by occlusal wear, *J Forensic Sci* 45:303-309, 2000.

Lewis LM, Levine MD, Dribben WH: Bites and stings. In Dale DC, Federman DD, editors: *Interdisciplinary medicine*, New York, 2000, WebMD Inc.

Mincer HH, Harris EF, Berryman HE: The ABFO study of third molar development and its use as an estimator of chronological age, *J Forensic Sci* 38:379-390, 1993.

Moenssens AA, Inbau FE, Slam JE: *Scientific evidence in criminal cases*, ed 3, Mineola, NY, 1986, Foundation Press.

Myers SL, Williams JM, Hodges JS: Effects of extreme heat on teeth with implications for histologic processing, *J Forensic Sci* 44:805-809, 1999.

Oeschger MP, Hubar JS: Modified intraoral film holders for postmortem identification, *J Forensic Sci* 44:846-848, 1999.

Ohtani S, Yamamoto T: Strategy for the estimation of chronological age using the aspartic acid racemization method with special reference to coefficient of correlation between D/L ratios and ages, *J Forensic Sci* 50:1020-1027, 2005.

Pierce L: Early history of bite marks. In Averill D, editor: *Manual of forensic odontology*, ed 2, pp 127-128, Colorado Springs, 1991, American Society of Forensic Odontology.

Pitluck HM: *Bite mark case management and legal considerations update.* Presentation at the UNLV School of Dental Medicine, Bite Mark Course, Las Vegas, 1999.

Pretty IA: A web-based survey of odontologists' opinions concerning bite mark analysis, *J Forensic Sci* 48:1117-1120, 2003.

Pretty IA, Sweet D: The scientific basis for human bite mark analysis—a critical review, *Sci Justice* 41:85-92, 2001.

Ramsland K: *The C.S.I. effect*, New York, 2006, Berkley Publishing Group.

Regan JD, Parrish JA: *The science of photomedicine*, New York, 1982, Plenum Press.

Roberts D: The iceman: lone voyager from the copper age, *Natl Geogr Mag* 183:36-67, 1993.

Sanger RG, Bross DC: *Clinical management of child abuse and neglect: a guide for the professional*, Chicago, 1984, Quintessence Publishing.

Schrader BA, Senn DR: Dental identification of human remains from orthopedic metallic fixation devices, *Proceedings of the American Academy of Forensic Sciences* 7:198, 2006.

Scientific Working Group on Imaging Technology (SWGIT), International Association for Identification. Available at http://www.theiai.org/guidelines/swgit/index.php. Accessed February 7, 2008.

Sinclair K, McKechnie VM: DNA extraction from stamps and envelope flaps using QIA amp and QIA shredder, *J Forensic Sci* 45:229-230, 2000.

Smith ES, Rawson RD: *Proceedings of the First National Symposium on Dentistry's Role and Responsibility in Mass Disaster Identification*, Chicago, 1988, American Dental Association.

Soomer H, Ranta H, Lincoln MJ et al: Reliability and validity of eight dental age estimation methods for adults, *J Forensic Sci* 48:149-152, 2003

Spitz WU, Spitz DJ: *Spitz and Fischer's medicolegal investigation of death: guidelines for the application of pathology to criminal investigation*, ed 4, Springfield, Ill, 2006, Charles C Thomas.

Standish SM, Stimson PG: Forensic dentistry: legal obligations and methods of identification for the practitioner, *Dent Clin North Am* 21:1-196, 1977.

Sweet DJ, Bowers CM: Accuracy of bite mark overlays: a comparison of five common methods to produce exemplars from a suspect's dentition, *J Forensic Sci* 43:362-367, 1998.

Sweet D, Lorente M, Lorente JA et al: An improved method to recover saliva from human skin: the double swab technique, *J Forensic Sci* 42:320-322, 1997.

Vale GL: Identification by dental evidence: basic and beyond, *J Can Dent Assoc* 32:665-672, 2004.

Vale GL et al: Guidelines for bite mark analysis, *J Am Dent Assoc* 112:383-386, 1986.

Warnick AJ: *Forensic dental identification team manual*, Detroit, 1989, Detroit Dental Association.

Wright FD, Golden G: Forensic photography. In Stimson P, Mertz C, editors: *Forensic dentistry*, Boca Raton, Fla, 1997, CRC Press.

Zarkowski P: Bite mark evidence: its worth in the eyes of the expert, *J Law Ethics Dent* 1:47-57, 1988.

Differential Diagnosis of Oral and Maxillofacial Diseases

The most important aspect of patient care is the accurate diagnosis of the patient's disease. Unfortunately, the clinical presentation of many disease processes can be strikingly similar, despite their vast differences in etiology and pathogenesis. Because treatment and, ultimately, prognosis are based on the diagnosis, the diagnostic process is critical in optimal patient management. This appendix provides some guidelines for expediting and facilitating the diagnostic process from a clinical perspective.

The first step in gathering information is the acquisition of a thorough history of the disease process. This step typically includes items such as the onset, severity, location, duration, character, and course of the signs and symptoms being experienced by the patient. Additional information regarding medical, social, and family history may be necessary. With this information, the clinician can often start the process of formulating a list of possible diagnoses, even before performing an examination.

The information obtained during the clinical examination is also important because many lesions have characteristic appearances. By evaluating these characteristics in conjunction with the patient's history, often the clinician can narrow the list of diagnostic possibilities. This list, known as a *differential diagnosis*, essentially includes possible pathologic entities, usually ranked in order from most likely to least likely.

DEFINITIONS

To better describe the appearances of lesions and communicate these features to colleagues, the clinician should be familiar with the following terms:

Macule. Focal area of color change that is not elevated or depressed in relation to its surroundings.

Papule. Solid, raised lesion that is less than 5 mm in diameter.

Nodule. Solid, raised lesion that is greater than 5 mm in diameter.

Sessile. Describing a tumor or growth whose base is the widest part of the lesion.

Pedunculated. Describing a tumor or growth whose base is narrower than the widest part of the lesion.

Papillary. Describing a tumor or growth exhibiting numerous surface projections.

Verrucous. Describing a tumor or growth exhibiting a rough, warty surface.

Vesicle. Superficial blister, 5 mm or less in diameter, usually filled with clear fluid.

Bulla. Large blister, greater than 5 mm in diameter.

Pustule. Blister filled with purulent exudate.

Ulcer. Lesion characterized by loss of the surface epithelium and frequently some of the underlying connective tissue. It often appears depressed or excavated.

Erosion. Superficial lesion, often arising secondary to rupture of a vesicle or bulla, that is characterized by partial or total loss of the surface epithelium.

Fissure. Narrow, slitlike ulceration or groove.

Plaque. Lesion that is slightly elevated and is flat on its surface.

Petechia. Round, pinpoint area of hemorrhage.

Ecchymosis. Nonelevated area of hemorrhage, larger than a petechia.

Telangiectasia. Vascular lesion caused by dilatation of a small, superficial blood vessel.

Cyst. Pathologic epithelium-lined cavity, often filled with liquid or semi-solid contents.

Unilocular. Describing a radiolucent lesion having a single compartment.

Multilocular. Describing a radiolucent lesion having several or many compartments.

By using these terms, the clinician can describe the characteristics of lesions efficiently and uniformly. Applying these clinical descriptors to the lesions also can help categorize them with respect to the differential diagnosis. By adding additional characteristics such as prevalence, patient race or nationality, patient age at diagnosis, patient sex, and sites of predilection, the clinician can hone the differential diagnosis list considerably.

HOW TO USE THIS APPENDIX

This appendix is designed to help the clinician formulate a differential diagnosis by organizing and categorizing disease entities according to their most prominent or identifiable clinical features. Under each "clinical feature" heading is a list of lesions with that clinical feature as a prominent component. Diseases are listed according to estimated frequency relative to similar diseases or lesions.

The most common lesions are marked with triple asterisks (***), less common lesions are marked with double asterisks (**), and rare lesions are marked with a single asterisk (*). Such estimated frequency indicators should not be compared between lists; they are intended only for the single differential diagnosis list in which they occur.

Clinical features that most readily distinguish the lesions are listed with each disease process to help focus the clinician's search for the most accurate diagnosis. Finally, the corresponding page number in the book is provided for each disease entity so that the reader can refer to the text for a more detailed discussion.

INDEX TO THE APPENDIX: DIFFERENTIAL DIAGNOSIS LISTS

Frequency of Occurrence	Lesion or Condition	Comments or Special Characteristics	Page
A. WHITE LESIONS: CAN BE SCRAPED OFF			
***	White coated tongue	May be scraped off slightly, with difficulty	13
***	Pseudomembranous candidiasis	"Milk curd" or "cottage cheese" appearance; may leave red base when rubbed off	213
***	Morsicatio	Surface may appear to be peeling off	286
**	Thermal burn	Example: pizza burn	289
**	Sloughing traumatic lesion	Example: cotton roll "burn"	293
**	Toothpaste or mouthwash reaction	Filmy whiteness; leaves normal appearing mucosa when rubbed off	350
**	Chemical burn	Example: aspirin burn secondary to direct application for toothache	291
*	Secondary syphilis	Mucous patch; may be only partially scraped off	188
*	Diphtheria	Gray-white pseudomembrane of oropharynx	186
B. WHITE LESIONS: CANNOT BE SCRAPED OFF			
***	Linea alba	Buccal mucosa along occlusal plane	285
***	Leukoedema	Primarily in blacks; milky white alteration of buccal mucosa bilaterally; disappears when stretched	8
***	Leukoplakia	May show benign hyperkeratosis, epithelial dysplasia, or invasive carcinoma	388
***	Tobacco pouch keratosis	Usually in mandibular vestibule; associated with use of snuff or chewing tobacco	398
***	Actinic cheilosis	Pale, gray-white, scaly alteration of lower lip; usually in older men with history of chronic sun exposure; precancerous	405
***	Lichen planus	Wickham's striae; typically bilateral on buccal mucosa	782
***	Morsicatio	Most common on anterior buccal mucosa, labial mucosa, and lateral border of tongue; exhibits ragged surface	286
***	White coated tongue	Diffuse involvement of dorsal tongue	13
**	Nicotine stomatitis	Usually associated with pipe smoking; occurs on hard palate	403
*	Hairy leukoplakia	Usually lateral border of tongue; rough surface with vertical fissures; usually associated with HIV infection	268
*	Hyperplastic candidiasis	Most commonly affects anterior buccal mucosa	217
*	Lupus erythematosus	Most common on buccal mucosa; may mimic lichen planus or leukoplakia; associated skin lesions usually present	794
*	Skin graft	History of previous surgery	–
*	Submucous fibrosis	More common in South Asia; associated with betel quid chewing	401
*	White sponge nevus	Hereditary; onset in childhood; generalized lesions, especially buccal mucosa	743
*	Hereditary benign intraepithelial dyskeratosis	Hereditary; onset in childhood; generalized lesions, especially buccal mucosa; ocular involvement possible	744
*	Pachyonychia congenita	Hereditary; onset in childhood; most common on dorsal tongue and areas of trauma; nail, palmar, and plantar changes also present	745
*	Dyskeratosis congenita	Hereditary; onset in childhood; dystrophic nail changes	746
*	Tertiary syphilis	Syphilitic glossitis	190
*	Uremic stomatitis	Renal failure	851

Frequency of Occurrence	Lesion or Condition	Comments or Special Characteristics	Page
C. WHITE AND RED LESIONS			
***	Erythema migrans	Geographic tongue; continually changing pattern; rarely involves other oral mucosal sites	779
***	Candidiasis	White component may be rubbed off	213
***	Lichen planus	Atrophic or erosive forms; Wickham's striae; typically bilateral on buccal mucosa	782
**	Burns	Examples: pizza burn, aspirin burn, other chemical burns; white component may be rubbed off	289
**	Actinic cheilosis	Pale, gray-white and red alteration to lower lip; usually in older men with history of chronic sun exposure	405
**	Nicotine stomatitis	Usually associated with pipe smoking; occurs on hard palate	403
**	Erythroleukoplakia	Usually shows epithelial dysplasia or carcinoma	392
**	Cinnamon reaction	Related to cinnamon flavored gum; typically on buccal mucosa and lateral tongue	352
*	Lupus erythematosus	Most common on buccal mucosa; may mimic lichen planus or leukoplakia; associated skin lesions usually present	794
*	Scarlet fever	Secondary to β-hemolytic streptococcal infection; strawberry/raspberry tongue	184
*	Verruciform xanthoma	Most common on gingiva and hard palate; surface may be papillary	372
D. RED LESIONS			
***	Pharyngitis	Examples: strep throat, viral pharyngitis	183
***	Traumatic erythema	Caused by local irritation	—
***	Denture stomatitis	Denture-bearing palatal mucosa	216
***	Erythematous candidiasis	Example: central papillary atrophy (median rhomboid glossitis)	215
***	Erythema migrans	Geographic tongue (cases with absence of white borders); continually changing pattern; rarely involves other mucosal sites	779
***	Angular cheilitis	Erythema and cracking at labial commissures	216
**	Thermal burns	Example: caused by hot liquids	289
**	Erythroplakia	Usually shows epithelial dysplasia or carcinoma	397
*	Anemia	Atrophic, red tongue; can be due to pernicious anemia, iron-deficiency anemia, hypovitaminosis B	827
*	Hemangioma	Develops in younger patients; may blanch; may show bluish hue	538
*	Lupus erythematosus	Usually with associated skin lesions	794
*	Scarlet fever	Secondary to β-hemolytic streptococcal infection; strawberry/raspberry tongue	184
*	Plasma cell gingivitis	Allergic reaction usually related to flavoring agents	159
*	Radiation mucositis	Patient currently undergoing radiotherapy	294
E. PETECHIAL, ECCHYMOTIC, AND TELANGIECTATIC LESIONS			
***	Nonspecific trauma	History of injury to lesional site	305
**	Upper respiratory infections	Soft palate petechiae	306
*	Infectious mononucleosis	Soft palate petechiae; tonsillitis and/or pharyngitis may be present	253
*	Idiopathic thrombocytopenic purpura	Areas of trauma; gingival bleeding possibly present	585
*	Trauma from fellatio	Posterior palatal petechiae or ecchymosis	307
*	Hemophilia	Hereditary; childhood onset; gingival bleeding may be present	573
*	Leukemia	Caused by secondary thrombocytopenia; gingival bleeding may be present	587

Continued

Frequency of Occurrence	Lesion or Condition	Comments or Special Characteristics	Page
E. PETECHIAL, ECCHYMOTIC, AND TELANGIECTATIC LESIONS—cont'd			
*	Hereditary hemorrhagic	Multiple, pinhead-sized telangiectasias; possible history of nosebleeds or gastrointestinal bleeding	754
*	CREST syndrome	Multiple, pinhead-sized telangiectasias; **C**alcinosis cutis, **R**aynaud's phenomenon, **E**sophageal motility defect, **S**clerodactyly, **T**elangiectasias	801
F. BLUE AND/OR PURPLE LESIONS			
***	Varicosities	Especially after 45 years of age; most common on ventral tongue and lips	15
***	Submucosal hemorrhage	Also see Appendix List, Part 1, E. (previous topic) Petechial, Ecchymotic, and Telangiectatic Lesions	305
***	Amalgam tattoo	Most common on gingiva; blue-gray; radiopaque amalgam particles sometimes discovered on radiographs	308
***	Mucocele	Especially on lower labial mucosa; typically pale blue; cyclic swelling and rupturing often exhibited	454
**	Eruption cyst	Overlying an erupting tooth	682
**	Salivary duct cyst	Usually pale blue	457
**	Hemangioma	Usually red-purple; may blanch under pressure; onset in younger patients	538
**	Ranula	Pale blue, fluctuant swelling of lateral floor of mouth	456
**	Kaposi's sarcoma	Especially in AIDS patients; usually purple; most common on palate and maxillary gingiva	270
*	Nasopalatine duct cyst	Midline of anterior palate	28
*	Salivary gland tumors	Especially mucoepidermoid carcinoma and pleomorphic adenoma; usually pale blue; most common on posterior lateral palate	Chapter 11
*	Gingival cyst of the adult	Most common in mandibular bicuspid-cuspid region	692
*	Blue nevus	Most common on hard palate	386
*	Malignant melanoma	Most common on hard palate and maxillary gingiva; may show mixture of deep blue, brown, black, and other colors	433
G. BROWN, GRAY, AND/OR BLACK LESIONS			
***	Racial pigmentation	Most common on attached gingiva in darker complexioned patients	–
***	Amalgam tattoo	Most common on gingiva; usually slate-gray to black; opaque amalgam particles may be found on radiographs	308
***	Black/brown hairy tongue	Discoloration and elongation of filiform papillae	13
**	Melanotic macule	Brown; most common on lower lip	379
**	Smoker's melanosis	Most common on anterior facial gingiva	316
**	Non-amalgam tattoos	Example: graphite from pencil	308
*	Melanocytic nevus	Most common on hard palate; can be flat or raised	382
*	Malignant melanoma	Most common on hard palate and maxillary gingiva; may show mixture of deep blue, brown, black, and other colors	433
*	Oral melanoacanthoma	Rapidly enlarging pigmented lesion; usually occurs in blacks	380
*	Drug ingestion	Examples: chloroquine, chlorpromazine, minocycline; especially on hard palate	317
*	Peutz-Jeghers syndrome	Freckle-like lesions of vermilion and perioral skin; intestinal polyps; hereditary	753
*	Addison's disease	Chronic adrenal insufficiency; associated with bronzing of skin	841
*	Neurofibromatosis type I	*Café au lait* pigmentation; cutaneous neurofibromas	529
*	McCune-Albright syndrome	*Café au lait* pigmentation; polyostotic fibrous dysplasia; endocrine disorders	636
*	Heavy metal poisoning	Typically along marginal gingiva (e.g., lead, bismuth, silver)	313
*	Melanotic neuroectodermal tumor of infancy	Anterior maxilla; destroys underlying bone	533

Frequency of Occurrence	Lesion or Condition	Comments or Special Characteristics	Page
H. YELLOW LESIONS			
***	Fordyce granules	Sebaceous glands; usually multiple submucosal papules on buccal mucosa or upper lip vermilion	7
**	Superficial abscess	Example: parulis from nonvital tooth	136
**	Accessory lymphoid aggregate	Most common in oropharynx and floor of mouth; may exhibit orange hue	572
**	Lymphoepithelial cyst	Most common on lingual and palatine tonsils, and floor of mouth; may be yellow-white	37
**	Lipoma	Most common on buccal mucosa; soft to palpation	523
*	Jaundice	Generalized discoloration, especially involving soft palate and floor of mouth; sclera usually affected also	821
*	Verruciform xanthoma	Most common on gingiva and hard palate; surface may be rough or papillary	372
*	Pyostomatitis vegetans	"Snail-track" pustules; associated with inflammatory bowel disease	850

Frequency of Occurrence	Lesion or Condition	Comments or Special Characteristics	Page
A. VESICULOEROSIVE AND ULCERATIVE LESIONS: ACUTE (SHORT DURATION AND SUDDEN ONSET)			
***	Traumatic ulcer	Mild-to-moderate pain; history of local trauma	287
***	Aphthous stomatitis	Extremely painful; may be single or multiple; nonkeratinized movable mucosa; often recurs	331
***	Recurrent herpes labialis	Vermilion and labial skin; begins as multiple vesicles; often recurs	243
**	Primary herpetic gingivostomatitis	Fever and malaise; children and young adults; multiple vesicles; gingiva consistently affected	241
**	Necrotizing ulcerative gingivitis (NUG)	Painful destruction of gingival papillae; fetid odor; mostly in teenagers and young adults	157
**	Mucosal burns	Chemical or thermal	289
**	Recurrent intraoral herpes simplex	Gingiva or hard palate (except in immunocompromised); focal cluster of vesicles and shallow ulcers	244
**	Allergic reactions	Example: Caused by topical medications or dental materials; erythema and vesicles	350
**	Erythema multiforme	Predominantly in children and young adults; multiple blisters and ulcers; often crusting, hemorrhagic lip lesions; may have associated "target" skin lesions or involvement of ocular and genital mucosa (Stevens-Johnson syndrome)	776
**	Herpangina	Especially in children; multiple small ulcers on soft palate and tonsillar pillars	257
*	Varicella (chickenpox)	Associated with skin eruption; few oral vesicles and ulcers; usually in children	248
*	Herpes zoster	Unilateral involvement along nerve distribution; usually middle-aged and older adults; painful vesicles and ulcers	250
*	Hand-foot-and-mouth disease	Especially in children; multiple vesicles and ulcers; associated vesicles on hands and feet	257
*	Necrotizing sialometaplasia	Usually posterior lateral hard palate; prior swelling may be present; deep crater-like ulcer; may be only minimal pain	471
*	Anesthetic necrosis	Usually at site of palatal injection	303
*	Primary syphilis	Chancre at site of inoculation; usually painless with clean ulcer bed	188
*	Behçet's syndrome	Aphthous-like ulcers; genital ulcers and ocular inflammation	336
B. VESICULOEROSIVE AND ULCERATIVE LESIONS: CHRONIC (LONG DURATION)			
***	Erosive lichen planus	Associated with white striae; usually in middle-aged and older adults; most common on buccal mucosa and gingiva ("desquamative gingivitis")	785
**	Squamous cell carcinoma	Usually in middle-aged and older adults; usually indurated and may have rolled border; may be painless	409
**	Mucous membrane pemphigoid	Most common in middle-aged and older women; most commonly presents as a "desquamative gingivitis"; may involve ocular and genital mucosa	771
**	Traumatic granuloma	Solitary, non-healing ulcer	287
*	Lupus erythematosus	May have associated red and white change; usually with skin involvement	794
*	Pemphigus vulgaris	Usually in middle-aged and older patients; multiple oral blisters and ulcers usually precede skin lesions	765
*	Deep fungal infections	Examples: histoplasmosis, blastomycosis; may be painless	Chapter 6
*	Tuberculosis	Associated mass may be present; may be painless	195
*	Sarcoidosis	May be associated with erythematous macules or plaques; may be painless	338

Frequency of Occurrence	Lesion or Condition	Comments or Special Characteristics	Page
B. VESICULOEROSIVE AND ULCERATIVE LESIONS: CHRONIC (LONG DURATION)—cont'd			
*	Epidermolysis bullosa	Hereditary (except epidermolysis bullosa acquisita); onset in infancy and childhood; multiple skin and oral blisters or ulcers in areas of trauma; may result in extensive scarring	761
*	Pyostomatitis vegetans	Yellowish "snail-track" pustules; associated with inflammatory bowel disease	850
*	Wegener's granulomatosis	Usually palatal ulceration and destruction; associated lung and kidney involvement may be present; may show "strawberry gingivitis"	345
*	Extranodal NK/T-cell lymphoma, nasal-type (midline lethal granuloma)	Palatal lymphoma with ulceration and destruction of underlying bone; may be painless	602
*	Noma	Gangrenous necrosis secondary to necrotizing ulcerative gingivitis; usually in malnourished children or immunocompromised individuals	201
*	Tertiary syphilis	Gumma; associated mass may be present; may be painless; may perforate palate	190
C. PAPILLARY GROWTHS: FOCAL OR DIFFUSE			
***	Hairy tongue	Usually brown or black discoloration; hyperkeratotic elongation of filiform papillae on posterior dorsal tongue	13
***	Papilloma	Can be white or pink; most common on soft palate and tongue; usually pedunculated	362
***	Inflammatory papillary hyperplasia	Usually involves midportion of hard palate beneath denture	512
**	Verruca vulgaris	Common wart; especially in younger patients; most common on labial mucosa	364
**	Leukoplakia (some variants)	Examples: proliferative verrucous leukoplakia, granular or nodular leukoplakia	391
**	Squamous cell carcinoma	Examples with papillary surface changes	409
*	Hairy leukoplakia	Usually lateral border of tongue; rough surface with vertical fissures; usually associated with HIV infection	268
*	Giant cell fibroma	Usually in children and young adults; most common on gingiva	509
*	Verruciform xanthoma	Most common on gingiva and hard palate	372
*	Verrucous carcinoma	Especially in older patients with long history of snuff or chewing tobacco use; especially in mandibular vestibule and buccal mucosa; may be white or red	422
*	Condyloma acuminatum	Venereal wart; broad-based lesions with blunted projections; frequently multiple	366
*	Multifocal epithelial hyperplasia	Usually multiple, flat-topped papular lesions; usually in children; most common in Native Americans and Inuit; color may vary from normal to white	367
*	Darier's disease	Most commonly appears as pebbly appearance of hard palate; associated crusty, greasy skin lesions; hereditary	751
*	Acanthosis nigricans (malignant type)	Most commonly appears as generalized pebbly alteration of upper lip; pigmented, pebbly skin changes in flexural areas; associated gastrointestinal malignancy	803

Frequency of Occurrence	Lesion or Condition	Comments or Special Characteristics	Page
A. SOFT TISSUE MASSES (LUMPS AND BUMPS): LOWER LIP			
***	Mucocele	Typically pale blue; often exhibits cyclic swelling and rupturing; labial mucosa only	454
***	Fibroma	Usually normal in color	507
**	Squamous cell carcinoma	Tumor with rough, granular, irregular surface; usually on vermilion border	409
*	Other mesenchymal tumors	Examples: hemangioma, neurofibroma, lipoma	Chapter 12
*	Salivary duct cyst	May be bluish; labial mucosa only	457
*	Salivary gland tumor	Usually mucoepidermoid carcinoma	Chapter 11
*	Keratoacanthoma	Volcano-shaped mass with central keratin plug; rapid development; vermilion border only	406
B. SOFT TISSUE MASSES (LUMPS AND BUMPS): UPPER LIP			
**	Fibroma	Usually normal in color	507
**	Salivary gland tumor	Usually canalicular adenoma (older than age 40) or pleomorphic adenoma (younger than age 40)	Chapter 11
**	Salivary duct cyst	May be bluish	457
*	Minor gland sialolith	Small, hard submucosal mass; may be tender	459
*	Other mesenchymal tumors	Examples: hemangioma, neurofibroma, neurilemoma	Chapter 12
*	Nasolabial cyst	Fluctuant swelling of lateral labial vestibule	27
C. SOFT TISSUE MASSES (LUMPS AND BUMPS): BUCCAL MUCOSA			
***	Fibroma	Usually normal in color; along occlusal plane	507
**	Lipoma	May be yellow; soft to palpation	523
**	Mucocele	Typically pale blue; often exhibits cyclic swelling and rupturing	454
*	Hyperplastic lymph node	Usually buccinator node; movable submucosal mass	571
*	Other mesenchymal tumors	Examples: hemangioma, neurofibroma	Chapter 12
*	Squamous cell carcinoma	Tumor with rough, granular, irregular surface	409
*	Salivary gland tumor	Pleomorphic adenoma and mucoepidermoid carcinoma most common	Chapter 11
D. SOFT TISSUE MASSES (LUMPS AND BUMPS): GINGIVA/ALVEOLAR MUCOSA			
***	Parulis	Fistula from nonvital tooth	136
***	Epulis fissuratum	Ill-fitting denture	510
***	Pyogenic granuloma	Usually red, ulcerated, easily bleeding; increased frequency in pregnant women	517
***	Peripheral ossifying fibroma	May be red or normal in color; may be ulcerated	521
**	Peripheral giant cell granuloma	Reddish purple; frequently ulcerated	520
**	Fibroma	Usually normal in color	507
*	Squamous cell carcinoma	Tumor with rough, granular, irregular surface	409
*	Metastatic tumors	May be painful and destroy bone	563
*	Gingival cyst of the adult	Most common in mandibular bicuspid-cuspid region; may be blue	692
*	Traumatic neuroma	Edentulous mandible in mental foramen area; often painful to palpation	524
*	Kaposi's sarcoma	Especially in AIDS patients; usually purple	270
*	Peripheral odontogenic tumors	Example: peripheral ameloblastoma	710
*	Congenital epulis	Usually in females; especially anterior maxilla	537

Frequency of Occurrence	Lesion or Condition	Comments or Special Characteristics	Page
D. SOFT TISSUE MASSES (LUMPS AND BUMPS): GINGIVA/ALVEOLAR MUCOSA—cont'd			
*	Melanotic neuroectodermal tumor of infancy	Anterior maxilla; destroys underlying bone; may be pigmented	533
*	Other mesenchymal tumors	Examples: hemangioma, neurofibroma	Chapter 12
E. SOFT TISSUE MASSES (LUMPS AND BUMPS): FLOOR OF MOUTH			
**	Ranula/mucocele	Typically a pale blue, fluctuant swelling	456
**	Sialolith	Usually hard mass in submandibular duct; may be associated with tender swelling of affected gland; radiopaque mass	459
**	Squamous cell carcinoma	Tumor with rough, granular, irregular surface	409
**	Lymphoepithelial cyst	Small, yellow-white submucosal lesion	37
*	Epidermoid or dermoid cyst	Midline yellow-white submucosal lesion	33
*	Salivary gland tumors	Especially mucoepidermoid carcinoma	Chapter 11
*	Mesenchymal tumors	Examples: lipoma, neurofibroma, hemangioma	Chapter 12
F. SOFT TISSUE MASSES (LUMPS AND BUMPS): TONGUE			
***	Fibroma	Usually normal in color; most common on margins of tongue	507
**	Squamous cell carcinoma	Tumor with rough, granular, irregular surface	409
**	Mucocele	Usually anterior ventral surface; usually bluish or clear color	454
*	Granular cell tumor	Dome-shaped; usually on dorsum of tongue	536
*	Other mesenchymal tumors	Examples: lymphangioma, hemangioma, neurofibroma, osseous choristoma	Chapter 12
*	Pyogenic granuloma	Usually red, ulcerated, easily bleeding	517
*	Salivary gland tumors	Especially mucoepidermoid carcinoma and adenoid cystic carcinoma	Chapter 11
*	Lingual thyroid	Usually posterior midline of dorsal surface; usually in women	12
G. SOFT TISSUE MASSES (LUMPS AND BUMPS): HARD OR SOFT PALATE			
***	Palatal abscess	Associated with nonvital tooth	136
***	Leaf-like denture fibroma	Pedunculated hyperplastic growth beneath ill-fitting denture	511
**	Salivary gland tumors	Especially pleomorphic adenoma, mucoepidermoid carcinoma, adenoid cystic carcinoma, polymorphous low-grade adenocarcinoma; may have bluish hue	Chapter 11
**	Kaposi's sarcoma	Usually purple; may be multiple; usually associated with AIDS	270
**	Nasopalatine duct cyst	Fluctuant swelling of anterior midline palate	28
*	Other mesenchymal tumors	Examples: fibroma, hemangioma, neurofibroma	Chapter 12
*	Squamous cell carcinoma	Tumor with rough, granular, irregular surface; occasionally arises from maxillary sinus	409
*	Mucocele/salivary duct cyst	Usually has bluish hue	454
*	Lymphoma	Often boggy and edematous; may have bluish hue; may be bilateral	595
*	Melanocytic nevus/melanoma	Usually pigmented	382, 433
*	Necrotizing sialometaplasia	Early stage lesion; often associated with pain or paresthesia	471
*	Adenomatoid hyperplasia of minor salivary glands	Asymptomatic, painless mass	471

Continued

Frequency of Occurrence	Lesion or Condition	Comments or Special Characteristics	Page
H. SOFT TISSUE MASSES (LUMPS AND BUMPS): MULTIPLE LESIONS			
**	Kaposi's sarcoma	Usually purple lesions of palate and maxillary gingiva; usually associated with AIDS	270
**	Neurofibromatosis type I	Oral and skin neurofibromas; *café au lait* skin pigmentation	529
*	Multifocal epithelial hyperplasia	Usually flat-topped papular lesions; usually in children; most common in Native Americans and Inuit; color may vary from normal to white	367
*	Amyloidosis	Pale, firm deposits, especially in tongue; periocular cutaneous lesions frequently present; most often associated with multiple myeloma	822
*	Granulomatous diseases	Examples: sarcoidosis, Crohn's disease, leprosy	338
*	Multiple endocrine neoplasia type 2B	Mucosal neuromas of lips and tongue; adrenal pheochromocytomas; medullary thyroid carcinoma; marfanoid body build	532
*	Tuberous sclerosis	Small fibroma-like growths on gingiva; angiofibromas of face; epilepsy; mental retardation	757
*	Multiple hamartoma syndrome	Cowden syndrome; small fibroma-like growths on gingiva; multiple hamartomas of various tissues; breast cancer in affected women	760
I. SOFT TISSUE MASSES (LUMPS AND BUMPS): MIDLINE NECK LESIONS			
**	Thyroid gland enlargement	Examples: goiter, thyroid tumor	–
*	Thyroglossal duct cyst	May move up and down with tongue motion	35
*	Dermoid cyst	Soft and fluctuant	33
*	Plunging ranula	Soft and compressible	457
J. SOFT TISSUE MASSES (LUMPS AND BUMPS): LATERAL NECK LESIONS			
***	Reactive lymphadenopathy	Secondary to oral and maxillofacial infection; often tender to palpation	571
**	Epidermoid cyst	Soft and movable	32
**	Lipoma	Soft mass	523
**	Infectious mononucleosis	Fatigue; sore throat; tender lymph nodes	253
**	Metastatic carcinoma	Deposits from oral and pharyngeal carcinomas; usually indurated and painless; may be fixed	417
**	Lymphoma	May be unilateral or bilateral; usually painless; Hodgkin's and non-Hodgkin's types	592
*	Salivary gland tumors	Arising from submandibular gland or tail of parotid gland	Chapter 11
*	Submandibular sialadenitis	Example: secondary to sialolithiasis	461
*	Cervical lymphoepithelial cyst	Soft and fluctuant; most common in young adults	36
*	Granulomatous diseases	Examples: tuberculosis, sarcoidosis	197, 338
*	Cat-scratch disease	History of exposure to cat	205
*	Cystic hygroma	Infants; soft and fluctuant	547
*	Plunging ranula	Soft and compressible	457
*	Other mesenchymal tumors	Examples: neurofibroma, carotid body tumor	Chapter 12
K. GENERALIZED GINGIVAL ENLARGEMENT			
***	Hyperplastic gingivitis	Examples: associated with puberty, pregnancy, diabetes	156
**	Drug-related gingival hyperplasia	Examples: phenytoin, calcium-channel blockers, cyclosporine; may be fibrotic	163
*	Gingival fibromatosis	May be hereditary; onset in childhood	166
*	Leukemic infiltrate	Usually boggy and hemorrhagic	587
*	Wegener's granulomatosis	"Strawberry" gingivitis; may have palatal ulceration and destruction; lung and kidney involvement	345
*	Scurvy	Vitamin C deficiency	826

Frequency of Occurrence	Lesion or Condition	Comments or Special Characteristics	Page
A. UNILOCULAR RADIOLUCENCIES: PERICORONAL LOCATION			
***	Hyperplastic dental follicle	<5 mm in thickness	680
***	Dentigerous cyst	>5 mm in thickness	679
**	Eruption cyst	Bluish swelling overlying erupting tooth	682
**	Odontogenic keratocyst	–	683
*	Orthokeratinized odontogenic cyst	–	687
*	Ameloblastoma	Especially unicystic type	702
*	Ameloblastic fibroma	Usually in younger patients	719
*	Adenomatoid odontogenic tumor	Usually in anterior region of jaws; most often with maxillary canine; usually in teenagers	713
*	Calcifying odontogenic cyst	Gorlin cyst	695
*	Carcinoma arising in dentigerous cyst	Mostly in older adults	700
*	Intraosseous muco-epidermoid carcinoma	Mostly in posterior mandible	490
*	Other odontogenic lesions	Examples: calcifying epithelial odontogenic tumor, odontogenic myxoma, central odontogenic fibroma	Chapter 15
B. UNILOCULAR RADIOLUCENCIES: PERIAPICAL LOCATION			
***	Periapical granuloma	Nonvital tooth	127
***	Periapical cyst	Nonvital tooth	130
**	Periapical cemento-osseous dysplasia (early)	Especially in black females; usually apical to mandibular anteriors; teeth are vital	641
*	Periapical scar	Usually endodontically treated tooth with destruction of cortical plate	130
*	Dentin dysplasia type I	Multiple periapical granulomas or cysts; shortened, malformed roots	108
C. UNILOCULAR RADIOLUCENCIES: OTHER LOCATIONS			
***	Developing tooth bud	Within alveolar bone	–
**	Lateral radicular cyst	Nonvital tooth; lateral canal	132
**	Nasopalatine duct cyst	Between and apical to maxillary central incisors; palatal swelling may occur	28
**	Lateral periodontal cyst	Especially in mandibular bicuspid-cuspid region	692
**	Residual (periapical) cyst	Edentulous area	132
**	Odontogenic keratocyst	–	683
**	Central giant cell granuloma	Especially in anterior mandible	626
**	Stafne bone defect	Angle of mandible below mandibular canal	24
*	Cemento-osseous dysplasia	Early stage; usually in young adult and middle-aged black women; usually in mandible	640
*	Central ossifying fibroma	Early-stage lesion	646
*	Ameloblastoma	Especially unicystic type	702
*	Other odontogenic cysts and tumors	Examples: ameloblastic fibroma, central odontogenic fibroma, calcifying odontogenic cyst	Chapter 15
*	Langerhans cell histiocytosis	"Histiocytosis X"; usually in children or young adults	590

Continued

Frequency of Occurrence	Lesion or Condition	Comments or Special Characteristics	Page
C. UNILOCULAR RADIOLUCENCIES: OTHER LOCATIONS—cont'd			
*	Melanotic neuroectodermal tumor of infancy	Anterior maxilla; may be pigmented	533
*	Median palatal cyst	Clinical midline swelling of hard palate	31
*	Neurilemoma/neurofibroma	Usually associated with mandibular nerve	528
D. MULTILOCULAR RADIOLUCENCIES			
***	Odontogenic keratocyst	—	683
***	Ameloblastoma	Especially in posterior mandible; often associated with impacted tooth	702
**	Central giant cell granuloma	Especially in anterior mandible	626
*	Ameloblastic fibroma	Especially in younger patients	719
*	Odontogenic myxoma	"Cobweb" trabeculation	729
*	Central odontogenic fibroma	—	726
*	Calcifying epithelial odontogenic tumor	Often associated with impacted tooth	716
*	Orthokeratinized odontogenic cyst	Often associated with impacted tooth	687
*	Lateral periodontal cyst (botryoid type)	Especially in mandibular bicuspid-cuspid region	692
*	Calcifying odontogenic cyst	Especially in cases with minimal or no calcifications; often associated with impacted tooth	695
*	Central hemangioma/ arteriovenous malformation	Especially in younger patients; may have honeycombed radiographic appearance; may pulsate	540
*	Aneurysmal bone cyst	Especially in younger patients	634
*	Cherubism	Hereditary; onset in childhood; multiple quadrants involved	629
*	Hyperparathyroidism (brown tumor)	Usually elevated serum calcium levels	838
*	Intraosseous muco-epidermoid carcinoma	Usually in posterior mandible	490
*	Fibrous dysplasia	Very rarely on panoramic films of mandibular lesions	635
E. RADIOLUCENCIES: POORLY DEFINED OR RAGGED BORDERS			
***	Periapical granuloma or cyst	Nonvital tooth	127
***	Focal osteoporotic marrow defect	Especially edentulous areas in posterior mandible; more common in females	619
**	Osteomyelitis	Usually painful or tender	141
**	Bisphosphonate-associated osteonecrosis	Exposed necrotic bone	299
*	Simple bone cyst	Mandibular lesion that scallops up between roots of teeth; usually in younger patients	631
*	Metastatic tumors	Painful; paresthesia; usually in older adults	669
*	Osteoradionecrosis	History of radiation therapy; painful	296
*	Multiple myeloma	May be painful; in older adults	604
*	Primary intraosseous carcinomas	Odontogenic or salivary origin	711
*	Osteosarcoma	Often painful; usually in young adults	660
*	Chondrosarcoma	—	664
*	Ewing's sarcoma	Almost always in children	667
*	Other primary bone malignancies	Examples: fibrosarcoma, lymphoma	—

Frequency of Occurrence	Lesion or Condition	Comments or Special Characteristics	Page

E. RADIOLUCENCIES: POORLY DEFINED OR RAGGED BORDERS—cont'd

*	Desmoplastic fibroma of bone	Especially in younger patients	658
*	Massive osteolysis	Phantom (vanishing) bone disease	622
*	NICO (neuralgia-inducing cavitational osteonecrosis)	Local or referred pain	866

F. RADIOLUCENCIES: MULTIFOCAL OR GENERALIZED

***	Cemento-osseous dysplasia	Early stage lesions; usually in black females; usually in mandible	640
**	Nevoid basal cell carcinoma syndrome	Odontogenic keratocysts	688
**	Multiple myeloma	Painful; in older adults; "punched-out" lesions	604
*	Cherubism	Usually multilocular; onset in childhood; hereditary	629
*	Hyperparathyroidism	Multiple brown tumors	838
*	Langerhans cell histiocytosis	"Histiocytosis X"; in children and young adults; teeth "floating in air"	590

G. RADIOPACITIES: WELL-DEMARCATED BORDERS

***	Torus or exostosis	Associated with bony surface mass	19
***	Retained root tip	Remnants of periodontal ligament usually seen	—
***	Condensing osteitis	Usually at apex of nonvital tooth	147
***	Idiopathic osteosclerosis	Most commonly associated with roots of posterior teeth; no apparent inflammatory etiology	620
**	Pseudocyst of the maxillary sinus	Homogeneous, dome-shaped relative opacity rising above bony floor of maxillary sinus	320
**	Odontoma, compound	Toothlike structures with thin, radiolucent rim at junction with surrounding bone; may prevent eruption of teeth; more common in anterior segments of jaws	724
**	Odontoma, complex	Amorphous mass with thin, radiolucent rim at junction with surrounding bone; may prevent eruption of teeth; more common in posterior segments of jaws	724
**	Cemento-osseous dysplasia	Late-stage lesions; especially in middle-aged and older black women; usually in mandible	640
**	Soft tissue radiopacity superimposed on bone	Examples: sialoliths, calcified nodes, phleboliths, bullet fragments, shotgun pellets, amalgam tattoos (See also Appendix List, Part 4, Q, page 933)	—
*	Intraosseous foreign body	—	—
*	Osteoma	Associated with bony surface mass	650
*	Enamel pearl	Furcation area of molar tooth	93
*	Osteoblastoma/osteoid osteoma/cementoblastoma	Late-stage lesions	653

H. RADIOPACITIES: POORLY DEMARCATED BORDERS

**	Cemento-osseous dysplasia	Late stage lesions; especially in middle-aged and older black women; usually in mandible	640
**	Condensing osteitis	Usually at apex of nonvital tooth	147
**	Bisphosphonate-associated osteonecrosis	Sclerosis of alveolar crestal bone; exposed necrotic bone	299
**	Sclerosing osteomyelitis	May be painful	144
**	Fibrous dysplasia	"Ground glass" appearance; onset usually in younger patients	635
*	Paget's disease of bone	"Cotton wool" appearance; late-stage lesions; in older patients	623
*	Proliferative periostitis	"Onion-skin" cortical change; in younger patients; often associated with nonvital tooth	148

Continued

Frequency of Occurrence	Lesion or Condition	Comments or Special Characteristics	Page
H. RADIOPACITIES: POORLY DEMARCATED BORDERS—cont'd			
*	Osteosarcoma	May have "sunburst" cortical change; frequently painful; usually in young adults	660
*	Chondrosarcoma	—	664
I. RADIOPACITIES: MULTIFOCAL OR GENERALIZED			
**	Florid cemento-osseous dysplasia	Late-stage lesions; especially in middle-aged and older black women; usually in mandible	641
**	Idiopathic osteosclerosis	—	620
**	Bisphosphonate-associated osteonecrosis	Multifocal sites of involvement; sclerosis of alveolar crestal bone; exposed necrotic bone	299
*	Paget's disease of bone	"Cotton wool" appearance; late-stage lesions; in older patients; more common in maxilla	623
*	Gardner syndrome	Multiple osteomas; epidermoid cysts; gastrointestinal polyps with high tendency toward malignant transformation; hereditary	651
*	Polyostotic fibrous dysplasia	"Ground glass" appearance; onset usually in younger patients; may be associated with *café au lait* skin pigmentation and endocrine abnormalities (McCune-Albright syndrome)	635
*	Osteopetrosis	Hereditary; recessive form may be associated with secondary osteomyelitis, visual and hearing impairment	615
J. MIXED RADIOLUCENT/RADIOPAQUE LESIONS: WELL-DEMARCATED BORDERS			
***	Developing tooth	—	—
**	Cemento-osseous dysplasia	Intermediate-stage lesions; especially in middle-aged black women; usually in mandible	640
**	Odontoma	Compound or complex type; in younger patients; may prevent eruption of teeth	724
*	Central ossifying fibroma	—	646
*	Ameloblastic fibro-odontoma	Usually in children	721
*	Adenomatoid odontogenic tumor	Usually in anterior region of jaws; most often with maxillary canine; usually in teenagers	713
*	Calcifying epithelial odontogenic tumor	Pindborg tumor; often associated with impacted tooth; may show "driven snow" opacities	716
*	Calcifying odontogenic cyst	Gorlin cyst; may be associated with odontoma	695
*	Osteoblastoma/osteoid osteoma	Intermediate-stage lesion; usually in younger patients; often painful	653
*	Cementoblastoma	Intermediate-stage lesion; attached to tooth root	655
K. MIXED RADIOLUCENT/RADIOPAQUE LESIONS: POORLY DEMARCATED BORDERS			
**	Osteomyelitis	With sequestrum formation or with sclerosing type; often painful	141
**	Bisphosphonate-associated osteonecrosis	Exposed necrotic bone	299
*	Metastatic carcinoma	Especially prostate and breast carcinomas; may be painful	669
*	Osteosarcoma/chondrosarcoma	May be painful	660

Frequency of Occurrence	Lesion or Condition	Comments or Special Characteristics	Page
L. MIXED RADIOLUCENT/RADIOPAQUE LESIONS: MULTIFOCAL OR GENERALIZED			
**	Florid cemento-osseous dysplasia	Intermediate-stage lesions; especially in middle-aged black women; usually in mandible	641
**	Bisphosphonate-associated osteonecrosis	Exposed necrotic bone	299
*	Paget's disease of bone	In older patients; more common in maxilla	623
M. UNIQUE RADIOGRAPHIC APPEARANCES: "GROUND GLASS" (FROSTED GLASS) RADIOPACITIES			
*	Fibrous dysplasia	Onset usually in younger patients	635
*	Hyperparathyroidism	May cause loss of lamina dura	838
N. UNIQUE RADIOGRAPHIC APPEARANCES: "COTTON WOOL" RADIOPACITIES			
**	Cemento-osseous dysplasia	Especially in middle-aged black women; usually in mandible	640
*	Paget's disease of bone	In older patients; more common in maxilla	623
*	Gardner syndrome	Multiple osteomas; epidermoid cysts; gastrointestinal polyps with high tendency toward malignant transformation; hereditary	651
*	Gigantiform cementoma	Hereditary; facial enlargement may be present	645
O. UNIQUE RADIOGRAPHIC APPEARANCES: "SUNBURST" RADIOPACITIES			
*	Osteosarcoma	Often painful; usually in young adults	660
*	Intraosseous hemangioma	Especially in younger patients	540
P. UNIQUE RADIOGRAPHIC APPEARANCES: "ONION-SKIN" RADIOPACITIES			
*	Proliferative periostitis	In younger patients; often associated with nonvital tooth; best seen with occlusal radiograph	148
*	Ewing sarcoma	In young children	667
*	Langerhans cell histiocytosis	"Histiocytosis X"; usually in children or young adults	590
Q. SOFT TISSUE RADIOPACITIES			
***	Amalgam tattoo	Markedly radiopaque; associated with surface discoloration	308
**	Other foreign bodies	Examples: bullet fragments, shotgun pellets	–
**	Sialolith	Glandular pain may be present while patient is eating	459
**	Calcified lymph nodes	Example: tuberculosis	197
**	Phlebolith	May occur in varicosities or hemangiomas	16
*	Tonsillolith	–	185
*	Osseous and cartilaginous choristomas	Most common on tongue	552
*	Calcinosis cutis	May be seen with systemic sclerosis (especially CREST syndrome)	801
*	Myositis ossificans	Reactive calcification in muscle	–

Frequency of Occurrence	Lesion or Condition	Comments or Special Characteristics	Page
J. ENLARGED PULP CHAMBER OR CANAL			
**	Internal resorption	Secondary to caries or trauma	65
**	Taurodontism	Enlarged pulp chambers; shortened roots	94
*	Dentinogenesis imperfecta	"Shell teeth"	106
*	Regional odontodysplasia	"Ghost teeth"	112
*	Vitamin D–resistant rickets	High pulp horns	847
*	Hypophosphatasia	–	845
*	Dentin dysplasia type II	"Thistle-tube" pulps; pulp stone formation	108
K. PULPAL CALCIFICATION			
***	Pulp stones	Asymptomatic radiographic finding	126
***	Secondary dentin	Response to caries	123
**	Calcific metamorphosis	Pulpal obliteration secondary to aging or trauma	123
*	Dentinogenesis imperfecta	Pulpal obliteration by excess dentin	106
*	Dentin dysplasia type I	Pulpal obliteration by excess dentin; "chevron"-shaped pulp chambers	108
*	Dentin dysplasia type II	Pulpal obliteration of primary teeth; pulp stones in permanent teeth	108
L. THICKENED PERIODONTAL LIGAMENT			
***	Periapical abscess	Focal thickening at apex of nonvital tooth; painful, especially on percussion of involved tooth	135
***	Current orthodontic therapy	–	–
**	Increased occlusal function	–	–
*	Systemic sclerosis (scleroderma)	Generalized widening	798
*	Sarcoma or carcinoma infiltration	Especially osteosarcoma; localized to teeth in area of tumor	661, 669
M. GENERALIZED LOSS OF LAMINA DURA			
*	Hyperparathyroidism	Calcium removed from bones; bone may have "ground glass" appearance	838
*	Osteomalacia	Vitamin D deficiency in adults	827
*	Paget's disease of bone	"Cotton wool" change hides lamina dura	623
*	Fibrous dysplasia	"Ground glass" change hides lamina dura	635
N. PREMATURE EXFOLIATION OF TEETH			
***	Trauma	Avulsed tooth	–
**	Aggressive periodontitis	Premature alveolar bone loss	173
**	Immunocompromised states	AIDS, leukemia, chemotherapy	272
**	Diabetes mellitus	Increased susceptibility to infection and severity of periodontitis	842
*	Osteomyelitis	Bone destruction loosening teeth	141
*	Cyclic or chronic neutropenia	Increased susceptibility to infection; premature alveolar bone loss	583
*	Langerhans cell histiocytosis	"Histiocytosis X"; eosinophilic granuloma; premature alveolar bone loss	590
*	Dentin dysplasia type I	"Rootless teeth"	108
*	Regional odontodysplasia	"Ghost teeth"	112
*	Papillon-Lefèvre syndrome	Palmar and plantar hyperkeratosis; premature periodontitis	176
*	Down syndrome	Premature periodontitis	–
*	Hypophosphatasia	Lack of cementum production in primary teeth	845
*	Scurvy	Vitamin C deficiency	826

Index

Page numbers followed by *f* indicate figures; *t*, tables; *b*, boxes.